Principles and Techniques of

Spine Surgery

Principles and Techniques of
Spine Surgery

Howard S. An, M.D.
The Morton International Professor of Orthopaedic Surgery
Department of Orthopaedic Surgery
Rush Medical College
Rush-Presbyterian St. Luke's Medical Center
Chicago, Illinois

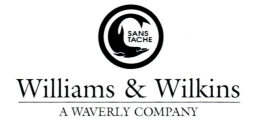

BALTIMORE • PHILADELPHIA • LONDON • PARIS • BANGKOK
BUENOS AIRES • HONG KONG • MUNICH • SYDNEY • TOKYO • WROCLAW

Illustrator: Carole A. Hilmer
Editor: Darlene Barela Cooke
Managing Editor: Frances M. Klass
Marketing Manager: Diane M. Harnish
Production Coordinator: Cindy Park
Project Editor: Kathy Gilbert
Designer: Elizabeth Sanders
Illustration Planner: Ray Lowman
Cover Designer: Randall J. Rogers
Typesetter: University Graphics, Inc.
Printer: Four Colour Imports, Ltd.
Digitized Illustrations: University Graphics, Inc.
Binder: Four Colour Imports, Ltd.

Copyright © 1998 Williams & Wilkins

351 West Camden Street
Baltimore, Maryland 21201-2436 USA

Rose Tree Corporate Center
1400 North Providence Road
Building II, Suite 5025
Media, Pennsylvania 19063-2043 USA

All rights reserved. This book is protected by copyright. No part of this book may be reproduced in any form or by any means, including photocopying, or utilized by any information storage and retrieval system without written permission from the copyright owner.

Accurate indications, adverse reactions and dosage schedules for drugs are provided in this book, but it is possible that they may change. The reader is urged to review the package information data of the manufacturers of the medications mentioned.

First Edition, 1998

Library of Congress Cataloging-in-Publication Data

Principles and techniques of spine surgery / [edited by] Howard S. An.
    p. cm.
    Includes bibliographical references and index.
    ISBN 0-683-30260-4
    1. Spine—Surgery. 2. Spinal cord—Surgery. I. An, Howard S.
    [DNLM: 1. Spine—surgery. 2. Spinal Diseases—surgery. WE 725
P9565 1997]
RD533.P75 1997
617.5'6059—dc21
DNLM/DLC
for Library of Congress   97-5525
                                                                                 CIP

The publishers have made every effort to trace the copyright holders for borrowed material. If they have inadvertently overlooked any, they will be pleased to make the necessary arrangements at the first opportunity.

To purchase additional copies of this book, call our customer service department at **(800) 638-0672** or fax orders to **(800) 447-8438**. For other book services, including chapter reprints and large quantity sales, ask for the Special Sales department.

Canadian customers should call **(800) 665-1148**, or fax **(800) 665-0103**. For all other calls originating outside of the United States, please call **(410) 528-4223** or fax us at **(410) 528-8550**.

Visit Williams & Wilkins on the Internet: http://www.wwilkins.com or contact our customer service department at **custserv@wwilkins.com**. Williams & Wilkins customer service representatives are available from 8:30 am to 6:00 pm, EST, Monday through Friday, for telephone access.

                                                                                                                    98 99 00
                                                                          2 3 4 5 6 7 8 9 10

To my wife (Sue), my daughter (Jennifer), and my son (Steven)

Preface

Principles and Techniques of Spine Surgery updates the scientific data and principles of spine surgery in a comprehensive fashion. In this text on surgery of the spine, an updated review of anatomy, surgical approaches, biomechanics, imaging techniques, electrodiagnostic tests, and clinical evaluation is provided in the first section. Ensuing chapters cover specific disorders, including congenital anomalies of the cervical spine, scoliosis, kyphosis, spondylolisthesis, spinal trauma, and degenerative cervical, thoracic, and lumbar disorders. Special chapters on spinal tumors, infections, inflammatory disorders, and sacral lesions make this text a complete book on the spine. Additionally, chapters on specific surgical techniques add to the value of the text. Specifically, surgical and instrumentation techniques of the cervical spine, posterior thoracolumbar spine, and anterior thoracolumbar spine are discussed fully. Finally, minimally invasive techniques, such as microsurgery and percutaneous procedures and bone grafting techniques, are well covered. The editor was blessed with dedicated contributing authors who have articulately expressed their experiences in the field of spine surgery.

Apart from outstanding contributing authors, unique features of this text are that the editor organized the book in a succinct manner to cover the various areas of spine surgery in one volume text and that the text is full of outstanding illustrations and photographs. The reader will find this book easy to comprehend and even enjoy with extensive illustrations. This book is primarily written for spine surgeons who can renew the current information on various aspects of spine surgery. This book is also useful for trainees as a study guide, and for nonsurgical physicians as a reference source.

I wish to extend thanks to the contributing authors. This text could not have been completed without their contributions. I extend great thanks to my medical illustrator, Carole Hilmer, for many of the outstanding illustrations in this book. I also thank the staff at Williams & Wilkins for their help. Finally, I express my deep appreciation to my family, particularly my wife who has followed my career with continued sacrifice but with endless support and encouragement.

Howard S. An, MD

Contributors

Howard S. An, MD
The Morton International Professor of
  Orthopaedic Surgery
Department of Orthopaedic Surgery
Rush-Presbyterian-St. Luke's Medical Center
Chicago, Illinois

Todd J. Albert, MD
Assistant Professor, Department of Orthopaedic Surgery
Jefferson Medical College of Thomas Jefferson University
Philadelphia, Pennsylvania

Paul A. Anderson, MD
Clinical Associate Professor
Orthopaedic Surgery
University of Washington
Seattle, Washington

Thomas G. Andreshak, MD
Clinical Instructor
Medical College of Ohio
Toledo, Ohio

Richard A. Balderston, MD
Clinical Professor of Orthopaedics
Jefferson Medical College
Chief of Orthopaedics
Thomas Jefferson University Hospital
Co-Associate Director
Regional Spinal Cord Injury Center of the Delaware
  Valley
Associate Director
Rothman Institute
Philadelphia, Pennsylvania

Paul E. Barkhaus, MD
Associate Professor of Neurology
Medical College of Wisconsin
Milwaukee, Wisconsin

Scott D. Boden, MD
Associate Professor of Orthopaedic Surgery
Director, The Emory Spine Center
Emory University School of Medicine
Decatur, Georgia

Henry Bohlman, MD
Professor, Department of Orthopaedics
Case Western Reserve University School of Medicine
Chief of the Reconstructive and Traumatic Spine Surgery
  Center
University Hospital - Cleveland
Chief of the Acute Spinal Cord Injury Service
Veterans Administration Medical Center
Cleveland, Ohio

David S. Bradford, MD
Professor and Chairman
Department of Orthopaedic Surgery
University of California, San Francisco
San Francisco, California

Keith H. Bridwell, MD
Professor of Orthopaedic Surgery
Washington University School of Medicine
St. Louis, Missouri

Lysa M. Charles, MD
Resident, Section of Orthopaedic Surgery
University of Michigan Medical Center
Ann Arbor, Michigan

Mark Coppes, MD
Orthopaedic Surgeon
South County Orthopaedics and Physical Therapy, Inc.
South County Hospitals
Wakefield, Rhode Island

Jerome M. Cotler, MD
The Everett J. and Marian Gordon Professor and Vice Chairman
Department of Orthopaedic Surgery
Jefferson Medical College of Thomas Jefferson University
Philadelphia, Pennsylvania

Bradford L. Currier, MD
Assistant Professor, Orthopaedic Surgery
Mayo Medical School
Consultant, Department of Orthopaedics
Mayo Clinic
Rochester, Minnesota

Sanford E. Emery, MD
Assistant Professor
Department of Orthopaedics
Case Western Reserve University School of Medicine
Cleveland, Ohio

Stephen I. Esses, MD
Professor, Clinical Orthopaedic Surgery
Baylor College of Medicine
Houston, Texas

Christopher Formal, MD
Magee Rehabilitation Hospital
Philadelphia, Pennsylvania

Bruce E. Frederickson, MD
Professor of Orthopaedic and Neurologic Surgery
Department of Orthopaedic Surgery
SUNY Health Science Center
Syracuse, New York

Steven R. Garfin, MD
Professor and Chairman of Orthopaedic Surgery
University of California, San Diego Medical Center
San Diego, California

J. Michael Glover, MD
Clinical Assistant Professor of Surgery
Uniformed Services University of the Health Sciences
Bethesda, Maryland

Gregory P. Graziano, MD
Associate Professor
Section of Orthopaedic Surgery and Neurosurgery
University of Michigan Medical Center
Ann Arbor, Michigan

Harry N. Herkowitz, MD
Chairman, Department of Orthopaedic Surgery
William Beaumont Hospital
Royal Oak, Michigan

Quinn Hogan, MD
Associate Professor
Medical College of Wisconsin
Milwaukee, Wisconsin

Serena S. Hu, MD
Assistant Professor
Department of Orthopaedic Surgery
University of California, San Francisco
San Francisco, California

S. Craig Humphreys, MD
Spine Fellow
Department of Orthopaedic Surgery
Medical College of Wisconsin
Milwaukee, Wisconsin

Roger P. Jackson, MD
Clinical Assistant Professor
University of Kansas School of Medicine
Kansas City, Missouri

Safwan S. Jaredeh, MD
Associate Professor of Neurology
Department of Neurology
Director, Autonomic Testing Laboratory and Muscle and Nerve Laboratory
Medical College of Wisconsin
Milwaukee, Wisconsin

Lawrence T. Kurz, MD
Staff Spine Surgeon
Department of Orthopaedic Surgery
William Beaumont Hospital
Royal Oak, Michigan

Marc Levine, MD
Spine Fellow
The Emory Spine Center
Emory University School of Medicine
Decatur, Georgia

Tae Hong Lim, PhD
Associate Professor, Director of Orthopaedic Biomechanics Laboratory
Department of Orthopaedic Surgery
Medical College of Wisconsin
Milwaukee, Wisconsin

Randall T. Loder, MD
Associate Professor, Section of Orthopaedic Surgery
University of Michigan Medical Center
Ann Arbor, Michigan

Donlin M. Long, MD, PhD
Professor and Director, Neurosurgery
Johns Hopkins University School of Medicine
Baltimore, Maryland

John E. Lonstein, MD
Clinical Associate Professor
Department of Orthopaedics
University of Minnesota and Minnesota Spine Center
Minneapolis, Minnesota

Roger M. Lyon, MD
Assistant Professor
Department of Orthopaedic Surgery
Medical College of Wisconsin
Milwaukee, Wisconsin

Bruce E. Mathern, MD
Clinical Assistant Professor
Department of Surgery - Division of Neurosurgery
Medical College of Virginia
Mid Atlantic Spine Specialists
Richmond, Virginia

Hallett H. Mathews, MD
Associate Professor
Orthopaedic Surgery
Medical College of Virginia
Mid Atlantic Spine Specialists
Richmond, Virginia

Tom G. Mayer, MD
Medical Director, PRIDE and PRIDE Research Foundation
Clinical Professor
Department of Orthopaedic Surgery
University of Texas Southwestern Medical Center
Dallas, Texas

Geoffrey M. McCullen, MD
Spine Fellow
SUNY Health Science Center
Syracuse, New York

John A. McCulloch, MD
Professor of Orthopaedics
Northeastern Ohio Universities College of Medicine
Akron, Ohio

Robert F. McLain, MD
Associate Professor
Department of Orthopaedics
University of California, Davis Medical Center
Sacramento, California

Lee H. Riley, III, MD
Assistant Professor
Department of Orthopaedic Surgery
The Medical College of Wisconsin
Milwaukee, Wisconsin

Todd E. Siff, MD
Orthopaedic Resident
Baylor College of Medicine
Houston, Texas

Christopher P. Silveri, MD
Clinical Instructor
Department of Orthopaedics
George Washington University
Washington, D.C.
Director of Spine Surgery
Fair Oaks Orthopaedic Associates
Fairfax, Virginia

Frederick A. Simeone, MD
Professor and Chairman of Neurosurgery
Thomas Jefferson University
Chief Of Neurosurgery
Pennsylvania Hospital
Philadelphia, Pennsylvania

J. Michael Simpson, MD
Clinical Assistant Professor
Department of Orthopaedic Surgery
The Medical College of Virginia
Director of Spine Surgery
Tuckahoe Orthopaedic Associates, Ltd.
Richmond, Virginia

Michael D. Smith, MD
Staff Surgeon
Minnesota Spine Center
Minneapolis, Minnesota

John G. Thometz, MD
Associate Professor
Medical College of Wisconsin
Chief, Pediatric Orthopaedics
Children's Hospital of Wisconsin
Department of Orthopaedic Surgery
Milwaukee, Wisconsin

Alexander R. Vaccaro, MD
Associate Professor
Department of Orthopaedic Surgery
Jefferson Medical College of Thomas Jefferson University
Philadelphia, Pennsylvania

Chun-sing Yu, MD
Visiting Spine Fellow
University of California, San Diego Medical Center
San Diego, California

Hansen A. Yuan, MD
Professor of Orthopaedic and Neurological Surgery
SUNY Health Science Center
Syracuse, New York

Contents

SECTION I: Principles and Diagnostic Tests

1. Anatomy of the Spine *Howard S. An* 1
2. Surgical Exposure and Fusion Techniques of the Spine *Howard S. An* 31
3. Spine Biomechanics *Tae-Hong Lim; Howard S. An* 63
4. History and Physical Examination of the Spine *Lee H. Riley* 91
5. Diagnostic Imaging of the Spine *Marc J. Levine; Scott D. Boden* 103
6. Electrodiagnosis and Intraoperative Monitoring in Disorders of the Spinal Cord and Nerve Roots *Paul E. Barkhaus; Safwan S. Jaradeh* 129

SECTION II: Pediatric Spine

7. Congenital Anomalies of the Cervical Spine *Randall T. Loder* 157
8. Neuromuscular Scoliosis *John G. Thometz* 173
9. Surgical Treatment of Pediatric Idiopathic Scoliosis *Keith H. Bridwell* 187
10. Congenital Spine Deformities *John E. Lonstein* 213
11. Juvenile Kyphosis *Serena S. Hu; David S. Bradford* 239
12. Lumbar Spondylolisthesis *Chun-sing Yu; Steven R. Garfin* 249
13. Pediatric Spine Injuries *Roger M. Lyon* 267

SECTION III: Spinal Trauma

14. Spinal Cord Injury and Lower Cervical Spine Injuries *Paul A. Anderson* 295
15. Upper Cervical Spine Injuries in the Adult *Alexander R. Vaccaro; Jerome M. Cotler* ... 331

xiii

16. Thoracolumbar Spine Injuries *Geoffrey M. McCullen; Hansen A. Yuan; Bruce E. Fredrickson* 359

17. Rehabilitation of Traumatic Spinal Cord Injury *Christopher Formal* 385

SECTION IV: Degenerative Disorders

18. Cervical Disc Disease and Cervical Spondylosis *Sanford E. Emery* 401

19. Thoracic Disc Disease *Michael D. Smith* 413

20. Lumbar Disc Disease *Christopher P. Silveri; Frederick A. Simone* 425

21. Spinal Stenosis *Howard S. An; Thomas G. Andreshak* 443

22. Functional Restoration of Back and Neck Work-Related Injuries *Tom G. Mayer* 461

SECTION V: Adult Deformities and Miscellaneous Disorders

23. Adult Scoliosis *Richard A. Balderston; Todd J. Albert; Alexander R. Vaccaro* 475

24. Sagittal Plane Abnormalities in Disorders of the Adult Spine *Roger P. Jackson* 489

25. Degenerative Lumbar Spondylolisthesis *Harry N. Herkowitz* 517

26. Spinal Neoplasms *Robert F. McLain* 527

27. Intradural Lesions of the Spine *Don M. Long* 551

28. Spinal Infections *Bradford L. Currier* 567

29. Rheumatoid Arthritis and Ankylosing Spondylitis *J. Michael Simpson; Howard S. An* 605

30. Sacral Disorders *Todd E. Siff; Stephen Esses* 629

SECTION VI: Spinal Procedures and Instrumentations

31. Spinal Orthoses *Gregory P. Graziano; Lysa M. Charles* 641

32. Cervical Spine Instrumentation *Howard S. An; Mark Coppes* 653

33. Posterior Instrumentation of the Thoracolumbar Spine *S. Craig Humphreys; Howard S. An* 675

34. Anterior Instrumentation of the Thoracolumbar Spine *Howard S. An; J. Michael Glover* 693

35. Injection for Diagnosis and Therapy of Back Disease *Quinn Hogan* 707

36. Percutaneous Procedures in the Lumbar Spine *Hallet H. Mathews; Bruce E. Mathern* .. 731

37. Microsurgery for Lumbar Disc Disease *John A. McCulloch* 747

38. Bone Grafting Procedures *Lawrence T. Kurz* 765

SECTION 1
Principles and Diagnostic Tests

CHAPTER ONE

Anatomy of the Spine

Howard S. An

Introduction

The human spine is a complex columnar structure, spanning from the occiput to the sacrum. In addition to protecting the spinal cord and nerve roots, the spine provides motions in three dimensions and maintains the balance of the head, trunk, and the pelvis through the muscles, ligaments, intervertebral disc, and facet joints (Fig. 1.1 A,B,C). The understanding of the normal spinal anatomy, alignment, and function is critical in the planning and execution of various surgical procedures. The normal thoracic kyphosis is in the range of 20 to 50°, and the normal lumbar lordosis is about 40 to 60°. In stance, the sagittal vertical axis falls from the odontoid process through the C7-T1 intervertebral disc and anterior to the thoracic vertebrae. The axis crosses the spinal column at T12-L1 intervertebral disc and falls posterior to the lumbar spine. The axis again crosses the spine the lumbosacral articulation and is located anterior to the second vertebra. This concept of the sagittal vertical axis is important in the realignment of sagittal-plane deformities.

In this chapter, the basic anatomy of the spine will be presented, emphasizing surgically related structures. The anatomy of the osseous structures, joints, intervertebral disc, ligaments, muscles, neurovascular structures, and related soft tissue structures will be described.

Neuroanatomy

Spinal Cord

The spinal cord emerges from the foramen magnum as a continuation of the medulla oblongata and ends in a cone-shaped structure known as the conus medullaris. The location of the conus medullaris is usually at the L1-2 intervertebral disc in adults (Fig. 1.2A). However, it may be as high as T12 or as low as L2-3, and in newborn infants, the conus is at the L2-3 region. The cervical cord enlarges maximally at C6 vertebra to provide C3-T2 nerve supplies to the upper limbs, and the lumbosacral enlargement is present at T11 to L1 vertebral segments to provide L1 to S3 cord segments to the lower extremities. It is important to remember the corresponding vertebral segment to the cord segment (Fig. 1.2). For example, the L1 vertebral segment corresponds to the sacral conus medullaris cord segment as well as traverses lower lumbar roots.

The spinal cord includes the outer white matter and the inner gray matter (Fig. 1.3) (10). The white matter of the spinal cord contains nerve fibers and glia and is divided into three columns: posterior, lateral, and anterior. The posterior column includes the fasciculus cuneatus laterally and fasciculus gracilis medially, mediating proprioceptive, vibratory, and tactile sensations. The lateral column contains the descending motor lateral corticospinal and lateral

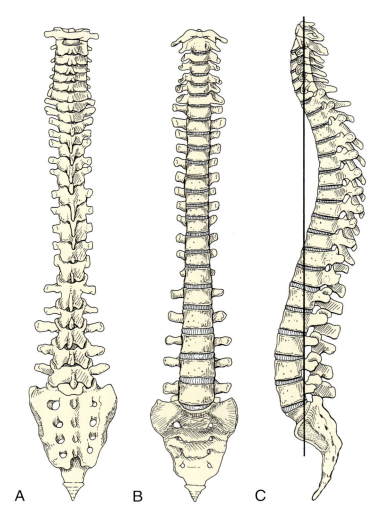

FIGURE 1.1.
The human spine. **A.** Posterior view of the entire spine. **B.** Anterior view of the spine. **C.** Lateral view of the spine; the vertical line illustrates a plumb line that starts from the odontoid process and crosses the C7 vertebra and T12-L1 junction and to the posterior aspect of the sacrum. This plumb line is used to assess sagittal imbalance clinically.

spinothalamic fasciculi, and the anterior funiculus contains the ascending anterior spinothalamic tract and other descending tracts. The lateral spinothalamic tracts cross through the ventral commissure to the contralateral side of the cord, conveying pain and temperature sensations. The anterior spinothalamic tract conveys the crude touch sensation. The gray matter of the spinal cord contains cell bodies of efferent and internuncial neurons. The somatosensory neurons are located in the posterior horn, and the somatomotor neurons are found in the anterior horn of the gray matter. The visceral center of the gray matter is found in the intermediolateral horn. The center of the spinal cord houses the central ependymal canal for the passage of cerebrospinal fluid.

The spinal cord is covered by the pia mater, which is the outer lining of the cord, and transparent arachnoid mater, which contains the cerebrospinal fluid (Fig. 1.4A). The dura mater is the outer covering of the spinal cord, which is continuous at the foramen magnum with the inner layer of the cranial dura. The spinal cord is anchored to the dura by the dentate ligaments that project laterally from the lateral side of the cord to the arachnoid and dura at points midway between exiting spinal nerves (Fig. 1.4B). By suspending the spinal cord in the cerebrospinal fluid, the dentate ligament cushions and protects the cord while minimizing the movement of the cord during ranges of motion. The epidural space contains fat, internal vertebral venous plexus and loose connective tissue. This venous plexus may be involved in spreading infection or neoplasm. The epidural space is about 2 mm at L3-4, 4 mm at L4-5, and 6 mm at L5-S1. Because of this relatively larger epidural space at L5-S1, spinal stenosis is less common at the lumbosacral junction. The plica mediana dorsalis durae matris is a delicate median fold at the lumbosacral epidural region that often blends with the epidural fat. A potential space exists between the dura and arachnoid, and the subarachnoid space lies between the arachnoid and pia. The subarachnoid space contains the cerebrospinal fluid, spinal blood vessels, and nerve rootlet from the spinal cord. The dural and arachnoid envelop may terminate between the S1 and S4 regions, but mostly at the S2 region. Distal to the S2 region, the dura invests the filum terminale and attaches to the coccyx.

The vessels supplying the spinal cord are derived

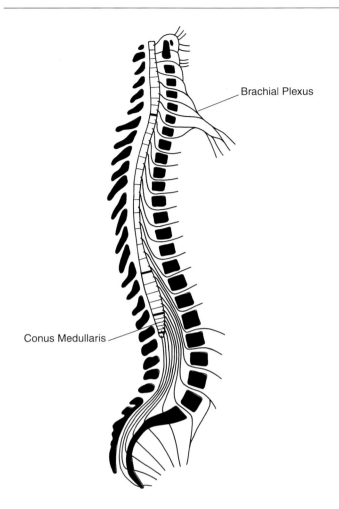

FIGURE 1.2.
Diagram of the spinal cord and nerve roots. The spinal cord emerges from the foramen magnum as a continuation of the medulla oblongata and ends in a cone-shaped structure known as the conus medullaris. The location of the conus medullaris is usually at L1–2 intervertebral disc in adults. The cervical cord enlarges maximally at C6 vertebra to provide C3-T2 nerve supplies to the upper limbs, and the lumbosacral enlargement is present at T11 to L1 vertebral segments to provide L1 to S3 cord segments to the lower extremities.

from branches of the vertebral, deep cervical, intercostal, and lumbar arteries (15). The arteries of the spinal cord include the anterior spinal artery lying in the anterior median fissure, and the two posterior spinal arteries running along the posterolateral sulci. These vessels are reinforced by segmental or radicular arteries. The anterior spinal artery in the cervical spine arises from the vertebral artery, which originates from the subclavian arteries and courses through the C6 transverse foramen in most cases. The vertebral artery courses cephalad within the transverse foramen of each vertebra, winds around the lateral mass and posterior arch of the atlas, and passes through the posterior atlantooccipital membrane into the foramen magnum. The vertebral arteries join together to form the basilar artery beyond the foramen magnum. In the foramen magnum region, the vertebral arteries give branches anteriorly that join together to form the single anterior spinal artery. The posterior spinal arteries arise from either the inferior cerebellar artery or the vertebral artery. The anterior and posterior spinal arteries are the major blood supply to the spinal cord. The anterior spinal artery supplies the majority of the spinal cord except the posterior columns. The posterior spinal artery and its branches supply the posterior funiculus, most of the posterior gray columns, and superficial lateral funiculus. The spinal cord also receives blood supplies from radicular arteries and medullary feeders from the vertebral, ascending cervical, posterior intercostal, lumbar, and lateral sacral arteries. These radicular arteries enter the vertebral canal through the intervertebral foramen and divide into anterior and posterior radicular arteries. The anterior radicular arteries supply the anterior spinal artery, and the posterior radicular arteries contribute blood to the posterior spinal arteries.

The most significant radicular artery to the cervical cord is an artery originating from the deep cervical artery, accompanying the left C6 spinal nerve root. Other medullary feeders to the cervical cord are commonly present at C3 from the left and C5 and T1 from the right. The radicular artery of Adamkiewicz supplies the thoracolumbar spinal cord and usually accompanies the left ventral root of T9-11, but it may be found anywhere from T5 to L5. This artery makes a major contribution to the anterior spinal artery and provides the main blood supply to the lower spinal cord. Venous blood returns from the cord through three veins posteriorly and three veins anteriorly. The venous system within the spinal canal consists of valveless sinuses in the epidural space. The venous plexus is most apparent anteriorly just medial to the pedicles over the midportion of the vertebral bodies, and anastomose with the veins from the opposite as well as with the basivertebral sinus, which is located in the space between the posterior longitudinal ligament and the posterior aspect of the vertebral body. The spinal venous circulation drains primarily into the azygos system and joins directly into the vena cava.

Spinal Nerves

The spinal nerve roots include 8 cervical, 12 thoracic, 5 lumbar, 5 sacral, and 1 coccygeal. The dorsal and ventral roots join to form the spinal nerve. The ventral root and the dorsal root ganglion are within the intervertebral foramen. Fascicles emerge from the spinal ganglion and from the ventral roots and converge to form the ventral and smaller dorsal rami of the spinal nerve proper (12, 18). A pair of spinal

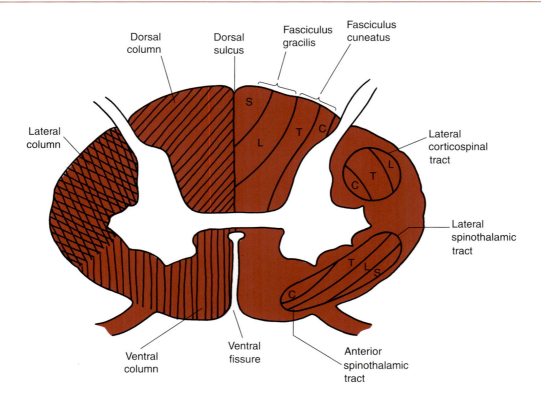

FIGURE 1.3.
Cross-section of the spinal cord with the outer white matter and the inner gray matter. The white matter of the spinal cord contains nerve fibers and glia and is divided into three columns: posterior, lateral, and anterior. The posterior column includes the fasciculus cuneatus laterally and the fasciculus gracilis medially. The lateral column contains the descending motor lateral corticospinal and lateral spinothalamic fasciculi, and the anterior funiculus contains the ascending anterior spinothalamic tract and other descending tracts. The lateral spinothalamic tracts cross through the ventral commissure to the contralateral side of the cord. The gray matter of the spinal cord contains cell bodies of efferent and internuncial neurons.

nerve roots leaves the dural sac by penetrating the dural sac in an inferolateral direction. This dural sleeve contains both the dura mater and arachnoid mater and extends as far as the intervertebral foramen and the spinal nerve. It becomes the epineurium of the spinal nerve.

In the cervical spine, the dorsal sensory rootlets enter the cord through the lateral longitudinal sulcus, and the ventral motor rootlets exit the cord through the ventral lateral sulcus (Fig. 1.5). The six or eight rootlets at each level leave the spinal cord laterally to lie in the lateral subarachnoid space bathed in the cerebrospinal fluid. The rootlets join to form the dorsal and ventral root, which together enter a narrow sleeve of arachnoid and pass through the dura to become a nerve root at each level. The cervical nerve roots that form from the ventral and dorsal nerve rootlet extend anterolaterally at a 45° angle to the coronal plane and inferiorly at about 10° to the axial plane. The C5 ventral rootlets are shorter and exit in a more horizontal direction; they may become easily taut and overstressed and predispose C5 palsy after decompressive procedures (39). The cervical nerve roots enter the intervertebral foramina by passing directly laterally from the spinal canal adjacent to the corresponding disc and over the top of the corresponding pedicle (Fig. 1.6A). The anterior root lies anteroinferiorly adjacent to the uncovertebral joint, and the posterior root is close to the superior articular process (Fig. 1.6B). The cervical nerve root is positioned at the tip of the superior articular process in the medial aspect of the neural foramen, and it courses more inferiorly to position over the pedicle in the lateral aspect of the neural foramen. The cervical roots occupy approximately one-third of the foraminal space in the normal spine, but occupy much more space in the degenerative spine. The roots are located in the inferior half of the neural foramen normally, but the nerve roots occupy a more cranial part of the foramina, and the size of the foramen is diminished if the neck is extended fully. The upper half of the neural foramen contains fat and small veins. The cervical neural foramen is approximately 9 to 12 mm in height, 4 to 6 mm in width, and 4 to 6 mm in length (8, 9). The neural foramen is bounded superiorly and inferiorly by pedicles; anteriorly by the uncinate process, the posterolateral aspect of the intervertebral disc, and the inferior portion of the vertebral body above the disc level; and posteriorly by the facet joint and superior articular process of the vertebral body

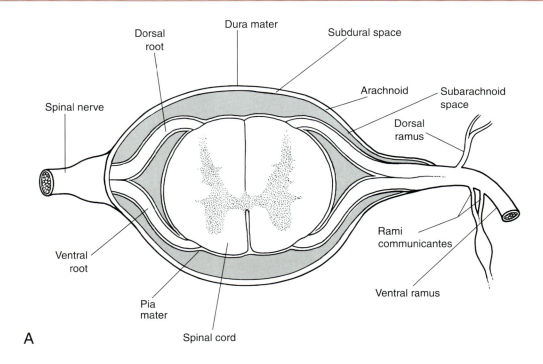

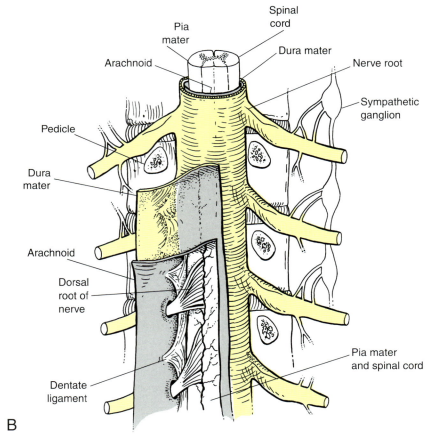

FIGURE 1.4.
Cross-section of the spinal cord and meninges. **A.** The spinal cord is covered by the pia mater, which is the outer lining of the cord, and transparent arachnoid mater that contains the cerebrospinal fluid. The dura mater is the outer covering of the spinal cord. **B.** The spinal cord is anchored to the dura by the dentate ligaments that project laterally from the lateral side of the cord to the arachnoid and dura at points midway between exiting spinal nerves.

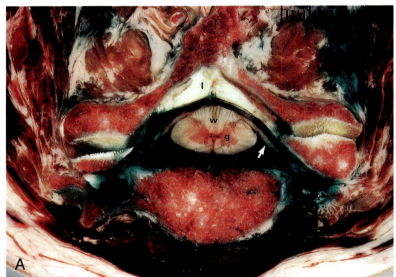
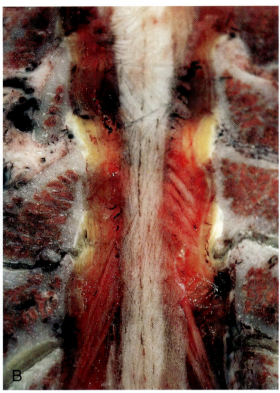

FIGURE 1.5.
A. A cryomicrotome section of the cervical spine showing the dorsal root (arrow) and the spinal cord with white matter (w), gray matter (g), ligamentum flavum (l). **B.** Dorsal view of the multiple dorsal rootlets at each level. The rootlets join to form the dorsal and ventral root, which together enter a narrow sleeve of arachnoid and pass through the dura to become a nerve root at each level.

below. Degenerative changes of these structures that bound the intervertebral foramen may compromise the spinal nerve.

In the thoracic spine, the thoracic spinal nerves are small and occupy about 20% of the intervertebral foramen. Each thoracic and lumbar spinal nerve exits below the pedicle that bears the same name. The ventral rami of the thoracic nerves do not form plexuses, but each pair runs inferior to the rib as the intercostal nerves. The intercostal nerves give off muscular and cutaneous branches around the back, thorax, and abdomen.

Within the lumbar dural sac, the nerve roots are arranged loosely with the sacral and coccygeal nerve roots to form the cauda equina. Each root is covered with its own sleeve of pia mater that is continuous with the pia mater of the spinal cord. The nerve roots within the cauda equina are well organized in a symmetric layering pattern (Fig. 1.7B). The most posterior nerve elements are the S5 roots, progressing anteriorly to S4, S3, S2, and S1 at L5-S1 level. This arrangement varies at different levels. For example, at L2-3 level, the L3-S1 roots form an oblique layered pattern with the S2-S5 roots occupying the dorsal aspect of the thecal sac. In the lumbar spine, the spinal nerves are larger and occupy about one-third of the foramen. Within the dural sac, the lumbar nerve roots are arranged loosely with the sacral and coccygeal nerve roots to form the cauda equina. The angle formed by each pair of spinal nerve roots and the dural sac becomes gradually more acute in the lower lumbar region. The angles formed by the L1 and L2 roots are about 40° and 32° respectively, whereas the angles of the L3 root are each approximately 30° and those of the L4 and L5 roots are 27° (6). The angle for the S1 root is more acute at 18°. The length of the nerve roots or the distance from the emerging point of the nerve root from the thecal sac to the dorsal root ganglion increases progressively to a maximum at L5 and decreases at S1. The dorsal root ganglion that contains the cell bodies of the sensory fibers in the dorsal root usually lies within the upper, medial part of intervertebral foramen (Fig. 1.7C,D). The S1 dorsal root ganglion is more frequently located intraspinally (26). The average dimension of the dorsal root ganglions gradually increase from L1 to S1. Using coronal MRI sections, Hasegawa et al. describes the locations of the lumbar dorsal root ganglions in asymptomatic individuals (22). The nerve root origin is noted to be more cephalad for the caudad nerve

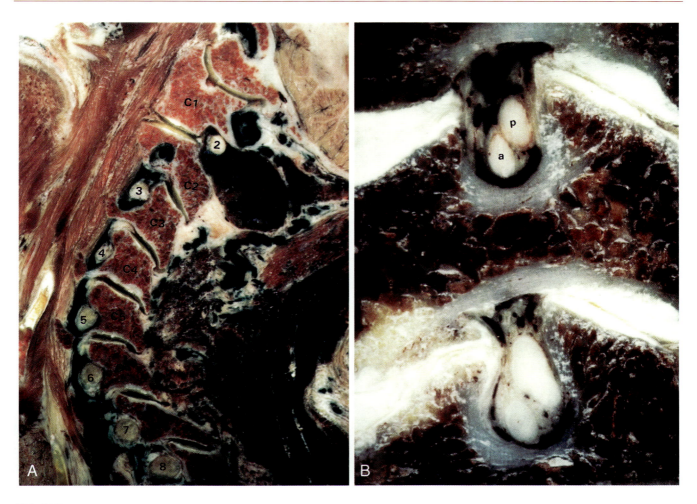

FIGURE 1.6.
Cryomicrotome sections of the cervical foramen **A.** The cervical nerve roots enter the intervertebral foramina by passing directly laterally from the spinal canal adjacent to the corresponding disc and over the top of the corresponding pedicle. **B.** The anterior root lies anteroinferiorly adjacent to the uncovertebral joint, and the posterior root is close to the superior articular process.

roots, particularly the S1. The length of the nerve roots increases progressively to a maximum at L5 and decreases at S1. The S1 nerve root is most unique in that it takes off more cephalad, at a more vertical angle, and is shorter. The S1 dorsal root ganglion is also unique in that it is the largest ganglion and is located intraspinally more frequently than other ganglions.

The lumbar intervertebral foramen, which is shaped like an inverted teardrop, forms a tunnel that connects with the spinal canal. It is bounded superiorly and inferiorly by the pedicle of the adjacent vertebrae. The posterior boundary is formed by the pars interarticularis and ligamentum flavum. The anterior boundary is formed by the posteroinferior margin of the superior vertebral body, the posterior margin of the intervertebral disc, and the posterosuperior margin of the inferior vertebral body. The nerve root is normally surrounded by fat (Fig. 1.7D). Additionally, various types of transforaminal ligaments may traverse within the foramen (31) (Fig. 1.7D). The nerve roots may have aberrant courses to give various anomalies (Fig. 1.8). These anomalies do not usually produce symptoms; however, the recognition of these anomalies is important in the diagnosis and treatment of patients with other pathologies associated with anomalies of the nerve roots. Based on Kadish and Simmons, there are four types of nerve root anomalies with an incidence of 14%: Type I: intradural anastomosis between rootlets; Type II: anomalous origin of nerve roots that are further divided into cranial origin, caudal origin, combination of cranial and caudal origins, and conjoined nerve roots; Type III: extradural anastomosis; and Type IV: extradural division of the nerve root (25). The conjoined roots and intradural anastomosis are most common.

The spinal nerve divides into dorsal primary rami and ventral primary rami branches. The dorsal primary rami gives medial, lateral, and occasionally intermediate branches to innervate the zygapophysial

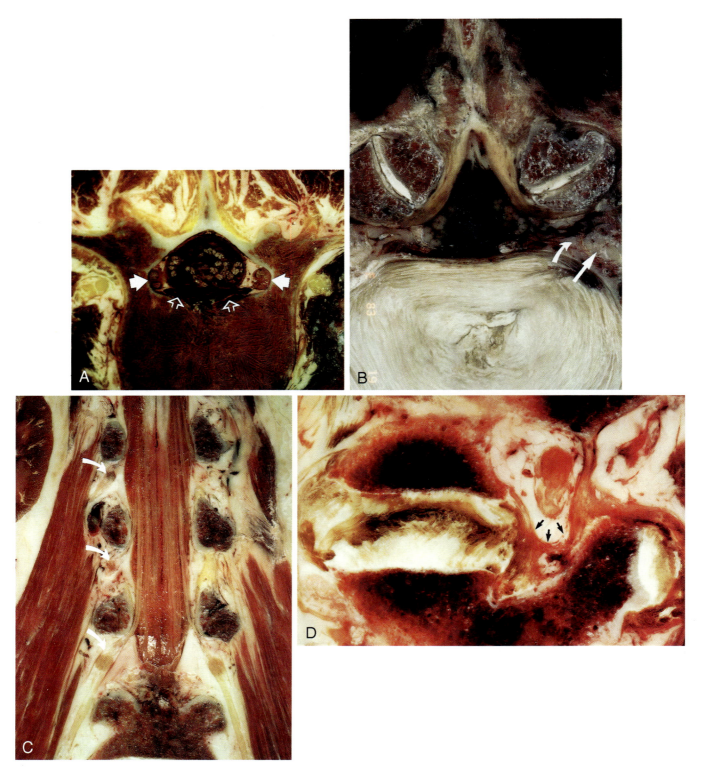

FIGURE 1.7.
Cryomicrotome sections of the lumbar spine. **A.** This cross-section shows the dural sac with the nerve roots that are arranged loosely with the sacral and coccygeal nerve roots to form the cauda equina. The exiting nerve root is shown medial to the pedicle (large arrows). Epidural space contains venous plexus anteriorly (open arrows). **B.** A cross-section of the lumbar spine at the intervertebral disc level. Nerve roots are arranged in a symmetrical pattern. The nerve root in the foramen (large arrow) is normally surrounded by fat (curved arrow). The facet joints are asymmetrical and are also known as facet tropism. **C.** Coronal section shows the course of nerve roots exiting below the pedicle and joining the dorsal root ganglion (arrows) in the intervertebral foramen. **D.** A sagittal section of the intervertebral foramen with the nerve root surrounded by fat and vascular structures inferiorly. The intervertebral foramen is bounded superiorly and inferiorly by the pedicle of the adjacent vertebrae. The posterior boundary is formed by the pars interarticularis and ligamentum flavum. The anterior boundary is formed by the posteroinferior margin of the superior vertebral body, the posterior margin of the intervertebral disc, and the posterosuperior margin of the inferior vertebral body. Inferiorly, the transforaminal ligament (arrows) extends from the posterior margins of the intervertebral disc and superior articular facet.

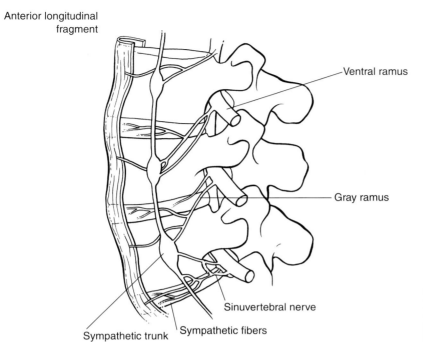

FIGURE 1.8.
Diagram of the ventral primary rami, sympathetic trunk, sinuvertebral nerve, and branches in the lumbar spine.

joints and the paraspinal musculature (20). The lateral branches of the lumbar dorsal rami innervate the iliocostalis muscle, while the intermediate branches supply the longissimus muscle. The medial branches play an important role in the distribution of the zygapophyseal joints. Each medial branch supplies the zygapophyseal joints above and below it. For example, the L4-5 zygapophyseal joints are innervated by the L4 posterior primary rami and the descending branches from the L3 posterior primary rami. The medial branches of the posterior primary rami also supply the segmental muscles and interspinous ligaments arising from the spinous process and lamina of the vertebra with the same segmental number as the nerve. For example, the L2 nerve supplies only those muscles and interspinous ligaments from the L2 vertebra.

The anterior aspect of the dura and the posterior longitudinal ligament are innervated by the sinuvertebral nerve (4, 5). This nerve receives contributions from the ventral rami and the grey ramus communicans (Fig. 1.8). The sinuvertebral nerve runs back into the spinal canal throughout the foramen, running somewhat cranial to the disc. The gray rami from the sympathetic ganglion join the ventral primary rami (Fig. 1.8). The anterior portion of the lumbar intervertebral discs is innervated by sympathetic fibers, whereas the posterior portion of the disc is innervated by the sinuvertebral nerve. In the lumbar spine, the sinuvertebral nerves are branches of the ventral rami but also receive contributions from the autonomic grey rami. The sinuvertebral nerves innervate the posterior longitudinal ligament, the posterior part of the anulus, and the ventral part of the dura. The sinuvertebral nerves typically ascend to innervate the superior disc as well. In other words, the sinuvertebral nerves arising from the L4 ventral rami innervate the posterolateral part of the L4-5 anulus but also course superiorly to innervate the L3-4 anulus. Sinuvertebral nerves are believed to derive from recurrent branches of the spinal nerve and the sympathetic nerve. The posterior portion of the disc seems to be dually innervated (30).

In the cervical spine, interconnections exist between gray rami, the perivascular plexus around the vertebral artery, and the sympathetic trunk, all of which give contributions to the ventral nerve plexus that innervates the anterior longitudinal ligament, outer anulus fibrosus, and the anterior vertebral body (20). The dorsal nerve plexus receives contributions from the sinuvertebral nerves, which originate from the gray rami and perivascular plexus of the vertebral artery in the cervical spine. The first cervical nerve, or suboccipital nerve, exits the vertebral canal above the posterior arch of the atlas and posteromedial to the lateral mass, and it lies between the vertebral artery and the posterior arch. The posterior primary ramus of the first cervical nerve enters the suboccipital triangle and sends motor fibers to the deep muscles. The anterior primary ramus of the first cervical nerve forms a loop with the second anterior primary ramus and sends fibers to the hypoglossal nerve. The cervical plexus receives fibers from anterior primary rami of C1-C4. The cervical plexus is located opposite C1-C3, ventral and lateral to levator scapulae and middle scalene muscles. The cervical plexus has distributions to the skin and muscles, such as rectus capitis anterior and lateralis, longus capitis and cervicis, levator scapulae, and middle scalene. The cervical plexus forms loops and branches to supply sternocleidomastoid and trapezius muscles. The cervical plexus communicates with the hypoglossal nerve from C1 and C2 and leaves this trunk as the superior root of the ansa cervicalis, which forms a loop called the ansa cervicalis with the inferior root from C2 and C3.

The second cervical nerve lies on the lamina of the axis posterior to the lateral mass, and the posterior primary ramus, or the greater occipital nerve, pierces the trapezius about 2 cm below the external occipital protuberance and 2 to 4 cm from the midline (Fig. 1.9). Cutaneous branches of the posterior primary rami of C2-C5 are consistently present in the skin of nuchal region, and the largest cutaneous nerve in this region is the greater occipital nerve. The lesser occipital nerve branches from the anterior cervical plexus

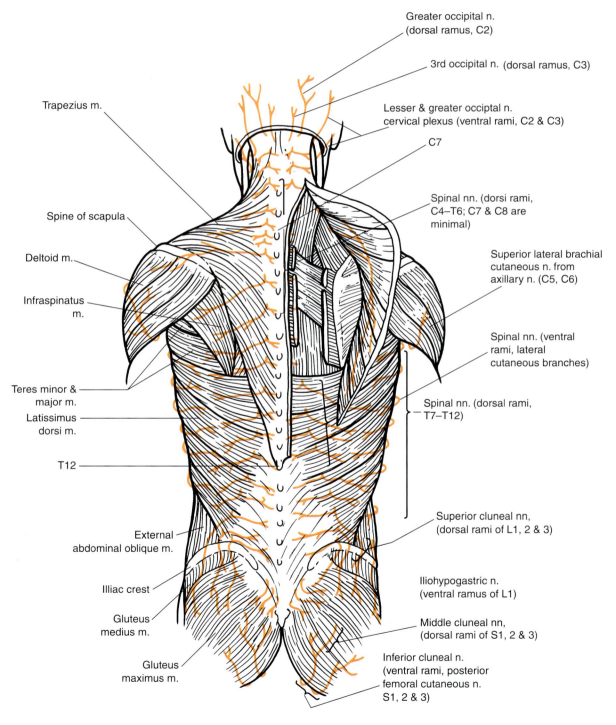

FIGURE 1.9.

Cutaneous nerves on the posterior aspect of the neck and back.

and runs upward and lateral to the greater occipital nerve (Fig. 1.9). The posterior primary ramus of C3, or third occipital nerve, pierces the trapezius more inferiorly and approximately 1 cm medial from the midline (Fig. 1.9). The cervical nerve exits over the pedicle that bears the same number, except C8 cervical nerve lies between the C7 and T1 vertebrae. The posterior primary rami of cervical nerves send motor fibers to the deep muscles and sensory fibers to the skin, but the first cervical nerve has no cutaneous branches. The anterior primary rami of C1-C4 form the cervical plexus, and C5-T1 form the brachial plexus. The lower cervical spinal nerves give specific dermatomal and motor distributions of the upper extremity, which are essential in the evaluation and treatment of patients with cervical radiculopathy (Fig. 1.10).

In the lumbar region, the ventral rami of the lumbar spinal nerves pierce the intertransverse ligament and continue to form lumbar and lumbosacral plexus. The L1 to L4 ventral rami form the lumbar plexus, and the L4 and L5 ventral rami join to form the lumbosacral trunk that enters the lumbosacral plexus. The dorsal rami of L1, or sometimes L2 and L3, furnish cutaneous branches that cross the posterior iliac crest about 7 to 8 cm from the midline (Fig. 1.9). The cutaneous branches are the superior cluneal nerves that should be preserved in surgical approaches. Kurz et al. reported that the cluneal nerves emerge about 7 to 8 cm lateral to the posterior superior iliac spine (28). More recently, Xu et al. reported that the average distances from the posterior superior iliac spine to the superior cluneal nerves, gluteal line, and superior gluteal vessels are 68.8, 26.6, and 62.4 mm, respectively (45). For posterior iliac crest bone harvesting, the incision should therefore stay

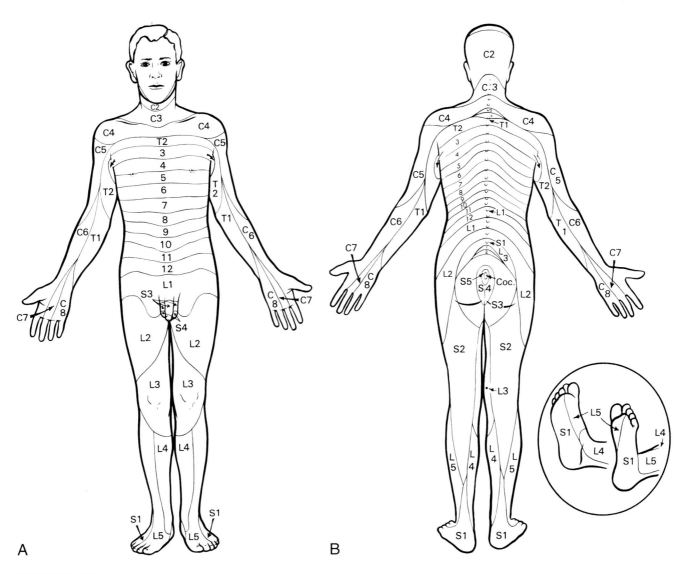

FIGURE 1.10.

Illustrations of dermatomes. **A.** Anterior dermatomes. **B.** Posterior dermatomes.

within 6.8 cm from the posterior superior iliac spine. The cutaneous branches from both dorsal rami and ventral rami provide consistent sensations that are useful clinically. Cutaneous nerves are arranged in a consistent dermatomal pattern. (Fig. 1.10) In evaluating patients with cervical spine disorders, the clinician should remember the C5 dermatome over the deltoid muscle, C6 dermatome of the thumb, C7 dermatome of the long finger, and C8 dermatome of the small finger. The nipple line corresponds to the T4 dermatome, and the umbilicus corresponds to the T8 dermatome. In evaluating lumbar spine disorders, the clinician should also remember that the L1 corresponds to the groin, L2 over the anterior thigh, L3 over the knee, L4 over the medial malleolus, L5 over the great toe, and S1 over the small toe and bottom of the foot. Sacral dermatomes are located around the perineum, which is important to remember when assessing patients with cauda equina or conus medullaris syndromes and also when evaluating sacral sparing incomplete spinal cord syndromes.

Osseous Structures and Articulations

The osseous structures in different regions of the vertebral column have different characteristics aside from the obvious differences in the size. The bony anatomy of the atlas and axis in the cervical spine is unique (Fig. 1.11). The atlas is a ring-like structure, in which the thick anterior arch blends into the lateral masses. The occipital condyles articulate with the concave superior aspects of the lateral masses as a cup-shape joint (11, 17). The occipital condyles project downward and outward while the superior facet of the atlas faces upward and inward to support the occiput. This atlanto-occipital articulation is supported by anterior and posterior occipital membranes, which are continuations of anterior longitudinal ligaments and ligamentum flavums, respectively (Fig. 1.12). The atlanto-occipital joint mostly allows for flexion, extension, and lateral bending motions. The inferior facets of the atlas are flatter and more circular than are the superior facets and face downward and inward to articulate with the axis (Fig. 1.13 A,B). The atlas has no body, and the anterior tubercle of the anterior arch serves as an attachment of the longus colli muscle. The posterior tubercle of the atlas are the bony attachments for the rectus minor muscle and suboccipital membrane. The mean thickness of the posterior ring is 8 mm, and the cortical bone is thin (13). The atlas has large transverse processes where the superior and inferior oblique muscles attach. The transverse foramen is lo-

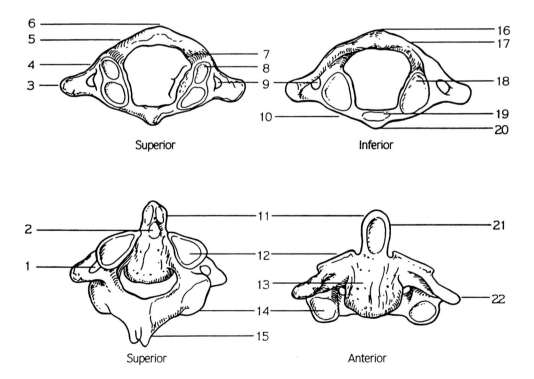

FIGURE 1.11.
The bony anatomy of the atlas and axis. 1. Transverse foramen, 2. Posterior articular facet, 3. Transverse process, 4. Lateral mass, 5. Posterior arch, 6. Posterior tubercle, 7. Groove for vertebral artery, 8. Superior articular facet, 9. Transverse foramen, 10. Anterior arch, 11. Dens, 12. Superior articular facet, 13. Body, 14. Inferior articular facet, 15. Spinous process, 16. Posterior tubercle, 17. Posterior arch, 18. Inferior articular process, 19. Fovea dentis, 20. Anterior tubercle, 21. Anterior articular facet, 22. Transverse process.

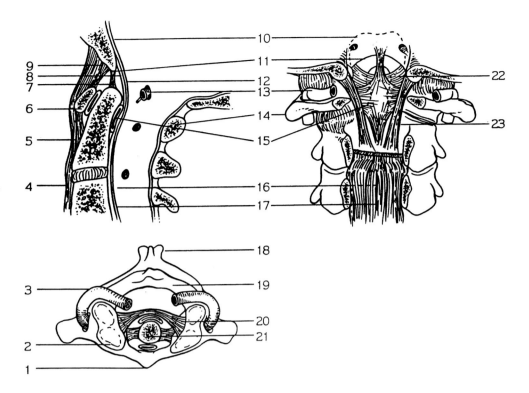

FIGURE 1.12.
Diagrams of ligamentous anatomy of the upper cervical spine: 1. Anterior tubercle, 2. Superior articular facet, 3. Vertebral artery, 4. Anterior longitudinal ligament, 5. Anterior atlas-axis membrane, 6. Anterior arch of atlas, 7. Apical ligament, 8. Vertical cruciform ligament, 9. Anterior atlas-occipital membrane, 10. Attachment of tectorial membrane, 11. Anterior edge of foramen magnum, 12. Tec torial membrane, 13. Vertebral artery, 14. Atlas, 15. Transverse ligament, 16. Origin of tectorial membrane, 17. Posterior longitudinal ligament, 18. Spinous process of C2, 19. Atlas, 20. Transverse ligament, 21. Dens, 22. Alar ligament, 23. Deep tectorial membrane.

cated within the transverse process, through which the vertebral artery passes.

The axis is also unique in its bony anatomy. The odontoid process project upward anteriorly, articulating with the posterior aspect of the anterior arch of the atlas as a synovial joint. The projection angle of the odontoid process varies from −2° to 42° with a mean of 13° (14). The average dens height is approximately 15 mm (44). The transverse ligament, which spans across the arch of the atlas, holds the odontoid process against the anterior arch of the atlas (Fig. 1.12). This transverse ligament is the principal stabilizing structure for the atlantoaxial articulation. The transverse ligament has superior and inferior extensions, which form the cruciated ligament of the atlas. Secondary stabilizers of this articulation are the alar ligament, which arises from the sides of dens to the condyles of the occipital bone, and the apical ligament, which arises from the apex of the dens to the foramen magnum as a remnant of the notochord. The tectorial membrane is a continuation from the posterior longitudinal ligament. Posteriorly, the axis has the large lamina and bifid spinous process, which serve as attachments for rectus major and inferior oblique muscles. The zone between the lamina and the lateral mass of axis vertebra is indistinct. The pedicle of axis is large and projects medially at 30° and superiorly at 20° (44). The atlantoaxial articulation provides approximately 50% of rotatory motion of the cervical spine. The spinal canal at the upper cervical spine is more capacious than is the lower cervical spine, with the sagittal diameters of 23 mm at C1 and 20 mm at C2. When approaching the posterior aspect of the atlas and axis, the surgeon should avoid injuries to the associated neurovascular structures such as the vertebral artery, spinal ganglion of C2, and the spinal cord.

The bony anatomy of the lower cervical spine from C3 to C6 is similar with slight dimensional increases from C3 to C6, but C7 is unique as the transitional vertebra. Posteriorly, spinous processes are bifid from C3 to C6 (Fig. 1.14A), which are projected inferiorly, and the C7 spinous process is large and not bifid; it often is called the vertebra prominens. A junction exists between the spinous process and lamina, although the transition is less distinct. This junction is anatomically important during spinous process wiring, in that when the wire penetrates beyond the spinolaminar line, it may impinge on the spinal cord. The lamina blends into the lateral mass, which

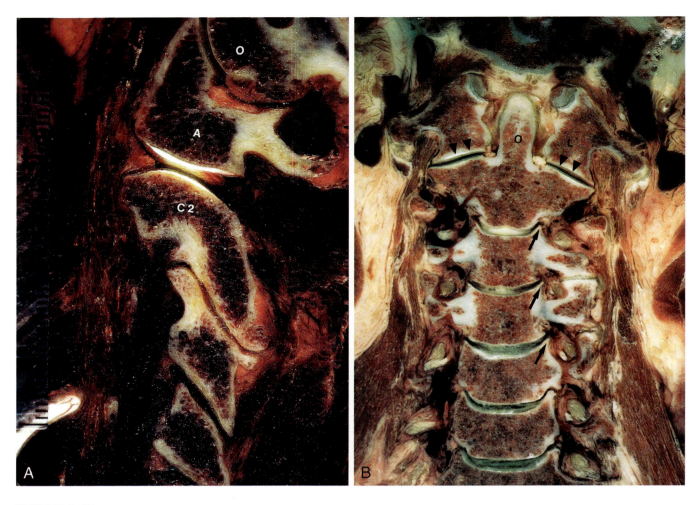

FIGURE 1.13.

A. A cryomicrotome of the upper cervical spine showing the occipital condyle (o) articulating with the concave superior aspect of the lateral mass of the atlas (A). The superior facet of the atlas has a cup-shape surface to support the occipital condyle, and the inferior facet is flatter to articulate with the axis (C2) below. **B.** A coronal cryomicrotome section of the cervical spine. The atlas articulate with the occipital condyle above and the axis below (arrow heads). The odontoid process (o) projects between the lateral masses (L) of the atlas. The uncovertebral joints are shown with arrows.

is the bone between the superior and inferior articular processes. The articular processes oppose each other to form the facet joint. The normal cervical facet joints have the articular cartilage and menisci that are surrounded by a capsular ligament and lined by a synovial membrane. Most adult cervical facet joints undergo changes with aging that consist of a thin layer of cartilage and irregularly thickened subarticular cortical bone (19, 48). The joint capsules are innervated richly by proprioceptive and pain receptors that may be important in the pathogenesis of neck pain.

From the posterior aspect, the facet joint line is horizontal and slightly circular inferiorly. The interfacet distances are relatively constant at different levels, but individual variations exist from 9 mm to 16 mm, with an average of 13 mm (1). For this reason, most posterior lateral mass plate-screw systems are designed to have screw holes distances at 13 mm. Important anatomic considerations during posterior plate-screw instrumentation are the landmarks of the facet joint lines, lateral mass margins, and joint inclination. There is a definite junction between the lamina and lateral mass, and the lateral edge of the lateral mass forms a ridge down to the transverse process. The facet joint itself is angled about 45° cephalad from the transverse plane (Fig. 1.14B). The lateral mass of C7 is more elongated from the superior-inferior aspect and is thinner than upper levels from the anterior-posterior aspect.

On the anterolateral aspect, a typical cervical vertebra consists of a body, transverse processes, and pedicles. The body is relatively small and oval, with the medial-lateral diameter greater than the anterior-posterior diameter (Fig. 1.14C). From the coronal plane, the superior surface of the vertebral body is

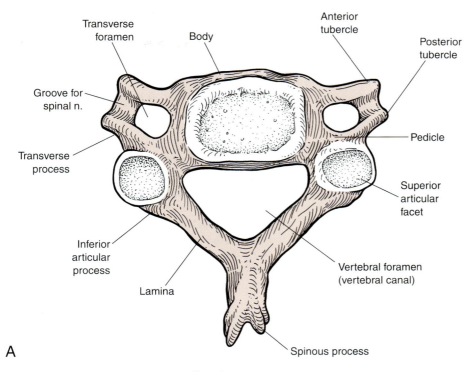
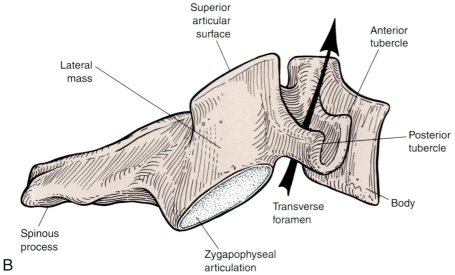
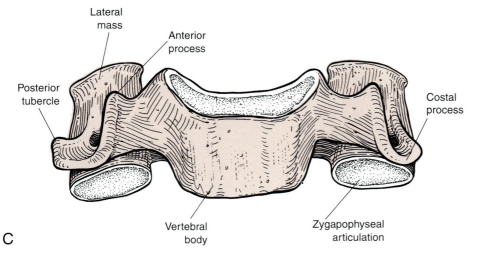

FIGURE 1.14.

The bony anatomy of the lower cervical spine. **A.** View from the top showing the vertebral foramen, superior articular facet, transverse process, transverse foramen, and the body. **B.** Side view showing the spinous process, superior and inferior articular surfaces, tubercles of the transverse process, and the body. **C.** Anterior view showing the vertebral body, transverse processes, lateral mass, and acicular processes.

concave, and the inferior surface of the body is correspondingly convex (Fig. 1.13). However, from the sagittal plane, the superior surface of the body is slightly convex to or straightly aligned with the corresponding concave inferior surface of the upper vertebral body.

The anteroinferior edge of the vertebral body is lipped inferiorly. The lateral surfaces of the superior vertebral body project upward, conforming to small grooves in the inferolateral borders of the cephalad vertebra, which forms the uncovertebral joints, or joints of Luschka (Fig. 1.13). The width and depth of the vertebral surfaces average 17 mm and 15 mm from C2 to C6, respectively, and increase to about 20 mm and 17 mm, respectively, at C7 (32). Vertebral heights on the posterior wall in the midsagittal plane range from 11 to 13 mm. Projecting laterally from the cephalad aspect of the vertebral body is the anterior tubercle of the transverse process, which joins the posterior tubercle of the transverse process. The anterior tubercle is a costal element, and the C6 anterior tubercle, also known as the carotid tubercle, is a prominent surgical landmark. Between the posterior tubercle and anterior tubercle is the groove or the costotransverse lamella, which projects inferiorly for the passage of the spinal nerve. The vertebral artery and venous system pass through the transverse foramen, which is located medial to the tubercles of the transverse process and lateral to the vertebral body. The transverse processes increase significantly in size at C6 and C7. The pedicles project posterolaterally from the vertebral body at a 30 to 45° angle and join the lamina to form the vertebral arch (Fig. 1.14A). The spinal canal or vertebral foramen is triangular with rounded angles, and the lateral width of the canal is significantly greater than is the anteroposterior depth at all levels. Normal sagittal diameters of the cervical spine are 17 to 18 mm at C3-C6,

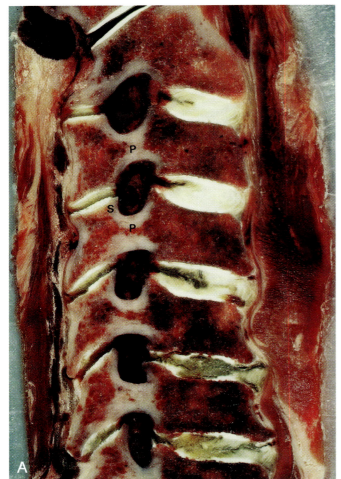
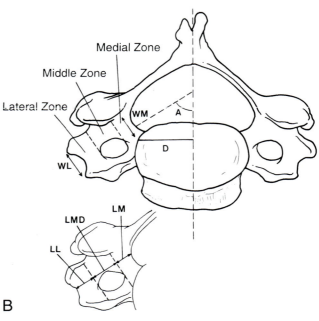

FIGURE 1.15.
A 45° oblique cryomicrotome section of the cervical spine. **A.** The intervertebral foramen is bordered by the uncinate process anteriorly, the superior facet posteriorly (s), and the adjacent pedicles superiorly and inferiorly (p) **B.** Zones of the cervical nerve root groove. Reprinted with permission from Ebraheim NA, An HS, Xu R, et al. The quantitative anatomy of the cervical nerve root groove and the intervertebral foramen. Spine 1996;21:1619–1623.

and 15 mm at C7 (32). The cross-sectional area of the spinal canal is largest at C2 and smallest at C7. The height of the pedicle is about 7 mm, and the width is about 5 to 6 mm with a slight increase from C3 to C7 (32). As mentioned before, the C2 pedicle is larger with the height of 10 mm and width of 8 mm. From C3 to C7, the angulation of the pedicles vary from 8° below to 11° above the transverse plane. The pedicle angle in the sagittal plane decreases from approximately 45 to 30° from C3 to C7.

The cervical nerve roots emerge from the vertebral canal via the intervertebral foramen. The intervertebral foramen is bordered by the uncinate process anteriorly, the superior facet posteriorly, and the adjacent pedicles superiorly and inferiorly (Fig. 1.15A) (34, 35). Ebraheim et al. measured the intervertebral foramen to be 7.5 to 8.5 mm in height and 4.5 mm to 7 mm in width on average (16). The foraminal height and width gradually increase from C3 to C7. Ebraheim et al. studied the cervical nerve root groove that extends approximately 1.5 to 2 cm from the medial aspect of the pedicle to the lateral end of the transverse process and associated costal process, where it is bounded by the anterior and posterior tubercles (16). The nerve root groove is divided into three zones, and the medial zone, or the intervertebral foramen, is important in the etiology of cervical radiculopathy (Fig. 1.15B).

The cervicothoracic junction is a transition region with C7 having similar anatomic characteristics at T1 and T2. The dimensions of the vertebral body is larger at C6 and C7 as are the sizes of the transverse processes and spinous processes. Additionally, dimensions of the spinal canal decrease at C6 and C7, representing a distinct transition to the thoracic region. The articulating facet joint between C7 and T1 resembles the thoracic facet joint, and the lateral mass of C7 is thinner than that of upper levels. Inner diameters of the pedicles at C7, T1, and T2 from the medial to lateral plane average 5.2 mm, 6.3 mm, and

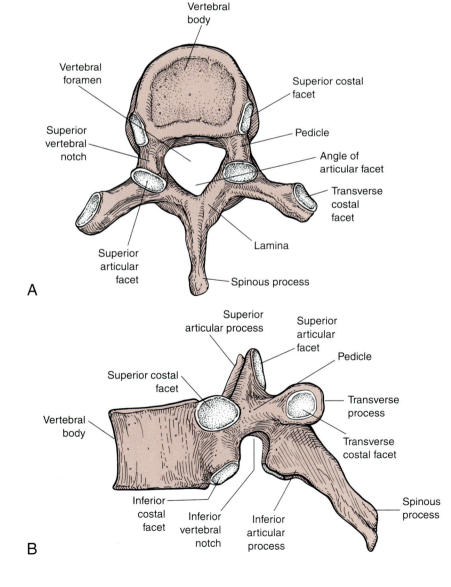

FIGURE 1.16.

Diagram of the thoracic vertebra. **A.** Top view shows articulation with the rib, heart-shaped body, and circular vertebral canal. **B.** Side view shows vertebral body, facets for the rib, pedicle, and the inferiorly projecting spinous process.

5.5 mm, respectively. Medial angulations of the pedicle are 34°, 30°, and 26° at C7, T1, and T2, respectively (1). These morphologic characteristics should be remembered when performing transpedicular procedures in the cervicothoracic region.

The thoracic vertebrae are unique in their articulation with the ribs and have heart-shaped bodies and circular vertebral canal (Fig. 1.16). The round spinal canal has less free space for the spinal cord than does the cervical and lumbar region. The articular facets for the ribs are located in the body and transverse process; the radiate and costovertebral ligaments are between the body and rib; and the costotransverse and intertransverse ligaments are between the transverse process and rib. The spinous processes are long and slender and overlap to the lower vertebral arches. The thoracic column is mechanically stiffer and less mobile because of the rib attachment. The upper and middle thoracic vertebrae have inherent stability against anteroposterior translation, and the lower thoracic vertebrae have greater stability against rotation caused by the orientation of the facet joint. T1 is atypical in that it has a long horizontal transverse process, and the size of the transverse processes gradually decrease from T1 to T10. The inferior T9 to T12 vertebrae have tubercles similar to the lumbar vertebrae. The pedicle of the thoracic vertebrae measures approximately 10 mm at T4 and 14 mm at T12 in height and approximately 4.5 mm at T4 and 7.8 mm at T12 in width (42). The pedicles incline anteromedially ranging from 0.3° at T12 to 13.9° at T4. The pedicle wall is thicker medially than it is laterally (27).

The vertebral body in the lumbar spine is largest at L5, which transmits the body weight to the base of the sacrum (Fig. 1.17). The pedicles connect between

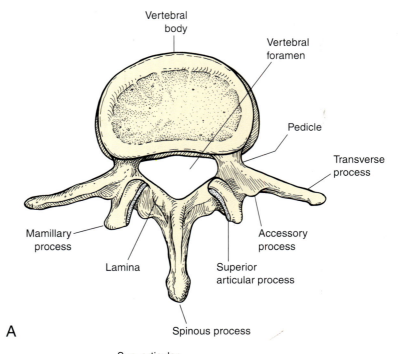

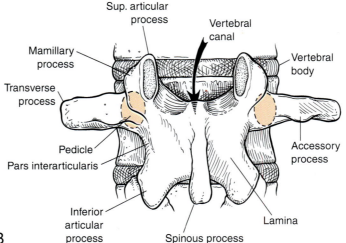

FIGURE 1.17.

Diagram of the lumbar vertebra. **A.** Top view shows the larger vertebral body, pedicles that connect between the body, and the posterior elements. The vertebral foramen is more triangular. **B.** Posterior view shows the lamina, pars interarticularis, transverse process, and articular processes. The pedicle region is outlined in oval shape.

the body and the posterior elements. The transverse pedicle width averages 18 mm at L5 and becomes smaller in the upper lumbar spine and averages 9 mm at L1. The medial angulation or transverse pedicle angle is about 30° at L5 and only 12° at L1 (49). From the posterior aspect, the pedicle is located about 1 mm inferior to the tip of the inferior articular process or in the middle of the transverse processes horizontally, and the posterior-most prominence of the superior articular process vertically. Near the transverse process and pedicle attachment, the accessory process is present as irregular bony prominence.

The facet joints in the lumbar spine is oriented more sagittally to resist axial rotation. The lumbosacral facet is oriented more coronally to resist anteroposterior translation. Mamillary processes are prominences on the posterior edge of the superior articular processes. The lumbar spinal canal is oval in the upper lumbar region and becomes triangular in the lower lumbar region.

The nerve root takes off from the thecal sac, courses under the lateral recess, and travels through a tubular canal or the intervertebral foramen (Fig. 1.18A,B) (2). The lateral lumbar spinal canal has been subdivided into three anatomic zones by Lee et al.: entrance zone, mid zone, and exit zone (29). The entrance zone is the subarticular area medial to the pedicle and is synonymous with the lateral recess area. The mid zone is located under the pars interarticularis and the pedicle, and the exit zone is synonymous with the intervertebral foramen.

The entrance zone is located underneath the superior articular process of the facet joint and medial to the pedicle. The entrance zone is the cephalad aspect of the more commonly known lateral recess, which begins at the lateral aspect of the thecal sac

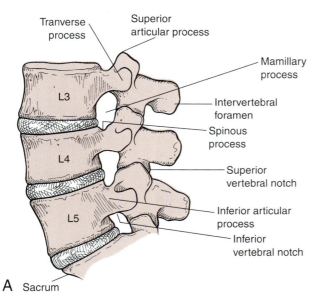

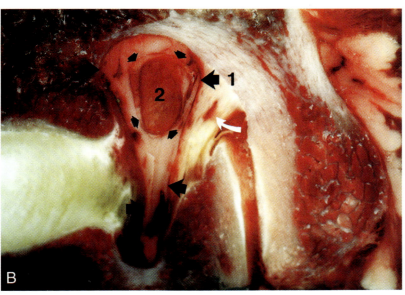

FIGURE 1.18.

Intervertebral foramen. **A.** Diagram of side view of the lower lumbar spine showing the intervertebral foramen. The foramen is shaped like an inverted teardrop and forms a tunnel that connects with the spinal canal. **B.** A sagittal cryomicrotome of the intervertebral foramen. The foramen is bounded superiorly and inferiorly by the pedicles of the adjacent vertebrae. The posterior boundary is formed by the pars interarticularis and the ligamentum flavum. The anterior boundary is formed by the postero-inferior margin of the superior vertebral body, the posterior margin of the intervertebral disc, and the postero-superior margin of the inferior vertebral body. The nerve root (2 and small arrows) is surrounded by fat (1). The soft tissue boundary of the foramen (large arrows) is smaller than the bony boundary. The bulging disc may narrow the foramen anteriorly, and the facet and ligamentum flavum (curved arrow) may narrow the foramen posteriorly.

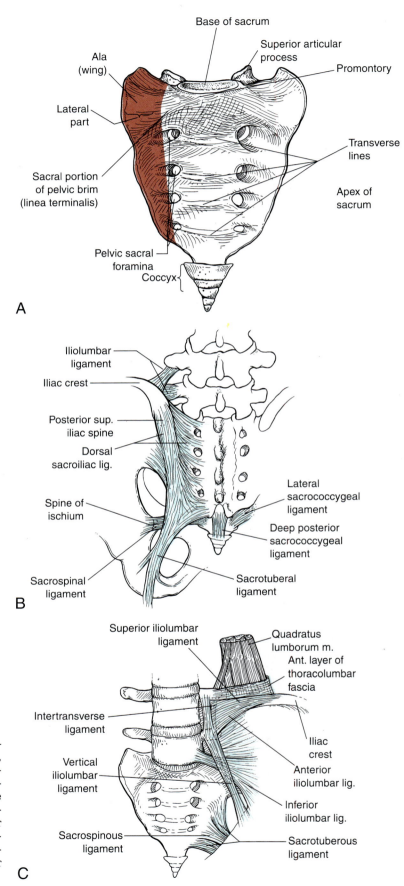

FIGURE 1.19.

Diagrams of the sacrum and sacroiliac articulation. **A.** Anterior view of the sacrum. The ala, promontory, sacral foramina, and articular surfaces are shown. The coccyx consists of four rudimentary vertebrae. **B.** Posterior view shows the iliolumbar ligament, posterior sacroiliac ligament, and sacrotuberous ligament. **C.** Anterior view of the sacroiliac articulation shows the anterior iliolumbar ligament, inferior iliolumbar ligament, vertical iliolumbar ligament, and superior iliolumbar ligament.

and runs obliquely downward and laterally toward the intervertebral foramen. Anatomically, the lateral recess is bordered laterally by the pedicle, posteriorly by the superior articular facet, and anteriorly by the posterolateral surface of the vertebral body and adjacent intervertebral disc. The medial border of the lateral recess is formed by the thecal sac. The narrowest portion of the lateral recess is between the superior border of the pedicle and the broad portion of the superior articular facet. The nerve root in this region is covered by the root sleeve and is surrounded by cerebrospinal fluid. The lateral margin of the nerve root sleeve contacts the medial cortical bone of the pedicle, and the medial margin of the nerve root is surrounded by epidural fat tissue. The normal lateral recess measurement has been well delineated by CT (7, 36, 41). A lateral recess height of 5 mm or more is normal. A height of 2 mm or less is pathologic, and a height of 3 to 4 mm suggests lateral recess stenosis.

The mid zone is located under the pars interarticularis and just below the pedicle. It is bounded anteriorly by the posterior aspect of the vertebral body and posteriorly by the pars interarticularis. The medial boundary is open to the central spinal canal. The nerve roots normally run obliquely downward through the lateral recess into the intervertebral foramen. The nerve root travels around the subpedicular notch and contacts posteriorly with the ventral wall of the pars interarticularis where the ligamentum flavum is attached. The exit zone is formed by the intervertebral foramen. The lumbar intervertebral foramen, which is shaped like an inverted teardrop, forms a tunnel that connects with the spinal canal. It is bounded superiorly and inferiorly by the pedicles of the adjacent vertebrae. The posterior boundary is formed by the pars interarticularis and the ligamentum flavum. The anterior boundary is formed by the postero-inferior margin of the superior vertebral body, the posterior margin of the intervertebral disc, and the postero-superior margin of the inferior vertebral body (Fig. 1.18A,B). The normal foraminal height varies from 20 to 23 mm, and the width at the upper foraminal area varies from 8 to 10 mm (22). The ventral and dorsal nerve roots occupy 23 to 30% of the area of the foramen and lie anterior to the dorsal root ganglion (DRG). The DRG normally lies within the superior lateral portion of the lumbar intervertebral foramen and directly below the pedicle in 90% of lumbar levels. Foraminal height of <15 mm and posterior disc height of <4 mm is associated with nerve root compression 80% of the time (21).

Bony structures of the sacrum include the ala, promontory, sacral crests, sacral foramina, and articular surfaces (Fig. 1.19A). The sacrum is composed of five fused sacral vertebrae, and it provides strength and stability to the pelvis, transmitting the body weight to the pelvis. The four pairs of sacral foramina contain ventral and dorsal divisions of the sacral nerves. The anterior sacral foramina are larger than the dorsal sacral foramina. The median sacral crest represents fused spinous processes, and S5 has no spinous process. The intermediate sacral crests represent the fused articular processes, and the lateral sacral crests are the tips of the transverse processes of the sacral vertebrae. The sacral hiatus leads to the sacral canal, which contains fatty connective tissue, the filum terminale, the S5 nerve, and the coccygeal nerve. The sacral cornua is the inferior articular process of the S5 vertebra and projects laterally. The coccyx consists of four rudimentary vertebrae. The coccygeal cornua articulates with the sacral cornua. The coccyx provides attachments for parts of the gluteus maximus and coccygeus muscles and anococcygeal ligament.

The sacroiliac joint consists of the sacral articular process with hyaline cartilage and the iliac surface with fibrocartilage. The sacroiliac joint is stabilized by the interosseous sacroiliac ligament, posterior sacroiliac ligament, and anterior sacroiliac ligament (Fig. 1.19B,C). Connecting ligaments in the lumbosacral junction and the pelvis include the sacrotuberous ligament from the sacrum to the ischial tuberosity, the sacrospinous ligament that divides the pelvis into greater and lesser sciatic notches, and the iliolumbar ligaments that connect the L5 transverse processes to the ala of sacrum. The iliolumbar ligaments connect the transverse process of the fifth lumbar vertebra to the ilium. The iliolumbar ligament can be divided into different parts based on the anatomic location, such as anterior, superior, posterior, inferior, and vertical. The iliolumbar ligament is important in resisting forward translation of the L5 vertebra on the sacrum.

Intervertebral Disc and Ligaments

The intervertebral disc is an avascular structure that includes the nucleus pulposus at the interior of the disc, the outer anulus fibrosus, and the cartilaginous endplates adjacent to the vertebral surfaces. The nucleus pulposus is derived from the primitive notochord and functions as a shock absorber, and the annulus fibrosus maintains the stability of the motion segment along with ligaments and articulations. The nucleus pulposus is clearly bordered by the annulus fibrosus in infancy, but the margin between the nucleus pulposus and annulus fibrosus becomes less distinct in the adult (Fig. 1.20A) (3). After 50 years of age, the nucleus pulposus becomes more difficult to distinguish from the annulus fibrosus, and the nucleus pulposus becomes a fibrocartilaginous mass similar to the inner zone of the annulus fibrosus (Fig. 1.20B). The annulus has an outer collagenous layer

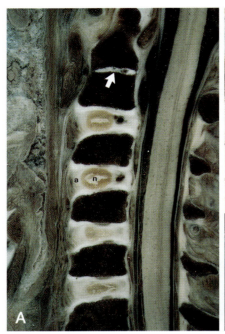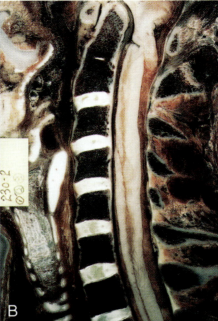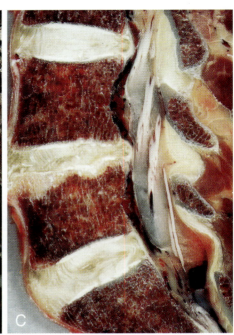

FIGURE 1.20.
Sagittal cryomicrotome sections of the spine. **A.** A sagittal cryomicrotome of a skeletally immature cervical spine shows the intervertebral disc with a clear margin between the nucleus pulposus and annulus fibrosus. The arrow shows the synchondrosis between the odontoid process and the body. **B.** Sagittal cryomicrotome in an adult shows an indistinct margin between the nucleus pulposus and the annulus fibrosus as the nucleus pulposus becomes a fibrocartilaginous mass similar to the inner zone of the annulus fibrosus. **C.** Sagittal cryomicrotome section of the lower lumbar spine shows the degenerative disc with bulging annulus fibrosus and loss of height at L4-L5.

in which the fibers are arranged in oblique layers of lamellae. The fibers of lamella run perpendicular to the fibers of the adjacent lamella. This oblique arrangement can offer resistance of movements in all directions. The collagen fibers in the posterior portion of the disc run more vertical than oblique, which may account for the relative frequency of anular tears seen clinically. The anulus fibrosus is attached firmly to the adjacent vertebral endplates. The cartilaginous endplate is a layer of hyaline cartilage resting on the subchondral bone, and it serves as a barrier between the pressure of the nucleus pulposus and the adjacent vertebral bodies. This cartilage is a growth plate and is responsible for endochoral ossification during growth. The cartilaginous endplates also allow the insertion of the inner fibers of the annulus fibrosus and the diffusion of nutrients from the subchondral bone to the disc.

The cervical intervertebral discs allow some translatory movement in the sagittal plane, but the lateral movement is resisted by the uncinate process. The uncinate process, which is located in the posterolateral aspect of the disc, may prevent disc herniation in this area. Degeneration of the anulus fibrosus in the cervical region is similar to the lumbar region in that concentric, transverse, and radial tears of the anulus occur, and the radial tear in the posterior aspect of the disc may be more clinically significant (Fig. 1.20C) (47, 38). The discs are thinnest in the thoracic region and thickest in the lumbar region, where they constitute a third of its length. The discs are thicker anteriorly in the lumbar spine because of the lordotic curvature, and the vertebral endplates of L3 are parallel and horizontal (Fig. 1.20C). The lumbar discs are normally concave or straight posteriorly, but the L5-S1 disc is normally slightly convex.

The outermost fibers of the annulus fibrosus are contiguous with the anterior and posterior longitudinal ligaments. The anterior longitudinal ligament is a strong band that attaches from the skull as the anterior atlantooccipital membrane and continues caudally over the entire length of the spine down to the sacrum. The anterior longitudinal ligament is thinner and more closely attached at the intervertebral disc margins than at the concave anterior vertebral surfaces. The posterior longitudinal ligament is wider in the upper cervical spine than the lower cervical spine, and wider over the intervertebral discs than over the vertebral bodies (33). In the cervical spine, the posterior longitudinal ligament is double-

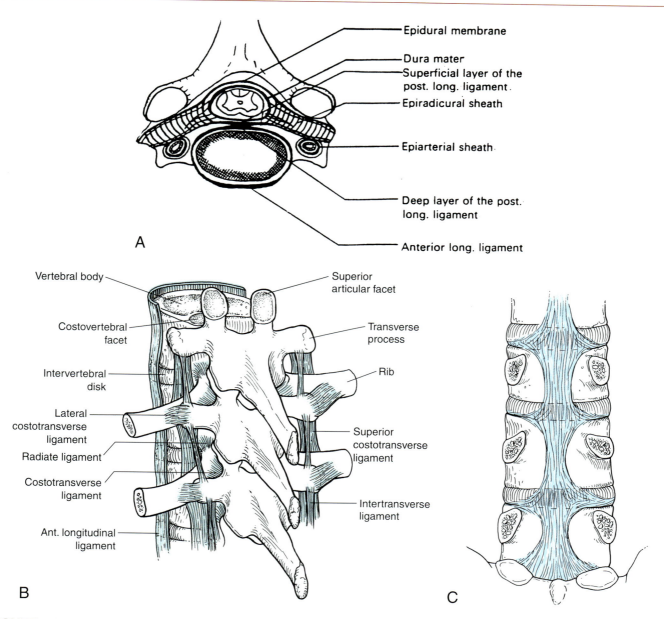

FIGURE 1.21.
Ligaments of the spine. **A.** Diagram of the cervical spine in cross-section showing the anterior longitudinal ligament, layers of the posterior longitudinal ligament, and perineural sheath. **B.** The thoracic spine has the articular facets for the ribs that are located in the body and transverse process. The radiate and costovertebral ligaments are between the body and rib, and the costotransverse and intertransverse ligaments are between the transverse process and rib. The spinous processes are long and slender and overlap to the lower vertebral arches. **C.** The posterior longitudinal ligament is broad in the thoracic and lumbar regions where it is attached to the intervertebral discs.

layered, and the deep layer sends fibers to the anulus fibrosus and continues laterally to the region of the intervertebral foramina (Fig. 1.21A) (23). The anterior longitudinal ligament also sweeps around and envelops the lateral aspects of the vertebral bodies under the longus collis muscle, and the lateral extension is continuous with the deep layer of the posterior longitudinal ligament in the region of the intervertebral foramina (23). The superficial, or more dorsal, layer of the posterior longitudinal ligament is adjacent to the dura mater and continues as a connective tissue membrane that envelops the dura mater, nerve roots, and the vertebral artery, suggesting that this membrane may serve as a protective barrier. In the thoracic spine, the transverse process and the body have articulations with the rib and connecting costotransverse ligaments and the radiate ligament (Fig. 1.21B). The thoracic spine is inherently more

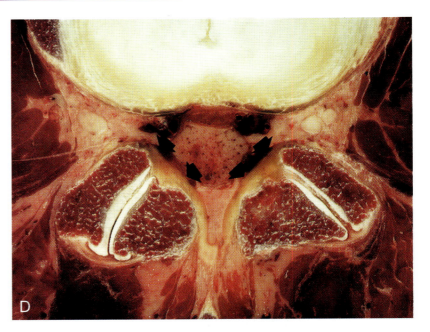

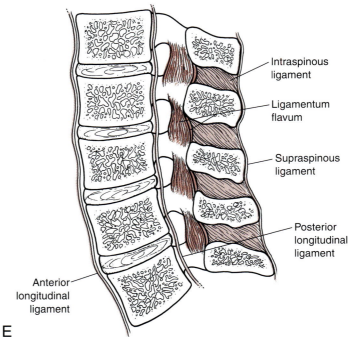

FIGURE 1.21—continued

D. The ligamentum flavum is a short ligament that joins the laminae of adjacent vertebrae. The ligamentum flavum attaches to the anterior surface of the lamina above and to the superior margin of the lamina below and extends laterally to the articular processes and contributes to the boundary of the intervertebral foramen (arrows). **E.** The ligaments between the vertebral arches include the interspinous ligament that connects adjacent spinal processes and the supraspinous ligament that stretches across the tips of the spinous process.

stable than the cervical or lumbar spine because of its attachment to the ribs. The posterior longitudinal ligament is broad in the thoracic and lumbar regions where it is attached to the intervertebral discs (Fig 1.21C). The posterior longitudinal ligament helps to prevent hyperflexion of the vertebral column and resist posterior protrusion of the intervertebral disc. In the lumbar spine, lumbar dural ligaments have been reported, namely the Spencer's ligament that courses from the dural tube to the posterior longitudinal ligament and the Hofmann's ligament that courses from the nerve root sheath to the inferior aspect of the pedicle within the neural canal (24, 40). Wiltse et al. also describe a peridural membrane that lies anterior to the posterior longitudinal ligament at the level of the vertebral body, and Yaszemski and White describe the discectomy membrane that is between the posterior longitudinal ligament and the nerve root at the level of the disc (43, 46). These membranes are important to recognize, particularly during surgical approaches.

The ligamentum flavum is a short ligament that joins the laminae of adjacent vertebrae. The ligamentum flavum attaches to the anterior surface of the lamina above and directly on the superior margin of the lamina below. It extends laterally to the articular processes and contributes to the boundary of the intervertebral foramen (Fig. 1.21D). The ligamentum flavum consists primarily of elastic fibers, but the elasticity weakens with aging, and anterior buckling or hypertrophy may contribute to spinal stenosis. A gap exists in the midline of the ligamentum flavum for the exit of veins.

The ligaments between the vertebral arches include the interspinous ligament that connects adjacent spinal processes and the supraspinous ligament that stretches across the tips of the spinous process (Fig. 1.21E). The interspinous ligament of the cervical spine is thin and less well developed than it is in the lumbar region. The interspinous ligaments attach in an oblique orientation from the posterior superior aspect to the anterior inferior aspect of the spinous process. The supraspinous ligament of the thoracolumbar spine extends in the cervical region as the ligamentum nuchae, which spans from the external occipital protuberance to the seventh cervical vertebra. The ligamentum nuchae is a fibroelastic septum for the attachment of adjacent muscles. The supraspinous ligament consists largely of tendinous fibers derived from the back muscles. It is better developed in the upper lumbar region and often is absent in the lower lumbar region.

Muscles, Fascia, and Related Structures

There are three groups of muscles in the back: superficial, intermediate, and deep (Fig. 1.22). The superficial group consists of the trapezius and latissimus dorsi muscles, and the intermediate group consists of the serratus posterior, which is involved in respiration. The trapezius originates from the external occipital protuberance and the medial nuchal line of C7 to T12 spinous processes, and it inserts on the spine of the scapula, the acromion, and the lateral aspect of the clavicle. The trapezius is innervated by the 11th cranial nerve and functions to extend the head. The latissimus dorsi arises from the lumbar aponeurosis, the posterior iliac crest, and the lower four ribs. It inserts on the bottom of the intertubercular groove of the humerus to extend, adduct, and rotate the arm medially. Its innervation is the thoracodorsal nerve.

The serratus posterior superior arises from the lower part of the ligamentum nuchae and the spinous processes of the seventh and upper thoracic vertebrae, and it inserts on the upper second to the fifth ribs. The serratus posterior inferior arises from the lower thoracic and upper two lumbar spinous processes and inserts on the lower four ribs. The serratus posterior muscles are innervated by the ventral rami of spinal nerves or intercostal nerves, and their function is to enlarge the thorax during respiration.

The intrinsic muscles are concerned with movements of the vertebral column. The intrinsic back muscles of the back are divided into superficial, intermediate, and deep layers. The posterior muscles of the back are innervated by the dorsal rami of the spinal nerves. The superficial muscles are longer, spanning many vertebrae; the deepest muscles span only one vertebral segment. In the cervical spine, deep to the trapezius and the rhomboids, the splenius capitis and splenius cervicis muscles, unlike the muscles in the thoracic and lumbar regions, arise medially and pass laterally as they are traced upward. These muscles comprise the superficial group of the intrinsic back muscles. These muscles originate from the spinous processes of the lower cervical and upper thoracic spines and insert on the transverse processes of the upper cervical spine and the mastoid process. These muscles aid in lateral bending and extension of the head and the cervical vertebral column.

In the intermediate layer of intrinsic deep muscles, the erector spinal muscles lie within a fascial compartment between the posterior and middle layers of the thoracolumbar fascia (Fig. 1.22B). The erector spinae is arranged in three vertical columns: iliocostalis laterally, longissimus intermediately, and spinalis medially. The erector spinae arises from the posterior part of the iliac crest, the posterior aspect of the sacrum, the sacroiliac ligaments, and the sacral and inferior lumbar spinous processes. The iliocostalis muscle is subdivided into lumbar, thoracic, and cervical portions. The intermediate longissimus arises from the transverse processes of the thoracic and cervical vertebrae and the mastoid process of the skull. The longissimus muscle is subdivided into longissimus thoracic, cervicis, and capitis. The spinalis muscle is narrow and insignificant, and extends from the spinous processes of the superior thoracic region. The erector spinae muscle is the primary extensor of the vertebral column.

In the deepest layer of the intrinsic back muscles, several short muscles are found between the transverse processes and spinous processes, namely semispinalis, multifidus, and rotatores (Fig. 1.22C). Collectively, this deep group of muscles is known as the transversospinalis muscle. The semispinalis muscle is divided into thoracis, cervicis, and capitis according to the insertion of the muscle bundles. Deep to the semispinalis are the multifidus that span from one to three vertebral segments. The muscle bundles run upward and medially from the transverse processes to the spinous processes, covering laminae of S4 to C2 vertebrae. The rotatores muscles arise from the transverse process of one vertebra and insert into the base of the spinous process of the second vertebra above. The interspinales and intertransversarii muscles, also known as short rotators, pass from one vertebra to the next vertebra above.

In the upper cervical spine, suboccipital muscles attach at the occiput to second vertebra. Rectus cap-

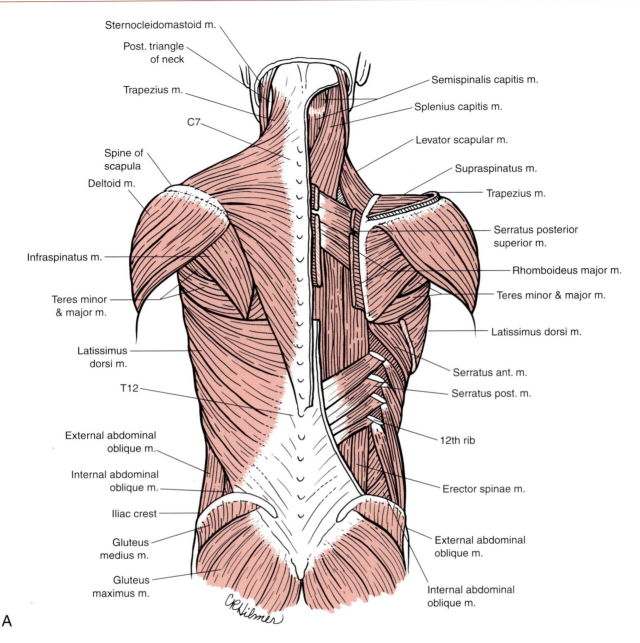

FIGURE 1.22.
Muscles of the back. **A.** Superficial layer.

itis posterior major originates from the C2 spinous process and inserts to the inferior nuchal line of the occiput, and rectus capitis posterior minor originates from the posterior tubercle of the atlas and inserts to the occiput. Obliquus capitis inferior originates from the C2 spinous process and inserts on the transverse process of the atlas, and obliquus capitis superior originates from the transverse process of the atlas and inserts on the occiput between the superior and inferior nuchal lines. Most posterior muscles are involved in producing extension of the neck and head, and some muscles produce rotation and lateral flexion. The posterior deep muscles are innervated by the posterior primary rami, and blood is supplied by the deep cervical vessels. The anterolateral muscles of the neck include platysma, sternocleidomastoid, hyoid muscles, strap muscles of the larynx, scalenes, longus colli, and longus capitis. The platysma is a thin muscle underneath the subcutaneous tissue that spans from the deltoid and upper pectoral fascia, crosses over the clavicle, and passes obliquely upward and medially to insert into the mandible, muscles of the lip, and the skin of the lower part of the face. The platysma depresses the lower jaw and the lip, and tenses and ridges the skin of the neck. The sternocleidomastoid originates from the sternum and the medial clavicle to the mastoid process and the lateral half of the superior nuchal line of the oc-

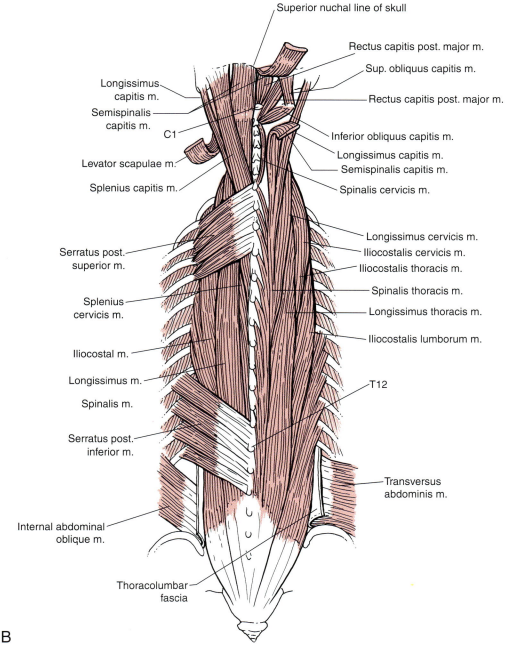

FIGURE 1.22—continued
B. Intermediate layer.

cipital bone. The sternocleidomastoid is innervated by the second cervical nerve and the spinal accessory nerve, and it serves to draw the head toward the shoulder and rotate it, pointing the chin cranially and to the opposite side. The sternocleidomastoids together flex the head and raise the thorax when the head is fixed. This muscle may be involved in the pathogenesis of the torticollic posture of the neck. Muscles that attach to the hyoid bone include the digastric, stylohyoid, mylohyoid, geniohyoid, and omohyoid muscles, and the strap muscles of the larynx include the sternohyoideus and sternothyroid muscles. These muscles do not control the cervical spine, but are important in controlling the movement of the hyoid and larynx and are important landmarks in the anterior approach to the cervical spine. The longus colli and longus capitis are the prevertebral muscles of the neck. The longus colli spans from C1 to T3 and extends laterally to attach at the anterior tubercles of the transverse processes of C3, C4, C5, and C6. The longus capitis originates from the anterior tubercles of the transverse processes of C3, C4, C5, and C6, and attaches on the inferior surface of the basilar part of the occipital bone. Underneath the lon-

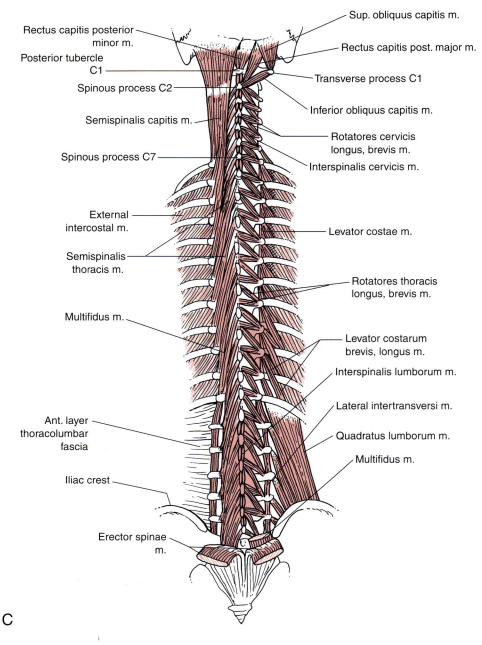

FIGURE 1.22—continued
C. Deep layer.

gus capitis, the rectus capitis anterior spans from the lateral mass of the atlas to the base of the occipital bone, and the rectus capitis lateralis spans laterally from the transverse process of the atlas to the inferior surface of the jugular process of the occipital bone. The scalenus anterior originates from the anterior tubercles of the transverse processes of C3 to C6 and inserts on the first rib, and the scalenus medius originates from the posterior tubercles of the transverse processes of C2 to C7 and inserts on the first rib. A vascular impingement of the subclavian artery may occur as it runs between the scalenus anterior and scalenus medius, as seen in the thoracic outlet syndrome. The scalenus posterior originates from the posterior tubercles of the transverse processes of C4 to C6 and inserts on the second rib. The muscles of the neck are also arranged in triangles. The posterior triangle is formed by the sternocleidomastoid, clavicle, and the trapezius muscles, and the omohyoid muscle divides it into the supraclavicular and the occipital triangles (33). The anterior triangle is bounded by the midline of the neck anteriorly, the lower border of the mandible superiorly, and the sternocleidomastoid posteriorly. The anterior triangle is subdivided by the submental triangle, the muscular triangle, the digastric triangle, and the carotid triangle. These triangles are important landmarks for making anterior approach to the cervical spine.

The fascia of the anterior part of the neck invest the muscles and viscera in separate compartments, and make the surgical approach much easier. The superficial fascia contains fat and areolar tissue, including the platysma muscle, external jugular vein, and the cutaneous sensory nerves. The structures deep to the superficial fascia are compartmentalized by the deep fascia, including the outer investing layer of deep fascia, middle cervical fascia, and the prevertebral fascia. The outer layer of the deep fascia extends from the trapezius muscle over the posterior triangle and splits to enclose the sternocleidomastoid muscle. The middle layers of the deep cervical fascia enclose the strap muscles and omohyoid and extend as far laterally as the scapula. The deeper middle layer is the visceral fascia that surrounds the thyroid gland, larynx, trachea, pharynx, and esophagus. The alar fascia spreads behind the esophagus and surrounds the carotid sheath structures laterally. The carotid sheath encloses the carotid artery, internal jugular vein, and vagus nerve. On the right side, the recurrent laryngeal nerve may leave the carotid sheath at a higher level, and the surgeon must take caution during dissection, especially below C6 (37). The recurrent laryngeal nerve usually enters the tracheoesophageal groove where the inferior thyroid artery enters the lower pole of the thyroid. It is also more common for the right inferior laryngeal nerve to be nonrecurrent where it travels directly from the vagus nerve and carotid sheath to the larynx. The incidence of nonrecurrent laryngeal nerve on the right side is reported as 1% (37). The deepest layer of the deep fascia is the prevertebral fascia, which covers the scalenus muscles, longus colli muscles, and the anterior longitudinal ligament.

The anterior muscles of the abdomen and the diaphragm are important structures in the anterior surgical approach to the thoracolumbar spine. The diaphragm is a dome-shaped musculofibrous septum that separates the thoracic cavity from the abdominal cavity. It originates from the xiphoid process, costal cartilage, lumbar vertebrae and inserts into the central tendon. Its innervation is from the phrenic nerve of the cervical plexus. The diaphragm is divided frequently for the thoracoabdominal approach to the thoracolumbar junction.

Abdominal muscles can be divided into posterior muscles, including the psoas major and minor, iliacus, quadratus lumborum, and the anterolateral muscles, including the rectus abdominis, external oblique, internal oblique, and transversus abdominis. These muscles are divided or separated for the anterior approaches to the lumbar spine.

The aorta bifurcates into the common iliac arteries at the L4-5 disc level. The right common iliac artery crosses the anterior surface of the L4-5 disc and fixes the left common iliac branch of the vena cava against the vertebral column. During the anterior exposure of the L4-L5 region, the iliolumbar vein should be identified and ligated to mobilize the great vessels. For the approach to L5-S1, the midline within the vascular bifurcation, in which the middle sacral vessels and the superior hypogastric plexus are located, should be exposed. The sacral artery runs down along the anterior aspect of the sacrum and is ligated frequently for distal sacral exposure. The presacral plexus of parasympathetic nerves must be preserved, which is important to sexual function. The left ureter crosses the left common iliac vessels over the sacroiliac joint.

In summary, this chapter outlines the anatomy of bone and joints, intervertebral discs, ligaments, muscles, and related structures of the spine. A short review of pertinent anatomic structures is presented here, and more detailed information is available in the literature. The knowledge of the anatomy is the first step toward a better understanding of pathology of the spine, imaging studies, and surgical approaches.

References

1. An HS, Gordin R, Renner K. Anatomic considerations for plate-screw fixation of the cervical spine. Spine 1991;16:S548–551.
2. An HS, Glover JM. Lumbar spinal stenosis: historical perspectives, classification, and pathoanatomy. Sem Spine Surg 1994;6:69–77.
3. Bland JH, Boushey DR. Anatomy and physiology of the cervical spine. Semin Arthritis Rheum 1990;20:1–20.
4. Bogduk N. The innervation of the lumbar spine. Spine 1983;8:286–293.
5. Bogduk N, Tynan W, Wilson A. The nerve supply to the human intervertebral discs. J Anat 1981;132:39–56.
6. Bose K, Balasubramaniam P. Nerve root canals of the lumbar spine. Spine 1984;9:16–18.
7. Ciric I, Mikael MA, Tarkington TA, et al. The lateral recess syndrome. J Neurosurg 1980;53:433–443.
8. Czervionke LF, Daniels DL. Cervical spine anatomy and pathologic processes. Applications of new MR imaging techniques. Radiol Clin North Am 1988;26:921–947.
9. Czervionke LF, Daniels DL, Ho PSP, et al. Cervical neural foramina: correlative anatomic and MR imaging study. Neuroradiology 1988;169:753–759.
10. Czervionke LF, Daniels DL, Ho PSP, et al. MR appearance of gray and white matter in the cervical spinal cord. Am J Neuroradiol 1988;9:557–562.
11. Daniels DL, Williams AL, Haughton VM. Computed tomography of the articulations and ligaments at the occipito-atlantoaxial region. Radiology 1983;146:709–716.
12. Daniels DL, Hyde JS, Kneeland JB, et al. The cervical nerves and foramina: local-coil MR imaging. Am J Neuroradiol 1986;7:129–133.

13. Doherty B, Heggeness MH. The quantitative anatomy of the atlas. Spine 1994;19:2497–2500.
14. Doherty B, Heggeness MH. Quantitative anatomy of the second cervical vertebra. Spine 1995;20:513–517.
15. Dommisse GF. The blood supply of the spinal cord. J Bone Joint Surg Br 1974;56:225.
16. Ebraheim NA, An HS, Xu R, et al. The quantitative anatomy of the cervical nerve root groove and the intervertebral foramen. Spine 1996;21:1619–1623.
17. Ellis JH, Martell W, Lillie JH, et al. Magnetic resonance imaging of the normal craniovertebral junction. Spine 1991;16:105–111.
18. Flannigan BD, Lufkin RB, McGlade C, et al. MR imaging of the cervical spine: neurovascular anatomy. Am J Radiol 1987;148:785–790.
19. Fletcher G, Haughton VM, Ho KC, et al. Age related changes in the cervical facet joints: studies with cryomicrotomy, MR, and CT. Am J Neuroradiol 1990;11:27–30.
20. Gerbrand JG, Baljet B, Drukker J. Nerves and nerve plexuses of the human vertebral column. J Anat 1990;188:282–296.
21. Hasegawa T, An HS, Haughton VM, et al. Lumbar foraminal stenosis: critical heights of the intervertebral discs and foramina. J Bone Joint Surg Am 1995;77:32–38.
22. Hasegawa T, Mikawa Y, Watanabe R, et al. Morphometric analysis of the lumbosacral roots and dorsal root ganglia by magnetic resonance imaging. Spine 1996;21:1005–1009.
23. Hayashi K, Yabuki T, Kurokawa T, et al. The anterior and the posterior longitudinal ligaments of the lower cervical spine. J Anat 1977;633–636.
24. Hoffmann M. Die befestignung der dura mater im wirbelcanal. Arch F Anat Physio (Anat Ab) 1898;403.
25. Kadish LJ, Simmons EH. Anomalies of the lumbosacral nerve roots. J Bone Joint Surg Br 1984;66:411–416.
26. Kikuchi S, Sato K, Konno S, et al. Anatomic and radiographic study of dorsal root ganglia. Spine 1994;19:6–11.
27. Kothe R, O'Holleran JD, Liu W, et al. Internal architecture of the thoracic pedicle. Spine 1996;21:264–270.
28. Kurz LT, Garfin SR, Booth RE. Harvesting autogenous iliac bone grafts: a review of complications and techniques. Spine 1989;14:1324–1331.
29. Lee CK, Rauschning W, Glenn W. Lateral lumbar spinal canal stenosis: classification, pathologic anatomy, and surgical decompression. Spine 1980;13:313–320.
30. Nakamura S, Takahashi K, Takahashi Y, et al. Origin of nerves supplying the posterior portion of lumbar intervertebral discs. Spine 1996;21:917–924.
31. Nowick BH, Haughton VM. Ligaments of the lumbar neural foramina. Clin Anat 1992;5:126–135.
32. Panjabi MM, Duranceau J, Goel V, et al. Cervical human vertebrae. Quantitative three-dimensional anatomy of the middle and lower regions. Spine 1993;16:861–874.
33. Parke WW, Sherk HH. Normal adult anatomy. In: Sherk HH, et al., eds. Cervical spine, 2nd ed. Philadelphia: JB Lippincott, 1989:11–32.
34. Pech P, Daniels DL, Williams AL, et al. The cervical neural foramina: correlation of microtomy and CT anatomy. Radiology 1985;155:143–146.
35. Rauschning W. Anatomy and pathology of the cervical spine. In: Frymoyer JW, ed. The adult spine. St Louis: C.V. Mosby Inc., 1991:907–929.
36. Rauschning W. Normal and pathologic anatomy of the lumbar root canals. Spine 1987;12:1008–1019.
37. Sanders G, Uyeda RY, Karlan MS. Nonrecurrent inferior laryngeal nerves and their association with a recurrent branch. Am J Surg 1983;146:501–503.
38. Sether LA, Yu S, Haughton VM, et al. Ruptures of the anulus fibrosus of cervical intervertebral discs studied by cryomicrotomy and magnetic resonance. Clin Anat 1989;2:1–8.
39. Shinomiya K, Okawa A, Nakao K, et al. Morphology of C5 ventral nerve rootlets as part of dissociated motor loss of deltoid muscle. Spine 1994;19:2501–2504.
40. Spencer DL, Irwin GS, Miller JAA. Anatomy and significance of the lumbosacral nerve roots in sciatica. Spine 1983;8:672.
41. Ullich CG, Binet EF, Sanecki MG, et al. Quantitative assessment of the lumbar spinal canal by computed tomography. Radiology 1980;134:137–143.
42. Vaccaro AR, Rizzolo SJ, Allardyce TJ, et al. Placement of pedicle screws in the thoracic spine. J Bone Joint Surg Am 1995;77:1193–1199.
43. Wiltse LL, Fonseca AS, Amster J, et al. Relationship of the dura, Hoffmann's Ligaments, Batson's plexus, and a fibrovascular membrane lying on the posterior surface of the vertebral bodies and attaching to the deep layer of the posterior longitudinal ligament: an anatomical, radiologic, and clinical study. Spine 1993;18:1030.
44. Xu R, Naudaud MC, Ebraheim NA, et al. Morphology of the second cervical vertebra and the posterior projection of the C2 pedicle axis. Spine 1995;20:259–263.
45. Xu R, Ebraheim NA, Yeasting RA, et al. Anatomic consideration for posterior iliac bone harvesting. Spine 1996;21:1017–1020.
46. Yaszemski M, White AA. The discectomy membrane (nerve root fibrovascular membrane): its anatomic description and its surgical importance. J Spinal Disord 1994;7:230–235.
47. Yu S, Haughton VM, Sether LA, et al. Anulus fibrosus in bulging intervertebral disks. Radiology 1988;169:761–763.
48. Yu S, Sether L, Haughton VM. Facet joint menisci of the cervical spine: correlative MR imaging and cryomicrotomy study. Radiology 1987;164:79–82.
49. Zindrick, Wiltse LL, Doornik A. Analysis of the morphometric characteristics of the thoracic and lumbar pedicles. Spine 1987;12:160–166.

CHAPTER TWO

Surgical Exposure and Fusion Techniques of the Spine

Howard S. An

Introduction

Successful spinal surgery depends significantly on the techniques of surgical exposure and fusion. Good exposure is the first step in performing any spinal operation and includes decompressive procedures, fusion, and various instrumentation. Many potential complications are avoided with careful and meticulous surgical approaches to the spine. The surgical exposure depends on the nature of the lesion, its location, and the extent of the pathology. In this chapter, operative techniques of surgical exposure and fusion of the cervical spine, thoracic spine, and lumbar spine are discussed.

The Cervical Spine

Posterior Exposure of the Upper Cervical Spine

The upper cervical spine can be approached either anteriorly or posteriorly, depending on the pathoanatomy of the lesion. Several posterior occipitocervical fusion techniques of the upper cervical spine have been described in the literature (38, 40, 41, 66, 75, 85). Posterior atlantoaxial stabilization and fusion can also be accomplished with wires and iliac bone graft in the majority of cases (14, 37, 39). Newer techniques use screw fixation between the lateral mass of C1 and C2 (40, 41, 54). Complications associated with posterior occipitocervical or atlantoaxial fusion may be devastating. Care is required during passage of the wires to prevent injuries to the brainstem or spinal cord. The vertebral artery must be protected during exposure and instrumentation. The use of somatosensory evoked potential monitoring is routine in myelopathic cases. Postoperative halo-vest external support is recommended in the majority of wiring cases.

A halo-vest is generally applied preoperatively. Anesthesia and intubation must be done cautiously; awake intubation using fiberoptic light is recommended in all unstable cases to minimize neck manipulation. If traction is not required and preoperative alignment is acceptable, surgery can be performed in the halo-vest on the routine operating table. If traction is required, or if spinal realignment is necessary during the procedure, the halo ring should be attached to a traction device on the Stryker table. To facilitate the exposure of the occiput and the upper cervical spine, a halo ring with a posterior opening is recommended.

A reverse Trendelenburg position allows venous drainage and less bleeding during the procedure (Fig. 2.1) (5). A midline incision is made from the external occipital protuberance to the spinous process of C2.

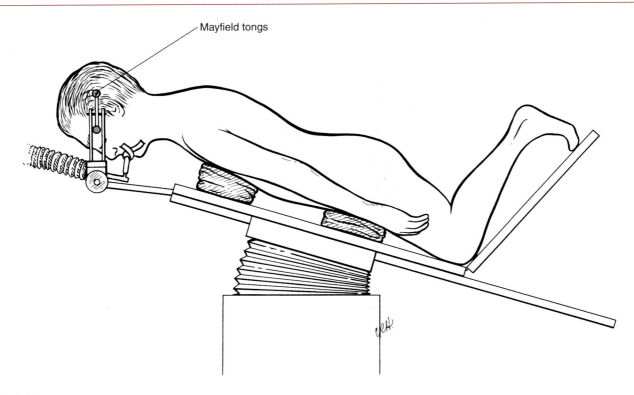

FIGURE 2.1.
Diagram of operating position for posterior cervical procedures. The Mayfield tongs and frame secure the head in position, and the reverse Trendelenburg position allows venous drainage and less bleeding during the procedure.

Surgical dissection on the occiput and the ring of the atlas must be done in a gentle manner because excess pressure may result in a fracture or slippage of the instrument. The ring of the atlas should not be dissected more than 1.5 cm laterally because the vertebral artery is at risk beyond this margin. One should avoid dissecting the foramen magnum from the inferior edge of the foramen to prevent uncontrollable venous bleeding. Wiring and other methods for stabilization will be discussed in the chapter on cervical spinal instrumentation (61).

Posterior Exposure of the Lower Cervical Spine and Fusion

Exposure of the posterior elements of the lower cervical spine is simple. Either Mayfield tongs or Gardner Wells tongs are used for positioning. A reverse Trendelenburg positioning is utilized. A midline incision is followed by subperiosteal dissection, exposing the spinous processes, lamina, and facet joints. One should expose only the levels to be fused because creeping fusion extension is common. For cervical laminectomy procedure, the junction between the lamina and facet is thinned with a power burr, and a small curette is used to finish the cut. Meticulous hemostasis is mandatory to prevent hematoma formation. Posterior fusion and stabilization of the cervical spine is a well-established procedure (11, 59, 65). The standard triple wiring and fusion with bone graft is performed in the majority of cases. If laminectomy has been performed, a lateral facet wiring, Luque rodding, or lateral mass plating can be performed (1, 9, 18, 30, 39, 59, 66).

Anterior Exposure to the Upper Cervical Spine

Anterior approaches to the upper part of the cervical spine include dislocation of the temporomandibular joint (63), osteotomy of the mandible (42), transoral approach (24, 25, 26, 34), and anterior retropharyngeal approaches (28, 57, 89). Each procedure has advantages and disadvantages, and the surgeon should be thoroughly familiar with the anatomy and potential complications associated with the particular procedure before undertaking this formidable task.

The transoral approach allows exposure of the midline between the arch of the atlas and C2 (24, 25). The exposure may be extended cephalad by dividing the soft and hard palate to allow access to the foramen magnum and lower half of the clivus (Fig. 2.2). The transoral procedure is a technically demanding operation with limited surgical indications. Any oropharynx or dental infections must be treated before elective transoral surgery. Somatosensory evoked potential monitoring, fiberoptic nasotracheal intubation, and a nasogastric tube are used. The patient is placed in the supine position with the head held in slight extension using the Mayfield frame. The oral cavity is cleansed with chlorhexidine, and perioperative antibiotics with an intravenous cephalosporin and metronidazole is instituted for 72 hours as prophylaxis against wound infection. The key surgical landmark is the anterior tubercle on the atlas to which the anterior longitudinal ligament and longus colli muscles are attached. The vertebral artery is at a minimum of 2 cm from this point in the midline. The transoral retractors are then inserted, exposing the posterior oropharynx. The area of the incision is infiltrated with 1:200,000 epinephrine. A midline, 3-cm vertical incision centered on the anterior tubercle is made through the pharyngeal mucosa and muscle. The mucosa and muscle are later closed in separate layers. The tubercle of the atlas and anterior longitudinal ligament are exposed subperiosteally, and the longus colli muscles are mobilized laterally. A high speed burr may be used to remove the anterior arch of the atlas to expose the odontoid process.

DeAndrade and Macnab described an anteromedial retropharyngeal approach to the upper cervical spine, which is an extension of Smith-Robinson approach to the lower cervical spine (28) (Fig. 2.3). The neck is hyperextended, and the chin is turned to the opposite side. The degree of neck hyperextension should be assessed preoperatively because too much hyperextension may produce myelopathic signs and symptoms. A skin incision is made along the anterior aspect of the sternocleidomastoid muscle and is curved toward the mastoid process. The platysma and the superficial layer of the deep cervical fascia are divided in the line of the incision to expose the

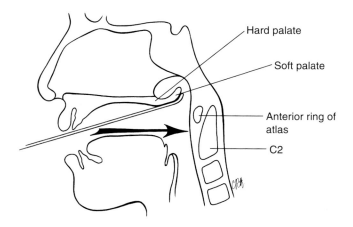

FIGURE 2.2.
Diagram of the transoral approach, which allows exposure of the midline between the arch of the atlas and C2. The exposure may be extended cephalad by dividing the soft and hard palate to allow access to the foramen magnum and the lower half of the clivus.

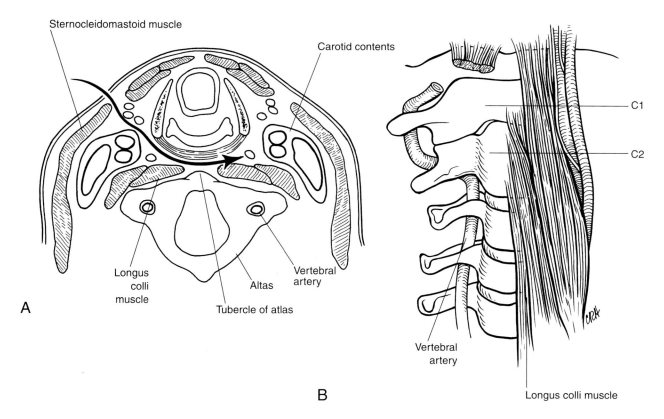

FIGURE 2.3.
The anteromedial approach to the upper cervical by DeAndrade and Macnab. **A.** The dissection is a retropharyngeal approach as an extension of the Smith-Robinson approach to the lower cervical spine. **B.** The longus collis muscle is retracted to expose the anterior tubercle of the atlas and body of the axis.

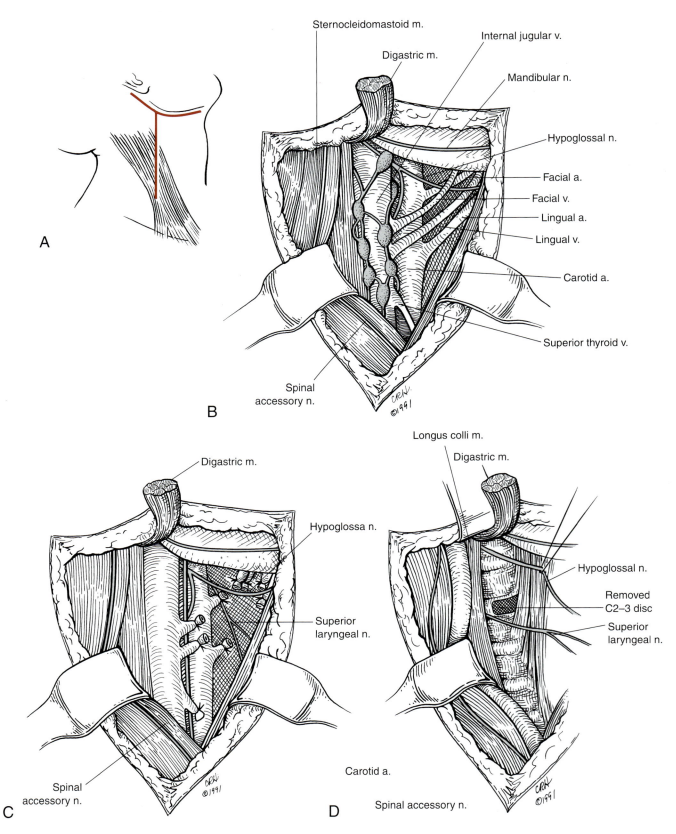

FIGURE 2.4.

Diagrams of the McAfee's retroperitoneal approach to the upper cervical spine. **A.** A right-sided submandibular T-shape incision is made. **B.** Division of the platysma leads to the sternocleidomastoid muscle and its deep cervical fascia. The mandibular branch of the facial nerve should be preserved. The digastric tendon is divided and tagged for later repair. Next, the hypoglossal nerve is identified and mobilized. **C.** The carotid contents are mobilized laterally by ligating arterial and venous branches. These include the superior thyroid artery and vein, lingual artery and vein, ascending pharyngeal artery and vein, and facial artery and vein, beginning inferiorly, progressing superiorly. The superior laryngeal nerve also is identified and mobilized. **D.** The prevertebral fasciae are transected longitudinally to expose and dissect the longus colli muscles.

anterior border of the sternocleidomastoid. The sternocleidomastoid muscle is retracted anteriorly, and the carotid artery is retracted laterally. The superior thyroid artery and lingual vessels are ligated. The facial artery is identified at the upper portion of the incision, which helps to find the hypoglossal nerve adjacent to the digastric muscle. The superior laryngeal nerve is in close proximity to the superior thyroid artery, and excessive retraction of this nerve causes hoarseness or inability to sing high notes. Stripping of the longus colli muscle exposes the anterior aspect of the upper cervical spine and basiocciput.

Another technique of retropharyngeal anterior exposure of the upper cervical spine has been described by McAfee et al. (57) (Fig. 2.4). A right-sided submandibular transverse incision and division of the platysma leads to the sternocleidomastoid muscle and its deep cervical fascia. The mandibular branch of the facial nerve should be identified with the aid of a nerve stimulator, and the retromandibular vein is ligated during the initial stage of dissection. The anterior border of the sternocleidomastoid muscle is mobilized. The submandibular salivary gland and the jugular digastric lymph nodes are resected. Care should be taken to suture the duct in the salivary gland to prevent a salivary fistula. The digastric tendon is divided and tagged for later repair. The hypoglossal nerve is next identified and mobilized. To mobilize the carotid contents laterally, the carotid sheath is opened, and arterial and venous branches are ligated. These branches include the superior thyroid artery and vein, lingual artery and vein, ascending pharyngeal artery and vein, and facial artery and vein, beginning inferiorly, progressing superiorly. The superior laryngeal nerve also is identified with the aid of a nerve stimulator and is mobilized. The prevertebral fasciae are transected longitudinally to expose and dissect the longus colli muscles.

The anterolateral retropharyngeal approach described by Whitesides and Kelley also provides exposure of the upper cervical spine but not of the basiocciput (89) (Fig. 2.5). This approach involves dissection anterior to the sternocleidomastoid but posterior to the carotid sheath. The skin incision is made from the mastoid along the anterior aspect of the sternocleidomastoid. The external jugular vein is ligated, and the greater auricular nerve is spared if possible. The sternocleidomastoid and splenius capitus muscles are detached from the mastoid, leaving a fascial edge for later repair. The spinal accessory nerve should be identified and protected. Retract the carotid contents along with the hypoglossal nerve anteriorly, while retracting the sternocleidomastoid posteriorly. Blunt dissection leads to the transverse processes and anterior aspect of C1 to C3. Potential complications of this approach include injuries to the spinal accessory nerve, the sympathetic ganglion, and the vertebral artery.

Anterior Exposure of the Lower Cervical Spine

The anterior approach to the lower cervical spine has been well described in the literature (21, 63, 64). The patient is placed in a supine and slight reverse Trendelenburg position to minimize venous pooling in the surgical area (Fig. 2.6). Traction is applied to the head using Gardner Wells tongs or halter device, and caudally directed traction to the shoulders is applied using adhesive tape. The right-handed surgeon prefers the right-sided approach, but to minimize injury to the recurrent laryngeal nerve, the cervical spine often is approached from the left, particularly for the C6-T1 region.

On the right side, the recurrent laryngeal nerve may leave the carotid sheath at a higher level, and the surgeon must take caution during dissection, especially below C6. A horizontal incision is used depending on the level. The hyoid bone overlies the third vertebra and the thyroid cartilage over the C4-5 intervertebral disc space, and the cricoid ring is located at the C6 vertebra (Fig. 2.7A). Placement of a needle on the skin with intraoperative radiograph or fluoroscopy may also guide the skin incision in the correct place. A vertical incision anterior to the sternocleidomastoid may be necessary in cases in which multiple levels need to be exposed. The transverse incision usually is made in line with the skin crease from the midline to the middle of the sternocleidomastoid muscle. The skin and subcutaneous tissue are undermined, followed by division of the platysma muscle. The sternocleidomastoid muscle is retracted laterally and strap muscles are retracted medially. The deep cervical fascia is divided between the sternocleidomastoid muscle and strap muscles, and blunt finger dissection is performed through the pretracheal fascia along the medial border of the carotid sheath (Fig. 2.7B). A self-retaining retractor is then positioned to expose the prevertebral fascia and longus colli muscles (Fig. 2.7C).

One must be careful not to enter the carotid sheath laterally to avoid injury to the carotid artery, internal jugular vein, or vagus nerve. Great caution should also be taken medially because the strap muscles surround the thyroid gland, trachea, and esophagus. The surgical dissection should not enter the plane between the trachea and esophagus because the recurrent laryngeal nerve is at risk. A sharp self-retaining retractor should be avoided to prevent perforation of the esophagus medially. It is also important to check for the temporal arterial pulse when the retractor is spread. Prolonged occlusion of the carotid artery may cause brain ischemia and stroke. The superior thyroid artery is encountered above C4 and the inferior thyroid artery is seen below C6. These vessels should

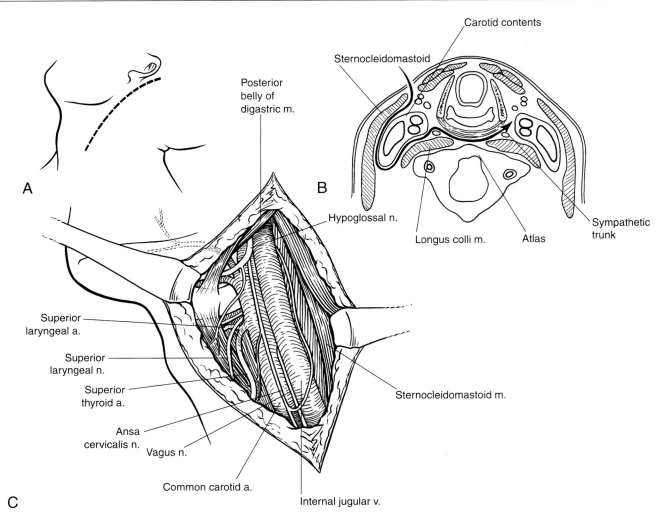

FIGURE 2.5.
Diagram of the anterolateral retropharyngeal approach (Whitesides and Kelley). **A.** The skin incision is made from the mastoid along the anterior aspect of the sternocleidomastoid. **B.** This approach involves dissection anterior to the sternocleidomastoid but posterior to the carotid sheath. **C.** Neurovascular structures that are encountered in this approach include the carotid contents and branches, superior laryngeal nerve, hypoglossal nerve, and ansa cervicalis.

be identified and ligated as necessary. One should also be aware of the thoracic duct below C7 during the left-sided approach (Fig. 2.7D). Further dissection is performed by palpating the prominent disc margins ("hills") and concave anterior vertebral bodies ("valleys"). A bent, 18-gauge needle is placed in the disc space, and a lateral radiograph is taken to confirm the correct level (Fig. 2.7E). The bent needle prevents inadvertent penetration to the spinal cord. To minimize bleeding and prevent injury to the sympathetic chain, the prevertebral fascia and the anterior longitudinal ligament must be divided in the midline, and subperiosteal mobilization of the longus colli muscles are completed.

This anteromedial approach to the cervical spine is used in the majority of cases. However, in special circumstances, lateral approaches described by Hodgson and Verbiest may be used (47, 82). Hodgson described an approach to the lower cervical area, dissecting posterior to the carotid sheath to expose the anterior and lateral aspect of the cervical spine (47). This approach avoids the thyroid vessel, vagus nerve, and superior laryngeal nerve. Verbiest modified the approach for the exposure of the vertebral artery; it involves dissecting anteriorly to the carotid sheath and exposing the vertebral artery and nerve roots posterior to the transverse processes (82). These lateral approaches may be better in cases in which the lesion is localized laterally or in which the vertebral artery must be exposed (Fig. 2.8).

Anterior cervical fusion may involve interbody fusion at one or more levels or vertebrectomy with strut fusion. The proper techniques of discectomy and fusion are crucial to successful outcomes. Neurologic consequences may be devastating, and bone graft complications are common. Proper lighting and loupe magnification of the surgical field are essential during discectomy. All of the disc material is removed, but the posterior longitudinal ligament is usually left alone. When the posterior longitudinal ligament is perforated by the offending disc material, further decompression should be performed up to the dura. Use of an operating microscope or loupe magnification and microsurgical instruments is important during dissection around the posterior longitudinal ligament and the dura.

The Smith-Robinson interbody fusion is found to be biomechanically superior compared with other counterparts, and clinically successful (10, 12, 74, 86, 87). The graft should be about 8 to 9 mm in height or 2 mm greater in height than the degenerated disc space to obtain maximal compressive strength and to

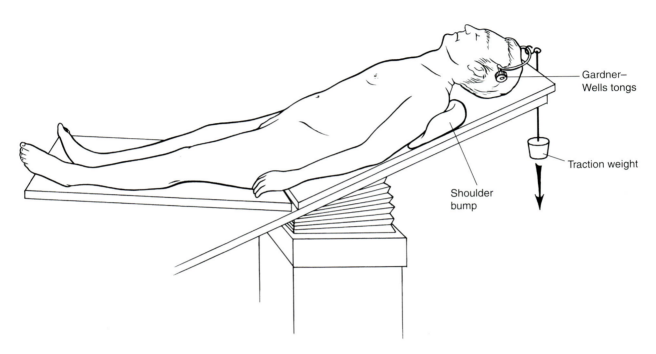

FIGURE 2.6.
Diagram of the supine position for the anterior cervical procedures. The patient is placed in a supine and slight reverse Trendelenburg position to minimize venous pooling in the surgical area. Traction is applied to the head using Gardner Wells tongs or halter device, and a bump in the upper thoracic area is placed to extend the cervical spine.

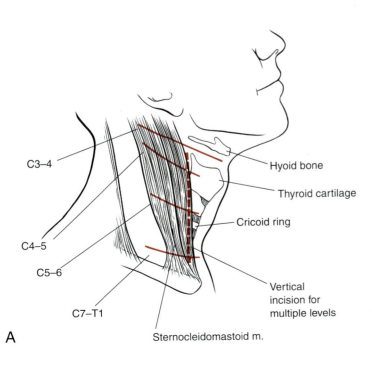

FIGURE 2.7.
The Smith-Robinson anteromedial approach to the lower cervical spine. **A.** Diagram of skin incisions for anterior cervical approaches. A horizontal incision is used at the level of the hyoid bone for C3–4, the thyroid cartilage for C4–5, and the cricoid ring for C6.

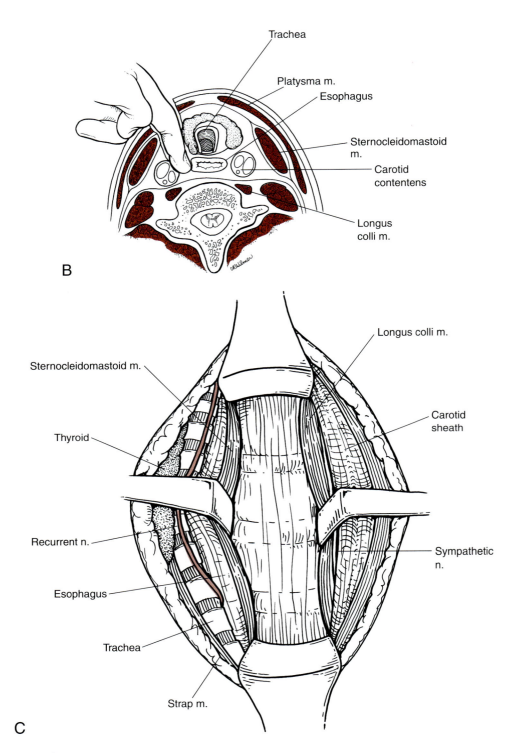

FIGURE 2.7—*continued*

B. Division of the platysma muscle is followed by lateral retraction of the sternocleidomastoid muscle. The deep cervical fascia is divided between the sternocleidomastoid muscle and strap muscles, and blunt finger dissection is performed through the pretracheal fascia along the medial border of the carotid sheath. **C.** A self-retaining retractor is then positioned to expose the prevertebral fascia and longus colli muscles.

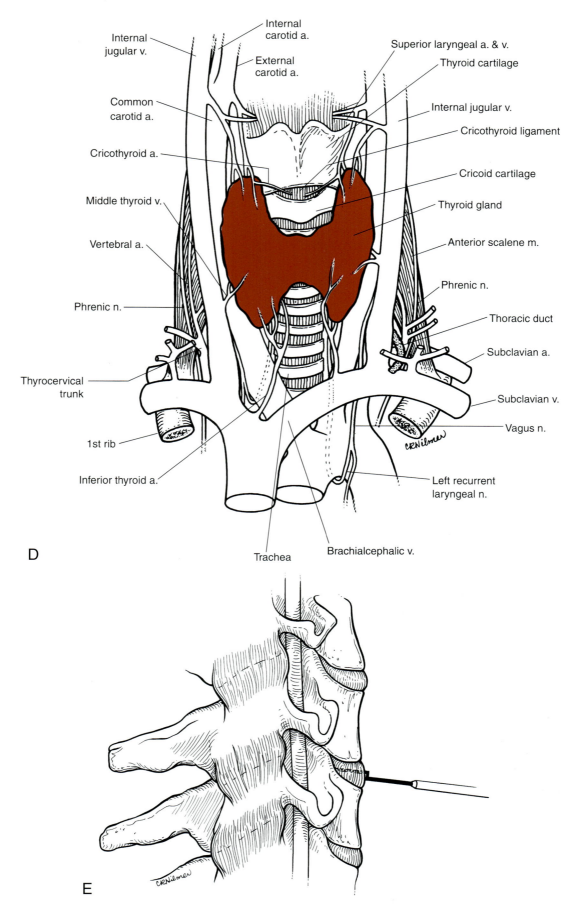

FIGURE 2.7—*continued*

D. Vital structures that are vulnerable to injury during this approach include recurrent laryngeal nerve, carotid contents and branches, thoracic duct, trachea, thyroid, and esophagus. **E.** Diagram of the needle placement for intraoperative radiographic confirmation of the level.

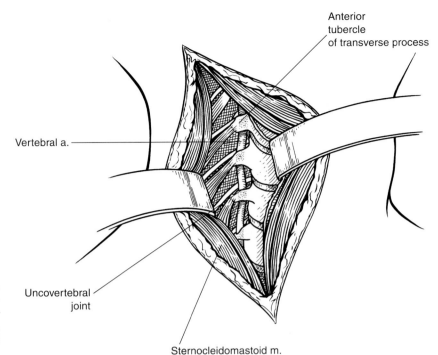

FIGURE 2.8.
Diagram of the lateral approach by Verbiest. This approach exposes the transverse processes and the vertebral artery. The dissection is done anterior to the carotid sheath, exposing the vertebral artery and nerve roots posterior to the transverse processes.

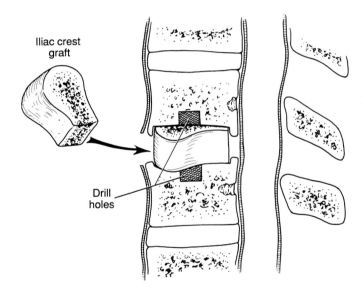

FIGURE 2.9.
Diagram of the Smith-Robison technique of anterior cervical fusion. The graft should be about 2 mm greater in height than the degenerated disc space to obtain maximal compressive strength and to enlarge the neural foramina. The endplates should be flattened with a power burr to maximize the contact area with the graft and to enhance vascularity and healing of the graft. Drill holes can be made in the middle of the endplate to enhance vascular flow.

enlarge the neural foramina (4). The endplates should be flattened with a power burr to maximize the contact area with the graft and to enhance vascularity and healing of the graft (33). Drill holes can be made in the middle of the endplate to enhance vascular flow without jeopardizing the strength of the endplate (Fig. 2.9) (2, 3). Distraction of the intervertebral space can be achieved by skull traction and laminar spreader. Graft extrusion can be avoided if the graft is countersunk 2 mm under the anterior cortical margin of the vertebral body (Fig. 2.9). Exact measurement of width and depth of the bone graft slot should be made using a caliper or ruler in each case. The tricortical iliac crest graft may be inserted with the cortical margin posteriorly (the so-called reverse Smith-Robinson technique). This construct may enhance distraction of the middle column, and clinical results have been favorable (13).

Vertebrectomy with strut grafting is performed frequently for patients with cervical spondylotic myelopathy, tumors, or burst fractures (Fig. 2.10) (10). The iliac crest bone is adequate in most cases, but the fibula may be used in more than three level vertebrectomy cases (Fig. 2.10F) (88). A power burr is used to remove bone down to the posterior longitudinal ligament (Fig. 2.10B). The body is prepared with slots for the ends of the strut graft (Fig 2.10C). The strut graft must be countersunk to prevent graft dislodgement (Fig. 2.10D). The graft may be slotted by making a window during insertion (Fig. 2.10E). The bone graft is placed against the endplates to achieve greater stability and to prevent kyphosis and collapse (Fig. 2.10E). If plating is used, the graft should span from the lower endplate of the cephalad vertebra and the upper endplate of the lower vertebra so that the vertebral body is intact for screws.

Potential complications associated with anterior exposure of the cervical spine are numerous (Table

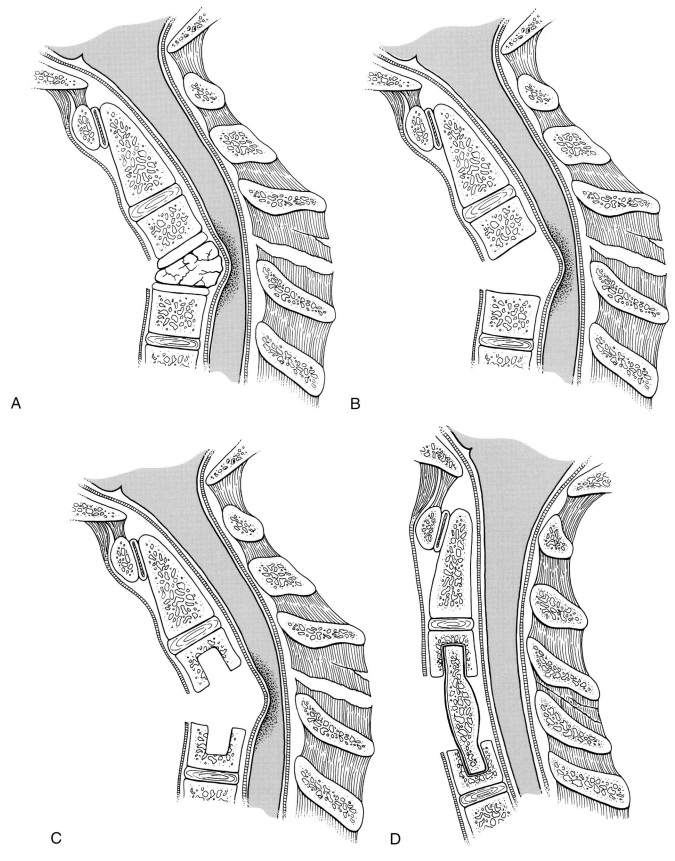

FIGURE 2.10.
Corpectomy and fusion techniques of the cervical spine. **A.** Diagram of burst fracture and spinal cord compression. **B.** Corpectomy is performed by removing bone down to the posterior longitudinal ligament or dura. **C.** The body is prepared with slots for the ends of the strut graft. **D.** The strut graft must be countersunk to prevent graft dislodgement.

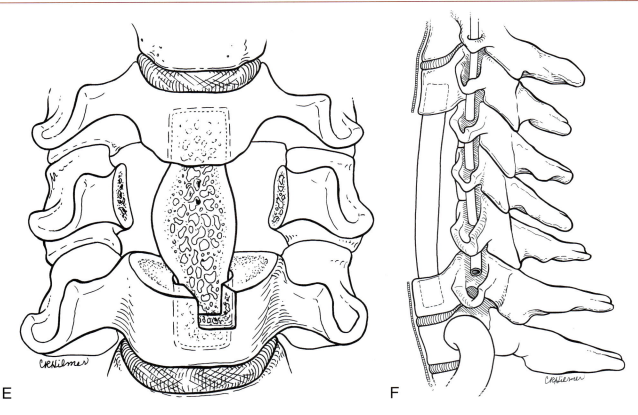

FIGURE 2.10—*continued*
E. The graft may be slotted by making a window during insertion. The bone graft is placed against the endplates to achieve greater stability and to prevent kyphosis and collapse. F. The fibular is used for more than three level construct.

TABLE 2.1.
Potential Complications of Anterior Cervical Fusion

Neural injury
    Spinal cord injury
    Nerve root damage
    Dural tear
Vascular injury
    Carotid artery
    Internal jugular vein
    Vertebral artery
Vocal cord damage (recurrent laryngeal nerve injury)
Esophageal perforation
Tracheal injury
Homer's syndrome
Thoracic duct injury
Pneumothorax
Bone graft complications
    Extrusion
    Collapse
    Nonunion
    Donor site complications
Infection
Wound problems (hematoma, drainage, dehiscence)

2.1). The most devastating complication is neurologic deterioration. Most spinal cord or nerve root injuries are associated with technical mishaps. The first consideration is anesthesia and positioning. Awake intubation with the aid of a fiberoptic light is helpful to prevent excessive manipulation during intubation. Awake intubation and somatosensory evoked potential monitoring should be routine in all myelopathic cases. Utmost care should be taken when removing osteophytes and disc material in the lateral corner near the uncovertebral joint to avoid nerve root injury. The depth of the graft should be measured carefully, and gentle tapping is all that is necessary for graft insertion. The stability of the graft should be maintained by compressive force on the graft. If neurologic complications are discovered postoperatively, one should administer dexamethasone and take a lateral radiograph to determine the position of the bone graft. Computed tomography or magnetic resonance imaging may be valuable in determining hematoma or cord contusion. If hematoma or bone graft is suspected to be the culprit of postoperative myelopathy, expeditious reexploration is required.

Dysphagia after an anterior cervical surgery may be caused by postoperative edema, hemorrhage, denervation, or infection (84). If persistent dysphagia is present, barium swallow or endoscopy should be considered. Esophageal perforation is a rare but serious complication of anterior cervical spine fusion. Sharp retractors must be avoided, and gentle handling of the medial soft structures is mandatory. Use of a nasogastric tube may be helpful in identifying the esophagus during surgery. If esophageal perforation is suspected during surgery, methylene blue can be injected for better visualization. The perforation is frequently not recognized until the patient develops an abscess, tracheoesophageal fistula, or mediastinitis in the postoperative period. The usual treatment consists of intravenous antibiotics, nasogastric feeding, drainage, debridement, and repair. Early consultation with head and neck surgeons is recommended.

Minor hoarseness or sore throat after anterior cervical fusion may be caused by edema or endotracheal intubation and occurs in nearly one-half of such patients. However, recurrent laryngeal nerve palsy may be the culprit of persistent hoarseness in a small number of patients (17). The incidence may be as high as 11% (44). The superior laryngeal nerve is a branch of the inferior ganglion of the vagus nerve and travels along with the superior thyroid artery to innervate the cricothyroid muscle. Damage to this nerve may result in hoarseness, but often produces symptoms such as easy fatiguing of the voice. The inferior laryngeal nerve is a recurrent branch of the vagus nerve that innervates all laryngeal muscles except the cricothyroid. On the left side, the recurrent laryngeal nerve loops under the arch of the aorta and is protected in the left tracheoesophageal groove. On the right side, the recurrent nerve travels around the subclavian artery, passing dorsomedially to the side of the trachea and esophagus. It is vulnerable as it passes from the subclavian artery to the right tracheoesophageal groove. The recurrent laryngeal nerve should be located when working from C6 downward. The best guideline to its location is the inferior thyroid artery. The nerve usually enters the tracheoesophageal groove where the inferior thyroid artery enters the lower pole of the thyroid. It is also more common for the right inferior laryngeal nerve to be nonrecurrent where it travels directly from the vagus nerve and carotid sheath to the larynx. The incidence of nonrecurrent laryngeal nerve on the right side is reported as 1% (68). If hoarseness persists for more than 6 weeks after anterior cervical surgery, laryngoscopy should be done to evaluate the vocal cord and laryngeal muscles. Treatment of inferior laryngeal nerve should include waiting at least 6 months for spontaneous recovery of function to occur. Further treatment or surgery by the otolaryngologist may be necessary in persistent cases.

Injury to the sympathetic chain may result in Horner's syndrome. The cervical sympathetic chain lies on the anterior surface of the longus colli muscles posterior to the carotid sheath. Subperiosteal dissection is important to prevent damage to these nerves. Horner's syndrome is usually temporary but may be permanent in some cases. The incidence of permanent Horner's syndrome is less than 1% (36). Ophthalmologic consultation may be needed for treatment of ptosis.

Serious bleeding complications after anterior cervical surgery is fortunately rare. Hematoma may be responsible for airway obstruction or spinal cord compression (69). The patient's head should be elevated in the immediate postoperative period because the source of bleeding is frequently venous. Meticulous hemostasis and placement of a drain should be routine to prevent these complications. Arterial bleeding from either the superior or inferior thyroid artery can be prevented by careful identification and ligation during surgery. Great caution should be taken not to dissect too far laterally because the vertebral artery is in danger along with the nerve roots (73). The transverse foramen of the more cephalad cervical vertebrae are more medial and more dorsal than the foramina of the lower cervical vertebrae. Hence, the vertebral artery is more susceptible to injury in the mid-cervical region than in the lower cervical region (81). Tears of the vertebral artery should be repaired by direct exposure of the vessel in the foramen rather than merely packing the bleeding site. Injuries to the carotid artery or internal jugular vein are exceedingly rare.

Airway obstruction after extubation may occur in the postoperative period. One must be certain that the patient can exchange air prior to extubation. In cases in which multiple vertebrectomy has been performed with retraction of soft tissues for a prolonged period of time, intubation should continue for a few days until retropharyngeal edema subsides. Corticosteroids may be used to decrease edema in those cases.

Complications associated with bone grafting and fusion are more common. Extrusion of graft usually occurs anteriorly away from the spinal cord and can be associated with dysphagia, tracheal obstruction, kyphotic deformity, or neurologic symptoms. In this situation, the graft should be repositioned and better stabilized. Graft collapse is another complication that may or may not require active treatment. The incidence of graft collapse appears to be slightly higher for allograft than for autograft (5, 15, 90). If graft collapse results in a significant kyphosis, revision surgery may be required. Failure of fusion is reported to be greater using the dowel technique, whereas the keystone method described by Simmons had no cases of nonunion in one series (72). Multiple-level fusion has also been associated with a higher rate of nonunion compared with single-level fusion (5, 86). Many of these patients are asymptomatic despite radiographic evidence of nonunion and require no treatment. Those with symptomatic nonunions may benefit from prolonged immobilization or revision surgery. Posterior foraminotomy with posterior fusion is a good procedure following failed anterior cervical fusion for unilateral radiculopathy. Repeat anterior fusion may also be done in these cases with good success.

Cervicothoracic Junction

Surgical approaches to the upper thoracic vertebrae present a challenge to the spinal surgeon. Anterior exposure of the upper thoracic vertebrae may be accomplished through the low cervical, supraclavicular approach, sternum-splitting approach, or transthoracic approach (7, 19). Low cervical approach is an extension of the anteromedial approach to the lower cervical spine (35). An oblique cervical incision is made, beginning 4 cm below the mastoid process and extending to the sternoclavicular joint or horizontal incision at the base of the neck. After division of the platysma muscle, the dissection is taken between the sternocleidomastoid muscle laterally and the esophagus and trachea medially to reach the spine. The inferior thyroid artery and vein are ligated. The recurrent laryngeal nerve muscle must be identified from the right-sided approach, whereas the thoracic duct must be spared from the left-sided approach.

The supraclavicular approach entails a transverse incision above the clavicle and a dissection posterior to the carotid sheath. After incision of the platysma muscle, division of the clavicular head of the sternocleidomastoid is done (51). The internal jugular and subclavian veins as well as the carotid artery must be protected from injury during division of the sternocleidomastoid muscle. After division of the sternocleidomastoid muscle, the fascia beneath is divided to release the omohyoid from its pulley. The subclavian artery and its branches, which include the thyrocervical trunk, suprascapular artery, and transcervical artery, must be identified. The suprascapular artery and transcervical arteries must be identified. The suprascapular and transcervical arteries should be ligated as necessary. The dome of the lung and the phrenic nerve are in close proximity to the scalenus anterior muscle. The phrenic nerve should be identified and retracted before the scalenus anterior muscle is divided. The brachial plexus and supraclavicular nerves are more superficial at the lateral border of the scalenus anterior muscle. Division of the scalenus anterior muscle exposes the Sibson's fascia in the floor of the wound, which covers the dome of the lung. Sibson's fascia is divided transversely using scissors, and the visceral pleura and lung should be retracted inferiorly. The trachea, the esophagus, and the recurrent laryngeal nerve must be protected during medial retraction. The posterior thorax, stellate ganglion, and upper thoracic vertebral bodies are now visible looking from above downward through the thoracic inlet. The recurrent laryngeal nerve should be identified and protected. Likewise, the inferior thyroid artery and vertebral artery should be identified. The thoracic duct should be identified if approached from the left. If damaged, the thoracic duct should be doubly ligated, both proximally and distally, to prevent chylothorax.

The low cervical or supraclavicular approaches usually allow exposure of the lower cervical spine and the first and second thoracic vertebrae, but the distal extent of the exposure may be limited by the size and position of the anterior thorax. Additionally, obese or muscular patients with short necks would be poor candidates for these approaches because of limited distal extent of the exposure. Low cervical or supraclavicular approaches generally do not provide an extensile exposure of the upper thoracic spine. All the complications discussed in the anteromedial approach to the low cervical spine apply to these approaches, particularly the injury to the recurrent laryngeal nerve, the thoracic duct, the lung, or the great vessels.

Upper thoracic vertebrae may also be approached through a standard thoracotomy that enters the chest through the bed of the third rib, but access to the low cervical region is restricted by the scapula and remaining ribs. Turner et al. described a surgical approach to the upper thoracic spine from T1 to T3 (80). The right-sided approach is preferred to avoid the left subclavian artery, which is more curved than the right brachiocephalic artery. The incision is medial and inferior to the scapula. The scapula is retracted laterally by dividing the trapezius, latissimus dorsi, rhomboids, and levator scapulae muscles. The posterior 7 to 10 cm of each of the second, third, fourth, and fifth ribs are removed. If T1 is involved, 2 to 3 cm of the first rib are also excised. Exposure of the vertebrae is made with an L-shape incision in the pleura and intercostal muscles. Potential complications of this approach may be restriction of scapular movement and paralysis of intercostal muscles caused by the muscle-splitting aspects of this dissection.

The sternum-splitting approach provides better access to the cervicothoracic junction from C4 to T4, particularly in the obese patient (7, 46) (Fig. 2.11). The skin incision is made anterior to the left sternocleidomastoid muscle and extends along the midsternal area down to the xiphoid process. After division of the platysma muscle and superficial cervical fascia, blunt dissection is done between the laterally situated neurovascular bundle and medial visceral structures. The retrosternal adipose and thymus tissues are retracted from the manubrium. Median sternotomy should be performed carefully to prevent injury to the pleura. Sternohyoid, sternothyroid, and omohyoid muscles are identified and transected as necessary. The inferior thyroid artery is ligated and transected. Blunt dissection is performed

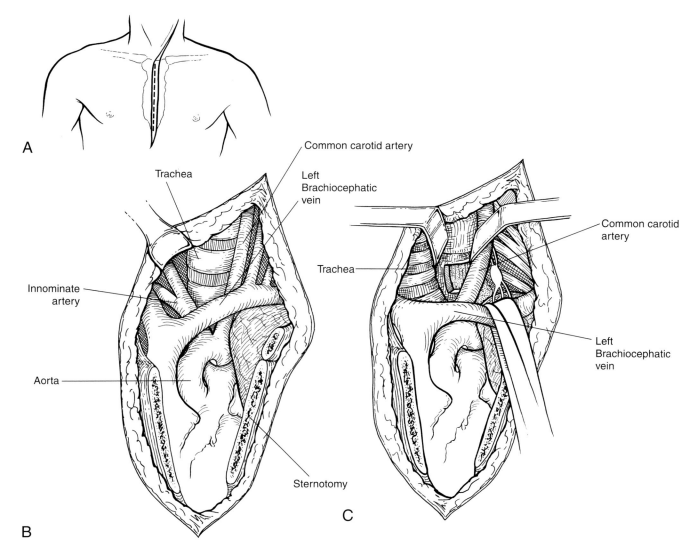

FIGURE 2.11.
Diagrams of the sternum-splitting approach. **A.** The skin incision is made anterior to the left sternocleidomastoid muscle and extends along the midsternal area down to the xiphoid process. **B.** The neck dissection is same for the Smith-Robison approach. The retrosternal adipose and thymus tissues are retracted from the manubrium. Median sternotomy exposes the left brachiocephalic vein and the common carotid artery. **C.** Retraction of the left brachiocephalic vein and common carotid exposes from C4-T4.

from the cranial portion toward the caudal portion until the left brachiocephalic vein is exposed. This vein may be ligated and transected if necessary, but postoperative edema of the left upper extremity may be a problem.

Great caution should be taken to avoid injuries to the sympathetic nerves, the cupola of the pleura, the great vessels, and the thoracic duct, which passes into the left venous angle between the subclavian artery and the common carotid artery. Because there is a significant perioperative mortality associated with this approach, modified approaches to the cervicothoracic junction have been reported (27, 50, 79). Sundaresan reported a less aggressive, T-shaped incision on the anterior chest wall (Fig. 2.12) (79). Dissection is taken down to the level of the body ma-

nubrium and clavicle with ligation of the anterior jugular venous arch and medial supraclavicular nerves. The left-sided approach is preferred because the recurrent laryngeal nerve is less variable on the left and is farther from the midline than from the right. At the level of the manubrium and clavicle, the sternal and clavicular heads of the sternocleidomastoid muscle are detached and retracted. The strap muscles on the ipsilateral side of approach are similarly detached and retracted. After clearing the fatty and areolar tissues in the suprasternal space, the sternal origin of the pectoralis major is stripped laterally. The medial half of the clavicle is then stripped subperiosteally with removal of the medial third of the clavicle with a Gigli saw. A rectangular piece of the manubrium is removed along with its posterior peri-

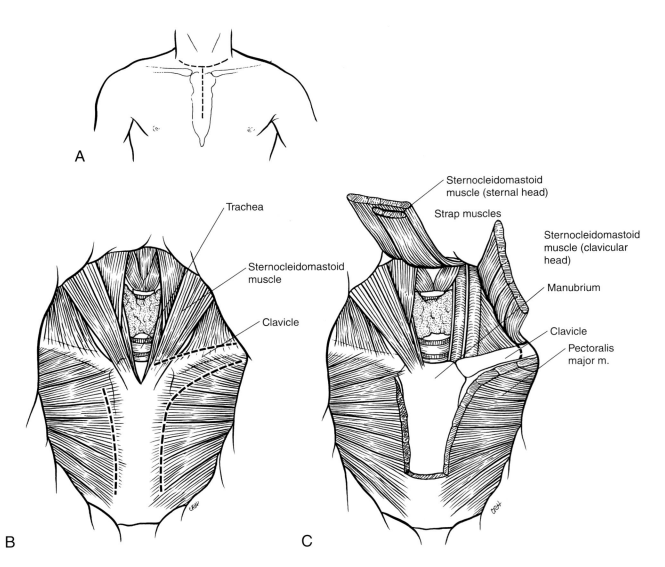

FIGURE 2.12.
Modified approach to the anterior cervico-thoracic junction by Sundaresan. **A.** T-shaped incision on the anterior chest wall. **B.** Dissection is taken down to the level of the body manubrium and clavicle. **C.** The sternal and clavicular heads of the sternocleidomastoid muscle are detached and retracted. The strap muscles on the ipsilateral side of approach are similarly detached and retracted.

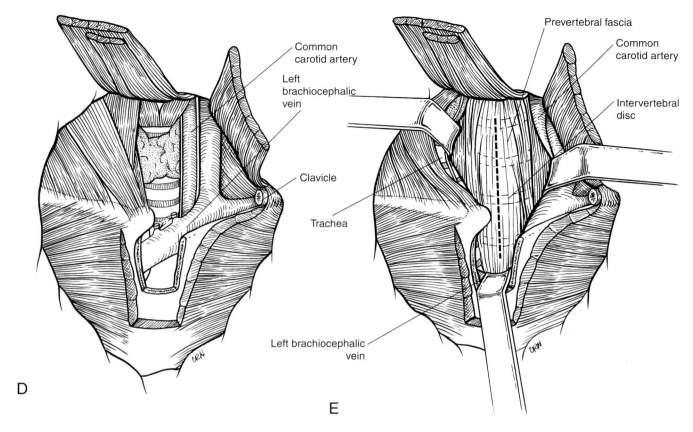

FIGURE 2.12—*continued*
D. The sternal origin of the pectoralis major is stripped laterally, and the medial third of the clavicle and a rectangular piece of the manubrium are removed. **E.** Dissection is continued between the left carotid artery on the left and the innominate artery, trachea, and esophagus on the right.

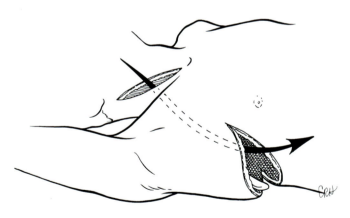

FIGURE 2.13.
Diagram of the combined low cervical and transthoracic approach to the cervicothoracic junction for severe kyphoscoliosis.

osteum. At this point, the exposed inferior thyroid vein and, if necessary, the innominate vein may be ligated. Dissection is then continued between the left carotid artery on the left, and the innominate artery, trachea, and esophagus on the right. Special attention must be given to protection of the thoracic duct and left recurrent laryngeal nerve. Kurz and Herkowitz presented a modified anterior approach to the cervicothoracic junction by removing the medial one third of the clavicle (50). They reported no complications in four patients with tumors, but one patient had recurrence of tumor. A combined low cervical and transthoracic approach has also been described to gain greater access to the cervicothoracic junction in patients with severe kyphoscoliosis (Fig. 2.13) (58).

Thoracic and Thoracolumbar Spine

Posterior Approaches to the Thoracic and Thoracolumbar Spine

Posterior exposure of the thoracic and thoracolumbar spine is relatively simple, but meticulous techniques are required to avoid pseudarthrosis. The patient is usually positioned on the four-poster or Relton-Hall frame (Fig. 2.14). By adjusting all posters with regard to the patient's width and height, pressure points are distributed evenly on the chest and proximal thighs, while obtaining some reduction of the deformity. One must avoid pressure on the brachial plexus and ulnar nerves for obvious reasons. The abdomen must be free of pressure to allow venous drainage of the

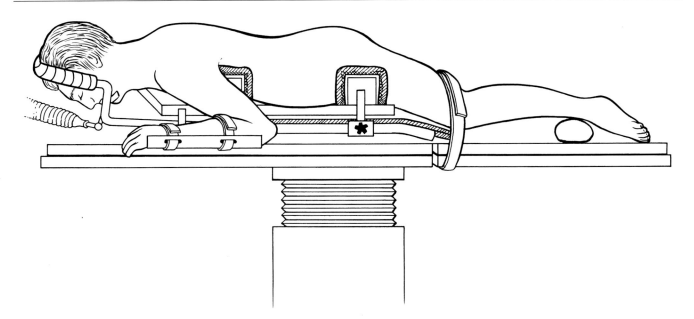

FIGURE 2.14.
Diagram of the prone post for the posterior approaches to the thoracolumbar spine. The four-poster, or Relton-Hall, frame has adjustable posters so that pressure points are distributed evenly on the chest and proximal thighs.

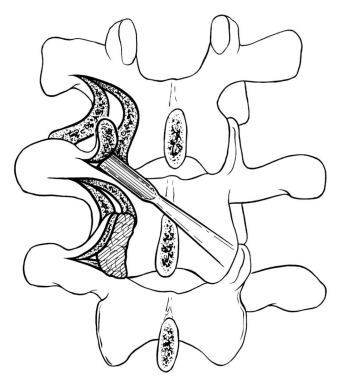

FIGURE 2.15.
Diagram of decortication of the posterior element using a gouge.

lower extremities and to decrease blood loss during surgery. Initial subperiosteal dissection is done with the Cobb elevator, exposing the spinous processes, lamina, facets, and the tips of the transverse processes. Facet excision can be done with instruments such as the osteotome, Lexcel rongeur, or power burr. Decortication should also be done meticulously using gouges, a rongeur, or a power burr (Fig. 2.15). Power instruments should be held in both hands, resting both wrists or forearms on the patient to provide proprioceptive feedback to the surgeon and to minimize the risk of an unexpected wayward deviation of these instruments.

Occasionally, laminectomy may be indicated for epidural lesions or intradural tumors. Thoracic laminectomy should be done by thinning the lateral margins of the lamina using a power burr and finishing the cut using a curet. Transpedicular approach is also useful for biopsy or decompression in the thoracic and thoracolumbar spine. Transpedicular biopsy or decompression requires a thorough knowledge of the anatomy of the thoracic pedicle. The thoracic pedicle is located by crossing a horizontal line at the midportion of the transverse process and a vertical line at the junction between the lamina and transverse process (Fig. 2.16). A power burr is used to remove the outer cortex. A pin is placed to confirm the location of the pedicle with a roentgenogram. An angle-tipped curette can be used to remove tissues from the vertebral body. Decompression of the spinal cord can be done by excising the pedicle and by removing tissues from a posterolateral direction.

Another posterior approach to the anterior and lateral aspect of the thoracic vertebra is the posterolateral costotransversectomy technique (49) (Fig. 2.17). This approach is less extensive than a formal thoracotomy and may be preferred for lesions in the lateral aspect of the vertebral body, lesions that do not re-

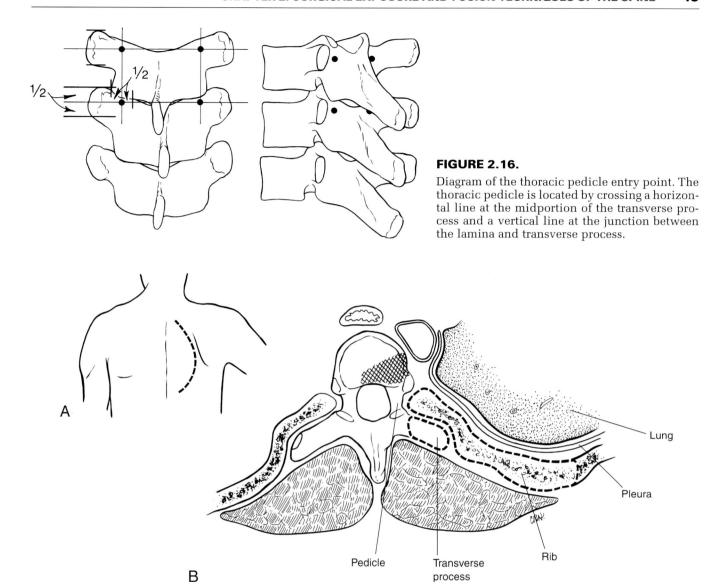

FIGURE 2.16.
Diagram of the thoracic pedicle entry point. The thoracic pedicle is located by crossing a horizontal line at the midportion of the transverse process and a vertical line at the junction between the lamina and transverse process.

FIGURE 2.17.
Diagram of the posterolateral costotransversectomy technique. **A.** A "C"-shaped curved skin incision is made along the paraspinous muscles, spanning approximately four to five ribs. **B.** The rib and transverse process are resected at one to four levels, depending on the extent of the lesion. The rib is excised approximately 3.5 inches lateral to the vertebra and is disarticulated at the costovertebral junction. Careful retraction of the pleura expose the vertebral bodies, pedicles, neural foramina, and spinal nerves.

quire a long strut graft, or for patients who cannot tolerate a formal thoracotomy. The patient is placed halfway between a lateral decubitus and prone position with a pad in the axilla, and the upper arm is extended slightly and supported securely. A "C"-shape curved incision is made along the paraspinous muscles, spanning about four to five ribs. The middle part of the incision should be about 2.5 inches from the midline at the paraspinal depression. By undermining the skin and subcutaneous tissue, exposure of the paraspinous muscles and posterior elements of the spine is completed. The trapezius and latissimus dorsi muscles are divided either longitudinally or transversely. The rib and transverse process are resected at one to four levels, depending on the extent of the lesion. The rib is exposed subperiosteally and excised approximately 3.5 inches lateral to the vertebra and is disarticulated at the costovertebral junction. Careful retraction of the pleura leads to the vertebrae. The pedicles, neural foramina, and spinal nerves should be identified. For neural decompression, the pedicles may be widened or excised to expose the dura. A strut bone graft may be applied if necessary.

Similarly, a posterolateral approach can be used to expose the anterolateral aspect of the vertebral body in the thoracolumbar region (52, 53) (Fig. 2.18). The patient is placed prone or in the lateral decubitus and

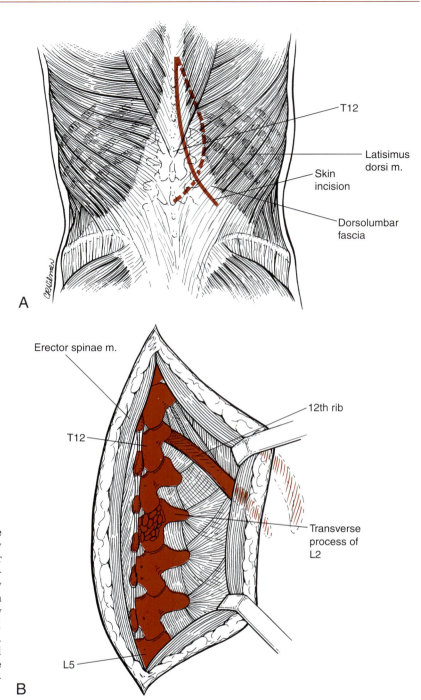

FIGURE 2.18.

Diagrams of the posterolateral approach to the thoracolumbar spine **A.** The skin incision may be in a C or J shape to expose the dorsolumbar fascia and latissimus dorsi fascia. **B.** The erector spinae muscle group is retracted medially from the surface of the eleventh and twelfth ribs. These ribs are isolated subperiosteally and resected. The transverse processes of L1 and L2 may also be resected to gain exposure. The twelfth, or L1, nerve is identified and traced back to its foramen. The pedicle of the appropriate vertebra is resected for the exposure of the dura laterally.

is rolled slightly toward the anterior side. A left- or right-sided approach can be done, depending on the pathoanatomy of the lesion. The skin incision may be in a C or J shape to expose the dorsolumbar fascia and latissimus dorsi fascia. These fascia are incised, and the erector spinae muscle group is retracted medially from the surface of the eleventh and twelfth ribs. These ribs are isolated subperiosteally and resected. The transverse processes of L1 and L2 also may be resected to gain exposure. The twelfth, or L1, nerve is identified and traced back to its foramen. The pedicle of the appropriate vertebra is resected using a Kerrison punch, and the dura is exposed laterally. Discectomy or vertebrectomy and fusion is then performed.

Total spondylectomy through the posterolateral approach has been described for lesions that require en bloc excision (67, 76, 77). This operation is a formidable procedure and should be performed by those with prior experience.

For the posterior exposure of the lumbar spine, a kneeling position is preferred to lessen blood loss by reducing the intra-abdominal venous pressure (Fig. 2.19A). For lumbar fusion cases, a midline incision is made and subperiosteal dissection of the paraspinous muscles is done, exposing the spinous process, lamina, facet joint capsules, pars interarticularis, and transverse processes. One must be careful not to destroy the facet capsule above the planned fusion site. The facet joints to be fused should be prepared meticulously by excising the cartilage from the joints and removing the cortical bone from the lateral portion of the superior articular process (Fig. 2.19B). Decortication of the transverse process, the lateral gutter, and the sacral ala are performed carefully using a power burr. Morselized bone from the iliac crest is placed in the prepared gutter. Posterior lumbar interbody fusion is a technique that involves insertion of the bone grafts into the disc space by retracting the nerve roots. Great care must be taken to avoid damage to the nerve roots.

The transpedicular approach is useful for biopsy, decompression, or screw insertion. Knowledge of the anatomy of the pedicle in relation to neural structures is crucial. The pedicle entrance point is located at the crossing of two lines (Fig. 2.19C). The vertical line is the extension of the facet joint in line with the bony crest coming from the inferior articular facet. The horizontal line passes through the middle of the insertion of the transverse process, or 1 mm below the joint line. The sacral entrance point is at the lower point of the L5-S1 articulation. The nerve root is situated just medial and inferior to the pedicle as it exits into the intervertebral foramen. Therefore, one must avoid the area medial and inferior to the pedicle to prevent damage of the nerve root. A small rongeur or burr is used to decorticate the pedicle entrance. A Steinmann pin with roentgenographic im-

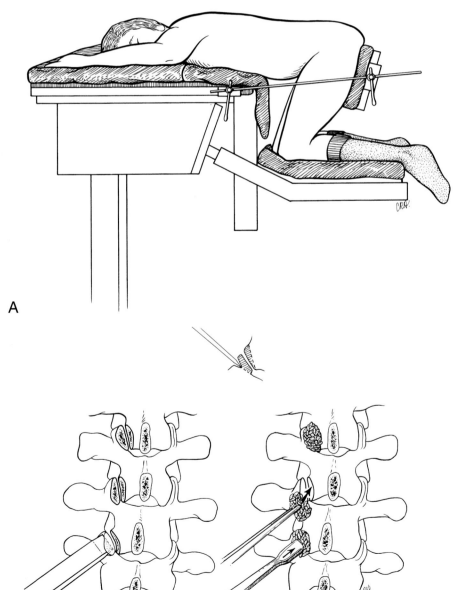

FIGURE 2.19.

Posterior approach to the lumbar spine. **A.** The kneeling position lessens blood loss by reducing the intra-abdominal venous pressure. **B.** For facet joint fusion, cartilage should be excised from the joints and packing with bone graft.

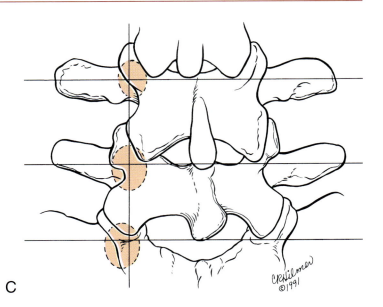

FIGURE 2.19—*continued*

C. The pedicle entrance point of the lumbar spine is located at the crossing of two lines. The vertical line is the extension of the facet joint in line with the bony crest coming from the inferior articular facet. The horizontal line passes through the middle of the insertion of the transverse process, or 1 mm below the joint line. The sacral entrance point is at the lower point of the L5-S1 articulation.

aging can be used to confirm the location of the pedicle. A blunt instrument is advanced carefully through the pedicle into the vertebral body. The amount of medial angulation varies, depending on the level and on the entry point. Preoperative imaging studies should be used to determine the exact angulations, depth, and size of the pedicle. Posterior exposure of the sacrum and coccyx is done through a vertical midline incision. One must be careful to avoid dural tear in the midline, particularly in patients with occult spina bifida. Posterior sacral foramina are surrounded richly by venous structures and can be sources of significant bleeding. Subperiosteal dissection around the coccyx should be done carefully to avoid injury to the rectum anteriorly. Posterior laminectomy of the sacrum for exposures of the nerve roots along with anterior exposure of the sacrum may be necessary for resection of certain sacral tumors.

Operative complications associated with posterior and posterolateral approaches of the thoracic and thoracolumbar spine include spinal cord injury, dural tear, vascular injury, visceral damage, and pseudarthrosis (8). Again, somatosensory evoked potential monitoring is recommended for scoliosis surgery or if decompression of the spinal cord is planned. Power drills, curettes, or rongeurs should be used in a cautious manner because neurovascular injury from use of these instruments can be devastating. Perforations of the dura can lead to neurologic impairment, pseudomeningocele formation, cerebrospinal fluid fistula, meningitis, or wound healing problems. Dural tears may occur during excision of the ligamentum flavum, but they occur more commonly during manipulation of the dural sac to free adhesions, particularly in a stenotic canal. Gentle handling of the dural sac largely avoids this complication. Dural tears should be primarily closed using a 6:0 or 7:0 nonabsorbable suture in such a way as to avoid constriction of the cauda equina. A fascial or free fat graft may be used to augment the repair (32). The paraspinous muscle, overlying fascia, subcutaneous tissue, and skin should be closed in multiple layers in a water-tight manner. Drains should be avoided.

New instrumentation systems have reduced the incidence of pseudarthrosis, but fusion procedures still require sound surgical techniques. A long-term good result depends primarily on patient selection. The incidence of pseudarthrosis may be decreasing with the current surgical devices, but it still remains a major problem in spinal fusion surgery. Thorough decortication, facet cartilage excision, use of copious amount of autogenous bone grafts, and stable instrumentation are essential in achieving a solid arthrodesis. Cigarette smoking has been associated with pseudarthrosis (16).

The abdominal structures anterior to the intervertebral disc are at risk of damage if the anterior annulus is violated during disc removal (43, 48, 60) or if the pedicle screw penetrates the anterior cortex of the vertebral body or the sacrum. The aorta bifurcates into the common iliac arteries at the L4-5 disc level. The right common iliac artery crosses the anterior surface of the L4-5 disc and fixes the left common iliac branch of the vena cava against the vertebral column. In addition to this vessel, the bowel and ureter are also in danger. The L5 nerve root courses anterior to the ala of the sacrum, and thus the pedicle screw should avoid this area. Great caution must be taken to avoid damage to these vital structures. During discectomy, the surgeon should always be aware of the depth of the instrument in the disc space. By maintaining contact with the vertebral endplates, the surgeon has better depth perception. The pituitary rongeur with a depth marking is helpful in avoiding excessively deep penetration. Preoperative radiographs and imaging studies should also be reviewed carefully to measure the depth of the intervertebral disc space.

Anterior Approaches to the Thoracic and Thoracolumbar Spine

Anterior Exposure of the Thoracic Spine

Exposure of the thoracic vertebral bodies is best accomplished by the anterior transthoracic approach (Fig. 2.20) (83). A right-sided thoracotomy is preferred because the exposure of the upper thoracic spine enables the surgeon to avoid the subclavian and carotid arteries in the left superior mediastinum. In the lower thoracic spine, a left-sided thoracotomy is preferred to avoid the liver. Because dissection is easier from above downward, the rib at the one or two upper levels should be removed, particularly if multiple levels are involved. For the thoracotomy approach, place the patient in the lateral decubitus position, moving the arm forward (Fig. 2.20A). Insertion of a double-branched endotracheal tube into the right and left mainstream bronchi helps allow selective collapse of the lung. An axillary roll under the down arm is important in preventing compression of axillary neurovascular structures. The skin incision is made along the rib intended for removal from the anterior margin of the latissimus muscle anteriorly to the costochondral junction. The anterior aspect of the latissimus muscle can be undermined or minimally incised, and the posterior border of the serratus anterior muscle is mobilized or transected (Fig. 2.20B).

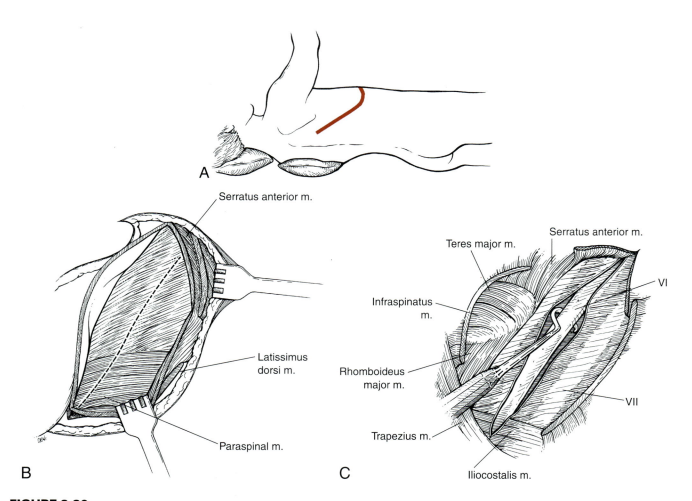

FIGURE 2.20.
Anterior exposure of the thoracic spine. **A.** The patient is in the lateral decubitus position with a roll under the axilla. The skin incision is made along the rib intended for removal from the anterior margin of the latissimus muscle anteriorly to the costochondral junction. **B.** The anterior aspect of the latissimus muscle can be undermined or minimally incised, and the posterior border of the serratus anterior muscle is mobilized or transected. **C.** Rib resection is performed by incising the overlying periosteum and using a rib stripper to dissect off the intercostal musculature. Care is taken to not damage the neurovascular bundle that travels along the inferior margin of the rib.

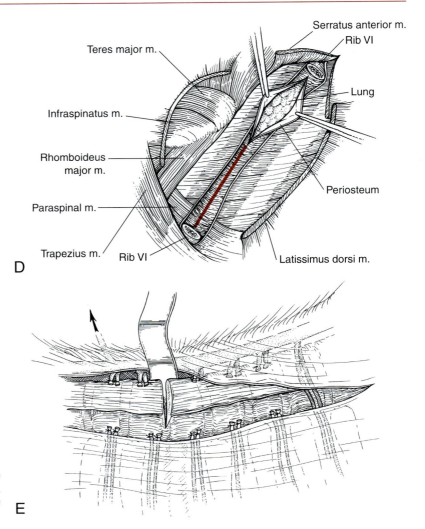

FIGURE 2.20—*continued*
D. Rib resection is followed by division of the pleura in the thoracic cavity. **E.** The segmental vessels ligated as needed in the middle of the vertebral bodies.

The lateral margin of the trapezius muscle is mobilized and transected if necessary (Fig. 2.20C). To verify the correct rib level, palpation of the ribs is done between the rib cage and serratus anterior muscle. Rib resection is then performed by first incising the overlying periosteum in the mid portion of the rib using electrocautery (Fig. 2.20C). A rib stripper is then used to dissect off the intercostal musculature, and care is taken not to damage the neurovascular bundle that travels along the inferior margin of the rib (Fig. 2.20D). Once the rib has been exposed, it is divided at the costochondral junction anteriorly, elevated, and resected as far posteriorly as the exposure will allow. This rib can then be saved for bone grafting. The chest is then entered sharply in the center of the rib bed, and the lung is retracted anteriorly and inferiorly. The pleura overlying the vertebral bodies is then incised and the segmental vessels are ligated as needed in the middle of the vertebral bodies (Fig. 2.20E). A blunt dissection is then performed beginning over the disc spaces, and a plane is developed that includes the ligated segmental vessels to the opposite pedicle. A moist lap and malleable retractor are placed on the opposite side of the vertebral body to retract and protect the great vessels and esophagus (Fig. 2.20E).

Anterior Exposure of the Thoracolumbar Junction

Exposure of the thoracolumbar junction is best achieved by a thoracoabdominal approach, which entails circumferential incision in the muscular portion of the diaphragm adjacent to the costal margin (Fig. 2.21) (83). The patient is placed in a lateral decubitus position with the left side up. The left-sided approach is preferred to avoid the liver and vena cava on the right side. A skin incision is made over the tenth rib from the lateral border of the paraspinous musculature to the costal cartilage. The incision is curved anteriorly to the edge of the rectus sheath (Fig. 2.21A). The dissection is extended down to the muscle layers to the periosteum of the tenth rib (Fig. 2.21B). The key is to access the retroperitoneal space by splitting the costal cartilage after removal of the tenth rib. After removing the rib, the pleura is incised and the lung is retracted. The costal cartilage is then split along its length. Under the retracted split tips of

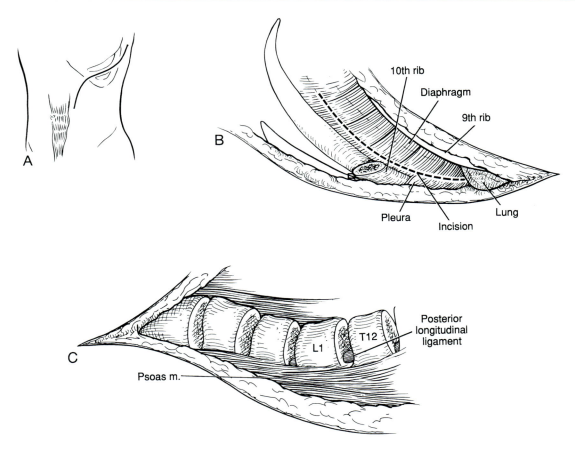

FIGURE 2.21.
The thoracoabdominal approach for the exposure of the thoracolumbar junction. **A.** The skin incision is over the tenth rib and is curved anteriorly to the edge of the rectus sheath. **B.** The dissection is extended down to remove the tenth rib. After removing the rib, the pleura is incised and the lung is retracted. The costal cartilage is then split along its length, and the retroperitoneal space is dissected bluntly to mobilize the peritoneum from the undersurface of the diaphragm and abdominal wall. The diaphragm is incised circumferentially 1 inch from its peripheral attachment to the chest wall. **C.** The exposure can be extended from T10 to L5.

costal cartilage, the retroperitoneal space is identified by the light areolar tissue. Blunt dissection is performed to mobilize the peritoneum from the undersurface of the diaphragm and abdominal wall. After the peritoneum is retracted, the external oblique, internal oblique, and the transverse abdominis muscles of the abdomen are divided one layer at a time. The next step entails circumferential incision in the muscular portion of the diaphragm adjacent to the costal margin. The diaphragm is incised circumferentially 1 inch from its peripheral attachment to the chest wall. Marker stitches or clips are placed for resuturing the diaphragm later. For the exposure of the T12-L1 region, the crus of the diaphragm is cut and mobilized. The segmental vessels are tied and ligated as necessary to mobilize the aorta. Malleable retractors are positioned to expose the thoracolumbar junction.

For the exposure of the thoracolumbar junction, either the eleventh rib or twelfth rib approach may be used while remaining in the extrapleural and retroperitoneal spaces (55). These exposures entail splitting the tip of the costal cartilage, and the parietal pleura is mobilized carefully from the undersurface of the rib bed. The peritoneum is mobilized anteriorly, and the retroperitoneal space is bluntly dissected toward the spine. These approaches give less extensile exposure of the thoracolumbar junction compared with the thoracoabdominal approach.

Anterior Exposure of the Lumbar Spine

In the lower lumbar region, a standard retroperitoneal flank approach is used (Fig. 2.22A) (83). The patient is placed in the right lateral decubitus position with the left side up. The retroperitoneal exposure uses the division of the abdominal muscles and blunt dissection through the retroperitoneal space toward the psoas muscles and the spine (Fig. 2.22B). The incision extends from the midaxillary line to the edge of the rectus sheath. The level of the incision varies according to the level of the spine approached. Dissection is through the external oblique, internal oblique, and transversus abdominis muscles. The ret-

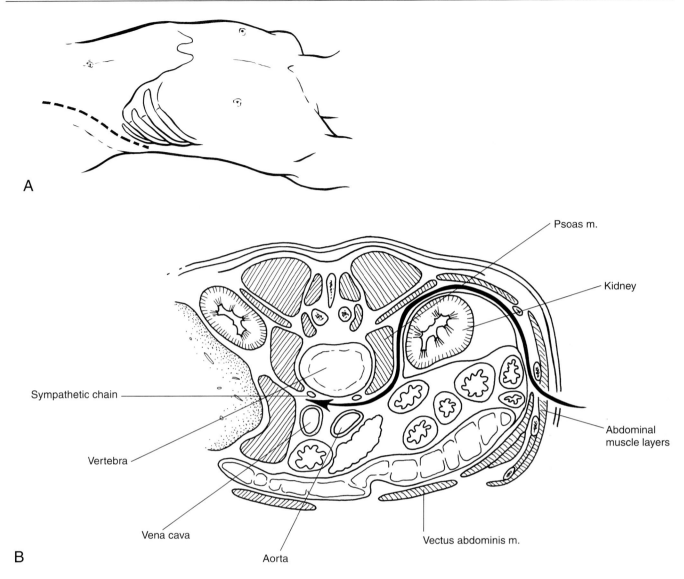

FIGURE 2.22.
The retroperitoneal flank approach to the lumbar spine. **A.** The patient is placed in the right lateral decubitus position, and the incision depends on the level of exposure required. **B.** The retroperitoneal exposure uses the division of the abdominal muscles and blunt dissection through the retroperitoneal space toward the psoas muscles and the spine.

roperitoneal space is entered laterally by identifying the retroperitoneal fat, taking care to avoid penetration of the peritoneum just lateral to the rectus sheath. Blunt finger dissection anterior to the psoas muscle should lead to the spine. One should identify the genitofemoral nerve on the anterior surface of the psoas muscle and the sympathetic chains medial to the muscle. Extreme caution must be used to avoid injuries to the ureter, which can be identified medially along the undersurface of the peritoneum, and the pulsating aorta, which is easily palpated. The aorta is mobilized and a retractor is positioned around the vertebral body. The segmental vessels are ligated to expose the valleys of the vertebral bodies. At the L4-L5 region, the iliolumbar vein should be identified and ligated to mobilize the great vessels. For the approach to L5-S1, the midline within the vascular bifurcation should be palpated by passing the finger over the left common iliac artery. The left common iliac vein is retracted to the left and cephalad, while the middle sacral vein and the superior hypogastric plexus are retracted to the right bluntly.

The paramedian retroperitoneal approach may be used for the exposure of the anterior aspect of the L3 to S1 vertebrae. This approach is done in the supine position. The anterior exposure of the lower lumbar vertebrae and the sacrum is better with this technique than the lateral approach. The lateral edge of the rectus abdominal muscle is palpated, and a vertical incision is made (Fig. 2.23). The length of the

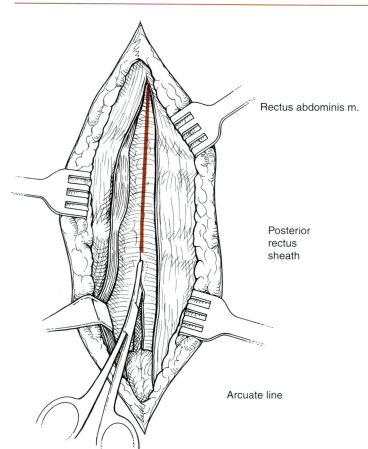

FIGURE 2.23.

The paramedian retroperitoneal approach is used for the exposure of the anterior aspect of the L3 to S1 vertebrae. This approach is done in the supine position. The skin incision is made on the lateral edge of the rectus abdominal muscle, and the rectus sheath is divided and the rectus abdominal muscle is retracted medially. The posterior rectus sheath is divided carefully from the arcuate line toward the top.

incision depends on the number of vertebrae needed to be exposed. The dissection is made to the level of abdominal fascia. The lateral border of the rectus abdominal muscle is palpated, and an incision is made in the anterior rectus sheath along the lateral edge of the muscle. The fibers of the rectus muscle are retracted medially to expose the posterior rectus sheath and the arcuate line (Fig. 2.23). The inferior aspect of exposure should not go beyond to the level of inferior epigastric vessels. Great caution is taken to preserve these vessels and to preserve any innervation to the rectus abdominal muscle. The arcuate line divides the posterior rectus fascia proximally and the transversalis fascia distally. The preperitoneal space can then be entered, and blunt dissection leads to the retroperitoneal space and the anterior aspect of the spine. The peritoneum is mobilized medially, and the dissection is carried down to the iliac vessels. The surgeon should identify the psoas muscle, aorta, iliac artery and vein, genitofemoral nerve, ureter, sympathetic chain, and the superior hypogastric plexus. For the exposure of L3-L5, the psoas muscle is mobilized laterally off the vertebral bodies, the left segmental vessels are identified and ligated, and the aorta and iliac vessels are mobilized medially. The iliolumbar vein should be ligated for the exposure of L4-L5. For the exposure of L5-S1, the aortic bifurcation at the L4-L5 is dissected further and the vessels are retracted laterally to enter the L5-S1 disc.

A transperitoneal approach through a vertical or transverse incision in the lower abdomen also provides an excellent exposure to the lumbosacral junction (Fig. 2.24A). The patient is in the supine position with the lumbosacral spine hyperextended. The transverse incision requires transection of the rectus abdominis muscle, and the vertical incision splits the rectus abdominis muscles in the midline linea alba. After division of the anterior rectus sheath, the conjoined fascia of the posterior rectus sheath and abdominal fascia is opened to the peritoneum. The peritoneum is divided carefully, and the bowel contents are mobilized away from the aorta and iliac vessels. The aortic bifurcation is palpated at the L4-L5 region (Fig. 2.24B).

Saline infiltration of the tissue over the anterior surface of the sacral promontory may be done to elevate the posterior peritoneum off the vascular structures. The posterior peritoneum is opened and the L5-S1 disc identified. The sacral artery runs down along the anterior aspect of the sacrum and may be ligated for distal exposure. Great caution should be taken to protect the left iliac vein in the aortic bifur-

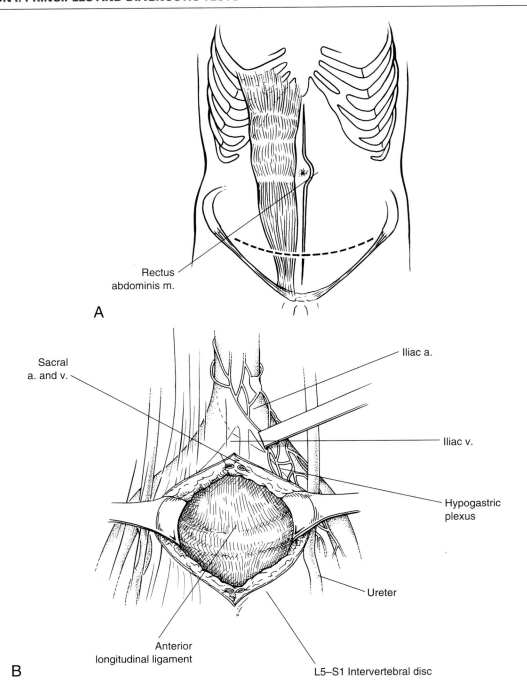

FIGURE 2.24.
The transperitoneal approach to the lower lumbar spine and the sacrum. **A.** The skin incision is through a vertical or transverse incision in the lower abdomen. **B.** After division of rectus sheaths, the perineum is divided carefully. The bowel contents are mobilized away from the aorta and iliac vessels. The aortic bifurcation is palpated and mobilized for the exposure of the L5-S1 intervertebral disc.

cation and to preserve the superior hypogastric plexus, which is important to sexual function. The electrocautery must be avoided to prevent damage to the hypogastric plexus. The left common iliac artery and left common iliac vein are retracted to the left, and the hypogastric plexus and right iliac vessels are retracted to the right. Retractors or Steinmann pins can be used to expose the L5-S1 region. Exposure can be extended to the L4-L5 region by mobilizing the great vessels to the right after ligating the L4-5 vessels, including the iliolumbar vein. Care must be taken not to injure the left ureter, which crosses the left common iliac vessels over the sacroiliac joint.

The techniques of anterior interbody fusion in the lower lumbar spine vary widely among different authors (24, 91). Nonetheless, the technique should consist of meticulous excision of the entire disc material, preparation of the endplates to provide stability and vascularity, and insertion of biomechanically sound bone graft or spacer. The graft or spacer should be biologically compatible to provide fusion of the construct.

After discectomy or corpectomy, the defect must be reconstructed with a tricortical iliac crest bone graft or other graft materials that provide good axial stability and bone healing. If the bone graft is used alone without a fixation device, the graft should span from the upper endplate above and lower endplate below with a countersinking technique. If a fixation device is used anteriorly, the graft should extend from the lower endplate above and upper endplate below, and screws are inserted into the vertebral bodies. Before inserting the graft, the operating room table should be flexed at the level that corresponds to the corpectomy site. This technique provides more space for the graft to be inserted, and the table should be flexed back to the neutral position to lock the graft in the interspace.

Potential complications during anterior dissection along the thoracolumbar spine include hemorrhage from great vessel injury, retrograde ejaculation and sterility from superior hypogastric sympathetic plexus injury, splenic injury, ureteral injury, sympathectomy effect, chylous leakage, and bowel injury (20, 22, 31, 45, 70, 71). Penile erection is predominantly under the parasympathetic system, and impotence is not anticipated after superior hypogastric sympathetic plexus injury, unless the patient also has advanced peripheral vascular disease. The aorta or vena cava is at risk of injury during the anterior exposure of the thoracolumbar spine. Thorough familiarity of the patient's anatomy is obviously important. Great caution should be taken when removing the annulus. To protect these vessels, an assistant should hold a malleable retractor between the vessels and the spinal column during disc removal. Late hemorrhage caused by erosion, leakage, or false aneurysm formation of the vessel is known, but this complication usually is associated with prominent metal implants (29).

Thoracoscopic and Laparoscopic Exposures of the Thoracic and Lumbar Spine

Thoracoscopic diagnostic procedures have been used for many years, and in recent years, more complex therapeutic procedures have been performed by the thoracic surgeon. Thoracoscopic procedures can reduce postoperative pain, minimize respiratory difficulties, shorten hospital stays, and improve shoulder girdle function early as compared to the formal thoracotomy procedures. These video thoracoscopic surgery techniques have been applied to treat multiple diseases of the thoracic spine, such as disc herniation, vertebral abscess, tumor, fractures, and spinal deformities (62). The availability of an experienced thoracic surgeon and modern thoracoscopic equipments are essential in performing these procedures.

Surgical techniques include general anesthesia with a double lumen intubation. The patient is placed in a lateral position, and the ipsilateral lung is collapsed. The table is flexed to widen the intercostal spaces. The entire chest should be prepped to allow conversion to an open thoracotomy should the need arise during the procedure. Typically, a 10-mm incision is made in the mid-axillary line over the sixth intercostal space. The skin and the intercostal muscles are spread using a hemostat. Blunt dissection with a finger creates an opening into the pleural space. Any pleural adhesions should be released before insertion of the trochar. A 10-mm trochar is placed through the intercostal opening for insertion of the thoracoscope into the chest cavity. Placement of the initial trochar is variable depending on the level of the thoracic spine to be accessed. A 10-mm rigid 30° angled scope is placed, and exploratory thoracoscopy is then performed. In those patients in whom complete resorptive atelectasis and lung collapse does not occur, temporary CO_2 insufflation can expedite and enhance collapse for better visualization. Gravity by Trendelenburg or reverse Trendelenburg, or tilting the table forward, can also enhance retraction of the lung. A fan retractor may be placed through a separate portal to retract the lung.

Once the thoracic spine is visualized through the parietal pleura, the correct level is ascertained by counting the ribs and by radiograph with a laparoscopic needle into the disc space. The pleura is divided over the spine to be exposed. Thoracoscopic electrocautery is used to divide the pleura. The segmental vessels are mobilized, clipped, and ligated. Thoracic discectomy, corpectomy, fusion, and even instrumentation may be performed through this thoracoscopic approach.

Laparoscopic procedures are common in general surgery, but laparoscopic lumbar spinal surgery is relatively new (91). The lower lumbar discs may be excised and fused through the laparoscopic technique, and it may be advantageous in preventing posterior muscular dissection and fibrosis-associated posterior fusion procedures. The upper lumbar spine may also be approached with an expandable balloon that dilates the potential retroperitoneal space. The technique of laparoscopic spinal surgery is exacting, and complications may be devastating. Furthermore, the long-term results of laparoscopic spinal procedures are not available, and strict indications for these procedures should be followed.

The patient is supine in a 20- to 30° Trendelenburg position on the radiolucent table with a C-arm fluoroscope ready. Lumbar lordosis should be maintained, and draping is done widely. Necessary equipment include CO_2 insufflation, 30° endoscope, and laparoscopic trocars with adaptors. The first portal is typically placed at the umbilicus. The incision is made with direct visualization, and CO_2 insufflation to 15 mmHg is maintained. The 30° scope is entered safely. Working portals are lateral to the epigastric vessel. The left trochar is used to mobilize the sigmoid colon from right to left, and two right-sided trocars are inserted in a way to avoid instrument crowding.

The dissection proceeds with monopolar endoshears to incise the peritoneum along reflection. The sigmoid colon mesentery is approached from the right side and incised longitudinally. The ureters are identified and protected. Blunt spreading technique is used to expose the aortic bifurcation. The middle sacral artery is mobilized and ligated with hemoclips and divided. The bifurcation of the inferior vena cava and inferior hypogastric sympathetic plexus must be protected to avoid retrograde ejaculation in males. Monopolar coagulation must be avoided in this area. Retraction of the right iliac vein and left iliac artery exposed the L5-S1 disc. The suprapubic portal is directed to the L5-S1 disc space. The access to L4-5 disc is more difficult, but the left common iliac artery and vein can be mobilized from left to right. The iliolumbar vein on the left must be identified, ligated, and divided for mobilization of the great vessels. Fluoroscopic discectomy and instrumentation can be performed in the disc spaces with the aid of the fluoroscope.

When the procedure is complete, the surgical field should be inspected thoroughly for bleeding as the CO_2 insufflation is reduced to 10 mmHg. The posterior peritoneum is closed with a running laparoscopic suture. The portals are examined for any bleeding and then closed with sutures.

Complications associated with thoracoscopic and laparoscopic procedures include great vessel injuries, trocar site bleeding, injuries to the visceral structures, and spine-related problems including epidural bleeding, dural tear, spinal cord injury, inadequate discectomy, and poor fusion constructs. Postoperatively, hypotensive episodes, ileus, hemorrhage, and construct failure may occur.

References

1. An HS, Gordin R, Renner K. Anatomic considerations for plate fixation to the cervical spine. Spine 1988; 13:813–816.
2. An, HS, Cotler JM. Spinal instrumentation. Baltimore: Williams & Wilkins, 1992.
3. An HS, Simpson JM, ed. Spinal instrumentation of the cervical spine. In: Surgery of the cervical spine. London: Martin-Dunitz, 1994;379.
4. An HS, Evanich C, Nowicki B, et al. Ideal thickness of Smith-Robinson/anterior cervical interbody graft. Spine 1993;18:2043–2047.
5. An HS, Simpson JM, Glover JM, et al. Comparison between allograft plus demineralized bone matrix vs. autograft in anterior cervical fusion. A prospective randomized multi-center study. Spine 1995;20:2211–2216.
6. An HS, Lynch K, Toth J. Comparison between allograft and autograft in adult posterolateral lumbar spine fusion. J Spinal Disord 1995;8:131–135.
7. An HS, Vaccaro A, Cotler JM. Spinal disorders at the cervico-thoracic junction. Spine 1994;15:2557–2564.
8. An HS, Balderston RA. Complications in scoliosis, kyphosis, and spondylolisthesis surgery. In: Balderston RA, An HS, eds. Complications in spine surgery. Philadelphia: WB Saunders, 1991;540.
9. Anderson PA, Henley MB, Grady MS, et al. Posterior cervical arthrodesis with AO reconstruction plates and bone graft. Spine 1991;16:S72–S79.
10. Bohlman HH. Cervical spondylosis with moderate to severe myelopathy. Spine 1977;2:15 1–162.
11. Bohlman HH. Acute fractures and dislocations of the cervical spine: an analysis of 300 hospitalized patients and review of the literature. J Bone Joint Surg Am 1979; 61:1119–1142.
12. Bohlman HH, Emery SE, Goodfellow DB, et al. Robinson anterior cervical discectomy and arthrodesis for cervical radiculopathy. J Bone Joint Surg Am 1993; 75:1298–1307.
13. Brodke DS, Zdeblick TA. Modified Smith-Robinson procedure for anterior discectomy and fusion. Spine 1992;17:S428–430.
14. Brooks AL, Jenkins EB. Atlanto-axial arthrodesis by the wedge compression method. J Bone Joint Surg Am 1978;60:279–284.
15. Brown MD, Malinin TI, Davis PB. A roentgenographic evaluation of frozen allografts versus autografts in anterior cervical spine fusions. Clin Orthop 1976; 119:231–236.
16. Brown CW, Orme TJ, Richardson HD. The rate of pseudoarthrosis (surgical nonunion) in patients who are smokers and patients who are nonsmokers: a comparison study. Spine 1986;11:942–943.
17. Bulger RF, Rejowski JE, Beatty RA. Vocal cord paralysis associated with anterior cervical fusion: consideration for prevention and treatment. J Neurosurg 1985; 62:657–661.
18. Callahan RA, Johnson KM, Margolis RN, et al. Cervical facet fusion for control of instability following laminectomy. J Bone Joint Surg Am 1977;59:991–1002.
19. Charles R. Anterior approach to the upper thoracic vertebrae. J Bone Joint Surg Br 1989;71:81–84.
20. Cleveland RH, Gilsanz V, Lebowitz RL, et al. Hydronephrosis from retroperitoneal fibrosis and anterior spinal fusion. J Bone Joint Surg Am 1978;60:996.
21. Cloward RD. Treatment of acute fractures and fracture dislocations of the cervical spine by vertebral body fu-

sion. A report of 11 cases. J Neurosurg 1961;18:205–209.
22. Coletta AJ, Mayer PJ. Chylothorax: an unusual complication of anterior thoracic interbody spinal fusion. Spine 1982;7:46–49.
23. Cotler HB, Cotler JM, Stoloff A, et al. The use of autograft for vertebral body replacement of the thoracic and lumbar spine. Spine 1985;10:748–756.
24. Crock HV. Anterior lumbar interbody fusion: indications for its use and notes on surgical technique. Clin Orthop 1982;165:157.
25. Crockard HA. Anterior approaches to lesions of the upper cervical spine. Clin Neurosurg 1988;34:389–416.
26. Crockard HA, Calder I, Ransford AO. One stage transoral decompression and posterior fixation in rheumatoid atlanto-axial subluxation. J Bone Joint Surg Br 1990;72:682–685.
27. Darling GE, McBroom R, Perrin R. Modified anterior approach to the cervicothoracic junction. Spine 1995; 13:1519–1521.
28. DeAndrade JR, Macnab I. Anterior occipitocervical fusion using an extra-pharyngeal exposure. J Bone Joint Surg ?? 1969;51A:1621–1626.
29. Dwyer AP. A fatal complication of paravertebral infection and traumatic aneurysm following Dwyer instrumentation. Proc Austral Orthop Assoc. J Bone Joint Surg 1979;61B:239.
30. Ebraheim NA, An HS, Jackson WT, et al. Internal fixation of the unstable cervical spine using posterior Roy-Camille plates: preliminary report. J Orthop Trauma 1989;3:23–28.
31. Eisenstein S, O'Brien JP. Chylothorax: a complication of Dwyer's anterior instrumentation. Br J Surg 1977; 64:339–341.
32. Eismont FJ, Wiesel SW, Rothman RH. The treatment of dural tears associated with spinal surgery. J Bone Joint Surg Am 1981;63:1132.
33. Emery SE, Bolesta MJ, Banks MA, et al. Robinson anterior cervical fusion. Comparison of the standard and modified techniques. Spine 1994;19:660–663.
34. Fang HSY, Ong GB. Direct anterior approach to the upper cervical spine. J Bone Joint Surg 1962;44:1588.
35. Fielding JW, Stillwell WT. Anterior cervical approach to the upper thoracic spine. A case report. Spine 1976;1:158–161.
36. Flynn TB. Neurologic complications of anterior cervical interbody fusion. Spine 1982;7:536–539.
37. Gallie WE. Fractures and dislocations of the cervical spine. Am J Surg 1939;46:495–499.
38. Grantham SA, Dick HM, Thompson KC, et al. Occipitocervical arthrodesis. Clin Orthop 1969;65:118.
39. Griswold DM, Albright JA, Schiffman E, et al. Atlantoaxial fusion for instability. J Bone Joint Surg Am 1978;60:285–292.
40. Grob D, Dvorak J, Panjabi M, et al. Posterior occipitocervical fusion. A preliminary report of a new technique. Spine 1991;16S:17–S24.
41. Grob D, Jeanneret B, Aebi M, et al. Atlantoaxial fusion with transarticular screw fixation. J Bone Joint Surg Br 1991;73:972–976.
42. Hall JE, Denis F, Murray J. Exposure of the upper cervical spine for spinal decompression. J Bone Joint Surg Am 1977;59:121–123.
43. Harbison SP. Major vascular complications of intervertebral disc surgery. Ann Surg 1954;140:342.
44. Heeneman H. Vocal cord paralysis following approaches to the anterior cervical spine. Laryngoscope 1973;83:17–21.
45. Hodge WA, DeWaid RL. Splenic injury, complicating the anterior thoracoabdominal surgical approach for scoliosis. J Bone Joint Surg Am 1983;65:396–397.
46. Hodgson AK, Stock FE, Fang HSY, et al. Anterior spinal fusion: the operative approach and pathologic findings in 412 patients with Pott's disease of the spine. Br J Surg 1960;48:172–178.
47. Hodgson AR. An approach to the cervical spine (C3-7). Clin Orthop 1965;39:129.
48. Holscher EC. Vascular and visceral injuries during lumbar disc surgery. J Bone Joint Surg Am 1968;50:383–393.
49. Johnson RM, McGuire EJ. Urogenital complications of anterior approaches to the lumbar spine. Clin Orthop 1981;154:114–118.
50. Kurz LT, Garfin SR, Booth RE. Harvesting autogenous iliac bone grafts. A review of complications and techniques. Spine 1989;14:1324–1331.
51. Johnson RM, Murphy MJ, Southwick WO. Surgical approaches to the spine. In: Rothman RH, Simeone FA, eds. The spine. Philadelphia: WB Saunders, 1992; 1607–1738.
52. Larson SJ, Hoist RA, Hemmy DC, et al. Lateral extracavity, approach to traumatic lesions of the thoracic and lumbar spine. J Neurosurg 1976;4S:628–637.
53. Lesoin F, Rousseaux M, Lozes G, et al. Posterolateral approach to tumours of the dorsolumbar spine. Acta Neurochir (Wien) 1986;81:40–44.
54. Magerl F, Seeman PS. Stable posterior fusion of the atlas and axis by transarticular screw fixation. In Kehr P, Weidner A, eds. Cervical spine. New York: Springer-Verlag, 1987;322–327.
55. McAfee PC, Bohlman HH, Yuan HA. Anterior decompression of traumatic thoracolumbar fractures with incomplete neurological deficit using retroperitoneal approach. J Bone Joint Surg Am 1985;67:89.
56. McAfee PC, Bohlman HH, Ducker T, et al. Failure of stabilization of the spine with methylmethacrylate: a retrospective analysis of twenty-four cases. J Bone Joint Surg Am 1986;68:1145–1157.
57. McAfee PC, Bohlman HH, Riley LH, et al. The anterior retropharyngeal approach to the upper pan of the cervical spine. J Bone Joint Surg Am 1987;69:1371–1383.
58. Micheli JJ, Hood RW. Anterior exposure of the cervicothoracic spine using a combined cervical and thoracic approach. J Bone Joint Surg Am 1983;65:992–997.
59. Meyer PR Jr. Surgical stabilization of the cervical spine. In: Meyer PR, ed. Surgery of spine trauma. New York: Churchill Livingstone, 1989;397–524.
60. Moore CA, Cohen A. Combined arterial venous and urethral injuries complicating disc surgery. Am J Surg 1968;115:574.
61. Newman P, Sweetnam R. Occipito-cervical fusion. J Bone Joint Surg Br 1969;51:423–431.

62. Regan JJ, Mack MJ, Picetti GD. A technical report on video-assisted thoracoscopy in thoracic spinal surgery. Spine 1995;20:831–837.
63. Riley LH Jr. Surgical approaches to the anterior structures of the cervical spine. Clin Orthop 1973;91:16–20.
64. Robinson RA, Walker E, Ferlic DC, et al. The results of anterior interbody fusion of the cervical spine. J Bone Joint Surg Am 1962;44:1569–1587.
65. Rogers WA. Treatment of fractures and dislocations of the cervical spine. J Bone Joint Surg Am 1942;24:245–248.
66. Roy-Camille IL, Saillant G, Mazel C. Internal fixation of the unstable cervical spine by a posterior osteosynthesis with plates and screws. In: Sherk HH, ed. The cervical spine. Philadelphia: JB Lippincott, 1989;390–421.
67. Roy-Camille R, Mazel C, Saillant G, et al. Treatment of malignant tumors of the spine with posterior instrumentation. In: Sudaresan N, Schmidek HH, Schiller AL, et al, eds. Tumors of the spine. Philadelphia: WB Saunders, 1990;473–487.
68. Sanders G, Uyeda RY, Karlan MS. Nonrecurrent inferior laryngeal nerves and their association with a recurrent branch. Am J Surg 1983;146:501–503.
69. Sang UH, Wilson CB. Postoperative epidural hematoma as a complication of anterior cervical discectomy. J Neurosurg 1978;49:288–291.
70. Shen YS, Cheung CY. Chylous leakage after arthrodesis using the anterior approach to the spine. Report of two cases. J Bone Joint Surg Am 1989;71:1250–1251.
71. Silber I, McMaster W. Retroperitoneal fibrosis with hydronephrosis as a complication of the Dwyer procedure. J Pediatr Surg 1977;12:255.
72. Simmons EH, Bhalla SK. Anterior cervical discectomy and fusion. A clinical and biomechanical study with eight-year follow up. J Bone Joint Surg Br 1969;51:225–232.
73. Smith MD, Emery SE, Dudley A, et al. Vertebral artery injury during anterior decompression of the cervical spine. J Bone Joint Surg Br 1993;75:410.
74. Smith GW, Robinson RA. The treatment of certain cervical spine disorders by anterior removal of the intervertebral disc and interbody fusion. J Bone Joint Surg Am 1958;40:607.
75. Smith MD, Anderson P, Grady S. Occipitocervical arthrodesis using contoured plate fixation. Spine 1993;18:1984–1990.
76. Stener B. Total spondylectomy in chondrosarcoma arising from the seventh thoracic vertebra. J Bone Joint Surg Br 1971; 53:288–295.
77. Stener B, Johnson OE. Complete removal of three vertebrae for giant cell tumor. J Bone Joint Surg Br 1971;53:278–287.
78. Stener B, Gunterberg B. High amputation of the sacrum for extirpation of tumors. Spine 1978;3:351–366.
79. Sundaresan N, Shah I, Foley KM, et al. An anterior surgical approach to the upper thoracic vertebrae. J Neurosurg 1984;61:686–690.
80. Turner PL, Webb JK. A surgical approach to the upper thoracic spine. J Bone Joint Surg Br 1987;69:542–544.
81. Vaccaro AR, Ring D, Scuderi G, et al. Vertebral artery location in relation to the vertebral body as determined by two-dimensional computed tomography evaluation. Spine 1994;19:2637–2641.
82. Verbiest H. Anterolateral operations for fractures and dislocations in the middle and lower parts of the cervical spine. J Bone Joint Surg Am 1969;51:1489–1530.
83. Watkins RG. Surgical approaches to the spine. New York: Springer-Verlag, 1983.
84. Welsh LW, Welsh JJ, Chinnici JC. Dysphagia due to cervical spine surgery. Ann Otol Rhinol Laryngol 1987;96:112–115.
85. Wertheim SB, Bohlman HH. Occipitocervical fusion. J Bone Joint Surg Am 1987;69:833–836.
86. White AA III, Southwick WO, DePonte RJ, et al. Relief of pain by anterior cervical fusion for spondylosis—a report of sixty-five patients. J Bone Joint Surg Am 1973;55:525–534.
87. White AA III, Jupiter J, Southwick WO, et al. An experimental study of the immediate load bearing of three surgical constructions for anterior spine fusions. Clin Orthop 1973;91:21–28.
88. Whitecloud TS, LaRocca H. Fibular strut graft in reconstructive surgery of the cervical spine. Spine 1976;1:33–43.
89. Whitesides TE Jr, Kelley RP. Lateral approach to the upper cervical spine for anterior fusion. South Med J 1966;59:879–883.
90. Zdeblick TA, Ducker TB. The use of freeze-dried allograft bone for anterior cervical fusions. Spine 1991;16:726–729.
91. Zucherman JF, Zdeblick TA, Bailey SA, et al. Instrumented laparoscopic spinal fusion: preliminary results. Spine 1995;20:2029–2035.

CHAPTER THREE

Spine Biomechanics

Tae-Hong Lim and Howard S. An

The spine is a flexible, yet relatively stable column with a multi-curved shape. It is straight and symmetrical in the frontal view. In the lateral view, the spine has four normal curves: cervical lordosis, thoracic kyphosis, lumbar lordosis, and sacral kyphosis. This curvature is due to the shape of the vertebrae and intervertebral discs. The kyphotic curves are primarily caused by the lesser height of the anterior vertebral borders compared with the posterior borders, whereas the lordotic curves are largely caused by the wedge-shaped intervertebral discs. This difference in anterior and posterior heights results in a greater degree of flattening of the cervical and lumbar lordosis compared with the thoracic kyphosis when the spine is distracted. The normal spinal curves are biomechanically important in that they increase the flexibility and energy absorption capacity of the spinal column.

The spine consists of essentially similar motion segments that can be considered in isolation. The motion segment, sometimes called a functional spinal unit (FSU), consists of two adjacent vertebrae and the connecting intervertebral disc and ligaments. Two vertebrae are connected by a compound joint that is made of a three joint complex. The posterior two joints are the facet joints, and the anterior joint is the intervertebral disc. These joints and ligaments are highly specialized to accommodate basic biomechanical functions of the spine.

Basic biomechanical functions of the spine are support, mobility, and protection of neural structures. The vertebral body, disc, and anterior and posterior longitudinal ligaments provide the major support for the spinal column and absorb impact, while the mobility is provided by the intervertebral joint complex. The spine architecture protects the spinal cord and nerves. Trunk muscles and ligaments also provide spinal stability and postural control. Normal spine functions depend on the interplay among spinal structure, stability, and flexibility, as well as on muscular strength and endurance. A disruption of this interplay may result in a spinal disorder.

The role of various components in a normal or diseased spine has been investigated using well-established engineering principles. The surgeon is confronted with more and more biomechanically related data as the surgical techniques are enhanced with the aid of advanced technologies, such as imaging, material instrumentation, and spinal instrumentation. A better understanding of the biomechanics of the spine is necessary to improve the diagnosis and treatment of spine disorders. This chapter reviews the biomechanical principles of surgery of the spine.

Kinematics of the Spine

Kinematics is a branch of mechanics that studies the motion of rigid bodies without consideration of influencing forces. A three-dimensional motion of a rigid body can be described as a combination of both translation and rotation with respect to a certain reference frame. Translation is a motion of a rigid body along an axis in which a straight line in the body always remains parallel to itself, and rotation is a spinning of rigid body about an axis. An orthogonal or Cartesian system is widely used for the kinematic analysis.

In the spine, a vertebra can translate along and/or rotate about three-orthogonal axes and thus have six degrees of freedom. These motions are usually coupled. For example, in a flexion/extension movement, the vertebra rotates in the sagittal plane with simultaneous anterior-posterior translation. The range of motion and the coupling characteristics are determined by the various anatomic elements, such as ligaments, facets, and intervertebral discs. Thus, the spinal kinematics can be described comprehensively by the range of motion for all six degrees of freedom, coupling characteristics, and functions of anatomic elements. A better understanding of kinematics is important for the diagnosis and treatment of spine pathology.

Kinematics of the Cervical Spine

Upper Cervical

RANGE OF MOTION AND COUPLING CHARACTERISTICS

The cervical spine can be divided into two regions: the upper cervical (occiput-C1-C2) and the lower cervical (C2-C7) region. In the upper cervical spine, as listed in Table 3.1, both occiput-C1 and C1-C2 segments demonstrate similar flexion/extension and lateral bending motions, whereas the lateral bending is less than flexion/extension in both segments. However, the axial rotation of the C1-C2 joint is much greater than that of the C0-C1 joint. In fact, more than half of the axial rotation of the entire cervical spine occurs at the C1-C2 level (135, 186). The deep fit of the convex occipital condyles in the concave facets of C1 is known to restrict the axial rotation. In contrast, a convex orientation of both articular surfaces of the C1-C2 lateral masses in the sagittal plane allows considerable mobility. The absence of taut yellow ligament connecting the posterior elements further enhances the axial rotational motion capacity. Instead, the posterior elements of the C1-C2 segment are connected by the loose, mobile atlanto-occipital membrane.

Translational motions in the upper cervical spine are small. There is insignificant translation between the occiput and C1. However, translation occurs between C1 and C2. The sagittal plane translations of the C1-C2 segment are minimal because of the snug fit of the ring of C1 about the dens. Normal translation is 2 to 3 mm measured based on the distance between the anterior portion of the dens and the posterior portion of the ring of C1. Jackson (73) found that the distance for adults was constant in full flexion and extension with a maximum of 2.5 mm, whereas a forward subluxation was often noted and the maximum distance was 4.5 mm for children. Lateral translation of the C1-C2 segment is controversial, but it is believed that lateral displacement of up to 4 mm between the dens and the lateral masses occurs during the axial rotation in the normal segment (186). C1 also can translate vertically while it rotates about the vertical axis. These translatory movements illustrate the coupling characteristics of the upper cervical spine.

FUNCTIONS OF ANATOMIC ELEMENTS

Skeletal contact between the anterior margin of the foramen magnum and the tip of the dens provide a check rein to flexion of the occiput-C1 joint, while the tectorial membrane limits the extension. The tectorial membrane is also known to limit the flexion and extension movements at the C1-C2 joint (183, 186). The ligaments limit the axial rotation of the occiput relative to C1. The alar ligaments provide a check rein to this motion (38). The alar ligaments also control the lateral bending motions. For example, the right upper portions of the alar ligament, connected to the occiput, and the left lower component, connected to the ring of C1, provide a check rein to the left lateral bending. The osseous anatomy of the up-

TABLE 3.1.

Representative (lower–upper limits) Values of Ranges of Rotational Motion of the Normal Spine

Region	Level	Flexion/Extension (deg)	One Side Lateral Bending (deg)	One Side Axial Rotation (deg)
Cervical	C0-C1	25 (10–45)	5 (2–13)	5 (0–11)
	C1-C2	20 (3–41)	5 (1–17)	40 (27–49)
	C2-C3	10 (5–16)	10 (11–20)	3 (0–10)
	C3-C4	15 (7–26)	11 (9–15)	7 (3–10)
	C4-C5	20 (13–29)	11 (0–16)	7 (1–12)
	C5-C6	20 (13–29)	8 (0–16)	7 (1–12)
	C6-C7	7 (6–26)	7 (0–17)	6 (2–10)
	C7-T1	6 (4–17)	4 (0–17)	2 (0–7)
Thoracic	T1-T2	4 (3–5)	5 (5)	9 (14)
	T2-T3	4 (3–5)	6 (5–7)	8 (4–12)
	T3-T4	4 (2–5)	5 (3–7)	8 (5–11)
	T4-T5	4 (2–5)	6 (5–6)	8 (5–11)
	T5-T6	4 (3–5)	6 (5–6)	8 (5–11)
	T6-T7	5 (2–7)	6 (6)	7 (4–11)
	T7-T8	6 (3–8)	6 (3–8)	7 (4–11)
	T8-T9	6 (3–8)	6 (4–7)	6 (6–7)
	T9-T10	6 (3–8)	6 (4–7)	4 (3–5)
	T10-T11	9 (4–14)	7 (3–10)	2 (2–3)
	T11-T12	12 (6–20)	9 (4–13)	2 (2–3)
	T12-L1	12 (6–20)	8 (5–10)	2 (2–3)
Lumbar	L1-L2	12 (5–16)	6 (3–8)	2 (1–3)
	L2-L3	14 (8–18)	6 (3–10)	2 (1–3)
	L3-L4	15 (6–17)	8 (4–12)	2 (1–3)
	L4-L5	16 (9–21)	6 (3–9)	2 (1–3)
	L5-S1	17 (10–24)	3 (2–6)	1 (0–2)

Data were obtained from White and Panjabi, 1990.

per cervical spine limits the upper cervical spine motion.

Lower Cervical

RANGE OF MOTION AND COUPLING CHARACTERISTICS

The ranges of rotational motion in three planes are listed in Table 3.1. Most of the flexion/extension motion occurs in the middle region, and the C5-C6 segment has the largest range. Lateral bending and axial rotation become smaller in the lower levels. However, no significant variation of the physical properties is found with respect to the vertebral level (115, 126).

The maximum anterior-posterior translation during flexion/extension was 2.7 mm with the representative value of 2.0 mm (184). In a more recent study, Panjabi et al. (127) measured an average anterior translation of 1.9 mm and posterior translation of 1.6 mm. White and Panjabi suggested 3.5 mm as guide for the upper limits of normal translation of the lower cervical spine. However, no data on the translational motions of the lower cervical spine in the other directions is available in the literature.

In contrast to the upper cervical spine, distinct coupling patterns exist in the lower cervical spine. The lateral bending of the lower cervical spine is coupled with the axial rotation. During the left lateral bending, for example, the spinous processes go to the right. Lysell (105) measured 2° of coupled axial rotation of C2 for every 3° of lateral bending as compared with 1° of axial rotation of C7 for every 7.5° of lateral bending. The axial rotations between C2 and C7 caused by lateral bending gradually decrease in the lower levels. Panjabi et al. (127) also noted a coupled lateral bending of 0.75° associated with a left axial rotation of 0.75°. Similarly, other investigators also observed coupled lateral bending to axial rotation (105, 115).

FUNCTIONS OF ANATOMIC ELEMENTS

The intervertebral disc provides the great resistance to horizontal translation. Its geometry and stiffness also dictate the rotational motion of the vertebra. For example, an intervertebral disc with greater height and smaller diameter allows a greater rotation. Ligaments also affect the kinematics of the cervical spine. The yellow ligament has a significant role in resisting flexion because of its elastic content (131). The ligamentum nuchae spans from the C7 spinous process to the external occipital protuberance. It is a dense, fibrous band and is believed to provide a major constraint to excessive flexion of the cervical spine. Facet joint capsule effectively limits the flexion, and greater than 50% resection of the C5-C6 capsule results in a hypermobility (196). Facet joint also prevents the horizontal translation of the vertebra (124).

Kinematics of the Thoracic Spine

RANGE OF MOTION AND COUPLING CHARACTERISTICS

The range of rotational motions of the thoracic motion segments are listed in Table 3.1. Average flexion/extension motions are about 4° in the upper levels (T1-T5) and 6° in the middle levels (T6-T10). In the lower segments (T11-T12 and T12-L1), each segment has 12° of flexion/extension motion. The lateral bending motions of the upper and middle segments are similar and increase in the lower segments to some extent (6° to 8–9°). In contrast, the axial rotational motions demonstrate a tendency for a smaller motion in the more caudal segments.

In the thoracic spine, lateral bending and axial rotation are coupled with each other as shown in the cervical spine. In the upper thoracic segments, the coupling of these rotations is strong. However, in the middle and lower thoracic spines, this coupling is not distinct, and the direction of coupling direction is not consistent as well. For example, the spinous processes rotate either to the right or to the left responding to the left lateral bending (186).

FUNCTIONS OF ANATOMIC ELEMENTS

The intervertebral joints and spinous processes limit the extension motion in the thoracic spine. The posterior ligaments, particularly the ligamentum flavum and facet capsules, are believed to be the major structures that resist axial rotational motion. The facet joint is not believed to resist the axial rotation in the thoracic spine because of the spatial alignment of the facet articulation.

Kinematics of the Lumbar Spine

RANGE OF MOTION AND COUPLING CHARACTERISTICS

The range of rotational motions of the lumbar motion segments are listed in Table 3.1. The range of flexion/extension motion shows a gradual increase from the cephalad to caudal direction in the lumbar spine. For lateral bending and axial rotation, the average range of motion is approximately the same at each level between L1 and L5, but becomes relatively smaller at the lumbosacral segment.

The sagittal plane translation that occurs during flexion/extension is an important component of lumbar spine motion because it has been used frequently to determine instability. Pearcy (132, 133) suggested 2 mm anterior translation as normal for the lumbar spine based upon the stereoradiographic measurement. Posner et al. (139) suggested 2.8 mm of anterior movement as the upper limit of normal translation based upon their in vitro study. Average posterior translation measured in extension is 1 mm (SD = 1) in all lumbar levels (11). In the in vitro studies, Panjabi et al. (130) observed that the application of the lateral bending moments produces lateral translations (average 1.1 mm) in the same direction and very small upward translation less than 1 mm for all levels. The authors also noted small translational motions (generally less than 1 mm) under axial rotational moment.

FUNCTIONS OF ANATOMIC ELEMENTS

The intervertebral disc permits considerable sagittal and frontal plane rotations and limits translational motion. The disc is also a major load-bearing structure in the lumbar spine. The anterior and posterior longitudinal ligaments check the flexion/extension of a motion segment, but their contribution is not significant in limiting axial rotation, lateral bending, and horizontal translation. The facet joints limit extension, axial rotation, and translation. The well-developed capsules of these joints resist the flexion and translational motions. The interspinous ligaments are not significant in controlling the segmental motion, whereas the supraspinous ligaments are more important in limiting flexion. The ligamentum flavum may slightly resist flexion and axial rotation; its exact role has not yet been determined.

Spinal Instability

The term "spinal instability" originates from Knutsson's radiologic observation of abnormal parallel displacements and tilting of the vertebra. Since then, spinal or segmental instability has been used as a clinical entity in the diagnosis of spinal disorders. The majority of spinal fusion and instrumentation is for the treatment of spinal instability associated with traumatic deformity and infectious, neoplastic, degenerative, and severely decompressed conditions. However, spinal instability is a very controversial topic among spine surgeons. For instance, there is no real consensus on the definition of spinal instability. It is also difficult to prove whether spinal instability generates back pain. The lack of consistent rules of measurement is another reason for the current controversial understanding of spinal instability. Thus, it is necessary to better understand the current knowledge of spinal instability for improving the diagnosis and treatment of spinal instability.

Definition of Spinal Instability

In an engineering sense, instability represents a specific state of a structure in which an addition of small load results in an excessively large displacement in an unpredictable or erratic manner. Accordingly, spinal instability should represent the condition in which a small load applied to the spine causes a catastrophically large displacement of the vertebrae. Such an unstable condition can be found in the spine after trauma or excessive surgical removal of supporting structures. In contrast, an abnormally large, but not catastrophic, segmental motion can be defined by the term "hypermobility," which represents a high flexibility or low stiffness as advocated by Ashton-Miller and Schultz (11).

Historically, however, the term spinal (or segmental) instability has been used by clinicians to describe the hypermobile segments as well as the catastrophic spinal conditions. The early definition of instability has focused on translation in the sagittal plane. Knutsson (82) described both abnormal displacement and tilting of the vertebra as a sign of disc degeneration and termed it as segmental instability. Hirsch and Lewin (72) defined subluxation of L5-S1 when the upper point of the superior facet of S1 was above the line along the inferior endplate of L5 in extension. Some investigators suggested abnormal anatomic features as a sign of instability. These anatomic features include disc space narrowing (175), osteophytes (spur) (106), and spondylo- or retro-listhetic deformities (76, 80, 106, 119, 144). Kirkaldy-Willis and associates (80) suggested four types of segmental instability. Type 1 is axial rotational instability, a fixed rotatory deformity and occasional translation that can be detected as malalignment of the spinous processes in AP radiograph. Type 2 instability includes abnormal translations and anatomic features as described by previous investigators (76, 82, 106). Approximately 3 mm subluxation was considered as a typical type 2 instability, particularly in female patients with L4-5 involvement. Type 3 is retrolisthetic instability that is observed most commonly at the L5-S1 level. Type 4 is postsurgical instability secondary to the excessive removal of supporting structures. Spinal instability in these studies does represent a hypermobile segment, except for the postsurgical instability, which can induce either hypermobile or catastrophic conditions.

Radiographs have been used most frequently to detect the presence of instability and its relation to symptoms. However, instability (i.e. hypermobility) appears to occur in asymptomatic subjects, and a question is raised whether the detected instability may be the source of pain. Kirkaldy-Willis and Farfan (81) postulated three stages of disc degeneration: temporary dysfunction, instability, and stabilization. They believed that instability is present when abnormal motion occurs due to the loss of stiffness as a result of damage beyond the capabilities of healing mechanism. The authors further specified cases in which pain results from the unstable motion segment as "clinical instability" because of the lack of correlation between abnormal motion and the presence of symptoms. Frymoyer and Selby (49) also defined spinal instability as a symptomatic condition in which a physiologic load causes abnormally large deformations of the intervertebral joint, emphasizing that instability may be an incidental finding unless it produces symptoms.

Clinical instability has been defined by White and Panjabi (186) as "the loss of the ability of the spine under physiological loads to maintain relationships between vertebrae in such a way that there is neither damage nor subsequent irritation to the spinal cord or nerve roots, in addition, there is no development of incapacitating deformity or pain due to structural changes." In this definition, incapacitating deformity is defined as a gross deformity that the patient finds intolerable, whereas incapacitating pain is pain unable to be controlled by non-narcotic drugs. As the authors commented, clinical instability can occur from trauma, disease, surgery, or some combinations of the three. Thus, clinical instability describes an abnormal (hypermobile) motion that produces incapacitating pain as well as a catastrophic motion of the spine caused by trauma under physiologic loads.

Although spinal instability has been defined in various ways in the literature (49, 81, 137, 186), its common feature is an abnormally large motion or abnormal patterns of motion. Abnormally large motions include not only erratic, catastrophic motions but also the substantial loss of segmental stiffness (or hypermobility). Particular controversy surrounds the diagnosis of hypermobility in the degenerated motion segments that is directly related to the pain or progressive deformity. Thus, a knowledge of normal behavior of the spine is a minimum requirement for detecting spinal instability.

In Vivo Spinal Motion Measurement Methods

Efforts have been made to quantify spinal motion, but precise assessment of complex three-dimensional spinal motion remains difficult. In vitro biomechanical studies (52, 53, 130) have characterized the displacement patterns (including coupled motions) under various types of loading. However, it is insufficient to establish a normal motion of the spine since in vivo loads resulting from muscular structures cannot be simulated properly in in vitro studies. As a result, several methods have been developed and used to quantify the spinal motion in vivo.

Dynamic flexion/extension radiographs have been used most frequently to assess the abnormal spine motion (13, 15, 37, 39–43, 105, 134, 139, 141). Plain radiographic findings that suggest segmental instability include disc space narrowing (175), osteophytes (spur) (107), and spondylo- or retro-listhetic deformities (76, 106, 119, 144). Greater importance has been placed on quantifying abnormal segmental motions in terms of rotation and translation. Methods for measuring segmental motion from lateral radiographs have been described by many investigators (8, 13, 15, 37, 39–43, 48, 92, 99, 105, 114, 141, 134, 180, 188).

These radiographs, however, provide a two-dimensional (2-D) representation of the true 3-D motion. Because actual spinal motion is three-dimensional and the instability may include significant changes in coupled motions, the accuracy of motion using planar radiographs is poor. Other potential sources of error include the location of anatomic landmarks in the radiographs, distortion of the radiographic image in central projection, quality of the roentgenograms, and techniques used to measure translation. Estimates of the measurement errors have been reported in previous spinal motion studies using 2-D lumbar spine lateral radiographs. The errors associated with sagittal plane translational motion measurement reported in the literature ranged from 1 to 4 mm (116, 129, 149) or 3 to 15% of the vertebral depth (33, 78, 181). In a series of experiments designed to assess the consistency and accuracy of various measurement protocols for measuring sagittal translation, Schaffer et al. (150) reported very high reliability across roentgenogram quality, raters, and measurement. In the same study, however, surprisingly high false-positive and false-negative rates (i.e., when normal translations are categorized outside of the normal range and vice versa) were found with significant differences between measurement methods. The method of using the anterior surface of the vertebra as a fundamental landmark (114) produced the fewest classification errors (up to 18% false-positive and 29% false-negative rates in high-quality roentgenograms) and was least affected by concomitant rotational motions. Significant increases in false-positive and false-negative rates with reduced film quality were also noted across all tested measurement methods.

Some investigators have developed 3-D measurement systems using biplanar roentgenograms. Bony landmarks have been used in these studies as reference points (18, 169, 171, 187). Optimization techniques have been employed in all of these reports to minimize errors in the localization of bony landmarks. Clinically valuable measurements have been made using these techniques (169, 187). The use of anatomical landmarks, however, is prone to error because of difficulties in accurately locating them in different radiographic views (169). Distortion of the radiographic image in central projection is also a potential error source.

In 1974, Selvik (156) developed a technique that avoided the inaccuracies inherent with the use of bony landmarks. He implanted biocompatible metallic markers into a subject's bone and then employed roentgen stereophotogrammetry to study longitudinal growth (157, 158). The use of small metallic markers permitted accuracy of 0.1 to 0.2 mm. Although the literature suggests that roentgen stereophotogrammetry combined with the use of radiopaque markers provides a superior method of motion analysis, the technique is invasive, which renders it impractical for routine clinical diagnoses.

In 1987, Penning and Wilmink (135) reported on the use of computed tomography (CT) for the measurement of in vivo axial rotation in the cervical spine of normal subjects. Rapid sequence, 9-mm sections and anteroposterior radiographs were used for the measurement of axial rotation, the degree of lateral flexion of the axis, and lateral displacement of the atlas. The pattern of motion was also investigated by trying to define an axis of rotation using CT scan slices. This method, however, had inherent inaccuracies associated with bony landmark location, and was not adequate for complete 3-D cervical motion description.

To avoid the limitations associated with radiographs, several methods for direct measurement of motion have been developed. Transducers or markers mounted on the skin or inserted in the spinous process have been used to measure vertebral motion (157, 126, 138). Panjabi et al. (126) and Pope et al. (138) used accelerometers mounted to pins inserted in the spinous processes to measure lumbar spine responses to vibration and impact. However, the use of skin-mounted transducers suffers from inaccuracies caused by skin motion artifact, whereas the placement of markers into the spinous processes is invasive. Alund and Larsson (5) reported a clinical method of 3-D motion analysis of neck motion using an electrogoniometric technique. This method provided good motion parameter description in 3-D space and afforded a more objective functional evaluation of common neck disorders for supplementing the radiographic examination. However, the data was only applicable to the spine as a unit and was incapable of providing motion assessment of each motion segment.

Current methods of in vivo spinal motion measurement are insufficiently sensitive, not specific, or invasive. An ideal in vivo spinal motion analysis system should be capable of providing sufficiently accurate 3-D motion data of each vertebra based on noninvasive measurements.

Diagnosis of Spinal Instability

Several factors need to be considered for the diagnosis of spinal instability. Structural integrity of anatomic elements must be evaluated because it plays a significant role in preserving stability of the spine. Anatomy is also significant in terms of position and space relationship between neural structures and potentially damaging structures. Motion characteristics of the spine also must be considered carefully in determining spinal instability. In the literature, many

TABLE 3.2.
Checklist for the Diagnosis of Clinical Instability

C0-C1-C2 Instability	• One side C0-C1 axial rotation $> 8°$ • C0-C1 translation (distance between the basin of the occiput and the top of the dens) > 1 mm increase with flexion/extension • Overhang C1-C2 (total right and left) > 7 mm • Oneside C1-C2 axial rotation $> 45°$ • C1-C2 translation (distance between the anterior border of the dens and the posterior border of the ring of C1) > 4 mm • Distance between the posterior body C2 and posterior ring C1 < 13 mm	

	Element	Points
Middle and Lower Cervical Instability	• Anterior elements destroyed or unable to function	2
	• Posterior elements destroyed or unable to function	2
	• Positive stretch test	2

	• Radiographic criteria
	  A. Flexion/extension x-rays
	    1. Sagittal plane translation > 3.5 mm or 20% (2 pts)
	    2. Sagittal plane rotation $> 20°$ (2 pts)
	  OR
	  B. Resting x-rays
	    1. Sagittal plane translation > 3.5 mm or 20% (2 pts)
	    2. Relative sagittal plane angulation $> 11°$ (2 pts)
		4

	• Abnormal disc narrowing	1
	• Developmentally narrow spinal canal (Sagittal dia. < 13 mm or Pavlov's ratio < 0.8)	1
	• Spinal cord damage	2
	• Nerve root damage	1
	• Dangerous loading anticipated	1
	Total of 5 or more pts = Unstable	

	Element	Points
Thoracic and Thoracolumbar Instability	• Anterior elements destroyed or unable to function	2
	• Posterior elements destroyed or unable to function	2
	• Disruptions of costovertebral articulations	1

	• Radiographic Criteria
	  1. Sagittal plane displacement > 2.5 mm (2 pts)
	  2. Relative sagittal plane angulation $> 5°$ (2 pts)
		4

	• Spinal cord or cauda equina damage	2
	• Dangerous loading anticipated	1
	Total of 5 or more pts = Unstable	

investigators have suggested several symptoms and signs that may indicate spinal instability. White and Panjabi (186) suggested the most comprehensive and objective system. They developed a checklist, giving point values to different individual criteria or components that can lead to the diagnosis of instability (Table 3.2).

At present, the diagnosis of spinal instability is limited by several issues. Detection of abnormal motion requires a more sensitive but noninvasive imaging technique for routine clinical usage. It is also important to determine if and when abnormal motion causes pain (88).

Effects of Surgical Decompression on Spinal Stability

Surgical decompression is indicated in the presence of spinal cord or nerve root impingement associated with tumors, trauma, infection, or degenerative changes. The goal of decompression is to remove the impinging structures to relieve pain and to prevent the neurologic problems. The extensive resection of spine structures may lead to spinal instability after surgical decompression, but the indication for fusion is controversial. For example, lumbar discectomy with a limited disc excision was found to be a safe, effective, and reliable method for the treatment of selected patients with herniated discs (167, 185). However, Frymoyer and Selby (49) found radiographic evidence of hypermobility of the segment with disc excision. Eie et al. (45) suggested posterior spinal fusion after discectomy because it provides better protection against recurrent low back pain compared with simple removal of the herniated disc material. This controversy raised a clinical question to surgeons: what extent of simple decompression procedures does not induce the instability that requires fusion? Consequently, controlled biomechanical studies have been performed to determine the effect of surgical decompression on the motion behavior of not only the involved level, but the levels adjacent to it as well. The results of these biomechanical studies are reviewed in this section.

Lumbar Region

In the lumbar spine, the decompression is less extensive than in the other regions of the spine, and the neural elements can be decompressed through a posterior approach in the large majority of situations. One of the decompression procedures in this region is discectomy with partial laminectomy and/or partial dissection of the medial aspect of the lateral overhang of the involved facet joint to remove herniated discs. Another common decompression procedure is bilateral laminectomy and facetectomy at the involved level(s) to relieve pain caused by spinal stenosis.

The effect of discectomy on spine stability has been investigated clinically and biomechanically. In a prospective study with biplanar radiography, Tibrewal et al. (173) observed flexion/extension motion of 15 patients before and after discectomy by fenestration and minimal resection of the lamina. Up to a 50% decrease in flexion/extension and increased coupled motions of lateral bending and axial rotation was found at the level above the discectomy in these patients. No change in the range of flexion/extension was caused by the surgery. Based on these results, they concluded that discectomy with minimal laminectomy did not produce instability. However, the evidence of hypermobility of the operated segment after disc excision at the L4-L5 level was found in the flexion/extension radiographs of patients, particularly in female patients with associated with traction spurs (48, 49).

The stabilizing role of the intervertebral disc has been investigated in many biomechanical studies (3, 52, 53, 79, 110, 125, 172). The major load-bearing role of the disc is in axial compression, flexion, and shear. The disc injury may significantly increase the major and coupled motions of the motion segment in all directions. However, the effect of most clinically significant disc injuries induced within a motion segment at the most common site of herniation was investigated by Goel and his colleagues (53).

The three-dimensional motion behavior was measured when the ligamentous lumbar spine with and without discectomy was subjected to a maximum pure moment of 6.9 Nm in flexion, extension, lateral bending, and axial torsion. The tested cases included 1) intact, 2) disc protrusion or herniation, an injury associated with low back pain prior to surgery, and 3) a partial discectomy. The disc herniation was simulated on the left side posterolaterally by cutting the left ligamentum flavum and the annulus horizontally. The nucleus pulposus was then gently teased out of the annulus so that the teased nucleus was not totally separated from its remaining part. The second simulated injury, partial discectomy, was created as suggested by Spengler (167). A small amount of nucleus pulposus was removed with a pituitary rongeur, which was inserted into the incision already made during the first injury. The percentage of primary motion changes caused by the injuries are shown in Figure 3.1. The flexion motion increased significantly with injury, whereas no significant motion change was found in extension. The response to the sequential injuries in lateral bending loads also increased compared with the intact motion, but at a reduced level of significance; similar motion changes

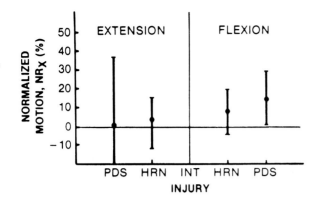
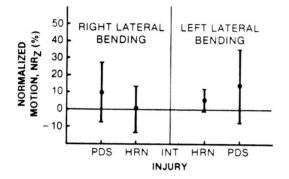
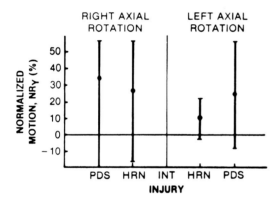

FIGURE 3.1.
The percentage motion changes corresponding to a 6.9Nm moment in various directions. The horizontal axis represents the sequential injuries investigated: INT = intact specimen; HRN = herniation; and PDS = partial discectomy. Adapted from Goel VK, et al. Mechanical properties of lumbar spinal motion segments as affected by partial disc removal. Spine 1986;11:1008–1012.

were observed in axial torsions. However, the secondary/coupled motion components did not show any significant changes in all loading modes. These results indicate that partial discectomy can significantly increase the segmental motion in flexion, lateral bending, and axial torsion mode.

Decompression procedures, such as laminectomy and facetectomy, disrupt the posterior spinal elements and can alter the load-bearing and kinematic characteristics of the lumbar spine. Numerous biomechanical studies have been performed to investigate the stabilizing role of the posterior elements. The facet joints play a major stabilizing role in the lumbar motion segment and, partial or complete removal of the facet joints can significantly destabilize the spine (1, 2, 36, 52, 54, 102, 139, 153, 170, 180). Abumi et al. (1) investigated the lumbar segmental instability after graded facetectomy using lumbar spinal functional units. Unilateral and bilateral medial facetectomy with division of supra- and interspinous ligaments increases the flexion motion, but not other motions. However, total facetectomy, even created unilaterally, resulted in significant motion increase in flexion and axial torsion. In an in vitro experiment, Goel et al. (54) observed an increasing trend of flexion, lateral bending, and axial torsion motions at the injured level (L4-L5) in the presence of hemilateral partial laminectomy and facetectomy. When the nucleus pulposus was removed totally in addition to these partial hemilateral decompressions, significant increases in major rotational motions and translational motions were noted in all loading modes as compared with the intact segments. Bilateral laminectomy and facetectomy also increased the flexion and axial torsional motion significantly at the injured level.

In clinical observations, spinal instability (or hypermobility) induced by laminectomy and facetectomy was not as clear as the results of biomechanical studies. No instability was found in 33 patients with discectomy and facetectomy in a 2- to 5-year follow-up, although there was a chance for a different outcome in the presence of multiple level decompression (67). In the observations of 45 patients with laminectomy and facetectomy for the treatment of spinal stenosis, Johnsson et al. (75) noted that postoperative slip of the vertebra was correlated with degenerative spondylolisthesis. However, this correlation did not affect operative outcome. They also showed that facetectomy in addition to laminectomy did not change the surgical outcome, although a tendency toward less slipping was noted after a more limited laminectomy. Sienkiewicz and Flatley (162) noted a distinct propensity to the forward slip of a L4 or L5 after laminectomy in the study of 8 women.

As described, it is unclear to what degree decompression procedures induce postoperative instability. However, it is clear that the segmental motion increase after decompression procedures is directly related to the extent and location of the spinal elements removal at the surgery. White and Panjabi (186), based on their own clinical experience and a review of the related clinical and biomechanical studies in the literature, suggest the following criteria for determining when to fuse decompression: 1) The patient is less than 75 years of age; 2) The decompression requires removal of more than 50% of the total facet joints at one level; or 3) The decompression required the removal of a significant portion (30 to 40%) of the annulus fibrosus.

Thoracic and Thoracolumbar Regions

In the thoracic spine, anterior decompression can be achieved through partial or total vertebral body resection. The anteriorly decompressed spine is unstable because the vertebral bodies are major load supporting elements. Stabilization of the decompressed spine using instrumentation for reduction and interbody fusion is recommended following anterior decompression.

Although highly controversial, laminectomies have been performed in the thoracic spine. Laminectomies may induce instability through the removal of supporting structures of the spinal column and also may be associated with additional neurologic deterioration (186).

Cervical Region

In the cervical spine, spinal cord and nerve roots can be decompressed through either an anterior or a posterior approach. Anterior approach involves discectomy and/or corpectomy. Reconstruction with an interbody bone graft is usually accomplished after anterior decompression, and this is sufficient if the posterior elements are intact. Otherwise, the posterior elements should also be fused (186). Thus, postoperative instability is not a controversial issue in an anterior decompression of the cervical spine.

In the posterior approach, laminectomy and foraminotomy are performed to decompress the spinal cord and nerve roots, respectively. The common complications after posterior laminectomy include development of kyphotic deformity, instability (spondylolisthesis), and inadequate decompression (21, 63, 69, 101, 189). Postlaminectomy kyphosis is seen most frequently in younger patients (21, 63, 101, 189). The greater tendency for ligamentous stretching and secondary vertebral body wedging in children is believed to lead to a higher incidence of deformity in this group compared with adults (189). However, in adults with normal preoperative alignment and stability, laminectomy usually is not associated with a significant rate of progressive kyphosis. Biomechanical studies using ligamentous cervical spines also demonstrated that the cervical laminectomy did not significantly change the load-displacement behavior of the injured level (55, 194).

When partial or total facetectomy is done during the posterior decompression procedures, it may induce acute instability of the cervical spine. Several biomechanical studies demonstrate the importance of facet joint integrity to cervical spine stability. Panjabi et al. (124) found that the cervical motion segment became unstable in flexion with disruption of all posterior structures and in extension with disruption of all anterior ligaments. They also noted a significant increase in the horizontal translation of the vertebra after removal of the facet joint. Zdeblic et al. (194) tested acute instability of the cervical spine after laminectomy and progressive staged foraminotomies using cadaveric cervical spines. They found acute hypermobility in flexion and axial torsion after resection of 75 or 100% of the facet, but no motion changes occurred after laminectomy alone or after resection of 25 or 50% of the facet for foraminotomy. Thus, they suggested a stabilization of the segment if more than 50% of the facet must be resected for adequate decompression. Zdeblic et al. (196) also investigated the effect of laminectomy and resection of the facet capsule alone without disruption of the bony facet to determine what degree of facet-capsule resection leads to acute instability. A significant motion increase was found in flexion and axial torsion after more than 50% facet-capsule resection after laminectomy, indicating a significant stabilizing role of the facet-capsule in the cervical segment with laminectomy. Based on these results, the authors of the study recommended great care in exposing an unfused facet to limit facet-capsule resection to less than 50% of the capsule.

The results of clinical and biomechanical studies demonstrate that fusion of the posteriorly decompressed cervical segment may be required at the time of surgery when there is disruption of greater than 50% of the facet joint integrity, or when the anterior elements are not intact. Immediate fusion of the injured segment may not be necessary in the posterior decompression with minimal disruption of the facet joint and with normal anterior structures. However, laminectomy alone, especially in the younger patient or in patients who require multiple foraminotomies, may lead to a deformity and instability.

Biomechanics of Fusion

Spinal fusion has been a commonly accepted procedure in spine surgery since Albee (4) reported the successful treatment of Pott's disease using a fusion technique with a bone grafting procedure. Spinal fusion is used for the following reasons: 1) to relieve pain by eliminating degenerated or unstable segments; 2) to stabilize the spinal segments after decompression; 3) to prevent progression of deformity of the spine, as in scoliosis, kyphosis, and spondylolisthesis; and 4) to maintain correction after mechanical straightening or osteotomy of the spine.

Several biomechanical factors need to be considered for the achievement of successful spinal fusion. Biomechanical considerations of spinal instability were described in previous sections. The adequate stabilization of the surgical construct is another important factor to prevent failure of fusion (pseudoarthrosis). Recently, numerous spinal fixation devices have been developed and used for this purpose. Details of this aspect will be discussed in the section on biomechanics of spinal instrumentation. The other factors that will be discussed in this section include biomechanical considerations of fusion in terms of material, strength, and size of fusion graft, enhancement of bone formation, and the evaluation of fusion constructs.

Biomechanical Considerations of Fusion Graft

Graft Materials

At present, autogenous bone graft is considered the best graft material. A bone graft can be obtained from fibula or tibia, but the small amount of cancellous bone and functional compromise of the mechanics of donor site may cause complications. Ribs are known as a good bone graft material, especially for arthrodesis of the anterior thoracic spine, because they are readily available (47). They also have the advantage of reasonable strength with a structure consisting of a modest cortex and porous cancellous bone. In general, however, the iliac crest has been used as the best donor for autogenous bone grafts because of a number of advantages: there is ample cortical and cancellous bone; it is expendable; it can be harvested with the patient in either the prone or supine position; the structure allows the removal and carpeting of a variety of useful shapes and sizes; and the potential for functional compromise of the mechanics of donor site is less than with the tibia and fibula. Autogenous bone grafts have been osteogenic and well tolerated by the body. However, complications associated with the use and harvest of autografts are also significant. Younger and Chapman (192) reported a complication rate of greater than 20%. Some of the complications associated with autografts include morbidity, pain, sepsis and/or reduced structural integrity at the donor site, and a lack of sufficient graft material, particularly in patients with poor bone quality (32, 59, 192).

Allografts obtained from a donor of the same species are useful in many situations with the advantage of having no complications at the donor site. In the literature, several studies suggest that the infection rate is not increased (174) and the fusion rate for spine surgery is approximately as good with freeze-dried allografts as it is with autografts (23, 117, 140, 198). However, allogeneic bone does not have the osteogenic potential of autogenous bone (20, 32, 59) and the graft may give only temporary structural support. Other disadvantages include the possible transmission of disease and the chances of an immunologic response to the allograft, which may cause complete resorption of the graft without concomitant deposition of bone.

The problems associated with bone grafts initiated much research focusing on developing synthetic bone graft substitutes, which are biocompatible and structurally sound. Of the materials that have been studied for use as bone graft substitutes, the class of calcium phosphate materials has shown superb biocompatibility over all others. Using a canine model, Hanely (64) studied the use of porous tricalcium phosphate (TCP), a resorbable biomaterial that supports bony ingrowth, as a synthetic bone graft for reconstruction of segmental spinal column defects. Experimental data indicates that TCP can promote osseous ingrowth and can subsequently be resorbed when placed within a segmental osseous defect in the thoracic vertebral column. The biomechanical effect of this implant was similar to that of a rib strut graft at six months. Pintar et al. (136) reported a 30% fusion rate for dense hydroxyapatite (HA) blocks and a 40% fusion rate for autograft in a goat model at 12 and 24 weeks. Also, encapsulation by new bone and maintenance of disc height occurred despite fracture of HA ceramic. In a similar study of a canine anterior cervical spine fusion model, bony apposition to the dense HA ceramic blocks was observed. The study also showed that the disc height was maintained with the dense HA ceramic, but significant height was lost with autograft (28). Zdeblic et al. (197) investigated the use of coral HA blocks in a goat model and noted a 48% incorporation rate at 3 months with the porous ceramic. Ceramic incorporation was increased significantly to 71% with the use of an anterior cervical plate. Most recently, Toth et al. (177) studied the use of 50/50 HA/β-TCP of 30, 50, and 70% porosity for the cervical interbody fusion in a goat model. Histological analysis showed a union rate of 0% for autograft and 30% ceramic, 67% for 50% ceramic, and 83% for 70% ceramic at 3 months after surgery. The union rate at 6 months was 67% for the 30, 50, and 70% porous ceramics, and 50% for autograft. These studies demonstrated the potential use of TCP ceramic for spinal fusion. However, no clinical results using TCP have been reported in the literature, and further investigation is required for its clinical application because of possible complications associated with the fracture of ceramics.

Mechanical Strength of Graft Materials

The spine supports the weight of upper body and external loads. Approximately 10% of total body weight is above T1 and approximately 50% is above T12 (68, 146). Biomechanical studies also suggest that a lumbar motion segment may experience axial compressive loads ranging from 400N during quiet standing to as high as 7000N during lifting (113, 155). With the introduction of these loadings, the load-bearing capacity of the grafts is required, particularly in the thoracic and lumbar regions. Inferior graft strength can lead to collapse, pseudoarthrosis, and recurrent symptoms.

Mechanical strength of bone grafts has been measured and has been correlated with bone mineral density in a few experimental studies (7, 165, 176). Toth et al. (176) tested the compressive strength of bone grafts obtained from three different regions in the anterior, middle, and posterior superior iliac crests. Measured compressive strength ranged from 7.1 to 40.9MPa with a mean of 16.2MPa. An et al. (7) reported a significant relationship between the compressive strength of tricortical iliac crest grafts and bone mineral density (BMD) of the iliac crest measured by dual energy x-ray absorptiometry (DEXA). In this study, BMDs were measured using DEXA in an area of 2×1 cm for typical anterior iliac strut graft (AIC graft) and in another area of 1×1 cm for the Smith-Robinson (SR) type graft within the anterior region of the iliac crest. The pelvis was rotated 70° from the supine posture to avoid bone overlap and to aim the beam more perpendicularly to the iliac bone. Afterward, the corresponding AIC and SR grafts were dissected from each hemipelvis and underwent the compressive failure test for the measurement of load to failure and compressive strength. Mean and standard deviation values of measured parameters are listed in Table 3.3, and the relationship between the load to failure and BMD of the iliac crest is illustrated in Figure 3.2. These results suggest that the mechanical strength of the iliac bone graft is very dependent on its bone mineral density, and DEXA has a potential clinical value in predicting iliac bone graft strength.

There are little data on the mechanical strength of bone graft substitutes, such as calcium phosphates and hydroxyapatite ceramics, although their osteogenic capability for fusion has been investigated as interbody grafts for spinal fusion. Toth et al. (176) measured the compressive strength of HA/β-TCP ceramics with various porosities of 15, 22, 27, 32, 40, 44, and 65% according to ASTM test C-773, which is a standardized test for ceramics. Mean compressive

TABLE 3.3.
Mean and Standard Deviations of the Measured Bone Mineral Density of the Iliac Crest and Load to Failure and Compressive Strength of the Tested Grafts

	Smith-Robinson (n = 12)		Anterior Iliac Crest (n = 12)	
	Mean	SD	Mean	SD
BMD (g/cm^2)	0.35	0.10	0.42	0.12
Load to Failure (N)	1368.41	438.10	2167.96	693.70
Compressive strength	9.61	2.02	14.74	6.54

Data obtained from An et al.

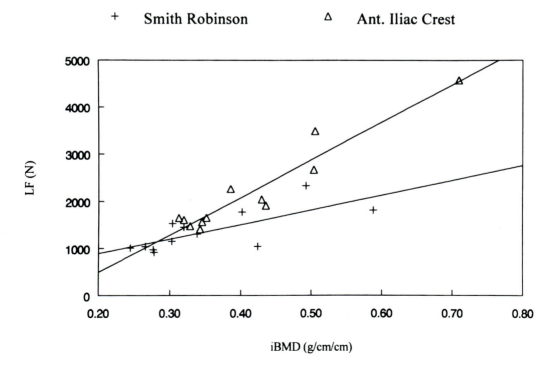

FIGURE 3.2.
Load to failure (LF) of Smith-Robinson and anterior iliac crest bone grafts was correlated with the bone mineral density of the iliac crest (R = 0.89). This correlation was positive for both SR (R = 0.78) and AIC types of graft (R = 0.90). Adapted from An et al. Prediction of bone graft strength using dual-energy radiographic absorptiometry. Spine 1994;19:2358–2363.

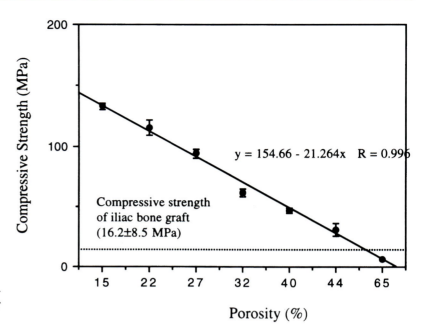

FIGURE 3.3.
Mean compressive strengths of the 50/50HA/b-TCP ceramics with various porosities. Error bar represents the standard deviations.

strengths of the ceramics are shown in Figure 3.3. The compressive strength of HA/β-TCP ceramic was found to decrease linearly (r = 0.96; p<0.05) as the porosity increased from 15 to 65%, and the mean compressive strengths of the ceramics with porosity less than 44% (32.2MPa) were significantly greater than that of the iliac bone grafts (16.2 MPa). The ceramics with 65% porosity was weaker than bone grafts.

However, the mechanical strength of ceramics needs to be studied further because of the fracture problems observed in animal studies. Shima et al. (159) reported ceramic fracture and anterior or posterior displacement of 70% of the β-TCP implants and spinal cord compression in 55% of the cases of anterior cervical interbody fusion attempted in canines. In the use of hydroxyapatite blocks for cervical interbody fusion in canines, Cook et al. (27) noted that most of the implants were fractured and 39% of the graft fracture was coupled with graft extrusion, which caused a loss of disc height and prevented fusion. Zdeblic et al. (197) reported a 29% collapse rate of coral hydroxyapatite used for anterior interbody fusion of goat cervical spines. Toth et al. (177) also noted the fracture in approximately 50% of HA/β-TCP ceramics with 30, 50, and 70% porosity used for anterior fusion in goat cervical spines, as well as a 50% fracture of autografts. As such, these ceramics may not have sufficient compressive strength for the immediate clinical use in spinal fusion. However, the major advantage of using these ceramics over autogenous bone graft is the elimination of surgery for harvesting bone grafts and thus eliminating the complications associated with the harvest at the donor sites. Further studies for enhancing the mechanical strength of these materials will increase the potential for clinical use in spine surgery.

Effect of Graft Size

Only a few studies of the effect of graft size in spine fusion are available in the literature. However, the results of these limited studies suggest that a careful determination of the graft size is important, particularly in an interbody fusion. Although anterior cervical discectomy and fusion is a well-established procedure used in the treatment of degenerative disc disease, the appropriate thickness for the interbody graft had been controversial. For example, Robinson and Smith (142) originally determined that a 10- to 15-mm graft was optimal, but White and Panjabi (185) and Rothman and Simeone (143) suggested smaller grafts (4 to 5 and 7 mm, respectively). Recently, however, An et al.(6) postulated that interbody grafts should not be an absolute thickness, but should reflect the original dimensions or preoperative baseline height of the affected interspace. They conducted an experimental study to establish the optimal thickness for Smith-Robinson anterior cervical fusion grafts. Anterior C4–5 discectomy and fusions were performed on six fresh, frozen cadavers. Plain radiographs and computed tomographic scans were then employed to correlate graft placement with changes in disc space height, foraminal height, and foraminal areas after 3-, 5-, 7-, and 9-mm interbody fusions. Moderate to high correlations existed between baseline disc height and foraminal height and between baseline disc height and foraminal area. Significant correlations also existed between disc space distractions with sequential graft placements and the change in foraminal height and area at the same level (Table 3.4). However, no correlation existed between

TABLE 3.4.
Correlation of Disc Space Distraction (DSD) at C4–5 and Change in Foraminal Height (FA) and ForaminalArea (FA) at the Same Level

Specimen	DSD vs. FH Right (R =)	Left (R =)	DSD vs. FA Right (R =)	Left (R =)
1	0.93	0.91	0.92	0.92
2	0.59	0.48	0.70	0.64
3	0.75	0.90	0.91	0.68
4	0.56	0.26	0.93	0.72
5	0.96	0.98	0.99	0.96
6	0.95	0.97	0.93	0.95
All	0.62	0.65	0.64	0.50

Data obtained from An et al. 1993.

disc space distraction at the C4–5 level and the effect on adjacent segments C3–4 and C5–6. The ideal graft thickness appeared to be directly related to the preoperative baseline disc height. For a preoperative disc height of 3.5 to 6.0 mm, an interbody graft of 2 mm above the baseline disc height was most appropriate. A thicker graft was required when the baseline disc height was smaller (2 mm), and a thinner graft was required when the disc height was larger (7.4 mm). In a similar experimental study of anterior interbody fusion in the lumbar spine, Chen et al. (22) noted significant increases in the neuroforamen areas (up to 29.0% at L4-L5 and 33.8% at L5-S1) caused by the anterior distraction of both levels with 13, 15, and 17-mm BAK implants (Spinetech Inc., Minneapolis, MN), providing adequate space for the nerve root and improving neuroforaminal stenosis. However, the ideal graft thickness for anterior lumbar interbody fusion was not determined in this study.

A critical bone graft area for interbody fusion was investigated by Closkey et al. (24) to better understand interbody fusion mechanics and the prevention of graft subsidence into the vertebral body that could cause serious problems, such as collapse of the disc space, recurrence of the spinal deformity, or failure of the fusion. First, the relationship between the vertebral body density determined by computed tomography and vertebral trabecular compressive strength was determined to predict minimum graft area based on the density measurements and anticipated physiologic loads. The relationship was $\sigma = 88.54 \times \rho^{1.6}$, where σ is the compressive strength (MPa) and ρ is the density (g/cm^3). End-plate decortication and placement of a graft block between 30 and 40% of total surface area was required to carry minimum thoracic physiologic loads (400 to 600 N) without trabecular subsidence.

Enhancement of Bone Formation

A double-blind study of pigs revealed that electric stimulation can significantly increase osteoblastic activity with bone formation (118). In a prospectively controlled clinical study, Kane (77) also showed that electrical stimulation improves the success rate in spine fusion. A fusion rate of 81% was observed in the group of 31 patients with electrically stimulated fusion as compared with 54% in the control group of 28 patients.

The use of bone morphogenetic proteins (BMP) in spine fusion has been studied recently by several investigators. Boden et al. (14) assessed the ability of bovine derived bone protein extract to serve as a bone graft substitute in a rabbit model for posterolateral lumbar spine fusion. The animals underwent bilateral intertransverse process fusion at L5–6 with one of three graft materials: 1) autogenous iliac graft; 2) BMP delivered in a carrier of rabbit demineralized bone matrix (DBM) and type I collagen; or 3) DBM/collagen carrier alone. A 100% fusion rate (10/10) was found in the BMP group, whereas the fusion rate was reduced significantly in the autograft group (62%) and DBM carrier alone group (17%). Uniaxial tensile testing results demonstrated that the BMP fusion was the strongest and stiffest after fusions with autograft and with DBM carrier alone. The histology also showed more mature fusions in the BMP animals with corticalization and more advanced remodeling and marrow formation. In a similar study using canine models, David et al. (34) tested the efficacy of recombinant human bone morphogenetic protein (rhBMP-2: Genetics Institute, Cambridge, MA) in intertransverse process fusion. Clinical and computed tomography (CT) evaluation of animals with various doses of rhBMP-2 (54, 215, 860μg) carried in a bovine type I collagen or a porous poly-lactic acid sponge demonstrated a 100% fusion rate (12/12) regardless of the type of carriers, compared with a 33% fusion in animals with autografts. CT images at 1 month postoperative showed the presence of large fusion masses whose dimension was proportional to the dose of rhBMP-2 delivered. Sandhu et al. (148) also reported that rhBMP-2 carried by an open cell poly-lactic acid (OPLA) vehicle is superior at both higher and lower doses (ranging from 57μg to 23mg) to autogenous iliac crest bone graft for inducing transverse process arthrodesis in the canine. Results of these studies clearly demonstrated an efficacy of using BMP in spinal fusion for enhancement of bone formation. However, the dose of BMP for clinical application needs to be investigated because a dose-dependent response to the osteoinductive growth factor was noted in the rabbit intertransverse process fusion model (14).

Biomechanical Evaluation of Fusion Constructs

Mechanical characteristics of the spinal column can vary in the presence of fused segments depending upon the location of the graft material. A spinal motion segment has five different anatomic sites at which spinal fusion can be attempted. They are the posterior spinous processes, the transverse processes, laminae, facet joints, and the disc space (46). Based on the site used for fusion, the fusion techniques can be termed anterior/posterior interbody fusion, bilateral fusion, or posterior fusion.

Lee and Langrana (90) investigated the altered kinematics and biomechanics of these three different types of spinal fusion through an in vitro test on cadaveric spine specimens (L3-sacrum). Fusion in the L5-S1 level of the specimens was achieved with the use of PMMA. They showed that all types of fusion have a stabilizing effect on the fused segment, implied by an increase in axial and bending stiffness compared with that of the intact spine. The axial stiffness increased by 10% in the posterior fusion, 40% in the bilateral fusion, and 80% in the interbody fusion compared with that of the normal intact specimen. In the flexion test, a loading frame attached to the L3 vertebra was rotated by 20°, and the resultant axial forces and moments at the bottom of the specimens were measured by a load cell. Compared with the intact specimen, the compressive load and bending moment increased, respectively, by 21% and 92% in posterior fusion, 11% and 48% in bilateral fusion, and 8% and 47% in the interbody fusion. In the extension test, the compressive load and bending moment increased by 31% and 13% in the posterior fusion, 20% and 25% in bilateral fusion, and 91% and 36% in the interbody fusion. Increased motion at the L3-L4 level and the L4-L5 level, caused by fusion at the L5-S1 level, was also observed during the testing. Furthermore, Lee and Langrana found through their mathematical model that the load on the facet joints increased when a fusion was performed. The posterior fusion caused a significant increase in the facet joint load compared with that of the anterior fusion. Based upon their investigations, they concluded that bilateral fusion presented the least amount of alteration in the mechanical properties of the adjacent, unfused segment, while it provided good stabilization on the fused segment.

Complications of Spinal Fusion

Complications associated with spinal fusion have been noted at both the fused and adjacent levels. A typical complication at the fused level is spinal stenosis. The incidence of spinal stenosis after spinal fusion has ranged from 11% to 41% (16, 107). Biomechanical fusion studies on human cadaveric spines and mathematical analysis of the stress distribution caused by the various types of spinal fusion procedures revealed abnormal stress increase within the fused segment, particularly within the posterior bony element and fusion mass (56, 90). These higher stresses may induce the abnormal growth of the graft after the solid fusion, and thus stenosis could ensue at the stabilized segments.

Junctional degeneration above a lumbar fusion is a clinically recognized complication in the treatment of degenerative spinal disorders. The reported complications include degenerated or prolapsed intervertebral disc (94, 103, 178), spinal stenosis (71, 91, 93), segmental instability (93, 152), and osteoarthritis of the facets (152). Although the pathomechanics of this phenomenon are not fully understood, some investigators have demonstrated that segmental immobilization can lead to increased motion and loads at the adjacent segment (90, 140, 160). Such a concentration of load can cause degeneration of the adjacent segment. Although these studies were performed using ex vivo models, the postulate was supported by the findings in clinical and in vivo animal studies of post-fusion mechanics of the lumbar spine (35, 48).

Biomechanics of Spinal Instrumentation

Over the last few decades, a number of spinal implants have been developed and have contributed to significant advancements in the field of spine fusion and instrumentation. These advances have improved the surgical techniques available to treat various spinal disorders, such as scoliosis, trauma, tumor reconstruction, and degenerative disease. A number of fixation devices have been developed and modified to achieve better treatment of spinal disorders by reducing the relevant complications. Each device has its own advantages and disadvantages, and it is crucial for the surgeon to choose a system based upon the particular needs and clinical situations. Selection of a proper fixation system requires a thorough knowledge of the capabilities of the fixation system and the disorder.

Review of Current Spinal Implants

Current spinal implants can be classified by the methods of attachment to the bony structure and by the implanting location. Based on these classifications, advantages and disadvantages of various implants are reviewed in this section.

Cervical Spine Implants

ANTERIOR INSTRUMENTATION

Anterior Screw for the Odontoid Fixation

Anterior screw stabilization of the odontoid is a procedure advocated by many for acute fractures of the dens. Particularly, for a widely displaced type II fracture, early surgical stabilization may be contemplated to enhance both the potential for fracture healing and the patient's functional recovery. The anterior screw fixation is useful in preventing unwanted translation of the fragment while preserving axial rotation about C1-C2 articulation. However, the anterior screw fixation is a technically demanding procedure and has a potential for serious complications.

Anterior Screw for C1-C2 Stabilization

Anterior C1-C2 screw or plate stabilization can be attempted for C1-C2 instability and fractures. This method can achieve relatively high stiffness fixation without passing laminar wire and is an alternative for patients with previously failed posterior procedures and for patients with absent posterior elements. Bilateral exposures required for this technique are time consuming and technically demanding compared with posterior arthrodesis techniques, and complications mostly include those inherent to the surgical approach.

Plate and Screw Fixation

Anterior cervical plating can be used in reconstruction of the spine after vertebral body resection or cases of fracture, spondylosis, tumor, or infection. Additional indications may include anterior ligamentous disruption secondary to hyperextension injuries with resulting instability and, less commonly, stabilization of interbody fusions after excision of the disc. Various types of plates, such as Caspar, Morscher, Orion™, and Ceri-lok™, are available for anterior cervical plating. Anterior plating potentially offers sufficient stability through a single surgical approach and minimizes patient morbidity, although additional posterior fixation may be needed to achieve it. Potential complications directly referable to anterior instrumentation include iatrogenic neural injury caused by overpenetration of posterior cortex with screw, misplacement of the screw into the adjacent disc space, and hardware loosening and subsequent injury to surrounding vital structures and organs.

POSTERIOR INSTRUMENTATION

Wiring for C1-C2 Stabilization

The indications for posterior atlantoaxial stabilization include traumatic atlantoaxial instability with rupture of the transverse ligament type II odontoid fractures with high risk of nonunion, as in older patients with a significant displacement, and late atlantoaxial instability caused by nontraumatic disorders, such as rheumatoid arthritis (89). Posterior atlantoaxial stabilization can be achieved using wires and bone graft according to either the Gallie, Brooks, or modified technique (17, 51, 58). These wiring methods can provide stable fixation in most loading modes but reduced stabilization against anterior translation. Additional disadvantages can include decreased axial rotation and risks of sublaminar wire passage.

Transarticular Screw for C1-C2 Fixation

Another method of posterior atlantoaxial stabilization is Magerl's transarticular screw fixation (109). This screw fixation provides better stabilization than the posterior wire fixation while avoiding sublaminar wire passage. However, this procedure requires thorough knowledge of surgical anatomy and meticulous technique to reduce risks of screw placement.

Interlaminar Clamp for C1-C2 Fixation

An interlaminar clamp is one method used for posterior atlantoaxial arthrodesis. These clamps may be used in selected cases in which sublaminar wiring would be difficult or dangerous to pass. The clamps have the advantage of easy application and stable posterior fixation. However, potential problems with interlaminar clamp fixation are implant slippage, difficulty with bone grafting, less extension stability, and pseudarthrosis.

Wiring for Occipitocervical Fixation

Occipitocervical fixation can be achieved by using wires with bone graft or implant. These techniques can provide stable internal fixation with high stiffness in all loading modes, particularly in segmental wiring with Luque rod. However, potential complications associated with sublaminar wiring in occipital and cervical regions prohibit routine use.

Plates and Screws for Occipitocervical Fixation

Screw fixation into the occiput has been described recently for occipitocervical fixation. The screw fixation provides stable internal fixation. This technique may be advantageous in patients who undergo decompressive laminectomy or who require multiple fixation from the occiput to the lower cervical spine.

Wiring for Lower Cervical Spine Fixation

Various cervical wiring techniques have been described in the literature. These wiring techniques have been shown to be safe and effective. The wiring procedure may provide adequate stability with effective prevention of flexion. However, the segmental stiffness provided by the wiring techniques is relatively lower. The most common complication associated with the wiring procedure is loss of fixation and recurrence of deformity. Sublaminar fixation is generally not recommended in the lower cervical spine because of a greater risk of neurologic injury.

Plate and Screws for the Lower Cervical Spine Fixation

Posterior stabilization of the cervical spine using screws and plates was pioneered by Roy-Camille (145). Louis uses a similar type of plate-screw fixation onto the lateral mass (103). Magerl devised a plate-screw system for the cervical spine in which the inferior portion of the plate is a hook configuration (109). The plate-screw fixation can provide more rigid fixation than the wiring procedures, especially in extension and torsion (29). This fixation technique can be used in the presence of extensive laminectomy and can achieve fixation without passage of laminar wires. However, potential problems associated with posterior plating with screws include injury of the vertebral artery or cervical nerve roots. Posterior plate-screw fixation must be done with thorough knowledge of lateral mass anatomy.

Thoracic and Lumbar Spine Implants

ANTERIOR INSTRUMENTATION

During the 1950s, experience was gained in anterior interbody fusion. Anterior spinal instrumentation was pioneered by Dwyer in the late 1960s (44). The indications for anterior implants remain somewhat controversial, but anterior spinal surgery has some potential advantages. In many clinical situations, the pathology is anterior, such as in most tumors and burst fractures. Decompression of the spinal cord and cauda equina is thus direct and more efficient, and it may be safer, particularly in the thoracic spine. The anterior approach permits single-stage decompression, segmental stabilization with adequate stability, and fusion of spinal injuries. However, anterior surgery is more extensive, and the risk of complications from operative trauma may be higher compared with the posterior approach. Considerable experience is also necessary before the surgeon can feel comfortable with anterior approaches (193). Loss of fixation caused by the loosening or breakage of the vertebral screw is a complication associated with anterior instrumentation, particularly in the three-column injuries and in the osteoporotic spine.

Rod and Vertebral Screws

The rod-screw systems immobilize the spinal segments with adequate rigidity and also permit either compressive or distractive forces to be applied across the injured segment. However, these rod-screw devices are somewhat bulky, making it difficult to obtain soft tissue coverage of the implant and increasing concerns of vascular injury.

Plate and Vertebral Screws

The plate-screw systems are of low profile and allow for nearly as rigid a stabilization as the rod-screw devices. A disadvantage of using these plate-screw devices is inability to employ reduction forces across the injured segment. However, recent devices, such as Z-plate and University Plate™, are designed to apply either compression or distraction forces.

POSTERIOR INSTRUMENTATION

The posterior approach of the spine is relatively simple and has less potential for serious complications compared with anterior approach. The first reported attempt of internal spinal fixation was Lange's use of interspinous process steel bars (87). Use of posterior instrumentation has been expanded widely for the surgical treatment of various spinal disorders, such as deformity, traumatic injuries, and degenerative disease, since the introduction of Harrington instrumentation in 1962 for the treatment of scoliosis (66).

Rods and Hooks

The rod and hook fixation devices were designed to apply distraction forces for the correction of the scoliotic spine. Rod and hook fixation can offer a broad range of stiffness, but most systems are rigid enough to achieve fusion. However, rod and hook systems require longer fusion and instrumentation than the anterior devices. Hook dislodgement can occur because of hook design and the lack of rotational control, especially when the rods extend below L3. Hook failure may cause a neurologic injury. Although supplemental use of sublaminar wires or compression rods improves the flexion and torsional stability (10, 50, 70), these modified constructs still cannot maintain lordosis and torsional control completely (111). Neurologic complication is also a potential problem of sublaminar wiring.

Rods and Wires

Posterior segmental fixation can be achieved with a wire that encircles the lamina and a portion of a metal rod. This rod and wire fixation can provide a strong stabilization, particularly in axial rotation. However, sublaminar wiring is dangerous to neural structures and is technically demanding. Compression or distraction force cannot be applied during this rod and wire fixation procedure.

Laminar Facet Screws

Fusion of the thoracolumbar spine can be obtained through a facet joint fixation using laminar facet screws that appear to be simple and easy to implant. This simple spine fusion construct rigidly immobilizes the spine (108), and it is associated with a better fusion rate (83). However, use of laminar facet screws is not common, and more laboratory and clinical studies are needed for a more reliable evaluation.

Pedicle Screw and Plates (or Rods)

Recently, various fixation devices using pedicle screws and plates (or rods) have been introduced. Regardless of the type of longitudinal linkage connecting the pedicle screws, intrapedicular fixation was known to provide sufficient rigidity to achieve short segmental instrumentation without involving fixation of additional segments. This high rigidity also may negate the need for anterior fusion and stabilization procedures. Other advantages of these intrapedicular fixation devices include universal application, ability to reduce abnormal translation, and ability to maintain normal sagittal contour. In contrast, potential complications associated with intrapedicular instrumentation are possibilities of neural injury, hardware failure, pseudoarthrosis, vascular injury, facet joint compromise, loss of correction, and infection.

Biomechanical Strength of Spinal Fixation

Hardware failure with a loss of fixation is a well-known complication that may result in pseudarthrosis, loss of correction, or subsequent injury to surrounding vital structures and organs. Hardware failure can occur in two ways: breakage of device components or loosening failure at bone-device interface or at a junction between device components, such as a screw-rod junction.

Mechanical strength and fatigue life of a device component depend on its material properties and geometry. The incidence of metal component failure has been reduced by the use of a stronger material and design changes for minimizing the stress concentration. A surface treatment using nitrogen-ion implantation was also found to inhibit crack initiation and thus to increase the fatigue life (100). However, careful fusion techniques are required to reduce metal fatigue susceptibility because all metal implants will eventually fail with failure of fusion.

On the other hand, failure at bone-implant interface can result from various reasons. For example, the wire fixation strength depends on wiring techniques. The bone-screw interface strength can be affected by screw design, screw insertion technique, and the bone quality. Many biomechanical studies of the fixation strength exist in the literature.

Strength of the Wire Fixation

Stainless steel wires have been used frequently in spine surgery to secure bone graft to the recipient site and to limit the motion of posterior elements. Various wire constructs are available, and a few biomechanical studies provide useful information for the surgeon when making a decision about stainless steel wires (60, 122, 154).

Important findings of these studies are as follows: fastening twists were found stronger than knots or the Association for Study of Internal Fixation (ASIF) bend techniques, although square knots are acceptable; two twists are enough and additional twists do not improve the strength; two single-wire loops are better than a continuous double-wire loop; fatigue resistance of wire can be reduced by 63% by notching 1% of the diameter, whereas bending, twisting, and knotting the wire had no serious effect; tension-equalizing loop opposite fastening loop weakened the system by 10 to 15%; the wire wrap and the ASIF loop techniques were unacceptable.

In many spinal surgical procedures, sublaminar wiring has been used and known as one of the most effective methods for achieving a very stable fixation. However, intrusion into the canal was noted more times than desired in both cases of implantation and removal of sublaminar wires (12, 120, 151). Observed complications associated with sublaminar wiring include hemorrhage, epidural adhesions, dural lacerations, cord indentations, and neurologic damage.

Strength of Screw Fixation

PEDICLE SCREW FIXATION STRENGTH

Effect of Screw Design

The pedicle screw design can differ in its major and minor diameters, pitch, and tooth profile. As expected, larger diameter screws can provide a greater pullout strength (104, 121, 163, 199). The effects of minor diameter, pitch, and the tooth profile on the pullout strength were insignificant (85, 163).

Effect of Screw Placement Methods

The method of screw insertion has a considerable effect on the fixation strength. There are several variables in insertion methods, such as depth of penetration, angulation, hole preparation, and insertion torque.

Biomechanical studies have shown that deeper insertion of the screw can provide a stronger screw fixation (85, 199). Particularly, Zindrick et al. (199) found a significant increase in pullout strength in "through cortex" insertion compared with "to cortex" and "50% depth" insertions. However, the penetration to the anterior cortex may increase the risk of damage to vital structures (84, 168).

The cephalad-caudal angulation of the pedicle screws was found not to significantly affect the fixation strength (163). In contrast, anteromedial angulation of the pedicle screws was recommended for improving the fixation strength (85, 108). The underlying concept was that convergence of the pedicle screws produces a "toe nailing" or triangulation effect that should substantially increase the pullout strength of a fully assembled construct. This concept was supported by a biomechanical study of triangulation of pedicle screw instrumentation (147).

The method of screw hole preparation, either probing or drilling, was found not to affect the screw insertion torque and ultimate pullout strength (31, 195). In contrast, a positive linear relationship exists between the screw insertion torque and pullout strength (31, 195). The maximum screw insertion torque was also correlated with the screw tilting moment and the cut-up force (123). These studies suggested an importance of screw insertion torque measurement in prediction of the fixation strength. However, a minimum screw insertion torque for an adequate fixation strength has not been determined yet.

Effect of Bone Quality

Advanced techniques, such as quantitative computed tomography (QCT) or dual energy x-ray absorptiometry (DEXA), are recently available for measuring bone mineral density. Subsequently, the studies of a relationship between the bone mineral density (BMD) of the lumbar vertebra and the pedicle screw pullout strength have recently been reported in the literature.

A positive linear correlation between BMD and the pedicle screw pullout strength has been demonstrated in many studies (26, 147, 166, 190). Soshi et al. (166) suggested the use of bone cement to enhance the fixation strength in cases with moderate osteoporosis, but the fixation was found to be poor in severe osteoporosis even with bone cement. Okuyama et al. (123) also conducted the tilting test to determine the load required to tilt the screw approximately 4° in the cranial direction and found a positive relationship between the tilting moment and BMD. These studies demonstrated the importance of assessing BMD before surgery to achieve a proper spinal fixation. However, these studies did not provide a threshold BMD value that indicates an early fixation failure at the screw-bone interface.

Anterior Vertebral Screw Fixation Strength

Lim et al. performed two biomechanical tests to investigate the relationship among the anterior vertebral screw fixation strength, BMD of the vertebral body, and screw insertion torque. The first test was a pullout test (97). A positive linear correlation was found between the screw pullout strength and the BMD. The relationship was $F = 1032.62 \times BMD - 360.265$ ($r = 0.85$; $p < 0.001$), where F = pullout strength (N) and BMD = bone mineral density of the vertebral body (g/cm^2). The pullout strength also was correlated with screw insertion torque ($r = 0.473$, $p < 0.001$). The stepwise regression revealed that the most significant predictor of the pullout strength was BMD.

The other test was a cyclic fatigue test in which fatigue loosening of a vertebral screw was induced (98). The screw loosening was defined as 1 mm displacement of the screw relative to bone, and the number of loading cycles to induce the loosening (NLC) was used as the screw fixation strength. NLC had a significant nonlinear relationship with the BMD values of the vertebral body measured using a DEXA unit (NLC = $-1190 \cdot BMD + 3168 \cdot BMD^2$, $p = 0.80$). NLC was also found to have a nonlinear relationship with the screw insertion torque ($p = 0.51$) but a weaker correlation than with BMD. Because of this nonlinear relationship, an attempt was made to determine a threshold value of BMD. For this purpose, the specimens were divided into two groups: one with larger BMD and the other with smaller BMD than the assumed threshold value. When the threshold value was 0.45 g/cm^2, a highly significant difference in mean NLCs was found (18 vs. 270, $p = 0.003$). These findings suggest that there may be a significantly higher risk of anterior vertebral screw loosening failure in the patients with grade III osteoporosis or severe grade II osteoporosis. However, testing a greater number of specimens as well as a clinical study would be recommended to determine a reliable threshold BMD value. Additionally, the magnitude of loading on the screw can vary depending on other factors. Thus, this threshold value of 0.45 g/cm^2 should not be used as a clinical value at this time.

Biomechanical Evaluation of Spinal Instrumentation

Spinal fixation devices can be evaluated biomechanically using three different types of biomechanical tests: strength, fatigue, and stability tests (128). Strength and fatigue tests are destructive in nature and usually are performed to evaluate the overall strength of the fixation device itself or the instrumented construct. Nondestructive stability tests have been performed to assess the stabilizing effect provided by a spinal instrumentation system under physiological loadings.

Great care must be taken in the interpretation of these biomechanical testing results. For example, a fixation device with a longer fatigue life does not necessarily provide a greater stabilizing effect. Thus, a complete understanding of each testing method and its own specific purpose is necessary for better evaluation of a spinal fixation device.

Strength and Fatigue Tests

In strength tests, the load is applied, using a material testing machine in most cases, until failure occurs. The strength test can provide the information of load to failure, energy absorbed to failure, and stiffness. For example, the fixation strength at the bone-screw interface has been evaluated in terms of the pullout strength (load to failure) using a strength test. Strength tests also have been performed to estimate the overall strength afforded by the use of a particular instrumentation (9, 19, 61, 62, 74, 86). In these studies, ligamentous spine segments were injured to mimic clinically relevant injuries and then were stabilized. The stabilized segments were subjected to various types of loading, such as flexion, extension, lateral bending, or axial torsion until failure. The load and resulting displacement at failure were compared with similar data obtained from the intact spines. The results of these studies showed that most of the tested devices were effective in restoring strength and stiffness over the intact specimens, although the degree of effectiveness varies among different devices. As such, strength tests help to characterize the overall stiffness and strength of the spinal construct as well as those of each component in an instrumentation system. Results of strength tests provided valuable information for the design and clinical application. Neither of these studies, however, provide an insight into the load-displacement behavior of the stabilized and adjacent levels separately.

In fatigue tests, the test specimen undergoes the load with cyclically varying magnitudes at a certain rate. The cyclic loading is continued until failure occurs. The number of loading cycles to failure defines the fatigue life of the device at that load magnitude. For example, Cunningham et al. (30) evaluated twelve different pedicle screw instrumentation systems implanted in polyethylene cylinders. The mean number of cycles to failure was significantly higher for the instrumentation systems employing longitudinal rods than those using plates under a 600 N compression load at 5 Hz. Cyclic loading tests using human cadaveric spines were also conducted to evaluate five different pedicle screw fixation systems (Zielke, VSP, AO Fixator Interne, Luque plate, and AO Notched plate) (10). Spinal constructs were subjected to axial loading of ± 450 N at 2 Hz until failure. Classic fatigue fractures occurred at the pedicle screw-plate junctions in all cases in which failure was noted, except in the Zielke system, which failed at the longitudinal threaded rod on the anterior aspect of the vertebra.

The fatigue characteristics of the implant should be evaluated because the implant must maintain its function without failure until a solid fusion occurs. However, the destructive nature of the tests also allows the test only a few selected loading modes. Furthermore, the fatigue tests cannot provide any information on biomechanical characteristics of the injured and stabilized site under various physiological loading modes, which may attract the most clinical concern.

Stability Tests

TESTING METHODS

Because the major purpose of spinal instrumentation is to stabilize the decompressed or injured spine until solid fusion occurs, the stabilizing effect of a spinal implant should be assessed under the nondestructive physiological loads. Stability tests have been used for this purpose. In the literature, stability tests were performed in two different methods: stiffness method and flexibility method. In the stiffness method, one end of the spinal construct is fixed to the test table while the other end is held fixed to the cross-head of a testing machine, e.g., Instron or MTS. In contrast, the flexibility method involves loading the superiormost vertebra of the spinal construct in an unconstrained manner so that the resultant displacements of the tested construct can be multidirectional. The resulting displacements of each vertebra are measured using a three-dimensional motion analysis system. In both methods, load-displacement curves were obtained and used to determine the stiffness (load/displacement) or the flexibility (displacement/load) for both the intact and the stabilized cases.

Although a standard protocol for the biomechanical test of spinal fixation devices has yet to be established, Panjabi (128) advocated the flexibility method for the stability test because, in this method, a load is applied to a free vertebra and the displacements are measured. This method allows natural multidirectional movement of the spine to take place, whereas the stiffness method allows the movement along the loading direction only. This multidirectional analysis addresses the importance of physiologic three-dimensional kinematics and kinetics of the patient's spine. The application of pure moments was also suggested for the stability tests because it provides constant bending moment at each level of the spine implant construct (Fig. 3.4). Such an application of constant bending moment is important because the weakest points in the construct can be identified.

Another concern is how to describe the stabilizing capability of an instrumentation system. Differences in measured flexibility (or displacements responding to the same load) between the intact and stabilized segments can be used to represent the stabilizing effect. However, the quality and biomechanical characteristics of intact cadaveric spine specimens vary, greatly depending upon size, age, or sex. Absolute values of the measured displacements may include these variations, and the direct comparison of these absolute values may decrease the statistical significance. These interspecimen variations can be reduced by normalizing the measured displacements of the stabilized spine with respect to those of the intact spine as suggested by Goel et al. (54). This normalized data are the percentage change of motion at a specific load that in fact represents the stabilizing effect. Thus, the use of this normalized data is recommended to evaluate the stabilizing capability of a spinal instrumentation system.

Experimental Studies

Numerous biomechanical studies of the stabilizing effect provided by various spinal fixation devices us-

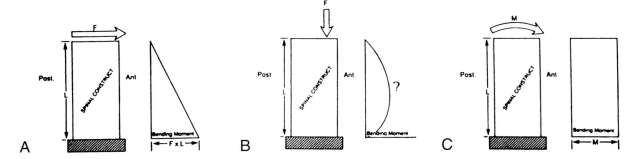

FIGURE 3.4.
Bending moment diagrams for three different methods of producing bending of the construct. **A.** Shear force applied at the free end produces increasing bending moment towards the fixed end. **B.** An anterior eccentric compression force produces variable bending moment as the construct deforms. **C.** A pure bending moment results in the most uniform loading of the construct. Adapted from Panjabi MM. Biomechanical evaluation of spinal fixation devices: I. A conceptual framework. Spine 1988;13:1129–1134.

ing either a stiffness or a flexibility method have been reported in the literature. The common findings of the biomechanical studies of thoracolumbar and lumbar spinal instrumentations can be summarized as follows: 1) Anterior and posterior fixation devices are similarly effective in providing sufficient stability beyond the intact spine in axial compression, flexion, extension, and lateral bending; 2) Pedicle screw instrumentation systems can provide greater stiffness than hook and rod systems; 3) Stabilizing effect of anterior and posterior segmental fixation systems are similar; and 4) None of the tested devices were found to restore the axial rotational stability beyond the intact level.

Biomechanical tests of cervical spinal instrumentation systems are relatively less than those of thoracolumbar fixation devices. Biomechanical studies of C1-C2 fixation showed that the Magerl bilateral screw fixation of the lamina of C2 to the lateral masses of C1 is stiffer than the C1-C2 Gallie type wiring technique in both flexion and axial rotation (65). Ulrich et al. (179) compared anterior and posterior cervical fixation procedures using cadaveric C5-C6 segments in flexion. The authors concluded that the hook plate alone appeared to provide stability, whereas the use of interlaminar alone or anterior plate alone did not provide adequate stability. Coe et al. (25) also observed that a posterior plate and screw fixation is more stable than anterior plate fixation.

Load Sharing Mechanism in Spinal Instrumentation

As reviewed in the previous section, most spinal instrumentation systems using screws and plates (or rods) provide a rigid fixation. However, these rigid devices may cause the stress-shielding of vertebral bodies within the stabilized segments, leading to stress-induced osteopenia. Although yet to be proven clinically, in vivo canine studies tend to support this

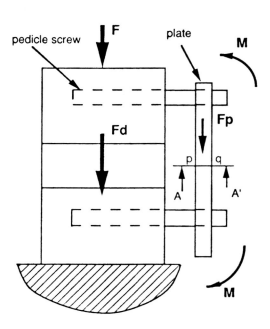

FIGURE 3.5.
A schematic diagram showing load shearing between spinal device and decompressed segment. Immediately after surgery, majority of the applied load (F) will be transmitted through the plate (F_p) because of the decreased segmental stiffness, but more load (F_d) will be shifted to the segment as it heals.

notion (95, 96, 112, 164). This hypothesis seems reasonable because the spinal instrumentation provides a bypass of the applied load on the stabilized segment as depicted in Figure 3.5. The amount of load transmitted through the decompressed segment varies as a function of the rigidity of the fixation device as well as the structural characteristics of the tissue in between the stabilized vertebral bodies, such as the interbody bone graft or a degenerated disc.

Knowledge of redistribution of loads enhances our understanding of the interaction between the spine and the spinal implant. In an experimental protocol,

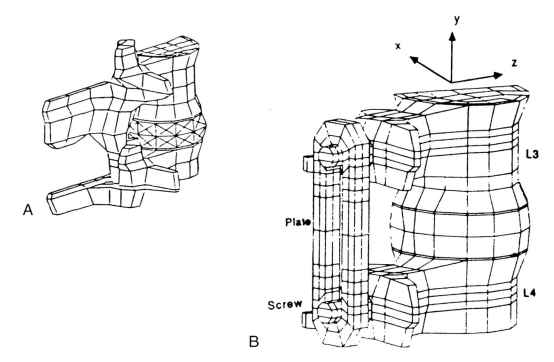

FIGURE 3.6.
Finite element models of the L3-L4 segment. **A.** Intact. **B.** The motion segment stabilized using a pedicle screw instrumentation after total laminectomy and facetectomy. A degenerated but intact intervertebral disc was simulated in the stabilized model.

however, it is almost impossible to address all the parameters that can be varied within a given system. It is also not realistic to quantify the loads being imposed on the spinal elements. In contrast, the finite element techniques have been used widely to analyze the mechanical behavior of complex structures like the spine. Lim (95) investigated the load sharing mechanism in the stabilized spinal segment using highly detailed finite element models (Fig. 3.6).

Load Sharing in the Intact and Stabilized Motion Segment

Load sharing characteristics of the intact motion segment can be explained by the facet contact force. In the compression mode, for 400 N or more of axial load, the total contact force (normal to the surface) across the two facet joints was computed to be approximately 13.7%. (The percentage was a bit higher at lower load magnitudes, and smaller for higher load values). This is in agreement with findings of Lorenz et al. (102) ($\approx$15%). In the intact model, the inclination of the facet to the horizontal axis is approximately 72°, and the axial component of total load on the facet would be approximately 4%. This is in agreement with Yang and King (19) and Shirazi-Adl and Drouin (161). These authors found the percentage to vary between 2 to 13%, depending on the magnitude of accompanying flexion rotation.

However, in response to the various axial compression loads of 200, 413, and 700 N, the axial forces transmitted through the VSP plates predicted from the stabilized model were 75.8, 157.3, and 264.3 N, respectively, when the degenerated intervertebral disc was assumed. These responses showed approximately 38% of the externally applied compressive loads.

Effect of Varying Axial Stiffness of the Spinal Segment

Changes in load sharing characteristics of the stabilized motion segment were investigated as the axial stiffness of the decompressed motion segment varies. The parametric changes in the axial stiffness were simulated by varying the material properties (elastic modulus, E) of the ground substances that had replaced the nucleus pulposus in the intervertebral disc of the stabilized model. E values used for the parametric study were 4.2, 8.4, 1000, and 2000 MPa. The extreme variations were E = 0 in case of a severe discectomy and E = 3500 MPa in case of interbody fusion. The severe discectomy, including total denucleation and excision of the disc annulus from the posterior aspect, was simulated by removing the corresponding elements from the stabilized model. The posterior interbody fusion was modeled by replacing these parts with the elements representing the bone graft, whose elastic modulus was assumed to be the same as that of the posterior bony elements.

Varying amounts of the axial forces transmitted through the VSP plates in response to the axial com-

TABLE 3.5.
Axial Compression Forces Transmitted Through the Plate as the Young's Modulus of the Disc Varies When an Axial Compression Force of 413 N is Applied on the Stabilized Motion Segment

Young's Modulus (MPa)	Axial Force (N)	Percentage Ratio
0.0 (Severe Discectomy)	413.0	100.0
4.2	178.9	43.4
8.4	157.3	38.0
1000.0	44.8	10.9
2000.0	41.8	10.1
3500.0 (PIBF)	37.5	9.1

PIBF = posterior interbody fusion with VSP system.
Data obtained from Lim.

TABLE 3.6.
Von-Mises Stresses (MPa) in Various Structures in the Stabilized Motion Segment When an Axial Compression Force of 413 N is Applied on the Stabilized Motion Segment

Structures		INTACT	ST	AL	PL
Cortical bone	Max	1.98	2.04	2.13	2.07
	Ave	1.83	1.51	1.67	1.82
Cancellous bone	Max	0.19	0.15	0.17	0.19
	Ave	0.11	0.07	0.09	0.09
Disc (ground substance)	Max	0.29	0.18	0.21	0.23
	Ave	0.21	0.12	0.14	0.16
plates	Max	—	29.23	15.65	2.49
	Ave	—	16.75	8.30	0.90
Superior screws	Max	—	39.62	12.68	2.94
	Ave	—	16.75	2.21	0.63
Inferior screws	Max	—	42.20	14.34	2.86
	Ave	—	7.24	2.86	0.62

Data obtained from Lim.

pression of 413 N (estimated load on the spine during quiet standing [155]) are listed in Table 3.5. These results show that the variations in the axial forces transmitted through the plates are large when the elastic modulus of the nucleus aspects of the disc is less than 1000 MPa. The values of the elastic modulus may vary depending on the actual condition of the intervertebral disc at surgery, but it should be less than those of the cancellous bone (100 MPa) if the intervertebral disc has no osteophytes. This may indicate that the load sharing characteristics may vary greatly from patient to patient unless the interbody fusion is indicated. Conversely, the variations were marginal (9.1% to 10.9%) when the elastic modulus was larger than 1000 MPa. Such a marginal variation may imply that the stiffness of the interbody graft material may not change the load sharing characteristics significantly. In the case of the posterior interbody fusion with the pedicle screw instrumentation, the collapse or the subsidence of the graft material should be of a greater concern than the load sharing characteristics because approximately 90% or more of the applied load would be transmitted through the vertebral column when the elastic modulus of the graft material is larger than 1000 MPa.

Effect of Varying Rigidity of the Posterior Instrumentation System

As depicted in Figure 3.5, the load sharing characteristics may be changed when the rigidity of the pedicle screw instrumentation system varies. Such variations are made by simulating the VSP system made of 316L stainless steel (ST), aluminum (AL), or Plexiglass® (PL). For this purpose, the material properties of the elements for the VSP system are replaced with those of each material, and a degenerated intervertebral disc is modeled in each case.

Use of AL and PL results in the 59% and 98% decrease in the flexural rigidity of the VSP system, respectively, as compared with the use of ST plates. The amount of axial force transmitted through the plates was predicted to decrease as the rigidity of the VSP system decreased (38.1% of the applied load through the ST plates, 27.3% through the AL plates, and 16.6% through the PL plates).

The stress distribution changes in the stabilized motion segment caused by the fixations with various rigidities also reflect the stress-shielding effect of the pedicle screw instrumentation (Table 3.6). As the rigidity of the VSP system decreased, average stresses in bone regions immediately inferior to the superior screws and the ground substance of the intervertebral disc were predicted to increase while the stresses in the plates and screws decreased, as expected. In particular, the maximum stress in the screws showed a steep decrease (42.2 MPa in ST screws, 14.3 MPa in AL screws, and 2.9 MPa in PL screws). In all stabilized models, however, the average stresses in these bone and disc regions were predicted to be still less than those in the intact model.

These studies of load-sharing mechanism clearly demonstrate that both the spinal segment and fixation devices are important load supporting components. Particularly, when the spinal segments are grossly unstable, the load on the implant may exceed its failure strength, and thus the proper use of graft material is important for the prevention of hardware failure. However, the use of an extremely rigid plate could result in failure of fusion because of the stress shielding that may cause too little load on the healing grafted area and subsequent resorption of the graft. There must be an optimum range of stiffness of the unstable spine-graft-implant construct for fast and solid fusion to occur, but this ideal stiffness is not known at present.

References

1. Abumi K, Panjabi MM, Kramer KM, et al. Biomechanical evaluation of lumbar spinal stability after graded facetectomies. Spine 1990;15:1142–1147.
2. Adams MA, Hutton WC, Stott JRR. The resistance to

flexion of the lumbar intervertebral joint. Spine 1985;5:245.
3. Adams MA, Dolan P, Hutton C. The lumbar spine in backwards bending. Spine 1988;13:1019–1026.
4. Albee FH. Transactions of a portion of the tibia into the spine for Pott's disease. JAMA 1911;57:885.
5. Alund M, Larsson S. Three-dimensional analysis of neck motion—a clinical method. Spine 1990;12:87–91.
6. An HS, Evanich CJ, Nowicki BH, et al. Ideal thickness of Smith-Robinson graft for anterior cervical fusion. Spine 1993;18:2043–2047.
7. An HS, Xu R, Lim TH, et al. Prediction of bone graft strength using dual-energy radiographic absorptiometry. Spine 1994;19:2358–2363.
8. Arkin AM. The mechanism of rotation in combination with lateral deviation in normal spine. J Bone Joint Surg Am 1950;32:180–188.
9. Ashman RB, Birch JG, Bone LB, et al. Mechanical testing of spinal instrumentation. Clin Orthop 1988; 227:113–125.
10. Ashman RB, Galpin RD, Corin JD, et al. Biomechanical analysis of pedicle screw instrumentation systems in a corpectomy model. Spine 1989;14:1398–1405.
11. Ashton-Miller JA, Schultz AB. Spine instability and segmental hypermobility biomechanics: a call for the definition and standard use of terms. Semin Spine Surg 1991;3:136–148.
12. Blackman R, Toton J. The sublaminar pathway of wires removed in SSI. Proc Scoliosis Res Soc 1984.
13. Boden SD, Wiesel SW. Lumbosacral segmental motion in normal individuals—have we been measuring instability properly? Spine 1990;15:571–576.
14. Boden SD, Schimandae JH, Hutton WC. In vivo evaluation of bovine-derived bone morphogenetic-link protein as a graft substitute for lumbar spine fusion. Proc Int Soc for the Studies of Lumbar Spine 1994;28.
15. Boxall D, Bradford DS, Winter RB, et al. Management of sever spondylolisthesis in children and adolescents. J Bone Joint Surg Am 1979;61:479–495.
16. Brodsky AE. Post-laminectomy and post-fusion stenosis of the lumbar spine. Clin Orthop 1970;115:130.
17. Brooks AL, Jenkins EB. Atlanto-axial arthrodesis by the wedge compression method. J Bone Joint Surg Am 1978;60:279–284.
18. Brown RH, Burstein AH, Nash CL, et al. Spinal analysis using a three-dimensional radiographic technique. J Biomech Eng 1976;9:355.
19. Brunski JB, Hill DC, Moskowitz A. Stresses in a Harrington distraction rod: their origin and relationship to fatigue fractures in vivo. J Biomech Eng 1983; 105:101–114.
20. Burchardt H. Biology of bone transplantation. Orthop Clin North Am 1987;18:187–196.
21. Cattle HS, Clark GL Jr. Cervical kyphosis and instability following multiple laminectomies in children. J Bone Joint Surg Am 1977;59:991–1002.
22. Chen D, Fay LA, Lok J, et al. Increasing neuroforaminal volume by anterior interbody distraction in degenerative lumbar spine. Spine 1995;20:74–79.
23. Cloward RB. New method of diagnosis and treatment of cervical disc disease. Clin Neurosurg 1962;8:93–132.
24. Closkey RF, Lee CK, Parsons JR, et al. Mechanics of interbody spinal fusion—analysis of critical bone graft area. Proc Ortho Res Soc 1993;65.
25. Coe JD, Warden KE, Sutterlin CE III, et al. Biomechanical evaluation of cervical spine stabilization methods in a human cadaveric model. Spine 1989;14:1122–1131.
26. Coe JD, Warden KE, Herzig MA, et al. Influence of bone mineral density on the thoracolumbar implants. Spine 1990;15:902–907.
27. Cook SD, Reynolds MC, Whitecloud TS, et al. Evaluation of hydroxyapatite graft materials in canine cervical spine fusion. Spine 1986;11:305–309.
28. Cook SD, Dalton JE, Tan EH, et al. In vivo evaluation of anterior cervical fusions with hydroxyapatite graft material. Spine 1994;19:1856–1866.
29. Cooper RP. Posterior stabilization of the cervical spine using Roy-Camille plates—a North American experience. Trans Orthop 1988;12:43.
30. Cunningham BW, Sefter JC, Shono Y, et al. Static and cyclical biomechanical analysis of pedicle screw spinal constructs. Spine 1993;18:1677–1688.
31. Daftari T, Horton W, Hutton W, et al. Factors in spinal screw pullout: Torque of insertion and screw hole preparation. Proc North Am Spine Soc 1992;7.
32. Damien CJ, Parsons JR. Bone graft and bone graft substitutes—a review of current technology and applications. J Appl Biomat 1991;2:187–208.
33. Danielson B, Frennerd K, Irstam L. Roentgenologic assessment of spondylolisthesis. I. A study of measurement variations. Acta Radiol 1988;29:345–351.
34. David SM, Murakami T, Tablor OB, et al. Lumbar spinal fusion using recombinant human bone morphogenetic protein (rhBMP-2)—a randomized, blinded and controlled study. Proc Int Soc for the Studies of Lumbar Spine 1995;14.
35. Dekutoski MB, Schendel MJ, Ogilvie JW, et al. Comparison of in vivo and in vitro adjacent segment motion after lumbar fusion. Spine 1994;19(15):1745–1751.
36. Dunlop RB, Adams MA, Hutton WC. Disc space narrowing and the lumbar facet joints. J Bone Joint Surg Br 1984;66:706–710.
37. Dupis PR, Yong-Hing K, Cassidy JD, et al. Radiologic diagnosis of degenerative lumbar spinal instability. Spine 1985;10:262–276.
38. Dvorak J, Panjabi MM, Gerber M. CT-functional diagnostics of the rotatory instability of the upper cervical spine; an experimental study on cadavers. Spine 1987; 12:197.
39. Dvorak J, Froehlic D, Penning L. Functional radiographic diagnosis of the cervical spine. Spine 1988; 13:748–755.
40. Dvorak J, Panjabi MM, Theiler R, et al. Functional radiographic diagnosis of the lumbar spine—Flexion/extension and lateral bending. Spine 1991;16:562–571.
41. Dvorak J, Panjabi MM, Novotny JE, et al. In vivo flexion/extension of the normal cervical spine. J Orthop Res 1991;9:828–834.
42. Dvorak J, Panjabi MM, Novotny JE, et al. Clinical validation of functional flexion/extension roentgenograms of the lumbar spine. Spine 1991;16:943–950.

43. Dvorak J, Panjabi MM, Grob D, et al. Clinical validation of functional flexion/extension radiographs of the cervical spine. Spine 1993;18:120–127.
44. Dwyer AF, Schafer MF. Anterior approach to Scoliosis. J Bone Joint Surg Br 1974;56:218–224.
45. Eie N, Solgaard T, Kepple H. The knee-elbow position in lumbar disc surgery: a review of complications. Spine 1983;8:897–900.
46. Evans JH. Biomechanics of lumbar fusion. Clin Orthop 1985;193:38–46.
47. Fang HSY, Ong BGB, Hodgson AR. Anterior spinal fusion—the operative approaches. Clin Orthop 1964;35:16.
48. Frymoyer JW, Hanley EN, Howe J, et al. A comparison of radiographic findings in fusion and non-fusion patients ten or more years following lumbar disc surgery. Spine 1979;4:435–440.
49. Frymoyer JW, Selby DK. Segmental instability: rationale for treatment. Spine 1985;10:280–286.
50. Gaines RW, Breedlove R, Monson G. Stabilization of thoracic and thoracolumbar fracture-dislocation with Harrington rods and sublaminar wires. Clin Orthop 1984;189:195.
51. Gallie WE. Fractures and dislocations of the cervical spine. Am J Surg 1939;46:495–499.
52. Goel VK, Goyal S, Clark C, et al. Kinematics of the whole lumbar spine—effect of discectomy. Spine 1985;10:544–554.
53. Goel VK, Nishiyama K, Weinstein JN, et al. Mechanical properties of lumbar spinal motion segments as affected by partial disc removal. Spine 1986;11:1008–1012.
54. Goel VK, Nye T, Clark CR, et al. A technique to evaluate an internal spinal device by the use of Selspot system—an application to the Luque closed loop. Spine 1987;12:150.
55. Goel VK, Clark CR, Harris KG, et al. Evaluation of effectiveness of a facet wiring technique—an in vitro biomechanical investigation. Ann Biomed Eng 1989;17:115–126.
56. Goel VK, Lim TH, Gwon J, et al. Biomechanics of fusion. In: Anderson GB, ed. Spinal stenosis. Chicago: Mosby, 1992;403–414.
57. Gregerson GG, Lucas DB. An in vivo study of the axial rotation of the human thoracolumbar spine. J Bone Joint Surg Am 1967;49:247.
58. Grob D, Dvorak J, Panjabi M, et al. Posterior occipito-cervical fusion—a preliminary report of a new technique. Spine 1991;16S:S17-S24.
59. Gross TP, Jinnah RH, Clarke HJ, et al. The biology of bone grafting. Orthopaedics 1991;14:563–568.
60. Guadagui JR, Drummond DS. Strength of surgical wire fixation—a laboratory study. Clin Orthop 1986;209:176.
61. Gurr KR, McAfee PC, Shih CM. Biomechanical analysis of posterior instrumentation systems after decompressive laminectomy: an unstable calf-spine model. J Bone Joint Surg Am 1988;70:680–691.
62. Guyer DW, Yuan HA, Werner F, et al. Biomechanical comparison of seven internal fixation devices for the lumbosacral junction. Spine 1987;12:569–573.
63. Haft H, Ransohoff J, Carter S. Spinal cord tumors in children. Pediatrics 1959;23:1152–1159.
64. Hanley EN. The suitability of porous tricalcium phosphate as a synthetic bone graft for reconstruction of segmental spinal column defects. Proc Int Soc for the Studies of Lumbar Spine 1985;111–112.
65. Hanson P, Sharkey N, Montesano PX. Anatomic and biomechanical study of C1/C2 posterior arthrodesis. Proc Cervical Spine Res Soc, 1988.
66. Harrington PR. Treatment of scoliosis. Correction and internal fixation by spine instrumentation. J Bone Joint Surg Am 1962;44:591–610.
67. Hazlett JW, Kinnard P. Lumbar apophyseal process excision and spinal instability. Spine 1982;7:171–177.
68. Henzel JH, Mohr GC, vonGierke HE. Reappraisal of biodynamic implications of human ejections. Aerospace Med 1968;39:231–240.
69. Herkowitz HN. A comparison of anterior cervical fusion, cervical laminectomy, cervical laminaplasty for the surgical management of multiple level spondylotic radiculopathy. Spine 1988;13:774–780.
70. Herring JA, Wenger DR. Segmental spinal instrumentation—a preliminary report of 40 consecutive cases. Spine 1982;7:285.
71. Hirabayashi K, Maruyama T, Wakano K, et al. Postoperative lumbar canal stenosis due to anterior spinal fusion. Keio J Med 1981;30:133–139.
72. Hirsch C, Lewin T. Lumbosacral synovial joints in flexion-extension. Acta Orthop Scand 1968;39:303–311.
73. Jackson H. The diagnosis of minimal atlanto-axial subluxation. Br J Radiol 1950;23:672.
74. Jacobs RR, Nordwall A, Nachemson A. Reduction, stability, and strength provided by internal fixation systems for thoracolumbar spinal injuries. Clin Orthop 1982;171:300–308.
75. Johnsson KE, Uden A, Rosen I. The effect of decompression on the natural course of spinal stenosis. A comparison of surgically treated and untreated patients. Spine 1991;16:615–619.
76. Junghans H. Spondylolisthesen ohne Spalt in Zwischengelenkstuck. Arch Orthop Unfall-Chir 1930;29:118–127.
77. Kane WJ. Direct current electrical bone growth stimulation for spinal fusion. Spine 1988;13:363–365.
78. Kälebo P, Kaziolka R, Swärd L, et al. Stress views in the comparative assessment of spondylolytic spondylolisthesis. Skeletal Radiol 1989;17:570–575.
79. Keller TS, Holm S, Hansson TH, et al. The dependence of intervertebral disc mechanical properties on physiological motion. Spine 1990;15:751–761.
80. Kirkaldy-Willis WH, Wedge JH, Young-Hing K, et al. Pathology and pathogenesis of lumbar spondylosis and stenosis. Spine 1978;3:319–328.
81. Kirkaldy-Willis WH, Farfan HF. Instability of the lumbar spine. Clin Orthop 1982;165:110–121.
82. Knutsson F. The instability associated with disc degeneration in the lumbar spine. Acta Radiol 1944;25:593–609.
83. Kornblatt MD, Casey MP, Jacobs RR. Internal fixation in lumbosacral spine fusion—a biomechanical and clinical study. Clin Orthop 1986;203:141.
84. Kostuik JP, Errico TJ, Gleason TF. Techniques of internal fixation for degenerative conditions of the spine. Clin Orthop 1986;203:219.

85. Krag MH, Beynnon BD, Pope MH, et al. An internal fixator for posterior application to short segments of the thoracic, lumbar, or lumbosacral spine. Clin Orthop 1986;203:75–98.
86. Laborde JM, Bahniuk E, Bohlman HH, et al. Comparison of fixation of spinal fractures. Clin Orthop 1980;152:303–310.
87. Lange F. Support for the spondylitic spine by means of burried steel bars attached to the vertebrae. Am J Orthop Surg 1910;8:344.
88. La Rocca H. Segmental instability: evolution of a concept. Semin Spine Surg 1991;3:94–104.
89. Larsson S, Toolan G. Posterior fusion for atlanto-axial subluxation in rheumatoid arthritis. Spine 1986;11:525–530.
90. Lee CK, Langrana NA. Lumbosacral spinal fusion—a biomechanical study. Spine 1984;6:574–581.
91. Lee CK. Clinical biomechanics of lumbar spine surgery. In: White AH, Rothman RH, Ray CD, eds. Lumbar spine surgery. St Louis: Mosby, 1987.
92. Lehmann TR, Brand RA. Instability of the lower lumbar spine. Orthop Trans 1983;7:97.
93. Lehmann TR, Spratt KF, Tozzi JE, et al. Long-term follow-up of lumbar fusion patients. Spine 1987;12:97–104.
94. Leong JC, Chun SY, Grange WJ, et al. Long term results of lumbar intervertebral disc prolapse. Spine 1983;8:793–799.
95. Lim TH. Design of a spinal fixation device and its evaluation—an analytical and experimental approach. Ph.D. Dissertation, The University of Iowa, Iowa City, 1990.
96. Lim TH, Goel VK, Park JB, et al. Comparison of stress-induced porosity due to conventional and a modified spinal fixation device. J Spinal Disord 1994;7:1–11.
97. Lim TH, An HS, Evanich C, et al. Strength of anterior vertebral screw fixation in relationship to bone mineral density. J Spinal Disord 1995;8:121–125.
98. Lim TH, An HS, Hasegawa T, et al. Prediction of fatigue screw loosening in anterior spinal fixation using dual energy x-ray absorptiometry. Spine 1995;20:2565–2568.
99. Lindahl O. Determination of the sagittal mobility of the lumbar spine. Acta Orthop Scand 1966;37:241–254.
100. Liu YK, Njus GO, Bahr PA, et al. Fatigue life improvement of nitrogen-ion-implanted pedicle screws. Spine 1990;15(4):311–317.
101. Lonstein JE, Winter RB, Bradford DB, et al. Postlaminectomy spine deformity. J Bone Joint Surg Am 1976;58:727.
102. Lorenz M, Patwardhan AG, Vanderby R. Load-bearing characteristics of lumbar facets in normal and surgically altered spinal segments. Spine 1983;8:122–130.
103. Louis RP. Surgery of the spine. Berlin: Springer-Verlag, 1983;49–83.
104. Lyon WF, Cochran JR, Smith L. Actual holding power of various screws in bone. Ann Surg 1941;114:376.
105. Lysell E. Motion in the cervical spine. Acta Orthop Scand Suppl 1969;123:1.
106. Macnab I. Spondylolisthesis with an intact neural arch-the so-called pseudo-spondylolisthesis. J Bone Joint Surg Br 1950;32:325–333.
107. Macnab I. The traction spur—an indication of segmental instability. J Bone Joint Surg Am 1971;53:663–670.
108. Magerl FP. Stabilization of the lower thoracic lumbar spine with external skeletal fixation. Clin Orthop 1984;189:125.
109. Magerl F, Seeman PS. Stable posterior fusion of the atlas and axis by transarticular screw fixation. In: Kerh P, Weinder A, eds. Cervical spine. Vienna, New York: Springer-Verlag, 1987;322–377.
110. Markolf KL, Morris JM. The structural components of the intervertebral disc. A study of their contributions to the ability of the disc to withstand compressive forces. J Bone Joint Surg Am 1974;56:675–687.
111. McAfee PC, Werner FW, Glisson RR. A biomechanical analysis of spinal instrumentation systems in thoracolumbar fractures. Spine 1985;10:204.
112. McAfee PC, Farey ID, Sutterin CE, et al. Device related osteoporosis with spinal instrumentation. Spine 1989;14:919–926.
113. McGill SM, Norman RW. Partitioning of the L4-L5 dynamic moment into disc, ligamentous and muscular components during ligating. Spine 1986;11:666–678.
114. Morgan FP, King T. Primary instability of lumbar vertebrae as a common cause of low back pain. J Bone Joint Surg Br 1957;39:6–22.
115. Moroney SP, Schultz AB, Miller AA, et al. Load-displacement properties of lower cervical spine motion segments. J Biomech 1988;21(9):769.
116. Nachemson A. The role of spine fusion. Spine 1981;6:306–307.
117. Nasca RJ, Whelchel JD. Use of cryopreserved bone in spine surgery. Spine 1987;12:222–227.
118. Nerubay J, Marganit B, Bubis JJ, et al. Stimulation of bone formation by electrical current on spinal fusion. Spine 1986;11:167.
119. Newman PH, Stone KH. The etiology of spondylolisthesis. J Bone Joint Surg Br 1963;45:35–39.
120. Nicastro JF, Harten CA, Traina J, et al. Intraspinal pathways of sublaminar wires during removal. An experimental study. J Bone Joint Surg Am 1986;68:1206.
121. Nunamaker DM, Perren SM. Force measurements in screw fixation. J Biomech 1976;9:669.
122. Oh I, Sander TW, Treharne RW. The fatigue resistance of orthopaedic wire. Clin Orthop 1985;192:228.
123. Okuyama K, Sato K, Abe E, et al. Stability of transpedicule screwing for the osteoporotic spine—an in vitro study of the mechanical stability. Spine 1993;18(15):2240–2245.
124. Panjabi MM, White AA, Johnson RM. Cervical spine mechanics as a function of transection of components. J Biomech 1975;8:327–336.
125. Panjabi MM, Krag MH, Chung TQ. Effects of disc injury mechanical behavior of the human spine. Spine 1984;9:707–713.
126. Panjabi MM, Anderson GB, Jorneus L, et al. In vivo measurements of spinal column vibrations. J Bone Joint Surg Am 1986;68:695.
127. Panjabi MM, Summers DJ, Pelker RR, et al. Three-dimensional load displacement curves of the cervical spine. J Orthop Res 1986;4:152.
128. Panjabi MM. Biomechanical evaluation of spinal fix-

ation devices: I. A conceptual framework. Spine 1988; 13:1129–1134.
129. Panjabi MM, Chang DC, Dvorak J. An analysis of errors in kinematic parameters associated with in vivo functional radiographs. Spine 1992;17(2):200–205.
130. Panjabi MM, Oxland TR, Yamamoto I, et al. Mechanical behavior of the human lumbar and lumbosacral spine as shown by three-dimensional load-displacement curves. J Bone Joint Surg Am 1994;76(3):413–424.
131. Parke WW, Sherk HH. Normal adult anatomy. In: Sherk HH, et al, eds. The cervical spine, 2nd ed. Philadelphia: JB Lippincott, 1989;15–18.
132. Pearcy MJ, Portek I, Shepher J. Three-dimensional x-ray analysis of normal movement in the lumbar spine. Spine 1984;9:294–297.
133. Pearcy MJ. Stereoradiography of lumbar spine motion. Acta Orthop Scand Suppl 1985;56:212.
134. Penning L. Normal movements of the cervical spine. Am J Roentgenol 1978;30:317–326.
135. Penning L, Wilmink JT. Rotation of the cervical spine. A CT study in normal subjects. Spine 1987;12(8):732–738.
136. Pintar FA, Maiman DJ, Hollowell, et al. Fusion rate and biomechanical stiffness of hydroxyapatite versus autogenous bone grafts for anterior cervical discectomy—an in vivo animal study. Spine 1994;19:2524–2528.
137. Pope MH, Panjabi MM. Biomechanical definitions of spinal instability. Spine 1985;10:255–256.
138. Pope MH, Wilder DG, Jorneus L, et al. The response of the seated human to sinusoidal vibration and impact. J Biomech Eng 1987;109:279.
139. Posner I, White AA, Edwards WT, et al. A biomechanical analysis of the clinical stability of the lumbar and lumbosacral spine. Spine 1982;7:374–389.
140. Quinnell RC, Stockdale HR. Some experimental observations of the influence of a simple lumbar floating fusion on the remaining spine. Spine 1981;6:263–267.
141. Quinnell RC, Stockdale HR. Flexion and extension radiography of the lumbar spine—a comparison with lumbar discography. Clin Radiol 1983;34:405–411.
142. Robinson RA, Smith GW. The treatment of certain cervical-spine disorders by anterior removal of the intervertebral disc and interbody fusion. J Bone Joint Surg Am 1958;40:608–622.
143. Rothman RH, Simeone FA. Anterior cervical fusion. In: The spine. 3rd ed. Philadelphia: WB Saunders, 1992;600–602.
144. Rosenberg NI. Degenerative spondylolisthesis—predisposing factors. J Bone Joint Surg Am 1975;57:467–474.
145. Roy-Camille R, Mazel C, Saillant G. Internal fixation of the unstable cervical spine by a posterior osteosynthesis with plates and screws. In: Sherk HH, Dunn EJ, Eismont FJ, et al, eds. The cervical spine, 2nd ed. The Cervical Spine Research Society. Philadelphia: JB Lippincott, 1989;390–403.
146. Ruff S. Brief acceleration—less than one second. German aviation medicine World War I. Department of the Air Force, Washington, 1950;1:584.
147. Ruland CM, McAfee PC, Warden K, et al. Triangulation of pedicular instrumentation—a biomechanical analysis. Spine 1991;16(6S):S270-S276.
148. Sandhu HS, Kamin MA, Kabo JM, et al. Comparison of various doses of rhBMP-2 and OPLA carrier in a canine spinal fusion model. Proc Int Soc for the Studies of Lumbar Spine 1995;16.
149. Saraste H, Broström LA, Aparisi T, et al. Radiographic measurement of the lumbar spine—a clinical and experimental study in man. Spine 1985;10:236–241.
150. Schaffer WO, Spratt KF, Weinstein J, et al. The consistency and accuracy of roentgenograms for measuring sagittal translation in the lumbar vertebral motion segment: an experimental model. Spine 1990;15:741–750.
151. Schrader WC, Bethem D, Scerbin V. The chronic local effects of sublaminar wires. Spine 1988;13:499.
152. Schultz KP, Assheuer J, Wehling P. Degeneration in the adjacent level above lumbar fusion. 21st Int Soc for the Study of the Lumbar Spine, Seattle, Washington, June 21–25, 1994;216.
153. Schultz AB, Warwick DN, Berkson MH, et al. Mechanical properties of human lumbar spine motion segments—Part I. J Biomech Eng 1979;101:46–57.
154. Schultz RS, Boger JW, Dunn HK. Stainless steel surgical wire in various fixation modes. Clin Orthop 1985;198:304.
155. Schultz AB. Loads on the lumbar spine. In: MIV, ed. The lumbar spine and back pain. New York: Churchill Livingstone, 1987;204.
156. Selvik G. A roentgen stereophotogrammetric method for the study of the kinematics of the skeletal system. Lund, Sweden; 1974. Thesis.
157. Selvik G, Alberins P, Aronson A. A roentgen stereophotogrammetric system construction, calibration and technical accuracy. Acta Radiol 1983;24:343–352.
158. Selvik G. RSA—a method for the study of the kinematics of the skeletal system. Ed 2. Acta Orthop Scand Suppl 1989;30:232.
159. Shima T, Keller JT, Alvira MM, et al. Anterior cervical discectomy and interbody fusion—an experimental study using a synthetic tricalcium phosphate. J Neurosurg 1979;51:533–538.
160. Shirado O, Zdeblick TA, McAfee PC, et al. Biomechanical evaluation of methods of posterior stabilization of the spine and posterior lumbar interbody arthrodesis—a calf-spine model. J Bone Joint Surg Am 1988;73(4):518–526.
161. Shirazi-Adl A, Drouin G. Load-bearing role of facets in a lumbar segment under sagittal plane loadings. J Biomech 1987;20:601–614.
162. Sienkiewicz PJ, Flatley TJ. Postoperative spondylolisthesis. Clin Orthop 1987;221:172–180.
163. Skinner MD, Maybee J, Transfeldt E, et al. Experimental pullout testing and comparison of variables in transpedicular screw fixation. A biomechanical study. Spine 1990;15(3):195–201.
164. Smith R, Hunt T, Asher MA, et al. The effect of a stiff implant on the bone-mineral content of the lumbar spine in dogs. J Bone Joint Surg Am 1991;73:115–123.
165. Smith MD, Cody DD. Load-bearing capacity of cortico-cancellous bone graft in the spine. J Bone Joint Surg Am 1993;75:1206.

166. Soshi S, Shiba R, Kondo H, et al. An experimental study on transpedicular screw fixation in relation to osteoporosis of the lumbar spine. Spine 1991;16:1335–1341.
167. Spengler DM. Lumbar discectomy results with limited disc excision and selective foraminotomy. Spine 1982;7:604–607.
168. Steffee AD, Biscup RS, Sitkowski DJ. Segmental spine plates with pedicle screw fixation. Clin Orthop 1986;203:45.
169. Stokes IAF, Wilder DG, Frymoyer JW, et al. Assessment of patients with low-back pain by biplanar radiographic measurement of intervertebral motion. Spine 1981;6:233–240.
170. Stokes IAF. Mechanical function of facet joints in the lumbar spine. Clin Biomech 1988;3:101–105.
171. Suh CH. The fundamentals of computer aided x-ray analysis of the spine. J Biomech 1974;7:161–169.
172. Tencer AF, Ahmed AM, Burke DL. Some static mechanical properties of the lumbar intervertebral joint, intact and injured. J Biomech Eng 1982;104:193–201.
173. Tibrewal SB, Pearcy MJ, Portek I, et al. A prospective study of lumbar spinal movements before and after discectomy using biplanar radiography. Correlation of clinical and radiographic findings. Spine 1985;10:455–460.
174. Tomford WW, Starkweather RJ, Goldman MH. A study of the clinical incidence of infection in the use of banked allograft bone. J Bone Joint Surg Am 1981;31:244.
175. Torgerson WR, Dotter WE. Comparative roentgenographic study of the asymptomatic and symptomatic lumbar spine. J Bone Joint Surg Am 1976;58:850–853.
176. Toth JM, Lim TH, An HS, et al. Comparison of compressive strength of iliac bone grafts and porous calcium phosphate ceramics for spinal fusion. Proc Ortho Res Soc 1994;719.
177. Toth JM, An HS, Lim TH, et al. Effect of porous biphasic calcium phosphate ceramics for anterior cervical interbody fusion in a caprine model. Spine 1995;20:2203–2210.
178. Unander-Scharin L. On low back pain. With special reference to the value of operative treatment with fusion. Acta Orthop Scand Suppl 1950;5:149.
179. Ulrich C, Woersdoerfer O, Claes L, et al. Comparative stability of anterior or posterior cervical plate fixation in vitro investigation. In: Kehr P, Weinder A, eds. Cervical spine I. Vienna-New York: Springer-Verlag, 1987;65.
180. Van Akkervecken PF, O'Brien JP, Park WM. Experimentally induced hypermobility in the lumbar spine: a pathologic and radiologic study of the posterior ligament and annulus fibrosis. Spine 1979;5:236–241.
181. Wall MS, Oppenheim WL. Measurement error of spondylolisthesis as a function of radiographic beam angle. J Pediatric Orthop 1995;15:193–198.
182. Weber H. Lumbar disc herniation: a controlled, prospective study with ten years of observation. Spine 1983;8:131–140.
183. Werne S. Studies in spontaneous atlas dislocation. Acta Orthop Scand Suppl 1957;23:1–150.
184. White AA, Johnson RM, Panjabi MM, et al. Biomechanical analysis of clinical instability in the cervical spine. Clin Orthop 1975;109:85.
185. White AA, Panjabi MM. Biomechanical considerations in the surgical management of cervical spondylotic myelopathy. Spine 1988;13:856–860.
186. White AA, Panjabi MM. Clinical biomechanics of the spine. 2nd ed. Philadelphia: JB Lippincott, 1990.
187. Wilder DG, Selgson D, Frymoyer JW, et al. Objective measurement of L4–5 instability. A case report. Spine 1980;5:7.
188. Wiltse LL, Winter RB. Terminology and measurement of spondylolisthesis. J Bone Joint Surg Am 1983;65:768–772.
189. Yasouka S, Peterson HA, Laws ER, et al. Pathogenesis and prophylaxis of postlaminectomy deformity of the spine after multiple level laminectomy—difference between children and adults. Neurosurgery 1981;9:145–152.
190. Yamagata M, Kitahara H, Minami S, et al. Mechanical stability of the pedicle screw fixation systems for the lumbar spine. Spine 1992;17(Suppl):S51.
191. Yang KH, King AI. Mechanism of facet load transmission as a hypothesis for low back pain. Spine 1984;9:557–565.
192. Younger EM, Chapman MW. Morbidity at bone graft donor sites. J Orthop Trauma 1989;3:192–195.
193. Yuan HA, Mann KA, Found EM, et al. Early clinical experience with the Syracuse I-Plate—an anterior spinal fixation device. Spine 1988;13:278–285.
194. Zdeblic TA, Zou D, Warden KE, et al. Cervical stability after foraminotomy—a biomechanical in vitro analysis. J Bone Joint Surg Am 1992;74:22–27.
195. Zdeblick TA, Kunz DN, Cooke ME, et al. Pedicle screw pullout strength—correlation with insertional torque. Spine 1993;18(12):1673–1676.
196. Zdeblic TA, Abitbol JJ, Kunz D, et al. Cervical stability after sequential capsule resection. J Spinal Disord 1993;18:2005–2008.
197. Zdeblic TA, Cooke ME, Kunz DN, et al. Anterior cervical discectomy and fusion using a porous hydroxyapatite bone graft substitute. Spine 1994;19:2348–2357.
198. Zhang ZH, Yin H, Yang K, et al. Anterior intervertebral disc excision and bone grafting in cervical spondylotic myelopathy. Spine 1983;8:16–19.
199. Zindrick MR, Wiltse LL, Widell EH, et al. A biomechanical study of intrapedicular screw fixation in the lumbosacral spine. Clin Orthop 1986;203:99–112.

CHAPTER FOUR

History and Physical Examination of the Spine

Lee H. Riley

Introduction

The history and physical examination are the first critical steps in the diagnosis and treatment of disorders of the spine. Attention to detail in this part of the process leads to a thoughtful, directed inquiry that is time and cost effective and thorough. Despite the seminal importance of these early steps, they are often compromised by the busy clinician who either delegates the task to others or relies more heavily on later diagnostic studies to fill in the gaps. The interview process itself can yield a wealth of information on the patient's concerns, limitations, expectations, and attitude that can have a critical impact on the overall outcome, but are not readily apparent and are more nuanced than the presenting problem. The high false positive rate of advanced imaging studies, such as MRI and CT, further underscores the need to use these studies only to confirm clinical suspicions based on a complete history and physical examination; it also emphasizes the folly of operations based on radiographic findings alone (2, 3, 13, 29). This chapter reviews the basic points of the history and physical examination of the cervical and thoracolumbar spine.

Cervical Spine

Degenerative Disorders

Presenting Symptoms

Neck pain is a common but nonspecific presenting problem in patients who have degenerative disorders of the cervical spine. Because neck pain itself occurs commonly in the general population (12), further inquiry is necessary to establish the diagnosis. Nonspinal causes include derangements of the shoulder, cardiothoracic abnormalities, and craniovertebral pathology (17, 26). Spinal causes include tumor, infection, degenerative disorders, and muscle and ligamentous strain (Table 4.1).

Pain can be described either by its character (mechanical or nonmechanical) or its location (axial or radicular). Mechanical pain tends to be associated with activity. It is relieved by rest and is progressive over the course of the day. Nonmechanical pain is independent of activity, is often worse at night, and is not relieved by rest or immobilization. Axial pain can occur from the base of the occiput to the shoulders and can extend down to between the scapulae.

TABLE 4.1.
Differential Diagnosis of Cervical Disc Disease

Neurologic
Multiple sclerosis
Amyotrophic lateral sclerosis
Hydrocephalus
Cervical cord tumors
Syringomyelia
Peripheral nerve entrapment neuropathies
Brachial plexus injury or Neuritis
Thoracic outlet syndrome
Inflammatory
Rheumatoid arthritis
Fibrositis (trigger point syndrome)
Polymyalgia rheumatica
Neoplastic
Metastatic disease
Primary bone tumors
Pancoast tumors
Infectious
Vertebral osteomyelitis/discitis
Primary shoulder and upper extremity problems
Subacromial bursitis
Calcific tendinitis
Biceps tendinitis
Impingement syndrome of the shoulder
Rotator cuff tear
Glenohumeral arthritis
Reflex sympathetic dystrophy
Cardiac ischemia

It is usually diffuse and associated with complaints of nonspecific shoulder or arm discomfort. It is not typically associated with paresthesia, numbness, or weakness in a radicular distribution.

Radicular pain is characterized by pain, dysesthesia, paresthesia, or numbness in a dermatomal distribution. A history of axial neck pain that proceeds and is superseded by arm symptoms is common in radiculopathy caused by disc herniation. Clinically evident weakness is often not noticed by patients at the time of presentation because of its insidious onset and one's unconscious accommodation to it (22).

Myelopathy presents with poorly characterized pain (5, 6). It can be associated with neck, arm or leg pain in a nondermatomal pattern or with pain in a cervical dermatome. Vague sensory and motor symptoms over a long period of time are also common. Difficulty with ambulation often begins subtly with difficulty walking over uneven ground and problems performing upper extremity fine motor functions, such as fastening buttons. Gait is slow and wide based (6). Lower extremity dysfunction and spasticity often precede upper extremity symptoms. Upper extremity involvement with little lower extremity findings, however, does occur, affecting touch, pain, proprioception, and motor function (9, 10, 16, 21).

Dysphasia is a less common problem associated with cervical spine disorders. It can be caused by an anterior osteophyte, tumor, or inflammatory mass irritating the esophagus as it passes the anterior aspect of the cervical vertebral bodies (11). A careful physical examination, including examination of the anterior neck for masses, tenderness, and lymphadenopathy, needs to be done when such symptoms are present.

Neurocentral joint osteophyte formation can lead to occlusion of the vertebral artery and Wallenberg's syndrome, which was first described in 1895 (28). This syndrome is characterized by symptoms of dysphasia and ipsilateral palatal weakness caused by involvement of the nucleus ambiguous; homolateral pain and temperature impairment of the face caused by involvement of the descending root of cranial nerve V; Horner's syndrome in the homolateral eye caused by involvement of the descending sympathetic fibers; cerebellar dysfunction in the ipsilateral arm and leg from restiform body and cerebellar involvement; and ipsilateral pain and temperature disorders of the trunk and limbs caused by spinothalamic tract involvement.

Physical Examination

Physical examination should begin with observation. Gait abnormalities can be grossly assessed as the patient is brought into the room. The patient's posture should also be examined for loss of normal cervical lordosis, torticollis, guarding of the cervical spine, or spontaneous posturing to relieve symptoms, such as the shoulder abduction relief position which is highly suggestive of a cervical radiculopathy (Fig. 4.1). Active range of motion of the neck should also be noted. Any adaptive behavior in response to weakness, such as using the opposite limb to position the arm, may also be evident at this time. This type of behavior can be particularly evident when shaking the patient's hand, an action that involves shoulder and elbow flexion, wrist and finger extension, and grip.

Asymmetry or spasm in paraspinal muscles and shoulder girdle, neck webbing, and atrophy of the neck, shoulder complex, arms, or hands should be documented. Surgical scars from previous spine or head and neck surgery and skin lesions should also be noted. Active range of motion should be recorded. A patient with normal range of motion should be able to place his or her chin near the chest, achieving approximately 45° of flexion, extension of 75°, axial rotation of 75°, which allows the patient to place the chin on either shoulder, and lateral bending of 40°. Range of motion should be checked for asymmetry, and specific positions of the neck that incite symptoms should be noted.

Physical examination should then proceed to palpation of the structures of the neck. The atlas is lo-

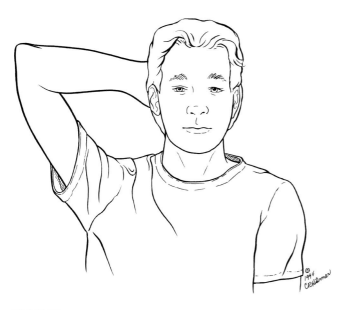

FIGURE 4.1.
Patients with cervical radiculopathy can obtain relief of their symptoms by holding their shoulder in an abducted position to relieve nerve root tension.

cated at the angle of the jaw and styloid. The hyoid is at the level of the C3 disk space, the thyroid is at the level of C4–5, and the cricoid is at the level of C6. The carotid tubercle is also palpable in most instances at C6 although some anatomic variation does exist. Anteromedial to the sternocleidomastoid muscle lies the anterior lymphatic chain. This chain may be tender or swollen with upper respiratory infections, but it can also be enlarged because of metastases. The supraclavicular region should also be palpated for masses, fullness, and cervical ribs.

Provocative Tests

Provocative and alleviating neck positions and maneuvers are useful in establishing the diagnosis. Positions that incite maximum neck discomfort and radicular symptoms, as well as positions that alleviate symptoms, should be documented.

Cervical spondylolysis often causes pain with extension and rotation to the affected side. Muscular and ligamentous strain causes pain with both passive stretch of the affected muscles as well as opposed firing of that muscle. Abnormalities of the atlantooccipital joint often present as pain with rotation and can be associated with an occipital headache.

Radicular symptoms can be increased with axial rotation of the neck and extension to the involved side (Fig. 4.2). This is known as the Spurling's sign, which narrows the involved foramen. Manual compression on the head that causes an increase in symptoms and a distraction that relieves arm pain is also highly suggestive of nerve root compression. The

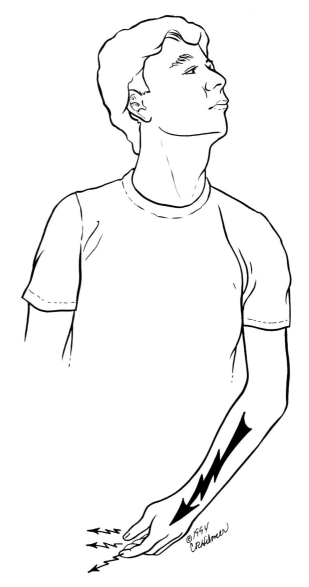

FIGURE 4.2.
Radicular symptoms can be reproduced or exacerbated by axial rotation and extension of the neck to the involved side (Spurling's sign) in cases of cervical radiculopathy.

shoulder abduction test or sign is often associated with cervical radiculopathy and is indicative of extradural compression of the cervical nerve roots (7). Patients report relief of their radicular symptoms by placing their hand behind their head and by flexing their neck. The Valsalva maneuver is thought to increase abdominal pressure, thereby increasing the cerebral spinal fluid pressure, which causes an increase in pressure about the nerve roots (11). This again will cause an increase in radicular symptoms.

The Adson test can be useful in distinguishing thoracic outlet syndrome from cervical radiculopathy. The shoulder is abducted and extended and the arm is rotated externally while the examiner palpates the radial pulse. The patient is then instructed to turn

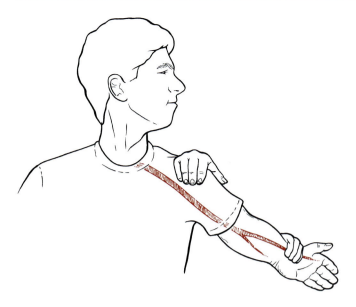

FIGURE 4.3.
A diminution or loss of the radial pulse occurs when the arm is abducted, externally rotated, and extended, and the patient turns his or her head to the involved side and takes a deep breath in a positive Adson test.

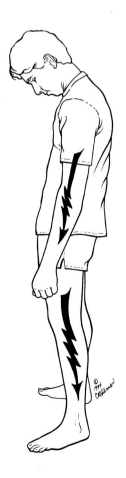

FIGURE 4.4.
An electric shock sensation is produced throughout the body with positioning of the head and neck, causing spinal cord compression.

his or her head toward the arm being tested and to take a deep breath (Fig. 4.3). Obliteration or diminution of the pulse is considered a positive test. This result suggests compression of the subclavian artery from an extra cervical rib, scalenus anticus and scalenus medius muscle compression, or other causes. Patients with subtle spinal cord irritation or compression may report an electric shock sensation through the body with neck flexion or extension. This shock is known as the L'Hermitte's sign (Fig. 4.4).

Neurologic Examination

The eight cervical nerve roots exit through a separate foramen. The first seven exit above the corresponding vertebral body. Cervical eight exits above the first thoracic vertebrae. An occasional cross-over innervation can occur, and variations in root contribution to sensory, motor, and reflex function does exist (1). Intrinsic muscles of the neck are innervated both by cranial nerves and by anterior primary rami from cervical roots. Their individual function can only be determined by EMG testing. Anterior strap muscles above the hyoid are innervated by the hypoglossal nerve. Anterior strap muscles below the hyoid are supplied by the ansa cervicalis. The trapezius and sternocleidomastoid muscles are supplied by the spinal accessory nerve.

Upper cervical nerve roots have less distinctive motor findings, and the diagnosis of upper cervical pathology is based more heavily on subjective reporting of radicular pain and the sensory findings on physical examination. Motor examination of the upper extremities involves testing of roots from C5 to T1, which form the cervical contribution to the brachial plexus.

Testing by Nerve Root

The C3 nerve root produces sensation in the distribution of the posterior neck to the mastoid. It has no reflex and nonspecific motor findings. The C4 root has a sensory distribution involving the posterior neck to the scapula and the anterior chest. It also has no reflex and nonspecific motor findings.

The C5 root has a sensory distribution involving the lateral arm to the elbow. There is some contribution to the biceps reflex; however, this reflex predominantly involves C6. Motor function is to the deltoid muscle, which should be tested with arms outstretched to each side to prevent contribution of the long head of the biceps.

C6 sensation involves the radial forearm to the thumb. The biceps and brachio-radialis reflexes involve primarily the C6 nerve roots. Motor function testing involves the biceps and wrist extensors. Extensor carpi ulnaris is innervated by C7, whereas the extensor carpi radialis longus and brevis are innervated by C6.

C7 sensation involves the mid radial forearm to the middle and possibly the index and ring fingers. The triceps reflex is primarily a C7 reflex. Motor function involves the triceps and wrist flexion. The flexion carpi radialis is C7 innervated, whereas the flexor carpi ulnaris receives C8 innervation. Extensor digitorum communis, extensor digitorum indicis, and extensor digiti quinti are all C7 distributed.

C8 sensation extends along the ulnar forearm to the little and ring fingers. There is no associated reflex. Motor function involves the intrinsics and finger flexors and is expressed most commonly in decreased wrist grip strength. T1 sensation involves the medial upper arm. There is no associated reflex, and motor distribution involves the hand intrinsics.

Reflex Testing

Deep tendon reflexes are an expression of the balance of upper and lower motor-neuron function of a specific segment (14). Anterior horn cell and lower motor neuron involvement abolishes or diminishes deep tendon reflexes to the involved segment. Involvement of the corticospinal tracts exaggerates the deep tendon reflexes below the level of the lesion.

The jaw reflex is a stretch reflex mediated by the trigeminal nerve that involves the masseter and temporalis muscles. With the mouth slightly open in the resting position, a finger is placed over the mental area of the chin and the finger is lightly tapped with a reflex hammer (Fig. 4.5). This maneuver normally causes the jaw to close. An absent or diminished reflex suggests fifth cranial nerve pathology. A brisk reflex suggests an upper motor neuron lesion at the level of the brainstem (11).

The Scapulohumeral Reflex (Shimizu) provides useful information about cord dysfunction cranial to the C3 body level (23). The major muscles involved in the reflex are the upper portion of the trapezius, the levator scapulae, and the deltoid. It is elicited by tapping at the tip of the spine of scapula or at the acromion in a caudal direction (Fig. 4.6). When there is elevation of the scapula and/or abduction of the humerus, the reflex is classified as hyperactive. There is no normal or hypoactive reflex response.

The inverted radial reflex is suggestive of compression at C5-C6. There is a depressed brachial radialis reflex with reciprocal spastic contractures of finger flexors when the distal brachioradialis tendon is struck (Fig. 4.7). This reflex is caused by involvement of the motor neuron fibers that are involved with the brachioradialis reflex; it is also caused by

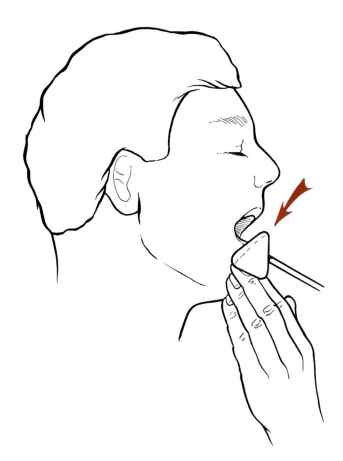

FIGURE 4.5.

The jaw reflex involves the masseter and temporalis muscles and the fifth cranial nerve. Hyperreflexia suggests an upper motor neuron lesion at the level of the brainstem.

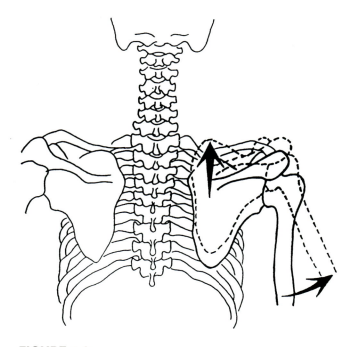

FIGURE 4.6.

Tapping the tip of the spine of the scapula and the acromion in a caudal direction elicits the scapulohumeral reflex.

involvement of the fibers of the corticospinal tract that mediate the tendon reflexes involved in the lower segment of the cord (14, 20, 24).

A positive Hoffmann's sign is another pathologic reflex suggestive of an upper motor neuron lesion in the cervical spine. It is positive if reflex finger flexion is elicited by sudden middle finger DIP joint extension (Fig. 4.8).

The cremasteric reflex is elicited by stroking the inner thigh with the back of a reflex hammer. This normally causes the scrotal sac to be pulled upward. Absence is abnormal when other upper motor neuron lesion pathologic reflexes are present. Unilateral absence is most indicative of lower motor neuron lesions between L1 and L2.

Other pathologic signs that can be elicited include the finger escape sign (21). This sign is positive if the patient is unable to hold the fingers in adduction and extension. The little and ring fingers falling into flexion and abduction in 30 seconds or less suggests cervical myelopathy (Fig. 4.9). The grip and release test is also suggestive of myelopathy (21). The patient is asked to make a fist and extend the fingers repetitively. This normally can be performed 20 times in 10 seconds. Patients who have cervical myelopathy often fumble or slow down rapidly after only a few attempts. A positive Babinski's sign is extension of the great toe with light plantar stimulation; this is also associated with an upper motor neuron lesion. Oppenheimer's sign also produces extension of the great toe when a finger is run along the crest of the tibia. This normally causes either no reaction or pain. Clonus can be elicited by a short upper thrust of the ankle and forefoot. This causes repetitive motion of the ankle joint.

Thoracolumbar Spine

Thoracolumbar spine deformity is a common reason for referral of an adolescent to a spine surgeon. The reason that the evaluation is being sought should be determined. Deformity and pain are the two most common problems reported at initial examination. Deformity is often discovered on routine school screening or physical examination in the absence of pain or other symptoms. A greater awareness of scoliosis as a result of formal school screening programs has led many parents to discover deformities themselves and bring them to medical attention.

Pain is another common presenting complaint. The circumstances surrounding its onset should be determined. Often, it will begin insidiously without any associated trauma, but any history of associated trauma should be determined. Other associated events, such as increased pain with menses, need to be elicited. Hematocolpos secondary to imperforate hymen (15) is an uncommon but reported source of pain in young women. Pain that is worse at night suggests a nonmechanical origin to the pain and suggests that investigation into other causes should be

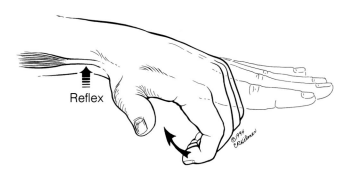

FIGURE 4.7.
Stretching of the brachioradialis tendon causes spastic finger flexor contraction in the inverted radial reflex.

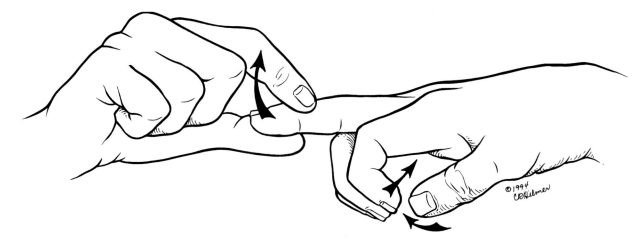

FIGURE 4.8.
Holding the middle finger extended and suddenly extending the distal interphalangeal joint produces reflex finger and thumb flexion. A positive Hoffman's sign is suggestive of spinal cord impingement, especially if asymmetric.

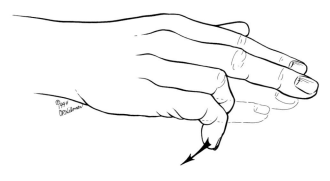

FIGURE 4.9.
A positive finger escape sign occurs when an individual cannot hold all of the fingers in an adducted and extended position and the ulnar two digits fall into flexion and abduction, usually within 30 seconds.

pursued. Any radicular component to the pain should be clearly elicited.

In general, childhood and adolescent deformity is not painful; therefore, pain is a more ominous sign in this age group and suggests spinal cord or bony tumor, Scheuermann's disease, or spondylolisthesis. In adulthood, when degenerative changes and pain are more common in the general population, deformity can be a unrelated finding. Pain associated with deformities tends to be present at the convexity early because of muscle fatigue and localizes to the concavity when degenerative changes have occurred. Exacerbating and relieving symptoms should also be elicited.

If the deformity alone is the reason for referral, characteristics of the curve should be determined. It is important to document when the curve was first noted and whether it has been followed by a local physician or other individuals prior to referral. Specifically ask the patient whether any change in the curve's characteristics has occurred. This change can manifest itself as a change in waistline or pant leg length, a new rotational prominence, or loss of height in an adult. It is also useful to ask specifically what concerns the patient or other family members have in association with the deformity. These concerns can range from cosmetic or obstetric concerns to misgivings over physical activity or progression.

In younger patients, the onset of menses and some idea of the recent growth history should be determined. All previous forms of treatment and their efficacy should be understood. If braces have been used in the past, the type, bracing schedule, duration, and compliance should be determined. Past surgery of the spine should also be documented, and attempts should be made to obtain the operative reports.

Past medical history of thoracotomies, closure of spina bifida, shunting of syrinx, or hydrocephalus are important to document. Medical conditions such as congenital heart disease, neurologic conditions, neo-

plasms, or radiation can predispose children and adolescents to deformities (4). Developmental history should also be obtained. Conditions of the birth, the presence or absence of normal milestones, and mental retardation should be documented.

Family history of myopathy or neurologic disorders can be useful in determining the specific disorders present and can aid in genetic counseling. Specific information regarding scoliosis, neurofibromatosis, and Marfan's syndrome should also be obtained.

Physical Examination

Patients must disrobe for a physical examination. Shorts are acceptable for men and a gown open at the back or two-piece bathing suits can be used for women. The overall appearance of the patient is important to note; often overlooked, it can provide valuable information. Neck webbing suggests Turner's syndrome. A high arched pallet is associated with a variety of syndromes, including Marfan's syndrome. Ear deformities are suggestive of a variety of congenital anomalies. Hemihypertrophy or hemiatrophy can also be noticed at this time, as can midline defects such as a hairy patch, hemangioma, and sinus or surgical scars. A search for café au lait spots should also be performed. Leg length discrepancies, chest deformities (either excavatum or carinatum), and high arched feet should also be noted.

Attention should then be directed to the patient's standing posture in both the frontal and sagittal planes. If a cervical component of the deformity is present, a plumb line from the C7 prominence or inion should be measured in centimeters from the gluteal crease. Shoulder asymmetry should also be estimated in centimeters from the acromioclavicular joints. Pelvis asymmetry is also important to note and document. If the iliac crest cannot be felt, then it should be measured in centimeters from the PSIS or ASIS.

The general nature of the curve should be noted. Is it short and severe, suggestive of congenital anomalies, or long, suggestive of neuromuscular disorder? Its location in the upper, mid, or lower thoracic spine and its cosmetic manifestations should also be determined.

A forward bending test should be performed. Have the patient place his or her feet together with knees straight and finger and palms opposed. The patient then flexes at the waist. The examiner looks from the back (Fig. 4.10). Rib prominence is measured from the area of maximum prominence in centimeters. A scoliometer can also be used as an objective measure of the deformity. Forward bending with consistent deviation to one side on repeated testing suggests irritative lesions such as a spinal cord tumor, a herni-

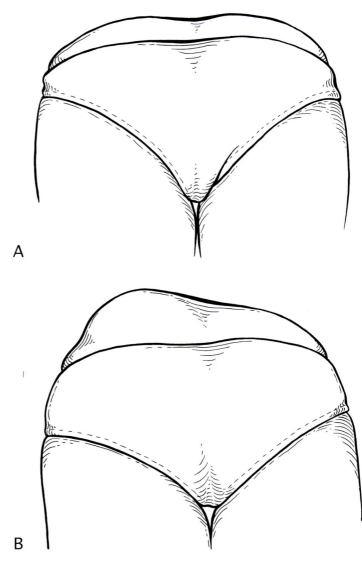

FIGURE 4.10.
Forward bending test. **A.** Normal. **B.** Rib or trunk prominence caused by scoliosis or rotational deformity.

ated disc, or an osteoid osteoma. Range of motion should also be documented, not only for its magnitude but for its effect on the curve itself and the pain it elicits. Normal range of motion of the thoracolumbar spine is 85° of flexion, 50° of extension, 40° of lateral bending, and 45° of rotation. Tanner stage should be noted and recorded (18, 19).

With the patient lying down, hip range of motion should be determined and any hip flexion contractures noted. Leg length should be measured. Abdominal examination should be performed to rule out any intra-abdominal cause of back pain. With the patient lying prone with arms at the sides, the flexibility of a kyphotic deformity can be assessed by asking the patient to raise the shoulders and head off the table. The examiner can also apply compression to the apex of the scoliotic deformity to get a rough estimation of its flexibility. A complete neurologic examination should also be performed and positive findings should be explored further. Any positive findings on the physical examination should guide subsequent diagnostic studies.

Lumbar Spine

Introduction

Over one-half of the population experiences at least one episode of low back pain that temporarily interferes with normal activities (25). Low back pain with two week or greater duration occurs cumulatively in 13.8% of the general population (8).

Although the precise cause of low back pain cannot be clearly delineated in most cases, a careful history and physical examination is necessary to identify a small sub-group of individuals who have a pathology that requires diagnostic evaluation and nonsurgical or surgical intervention. It is also important to consider other causes of low back pain as part of the differential (Table 4.2).

History

The history should focus on the onset, location, character, and associated factors related to the primary report of pain. Whether the pain occurred acutely or

TABLE 4.2.
Differential Diagnosis of Low Back Pain

Congenital defects
Facet tropism
Lumbarization or sacralization
Dysplastic spondylolithesis
Neoplasms
Metastatic tumors
Primary bone tumors (benign and malignant)
Intraspinal tumors (spinal cord and nerve root tumors)
Infections
Osteomyelitis
Epidural abscess
Discitis
Inflammations
Seronegative spondylitis (ankylosing spondylitis, Reiter's syndrome, psoriatic spondylitis, and inflammatory bowel diseases)
Sacroliliitis
Isolated disc resorption
Metabolic diseases
Osteoporosis or osteomalacia
Paget's disease
Hyperparathyroidism
Gout
Neurological diseases
Neuropathies
Demyelinating diseases
Transverse myelitis
Trauma
Muscle strain
Ligamentous sprain
Compression fractures
Spondylolysis and spondylolithesis
Degenerative diseases
Herniated disc
Spinal stenosis
Mechanical instability
Visceral diseases
Genitourinary disorders
Uterine and ovarian diseases
Gastrointestinal disorders
Vascular diseases and aortic aneurysm
Miscellaneous diseases
Piriformis syndrome
Iliolumbar syndrome
Facet syndrome
Quaratus lumborum syndrome
Meralgia paresthetica
Vertebral sclerosis
Postsurgical problems
Osteolysis
Arachnodinitis
Instability
Post-fusion stenosis
Recurrent disc herniation
Psychosocial problems
Compensation or litigation involvement
Drug addiction
Hysterical conversion state

insidiously should be determined. Its location—midline, paraspinous muscle region, buttocks, legs, or radicular—should be determined. Patients should be asked specifically about the distribution of pain, tingling, and numbness. Radicular pain occurs in specific dermatomal patterns of motor weakness, reflex, and sensory changes. Referred pain should not be confused with radicular symptoms. Sclerotomal pain can extend into the buttock, hips, groin, or distal thigh in a nonspecific pattern that needs to be distinguished from the dermatomal pattern of radicular pain. Whether the onset of pain was related to work or trauma, and whether the patient is involved in litigation or a Workman's Compensation claim, should also be elicited at this time. It is important to determine whether the pain is mechanical (which is associated with activity and relieved by rest), progressive over the course of the day, or nonmechanical.

Constitutional symptoms should also be determined. Any recent weight loss, history of fevers, chills, or recent infections should be elicited, because tumors or infection are common but frequently-missed sources of back pain. Relieving and exacerbating activities and all successful or unsuccessful prior attempts at conservative treatments should also be determined.

Physical Examination

The physical examination begins with an assessment of gait. A toe and heel walk should be performed. Toe walking can be used as a general assessment of S1 motor function, and heel walk is a gross measurement of L4 and L5 motor strength. A single knee bend is used to assess quadriceps strength, which can be decreased from L3 or L4 nerve root involvement. Subtle motor weakness or early fatiguing can often be elicited by repetitive muscle testing and can be a subtle sign of nerve root involvement.

Physical examination can then proceed to assessment of the overall alignment of the cervical, thoracic, and lumbar spine. Palpation, both in the midline and paraspinous muscle region, should be performed to elicit tenderness or note malalignment. Any tenderness or spasm in the paraspinous muscle region and sacroiliac region should be determined.

Forward flexion and extension and left and right lateral bending should be performed, both to assess the overall range of motion and to determine if pain is provoked by any of these maneuvers. The type of pain—low back, referred, or sciatic—should also be noted. Pain elicited in forward flexion suggests disc pathology, and extension suggests facet joint arthritis or spinal stenosis.

A thorough motor examination should be performed (10). S1 function is assessed by plantar flexion and eversion of the foot. Extensor hallucis longus strength is an indicator of L5 root function. Tibialis anterior strength is associated with L4 motor function. Quadriceps strength is decreased with L3 and L4 root involvement. Iliopsoas weakness suggests L1 and L2 nerve root dysfunction.

Light touch to pin prick deficits should be determined. There can be overlapping sensory distribution of lumbar nerve roots. The sensory distribution of the S1 nerve root involves the posterior calf, the lateral foot, and the sole. L5 root sensation is distributed over the lateral calf and the first dorsal web space. L4 root sensation involves the medial ankle and anterior aspect of the shin. Perianal and perineal sensation should be tested for S2, 3, and 4 nerve root function. Proprioception of both the lower and upper extremities should also be noted. Proprioception is often lost in both cervical spinal stenosis and neuropathy. A rectal examination should be performed to assess sphincter strength. Abnormal anal wink is suggestive of a sacral root involvement.

Reflexes should be tested for evidence of asymmetry and then compared to the upper extremities. Hyper-reflexia, clonus, and Babinski's sign are important indications of upper motor neuron involvement. L4 and S1 nerve root function affects the knee and ankle jerk, respectively. The posterior tibial reflex is the most specific for the L5 nerve, but it is difficult to elicit and is absent bilaterally in more than 50% of patients.

Provocative tests, such as the contralateral straight leg raise and reverse straight leg raise test, are also useful. The straight leg test can be performed either sitting or lying down, with the knees extended and the pelvis in a stable, fixed position. The degree at which the straight leg raise reproduces radicular symptoms is noted, as are the symptoms that are produced. The straight leg raise test is only positive if it elicits radicular symptoms; it should not be considered positive when back or thigh pain is provoked. The contralateral straight leg raise is a more sensitive measure of nerve irritability. The asymptomatic leg is elevated and elicits radicular pain in the contralateral symptomatic leg.

The bowstring test is tested on the symptomatic leg. The straight leg raise is performed until radicular symptoms are elicited. The knee is then flexed until the symptoms are relieved. Compression of the popliteal fossa is then performed, which should reproduce radicular symptoms if the test is positive.

The prone straight leg raise test or femoral stretch test is used to test specifically for nerve root irritation of L3 and L4. This test should be performed with the knee in extension and should reproduce pain in a radicular pattern. Peripheral pulses should also be noted. Their absence is suggestive of vascular claudication.

Nonorganic physical sign testing can be a useful adjunct in the overall assessment of patients who have low back pain. The Waddell signs provide a simple screening tool to identify individuals who require more formal psychologic testing as part of their overall assessment. These signs can be useful in recognizing individuals whose psychologic component to their disease may compromise their ultimate surgical outcome (27). The five types of physical signs are tenderness, simulation, distraction, regional, and overreaction. Three or more positive types of signs are suggestive of malingering, secondary gain, or a significant psychogenic component.

Nonorganic tenderness is defined as superficial or nonanatomic tenderness. The two simulation tests are the axial loading test and the rotation test. The axial loading test is positive when vertical loads applied to the top of the head elicit back pain. A positive rotation test occurs when rotation of the shoulders and pelvis in the same plane produces back pain. In the presence of root irritation, this maneuver may cause leg pain—this does not constitute a positive test for nonorganic pain. Findings that are present on formal examination but absent with casual observation or reexamination using a different provocative maneuver can suggest a nonorganic component. The "flip" test is employed commonly to elicit such findings. The straight leg raise test performed in a supine position will be substantially worse than when tested sitting.

Regional disturbances are widespread sensory or motor disturbances that do not correspond to specific neuroanatomic lesions. Often, both motor and sensory disturbances involve the same location, such as an entire limb or half of the body. Weakness on formal testing is give way or partial cogwheel weakness involving multiple muscle groups in a random non-neuroanatomic pattern. Sensory disturbances are characterized by light touch, pinprick, and other sensory modalities in a nondermatomal pattern that is commonly stocking-glove in nature.

Overreaction, the last of the physical signs during examination, can take the form of collapsing, sweating, tremor, disproportionate muscle tension, facial expression, and verbalization. Exaggerated response to venipuncture or myelography can also be significant. Overreaction is the physical sign most prone to observer bias and cultural variation. Therefore, its significance must be weighed evenly with the other nonorganic signs found on physical examination.

Conclusion

A careful, focused history and physical examination is critical to providing good, cost-effective health care. Imaging studies should be ordered only after a differential diagnosis has been generated to minimize unnecessary testing. Individual patient concerns and needs and nonorganic components should be recognized and addressed because these elements can have a significant influence on the overall outcome. Attention to detail throughout this process leads to thorough and efficient diagnosis and management of disorders of the spine.

References

1. Benmi A. Clinical features of cervical root compression C5-C8 and their variations. Neurol Orthop 1987;4:74–88.
2. Boden SD, Davis DO, Dina TS, et al. Abnormal magnetic resonance scans of the lumbar spine in asymptomatic subjects: a prospective investigation. J Bone Joint Surg Am 1990;72:403–408.
3. Boden SD, McCowin PR, Davis DO, et al. Abnormal magnetic resonance scans of the cervical spine in asymptomatic subjects: a prospective investigation. J Bone Joint Surg Am 1990;72:1178–1184.
4. Bradford DS, Lonstein JE, Moe JH, et al., eds. Moe's textbook of scoliosis and other spinal deformities, 2nd ed. Philadelphia: WB Saunders, 1987.
5. Bradshaw P. Pain caused by cervical spondylosis. Rheumatism 1961;17:2–7.
6. Clark CR. Cervical spondylitic myelopathy: history and physical findings. Spine 1988;13:847–849.
7. Davidson R, Dunn E, Metzmaker J. The shoulder abduction test in the diagnosis of radicular pain in cervical extradural compressive monoradiculopathies. Spine 1981;6:441–446.
8. Deyo RA, Tsai-Wu YJ. Descriptive epidemiology of low back pain and its related medical care in the United States. Spine 1987;12:264–268.
9. Good D, Couch J, Wascaster L. Numb clumsy hands and high cervical spondylosis. Surg Neurol 1984;22:285–291.
10. Gorter K. Influence of laminectomy on the course of cervical myelopathy. Acta Neurahiv 1976;33:265–281.
11. Hoppenfeld S. Physical examination of the cervical spine and temporomandibular joint. In: Hoppenfeld S, ed. Physical examination of the spine and extremities. Norwalk, CT: Appleton-Century-Crofts, 1976.
12. Hult L. The Munkforts investigation. Acta Orthop Scand Suppl 1959;16:1.
13. Kleiner JB, Donaldson WI, Lurd JG, et al. Extraspinal causes of lumbosacral radiculopathy. J Bone Joint Surg Am 1991;73:817–821.
14. Lestini WF, Weisel SW. The pathogenesis of cervical spondylosis. Clin Orthop 1989;239:69–94.
15. Letts M, Haasheck I. Hematocolpos as a cause of back pain in premenarchal adolescents. J Pediatr Orthop 1990;10:731–732.
16. Lunsford LD, Bissonette D, Zorub D. Anterior surgery for cervical disc disease. Part 2. J Neurosurg 1980;53:12–19.
17. Mackab I. Cervical spondylosis. Clin Orthop 1975;109:67–77.
18. Marshall WA, Tanner JM. Variations in pattern of pubertal changes in girls. Arch Dis Child 1969;44:291.
19. Marshall WA, Tanner JM. Variations in pattern of pubertal changes in boys. Arch Dis Child 1970;45:13.
20. Montgomery DM, Brower RS. Cervical spondylitic myelopathy. Clinical syndrome and natural history. Orthop Clin North Am 1992;23 487–493.
21. Ono K, Ebara S, Fijit. Myelopathic hand. J Bone Joint Surg Br 1987;69:215–219.
22. Rothman RH, Rashbaum RF. Pathogenesis of signs and symptoms of cervical disc degeneration. In: American Academy of Orthopaedic Surgeons, Instructional Course Lectures. Vol XXVII, 203–215. St. Louis: CV Mosby, 1978.
23. Shimizu T, Shimada H, Shirakura K. Scapulohumeral reflex (Shimizu). Its clinical significance and testing maneuver. Spine 1993;18:2182–2190.
24. Spellane JD, Lloyd GH. The diagnosis of lesions of the spinal cord in association with "osteoarthritic" disease of the cervical spine. Brain 1952;7S:177–186.
25. Svensson HO, Vedin A, Wilhelmson C, et al. Low back pain in relation to other diseases and cardiovascular risk factors. Spine 1983;8:277–285.
26. Sypert GW. Neck pain and cervical syndromes: Part I: Evaluation. Surgical Rounds for Orthopaedics 1990:36–44.
27. Waddell G, McCullough JA, Kummel E, et al. Nonorganic physical signs in low-back pain. Spine 1980;5:117–125.
28. Wallenberg A. Acute bulbür affection (Embolic der Art. Cerebellar Post, Inf. Sinistr.) Arch Psychriat (Berlin) 1895;27:504.
29. Wiesel SW, Bell GR, Feffer HL, et al. A study of computer assisted tomography: I. The incidence of positive CAT scans in an asymptomatic group of patients. Spine 1984;9:549–551.

CHAPTER FIVE

Diagnostic Imaging of the Spine

Marc J. Levine and Scott D. Boden

Introduction

Recent advances in diagnostic imaging have greatly enhanced the physician's ability to accurately diagnose and treat spine pathology. However, these very technical advances have also increased the potential for patient mismanagement. The temptation to "over" image the spine can be particularly dangerous in terms of leading to inappropriate treatment decisions. In worst case scenarios, unnecessary surgery is performed or subtle pathology is clouded by obvious but clinically incidental findings.

A thorough history and physical examination leads to a preliminary clinical diagnosis, which then predicates both the selection and timing of imaging tests. An appreciation of the sensitivity, specificity, and accuracy of various imaging modalities in conjunction with different disease processes can greatly refine interpretive skills. Efficient use of diagnostic imaging not only allows effective and timely patient management but also minimizes costly medical expenditures.

This chapter is separated into two sections. In the first, the strengths, weaknesses, and basic theory of the different imaging modalities are discussed. Specifically, these imaging modalities include plain films, plain film tomography, discography, myelography, computerized axial tomography, magnetic resonance imaging, and the bone scan. The second section addresses the rationale for ordering these tests based on a variety of clinical findings.

Imaging Modalities

Diagnostic tests should be used to confirm information ascertained during a comprehensive history and physical examination. One should not go "fishing" for a diagnosis by ordering multiple imaging tests, but instead carefully select studies based on a core of clinical findings. In addition, the temporal sequence in which each test is ordered must be tailored to a working diagnosis. Irresponsible testing can lead to unnecessary complications from invasive procedures. Furthermore, although difficult to measure, severe anxiety can occur when patients anticipate and undergo a diagnostic evaluation. It is therefore important to have a basic understanding of modalities that are commonly used and to appreciate their application in specific clinical settings.

Plain Radiographs

Plain radiographs remain the most commonly ordered modality for diagnosing spine pathology. It is estimated that over 4 million cervical and 7 million lumbar spine examinations are performed yearly in the United States (65). Unfortunately, many of these tests are prematurely obtained in patients who have self-limiting processes.

When used appropriately, the plain radiograph can be the first and only test needed to treat a patient or confirm the lack of injury. In many instances, it is used as an adjunct to additional modalities, such as the bone scan. Plain radiographs can adequately be used to follow diseases that affect the bony structure or alignment of the spinal column.

The main limitation of plain radiographs is its inability to demonstrate intraspinal or extraspinal soft tissue pathology. Another limitation is the inability to display early bone destruction from a pathologic process. It has been estimated that bone destruction must exceed 30 to 40% to be detected by plain radiographs.

Although no immediate complications result from routine radiography, axial skeletal radiographs do incur a significant amount of radiation exposure compared with studies of other areas. Radiographic examination of the lumbosacral region delivers one of the highest doses of radiation to the skin, bone marrow, and reproductive organs (19, 33, 110). Gonadal radiation exposure from lumbarsacral films is exceeded only by colon and urologic examinations (19). Radiation exposure to the bone marrow and lungs for examination of the cervical, thoracic, and lumbar regions is equivalent in men and women. However, gonadal exposure is significantly greater in females during examination of the lumbar and lumbosacral spine (65). Proper technique with careful attention to centering, coning, and calibration can reduce the number of "repeated" films performed and can decrease patient exposure. Specific views that the examiner needs should be ordered clearly; use of terms such as "routine series" should be avoided. For instance, in following a child with scoliosis in the absence of a severe sagittal deformity, follow-up radiographs should consist only of PA films, which require 25% of the radiation used to obtain a lateral view (87).

Plain Film Tomography

Conventional pluridirectional tomography (CPT) represents one of the earliest advances of routine radiography for imaging the spine (4, 71). Although rectilinear tomography is considered inferior to pluridirectional tomography, CPT is more readily available because of economic factors. Both types of tomography allow for multisegmental displays of images in the sagittal and coronal planes. Traditionally, plain film tomography is oriented parallel to a longitudinal axis and is superior to computerized axial tomography (CT) for evaluating axially oriented structures such as the dens (50). Littleton points out possible indications for plain film tomography to include evaluation of: 1) the longitudinal plane; 2) fine details; 3) subtle fractures; 4) fractures believed to be in the same plane as a CT section; and 5) a fusion mass in follow-up (72). In the absence of CT and magnetic resonance imaging (MRI), plain film tomography may be the only alternative available for cross-sectional imaging.

Tomographic images are based on an x-ray source moving in one direction and a receiver moving in the opposite direction. Successful image production largely depends on the anatomic knowledge and expertise of the technician. As with plain x-rays, plain film tomograms are unable to define intraspinous and extraspinous structures. The resolution capacity of tomography is approximately five lines per millimeter, which is slightly less than routine radiographs but superior to reconstructed CT and MRI images (72). Characteristic "blurs" seen with tomography require an experienced interpreter to avoid overreading normal images.

Discography

A discogram is an injection of dye into the intervertebral disc space, usually performed under local anesthesia. An abnormal discogram occurs when the dye is not contained within the confines of the disc space on the radiograph and when the injection reproduces the patient's typical back or neck pain, both in character and distribution. Discography has been used in the cervical spine since 1957, in the lumbar spine since 1948, and it remains a controversial diagnostic modality. Proponents of discography claim that it is sensitive and accurate for identifying patients who have axial pain caused by intrinsic disc pathology (so-called "internal disc derangement" or "discogenic pain"). Others question the validity of this diagnosis or, more accurately, question the ability of their being able to make the diagnosis reliably. Even if this test is considered valid, the treatment remains somewhat uncertain and the results somewhat unpredictable, thus the continued controversy of discography (12). Generally, cervical discography is less reliable than lumbar discography. Particularly in the older population, the relative weakness of the cervical annulus compared with the lumbar annulus becomes compounded and may be responsible for an increase in false positive results. The indications for obtaining a discogram are few and may be limited to persistent low back or neck pain with or without radicular symptoms in the face of a negative myelogram.

Discography is a provocative test, reflecting symptomatic morphologic changes of the disc resulting from various pathophysiologic processes. The interpretation and reporting of results are critical for properly incorporating findings into a treatment plan. The following information should be included in all reports; injection volume and endpoints, concordance or nonconcordance to clinical symptoms, location and intensity of pain, and information regarding disc morphology (97).

As with any invasive procedure, there are inherent risks for complications. These risks include infection, headaches, radicular pain, and needle breakage.

Low back pain post-discography is a self-limiting condition that may persist for up to 10 days (42).

Myelography

Myelography has long been the "gold standard" for measuring neural compression in both the cervical and lumbar spine. Dye is injected into the dural sac and mixes with the cerebrospinal fluid (CSF). The outline of the contents of the dural sac can be visualized on x-ray film. Any extradural mass, such as a herniated disc, shows up as an impression in the dye column, whereas an intrathecal mass may appear as an outwardly protruding filling defect. Myelography is unable to differentiate disc protrusion from bony, malignant, infectious, or other extradural encroachments of the dural sac. The diagnostic accuracy of myelography is also questionable in cases of far lateral disease and in the lumbar spine at the L5-S1 level where the epidural space may be large.

Originally, myelography was performed with oil-based dyes, introduced in 1921, that had a relatively high complication rate, including headache, nausea, vomiting, seizures, arachnoiditis, and intrathecal scarring of the nerve roots (66). More recently, water soluble dye and nonionic contrast materials have allowed the detection of subtle changes in the contour and location of nerve roots with a decreased risk of complication (Fig. 5.1).

The primary advantage of myelography over other modalities, such as CT and MRI, is that myelography is a dynamic test that measures the ability of CSF to flow around any potential extradural lesion. In other words, when there is a block on the myelogram, it implies a functional block in the ability of CSF to pass by the lesion and it raises the level of severity of neural compression. It is difficult to ascertain this dynamic information on static examinations, such as CT or MRI.

Complications from myelography can occur as a result of either dye reactions or technical considerations. Iophendylate (Pantopaque), a formerly used

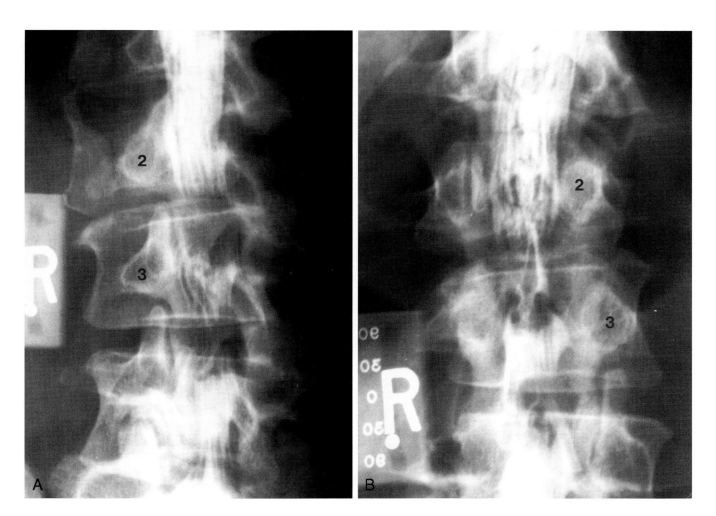

FIGURE 5.1.

A. Post-myelogram oblique radiograph of lumbar spine demonstrating a block of dye at the L2-L3 and L3-L4 levels with reconstitution of the dye pool cranially. **B.** An anteroposterior radiograph of the same patient also showing blocks at the L2-L3 and L3-L4 levels. The etiology of this block cannot be determined by this study.

oil-based contrast agent, was associated with a 25% risk of arachnoiditis (48). Complications from metrizamide (Amipaque), which until recently was the most commonly used nonionic water soluble contrast agent, are a result of pathophysiologic processes. Meningeal irritation may cause nausea, vomiting, dizziness, and headache (52). Radicular pain, hyperesthesias, and retention may result from nerve irritation. Catastrophic complications, including quadriplegia and death, have also been reported (74, 94). Newer nonionic water soluble contrast agents, such as iohexol, have even fewer complications.

Computed Tomography

Computed tomography (CT) is currently the most versatile and widely available noninvasive modality for evaluating abnormalities of the spine. Multiple cross-sectional (axial) images of the spine are made at various levels, and with reformatting, coronal, sagittal, and three-dimensional images may be created. The CT scan demonstrates not only the bony configuration, but also the soft tissue in graded shadings, so that ligaments, nerve roots, free fat, and the intervertebral disc protrusions can be evaluated as they relate to their bony environment.

The CT scan is particularly useful for distinguishing between hard discs (osteophytes) and soft discs (herniated nucleus pulposus). In addition, CT is useful for localizing and finding the extent of neoplastic or infectious involvement in the spine, particularly as it relates to bony destruction and residual stability. The primary weakness of CT scanning remains its unreliability in demonstrating intrathecal pathology without the introduction of an intrathecal contrast agent (Fig. 5.2).

A post-myelogram CT may be performed to give better visualization of the spinal canal and its contents. Extradural tissues are also better delineated with this technique. Overall, a post-myelogram CT scan provides a more detailed picture of neuroanatomic structures in relation to bony structures and soft tissue pathology.

The risks associated with CT/myelograms are dictated by the introduction of contrast dyes as previously discussed.

Magnetic Resonance Imaging

Magnetic resonance imaging (MRI) is the newest and most technically advanced modality currently available. The strengths of MRI lie in its ability to provide excellent soft tissue resolution and to characterize tissue pathology. MRI provides multiplanar images and avoids complications that may be associated with ionizing radiation and contrast injections. Despite its universal acceptance and casual use, it remains the least understood spinal imaging technique.

Fundamentally, an image is obtained by detection of extremely small differences in proton density in a magnetic field bombarded with short pulses of radio waves, which cause atoms to vibrate in a specific manner. More specifically, hydrogen atoms (protons) align themselves uniformly once a magnetic field is applied. A radiofrequency is then applied, which causes excitation of the protons to a higher energy state. Once the radiofrequency pulse is discontinued, the protons return to their previous state and in doing so release energy. This energy release is detected as the magnetic resonance signal (29). Still aligned to the applied magnetic field, the delivery of a pulsed radiofrequency can be repeated or altered. Numerous advances have been made since the inception of MRI. A rudimentary understanding of the physics upon which MRI is based allows a physician to better interpret and use MRI.

As already outlined, an MRI image is based on the energy released during the transition of a proton from

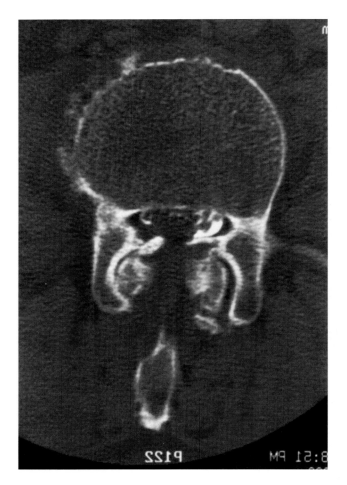

FIGURE 5.2.
Post-myelogram computerized axial tomogram showing central canal stenosis at L3 secondary to degenerative osteophyte formation.

an excited state, secondary to a pulsed radiofrequency, to a baseline state. The absorption and release of energy between states is termed nuclear magnetic resonance. The transition from a higher energy state to a baseline state is termed relaxation and is characterized by two independent time constants; T1 and T2. T1 reflects the longitudinal relaxation time, and T2 reflects the transverse relaxation time. The exact physics behind T1 and T2 relaxation time are not as important as the appreciation that these are both intrinsic properties of biologic tissue (18). The magnetic resonance image is therefore dependent on these intrinsic properties and on the proton density, another intrinsic property.

Once the magnetic field strength has been determined (typically either a high field strength magnet of 1.5 Telsa or a mid field strength 0.4 Telsa), exploitation of the differences between the T1 and T2 intrinsic properties of imaged tissue is accomplished in two ways. The repetition time (TR), or time between radiofrequency pulses, and the echo time (TE), or the time between application of the radiofrequency pulse and the time of recording the MR signal, can be altered. Both TR and TE times are determined at the time of image acquisition. Therefore, by varying the TR and TE intervals, images can be "T1-weighted," "T2-weighted," or any combination in between.

T1-weighted sequences show fat-related structures with high signal intensity (bright) on images. They are produced with short TR (400 to 600 milliseconds) and short TE (5 to 30 milliseconds) intervals. T2-weighted sequences show hydrated structures with high signal intensity (bright) on images. They are produced with long TR (1,500 to 3,000 milliseconds) and long TE (60 to 120 milliseconds) intervals. Structures that are bright on T1-weighted sequences will be dark on T2-weighted sequences, the converse of which is also true (Table 5.1) (Fig. 5.3).

Spatial resolution, signal to noise (S/N) ratio, and contrast resolution are the three parameters that determine the quality of an MR image. Any improvement in image quality represents a combination of increased spatial resolution, increased S/N ratio, or enhanced contrast resolution.

Contrast resolution is the ability to discriminate between different tissue based on the intrinsic T1 and T2 properties and on the proton density of dif-

TABLE 5.1.
Tissue and Body Fluid Signal Intensity on MRI

Tissue or Body Fluid	T1-Weighted	T2-Weighted
Cortical bone	Low	Low
Tendons and ligaments	Low	Low
Fibrocartilage	Low	Low
Hyaline cartilage	Intermediate	Intermediate
Muscle	Intermediate	Intermediate
Free water (CSF)	Low	High
Abscess	Intermediate	High
Adipose tissue	High	Intermediate-High
Hemorrhage	Variable	Variable

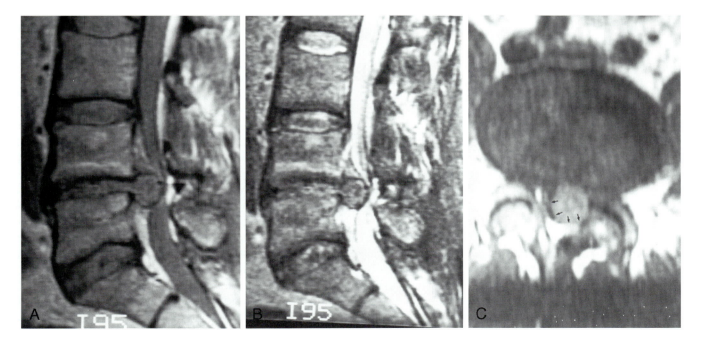

FIGURE 5.3.

A. Large L4-L5 herniated nucleus pulposus seen on T1-weighted sagittal MRI sequence. **B.** Same lesion visualized with a T2-weighted sequence. **C.** Axial MRI image showing large amount of disc material (arrowheads) in the canal compressing the cord.

ferent tissue. This is accomplished by adjusting the TR and TE intervals (Table 5.1).

Spatial resolution is the ability to delineate fine detail. The smallest size detectable is determined by slice thickness, field of view (FOV), and the size of the acquisition and display matrices. Spatial resolution is defined in pixel units. To achieve improved spatial resolution, thin slices (3 mm) should be used with a large matrix. Generally, an inverse relationship exists between improved spatial resolution and S/N ratio. One exception occurs with the use of posterior surface coils, which, because of the relatively superficial position of the spine, allow for improved spatial resolution without decreasing the S/N ratio.

The S/N ratio is the relatively useful signal divided by the extraneous and distorted signal present during image acquisition. One way to improve the S/N ratio is to image larger volumes that have greater proton densities; however, this inevitably decreases spatial resolution. Again, posterior surface coils allow for an improved S/N ratio without negatively affecting the spatial resolution. In fact, surface coils allow for MR imaging of almost the entire spine (48 cm in length) with an adequate spatial resolution and S/N ratio on a single image acquisition (70). Therefore, surface coils improve the S/N ratio by affecting the numerator. By decreasing the time to image acquisition artifact, patient motion can be minimized, leading to a reduction in noise and an improved S/N ratio. Significant advances have been made in this area of magnetic resonance imaging since its inception; these advances are known as fast-scanning techniques.

Gradient-echo imaging was the first of the fast-scanning techniques developed. The technique is based on gradients rather than a 180° radiofrequency to refocus spins. Both flip time and TR intervals are decreased (70). Besides the rapidity of image production, its greatest advantage is the ability to obtain thin images (1 mm) and 3D-volumetric thin-section axial images that are particularly useful in the cervical spine. Conventional 2D spin echos provide only 3-mm slices. In the absence of 180° radiofrequency refocusing, gradient echo is more susceptible to artifacts from tissue and motion.

Fast spin-echo (FSE) imaging is another fast scanning technique. First proposed by Hennig and refined by Melki in 1990, it has had a significant impact on MR imaging (68, 69, 84). Also known as RARE (Rapid Acquisition Relaxation Enhanced), sequence variations include fast spin-echo and turbo-spin-echo. FSE/RARE provides good T2-weighted contrast in a fraction of the time required for a true spin-echo acquisition, with better resolution and S/N ratios than previously possible. This image sequence takes only a few minutes to yield images that require 10 minutes if formatted with conventional T2-weighted techniques.

Before undergoing the MRI examination, each patient must be questioned to determine if any contraindications to the study exist. Absolute contraindications include ferromagnetic cerebral aneurysmal clips, cardiac pacemakers, metallic foreign bodies in the orbit, and ferromagnetic cochlear or ocular implants (62, 63). Artifact can be predicted from any metallic implant and is minimized most with titanium implants when compared with steel. Patients should be counseled and prepared to lie motionless for long periods of time in what many consider a claustrophobic environment. Sedation is often needed, particularly when imaging the pediatric population.

Radionuclide Imaging

Radionuclide imaging, or bone scintography, is a good technique for imaging bone abnormalities. This noninvasive process detects pathophysiologic disturbances based on variations of blood flow and bone metabolism. Any process that disturbs the balance and results in an increased bone turnover is associated with a greater concentration of radionuclide tracer on the bone scan. Interruption of blood flow to the bone results in an absence (cold spot) of tracer on the scan. A number of radiotracers have been used, including technetium-99m phosphate, gallium, and indium.

Technetium-99m remains the most commonly used radiotracer. A triple bone scan classically consists of two early phase readings and a final delayed reading. Image acquisition generally begins 2 to 4 hours after an intravenous bolus. The early phase images represent a dynamic state based on blood flow and blood pooling to an area. Changes in these early phases often are secondary to inflammatory or neoplastic processes. The final and delayed image phase represents a more static state based on the metabolic activity of bone. Processes such as degenerative joint disease, healing fracture, and well treated osteomyelitis may have increased uptake on the delayed phase image with little or no activity on the two earlier phase images. The exact mechanism by which technetium-99m binds is largely unknown, although uptake has been seen with both immature collagen and metabolically active bone (Fig. 5.4).

Gallium-67 citrate was the first agent used to specifically diagnose infection. When used as an adjunct to bone scintography, gallium presents diagnostic difficulties because of its somewhat nonspecific binding characteristics. Sites of accumulation include serum proteins, bacterial cell surfaces, leukocytes, liver, spleen, bone, hematopoietic marrow,

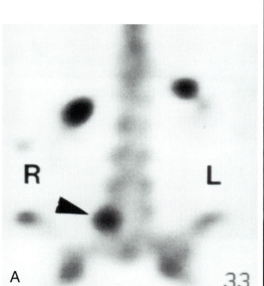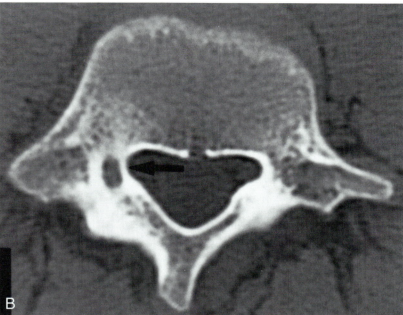

FIGURE 5.4.
A. Technetium bone scan with focal uptake in the right lumbar L5 region (arrowhead) B. CT scan with classic appearance of an osteoid osteoma (arrow).

breasts, and salivary and lacrimal glands (111). The primary disadvantage of gallium is its nonspecificity, which causes particular difficulty in distinguishing hepatosplenic pathology from neighboring spine pathology.

The indium-111-labeled leukocyte scan is commonly used to help differentiate pyogenic states. Indium-WBC preparation requires approximately 50 mL of autologous blood with a white blood cell count of at least 5000 cells/mm^3. The preparation time is approximately 2 hours, after which the labeled white blood cells are injected intravenously. The specificity and sensitivity of this technique is generally superior to the gallium scan for determining acute infections. The only difficulty in diagnosing spine infections occurs in the presence of red bone marrow, which also has an affinity for the indium-labeled leukocytes (111). Indium scans should be performed before antibiotic therapy is instituted, and they may be difficult to perform in immunocompromised individuals.

General Imaging Considerations

The decision of when to order an imaging test is almost as important as the decision of which test to order. The reason is that the vast majority of causes of acute neck pain, back pain, or radiculopathy tend to have a favorable natural history resulting in improvement with nonoperative management within 6 to 8 weeks. Accordingly, with the exception of acute trauma or presence of a progressive neurologic deficit, most degenerative conditions should be treated for at least six weeks before examination with more aggressive imaging modalities. In fact, plain radiographs are not necessary for most neck and back strains, or even in cases of sciatica, for at least 4 to 6 weeks. The exception to this rule would be in patients less than age 20 or older than 50. Other exceptions include patients with a history of malignancy or a clinical examination consistent with tumor or infection.

To assess the true clinical performance of any diagnostic study, the physician must know its sensitivity, which is a reflection of the false negative results, or the ability of the test to detect disease when it is present. More relevant to the avoidance of overtreatment is the specificity of a test, which is a reflection of the false positive results, or the ability of the test to remain negative in the absence of disease. The remainder of this chapter addresses the authors' rationale of using the various modalities based on clinical symptom groups.

Cervical Spine

Axial Neck Pain

Neurologic sequelae secondary to cervical spine pathology can be divided into three categories: axial neck pain, radiculopathy, and myelopathy. In the absence of clinical findings suggestive of infection, tumor, inflammatory arthritides, and trauma, most cases of axial neck pain arise from degenerative changes of the disc and facet joints. The differential diagnosis for axial neck pain includes a multitude of referred sources, including tension headaches and localized muscle strains. For this reason, the clinician must be cautioned about the overimaging of axial neck pain.

After an unsuccessful 6- to 8-week trial of nonoperative therapy, the initial radiographic evaluation of the cervical spine should begin with plain radiographs. Anteroposterior, lateral, open mouth, and oblique films provide an adequate look at the cervical spine. This study is often sufficient to rule out any missed underlying pathologies. Destructive processes, including tumor and infection, may be revealed. If there is any concern regarding instability by history or from the initial plain radiographs, flexion/extension films should be the next test ordered.

Each sub-axial cervical spinal motion segment consists of five articulations, two uncovertebral joints, two facet joints, and the intervening cervical disc. As seen in other joints in the body, degenerative changes of cervical articulations can cause pain. The continuum of degenerative cervical disease may result in both disc and bony pathology. Degenerative disc disease is seen on plain radiographs by a decrease in disc space. A "vacuum disc" is the phenomena of gas production (92% nitrogen) by degenerating discs represented by lucencies in the disc space on plain radiographs (92). The pathophysiology associated with disc degeneration includes a decrease in proteoglycans and, more specifically, a decrease in the chondroitin sulfate:keratin sulfate ratio. This decrease in proteoglycans contributes to disc dehydration, which is characteristic of the elderly population. On MRI, corresponding changes include a decrease signal intensity on T2-weighted images and an increase on T1-weighted images.

Osteophyte formation, sclerosis, and deformity are common findings in degenerative cervical spine disease. Erosive endplate changes are suggestive of inflammatory arthritides. Careful assessment of osteophytes may aid in the diagnosis of nondegenerative arthritides. The marginal syndesmophytes of ankylosing spondylitis should not be confused with the nonmarginal syndesmophytes of diffuse idiopathic sclerosing hyperostosis (DISH), or Forestier's disease.

Although plain radiographs may indicate degenerative disease, it is dangerous to rely on this test for determining the etiology of axial neck pain. Gore et al. used lateral radiographs to study 200 asymptomatic men and women between the ages of 20 and 65. Subjects were divided into five age groups, and 95% of men and 70% of women had evidence of degenerative changes on x-ray. The authors concluded that although degenerative changes may be seen on x-ray, these changes do not necessarily correlate with symptoms (46).

In the absence of myelopathy or radiculopathy, MRI plays a limited role in the evaluation of general axial neck pain. The inherent oversensitivity and high false positive rate of this test often complicates appropriate management. Boden et al. prospectively studied cervical MRIs obtained from 63 asymptomatic volunteers and compared them to scans of 37 symptomatic patients. In 19% of asymptomatic patients, an abnormality of either a herniated nucleus pulposus, bulging disc, or stenosed foramina was found. This finding occurred in 19% of volunteers younger than age 40 and 28% of volunteers older than age 40. A degenerated disc, as evidenced by decreased signal on T2-weighted sequences, was seen in 25% of those younger than 40 and in 56% of those older than 40 (14).

A thorough clinical examination, a careful management plan, and an appreciation of surgical clinical outcomes helps prevent the treatment of incidental findings or self-limiting processes. This is not to say that an MRI is never indicated for axial neck pain. For instance, in the presence of persistent nonradiating axial neck pain despite appropriate management often up to 6 months, an MRI may help rule out any soft tissue pathology or insidious bony process. However, a slightly bulging disc without radicular distribution should not prompt a surgical procedure.

Cervical Radiculopathy

Cervical radiculopathy is a clinical diagnosis based on a dermatomal distribution of pain, motor, and/or sensory changes. Any process that causes nerve root compression may lead to a cervical radiculopathy. Impingement may be brought about by retropulsed disc material, osteophytes, facet hypertrophy, or tumor, as well as by soft tissue pathology. Numerous studies have been used to diagnose this problem. After appropriate physical examination and initial management, a physician needs to intelligently choose an imaging test that will aid in designing a comprehensive treatment plan.

The role of plain radiographs in cervical radiculopathy is somewhat limited because they do not allow for visualization of neurologic structures. However, plain films may confirm the presence of degenerative changes seen as osteophyte formation or a decreased disc space. Dynamic lateral flexion/extension films may help diagnose radicular symptoms secondary to instability. The oblique cervical radiograph is useful in visualizing osteophyte formation that causes foraminal stenosis. Although plain radiographs are accepted widely as an initial screening imaging modality, Friedenberg and Miller showed that by the fifth decade, 25% of their asymptomatic patients had evidence of degenerative changes, and by the seventh decade this number rose to 75%. In fact, when comparing 92 asymptomatic patients to a group of age-matched symptomatic patients, the only radiographic difference was a higher rate of degenerative changes at the C5–6 and C6–7 spaces in the symptomatic population (36).

The most informative imaging studies for evaluation of cervical radiculopathy are myelography, computerized axial tomography, and magnetic resonance imaging. A cervical myelogram is performed by introducing dye into the thecal sac. The radiopaque contrast agent may be injected at the C1-C2 interspace, which allows for visualization of the cervical neural elements as the dye progresses caudally by gravity.

Easy visualization can be complicated by inherent risks of improper needle placement at this level, which may be either neurologic or vascular. If dye is injected at the lumbar region, patients must be positioned in such a fashion so that the dye is able to overcome gravity and flow cranially. The complications from improper lumbar needle placement are normally less catastrophic than with the cervical approach; however, timely visualization is more difficult. There is also a risk of neural toxicity if cranially flowing agents pass through the foramen magnum (9). As with all imaging modalities, abnormal findings must be clinically correlated. Hitselberger and Witten reported a 21% incidence of a cervical spine filling defects in 300 asymptomatic patients undergoing myelography for evaluation of acoustic tumors (55).

Myelography provides for adequate visualization of neuroanatomic structures but has little value when used alone for determining the etiology of nerve root impingement. Disc disease and osteophyte formation lead to mechanical obstruction of the nerve roots and spinal cord but often are indistinguishable by this modality. The accuracy of the cervical myelogram has been reported in the literature to range from 67% to 92% (9). For these reasons, myelography is often combined with CT scanning. Axial images of dye-injected neural elements allow for excellent visualization of nerve roots in relation to their bony encasement. CT scan also allows for some soft tissue visualization, including disc material. By itself, CT scan may give adequate bony and soft tissue images. Compared with myelography, CT scan provides images beyond dye blocks and localizes hypertrophic changes that may lead to foraminal stenosis. Combining these two techniques can help clarify clinical findings and often are integral to preoperative planning.

Magnetic resonance imaging has had a significant effect on the radiographic evaluation of cervical radiculopathy. Immediate advantages include its noninvasive protocol and its ability to image the entire cervical spine in one sitting. The disadvantage is the relative decreased image quality when compared with the lumbar spine. The inadequate visualization of lateral foraminal stenosis is perhaps the biggest shortcoming of cervical MRI.

MRI examination of the cervical spine should include both T1-weighted and T2-weighted sequences. T1-weighted sagittal examination of the cervical spine provides an excellent survey of the cervical spine. Intervertebral discs, spinal cord, thecal sac, and posterior elements are seen with clarity. The axial T1-weighted image emphasizes paraspinal and intraspinal pathology, including spinal cord morphology, intrathecal nerve root anatomy, vertebral bodies, and posterior elements. Low signal intensity on T1-weighted images makes differentiation of the following structures difficult: the vertebral body cortex, the posterior annular-posterior longitudinal ligament complex, and the CSF in the adjacent thecal sac. Associated pathology, including small disc herniations, calcified ligaments, and small posterior bony vertebral body spurs, may be obscured by this technique. T2-weighted images in which the CSF has high signal intensity provide excellent delineation of these structures. The result is an MRI scan with a "myelographic" view of the spinal cord. Specifically, a RARE (fast spin echo), T2-weighted sequence is commonly used to reduce artifact/noise, which often complicates the longer T2-weighted image sequence.

Numerous studies have compared the accuracy of myelography, CT scan with or without dye, and MRI. Modic et al. prospectively compared the accuracy of MRI, myelography, and CT-myelography in evaluating patients with cervical radiculopathy. In this study, MRI was as sensitive as CT/myelography in the identification of a diseased segment but not as accurate in the exact identification of the disease process. Myelography alone was inferior to both studies. The authors concluded that an MRI accompanied by a plain CT scan provides excellent visualization of the cervical spine (81).

In summary, the authors believe that radiographic examination of cervical radiculopathy should begin with plain radiographs and then proceed to the appropriate noninvasive MRI sequences for preoperative evaluation. If there is any question as to the magnitude of lateral stenosis, quality of MRI, or extent of bony changes, a myelogram with a post-myelogram CT scan is warranted for preoperative planning. There is little role for tomography, discography, or bone scan in the evaluation of cervical radiculopathy.

Cervical Myelopathy

The etiology of cervical myelopathy is often multifactorial. Congenital narrowing may be associated with degenerative changes of the disc or thecal impingement from osteophyte formation and instabil-

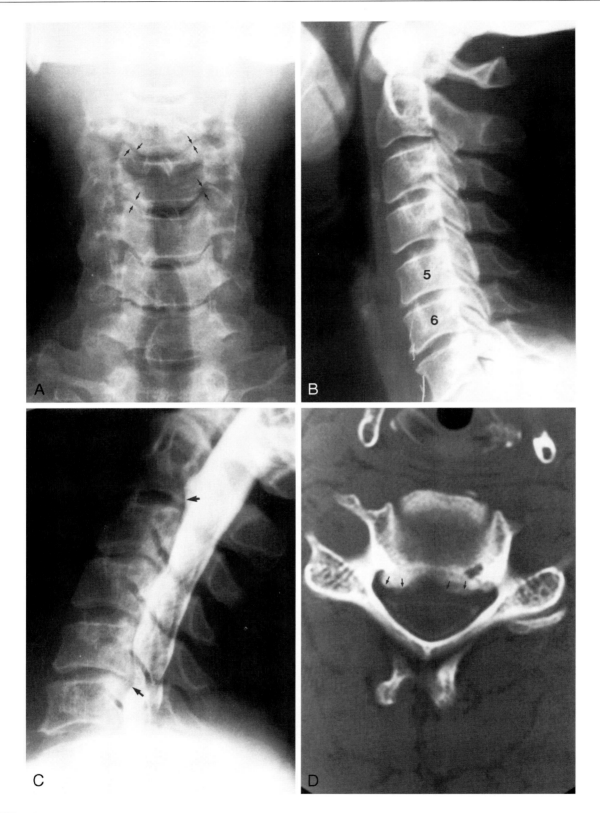

FIGURE 5.5.

A. AP radiograph of cervical spine with evidence of degenerative facet changes (arrowheads). **B.** Lateral radiograph of cervical spine with decreased disc space at the C5-C6 level. **C.** Cervical myelogram with narrowing of the dye pool at both the C3-C4 and C5-C6 levels. **D.** Post-myelogram CT scan with a spondylotic bar causing central stenosis and compression of the spinal cord at C5-C6.

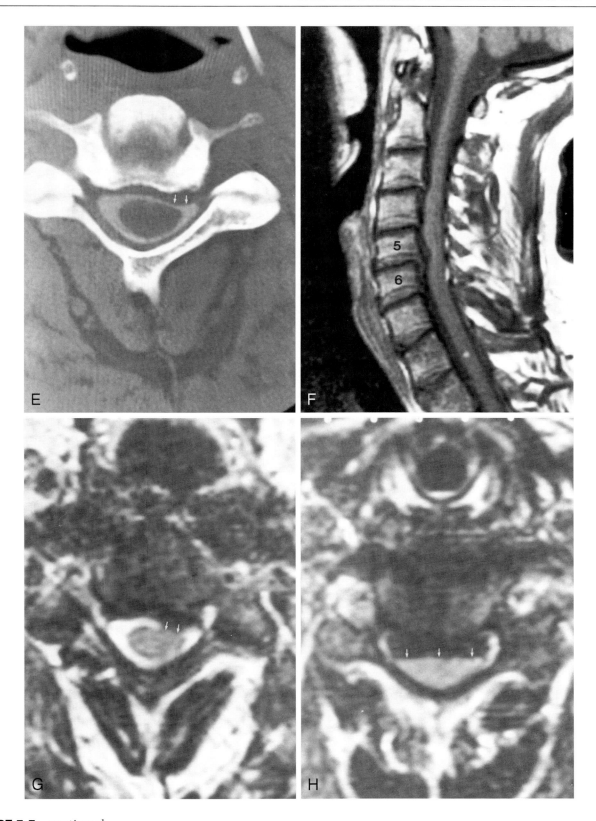

FIGURE 5.5—*continued*
E. Post- myelogram CT scan with soft disc protrusion causing impingement of contrast dye at the C3-C4 level. F. Sagittal MRI showing a small herniated disc at the C3-C4 level. There is a herniation at the C5-C6 level consisting of a free fragment. G. Axial MRI at the C3-C4 level showing a bulging soft disc on the left. H. Axial MRI at the C5-C6 level showing a large fragment of disc material compressing the spinal cord.

ity. Compression of the cord is the common finding in any mechanical cause of myelopathy, although vascular compromise should also be ruled out.

The entity of degenerative cervical myelopathy represents a continuum of cervical changes known as cervical spondylotic myelopathy (CSM). Brain and Wilkinson defined CSM as a progressive degeneration of the cervical disks and all of the surrounding structures, including the zygapophyseal joints and the joints of Luschka, as well as the formation of chondro-osseous spurs and thickening with infolding of the ligamentum flavum (16).

Plain radiographs, including flexion and extension views of patients with cervical myelopathy, are helpful for screening malalignment and instability. In addition, a decrease in disc space may be suggestive of degenerative disc disease. Evaluation of the AP canal diameter may be assessed by plain radiographs. With a 72-inch target-film distance, the commonly accepted canal diameter is roughly 17 to 18 millimeters (43). A measurement less than 13 millimeters is considered stenotic by definition. Oblique views may reveal posterior osteophytic spurs, which can narrow the space available for the cord and lead to stenosis.

After plain radiographs, CT/myelography or MRI may be used to determine stenotic changes leading to myelopathy. Visualization of degenerative changes, which include hyperostotic spurring of the vertebral body end-plates, uncinate processes, facet joints along with hypertrophied ligamentum flavum, and anterior facet capsules, allows for precise surgical and nonsurgical management. Many patients presenting with myelopathic findings also have a radicular component to their examination. The next test chosen to evaluate either myelopathy or myeloradiculopathy should have the capability to illustrate these cervical changes with bony and soft tissue components.

Before the development of MRI, myelography and CT-myelography were the gold standard for evaluation of cervical radiculopathy, myelopathy, and myeloradiculopathy. In an effort to avoid the invasive nature of CT-myelography, much attention in recent years has been aimed at improving the accuracy of MR sequences. Some studies suggest that MRI has been as effective as CT-myelography in evaluating cervical myelopathy (21, 57). Brown et al. looked at 256 patients who were screened for cervical radiculopathy and myelopathy by MRI. 34 patients with 50 diseased segments subsequently underwent surgery with a preoperative evaluation that included CT, myelography, and CT myelography. Disease defined as herniated discs, bony canal stenosis, and intradural lesions was predicted accurately by MRI in 88% of patients compared with 81% for CT myelography, 58% for myelography, and 50% for CAT scan. The authors pointed out that in two patients, herniated discs in the lateral root canals were visualized more readily by CT myelography than by MRI. The authors concluded that plain films along with MRI should be the first studies performed for surgical evaluation of cervical radiculopathy and myelopathy, while CT myelography is preferred for follow-up examination (20).

MRI evaluation of the cervical spine is more difficult than imaging of the lumbar spine. Standard sagittal T1- and T2-weighted sequences accompanied by newer axial 3D thin-section gradient echo sequences have provided improved insight into the exact etiology of cervical stenosis. MRI provides an unparalleled image of the spinal cord, allowing for measurement of cord volume, which many site as the best predictor of surgical outcome (37, 38). Shortcomings of MRI, particularly in the cervical spine, include difficulty delineating structures at the interface of the posterior vertebral body and thecal sac as well as inferior bony definition (Fig. 5.5).

The radiographic approach to cervical myelopathy is difficult and somewhat dependent upon the quality of imaging modalities available. Initial plain radiographs are typically followed by MRI studies. If the treatment regimen requires surgery, computerized axial tomography should be performed to better define bony structures. Furthermore, in the event that an MRI is unable to establish a precise diagnosis, myelography may be added to the CAT scan study to clarify soft tissue and bony relationships. A physician should not confuse health care cost containment with compromised patient care. If surgery is warranted, the precise approach and diagnosis must be established preoperatively because there is little or no role for exploratory surgery.

Lumbar Spine

The lifetime incidence of low back pain has been estimated at 60 to 80% and that of sciatica estimated at 40% (8). Roughly 50% of low back pain patients recover in two weeks and 90% recover in three months. Similarly, 50% of patients with sciatica recover in 1 month, and 95% recover in 6 months (8). With these promising recuperative statistics, the temporal sequence of ordering tests is as important as which test to order. The discussion of low back pain imaging is divided into evaluation of low back pain predominant (both acute and chronic) and leg pain predominant.

Acute Low Back Pain

As previously mentioned, the natural history of acute low back pain precludes early radiographic imaging. Except in patients less than 20 year of age or greater than 50 years of age, the relative indications for plain radiographs at the time of first presentation include history of; malignancy, trauma, neurologic deficits, infection, or constitutional symptoms. After 6 weeks of persistent symptoms, despite appropriate nonoperative management, plain radiographs, including anteroposterior and lateral, are obtained. At this point, tumor, infection, spondyloarthropathy, instability, hip disease, and pars interarticularis defects should be ruled out. If a pars defect is suspected, appropriate studies include oblique radiographs followed by a CT scan. Although degenerative changes including osteophyte formation, disc space narrowing, and facet hypertrophy are commonly found on plain radiographs, numerous studies have shown a poor correlation of these findings with clinical symptoms (102, 105, 107).

Mechanical low back pain caused by instability may be identified on lateral flexion and extension plain radiographs. The ability to accurately identify instability by this modality is confounded by the limitations of biplanar radiography. In fact, many believe that plain radiographs are unable to identify lumbar instability (1). The currently accepted definition of lumbar instability based on sagittal translation on flexion and extension views is instability greater than 3 mm (15, 88). Excessive angular rotatory change also can be identified on radiograph, although this may be more difficult.

After plain radiographs, radionuclide (technetium 99) bone scan may be helpful in finding infection, tumor, or fracture not identified on x-ray. In a study by De Nardo et al., 40% of patients with known metastatic disease had positive bone scan in the face of normal x-rays (31). Other studies have shown the value of a bone scan in the face of negative x-ray exams, particularly for tumor and fractures of osteoporotic bone (95, 96). The sensitivity of bone scan relies on its ability to detect bone turnover, which also makes it a very nonspecific test.

In the presence of acute low back pain with negative bone scan and radiograph, further diagnostic imaging should be performed only when a specific clinical diagnosis is suspected. MRI is often overused for the evaluation of acute low back pain. In fact, because most surgical procedures for degenerative causes of low back pain are not performed until after at least 6 months of nonoperative treatments, early MRI scans are discouraged because findings can change drastically over time and therefore alter preoperative planning or discogram level selection.

Chronic Low Back Pain

If the patient fails to improve after 6 to 10 weeks of treatment, the physician can rule-out occult tumor or infection by bone scan. After 4 to 6 months of low back pain, the physician may evaluate extraspinal causes of low back pain and the presence of disc degeneration. A noninvasive MRI with its capability for intraspinal and extraspinal imaging is the modality of choice. Fractures of the pars interarticularis are best seen on T1-weighted images, on which they are apparent long before detection by conventional radiographs or computerized axial tomography (61, 115). The T1-weighted image shows a hypotense signal in the area of the pars interarticularis. In addition, a marrow signal intensity may be seen in the marrow of the pedicle adjacent to the spondylitic defect. Instability of the lumbar spine despite a normal appearing disc space is represented by more subtle marrow MRI changes. Toyone et al. reviewed 74 patients who had degenerative lumbar disc disease and identified two types of marrow changes in patients with hypermobility; 70% had a decreased marrow signal, whereas 16% had an increased signal (104).

The magnetic resonance scan is now regarded as the best modality for visualization of degenerative disc disease. The T2-weighted image will have decreased intensity at the levels of degenerative discs because of relative dehydration. The most common level for degenerative disc changes is between the fourth and fifth lumbar levels, followed by fifth lumbar and sacrum. A young healthy disc appears bright on T2-weighted images and progressively darkens and loses height as the degenerative process advances (116). Clinical correlation of symptoms and MRI findings is imperative when planning care for degenerative disc disease. The incidence of MRI positive disc disease in asymptomatic patients is age-specific but ranges from 35 to 93% (14, 59). The degenerative disc changes seen on MRI often are accompanied by changes in the bone marrow of adjacent vertebral bodies. Modic et al. identified three patterns: Type 1-decreased signal intensity on T1-weighted spin echo images and increased signal intensity on T2-weighted images; Type 2-increased signal intensity on T1-weighted images and a normal or slightly increased intensity on T2-weighted images; and Type 3-hypotense signals on both T1- and T2-weighted images (82, 83).

If MRI reveals one or two isolated degenerative disc levels, the physician must determine if provocative tests, such as discography, will aid in managing the patient with chronic low back pain. Discography is superior to CT scan without contrast or myelography for the identification of disc degeneration and annular tears, and it may be superior to MRI for identification of annular tears (6, 47, 78, 117). Because discography is a provocative test, the most important reporting criteria is the concordance of pain with diseased segments and the absence of pain during injection of normal disc spaces. Studies by both Holt and Walsh have emphasized the importance of pain concordance when interpreting discography (99, 109). There are no prospective studies that have correlated the incidence of positive discograms to successful lumbar fusions.

Leg Pain Predominant

The patient with sciatica, regardless of the presence of low back pain, is approached differently than is the patient with predominantly low back pain. The need for emergent imaging is based on clinical findings suggestive of tumor, infection, trauma, or cauda equina syndrome with bowel or bladder symptoms. Most patients can be treated without imaging for 6 to 8 weeks. Clearly, the majority of sciatic symptoms occur as a result of a herniated nucleus pulposus (HNP) or spinal stenosis.

Aside from ruling out other etiologies, plain radiographs add little to the evaluation of leg pain secondary to either stenosis or HNP. In the 1980s, computed tomography replaced myelography as the modality of choice for diagnosing a lumbar HNP (51). Schipper et al. reviewed over 450 patients and found the sensitivity and specificity of CT scan to be roughly 10% better than myelography. Computed tomography has proven particularly useful in diagnosing far lateral disc herniations (44, 101). The combination of myelography and computed axial tomography has exceeded that of either study alone (45, 54, 108).

MRI is now considered to be the most sensitive test for diagnosing herniated discs. The importance of clinical correlation has been brought out in work by Boden et al. who showed a 28% prevalence of disc herniations in asymptomatic volunteers (14). The possibility of distinguishing symptomatic from asymptomatic discs by visualizing gadolinium enhancement of nerve roots is currently under investigation (30, 60, 103). MRI is superior to other modalities not only for identifying herniated discs but also for distinguishing between sequestered and contained fragments (64, 75, 98). This added information may assist the surgeon in removing offending disc material (Fig. 5.6).

Evaluation of neurogenic claudication associated with leg pain may be accomplished best by a post-myelographic CT scan or MRI. The CT/myelogram study allows for optimal visualization of bony structures in patients who have stenosis. Hard discs and hypertrophic spurs are displayed readily along with the secondary compression of the neural elements. In addition, pedicle anatomy can be studied for potential intraoperative instrumentation. The severity of stenosis may be ascertained by the presence of complete blocks on myelography. With respect to MRI and stenosis, some feel this modality overexaggerates thecal sac impingement.

Two less common causes of predominant leg pain with or without low back symptoms are facet cysts and isthmic spondylolisthesis. MRI provides adequate images of both processes. Facet cysts most

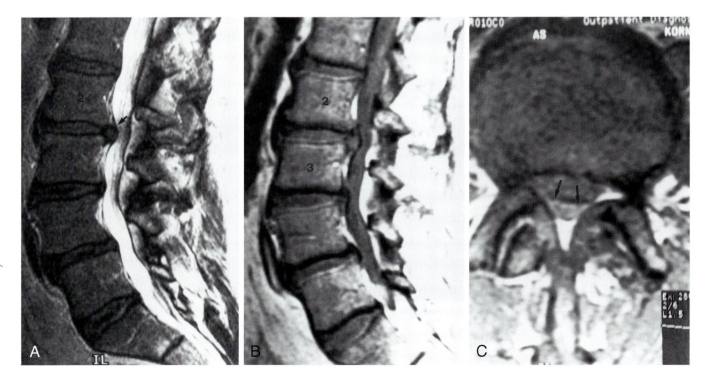

FIGURE 5.6.

A. T2-weighted image of a herniated nucleus pulposus at the L2-L3 level. **B.** T1-weighted image of a herniated nucleus pulposus at the L2-L3 level. **C.** Axial MRI image of the L2-L3 HNP (arrowheads).

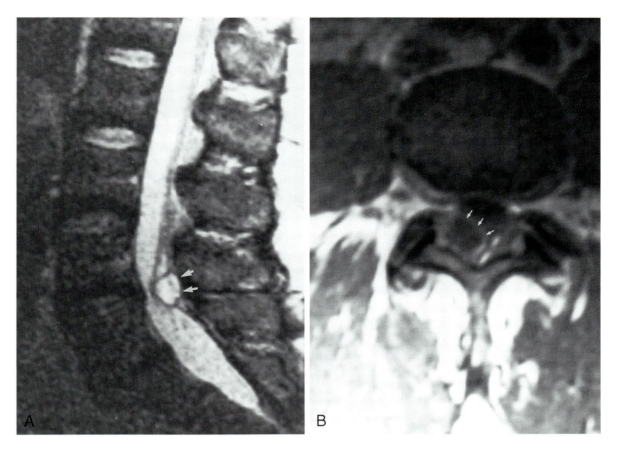

FIGURE 5.7.
A. T2-weighted sagittal MRI with a typical high signal facet cyst (arrow) at the L4-L5 level. **B.** Large right facet cyst (closed arrow) and smaller left facet cyst (open arrow) seen on T1-weighted axial MRI.

commonly occur at the junction of the fourth and fifth lumbar vertebrae. On MRI they appear as a dorsal epidural mass of varying intensity (58, 73, 114). In one study of 17 patients with isthmic spondylolisthesis, the parasagittal MRI showed abnormal images in all patients (5) (Fig. 5.7).

The role of discography in patients who predominantly report leg pain is limited. A tear in the annulus without herniation of disc material may allow for extravasation of enzymatic fluids leading to a radiculitis. In this situation, a discogram may show injected dye leaking through an annular tear near the affected nerve root (76).

Imaging of the Postoperative Lumbar Spine

The failure rate after initial lumbar spine surgery has been estimated to be between 15 and 40%, representing 25,000 to 50,000 failures per year (56). The constellation of postoperative symptoms, including persistent low back pain sciatica and impairment, is known as failed back surgery syndrome (FBSS). Imaging of the postoperative spine presents a set of unique obstacles that must be overcome to properly manage this challenging patient population.

Leg Pain Predominant

Once mechanical instability, bony stenosis, and arachnoiditis have been ruled out, the two most common causes of leg pain in FBSS are secondary to residual or recurrent disc and scar formation. It is therefore imperative to distinguish adequately these two entities because the surgical outcome of each is drastically different. Whereas patients with retained fragments may benefit from further surgery, those with scar formation tend to do poorly (35).

Computed axial tomography with and without intravenous contrast has been used to image the postoperative lumbar spine. The distinction between scar and disc has been shown to be approximately 75% with a range in the literature from 67 to 100% (23, 56). On CT scan examination, discs are seen as areas of decreased attenuation frequently with a rim of enhancement. Epidural fibrosis demonstrates homogeneous enhancement with intravenous contrast agents. In general, the unenhanced CT scan can be used to study mass effects, morphology, location, and density of offending tissue. Abnormal tissue that is seen above or below a disk space with evidence of thecal retraction and a linear pattern is more likely to represent scar formation (56).

MRI has quickly become the modality of choice for distinguishing between scar and disk in the postoperative spine. Unenhanced MRI is reported to have an accuracy equivalent to contrast enhanced CT scanning (76 to 89%) (22, 23, 100). The diagnostic accuracy of enhanced MRI has been reported to be as high as 100% with a range of 96 to 100% (27, 56).

Postoperative scarring typically presents on MRI as an extradural mass of irregular configuration with unsharp margination and without disc space continuity (41). As Genant points out, signal intensity depends on a number of factors, including scar morphology, fat content, age of the scar, vascularity, location, and inflammation. Initially, scars appear hyperintense on T2-weighted images because of inflammatory factors leading to a relatively high water content. As the scar matures, the T2 signal becomes less intense as the amount of fibrosis increases. With maturity, scars become hypointense on both T1- and T2-weighted images. Non-ionic contrast agents such as Gadolinium-DTPA/dimeglumine enhance abnormal soft tissue changes. Early images (those taken within 10 minutes of injection) tend to highlight scar formation. Delayed images tend to have a more homogeneous signal. It is postulated that the increased vascularity of scar allows for an early pooling of the contrast agent followed by an equilibration phase. This would explain the benefit for early phase imaging of scar formation after the introduction of a contrast media. Both human and animal investigations have shown that the optimal time for early phase imaging is within 5 to 6 minutes of contrast introduction (39).

Unlike postoperative scar, the morphology of residual disc material includes sharply marginated globules contiguous with the index disc space. Furthermore, in contrast to scar, residual disc material is relatively avascular and behaves as such when imaged with MRI. On T1-weighted images, contrast is seen between residual disc and the hyperintense epidural fat and hypointense thecal sac. On T2-weighted image, contrast is seen next to the hyperintense thecal sac. A mass effect with compression of the thecal sac is more typical for recurrent disc material than for scarring. Early post-gadolinium images usually appear isotense or hypointense because of the relative avascularity of disc material. Delayed-phase imaging, greater than 30 to 40 minutes, generally shows an increase in signal intensity most likely from the eventual equilibration of contrast agents (41).

The incidence of abnormal findings in asymptomatic postoperative patients is unfortunately high for both computed tomography and MRI. CT studies have shown a 44% incidence of postoperative changes consistent with preoperative pathology in both symptomatic and asymptomatic individuals (28). Work by Boden et al. demonstrated the progression of image changes on MRI that occur within the first 6 months following lumbar surgery. The authors concluded that despite the use of gadolinium, management decisions based on MRI findings obtained within the first 3 to 6 months after surgery should be done carefully. There is a series of normal postoperative changes in asymptomatic patients after successful discectomy which may demonstrate a mass effect initially and then resolve over time (13).

Arachnoiditis, another postoperative finding which complicates lumbar spine surgery, may be visualized by gadolinium-enhanced MRI. Three distinct patterns have been described by Delamarter et al. (32). Contrast enhancement of thickened nerve roots in the dural sac is seen in patients who have documented arachnoiditis.

Back Pain Predominant

It is estimated that of the many spinal fusions performed each year for instability, as many as 30 to 40% have recurrent pain (25). The diagnosis of pseudoarthrosis is often very difficult to make using conventional imaging modalities. Plain radiographs, conventional pluridirectional tomography (CPT), and CT scan may be useful for imaging gross structural patterns but have a limited role in determining the functional stability of an arthrodesis. Careful interpretation of coronal CPT and 3-D CT scan images have at times offered supportive findings in the clinically suspect pseudoarthrosis. Only MRI has the potential to indicate the functional stability of an arthrodesis. The initial source of a bone graft determines its appearance on early MRI images. Because of their high fat content, autogenous bone grafts appear bright on T1-weighted images, whereas allografts show low signal intensity on both T1- and T2-weighted images. In a structurally intact arthrodesis, the subchondral bone of adjacent vertebral bodies has an increased signal intensity on T1-weighted sequences. As the transmission of load is circumvented through the fusion mass, the decrease in load bearing of the adjacent vertebra allows for fat replacement and this characteristic MRI imaging pattern (41). MRI characteristics for an unstable spine secondary to pseudoarthrosis include neighboring endplates with a low signal intensity on T1-weighted images and high signal intensity on T2-weighted images. These characteristics occur as a result of a constant inflammatory cycle secondary to lumbar spine instability (67). Unfortunately, diagnostic imaging of a failed arthrodesis remains a difficult problem for even experienced physicians and often requires surgical exploration to obtain a definitive diagnosis.

Infection

Infections of the spine have for many years posed a complex issue for both diagnosis and treatment. Along with the rising number of cases of acquired immunodeficiency disease syndrome (AIDS) has come an increase in the number of reported spine infections. Ninety-two percent of infected spines will present with a history of back pain, and the most common location is the lumbar spine (85).

Plain radiography often does not show any evidence of infection for the first 2 to 8 weeks of the disease process. Often the earliest sign of pyogenic osteomyelitis is evidence of paravertebral soft tissue swelling. The temporal sequence of findings on plain radiographs according to Wisneski include the following: end plate erosion and decreased bone density adjacent to disc spaces in the early stage; bony destruction at 3 to 6 weeks; and destruction and narrowing with sclerosis of the endplates at 8 weeks (112). Modic et al. found plain radiographs to have a sensitivity of 82%, a specificity of 57%, and an accuracy 73% for diagnosing spinal infections (79).

Radionuclide studies can be very helpful in diagnosing early spine infection. The sensitivity and specificity of bone scan for detection of infection has been as high as 95% and 92%, respectively, compared with 32% and 89% for plain radiography (86). In the two early phases of a technetium scan, representing blood flow and blood pooling hot spots are seen in the hyperemic infected vertebral bodies. In the third phase, diffuse patterns seen on earlier phases become more focal. Patients who are clinically suspected of having a spine infection with a negative technetium scan should undergo a gallium scan. As discussed earlier, gallium-67 citrate has an affinity for polymorphonuclear leukocytes and bacteria. This modality is particularly useful for following infection because images will return to normal with the eradication of infection. Finally, indium labeled white blood cell scans are particularly useful for detecting infection penetrance into surrounding soft tissue (112).

Magnetic resonance imaging has become the modality of choice for diagnosing spine infections. MRI has been shown to have a sensitivity of 96%, a specificity of 92%, and an accuracy of 94%, which is roughly equivalent to technetium and gallium scans when used together (80). However, the soft tissue visualization that MRI affords is unparalleled. These details unique to MRI may dictate treatment protocols and predict neurologic sequelae. Standard MRI sequences should include T1- and T2-weighted images as well as T1 post-gadolinium imaging. On T1-weighted images, signal intensity of disc and vertebrate decreases in the presence of osteomyelitis. Conversely, on T2-weighted images, both disc and involved vertebrate appear hyperintense. Gadolinium adds to the sensitivity of diagnosing infection and plays a useful role in following the infectious process once therapy has begun (91). In addition, gadolinium-enhanced MRI is the modality of choice for imaging intraspinal cord infections. An enhanced and enlarged discreet lesion is visualized readily with the help of gadolinium. Finally, gadolinium-enhanced MRI has become recognized as the modality of choice for imaging spinal cord diseases in patients with AIDS (90) (Fig. 5.8).

Although most of the necessary information is available from MRI, typical bone changes and gas formation from abscesses are seen more readily on CT scan (17). CT scan changes consistent with tubercu-

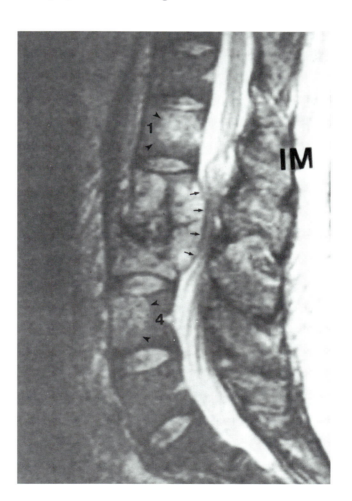

FIGURE 5.8.

Destruction of L2 and L3 with involvement of the intervening disc space secondary to tuberculosis (Pott's disease). Extension of lesion has lead to cauda equina compression (arrows) and neurologic deficits. Also found incidentally were hemangiomas of L1 and L4 (arrowheads).

losis include anterior vertebral body destruction with disc space involvement resulting in narrowing along with calcification of paravertebral masses (24). In comparison to pyogenic infections, tuberculous spondylitis is less likely to be sclerotic or osteophytic but more apt to have multiple vertebral segments involved with calcification of paraspinal abscesses (65). Fungal infections of the spine are typically found in the immunocompromised population. Early in the clinical course there is involvement of the vertebral body that usually spares disc spaces. Paraspinal abscesses are common late in the course, whereas epidural lesions are relatively rare (93). Findings on post-myelogram computerized axial tomography suggestive of arachnoiditis include a loss of nerve root sleeve filling with a matting of nerve roots. An "empty sac" appearance in the lumbarsacral region may occur as a result of nerve roots adhering to the thecal sac (93). CT scan can be used to assess the degree of bone destruction when making decisions about potential instability and reconstructive options.

Tumor Imaging

The spine is the most common place for skeletal metastases to occur. Roughly 5% of all patients with a malignancy will have metastatic disease to the spine (11). The most common metastatic tumors of the spine metastasize from the breast, lung, prostate, and lymphatic system. Along with multiple myeloma, these metastatic diseases represent 60% of metastatic disease in one review of 2800 cases (77).

The evaluation and staging of spine tumors generally include up to four imaging modalities. Plain radiographs, radionuclide scans, CT scan, and MRI all play a role in diagnosing and treating tumors of the spine. The pathophysiology, clinical workup, and treatment protocol for specific tumors will be discussed in a later chapter.

Although the value of plain radiographs in spine tumor evaluation may be argued, it is typically the first imaging modality to be obtained. In the presence of gross vertebral destruction, plain radiographs may be helpful in making a diagnosis. Plain radiographs show spinal deformity such as progressive kyphosis resulting from collapse of vertebral bodies and can be monitored on serial studies. This information may be helpful in formulating a treatment plan; however, these changes occur later in the clinical course of metastatic disease. It has been theorized that because of the relatively rich vascular supply of the vertebral body, the preponderance of metastatic disease is found anteriorly. In contrast, most tumors of the posterior elements are benign or have primary characteristics. Osteoblastomas, aneurysmal bone cysts, and osteoid osteomas are three of the more common benign tumors found in the posterior elements. The general guidelines presented here concerning anterior versus posterior lesions have many exceptions and should not supersede clinical suspicions. Radiographically, pedicle destruction and not vertebral body destruction is often the first radiographic evidence of metastatic disease. On an AP view of the spine, destruction of a single pedicle results in the "winking owl sign." Because destruction of 30 to 40% of the vertebral body is needed before detection by routine radiographs, the "winking owl" sign often is the first clue to the presence of metastatic disease (49).

In the absence of a neurologic deficit, the first two modalities ordered may be plain radiographs and radionuclide imaging. Radionuclide imaging is a sensitive test that is part of the preliminary evaluation of persistent back pain in the absence of radiculopathy and myelopathy. Patients suspected of having a spinal tumor, whether it be from a primary posterior element tumor (i.e., osteoid osteoma) or a metastatic process of the anterior column, are screened adequately with a technetium-99 bone scan. Focal uptake is seen in regions with an increase in bone turnover, particularly in areas that have new bone being laid. This blastic process and the associated increased local vascularity produce "hot" scans (49). The focal uptake seen on the initial phase of bone scanning directly reflects this increased vascularity.

The formation of woven bone in response to tumor infiltration is responsible for the increased uptake seen in the second or delayed phase of technetium scintography. This pathophysiology on which technetium-99 scans are based allows for detection of tumors up to 18 months earlier than with routine radiographs (40). The false negative rate of radionuclide imaging has been as low as 2% compared with 50% for plain radiographs. This highly sensitive test not only enables the physician to evaluate patients with back pain, but also, through serial scans, allows the physician to follow patients with known primary malignancies predisposed to axial and appendicular metastases. Initial bone scanning for back pain may also show focal uptake at the site of the primary organ malignancy, expediting comprehensive care of the patient and making technetium scans an excellent first line imaging modality.

Unfortunately, the very mechanism that provides bone scans with a high sensitivity is also responsible for the relative nonspecificity of this test. Any condition that is associated with an increased osteoblastic process and vascularity may portray a "hot scan." Bone scans are therefore unable to differentiate between tumor, infection, osteoarthritis, and fracture. Another disadvantage of bone scan is its inability to emphasize a specific "hot spot" as the source of pain or neurologic deficit when multiple areas of the spine show an increased uptake. Similarly, technetium scans cannot be used to follow the progression of a destructive process. False negative bone scans may occur despite the presence of a tumorous condition if there is little reactive bone formation or little increase in vascularity, which may occur with slow growing lesions. Certain malignancies routinely have a negative or "cold" scan. Multiple myeloma is the most common primary malignancy of the spine but has a cold scan in an estimated 40% of lesions. A disproportionately greater amount of osteoclastic versus osteoblastic activity is responsible for this phenomenon (113).

Before the development of MRI, post-myelography CT scans were instrumental for evaluating spine tumors. The ability to delineate both destructive and reactive bony structures perhaps remains its biggest contribution in imaging spine tumors. Preoperatively, a CT scan with axial and 3D reconstruction images is often useful for planning both surgical resection and reconstruction. The limited field of view inherent to CT scan studies remains one of its biggest drawbacks. In a review of 62 patients with myelographic evidence of cord compression, 6 patients had a second site of compression separated by an average of 12 vertebral segments (10).

MRI has become the modality of choice for localizing spine tumors. For radiographic purposes, these tumors may be organized into four categories based on location: 1) intramedullary, 2) intradural-extramedullary, 3) extradural, and 4) osseous. Numerous studies have shown MRI to be the most accurate study for intramedullary pathology (53, 89). Because of differences between signal intensity of blood, cyst, and tumor, MRI is able to provide insight into the character of the lesion. Intramedullary cord tumors may be isointense or hypointense on T1-weighted images and isointense or hyperintense on T2-weighted images. Intradural-extramedullary lesions are best imaged with the addition of gadolinium. Carmody et al. found the specificity and accuracy of MRI and myelography to be approximately equal for intradural-extramedullary lesions. In the same study, however, a significant difference was seen between myelography and MRI when imaging extradural masses. The sensitivity and specificity of MRI was 73% and 90%, respectively, versus 49% and 88% respectively for myelography. The authors suggested MRI to be the preferred first imaging modality for studying cord compression (26).

MRI imaging of osseous lesions of the spine largely depends on the replacement and destruction of red and yellow marrow components. Red marrow is composed of 40% water, 40% fat, and 20% protein, whereas yellow marrow is composed of 15% water, 80% fat, and 5% protein. T1-weighted images become hypointense in fat depleting processes. However, it is the T2-weighted sequences that are used to

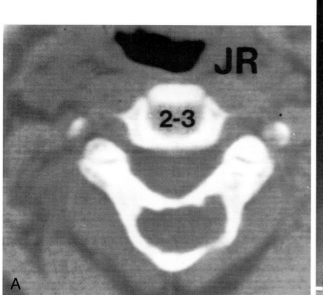
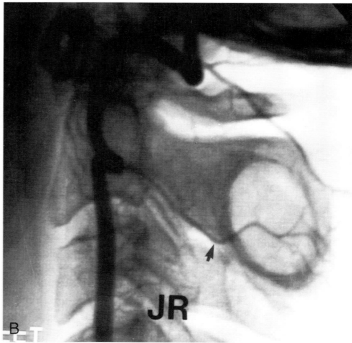

FIGURE 5.9.
A. CT scan of a well circumscribed lytic lesion of the posterior elements of C2 consistent with an aneurysmal bone cyst.
B. Arteriogram of lesion revealing a prominent vascular supply (arrow).

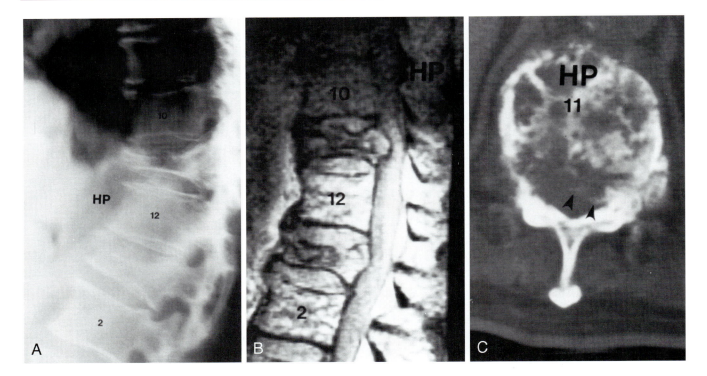

FIGURE 5.10.
A. Atraumatic compression fractures of T11 and L1. **B.** Sagittal MRI with nonhomogeneous signals at the T11 and L1 levels. **C.** CT scan of T11 revealing a destructive lesion causing cord compression (arrowheads) consistent with multiple myeloma.

best image pathologic tissue usually with a relative increased water content from inflammatory processes or increased vascularity. If the degree of bone destruction is not clear on the MR scan, then a CT scan will provide complementary information necessary for decisions about spine structural stability and reconstructive options.

The distinction between a simple compression fracture and a pathologic fracture secondary to tumor is particularly difficult. No current consensus exists as to the value of MRI for making this diagnosis. One study reported chronic benign fractures as having a homogeneous isotense signal on both T1 and T2 weighted sequences. Pathologic vertebral fractures had a decreased signal intensity on T1 images and an increased signal on T2 images. Acute benign fractures were also found to have increased signal intensity on T2 images but were inhomogeneous in their signal (7).

The differentiation between tumor and infection is another often difficult clinical and radiographic diagnosis. An et al. reviewed the radiographic studies of patients who had proven spine infection or tumor and found MRI to be superior to other modalities for making this distinction. Based on their work, the authors made five observations regarding the use of MRI for distinguishing between tumor and infection. Involvement of disc space and adjacent vertebral bodies with decreased signal intensity on T1-weighted images and increased signal intensity on T2-weighted images was the most consistent finding for vertebral osteomyelitis. End plate destruction was more common with infection than with tumor. Infection processes were more apt to have contiguous vertebral involvement. Fat planes were regionally disrupted with infection while only focally disrupted or intact with tumor (3) (Figs. 5.9, 5.10).

Spine Trauma Imaging

Patients that present with an apparent traumatic spine fracture should have plain films obtained of their entire spine, including the sacral region. Several studies have shown an incidence of noncontiguous fractures in patients who have apparent isolated traumatic vertebrate injuries (2, 106). The standard cervical spine films include anteroposterior, lateral, and open mouth views; some physicians prefer to add oblique views, particularly if facet disruption has occurred. It is important to visualize the entire cervical spine, from the occiput-C1 articulation to the C7-T1 articulation. If imaging of the cervicothoracic junction is difficult, a swimmer's view or Twinning view allows evaluation of this region. Visualization of the thoracic and lumbar region is obtained adequately with anteroposterior and lateral radiographs. Again, some institutions advocate oblique films of the lumbar region. The role of dynamic plain radio-

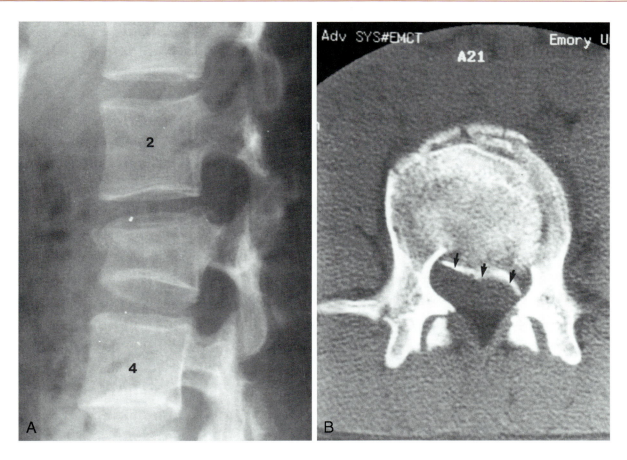

FIGURE 5.11.

A. Lateral radiograph of an L3 burst fracture. **B.** CT scan of burst fracture with retropulsed bone resulting in canal compromise (arrows).

graphs in the setting of acute trauma is somewhat dependent on the judgment of the physician. Without evidence of cervical injury on plain radiographs and a low energy of injury, erect flexion/extension films may be obtained. However, if there is a moderate question as to cervical stability, despite normal radiographs, flexion/extension films can be obtained with the patient supine while sequentially altering head position with pillows. Alternatively, in patients with significant neck pain and a normal neck series, patients may be maintained in a cervical collar and imaged with flexion/extension views in 2 weeks during an office follow-up. In the absence of a neurologic deficit, the next modality obtained should be a CT scan with 3-mm slices. CT scan examination should be performed as dictated based on plain radiographs and physical examination. These axial images along with 3D reconstruction are often the basis for nonoperative and preoperative treatment protocols. Fractures of the dens often are better visualized with longitudinal conventional pluridirectional tomography. In the presence of a neurologic deficit, MRI is the modality of choice for imaging the spinal cord. Cord compression from bony or soft tissue structures can be identified readily. Spinal cord pathology is best visualized with T2-weighted sequences, although both T1 and T2 sequences should be obtained. Gradient echo sequences are the most sensitive for detecting hemosiderin deposits. In patients requiring a cervical reduction, some studies advocate MRI imaging of the spine before any attempted reduction. MRI allows for the identification of traumatic herniated discs that may cause catastrophic complications if unrecognized before cervical reduction (34) (Fig. 5.11).

Summary

Diagnostic imaging of the spine is perhaps second in importance only to taking a history and performing a physical examination for evaluating spinal pathology. The development and refinement of advanced modalities have provided for a vast improvement in the visualization of spine anatomy. In some cases, this very advancement has caused confusion as to what and when to order which test. To maximize imaging of pathology and minimize unnecessary testing, it behooves the physician to have a basic understanding of the advantages and limitations of each study ordered. The choice and temporal sequence of

TABLE 5.2.
Suggested Imaging Modality Utilization

Modality Pathology	X-ray	Tomos	Myelo	CT	CT/Myelo	MRI	Disco	BS
Neck pain	1					3	4	2
Cerv radic	1			3		2		
Cerv myel	1			3		2		
LBP (acute)	1							
LBP (chron)	1					2	3	2
LBP/Leg	1					2		
Postop			1	1		1(gad)		
Infect	1		3		2			
Tumor	1		3		2			2
Trauma	1	2	2		3			

Suggested order in which modalities are ordered until a diagnosis is made. The temporal sequence has been well outlined in this chapter. Certain choices depend on specific clinical scenarios and presumed diagnoses. For example, in the case of an odontoid fracture identified on plain films, the physician may order tomograms, particularly if CT scan 3-D reconstructions are not available. In other cervical spine fractures, the CT scan is consistently the second image modality obtained.

study is based on the clinician's well thought out working diagnosis based on patient symptomatology. By having a general understanding of imaging modalities and selectively ordering tests, the physician can expedite efficient patient care in an economic fashion (Table 5.2).

References

1. Abe M, Shinomiya K, Nakai O, et al. A study of validity of recumbent roentgenograms of the lumbar spine on forward flexion as used to measure mobility in patients with low back pain. Presented at the 21st Annual Meeting of the International Society for Study of the Lumbar Spine, June 21–25, 1994, Seattle, WA. Spine 1994.
2. Albert TA, Levine MJ, Balderston RA, et al. Concomitant noncontiguous thoracolumbar and sacral fractures. Spine 1993;18:1285–1291.
3. An HS, Vaccaro AR, Dolinskas CA, et al. Differentiation between spinal tumors and infections with magnetic resonance imaging. Spine 1991;16(Suppl):334–338.
4. Anderson PE. Relative effectiveness of computed and conventional tomography in lesions of the spine. In: Littleton JT, Durizch ML, eds. Sectional imaging methods: a comparison. Baltimore: University Park Press, 1983:235–243.
5. Annertz M, Holtas S, Cronqvist S, et al. Isthmic lumbar spondylolisthesis with sciatica. MR imaging vs. myelography. Acta Radiol 1990;31:449–453.
6. Antti-Poika I, Soini J, Tallroth K, et al. Clinical relevance of discography combined with CT scanning. A study of 100 patients. J Bone Joint Surg Br 1990;72:480–485.
7. Baker LL, Goodman SB, Perkash I, et al. Benign versus pathologic compression fractures of vertebral bodies: assessment with conventional spin-echo, chemical-shift, and STIR MR imaging. Radiology 1990;174:495–502.
8. Bell GB. Lumbar spine. In: Frymoyer JW, ed. Orthopaedic knowledge update 4. Rosemont: AAOS, 1993:491–501.
9. Bell GR, Ross JS. Diagnosis of nerve root compression. Orthop Clin North Am 1992;23:405–419.
10. Bernat JL, Greenberg ER, Barrett J. Suspected epidural compression of the spinal cord and cauda equina by metastatic carcinoma; clinical diagnosis and survival. Cancer 1957;51:1953–1957.
11. Black P. Spinal metastasis: current status and recommended guidelines for management. Neurosurgery 1979;5:726–746.
12. Boden SD. Diagnostic imaging of the spine. In: Weinstein JN, Rydevik BL, Sonntag VKH, eds. Essentials of the spine. 2nd ed. New York: Raven Press, 1995:97–110.
13. Boden SD, Davis DO, Dina TS, et al. Contrast-enhanced MR imaging performed after successful lumbar disk surgery: prospective study. Radiology 1992;182:59–64.
14. Boden SD, Davis DO, Dina TS, et al. Abnormal magnetic-resonance scans of the lumbar spine in asymptomatic subjects. A prospective investigation. J Bone Joint Surg Am 1990;72:403–408.
15. Boden SD, Wiesel SW. Lumbosacral segmental motion in normal individuals: have we been measuring instability properly? Spine 1990;15:571–576.
16. Brain L, Wilkinson M, eds. Cervical spondylosis and other disorders of the cervical spine. Philadelphia: WB Saunders, 1967.
17. Brant-Zawadzki M, Burke VD, Jeffrey RB. CT in evaluation of spine infection. Spine 1983;8:358–364.
18. Breger RK, Rimm AA, Fischer ME, et al. T1 and T2 measurements on a 1.5 T commercial MR imager. Radiology 1989;17:273–276.
19. Brekkan A. A radiographic examination of the lumbosacral spine: an "age stratified" study. Clin Radiol 1983;34:321–324.
20. Brown BM, Schwartz AH, Frank E, et al. Preoperative evaluation of cervical radiculopathy and myelopathy by surface-coil MR imaging. AJR Am J Roentgenol 1988;151:1205–1212.
21. Brown BM, Schwartz RH, Frank E, et al. Preoperative evaluation of cervical radiculopathy and myelopathy by surface-coil MR imaging. AJR Am J Roentgenol 1988;151:1205–1212.
22. Bundschuh CV, Modic MT, Ross JS. Epidural fibrosis

and recurrent disk herniation in the lumbar spine: MR imaging assessment. AJNR Am J Neuroradiol 1988; 90:169–178.
23. Bundschuh CV, Stein L, Slusser JH. Distinguishing between scar and recurrent herniated disk in postoperative patients: value of contrast-enhanced CT and MR imaging. AJNR Am J Neuroradiol 1990;11:949–958.
24. Burke DR, Brant-Zawadzki MB. CT of pyogenic spine infection. Neuroradiology 1985;27:131–137.
25. Burton CV. Causes of failure of surgery on the lumbar spine: Ten-year follow-up. Mt Sinai J Med 1991; 58:183–187.
26. Carmody RF, Yang PJ, Seley GW, et al. Spinal cord compression due to metastatic disease: diagnosis with MR imaging versus myelography. Radiology 1989; 173:225–229.
27. Cervellini P, Curri D, Bernardi L, et al. Computed tomography after lumbar disc surgery: a comparison between symptomatic and asymptomatic patients. Acta Neurochir Suppl (Wien) 1988;43:44–47.
28. Cervellini P, Curri D, Volpin L, et al. Computed tomography of epidural fibrosis after discectomy: a comparison between symptomatic and asymptomatic patients. Neurosurgery 1988;23:710–713.
29. Chafetz N, Genant HK, Gillespy T, et al. Magnetic resonance imaging. In: Kricun ME, ed. Imaging modalities in spinal disorders. Philadelphia: WB Saunders, 1988:478–502.
30. Crisi G, Carpeggiani P, Trevisan C. Gadolinium-enhanced nerve roots in lumbar disk herniation. AJNR Am J Neuroradiol 1993;14:1379–1392.
31. De Nardo GL, Jacogson SJ, Raventos A. 85-Sr bone scan in neoplastic disease. Semin Nucl Med 1972; 2:18–25.
32. Delamarter RB, Ross JS, Masaryk TJ, et al. Diagnosis of lumbar arachnoiditis by magnetic resonance imaging. Spine 1990;15:304–310.
33. Eisenberg RL, Akin JR, Hedgcock MW. Single, well-centered lateral view of lumbosacral spine: Is coned view necessary? AJR Am J Roentgenol 1979;133:711–713.
34. Eismont FJ, Arena MJ, Green BA. Extrusion of an intervertebral disc associated with traumatic subluxation or dislocation of cervical facets. J Bone Joint Surg Am 1991;73:1555–1556.
35. Finnegan WJ, Fenlin JM, Marvel JP. Results of surgical intervention in the symptomatic multiply-operated back patient. J Bone Joint Surg Am 1979;61:1077–1082.
36. Friedenberg ZB, Miller WT. Degenerative disc disease of the cervical spine. J Bone Joint Surg Am 1963; 45:1171–1178.
37. Fujiwara K, Yonenobu K, Ebara S, et al. The prognosis of surgery for cervical compression myelopathy: an analysis of the factors involved. J Bone Joint Surg Br 1989;71:393–398.
38. Fujiwara K, Yonenobu K, Hiroshima K, et al. Morphometry of the cervical spinal cord and its relation to pathology in cases with compression myelopathy. Spine 1988;13:1212–1216.
39. Gabrielsen TO, Gebarski SS, Knake JE, et al. Iohexol versus metrizamide for lumbar myelography: double-blind trial. AJR Am J Roentgenol 1984;142:1047–1049.
40. Galasko CSB. The significance of occult skeletal metastases detected by skeletal scintigraphy, in patient with otherwise apparently 'early' mammary carcinoma. J Bone Joint Surg Br 1975;62:694–696.
41. Genant HK. Magnetic resonance imaging of the postoperative spine. In: Schafer M, ed. Instructional course lectures; volume 43. Rosemont: AAOS, 1994: 471–473.
42. Ghelman B. Discography. In: Kricun ME, ed. Imaging modalities in spinal disorders. Philadelphia: WB Saunders, 1988:538–556.
43. Gibson G. Radiographic evaluation of the cervical spine. Spine:State Art Rev 1991;5:177–187.
44. Godersky JC, Erickson DL, Seljeskog EL. Extreme lateral disc herniation: diagnosis by computed tomographic scanning. Neurosurgery 1984;14:549–552.
45. Goldberg AL, Soo MS, Deeb ZL, et al. Degenerative disease of the lumbar spine. Role of CT-myelography in the MR era. Clin Imaging 1991;15:47–55.
46. Gore DA, Sepic SB, Gardner GM. Roentgenographic findings of the cervical spine in asymptomatic people. Spine 1986;11:521–525.
47. Grubb SA, Lipscomb HJ, Guilford WB. The relative value of lumbar roentgenograms, metrizamide myelography, and discography in the assessment of patients with chronic low-back syndrome. Spine 1987; 12:282–286.
48. Hansen EB, Fahrendrug A, Praestholm J. Late meningeal effects of myelographic contrast media with special reference to metrizamide. Br J Radiol 1978;5:321–327.
49. Harrington KD. Metastatic disease of the spine. J Bone Joint Surg Am 1986;68:1110–1115.
50. Harris JH, Edeiken-Monroe B. Radiographic examination. In: Harris JH, Edeiken-Monroe B, eds. The radiology of acute cervical trauma. 2nd ed. Baltimore: Williams & Wilkins, 1987:45–64.
51. Hashimoto K, Akahori O, Kitano K, et al. Magnetic resonance imaging of lumbar disc herniation. Comparison with myelography. Spine 1990;15:1166–1169.
52. Hauge O, Falkenberg H. Neuropsychologic reactions and other side effects after metrizamide myelography. AJNR Am J Neuroradiol 1982;3:229–232.
53. Heilbronner R, Fankhauser H, Schnyder P, et al. Computed tomography of the postoperative intervertebral disc and lumbar spinal canal: serial long-term investigation in 19 patients after successful operation for lumbar disc herniation. Neurosurgery 1991;29:1–7.
54. Herkowitz HN, Garfin SR, Bell GR, et al. The use of computerized tomography in evaluating non-visualized vertebral levels caudad to a complete block on a lumbar myelogram. A review of thirty-two cases. J Bone Joint Surg Am 1987;69:218–224.
55. Hitselberger WE, Witten RM. Abnormal myelograms in asymptomatic patients. J Neurosurg 1968;28:204–206.
56. Hueftle MG, Modic MT, Ross JS, et al. Lumbar spine: postoperative MR imaging with Gd-DTPA. Radiology 1988;167:817–824.
57. Hyman RA, Edwards JH, Vacirca SJ, et al. 0.6 T MR imaging of the cervical spine: multislice and multi-echo techniques. AJNR Am J Neuroradiol 1985;6:229–236.

58. Jackson DE Jr, Atlas SW, Mani JR, et al. Intraspinal synovial cysts: MR imaging. Radiology 1989;170:527–530.
59. Jensen MC, Brant-Zawadzki MN, Obuchowski N, et al. Magnetic resonance imaging of the lumbar spine in people without back pain [see comments]. N Engl J Med 1994;331:69–73.
60. Jinkins JR. MR of enhancing nerve roots in the unoperated lumbosacral spine. AJNR Am J Neuroradiol 1993;14:193–202.
61. Jinkins JR, Matthes JC, Sener RN, et al. Spondylolysis, spondylolisthesis, and associated nerve root entrapment in the lumbosacral spine: MR evaluation. [Review]. AJR Am J Roentgenol 1992;159:799–803.
62. Kanal E, Shellock FG. MR imaging of patients with intracranial aneurysm clips. Radiology 1993;187:612–614.
63. Kelly WM, Paglan PG, Pearson JA, et al. Ferromagnetism of intraocular foreign body causes unilateral blindness after MR study. AJNR Am J Neuroradiol 1986;7:243–245.
64. Kim KY, Kim YT, Lee CS, et al. Magnetic resonance imaging in the evaluation of the lumbar herniated intervertebral disc. Int Orthop 1993;17:241–244.
65. Kricun ME. Conventional radiography. In: Kricun ME, ed. Imaging modalities in spinal disorders. Philadelphia: WB Saunders, 1988:59–288.
66. Kricun R, Kricun ME. Computed tomography. In: Kricun ME, ed. Imaging modalities in spinal disorders. Philadelphia: WB Saunders, 1988:376–467.
67. Lang P, Chafetz N, Genant HK, et al. Lumbar spinal fusion. Assessment of functional stability with magnetic resonance imaging. Spine 1990;15:581–588.
68. LeBihan D, Breton E, Lallemand D. MR imaging of intra-voxel incoherent motions: applications to diffusion and perfusion in neurologic disorders. Radiology 1986;161:401–407.
69. LeBihan D, Breton E, Lallemand D. Separation of diffusion and perfusion in intra-voxel incoherent motion MR imaging. Radiology 1988;168:497–505.
70. Lee RR. Recent advances in magnetic resonance imaging of the spine. Spine:State Art Rev 1995;9:45–60.
71. Littleton JT. The spine. In: Littleton JT, ed. Tomography: physical principles and clinical applications. Baltimore: Williams & Wilkins, 1976:324–429.
72. Littleton JT. Conventional pluridirectional tomography. In: Kricun ME, ed. Imaging modalities in spinal disorders. Philadelphia: WB Saunders, 1988:289–324.
73. Liu SS, Williams KD, Drayer BP, et al. Synovial cysts of the lumbosacral spine: diagnosis by MR imaging. AJR Am J Roentgenol 1990;154:163–166.
74. Mapstone TB, Redate HL, Shurin SB. Quadriplegia secondary to hematoma after lateral C1, C2 puncture in a leukemic child. Neurosurgery 1983;12:230–231.
75. Masaryk TJ, Ross JS, Modic MT, et al. High-resolution MR imaging of sequestered lumbar intervertebral disks. AJR Am J Roentgenol 1988;150:1155–1162.
76. McCutcheon ME, Thompson WC. CT scanning of lumbar discography. A useful diagnostic adjunct. Spine 1986;11:257–259.
77. Mclain RF, Weinstein JN. Tumors of the spine. Semin Spine Surg 1990;2:157–180.
78. Milette PC, Raymond J, Fontaine S. Comparison of high-resolution computed tomography with discography in the evaluation of lumbar disc herniations. Spine 1990;15:525–533.
79. Modic MT, Feighlin DH, Piraino DW. Vertebral osteomyelitis: assessment using MR. Radiology 1985;157:157–166.
80. Modic MT, Feighlin DH, Piraino DW, et al. Vertebral osteomyelitis: assessment using MR. Radiology 1985;157:157–166.
81. Modic MT, Masaryk TJ, Mulopulos GP, et al. Cervical radiculopathy: prospective evaluation with surface coil MR imaging, CT with metrizamide, and metrizamide myelography. Radiology 1986;161:753–759.
82. Modic MT, Masaryk TJ, Ross JS. Imaging of degenerative disk disease. Radiology 1988;168:177–186.
83. Modic MT, Steinberg PM, Ross JS, et al. Degenerative disk disease: assessment of changes in vertebral body marrow with MR imaging. Radiology 1988;166:193–199.
84. Mulkeren RV, Wong ST, Winalski C, et al. Contrast manipulation and artifact assessment of 2D and 3D RARE sequences. Magn Reson Imaging 1990;8:557–566.
85. Musher DM, Thorsteinsson SB, Minuta JN. Vertebral osteomyelitis still a diagnostic pitfall. Arch Intern Med 1976;136:105–110.
86. Nelson HT, Taylor A. Bone scanning in the diagnosis of acute osteomyelitis. Eur J Nucl Med 1980;5:267–269.
87. Pizzutillo PD. Idiopathic scoliosis and kyphosis. In: Schafer M, ed. Instructional course lectures volume 43. Rosemont: AAOS, 1994:185–192.
88. Posner I, White AA, Edwards WT. A biomechanical analysis of the clinical stability of the lumbar and lumbosacral spine. Spine 1982;7:374–389.
89. Post MJ, Quencer RM, Green BA, et al. Intramedullary spinal cord metastases, mainly of nonneurogenic origin. AJR Am J Roentgenol 1987;148:1015–1022.
90. Post MJ, Sheldon JJ, Hensley GT. Central nervous system disease in acquired immunodeficiency syndrome: prospective correlation using CT, MR imaging, and pathologic studies. Radiology 1986;158:141–148.
91. Post MJ, Sze G, Quencer RM. Gadolinium enhanced MR in spinal infection. J Comput Assist Tomogr 1990;15:721–729.
92. Rahim KA, Stambough JL. Radiographic evaluation of the degenerative cervical spine. Orthop Clin North Am 1992;23:395–404.
93. Reddy S, Leite CC, Jinkins JR. Imaging of infectious disease of the spine. Spine:State Art Rev 1995;9:119–140.
94. Rogers LA. Acute subdural hematoma and death following lateral cervical spinal puncture: case report. Neurosurgery 1983;58:284–286.
95. Ryan PJ, Evans P, Gibson T. Osteoporosis and chronic back pain: a study with single photon emission computed tomography (SPECT) bone scintigraphy. J Bone Miner Res 1993;7:1455–1460.
96. Ryan PJ, Evans PA, Gibson T, et al. Chronic low back pain: comparison of bone SPECT with radiography and CT. Radiology 1992;182:849–854.

97. Schellas KP. Diskography. Spine:State Art Rev 1995; 9:27–44.
98. Silverman CS, Lenchik L, Shimkin PM, et al. The value of MR in differentiating subligamentous from supraligamentous lumbar disk herniations. AJNR Am J Neuroradiol 1995;16:571–579.
99. Simmons JW, Aprill CN, Dwyer AP, et al. A reassessment of Holt's data on: "The question of lumbar discography". [Review]. Clin Orthop 1988;120–124.
100. Soitropoulos S, Chafetz N, Lang P. Differentiation between postoperative scar and recurrent disk herniation: prospective comparison of MR, CT, and contrast-enhanced CT. AJNR Am J Neuroradiol 1989;10:639–643.
101. Spanu G, Rodriguez, Rainoldi F. Reliability of clinical examination and computed tomography in the diagnosis of extreme lateral disc herniation. Neurochirurgia (Stuttg) 1987;30:112–114.
102. Torgenson WR, Dotter WE. Comparative roentgenographic study of the asymptomatic and symptomatic lumbar spine. J Bone Joint Surg Am 1976;58:850–853.
103. Toyone T, Takahashi K, Kitahara H, et al. Visualization of symptomatic nerve roots. Prospective study of contrast-enhanced MRI in patients with lumbar disc herniation. J Bone Joint Surg Br 1993;75:529–533.
104. Toyone T, Takahashi K, Kitahara H, et al. Vertebral bone-marrow changes in degenerative lumbar disc disease. An MRI study of 74 patients with low back pain. J Bone Joint Surg Br 1994;76:757–764.
105. Tress BM, Hare WS. CT of the spine: are plain spine radiographs necessary? Clin Radiol 1990;41:317–320.
106. Vaccaro AR, An HS, Lin SS, et al. Noncontiguous injuries of the spine. J Spinal Disord 1992;5:320–329.
107. Vanharanta H, Sachs BL, Spivey M, et al. A comparison of CT/discography, pain response and radiographic disc height. Spine 1988;13:321–324.
108. Voelker JL, Mealey J Jr., Eskridge JM, et al. Metrizamide-enhanced computed tomography as an adjunct to metrizamide myelography in the evaluation of lumbar disc herniation and spondylosis. Neurosurgery 1987;20:379–384.
109. Walsh TR, Weinstein JN, Spratt KF, et al. Lumbar discography in normal subjects. A controlled, prospective study. J Bone Joint Surg Am 1990;72:1081–1088.
110. Webster EW, Merrill OE. Radiation hazards. II. Measurements of gonadal dose in radiographic examinations. N Engl J Med 1957;27:811–819.
111. Wegener WA, Alavi A. Diagnostic imaging of musculoskeletal infection: roentgenography; gallium, indium-labeled white blood cell, gammaglobulin, bone scintography, and MRI. Orthop Clin North Am 1991;22:401–418.
112. Wisneski RJ. Infectious disease of the spine, diagnostic and treatment considerations. Orthop Clin North Am 1991;22:491–501.
113. Woolfenden JM, Pitt MJ, Durie BGM. Comparison of bone scintography and radiography in multiple myeloma. Radiology 1980;134:723–728.
114. Xu GL, Haughton VM, Carrera GF. Lumbar facet joint capsule: appearance at MR imaging and CT. Radiology 1990;177:415–420.
115. Yamane T, Yoshida T, Mimatsu K. Early diagnosis of lumbar spondylolysis by MRI. J Bone Joint Surg Br 1993;75:764–768.
116. Yu SW, Haughton VM, Ho PS, et al. Progressive and regressive changes in the nucleus pulposus. Part II. The adult. Radiology 1988;169:93–97.
117. Yu SW, Haughton VM, Sether LA, et al. Comparison of MR and diskography in detecting radial tears of the anulus: a postmortem study. AJNR Am J Neuroradiol 1989;10:1077–1081.

CHAPTER SIX

Electrodiagnosis and Intraoperative Monitoring in Disorders of the Spinal Cord and Nerve Roots

Paul E. Barkhaus and Safwan S. Jaradeh

Electrodiagnosis

Introduction

Electrodiagnosis (EDX) is a general term that includes evoked potentials (EPs), electroneurography (nerve conduction studies) and electromyography (EMG). Strictly speaking, EMG is the needle electrode examination of the muscles. In current parlance, however, the term has also come to include electroneurography and is referred to as such in this chapter. Collectively, these techniques are used in the electrophysiologic evaluation of diseases of the spinal cord, nerve, and muscle. EDX procedures have been in clinical use for over 40 years and have continued to evolve with advances in instrumentation and computerization.

Intraoperative monitoring (IOM) is not a diagnostic procedure per se. IOM is an EDX technique that most commonly uses somatosensory evoked potentials (SEPs) to monitor the electrophysiologic integrity of the nervous system (for our purposes here, the spinal cord and nerve roots) during surgery. Additional monitoring techniques of the motor tracts may also be used, including magnetic stimulation and direct stimulation of the spinal cord. IOM is considered in more detail in a separate, final section.

The purpose of this chapter is to highlight the essential aspects of EDX techniques along with their clinical applications and limitations. For more information on methodological details, basic anatomy, and physiology, the reader is referred to one of several comprehensive reference texts on EDX (4, 13, 14, 27, 54). Many abbreviations commonly used in EDX are used in this chapter. They are discussed in the text and are listed again at the end of the chapter.

Usage of EDX in Clinical Practice

Before discussing the traditional anatomy and physiology involved in EDX, a review the application of EDX in clinical practice is appropriate. Physicians, even within the same specialty, may vary in their approach to the evaluation of clinical problems. EDX is no exception. Like any other test, maximum benefit is obtained when the physician who is managing the patient has reasonable knowledge of how EDX can improve his/her understanding of the clinical problem. This becomes very important as external economic pressures on the physician increase to resolve clinical problems in the most cost-efficient manner possible, yet to maintain a high standard of care.

As a general principle, EDX should not be used to subsidize or supplant an incomplete history or physical examination of the patient. This only compounds the original incomplete understanding of the patient's problem. The exception would be the patient who, for whatever reason, cannot give an accurate history or on whom the physical examination is "non-physiologic" (e.g., apparent weakness on formal resistance testing yet reflexes are normal and observation of the patient's functional motor movements appear uncompromised) (95).

To further consider the use of EDX in clinical practice, it may be helpful to fall back on the poet Rudyard Kipling's "six honest serving men" (55):

1. **What** specific EDX tests should be ordered? This answer varies with the clinical problem and the experience of the referring physician. For radiculopathies and similar lesions in which other processes such as neuropathies need to be excluded, a thorough EMG should be sufficient. In some laboratories, other EDX testing, such as EPs, may be employed (3, 4). In diagnostic testing, SEPs tend to be employed more in central disorders (i.e., spinal cord and brain). Anatomic structures with their EDX correlate are shown in Table 6.1.

   In ordering an EMG, it is important for the physician to specify precisely the clinical problem. Succinct requests such as "right arm" are not very helpful. Taken literally, this problem requires simple observation rather than an EMG! On the reverse end of the spectrum, there are the rare physicians who meticulously specify every nerve conduction and muscle they wish studied. The findings on an EMG study cannot always be predicted, and the electromyographer must have flexibility to formulate a complete study. A common example is when an EMG for a cervical radiculopathy is requested. In performing the pre-procedure clinical examination and the actual procedure, evidence for a polyneuropathy may be found and additional nerves outside of the extremity in question might need evaluation. Finally, the referring physician should consult with the electromyographer before requesting uncommon studies (e.g. nerve root stimulation): this is to ascertain whether the study requested can be done in that particular laboratory, and if so, whether reference (i.e., normal) data are available to allow adequate interpretation.

2. **Why** use EDX? The remarkable advances in imaging procedures of the spine and spinal cord would seem to relegate the use of EDX to disorders of the nervous system other than radiculopathy and myelopathy caused by spine disease. Each has its unique niche: imaging elucidates the structural aspects of the anatomy in question while EDX addresses the functional or physiologic aspects of the spinal cord and nerve roots. Each is complementary to the other. Apparent "abnormalities" are common in the spine, such as asymptomatic herniated discs occurring as incidental findings (49, 90). These incidental findings have prompted caution in correlating structural findings with clinical symptoms. In other words, a "picture" of a pager does not necessarily imply that it is "beeping." Finding evidence for active denervation in the myotome supplied by a structural spine abnormality, however, lends weight to the suspicion that the lesion is clinically significant.

   EMG has another important role. EDX can also quantitate or determine the severity of the neurologic condition. For example, the presence of a herniated disc does not necessarily mean that a completely physiologically compromised root exists. There is a spectrum of physiologic nerve dysfunction ranging from mild neurapraxia to varying degrees of axonal loss. Such information can enable the treating physician to better "quantify" or gauge the severity of the lesion and determine appropriate treatment options.

3. **When** should EDX testing be ordered? This depends on the questions being posed in light of the pathophysiology of the injury (67). Abnormalities in the needle electrode examination follow a fairly predictable course after a nerve or nerve root injury (see upcoming section on pathophysiology of denervation/reinnervation of motor nerve fibers). Based on the expected evolution of changes, one can approximate the chronicity of a lesion. Nerve conductions and SEPs are less helpful in dating lesions with respect to chronicity (see same section). If an axon is focally interrupted along its length, the distal segment may remain excitable for approximately 5 days depending on the length of the truncated segment. Excitability may remain slightly longer in proximal lesions and slightly less in distal ones (67). In otherwise uncomplicated

TABLE 6.1.
Anatomic Structural Levels of the Peripheral Nervous System and Their Electrodiagnostic Correlate

Anatomic Structure	Corresponding Electrodiagnostic Methods of Assessment
Motor units	Needle electrode examination
• Motor axons	Motor nerve distal latencies and conductions (distal segments), F waves, H waves (proximal segments)
• Neuromuscular Junctions	Repetitive motor nerve stimulation, single fiber electromyography (jitter or stability)
• Muscle fibers	Needle electrode examination
Sensory axons	Sensory nerve distal latencies and conductions (distal segments), H waves (proximal segments), somatosensory evoked potentials (proximal segments and central pathways)

cases (e.g., no polyneuropathy present), nerve conduction studies should be delayed for 5 to 7 days to avoid spurious normal results.

In patients with a discrete injury, the clinician can time the EDX study apropos to the clinical questions posed. In a patient without a history for a discrete injury or cause, it may be more useful to wait until definite evidence for denervation (i.e., fibrillation potentials) would be anticipated so that only one EMG study need be done to provide optimal localization. Some patients may be complicated by the presence of other disorders of the peripheral nervous system (e.g., polyneuropathy). In such cases, it may be preferable to perform a baseline study immediately after injury because the "baseline study" is expected to be abnormal for other reasons. When, for instance, denervation from a new lesion is expected to manifest, a limited repeat EDX examination can focus on "newer" changes among the "established" or chronic abnormal findings.

Repeat studies in radiculopathy are seldom indicated. Such circumstances include the presence of other complicating neurologic disease as previously mentioned, uncertainties in timing of onset of the process (i.e., when did the denervation begin . . . at time of injury?), or changes in the patient's clinical status. Serial studies to "monitor" the progression of a radiculopathy are uncommonly indicated. In lesions of a plexus or peripheral nerves, however, repeat studies may be indicated to assess reinnervation. This in turn may have important implications in management, i.e., timing of surgical exploration. The electrophysiologic changes expected in denervation/reinnervation and how the motor unit remodels (84) are described later in the chapter and in Table 6.2.

4. *How* should EDX studies be ordered? The longer the chain of communication from the ordering physician to the EDX laboratory, the greater the chance for error or omission. If consult forms are used, the physician ordering the procedure should take the responsibility for completing it or perhaps cross copy the EDX laboratory his/her written evaluation of the patient, which could include details of the EDX testing desired.

5. *Where* should the laboratory for EDX studies be located? Current use of improved instrumentation makes the site of laboratory less prone to the idiosyncrasies of an institution's electrical system. If possible, EDX studies are best performed in an experienced laboratory that has its own reference data (1). This also tends to reduce technical artifact and potential damage to equipment from unnecessary movement.

"Portable" EMG studies can be performed at the bedside of a hospitalized patient. They should be avoided if at all possible to reduce technical problems and potential damage to equipment. In cases in which a patient is bedridden and/or in traction, it may be better to request that the electrodiagnostic physician clinically evaluate the patient first to determine whether the timing of the study is optimal vis-a-vis the questions posed and to ensure that the anatomy to be studied is accessible. Limitations in the latter situation caused by body position, casting, or presence of other orthopedic instrumentation may impose significant limitations on a proposed EMG study.

6. *Who* should perform EDX studies? The authors of this chapter defer to the guidelines as outlined by the American Association of Electrodiagnostic Medicine (1). The EDX study should be planned by a physician who has appropriate training and experience in EDX after the request/clinical information has been reviewed and the patient examined.

Although technicians may assist in procedures such as the nerve conductions and EPs, the needle electrode examination should be performed by a physician with appropriate training in EDX. EDX,

TABLE 6.2.
Chronology of Neurogenic Changes (i.e., denervation/reinnervation) in the Needle Electrode Examination (EMG) of Muscle in Acute Radiculopathy with Axonal Loss

Time after Lesion	Insertional Activity	Fibrillation Potentials	Fasciculation Potentials	Recruitment	Motor Unit Action Potentials Amplitude/Area/ Duration	Complexity	Stability
Preinjury	Normal	Absent	Absent	Normal	Normal	Normal	Stable
Acute (14–21 days)	Increased	Absent	Rare	Reduced	Normal	Normal	Usually stable
Subacute (>21 days)	Increased	Present: Maximal number	Rare	Reduced	Normal	Normal	Mildly unstable
Recent (1–3 months)	Normal to increased	Present: Maximal Number	Rare	Reduced	May see mild increases	Mild increase	Unstable
Chronic (>6 months)	Usually normal	Present: ↓ Number and ↓ Amplitude	Rare	Reduced	Variable increase in size depending on severity	Increase	Mildly unstable to stable

particularly the needle electrode examination, is not the same as other electrodiagnostic tests where recordings can be placed on hard copy (e.g., paper print out) in a highly standardized manner for off line analysis by a physician. The EDX physician must be present to continually monitor the quality of the data acquired. EDX requires a constant assessment of the diagnostic hypothesis as each new piece of data is acquired. EDX may be considered an extension of the physical examination, and as such, within the purview of the practice of medicine.

The synthesis of the data obtained to generate a report and interpretation presumes a detailed understanding of the normal anatomy and physiology of the nervous system and an understanding of the pathologic processes involved. In the authors' experience, the most common reason for being asked to "repeat" a study has been that the original study was incomplete, with artifacts posing as apparent pathology being a close second.

Applied Anatomy and Physiology

From an electrodiagnostic perspective, the fundamental anatomic unit studied on the needle electrode examination is the motor unit (MU). The MU is composed of the anterior horn cell, its axon, the neuromuscular junctions its terminal axonal branches form, and all the muscle fibers that these terminal branches innervate (2). The number of muscle fibers supplied by a single motor neuron is referred to as the innervation ratio. Estimates of this ratio vary widely between muscles. In extraocular muscles, it may be approximately 1:10 in contrast to proximal limb muscles, which have estimates of 1:500. There are also different functional types of MUs. In humans, there are three types of MUs based on recruitment threshold (16). In routine EMG, only the lower threshold MUs are typically recorded and measured except when describing the recruitment/interference pattern when the higher threshold MUs are activated.

A myotome refers to that group of motor axons emerging from a single spinal root that supply innervation to a number of muscles. Conversely, muscles typically receive variable numbers of motor efferent nerve fibers from 2 to 3 myotomes (i.e., roots) (53, 78). For purposes of clinical localization, Schliak (82) has proposed the concept of segmental pointer muscles. This concept involves the use of certain muscles, by virtue of their innervation, to precisely localize lesions. It is thought that the most precise and consistent segmental root innervations are to the multifidus (i.e., the deep medial paraspinal musculature) and thoracic intercostal muscles (82). In practice, however, neither of these muscle groups are segmentally identifiable by clinical examination, or by EMG study, because of the inevitable overlap in segmental (i.e. myotomal) innervation in these muscles.

Byrne and Waxman (17) have proposed a modification of Schliak's concept (82) using limb muscles. In addition to normal anatomic variations in myotomes (for a comparison chart on myotomes, see Kendall et al. [53]), there are also anatomic variations in peripheral nerve innervation to some muscles that can account for apparent atypical or "unusual" findings (40). For example, the brachial plexus may receive variable contributions from either the rostral spinal roots (e.g., C4) or the lower spinal roots (T1 and 2), in which case the plexus is said to be prefixed or postfixed, respectively (29). Remember that localizations (either by clinical examination or by EMG) should not be based exclusively on one muscle.

The area within which the muscle fibers of a MU are distributed is referred to as the motor unit territory. The muscle fibers within a MU's territory are not contiguous, but are distributed in a "patchy" or checkerboard fashion. Hence, there is great overlap between MUs. In a low power microscopic field of a cross section of muscle, muscle fibers representing 20 to 50 MUs may be present (16).

The motor unit action potential (MUAP) is the summation of the electrical activity of all of the single muscle fibers (i.e., their action potentials) comprising a MU as previously defined. This concept is more theoretical because the actual MUAP recorded on an electromyograph is actually defined by the recording electrode used. Different needle recording electrodes may record different electrical signals by nature of their physical characteristics, in addition to variations in instrumentation settings on the actual electromyograph. In routine EMG, most centers use either concentric or monopolar disposable needle electrodes. Because of their recording characteristics, these record from only a portion of the MU's territory (13, 14, 21, 27, 54).

Sensation is often clinically organized by modality (i.e., position sense, rapidly adapting mechanoreceptors [or vibration], pain [or sharp touch], temperature). The first two examples are mediated by large diameter afferent axons, which are measured in standard sensory nerve conduction studies. In a manner analogous to myotomes, peripheral nerves typically are composed of sensory fibers emanating from more than one dermatome. In addition to sensory nerve conductions, there is commercially available, dedicated equipment that quantifies such modalities as thermal threshold, tactile sensation, and vibration. This equipment is not widely used and there is no final consensus regarding its utility in EDX at present.

Although, conceptually, one should be able to record nerve conductions from any motor nerve or sensory nerve, there are relatively few nerves that are routinely studied. This is because most clinical questions can be addressed by assessing a set of standard nerves (complemented by the needle electrode examination), extensive reference values are available for the commonly done studies, and uncertainties caused by variations in innervation can be kept to a minimum.

The segmental spinal cord roots are paired (i.e., right/left). The segments commonly affected by structural spine disorders (i.e., radiculopathy) contain a dorsal (or afferent) root and a ventral (or efferent) root. Just distal to the emergence of the dorsal root, there is a dorsal root ganglion containing the soma or cell bodies of the sensory neurons. This observation is a point of EDX significance. In root avulsions, dense clinical sensory deficits may occur despite apparently "normal" peripheral sensory conductions (5). These deficits are caused by the preservation of the sensory neuron cell bodies within the dorsal root ganglia, allowing the peripheral processes of these neurons to remain physiologically intact.

The ventral roots contain the motor, or efferent, processes of the anterior horn cells. These merge with the dorsal roots to form the posterior and anterior rami. The former compose the sensorimotor nerve fibers supplying posterior axial sensation and motor innervation (i.e., the paraspinal musculature) with the latter composing what ultimately becomes the spinal nerves (i.e. compound mixed sensorimotor nerves) to the extremities, chest, and abdomen.

The autonomic nervous system is a diffuse, complex system that has recently been receiving more interest with respect to functional testing. The details of this are beyond the scope of this chapter and the reader is referred to more extensive reviews (65). Relatively few EDX laboratories offer extensive autonomic testing that assess function of the smaller diameter autonomic fibers mediating temperature, sweating, and vasomotor tone. Such testing may be useful in cases of reflex sympathetic dystrophy and other types of sympathetically mediated pain in which, in the absence of obvious nerve trauma, routine EMG studies may be normal.

The spinal cord is the caudal portion of the central nervous system. It is composed of grey (neuronal) and white (tracts) matter. The former contains the paired (i.e., right/left) segmental groupings of dorsal afferent (sensory) and ventral efferent (motor) neurons. The white matter portion of the spinal cord is organized into a number of paired (i.e., right/left) ascending (afferent) and descending (efferent) tracts (17, 23, 24). These tracts have an internal topographic organization (or "lamina") with the more caudal (e.g., lumbosacral) segments being represented laterally and the rostral (e.g., cervical) segments represented medially. The reader is referred to more extensive discussions (17, 27) of principles of spinal cord anatomy and physiology with respect to how particular constellations of neurological symptoms and signs are produced by lesions located at different spinal cord levels and at different loci within a segment (i.e., intramedullary, extramedullary).

Clinical neurophysiologic testing of spinal cord integrity is divided into two main categories: segmental testing and central conductions SEPs. The first deals with central segmental (i.e., myotome/dermatome) function, which is contingent on the presumed integrity of its afferent and efferent nerve fibers peripheral to the root level. Examples of segmental testing include H reflexes and F waves (36).

The H reflex is the electrophysiologic analog of the tendon "stretch" reflex. The "H" refers to Hoffman who first described it. It is recorded most commonly from the soleus or gastrocnemius muscles (i.e., S1 root segment). The H reflex differs from the tendon reflex in that it is elicited by external electrical stimulation of the afferent nerve fibers rather than by mechanical excitation of the spindles. Although it is technically more difficult to record H reflexes from the upper extremity, they may be recorded from the flexor carpi radialis muscle. H reflexes are recorded more easily in the presence of an upper motor neuron lesion.

The F wave is *not* a reflex. It is a long latency response mediated exclusively by the efferent motor fibers. The appellation "F" derives from the German *fuss* or foot, the anatomic site at which the response was first recorded. F waves result from the bidirectional (i.e., orthodromic or distal and antidromic or proximal) excitation of motor fibers upon external, supramaximal stimulation of a peripheral nerve. The F wave specifically results from the latter, i.e., antidromic, stimulus, which travels proximally to the pool of anterior horn cells of the root segment. No synapse is therefore involved centrally in the spinal cord.

This stimulus evokes a discharge from an anterior horn cell which in turn sends back an orthodromic impulse to the muscle where the earlier, direct orthodromic response has already been recorded. Because the impulse producing the F response is presumed to derive from a single anterior horn cell, the F wave is thought to represent the surface-recorded action potential of a single MU. The F wave is discussed further in the next section under techniques. F waves, like H reflexes, are useful in assessing conductions in the proximal segments of the peripheral nerves and nerve roots.

SEPs can be recorded by stimulating compound mixed (i.e., sensorimotor nerves), sensory nerves or dermatomes. They measure central conduction times within the spinal cord between the segment stimulated to the cerebral cortex. SEP responses may be affected by peripheral abnormalities. If there is uncertainty about the integrity of peripheral nerve conductions, they should be evaluated concurrently with the SEPs.

Techniques in Electrodiagnosis

Based on the preceding discussion, this section briefly reviews basic EDX techniques. For a complete discussion, the reader is referred to a more comprehensive basic EDX reference (4, 13, 14, 27, 54). Table 6.1 summarizes some of these techniques with their anatomic correlate. Motor and sensory nerve conductions are customarily performed first because they are less "intimidating" than the needle electrode examination. Also, potential focal or diffuse neuropathies can be identified, which may explain completely, or in part, the findings on the needle electrode examination. By doing the nerve conduc-

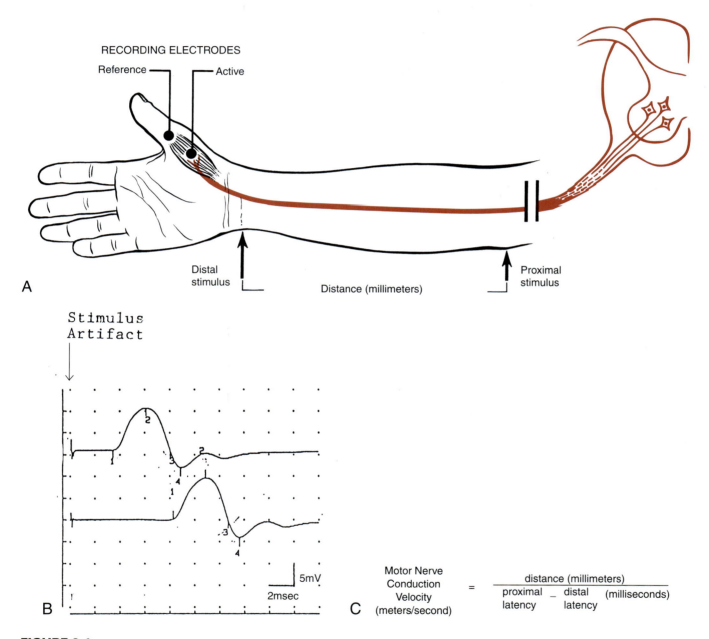

FIGURE 6.1.

A. Schematic for performing motor nerve conduction study. A pair of recording electrodes are placed over the muscle to be recorded and stimulation is performed at two points along the course of the nerve. The CMAPs are recorded (see **B**: tracings—the upper trace is the distal response to stimulation and the lower trace represents the proximal response) and measured for latency (time from the stimulus artifact to the onset of the CMAP) and for negative amplitude (vertical distance depending on the sensitivity setting on the amplifier display between marker "1" and marker "2"). **C.** The motor conduction velocity is calculated according to the previous formula. For example, if the distance between the two points of stimulation is 275 mm and the proximal and distal latencies are 8.8 msec and 3.8 msec, respectively, then the conduction velocity according to the above formula is 55 mm/msec (= 55 meters/sec).

tions first, the EDX physician usually can be more efficient in the number of muscles that need to be examined with the needle electrode. Because SEPs are usually done for reasons other than radiculopathy, they are customarily tested at a separate time from the routine EMG. An EDX laboratory should have established reference values for all of the procedures they perform.

Motor Conductions

The motor nerve conduction study is performed by placing an active recording electrode over the belly (and optimally the endplate zone) of a muscle that the nerve innervates. A reference electrode is placed over the tendinous insertion of the same muscle (Fig. 6.1). Despite variations in size of muscles, the recording territory of the surface electrode within the muscle is relatively limited (10). See Table 6.3 for common terminology. A bipolar stimulator is used which has a negative (cathode) and a positive (anode) tip. The cathode is always placed closest along the nerve trunk toward the active recording electrode (reversing them can cause hyperpolarization of the nerve, i.e. anodal block).

An electrical stimulus is applied at distal and proximal sites along the course of the nerve being studied. Examples include the wrist and elbow for the median or ulnar nerves or at the knee and ankle for the common peroneal or posterior tibial nerves. Most EDX laboratories use a standardized distance between the active recording electrode and the distal stimulating electrode (cathode) to allow easier pooling of reference data. A supramaximal electrical stimulus is used to avoid artifacts in the latency, size, and configuration of the evoked response.

Refer to Figure 6.1 for further description on how conduction velocity is calculated. The distance between the distal and proximal positions where the stimulating (cathode) electrode is applied is called the conduction distance. This distance is not standardized and will vary between patients because of limb length. It is the segment over which the conduction velocity is calculated. The conduction time for this segment is derived by subtracting the distal latency from the proximal latency. In subtracting the distal motor latency, the portion of the distal latency involving neuromuscular transmission time is eliminated.

The response evoked from the muscle is termed the compound muscle action potential (CMAP). The amplitudes of the CMAPs are quantitated and have a large range in values in normal subjects. Although motor fibers to other muscles and sensory nerve fibers within the nerve are also excited, their contribution to the recording is negligible because the recording is made exclusively from a single specified muscle (i.e., that muscle over which the recording electrode is placed). In doing motor conductions, additional segmental stimulations may be performed at other points along the course of a nerve, such as when focal conduction blocks may be suspected. More proximal motor stimulations can be used, including near-nerve root stimulation. Magnetic stimulation can also be employed to elicit nerve responses but is used in relatively few laboratories, primarily for EDX studies of the central nervous system (33).

Late Responses

Late responses include F and H waves (36). The F wave is typically easy to record from distal muscles. After the standard conductions for a motor nerve are performed, distal stimulation is again performed (Fig. 6.1B). At this time, the settings on the electromyograph are altered (i.e., slowing the sweep speed and increasing the sensitivity setting). In Figure 6.2, the CMAP recorded distally appears shifted to the left and enlarged. F waves may not necessarily be recorded with every stimulation, and the latencies of

TABLE 6.3.
Commonly Used Electrodiagnostic Terms (2, 4, 13, 24, 54)

Conduction distance	The distance between two points of stimulation along a nerve trunk.
Conduction time	The difference in latency values between two points of stimulation.
Conduction velocity	The common use is defined as maximum conduction velocity calculated by dividing the conduction time by the conduction distance; expressed in meters/second (m/s).
Compound muscle action potential (CMAP)	The summation of nearly synchronous muscle fiber action potentials recorded from a muscle by stimulating (directly or indirectly) the nerve supplying it.
Compound sensory action potentials (Compound SNAP)	The summation of sensory axonal action potentials which should be evoked by stimulating a sensory nerve. If derived from stimulating a mixed (i.e. motor and sensory) nerve, then either the stimulating or recording electrodes should be placed over a sensory branch of the nerve.
Motor latency	Time interval between onset of a stimulus and onset of the resultant evoked CMAP. When it refers to the distal position of the nerve (e.g., wrist to hand) it typically refers to the distal latency. If so, it must be specified as the distal motor latency.
Sensory latency	Time interval between onset of a stimulus and onset of the resultant evoked Compound SNAP. As in motor latency above, it typically refers to the distal latency, i.e., distal sensory latency.

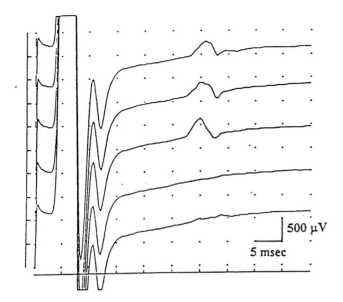

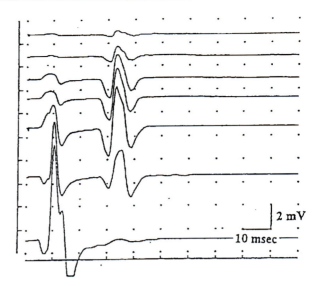

FIGURE 6.2.

F waves. There are 5 sequential stimuli using electrode positions similar to performing a distal motor latency as shown in the top tracing in Figure 6.1B. The difference for their appearance is that the amplifier is set to a higher sensitivity by a factor of 10 (0.5 mV versus 5.0 mV in Figure 6.1B.) and the time line is slowed (5 msec versus 2 msec per horizontal division: see calibration marker). Hence the CMAP appears enlarged in amplitude and shifted to the left. The smaller amplitude responses occurring at the midportion of the trace are the F waves. The first three sweeps show easily discernible responses (going top to bottom) with the latency being measured from the stimulus artifact (to the left of the CMAP) to the onset of the F wave. The fourth sweep shows no evoked F wave, and the fifth shows a very low amplitude distortion of the baseline that probably represents a response just outside the recording area of the active surface electrode. Note that the top three F waves differ slightly in shape and latency, indicating that they are recorded from different MUs. Such a difference is characteristic of F waves.

FIGURE 6.3.

H wave. The electrode configuration is similar to that for a motor nerve conduction as shown in Figure 1.B, but here the recording electrodes are placed over the soleus muscle and stimulation is applied to the tibial nerve in the popliteal fossa. Sequential stimuli from top to bottom show progressively increasing stimulus intensity. The H wave or H reflex is easily seen in the top 6 of the 7 traces. Despite variable amplitude, the downgoing or positive initial onset remains the same (compare to the F waves in Figure 6.3). With increasing stimulus intensity, more motor fibers are excited directly, producing an increasingly larger direct "M" or muscle response (i.e., CMAP) to the left as shown in traces 3–7. As the CMAP approaches maximum, the H wave becomes smaller. The bottom CMAP is large, so the barely discernible, small amplitude late response is most likely a F wave. To ensure that the desired response is a H wave, a series using increasing stimulus intensity as shown here should be recorded.

the F waves vary. There are different protocols for quantifying F waves, and the physician recording the F waves must be able to discriminate true F responses from random baseline noise, voluntary surface-recorded muscle activity, and other types of late responses.

As a true reflex, the H wave or H reflex uses both an afferent and efferent pathway. H waves can be elusive to record. Submaximal stimulation is used because the afferent fibers have a lower threshold to stimulation than the efferent fibers, and eliciting F waves will be avoided as much as possible. To be certain that a response is a true H wave, the EDX physician should record a series of responses at the same site, incrementally increasing the stimulus intensity to show the changes in H wave amplitude yet maintaining constant latency as the direct M wave amplitude increases (Fig. 6.3). The sine qua non of an H reflex is that it should be present when the direct response or CMAP is absent, or at least be larger than the CMAP at submaximal levels of stimulation. At supramaximal stimulation, F waves typically replace the H wave.

H waves are classically recorded from the gastrocnemius or soleus upon stimulation of the tibial nerve in the popliteal fossa. Therefore, this has practical application in processes affecting the S1 root. The cathode of the stimulating pair of electrodes is directed centrally (i.e., toward the spinal cord). In this protocol, the H wave is the EDX analog of the ankle jerk. Although technically more difficult, H waves can sometimes be recorded from the flexor carpi radialis muscle (upon median nerve stimulation at the elbow) in the upper extremity and from other muscles.

Sensory Conductions

Sensory conductions are made using surface or subcutaneous needle (i.e., "near-nerve") electrodes along the course of the sensory nerve to be studied (Fig. 6.4). Sensory nerve action potentials (SNAPs) are among the smallest responses recorded in routine EMG and may also be one of the more difficult to obtain in a reproducible, qualitative way. Special techniques such as signal averaging may be required in cases in which baseline noise is excessive and/or the amplitude of the evoked response is reduced, such as polyneuropathy (Fig. 6.4C).

A bipolar stimulator is used in the same manner described for motor nerves. Stimulation is made at one or two points proximal to the recording electrodes. Such recordings are "antidromic." Some laboratories prefer to make orthodromic sensory recordings in which the electrode placements are the reverse of those previously described. In either instance, a standardized distance between stimulating and recording electrodes is used to allow pooling of reference data. In addition to latency and amplitude of the SNAP, conduction velocity may also be calculated.

Needle Electrode Examination

The needle electrode examination is the most memorable, or perhaps the more notorious, of the EDX procedures (44). By performing the nerve conduc-

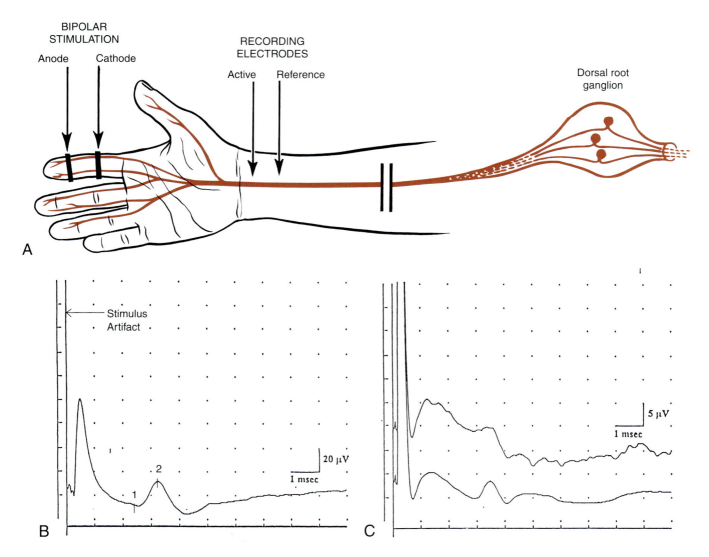

FIGURE 6.4.
A. Schematic for performing (e.g., median) orthodromic sensory nerve conduction study. A pair of stimulating electrodes are placed at the digital cutaneous branch of the index finger and a pair of recording electrodes are placed proximally over the course of the nerve at the wrist at a specified distance. In an antidromic recording, the positions of the stimulating and recording electrode pairs would be reversed. Tracing 6.2.B shows a normal evoked SNAP in which the latency is measured along the horizontal time line from the stimulus artifact to the peak of the SNAP at marker "2". The amplitude is measured along the vertical distance according to the sensitivity setting on the amplifier display between marker "1" and marker "2". Figure 6.2.C shows a low amplitude SNAP (compare calibration marker to that of 6.2.B) in which the signal in the top trace is difficult to discern from baseline noise. The result of averaging 16 stimuli as shown in the lower trace reveals a small, but high quality SNAP that can be measured easily.

tions first, experienced EDX physicians find that most patients will develop a rapport and sense of confidence in them. The MUAPs of a particular muscle are "surveyed" by inserting (i.e., moving) the needle recording electrode perpendicular to the skin surface from superficial to deep along linear tracks or corridors. The EDX physician tries to minimize overlap between the territories of those MUs activated at minimal effort. At least 20 different MUAPs are sampled per muscle.

At low voluntary activation, the various features of individual MUAPs are measured (Fig. 6.5), including the amplitude, area, duration, complexity, and recruitment (Fig. 6.6A) (21). Complexity refers to the number of phases and turns in the MUAP. A phase is defined as a deviation from, and return to, the baseline. A turn is a change in polarity of a segment of the MUAP (2). In most quantitative EMG methods, a MUAP having greater than 4 phases and/or greater than 5 turns is considered complex (69, 87). The acceptable maximum percentage of complex MUAPs recorded in a muscle varies with different muscles and measurement techniques.

The analysis of MUAPs in routine EMG is made subjectively by the EDX physician. In addition, there are several computer-assisted programs available for electromyographs that may objectively quantitate the features of the acquired MUAPs (26, 69, 87). Determination of whether the study of a muscle is "normal" is then based on the mean values of MUAP duration, amplitude, area, and percentage of complex MUAPs. This objective quantitation is helpful when the routine examination is ambiguous. Regardless of approach, accurate assessment of the MUAPs with the subjective or objective approach depends heavily on the skill and knowledge of the ED physician. He/she must be able to ensure the quality of the myogenic signal (i.e., that the MUAPs are recorded within their respective MU territory [11] and that cannula signals are excluded).

The EDX physician also evaluates the insertional and spontaneous activity, either of which may be increased (abnormal) in neuromuscular disorders. The former refers to that electrical activity which is generated by the insertion or movement of the needle electrode (2). Examples include runs of positive sharp waves seen in early denervation and myotonic discharges. Spontaneous activity refers to electrical activity recorded from a muscle at rest after the insertion activity has subsided and in the absence of voluntary activity (2). Fibrillation (Fig. 6.7) and fasciculation potentials would be examples of spontaneous activity (i.e., discharges) of single muscle fibers and single MUs, respectively.

Recruitment is defined as the number of different MUAPs activated, as well as the rate at which they are discharging, at a given level of voluntary effort (i.e., contraction) of the muscle being studied (Fig. 6.6A) (2). It is assessed using the needle recording electrode at different sites within the muscle under study concomitant with assessment of the size and shape of the individual MUAPs. Interference pattern is not synonymous with recruitment rate and is defined as the electrical activity of the muscle recorded at maximal effort (2).

Assessment of stability is essentially an assessment of jitter. The latter is a single fiber EMG term and generally refers to the integrity of neuromuscular transmission between a terminal motor axon and the muscle fiber it innervates. It is defined as "the variability with consecutive discharges in interpotential interval between two single muscle fiber action potentials belonging to the same MU" (2). It can be visualized subjectively or be quantitated (Fig. 6.8) by adjusting the standard settings on the electromyograph.

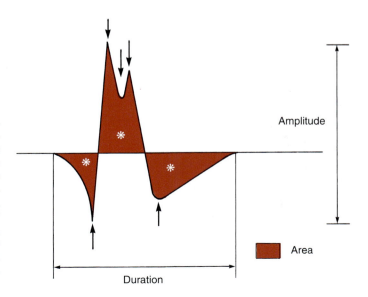

FIGURE 6.5.
Motor unit action potential (MUAP) showing its component features. Amplitude is the maximum negative (upgoing) to positive (downgoing) vertical distance. Duration is the initial deviation from, to the final return to, the baseline. The colored portion is defined as the area. Turns (arrows) are a change in polarity. Phases (asterisks) are defined as a deviation from, and return to, the baseline. When the number of turns and/or phases is increased, a MUAP is considered complex. Computer algorithms incorporated into some newer electromyographs can quantitate these features. The subjective (i.e., on-line visual) analysis on which most ED physicians base their impressions rely on amplitude, duration, and complexity.

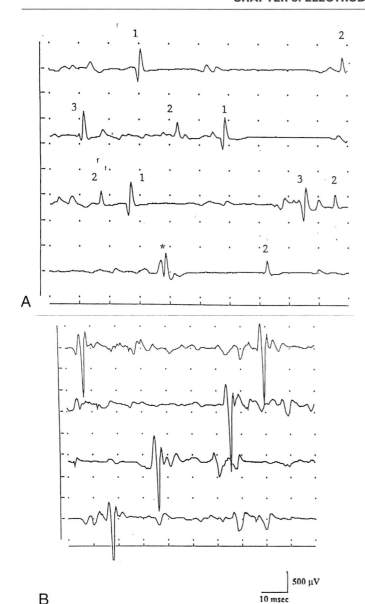

FIGURE 6.6.
A. Normal MUAPs from the biceps brachii firing at relatively low level of recruitment as shown at one needle electrode recording position on sequential traces (top to bottom). At least three different MUAPs can be seen. As MUAPs fire asynchronously, they may commonly overlap (see MUAP complex " * " on bottom trace which represents an overlap of MUAPs 2 and 3), hence the importance of visualizing them at low effort with adequate baseline between discharges. A MUAP discharge should be visualized at least three times before it is accepted for subjective analysis. MUAP "3," however, should be visualized at least two more times. Although it is seen twice, on trace three it overlaps with some low amplitude distant MUAPs so that the duration, phases, and turns cannot be resolved into their respective MUAPs. **B.** Neurogenic MUAPs from the same muscle and level of effort in a different patient using the same amplification display as in **A**. Note the prominent enlarged complex MUAP firing without other well-defined MUAPs within the recording area of the needle electrode.

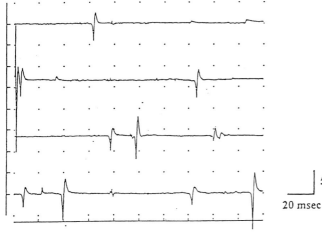

FIGURE 6.7.
Fibrillation potentials discharging at one site as recorded by a needle electrode and displayed on sequential traces (top to bottom). Note the higher sensitivity setting (50 μV/division) and slower sweep speed (20 msec/division) used to display these compared to Figure 6.6.

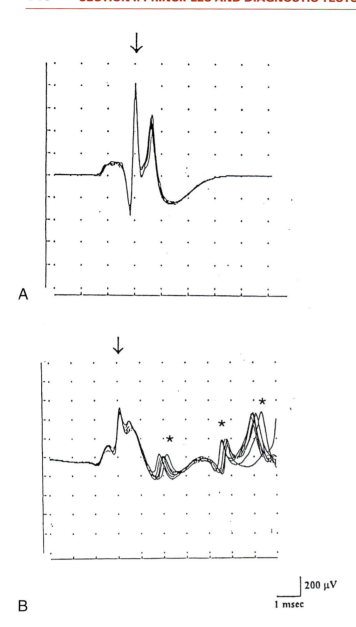

FIGURE 6.8.
MUAP stability. **A.** Normal stability. **B.** Instability or increased jitter. An amplitude trigger and delay line with filter modifications are used to allow the sequential superimpositions of the MUAP discharges. With such modification in recording, the MUAP is broken down or resolved into relatively sharp spikes representing single muscle fiber action potentials. See text for definition of stability. The triggering potentials are denoted by arrows in both **A** and **B**. In **A**, the superimpositions are more congruent with a minimal amount of variability or normal stability/jitter seen in the interpotential intervals (e.g., interval between the spike trigger and potential to the right). In **B**, the number of individual muscle fiber action potentials seen at one site is increased, suggesting a greater than normal number of muscle fibers within the immediate recording tip of the needle electrode. Greater interpotential variability is seen between the triggering spike (arrow) and the peaks to the right (marked with "*"), suggesting incomplete reinnervation.

Whereas the needle insertion is usually uncomfortable, the use of a sharp, high quality needle recording electrode in experienced hands requires only a few minutes to assess the MUAPs in most cases. Depending on the clinical question (e.g., radiculopathy, neuropathy), adequate sampling of muscles of a myotome/motor nerve, extremity, or contralateral extremity must be made. For example, if a fifth lumbar radiculopathy is suspected, then abnormalities should be noted in at least two muscles supplied by that myotome but innervated by different motor nerves (e.g., gluteus medius and anterior tibial muscles) (53). See the preceding section on segmental pointer muscles (17, 82).

The overlapping myotomes along the paraspinal muscles makes use of these for individual or segmental myotome localization difficult. The benefit from doing these muscles is to establish the process as being proximal (i.e., radicular) as opposed to distal (e.g., plexus) and to assess timing (Table 6.2). When a diffuse process such as motor neuron disease is suspected, abnormality should be observed in at least three muscles supplied by three different nerves or myotomes in three extremities (or two extremities and the bulbar muscles, the latter confirming the process to be rostral to the spinal cord).

Pathophysiology of Denervation/Reinnervation in Motor Nerve Fibers

In the acute phase of a lesion that disrupts the motor axon(s), there is a reduced number of normal appearing, rapidly firing MUAPs. Depending on the length of the motor axon to the muscle, increased membrane irritability followed by fibrillation potentials (56) (Fig. 6.7) occurs between 2 and 3 weeks. This proceeds in a proximal to distal direction. In a single level radiculopathy, the earliest changes would be focal changes in the paraspinal muscles followed by denervation changes in the extremity muscles in a centrifugal pattern (27, 67).

Reinnervation begins relatively soon (within weeks) depending on the severity of the lesion (Table 6.2). It usually is accomplished by collateral sprouting from terminal axons within the same muscle. These "sprouts" may derive from unaffected MUs from the same root in an incomplete lesion or from MUs supplied by a different root(s) within the same muscle. Depending on the specific etiology of a radicular lesion, axonal regrowth may be possible but slow and insignificant (67). Denervation and reinnervation may also be seen in chronic polyneuropathy or in focal entrapment neuropathy, but for different pathophysiologic reasons. In such cases, the nerve conduction studies help distinguish these from radiculopathy. Discussion of polyneuropathies and focal entrapment neuropathies is beyond the scope of this chapter, and the reader is referred to more detailed discussions elsewhere (4, 13, 14, 27, 29, 54, 81).

This "remodeling" of the MU via reinnervation means that the innervation ratio or number of muscles fibers being supplied by a motor axon increases proportionally to the degree of collateral sprouting (67, 84). When the number of single muscle fiber action potential generators increases for a given MU, the standard recording needle electrodes reflect these changes as MUAPs which are increased in amplitude, area, duration, and complexity (see Fig. 6.6A versus 6.6B). This remodeling is considered to be permanent. Once MUAPs are enlarged, they do not revert to normal amplitude, area, and duration values if the pathologic process is arrested or reversed.

In activating or contracting a muscle affected by a chronic neurogenic process, there are a reduced number of MUAPs firing rapidly for any given level of voluntary effort. This is referred to as a reduced or decreased recruitment rate (Fig. 6.6B). The degree of reduction in number of MUAPs that can be recruited is proportional to the severity and chronicity of the lesion. Clinical weakness is not necessarily present when chronic reinnervation changes are established or occurring. In a chronic process of ongoing denervation and reinnervation, it is estimated that approximately one third of the motor neurons supplying a muscle may be lost before clinical weakness becomes manifest (96).

A total loss of axons innervating a muscle is relatively uncommon in single nerve root lesions. This generally suggests a multiple radiculopathy or a more distal process, at the level of the plexus or peripheral nerve. If axonal growth proceeds, reinnervation of the muscle fibers will begin commensurate with the time required for those growing axons to traverse the linear distance from the site of the lesion (i.e., approximately 1 millimeter/day) (67).

The resulting "early reinnervation" or "nascent" MU has fewer muscle fibers than normal for that muscle (i.e., decreased innervation ratio). The MUAP reflecting this degree of reinnervation appears as reduced in amplitude, reduced in duration, complex, and unstable with a reduced recruitment pattern. Myopathies may show MUAPs of similar size and complexity, but the recruitment pattern shows an increased number of small MUAPs firing for level of effort (8). In the more chronic phase (many months or longer), neurogenic MUAPs increase in size, reflecting the increase in innervation ratio beyond normal for that muscle, with a persistently reduced recruitment pattern (84).

While instability or increased jitter is the hallmark of disorders of the neuromuscular junction (e.g., myasthenia gravis), they also arise from changes at the neuromuscular junction during denervation/reinnervation (Fig. 6.8). Because denervation is a relatively brief process (a few days, particularly when the insult is known to be a monophasic event, e.g., acute trauma), this type of instability more often reflects reinnervation and has two main causes. The first is instability resulting from reinnervation of motor end plates, which resolves after about 6 months. The second possibility for instability is the reduced conduction velocity along muscle fibers of smaller diameter such as occur in recently reinnervated muscle fibers (85). Stable, enlarged MUAPs of variable complexity would therefore suggest a remote (i.e., resolved) or slowly progressive process (84, 85). Such an observation may have management implications, for example, in the timing of the surgical exploration of a traumatic lesion.

SEPs

SEPs are a series of waveforms that can be recorded from the nervous system in response to repetitive afferent stimuli (4, 27). In this chapter, our discussion of SEPs is restricted to those obtained from repetitive electrical stimulation of mixed nerve trunks. As in nerve conductions studies, a bipolar stimulator delivering a square-wave pulse of either constant current (preferable) or constant voltage is used. Because the recorded signals are small in amplitude, repetitive stimuli are delivered to excite type I muscular and type II cutaneous afferent fibers. Because a mixed nerve is stimulated (e.g., median nerve at the wrist or tibial nerve at the ankle), the current intensity is adjusted to produce a visible motor twitch (e.g., median-innervated thenar or tibial-innervated toe flexors). Thus, the stimulus intensity is just suprathreshold to the motor fibers to ensure adequate stimulation of afferent nerve fibers. Many stimuli (hundreds) may be required to obtain a reproducible response that can be delineated from artifact or baseline noise.

These electric stimuli are transmitted proximally to the spinal cord where they travel through the posterior columns of the spinal cord towards the nuclei of the brainstem, thalamus, and ultimately the somatosensory cortex. Extralemniscal pathways may also make a small contribution to some of the waveforms. Recording electrodes are conventionally placed over more proximal nerve segments, the spinal cord, and the scalp. Various waveforms, both positive (downgoing) and negative (upgoing), are recorded. Table 6.4 describes the nomenclature of waveforms recorded with repetitive median and tibial nerve stimulation, and their accepted generator sources.

A recording electrode that is close to the source of the generated activity is termed "active." A recording electrode placed remote or distant to the site of the

TABLE 6.4.
Nomenclature of SEP Waveforms Recorded in Median and Tibial Nerve Stimulation and their Accepted Generator Sources (4)

Nerve	Waveform*	Generator
Median	N9/P9	Afferent volley at brachial plexus
	N11/P11	Spinal cord entry
	N13/P13	Cervical dorsal column interneurons
	P14	Caudal medial lemniscus
	N18	Upper brainstem/Thalamus
	N20	Parietal cortex
	P23	Frontoparietal cortex
Tibial	N9/P9	Afferent volley at popliteal fossa
	N21/P21	Spinal cord entry
	N22/P22	Lumbar dorsal column interneurons
	N31/P31	Caudal medial lemniscus
	N34/P34	Upper brainstem/Thalamus
	P37	Parietal cortex
	N45	Frontoparietal cortex

* N = negative-going wave, P = positive-going wave, numbers indicate latency value (msec) where waveform occurs.

electric activity is termed "reference." A recording is "bipolar" when the waveform is the difference between two active recording electrodes. A recording is termed "referential" when it measures the difference between an active electrode and a reference one. This latter pattern of recording is similar to how routine motor and sensory conductions are made.

Electric activity of biologic origin generated near and far from the recording electrodes is termed "near-field" and "far-field" potentials, respectively. Near-field potentials use an active recording electrode close to the area under study with a reference electrode placed over a more "electrically quiet" area some distance (centimeters) away. Far-field recording methods are used in which the biologic signal generators are remote from the recording electrodes. Although exact placement of the recording electrodes is less important, they must be reasonably far apart to discriminate small amplitude potential differences between them (i.e., $<1\mu V$).

The arrangements of various electrodes, referred to as montages, vary between laboratories. Ideally, a recording montage should be consistent for any particular laboratory, combining both referential and bipolar connections. Because the difference between the two electrodes are fed into a differential amplifier, signals common to both electrodes are subtracted and canceled out. Therefore, a bipolar montage reads the electrical activity generated near one of the recording electrodes, while referential montages read the entire electrical activity generated by both close and remote neural sources (Table 6.4 and Fig. 6.9).

There are two main types of neural events responsible for the generation of EPs. The first type is synaptic potentials that result from the summation of individual action potentials related to neurons clustered in groups. The second type is action potentials propagated through various pathways. These two types of neural events result in either a near field or a far field potential. Near field potentials usually have a regional distribution, their latencies increase at more distant sites, and they are present on both bipolar and referential montages. Far field potentials are stationary waveforms that are distributed widely, have latencies that usually are independent of the electrode position, and are seen only in referential montages because they tend to be canceled out in bipolar ones (70).

The amplitudes of most SEPs are under 5 μV. SEP amplitudes are therefore smaller than those obtained for SNAPs, which are recorded in routine sensory nerve conductions (typically $>5\mu V$). They are also substantially smaller than the amplitudes of surrounding "noise" generated by such volume conductors as muscle tissue and brain EEG activity. Therefore, the identification of SEPs requires the averaging of multiple recorded responses. The recorded waveforms are time-locked to a stimulus. To obtain a sufficient signal-to-noise ratio resolution, 250 to 500 responses usually are required to define and to amplify reliable waveforms. The signal-to-noise ratio is improved by a factor equal to the square root of the number of responses averaged, assuming no changes in the level of the random "electrical noise" present in the baseline.

The trial usually is repeated a second time to ensure consistency. If muscle activity is excessive, sedation before the test may be necessary. The reader is referred to more comprehensive sources for additional methodological details such as filtering (4, 27).

EP amplitudes tend to vary between subjects and from one trial to the next. The latencies of the major peaks are relatively constant and measurements of these are the values used for interpretation (Fig. 6.9). The waveforms are named for their polarity (N = negative or up-going; P = positive or down-going) and the latency at which they are recorded. For instance, the N9 potential is a negative waveform occurring at 9 msec after the stimulus artifact (see Table 6.4). Because the latencies of the SEP waveforms are unchanged using consistent montages, central and spinal conduction times can be calculated. Spinal conduction time for the tibial nerve is calculated by subtracting the N22 from the P31 wave latency (see Table 6.4). Central conduction time for the tibial nerve is calculated by subtracting the P31 from the P37 wave latency; that of the median nerve is calculated by subtracting the P14 from the N20 wave latency (Table 6.4) (32).

The initial portion of a SEP waveform is termed a short-latency sensory evoked response. It occurs within 25 msec of median nerve stimulation, 40 msec of common peroneal nerve stimulation, and 50 msec

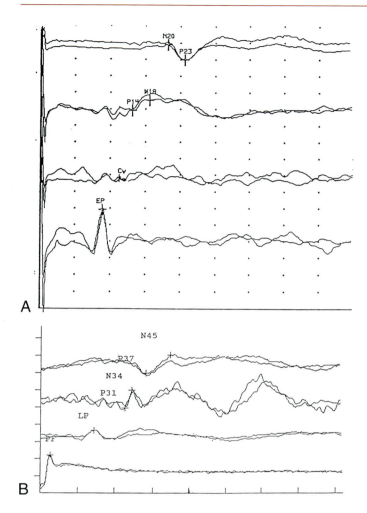

FIGURE 6.9.

A. Normal median SEPs. The top through bottom traces are channels 1 through 4, respectively. The following describes the montage used. Channel 1: contralateral parietal cortex referenced to the ipsilateral parietal cortex. Channel 2: ipsilateral parietal cortex referenced to the contralateral Erb's point. Channel 3: C5 spinous process referenced to contralateral Erb's point. Channel 4: Ipsilateral Erb's point referenced to contralateral Erb's point. (EP = Erb's potential; Cv = N13 Cervical potential; P14-N18 and N20-P23 are as described in the Nomenclature, Table 6.4). Division markers: horizontal = 5 msec; vertical = 2 μV. **B.** Normal tibial SEPs. Channels 1–4 correspond to the order of tracings as in Figure 6.5.A. The following describes the montage used. Channel 1: midline Centro-parietal (Cpz) referenced to midline Frontal (Fz). Channel 2: Fz referenced to Cv. Channel 3: LP = Lumbar potential at level of conus medullaris (T12 spinous process referenced to ipsilateral iliac crest). Channel 4: PF = Popliteal fossa (Ipsilateral popliteal fossa referenced to an adjacent point a few centimeters away). P31-N34 and P37-N45 are as in the Nomenclature, Table 6.4. Division markers: horizontal = 10 msec; vertical = 2.5 μV. Note that time division markers in **B** are longer than **A**.

of tibial nerve stimulation (4, 27). These short latency EPs are therefore the earliest portion of the total SEP waveform.

The segmental sensory nerve evoked potentials (SSEPs) are the EPs elicited from the stimulation of single cutaneous nerve trunks. Compared with mixed nerve SEPs, these have the advantage of isolating cutaneous nerve fibers emanating from specific dermatomes. Common nerves used in the lower extremity are sural, superficial peroneal, and saphenous nerves, which represent the S1, L5, and L4 dermatomes, respectively. In the upper extremity, the ulnar nerve branches of the fifth digit, median nerve branches of the third digit, and the median/radial branches from the thumb are stimulated to elicit responses from the C8, C7, and C6 dermatomes, respectively.

The montages for recording over the spine and scalp are similar to those for SEPs. In contrast to the latter, the latencies are slightly longer and the amplitudes smaller because of the fewer axons stimulated peripherally. These conditions necessitate the use of sensitive recording equipment and a higher number of averaged responses. SSEPs provide information similar to that obtained from SEPs, but because of their more restricted territorial derivations, and in turn, projections, they tend to be more reliable in determining the level of an affected root (31). When performed in a rigidly controlled manner, they have a higher sensitivity in diagnosing radiculopathies compared to SEPs (93) or in diagnosing primary sensory nerve injuries (e.g., lateral femoral cutaneous neuropathy) compared to nerve conduction studies (89).

Dermatomal evoked potentials (DEPs) differ from SEPs by virtue of the location of the stimulus, i.e., the skin of the dermatome to be studied is stimulated rather than a peripheral nerve. Recording montages are similar to those described for SEPs. DEPs may be technically more difficult to record than SEPs. Because SSEPs and DEPs bypass the motor fibers within the peripheral nerves and nerve roots, other techniques, such as SEPs and EMG, are needed if motor pathways must also be studied.

Electrodiagnostic Findings in Diseases of the Spinal Cord and Nerve Roots

Chronic myelopathy primarily affecting the white matter without associated radiculopathy has few EDX findings on routine EMG studies (7, 57, 66). The motor and sensory nerve conductions are typically normal. In other types of myelopathy, the F and H wave latencies may vary, depending on the structures affected and level of involvement (17, 27). F waves have been suggested to be of value in acute cervical myelopathy caused by anterior spinal artery syndrome (6).

In chronic spinal cord lesions affecting the anterior grey matter, F wave responses corresponding to that segment may be prolonged or absent. Where anterior grey matter (i.e., motor neurons) is affected, the amplitudes of the CMAPs on the motor conductions may be reduced and the needle electrode examination of muscles innervated by that myotome may show reinnervation changes. Study of adjacent, ipsilateral roots as well as that of the same root level on the contralateral side is necessary to optimally define localization. Unless the dorsal root ganglia are affected, the sensory nerve conductions are normal as discussed previously. EDX studies do not differentiate intramedullary from extramedullary spinal cord processes.

In some cases of spinal cord pathology, the etiology of neurogenic changes in the muscles may be less obvious. Wasting in hand muscles may be seen in high cervical cord lesions rostral to the myotomes supplying these muscles. This is thought to have an ischemic basis (38, 60, 86). In very rostral lesions, such as foramen magnum tumors, EMG of the high cervical paraspinal muscles may be helpful (45). In the authors' experience, study of the more rostral cervical paraspinal muscles is generally not helpful and can be a difficult exercise in localization of the level of the lesion because of overlap in the myotomes.

SEPs are helpful in the evaluation of cervical myelopathies, particularly those caused by cervical spondylosis. Changes in the lower extremity SEP tend to occur early in the course of the disease (70). The degree of involvement of cervical roots versus grey matter within the spinal cord can be determined from comparison of near and far field potentials (79, 80). Although not in widespread use, at our institution the authors also record cortical SEPs in neutral position of the cervical spine, followed by recording with the neck in flexion and in extension (20). The presence of significant changes (defined as an amplitude drop greater than 50% or latency increase greater than 10%) usually correlates with dynamic compromise to the cervical spinal cord as demonstrated on myelography.

In other nonstructural diseases of the spine affecting the spinal cord, such as in multiple sclerosis, median and tibial SEPs are important in detecting subclinical lesions, particularly when MR scan of the brain is within normal limits. Diagnostic information may be obtained from lower extremity SEPs in disorders such as lumbar spinal stenosis, spinal cord tumors, arteriovenous malformations, leukodystrophies, HIV myelopathy, transverse myelitis, and spinocerebellar degenerations (4).

Conus medullaris lesions show variable degrees of sensory and upper and lower motor findings on clinical examination. The electrodiagnostic findings usually show patchy, asymmetric involvement of the caudal lumbosacral nerve roots on needle electrode examination. The motor conductions are usually normal as in myelopathy, but the late responses (F and H waves) may be prolonged or absent. Sensory conductions are normal if the lesion(s) is proximal to the dorsal root ganglion. In lesions of the cauda equina, the EDX findings are again variable depending on which roots are involved and where along the course of the nerve root the pathology is located (17, 27).

Radiculopathy, assuming the lesion truly is at the nerve root level and affects only one segment or root, does not affect the distal motor and sensory conductions. This is due to the proximal location of the lesion and the multisegmental (i.e., greater than one dermatome/myotome) composition of most peripheral nerves. The F and H late responses may be prolonged or absent in muscles receiving significant innervation from the involved root. If a single root is severed or avulsed completely, one may assume that all sensorimotor nerve fibers within that root are affected equally, i.e., completely interrupted. In other lesions of the nerve roots, sensorimotor nerve fibers within a given root may be affected to varying degrees at the level of the lesion. Therefore, one should not assume that each sensorimotor nerve fiber is affected equally at the level of the lesion. Abnormal responses to repetitive motor stimulation suggesting myasthenia have been reported (37), emphasizing the importance of clinical interpretation of EDX tests and avoiding "phenomenological" interpretations independent of clinical findings.

Mixed nerve SEPs have not proven helpful in the routine evaluation of root lesions (3, 93). This finding is caused by the significant dermatomal overlap in the sensory fibers coursing within the nerve trunk. However, SSEPs may be beneficial in pure sensory radiculopathies because the sensory nerves stimulated have smaller territorial (i.e., dermatomal) projections centrally (93). SEPs complement conventional EDX studies in brachial plexus lesions, particularly those caused by trauma where root avulsion may also be suspected. The absence of consistent cervical responses, despite recordable, albeit small amplitude peripheral potentials, indicates root involvement (5, 50). Although SEPs theoretically should be of value in measuring conduction between the brachial plexus and cervical roots, its use in evaluating neurogenic thoracic outlet syndrome remains uncertain (3, 5).

The needle electrode examination is considered to

be the most helpful EDX study in radiculopathy (94). To establish this diagnosis, there should be neurogenic changes in the muscles of the affected myotome(s) commensurate with the presumed duration of the process (Table 6.3). Patients may have other, coexistent peripheral neurologic problems. For example, some older patients with presumed carpal tunnel syndrome have more severe and proximal symptoms than what would be expected with simple distal median neuropathy. These individuals may also have a concurrent C6 radiculopathy, which has been called the "double crush syndrome" (74). Therefore, in patients being evaluated for radiculopathy, it is useful to perform nerve conduction studies appropriate to that root(s).

In cases of structural spine disorders, interruption in the integrity of the nerve root is contingent on where the structural problem occurs. Hence, in the case of a ruptured intervertebral disc, the physiologic function of the disrupted root depends on the location of the lesion. In more laterally-placed lesions, the likelihood for acute compression with neurologic deficit is greater because the root is traveling in a more confined space. More medial lesions may show more of a pattern of subjective pain and sensory disturbance where the root may be mechanically distorted but without significant compression. In the latter situation, minimal to no axonal disruption may occur; consequently, denervation and related findings on the EMG may also be minimal to absent.

EMG studies in the patient who is already post-surgery (e.g., "failed back syndrome") present a special problem (63, 83). EMG studies performed preoperatively do not appear to help identify or predict such cases (35). Even so, it is helpful to have a reliable preoperative study when confronted with such a situation. If the postoperative EMG of limb muscles is normal, the conclusion is less problematic than if reinnervation changes, suggesting a chronic radiculopathy, are present. In the latter instance, the absence of fibrillation potentials and the presence of stable, enlarged MUAPs imply that the process is either slowly progressive, or more likely, remote (i.e. reinnervation completed).

Given the overlapping segmental innervation of paraspinal muscle, study of these muscles near an

TABLE 6.5.
Some Neurologic Conditions Not Associated with Structural Spine Lesions That May be Confused with Myelopathy or Radiculopathy due to Structural Spine Disease

Disorder	Comment
Acute transverse myelopathy (or myelitis)	This is a syndrome in adults with variable causes: infectious, dysimmune, paraneoplastic (17, 62).
Multiple sclerosis	May be seen in older individuals (>50 years) as a progressive myelopathy (72).
Vascular Myelopathy	Thought to be due to arteriosclerosis and may be difficult to diagnose (17, 48).
Lyme disease	May present as myelopathy, radiculopathy, and/or neuropathy (12, 41).
Old polio	Asymmetric involvement with the disease process allegedly stable. Needle electrode examination of such patients typically shows widespread involvement of clinically unaffected muscles; may need to differentiate from post-polio muscular atrophy (30, 46).
Traumatic brachial plexopathy	Motor and sensory conductions typically abnormal with sparing of paraspinal muscles. Caveat: cervical root avulsions and necessary cranial neuropathy may also be seen in traumatic plexopathy (5, 18).
Neuralgic amyotrophy (Parsonage Turner Syndrome)	Commonly an upper brachial plexopathy, hence nerve conductions commonly normal; paraspinal muscles usually spared; may see more subtle widespread involvement of muscles in same limb by needle electrode examination, as well as on the contralateral side (34).
Mononeuritis multiplex or multiple mononeuropathy	Nerve conductions abnormal giving a pattern of patchy, widespread involvement which may not be clinically obvious. Although uncommon, this pattern may occur in diabetes, vaculitides, etc. (29, 81).
Thoracic outlet syndrome	True neurogenic thoracic outlet syndrome is rare—characteristic nerve conduction findings are sensory involvement on the medial (ulnar) aspect of the hand and motor on the lateral (median) aspect. Needle electrode examination findings occur in the territory of the low cervical roots without paraspinal muscle involvement (19).
Motor neuron disease (ALS)	May present with subacute to chronic focal motor deficit with sensory sparing (e.g., foot drop); needle electrode examination shows widespread denervation in established cases (27).
Post-traumatic amyotrophy	Should have history of trauma. Weakness is typically limited to one or few myotomes. Process stabilizes in chronic phase (71).
Myopathy	Most myopathies are subacute to chronic symmetric processes; however, some, such as inclusion body myositis, may be asymmetric and effect distal upper extremity muscle more severely, thus suggesting nerve root disease (8, 9, 27, 64).
Focal entrapment neuropathy	Diagnosis depends on site: e.g., a common peroneal neuropathy should have sensory conduction abnormality of the peroneal nerve, slowing and conduction block would be expected at the compression site (fibular head?), and there should *only* be involvement of muscles supplied by this portion of the common peroneal nerve (i.e., distal to the lesion) and *none* in proximal or nonperoneal L5 innervated muscles (27, 88).

operative site may be an interpretative challenge. Even considering the possibility of secondary changes in the paraspinal muscles as a direct result of prior surgical manipulation, the absence of fibrillation potentials and presence of stable MUAPs augur a remote (radicular) process. Conversely, if such changes are diffusely present along the operative site bilaterally, one should suspect they resulted from direct surgical manipulation of the paraspinal muscle. These changes may persist for a few years after surgery (27, 56). Only highly focal findings compatible with ongoing reinnervation (e.g., fibrillation potentials and unstable MUAPs) correlated with clinical findings and abnormalities on imaging studies should be considered suspicious for an active radiculopathy.

The goal of this chapter is to deal with EDX findings in spine disorders. Patients may present, however, with neurologic problems and deficits suggesting a single or multiple root process but lacking correlative findings on imaging studies. These apparent "anatomic" lesions may have a structural basis, but not from spine disease. Diabetics may notoriously present with radicular lesions (lumbosacral in particular) which are thought to be caused by ischemia of the vaso nervorum (91). Other vasculitic processes (17) may show similar clinical patterns, as may herpes zoster (28). In zoster, the characteristic rash usually accompanies the sensorimotor deficit. Other neurologic nonradicular conditions that may be confused with myelopathy/radicular conditions are summarized in Table 6.5.

What To Do About a Normal EDX Study?

In general, the value of a test is contingent on the clinical acumen of the physician ordering it. Frustration may be generated by a referring physician over a "normal" study. To the referring physician, a "normal" EDX study may seem incompatible with the patient's clinical findings. Regardless of the results, the findings must be placed in the perspective of the patient's clinical problem.

If so, the referring clinician is recommended to review the study with the EDX physician. Clinicians often review scans and other imaging studies with the radiologist in the most minute detail. The authors have rarely had clinicians request to review their patients' EDX studies. The reasons for this may include: 1) a bias to place more confidence in anatomy over physiology; 2) training and practice patterns; 3) a relative lack of appreciation of the value of EDX studies, and 4) perhaps a combination of these and other factors.

In the case of suspected radiculopathy based only on pain and without evident neurologic deficit, EDX studies may be "normal." The implication is that the lesion is not producing compression or other mechanical disturbance of the nerve root(s). We reemphasize that a presumed clinically significant structural abnormality seen on imaging study of the spine should correlate with an electrophysiologic abnormality with respect to level and side to imply a relationship between them. Conversely, there may not be an electrophysiologic abnormality present for every structural finding ("abnormality"?) observed on imaging studies (49, 90). The precise etiology for pain in this situation is not completely clear and does not always presume radicular involvement. All spine "pain" should not be inferred to arise from the nerve root per se.

Other reasons for "normal" studies may not be readily evident to the referring physician. Based on the description of what was done during the procedure, the referring physician may be able to at least infer one of the more common problems for a "normal" or "inconclusive" study, which is an *incomplete* study. For example, an insufficient number of muscles may not have been studied because of a patient's intolerance of the procedure to reliably determine the presence or absence of a radiculopathy. Also, there may be an additional process present, such as a polyneuropathy, that precluded identification of the radiculopathy.

Another possibility for a "normal" EDX study is that the neurologic abnormality on clinical examination is not amenable to conventional, and possibly not unconventional, EDX study procedures. An example would be meralgia paresthetica, or lateral femoral cutaneous neuropathy. This is a sensory branch of the femoral plexus that is variable in location and in the manner in which it branches distally over the lateral thigh. It is possible to do sensory conductions of this nerve, but it may be difficult to obtain results even in control subjects. In our laboratory, we do the unaffected side first before attempting the involved side. The remainder of our strategy in such a patient is to perform conventional nerve conductions to exclude a neuropathy and to study enough muscles on the affected side to exclude an upper lumbar radiculopathy, femoral plexopathy, or neuropathy. In this specific example, SSEPs, if available, may be useful to identify the lesion (89).

Having excluded the preceding considerations, one may consider other possibilities. Is the clinical problem accurately defined? In some patients, the pattern of pain may be of neurologic origin but may be misleading (e.g., lower extremity pain secondary to a cervical process [58]). Can the symptoms be caused by a referred pain problem? For example, could a patient's hyperesthesia over the inferior portion of the right scapula be caused by cholecystitis (i.e., Boas' sign) rather than radiculopathy? Are the symptoms caused by a connective tissue problem (e.g., a myoligamentous strain) and therefore not a primary neurologic etiology? Careful inquiry into provocative factors, such as occupation, is often revealing (59).

If the preceding issues are considered and addressed adequately, then the referring physician should be confident of the integrity of the peripheral nervous system based on the EDX studies. In patients whose history cannot be relied upon or in cases in which functional overlay may be suspect, EDX studies are useful in reconciling dubious symptoms or "apparent" deficits. This is not always so easy to establish and must be done with great care by an experienced EDX physician (95). SEP studies may be useful in demonstrating the integrity of the somatosensory pathways in patients with hysterical sensory loss of one or more extremities.

In another example, a patient with a "foot drop" may offer no volitional activation in the anterior tibial muscle on direct examination, yet has no other convincing objective findings. This instance is suspicious for a nonphysiologic deficit. If so, the EMG would be expected to show normal sensorimotor peroneal nerve conductions with spontaneous normal volitional activation of anterior tibial MUAPs when distracted. The latter may be difficult to achieve. In one of the authors' cases, a recording needle electrode was placed in the nonfunctioning anterior tibial muscle. No MUAPs were recorded on volitional activation, but a normal recruitment pattern showing normal MUAPs was elicited easily as the patient went from a sitting to a standing position.

Intraoperative Monitoring of Evoked Potentials During Spine Surgery

Introduction

In the past one to two decades, EPs have been increasingly employed in the monitoring of spinal cord and other neural pathways during various surgical procedures. SEP monitoring is the most commonly used modality in spine surgery. Some of the many indications for IOM with EPs are summarized in Table 6.6. The main purpose of monitoring in these situations is to prevent injury to neural structures while the patient is under anesthesia. IOM becomes particularly important in the setting of a preoperative neurologic deficit. It is important for the EDX physician who is performing the monitoring to have adequate time to plan for the procedure. This planning includes the ability to obtain baseline SEPs and to address any other special technical problems before the start of surgery. IOM is almost as large a time com-

TABLE 6.6.

Common Indications for Intraoperative Monitoring with Evoked Potentials (modified from Harper and Daube, 42)

Spine Diseases	Spinal Cord Diseases	Other Conditions
Scoliosis	Arteriovenous malformations	Dorsal rhizotomy
Degenerative conditions	Syringomyelia	Aortic aneurysms
Trauma	Cauda equina surgery	Posterior fossa lesions
Tumors	Tumors	Peripheral nerve lesions
		Brachial/lumbosacral plexus lesions

mitment for the EDX physician as the procedure is for the surgeon.

Methodology

Despite the electrical noise inherent to the operating room, the monitoring technique should be reliable and offer minimal interference with the surgical procedure. Equipment with preamplifiers that can stand high current loads should be used. Table 6.7 lists several means to reduce the amount of noise and interference from surrounding equipment (73). The following paragraph emphasizes some points of methodology. The reader is also referred to more comprehensive reviews (4, 15, 22, 39, 42, 47).

Several factors may interfere with the signal to noise ratio of the responses, which in turn determines the quality of the recorded EPs. These factors include the primary disease, the subject's age, the depth of the anesthesia, the type of anesthetic agent (Table 6.8), how the agent is delivered, and the mean arterial pressure (42). Therefore, it is preferable to use recording equipment with the capability of concurrently monitoring different EPs and EMG responses (i.e., multichannel recordings). This permits greater confidence in the recordings with minimal interfer-

TABLE 6.7.

Strategies to Reduce Noise During Intraoperative Monitoring (modified from Nuwer, 73)

1. Glue electrodes to skin with collodion
2. Re-gel electrodes every few hours
3. Keep recording electrodes close together and away from the stimulator
4. Avoid crossing or passing electrode wires near power cables
5. Use separate power outlets for monitoring equipment
6. Use equipment that stops averaging during cautery
7. Adjust/reduce the amplifier sensitivity and increase the low frequency filter as necessary

TABLE 6.8.
Effects of Major Anesthetics on Evoked Potentials (42, 51, 52, 77, 97)

Anesthetic	Cortical SEP	Spinal SEP	CMAP	F or H Wave	Motor EP
Etomidate	0 or ⇑	0 or ⇑	0	0	⇑ / ⇓
Fentanyl	0 or ⇓	⇓	0	0	⇑ / ⇓
Halothane	0 or ⇓	0	0	0	⇓
Isoflurane	⇓	0 or ⇓	⇓	⇓	⇓
Ketamine	0 or ⇑	0 or ⇑	0	0	0 or ⇓
Midazolam	⇓	0	0	0	⇓
Morphine	⇓	⇓	0	0	0
N₂O	⇓	⇓	0	0	⇓
Propofol	⇑	⇑	0	⇓	⇓
Thiopental	⇓	0	0	0	0

(0 = no change; ⇑ = increase; ⇓ = decrease; ⇑ / ⇓ variable change)

ence with the surgical procedure. The duration of the surgery is also not unnecessarily prolonged from doing excessive repetitions of EPs.

The methods of stimulation are similar to those described previously in routine SEPs. It is especially important to stimulate nerves that are most likely to be compromised, even if their baseline recording is technically more difficult to obtain. Although any nerve can be monitored, ulnar nerve responses usually are more sensitive for cervical spine surgery (92). Tibial nerve responses are important for surgeries at any level below the cervical spine or for lesions adjacent to the midline in the cervical region. SEPs of both upper and both lower extremities may be recorded concurrently.

Monitoring the spinal EPs can be obtained using rapid rates of stimulation. The cortical SEPs, however, are usually more sensitive to the effects of anesthetics and to other changes in the systemic circulation. This is particularly noticeable in younger patients (less than 20 years) or in the elderly (Fig. 6.10B), in whom a slower rate of stimulation is necessary. Although baseline SEPs usually are obtained at motor threshold stimulation, the authors often increase the intensity of stimulation above this level during surgical monitoring. This increase ensures that all of the larger afferent fibers are being stimulated (i.e., supramaximal stimulation).

The scalp electrode montage for recording standard SEPs is customarily used in IOM. For prolonged surgeries (i.e., longer than 6 hours), or when there is the risk of significant displacement of these electrodes, disposable needle EEG electrodes may be used to record from the scalp. Though less commonly used, surface electrodes can be applied to the spine and to various peripheral locations. If there is a possibility of displacement of these electrodes, recordings should be obtained from monopolar needle electrodes inserted along the length of the nerve trunk and over the spinal cord between various spinous processes. To minimize interference from electrical "noise," it is important to have both recording and reference electrodes of the same material aligned in parallel.

Other types of recording electrodes include small wicks. These wicks can record directly from the spinal cord or the cortex. Another variety of electrode is small epidural plastic plates that have several metal electrodes embedded in them which can be applied to the surface of the cortex or spinal cord (42). Although epidural electrodes usually give large amplitude recordings (50), they often are in the way of the surgeon. There is also a risk, albeit small, of infection. Nevertheless, they may be useful in spinal cord tumors or arteriovenous malformations. Should the EPs become lost, they allow direct and focal localization of the area.

Esophageal electrodes (25, 42) are used in several centers to obtain cervical cord potentials during the posterior approach to cervical spine surgery. An alternative that we have used in our center is the placement of an anterior cervical electrode over the thyroid cartilage that records a cervical near field positive potential (P13). At some centers, including the authors', electrodes linking both mastoid regions referenced to Fz (i.e., frontal midline of the scalp) may be used to help record near and far field potentials traveling across the foramen magnum and brainstem. The authors have found the latter montage primarily helpful in high cervical surgery (i.e., above the C5 level).

IOM requires ongoing trains of stimuli to be applied. As in routine SEP studies, sufficient numbers of stimuli are acquired to produce a well-defined tracing. This process is repeated throughout the surgery in continuous cycles, alternating nerves and sides being monitored. Hard copies (i.e., printouts) of the EPs are made at regular intervals for the record. If the EPs show alteration during the procedure, the EDX physician must be able to immediately troubleshoot the problem, be it technical (e.g., loose electrode) or a true change in the physiologic status of the spinal cord requiring appropriate confirmation (see later text).

Interpretation of Findings in IOM

During surgical monitoring, it is common to observe variability in the SEPs from one run to the next. Several factors contribute to this variability: intercurrent artifacts (Fig. 6.10A), fluctuations in blood pressure, change in levels of anesthesia (Fig. 6.10B), body position (Fig. 6.11), and body temperature, to name a few. It is therefore critical to ascertain that a consistent alteration in the waveforms, *not caused by technical or physiologic factors*, is confirmed before unduly alerting the surgeon or anesthesiologist. A common rule of thumb is that any consistent drop of EP amplitude by greater than 50% or any increase in the EP latencies greater than 10% compared to pre-anesthesia baseline values, is alarming (39, 42). If waveforms recorded from one nerve or site become lost or abnormal, additional nerves and sites must be monitored. This ensures reproducibility in the monitoring before determination of abnormality is made with certainty.

The most common type of IOM abnormality is a fairly abrupt change in the SEP amplitudes with lessor frequent change in latencies occurring immediately, or within several minutes after, surgical manipulation (Fig. 6.12). The change in the response usually is caused by slowing of the neural impulses or by manipulation of conduction block in the neural tissue. Such changes are often reversible once the problem is identified and corrected (39).

A second type of abnormality is a gradual loss of the EP amplitude or a gradual prolongation of the EP latency beginning more than 15 minutes after manipulation (Fig. 6.13). These changes continue to progress, typically over the subsequent 30 minutes. This pattern of change suggests ischemia. If the pattern is identified quickly, recovery occurs in the majority of patients (39).

Abrupt and complete loss of SEPs independent of surgical manipulation is a worrisome sign and may indicate ischemia to the spinal cord. Should this occur, it is important to continue nerve stimulation while recording from needle electrodes along various spinal segments. This allows localization of the site where the EPs are lost. A partially reversible cause (e.g., hematoma) is discovered occasionally and can be corrected. Recovery in these situations, however, is often incomplete.

The EDX physician should continue to monitor patients until they are awake. Some surgeons perform a wake-up test in the middle of the procedure. Currently, however, the majority of surgeons rely solely on the IOM. After the surgeon closes and an-

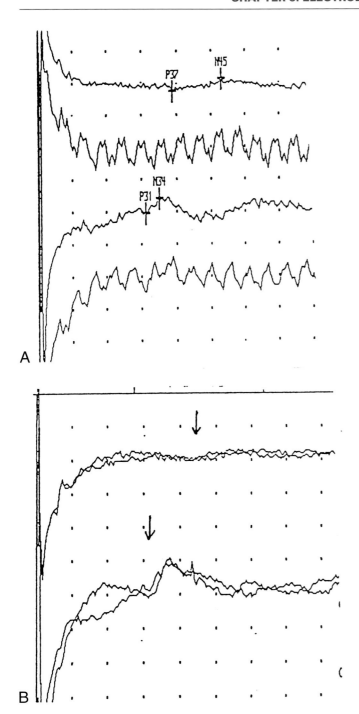

FIGURE 6.10.
A. Tibial SEP during IOM showing wide variability between recordings of the SEP. Trial 1 (top trace 1 and 3) compared to trial 2 (traces 2 and 4). Trial 2 shows marked artifact from electrical surgical equipment. Montages are as in Figure 6.5B. (Divisions markers: horizontal = 10 msec, vertical = 0.5 μV). **B.** Tibial SEP during IOM in an adolescent. There is marked suppression of the P37-N45 (cortical) potential (upper trace, arrow) immediately following anesthesia. The P31-N34 (cervical) potential is still clearly visible. Montages are as in Figure 6.5B. (Division markers: horizontal 10 msec, vertical = 0.5 μV.)

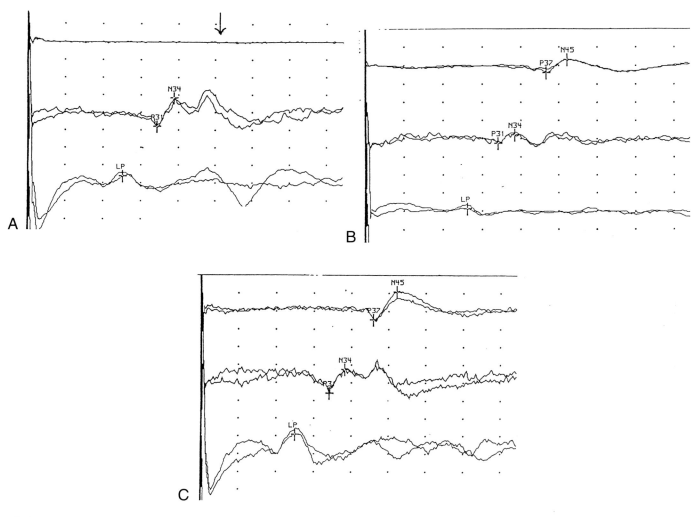

FIGURE 6.11.
Left tibial SEP during IOM monitoring. **A.** There is near absence of the P37-N45 (cortical) potential (top trace, arrow) after left side stimulation. In trace 2, the P31-N34 (cervical) potential is still visible as well as the LP (lumbar potential) in trace 3. **B.** The P37-N45 (cortical) potential is unremarkable after right side stimulation. This suggested compromise of spinal cord conduction is caused by excessive rotation of the patient's head and emphasizes the importance of confirming this observation with contralateral stimulation. **C.** Once head position had been corrected, the P37-N45 potential reappeared after left tibial stimulation. The montages are as in Figure 5.9B. (Division markers: horizontal = 10 msec; vertical = 0.5 μV [Figures 6.11A and C] and 1.0 μV [Figure 6.11B].)

esthesia has been reversed, patients are asked to move their extremities as a clinical confirmation of neurologic integrity.

Studies (39) have shown that IOM is important in preventing intraoperative injuries. Only rare cases are reported of postoperative deficit occurring despite the presence of otherwise normal EPs obtained from ostensibly uneventful IOM (61). In this setting, the neurologic damage has been located in pathways not directly monitored with the standard IOM techniques.

The use of SSEPs and DEPs follow the same guidelines as mixed nerve SEPs. Their responses have typically smaller amplitudes. In the authors' experience, they are somewhat more sensitive to various intraoperative changes compared with the mixed nerve SEPs. SSEPs and DEPs are not employed widely in IOM to date. Several centers, including the authors', are currently evaluating their specificity.

A shortcoming of current SEPs techniques is that they fail to reliably evaluate the motor pathways. Different techniques have been devised to monitor motor function. It is possible to insert nychrome wire electrodes into various muscles belonging to one or several myotomes that may be at surgical risk. These electrodes can be connected to special preamplifiers and the spontaneous or evoked EMG activity recorded during the surgery.

Of the variety of patterns on ongoing EMG activity that may be seen, the presence of neurotonic discharges is the most important one to recognize. These discharges are trains of impulses firing at a high rate;

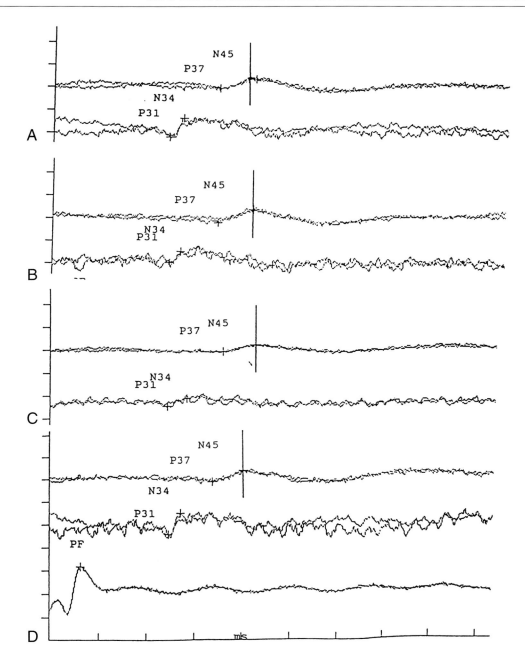

FIGURE 6.12.
A. IOM showing tibial SEP baseline run prior to rod and hook placement in the upper thoracic spine. **B.** During hook placement, there is a rapid, mild prolongation in the latencies and decrease in the amplitudes of the P37-N45 (cortical) and P31-N34 (cervical) potentials (approximately 10%). **C.** This decrease progressed as the hooks were tightened with an associated increase in their latencies. **D.** These abnormalities reversed within 6 minutes after the tight hooks were loosened, suggesting transient conduction block of the neural pathways being monitored. Montage as in Figure 6.9B. Division markers: horizontal = 10 msec; vertical = 1.2 μV.

they result from irritation or injury to the corresponding motor pathways. Although neurotonic discharges are an extremely valuable observation, their occurrence declines gradually with increasing levels of neuromuscular blockade (particularly when the latter exceeds 50%) (22).

Other means of monitoring motor pathways have therefore been devised. These include the assessment of the F and H waves in the manner described earlier in this chapter, recording both responses from the same electrodes. The F and H waves are sensitive markers for potential ischemia to the cord (6, 43). The advantage of the F and H waves is their relative resistance to neuromuscular blockade because they can be recorded even at 80% neuromuscular blockade. An important caveat is that F and H waves can be

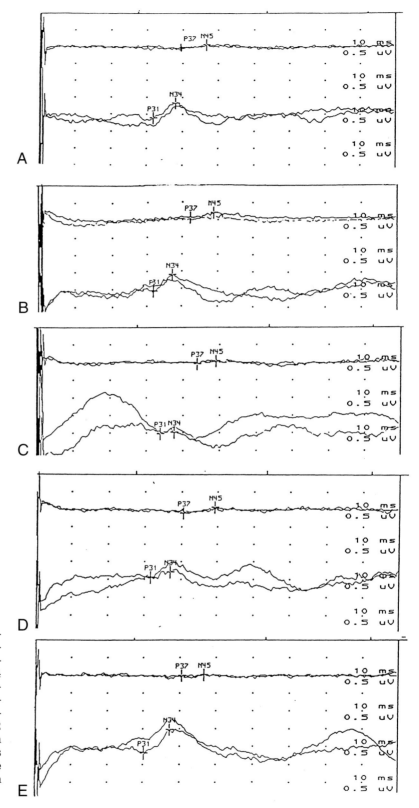

FIGURE 6.13.
A. Tibial SEP baseline run before ligation of midthoracic arteries for hemostasis. **B.** During ligation, there is a gradual decrease in the amplitudes of the P37-N45 (cortical) and P31-N34 (cervical) potentials. **C.** This progressed and became associated with an increase in their latencies 10 minutes post-ligation. **D.** The abnormalities gradually reversed over 20 minutes after 2 ligatures have been removed, with the bottom run (**E**) showing full recovery to baseline values (**A**). This is compatible with transient, reversible ischemia. Montages as in Figure 6.9B. Division markers: horizontal = 10 msec; vertical 0.5 μV.

sensitive to induction and inhalation anesthetics, especially in young or very old subjects. If they disappear during surgical manipulation when these agents are used, it may be necessary to reduce induction anesthesia and record the F and H waves on narcotics only. Table 6.8 summarizes the effect of various anesthetic agents on IOM modalities.

A final category of IOM involves responses elicited from direct stimulation of the motor pathways (33, 68, 75, 76). Magnetic or electric stimulation can be applied either to roots, spinal cord, or cortex. Magnetic stimulation uses a primary current to induce a secondary one in an adjacent neural structure. In the cerebral cortex, this generates direct and indirect waves. Magnetic stimulation in the spinal cord results in motor responses caudal to the level of stimulation. The recorded responses can be facilitated considerably by partial volitional activation of target muscles (68). This feature is useful in an awake patient but obviously not applicable during anesthesia.

Despite stable stimulus parameters, the latencies and amplitudes of the evoked responses may vary in magnetic stimulation. Even in normal subjects, the amplitudes of the evoked responses are small and tend to disappear at low levels of anesthesia. Magnetic stimulation is overall highly sensitive to the level of anesthesia: certain anesthetics tend to reduce or cancel the motor EP despite the integrity of the motor pathways (Table 6.8) (51, 52). Magnetic stimulation of the cortex or spinal cord is used infrequently and is considered experimental in most centers.

Direct electrical stimulation of the cortex or spinal cord also elicits direct motor responses from muscles caudal to the level of stimulation. The recorded responses are less variable than those evoked by magnetic stimulation. Recorded responses also disappear with increasing neuromuscular blockade (Table 6.8) (39, 68). Partial controlled neuromuscular blockade may still be necessary, however, to reduce the motor artifacts generated by the contraction of the paraspinal musculature. With cortical stimulation, there is a small risk of activating an epileptic focus (68).

The authors thank James M. Gilchrist, M.D., Gary P. Jacobson, Ph.D., Joan K. Kappes, M.S., and John C. Kincaid, M.D. for their review and comments.

List of Abbreviations Used:

CMAP	Compound Muscle Action Potential
Cpz	Centro-parietal (as in SEP montage)
DEP	Dermatomal Evoked Potential
EDX	Electrodiagnosis
EMG	Electromyography
EP	Evoked Potential, also Erb's Point in SEP montages
Fz	Frontal (as in SEP montage)
μV	microvolt
mm	millimeter
msec	millisecond
MU	Motor Unit
MUAP	Motor Unit Action Potential
mV	millivolt
SEP	Somatosensory Evoked Potential
SNAP	Sensory Nerve Action Potential
SSEP	Short-Latency Somatosensory Evoked Potential

References

1. American Association of Electromyography and Electrodiagnosis. Guidelines for electrodiagnostic medicine. Muscle Nerve 1992;15:229–253.
2. American Association of Electrodiagnostic Medicine. AAEM glossary of terms in clinical electromyography. Muscle Nerve 1987;10 (8S).
3. Aminoff MJ. The clinical role of somatosensory evoked potential studies: a critical appraisal. Muscle Nerve 1984;7:345–354.
4. Aminoff, MJ, Eisen A. Somatosensory evoked potentials. In: Aminoff MJ, ed. Electrodiagnosis in clinical neurology, 3rd ed. New York: Churchill Livingstone, 1992;571–603.
5. Aminoff MJ, Olney RK, Parry GJ, et al. Relative utility of different electrophysiologic techniques in the evaluation of brachial plexopathies. Neurology 1988; 38:546–550.
6. Amoiridis G, Poehlau D, Przuntek H. Neurophysiological findings and MRI in anterior spinal artery syndrome of the lower cervical cord: the value of F waves. J Neurol Neurosurg Psychiatry 1991;54:738–740.
7. Barkhaus PE, Morgan O. Jamaican neuropathy: an electrophysiologic study. Muscle Nerve 1988l1:380–385.
8. Barkhaus PE, Nandedkar SD, Sanders DB. Quantitative EMG in inflammatory myopathy. Muscle Nerve 1990; 13:247–253.
9. Barkhaus PE. Quantitative EMG in inclusion body myositis. J Neurol Sci 1990;98 (suppl):180.
10. Barkhaus PE, Nandedkar SD. Recording area of the surface electrode. Muscle Nerve 1994;17:1317–1323.
11. Barkhaus PE, Nandedkar SD. On the selection of concentric needle EMG motor unit action potentials for analysis: is the rise time criterion too restrictive? Muscle Nerve 1996;19:1554–1560.
12. Berlit P, Pohlman-Eden B, Henningsen H. Brown-Sequard syndrome caused by *Borrelia burgdorferi*. Eur Neurol 1991;31:18–20.
13. Brown WF. The physiological and technical basis of electromyography. Boston: Butterworths, 1984.
14. Brown WF, Bolton CF, eds. Clinical electromyography. Boston: Butterworths, 1987.
15. Brown WF, Veitch J. Intraoperative monitoring of peripheral and cranial nerves. Muscle Nerve 1994; 17:371–377.
16. Burke RE. Motor units in mammalian muscle. In: Sumner AJ, ed. The physiology of peripheral nerve disease. Philadelphia: WB Saunders, 1980;133–194.
17. Byrne TN, Waxman SG. Spinal cord compression. Philadelphia: FA Davis, 1990.
18. Coene LN. Mechanisms of brachial plexus lesions. Clin Neurol Neurosurg 1993;95(S):S24–29.
19. Cuetter AC, Bartoszek DM. The thoracic outlet syn-

drome: controversies, overdiagnosis, overtreatment, and recommendations for management. Muscle Nerve 1989;12:410–419.
20. Cusik JF. Neurosurgical considerations of cervical myelopathy. Semin Neurol 1989;9:193–199.
21. Daube JR. Needle electrode examination in clinical electromyography. Muscle Nerve 1991;14:685–700.
22. Daube JR, Harper CM. Surgical monitoring of cranial and peripheral nerves. In: Desmedt JE, ed. Neuromonitoring in surgery. Amsterdam: Elsevier, 1989;115–138.
23. Davidoff RA. The dorsal columns. Neurology 1989;39:1377–1385.
24. Davidoff RA. The pyramidal tract. Neurology 1990;40:332–339.
25. Desmedt JE. Somatosensory evoked potentials in neuromonitoring. In: Desmedt JE, ed. Neuromonitoring in surgery. Amsterdam: Elsevier, 1989;1–21.
26. Dorfman LJ, McGill KC. Automatic quantitative electromyography. Muscle Nerve 1988;11:804–818.
27. Dumitru D. Electrodiagnostic medicine. Philadelphia: Hanley & Belfus, 1995.
28. Dueland AN, Gilden DH. Neurologic aspects of *Varicella zoster* infections. In: Appel SH, ed. Current neurology, Volume 12. Chicago: Year Book Medical Publishers, 1992; 83–109.
29. Dyck PJ, Thomas PK, eds. Peripheral neuropathy, 3rd ed. Philadelphia: WB Saunders, 1993.
30. Einarsson G, Grimby G, Stalberg EV. Electromyographic and morphological functional compensation in late poliomyelitis. Muscle Nerve 1990;13:165–171.
31. Eisen A, Hoirch M, Moll A. Evaluation of radiculopathies by segmental stimulation and somatosensory evoked potentials. Can J Neurol Sci 1983;10:178.
32. Eisen A. Noninvasive measurement of spinal cord conduction: review of presently available methods. Muscle Nerve 1986;9:95–103.
33. Eisen A, Shtybel W. Clinical experience with transcranial magnetic stimulation. Muscle Nerve 1990;13:995–1011.
34. England JD, Sumner AJ. Neuralgia amyotrophy: an increasingly diverse entity. Muscle Nerve 1987;10:60–68.
35. Falck B, Nykvist F, Hurme M, et al. Prognostic value of EMG in patients with lumbar disc herniations—a five year follow up. Electromyogr Clin Neurophysiol 1993;33:19–26.
36. Fisher MA. H reflexes and F waves: physiology and clinical applications. Muscle Nerve 1992;15:1223–1233.
37. Gilchrist JM, Sanders DB. Myasthenic U-shaped decrement in multifocal cervical radiculopathy. Muscle Nerve 1989;12:64–66.
38. Good DC, Couch JR, Wacaser L. "Numb, clumsy hands" and high cervical spondylosis. Surg Neurol 1984;22:285–291.
39. Grundy BL. Intraoperative monitoring by evoked potential techniques. In: Aminoff MJ, ed. Electrodiagnosis in clinical neurology, 3rd ed. New York: Churchill Livingstone, 1992;649–682.
40. Gutmann L. Important anomalous innervations of the extremities. Muscle Nerve 1993;16:339–347.
41. Halperin J, Luft BJ, Volkman DJ, et al. Lyme neuroborreliosis: peripheral nervous system manifestations. Brain 1990;113:1207–1221.
42. Harper CM, Daube JR. Surgical monitoring with evoked potentials: The Mayo Clinic experience. In: Desmedt JE, ed. Neuromonitoring in surgery. Amsterdam: Elsevier, 1989;275–301.
43. Harper CM, Daube JR, Litchy WJ, et al. Lumbar radiculopathy after spinal fusion for scoliosis. Muscle Nerve 1988;11:386–391.
44. Heller J, Vogel S. No laughing matter. New York: GP Putnam & Sons, 1986.
45. Honch GW. Spinal cord and foramen magnum tumors. Semin Neurol 1993;13:337–342.
46. Howard RS, Wiles CM, Spencer GT. The late sequelae of poliomyelitis. Q J Med 1988;66(251):219–222.
47. Jacobson GP, Tew JM. Intraoperative evoked potential monitoring. J Clin Neurophysiol 1987;4:145–176.
48. Jellinger K. Spinal cord arteriosclerosis and progressive vascular myelopathy. J Neurol Neurosurg Psychiat 1967;30:195–206.
49. Jensen MC, Brant-Zawadski MN, Obuchowski N, et al. Magnetic resonance imaging of the lumbar spine in people without back pain. New Engl J Med 1994;331:69–73.
50. Jones SJ, Wynn Parry CB, Landi A. Diagnosis of brachial plexus traction lesions by sensory nerve action potentials and somatosensory evoked potentials. Injury 1981;12:376–382.
51. Kalkman CJ, Drummond JC, Patel PM, et al. Effects of propofol, etomidate, midazolam and fentanyl on motor evoked responses to transcranial electric or magnetic stimulation in humans. Anesthesiology 1992;74:502–509.
52. Kalkman CJ, Drummond JC, Patel PM, et al. Effects of droperidol, pentobarbital and ketamine on myogenic transcranial magnetic motor-evoked responses in humans. Neurosurgery 1994;35:1066–1071.
53. Kendall FP, McCreary EK, Provance PG. Muscles: testing and function. 4th ed. Baltimore: Williams & Wilkins, 1993;406–410.
54. Kimura J. Electrodiagnosis in diseases of nerve and muscle. 2nd ed. Philadelphia: FA Davis, 1989.
55. Kipling R. Just so stories. New York: Weathervane, 1978;66.
56. Kraft GH. Fibrillation potential amplitude and muscle atrophy following peripheral nerve injury. Muscle Nerve 1990;13:814–821.
57. Krauss WE, McCormick PC. Cervical spondylotic myelopathy. Semin Neurol 1993;13:343–348.
58. Langfitt TW, Elliott FA. Pain in the back and legs caused by cervical cord compression. JAMA 1967;200(5):112–115.
59. Lederer RJ. Neuromuscular problems in the performing arts. Muscle Nerve 1994;17:569–577.
60. Lesoin F, Rousseaux M, Martin HJ, et al. Astereognosis and amyotrophy of the hand with neurinoma of the second cervical root. J Neurol 1986;233:57–58.
61. Lesser RP, Raudzens P, Luders H, et al. Postoperative neurological deficits may occur despite unchanged intraoperative somatosensory evoked potentials. Ann Neurol 1986;19:22–25.

62. Lipton HL, Teasdall RD. Acute transverse myelopathy in adults. Arch Neurol 1973;28:252–257.
63. Long DM, Filtzer DL, BenDebba M, et al. Clinical features of the failed back syndrome. J Neurosurg 1988;69:61–71.
64. Lotz BP, Engel AG, Nishing H, et al. Inclusion body myositis. Brain 1989;112:727–747.
65. Low PA. Clinical autonomic disorders. Boston: Little, Brown, 1992.
66. MacFayden DJ. Posterior column dysfunction in cervical spondylotic myelopathy. Can J Neurol Sci 1984;11:365–370.
67. Miller RG. Injury to peripheral motor nerves. Muscle Nerve 1987;10:698–710.
68. Murray NMF. Motor evoked potentials. In: Aminoff MJ, ed. Electrodiagnosis in clinical neurology, 3rd ed. New York: Churchill Livingstone, 1992;605–626.
69. Nanadedkar SD, Barkhaus PE, Charles A. Multi-motor unit action potential analysis (MMA). Muscle Nerve 1995;18.
70. Noel P, Desmedt JE. Cerebral and far-field somatosensory evoked potentials in neurological disorders involving the spinal cord, brainstem, thalamus and cortex. In: Desmedt JE, ed. Clinical uses of cerebral, brainstem and spinal somatosensory evoked potentials: progress in clinical neurophysiology (Volume 7). Basel, Karger, 1980;205–230.
71. Norris FH. Benign post-traumatic amyotrophy. Arch Neurol 1972;27:269–270.
72. Noseworthy J, Paty D, Wonnacott T, et al. Multiple sclerosis after the age of 50. Neurology 1983;33:1537–1544.
73. Nuwer MR. Basic electrophysiology: evoked potentials and signal processing. In: Nuwer MR, ed. Evoked potential monitoring in the operating room. New York: Raven Press, 1986;5–48.
74. Osterman AL. The double crush syndrome. Orthopedic Clin North Am 1988;19:147–155.
75. Owen JH, Bridwell KH, Grubb R, et al. The clinical application of neurogenic motor evoked potentials to monitor spinal cord function during surgery. Spine 1991;16(8 Suppl):S385–390.
76. Owen JH. Intraoperative stimulation of the spinal cord for prevention of spinal cord injury. Adv Neurol 1993;63:271–288.
77. Peterson PO, Drummond JC, Todd MM. Effects of Halothane, Enflurane, Isoflurane and Nitrous oxide on somatosensory evoked potentials in man. Anesthesiology 1986;65:35.
78. Phillips LH, Park. Electrophysiologic mapping of the segmental anatomy of the muscles of the lower extremity. Muscle Nerve 1991;14:1213–1219.
79. Restuccia D, DiLazzaro V, Valeriani M, et al. Segmental dysfunction of the cervical cord revealed by abnormalities of the spinal N13 potential in cervical spondylotic myelopathy. Neurology 1992;43:1054–1063.
80. Restuccia D, DiLazzaro V, Valeriani M, et al. N24 spinal response to tibial nerve stimulation and magnetic resonance imaging in lesions of the lumbosacral spinal cord. Neurology 1993;43:2269–2275.
81. Schaumberg HH, Spencer PS, Thomas PK. Disorders of peripheral nerves, 2nd ed. Philadelphia: FA Davis, 1992.
82. Schliak H. Segmental innervation and the clinical aspects of nerve root syndromes. In: Vinken PJ, Bruyn GW, ed. Localization in clinical neurology, Volume 2. Handbook of clinical neurology. Amsterdam: North Holland Publishing Co., 1969;157–177.
83. Sihvonen T, Herno A, Paljärvi L, et al. Local denervation atrophy of paraspinal muscles in postoperative failed back syndrome. Spine 1993;18:575–581.
84. Stalberg EV. Electrodiagnostic assessment and monitoring of motor unit changes in disease. Muscle Nerve 1991;14:293–303.
85. Stalberg EV, Trontelj JV. Single fiber electromyography. Studies in healthy and diseased muscle. New York: Raven Press, 2nd ed. 1994;155–157.
86. Stark RJ, Kennard C, Swash M. Hand wasting in spondylotic high cord compression: an electromyographic study. Ann Neurol 1981;9:58–62.
87. Stewart CR, Nandedkar SD, Gilchrist JM, et al. Evaluation of an automatic method of measuring features of motor unit action potentials. Muscle Nerve 1989;12:141–148.
88. Stewart J. Focal peripheral neuropathies. 2nd ed. New York: Raven Press, 1993.
89. Synek VM, Cowan JC. Somatosensory evoked potentials from stimulation of cutaneous femoris lateralis nerve and their applications in meralgia paresthetica. Clin Electroencephalogr 1983;14:161–163.
90. Teresi LM, Lufkin RB, Reicher MA, et al. Asymptomatic degenerative disk disease and spondylosis of the cervical spine: MR imaging. Radiology 1987;164:83–88.
91. Thomas PK, Tomlinson DR. Diabetic and hypoglycemic neuropathy. In Dyck PJ, Thomas PK, eds. Peripheral neuropathy, 3rd ed. Philadelphia: WB Saunders, 1993.
92. Veilleux M, Daube JR. The value of ulnar somatosensory evoked potentials (SEPs) in cervical myelopathy. Electroencephalogr Clin Neurophysiol 1987;68:415–423.
93. Walk D, Fisher MA, Doundoulakis SH, et al. Somatosensory evoked potentials in the evaluation of lumbosacral radiculopathy. Neurology 1992;42:1197–1202.
94. Wilbourn AJ, Aminoff MJ. The electrophysiologic examination in patients with radiculopathies. Muscle Nerve 1988;11:1099–1114.
95. Wilbourn AJ. The electrodiagnostic examination with hysteria-conversion reaction and malingering. Neurol Clin North Am 1995;13:385–405.
96. Wohlfart G. Collateral reinnervation in partially denervated muscles. Neurology 1958;8:175–180.
97. Zentner J, Albrecht T, Heuser D. Influence of halothane, enflurane and isoflurane on motor evoked potentials. Neurosurgery 1992;31:298–305.

SECTION 2
Pediatric Spine

CHAPTER SEVEN

Congenital Anomalies of the Cervical Spine

Randall T. Loder

Congenital anomalies of the pediatric cervical spine are a result of aberrant growth and developmental processes. Understanding the normal embryology, growth, and development of the pediatric cervical spine is of paramount importance.

Normal Embryology, Growth, and Development

Embryology of the Occiput-Axis-Atlas Complex

The occiput is formed from four or five somites. All definitive vertebrae develop from the caudal sclerotome half of one segment and the cranial sclerotome half of the next succeeding segment (87). These areas of primitive mesenchyme separate from each other during fetal growth, chondrify, and then subsequently ossify. This chondrification and ossification is a passive process, following the blueprint laid down by the mesenchymal anlage. Because of this sequencing, the cranial half of the first cervical sclerotome remains as a half segment between the occipital and atlantal rudiments, and is known as the proatlas. The primitive centrum of this proatlas becomes the tip of the odontoid process, while its arch rudiments assist in the formation of the occipital condyles (102). The vertebral arch of the atlas separates from its respective centrum, becoming the ring of C1. The separated centrum fuses with the proatlas above and the centrum of C2 below to become the odontoid process and body of C2. The axis forms from the second definitive cervical vertebral mesenchymal segment. The odontoid process is the fusion of the primitive centra of the atlas and the proatlas half segment. The posterior arches of C2 form from only the second definitive cervical segment.

Thus, the atlas is made up of three main components: the body and two neural arches. The axis is made up of four main components: the body, two neural arches, and the odontoid (or five components if the proatlas rudiment is considered).

Embryology of Vertebrae C3–C7

These vertebrae follow the normal formation schema of all vertebrae (86). A portion of the mesenchyme from the sclerotomal centrum creates two neural arches which migrate posteriorly and around the neural tube. This forms the pedicles, laminae, spinous processes, and a very small portion of the vertebral body. The majority of the body is formed by the centrum. An ossification center develops in each of the two neural arches and one in the vertebral center, with a synchondrosis formed by the cartilage between the ossification centers.

Normal Growth and Development

Atlas

Ossification exists only in the two neural arches at birth (82). These ossification centers extend posteriorly toward the rudimentary spinous process to form the posterior synchondrosis, and anteriorly to form the facets. The neurocentral synchondroses form anteromedial to each facet, joining the neural arches and the body; this occurs on each side of the expanding anterior ossification center. The body starts to ossify between 6 months and 2 years, usually in a single center. By 4 to 6 years, the posterior synchondrosis fuses, followed by the anterior ones. The final internal diameter of the pediatric C1 spinal canal is determined by 6 to 7 years of age. Periosteal appositional growth on the external surface leads to thickening and an increased height, but does not change the internal size of the spinal canal.

Axis

The odontoid develops two primary ossification centers that typically coalesce within the first 3 months of life, and are separated from the C2 centrum by the dentocentral synchondrosis (83, 85). This synchondrosis is below the level of the C1–C2 facets. It contributes to the overall height of the odontoid and to the body of C2. It is continuous throughout the vertebral body and facets, and coalesces with the anterior neurocentral synchondroses. These synchondroses progressively close, starting first in the regions of the facets, next at the neurocentral synchondroses, and finally at the dentocentral synchondrosis. This closure occurs between 3 and 6 years of age. The tip of the dens is comprised of a cartilaginous region similar to an epiphysis, called the chondrum terminale. When it develops an ossification center between 5 to 8 years, it becomes the ossiculum terminale, which fuses to the remainder of the odontoid between 10 to 13 years of age.

The posterior neural arches are partially ossified at birth, joined by the posterior synchondrosis. By 3 months of age, posterior growth of these arches forms the rudimentary spinous process, which by 1 year of age becomes ossified. By 3 years of age, the posterior synchondrosis has fused. Similar to the axis, the posterior and anterior atlantal synchondroses close by age 6, and there is again no further increase in spinal canal size after this age.

C3–7

At birth, all three ossification centers are present (34, 184). The anterior synchondrosis (neurocentral synchondrosis) is slightly anterior to the base of the pedicle; it typically closes between 3 and 6 years of age. The posterior synchondrosis is at the junction of the two neural arches, and usually closes by 2 to 4 years of age. In the neonate and young child, the articular facets are quite horizontal, but become more vertically oriented as the child ages. They are also more horizontal in the upper cervical spine than in the lower cervical spine. The vertebral bodies enlarge circumferentially by periosteal appositional growth, whereas they grow vertically by endochondral ossification. Secondary ossification centers develop at the tips of the spinous processes and the cartilaginous ring apophyses of the bodies around the time of puberty. These ring apophyses are involved in the vertical growth of the body. These secondary ossification centers fuse with the vertebral body around age 25.

Normal Radiographic Parameters

Certain radiographic parameters indicate pathology of the cervical spine in adults but in children represent normal developmental processes. These parameters are the atlanto-occipital and atlanto-dens interval, pseudosubluxation and pseudoinstability, and normal cervical spine motion in children.

Atlanto-dens Interval (ADI) and Atlantooccipital Motion

These intervals are determined on lateral flexion/extension views, which should be conducted voluntarily with the patient awake. The ADI is the space between the anterior aspect of the dens and the posterior aspect of the anterior ring of the atlas (Fig. 7.1). An ADI of more than 5 mm on flexion/extension lateral radiographs indicates instability (58, 90). This

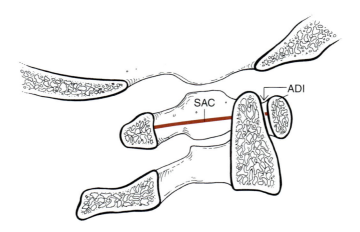

FIGURE 7.1.

(ADI) is the space between the anterior aspect of the dens and the posterior aspect of the anterior ring of the atlas. Space available for the spinal cord (SAC) is between the posterior aspect of the dens and the anterior aspect of the posterior ring of the atlas.

measurement is more than the 3-mm adult value because of the increased cartilage content of the odontoid and ring of the atlas in children, as well as increased ligamentous laxity in children. In extension, overriding of the anterior arch of the atlas on top of the odontoid can also be seen in up to 20% of children (15).

A mild increase in this interval may indicate a subtle disruption of the transverse atlantal ligament. In adults, this ligament ruptures around an interval of 5 mm (35). In chronic atlantoaxial conditions (e.g., rheumatoid arthritis, Down's syndrome, congenital anomalies) the ADI is less useful. In these children, who are frequently hypermobile but do not have a ruptured transverse atlantal ligament, the ADI is increased beyond the 3 to 5 mm range. It is here where the complement of the ADI, or the space available for the cord (SAC), is useful. This space is the distance between the posterior aspect of the dens and the anterior aspect of the posterior ring of the atlas inflexion, or between the posterior aspect of the dens and the anterior aspect of the C2 lamina or the foramen magnum in extension (Fig. 7.2). A decrease in the SAC to 13 mm or less may be associated with neurologic problems (107).

In these patients in whom there is an attenuation of the transverse atlantal ligament but without rupture, the alar ligament does provide some stability. It acts like a checkrein (110), first tightening up in rotation, and then becomes completely taut as the odontoid process continues to move posteriorly a distance equivalent to its full transverse diameter. This safety zone between the anterior wall of the spinal canal of the atlas and axis and the neural structures is an anatomic constant equal to the transverse diameter of the odontoid. This constant defines Steel's rule of thirds: one-third cord, one-third odontoid, and one-third space. The cord can move into this space (safe zone) when the odontoid moves posteriorly because of an attenuated transverse atlantal ligament. Here the alar ligament becomes taut, acting as a checkrein and secondary restraint, preventing further movement of the odontoid into the cord. In the chronic situation, it is important to recognize when this safe zone has been exceeded and the child enters the region of impending spinal cord compression. In the case of trauma, the alar ligament is insufficient to prevent a fatal cord injury in the event of another neck injury similar to the one that caused the initial interruption of the transverse atlantal ligament.

Normal ranges of motion at the atlantooccipital interval are not well defined. In a series of 40 normal college freshmen, the tip of the odontoid remained directly below the base of the skull in both flexion and extension (29). Thus, the joint should not allow

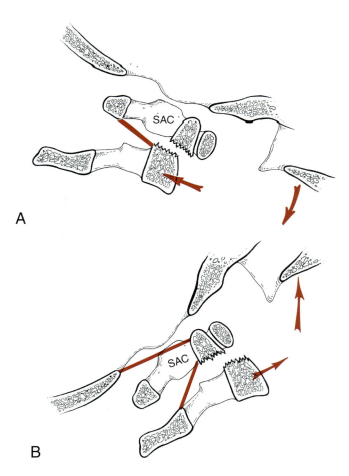

FIGURE 7.2.

A. In flexion, SAC may become less between the posterior aspect of the dens and the anterior aspect of the C1 posterior ring. **B.** In extension, SAC may become less between the posterior aspect of the dens and the anterior aspect of the C2 lamina or the foramen magnum.

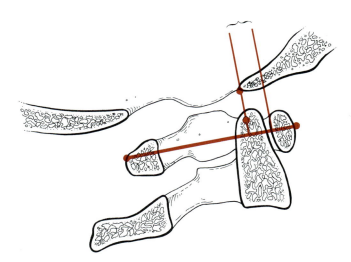

FIGURE 7.3.

The technique of Wiesel and Rothman: the vertical lines from the clivus and the posterior aspect of the anterior ring of the atlas should not translate > 1 mm.

any horizontal translation during flexion and extension. Tredwell et al. (116) feel that a posterior subluxation of the atlantooccipital relationship in extension of > 4 mm indicates instability. This subluxation can be measured as the distance between the anterior margin of the condyles at the base of the skull and the sharp contour of the anterior aspect of the concave joint of the atlas anteriorly, or as the distance between the occipital protuberance and the superior arch of the atlas posteriorly. Another method to measure this posterior subluxation of the atlantooccipital joint uses the technique of Wiesel and Rothman (122) (Fig. 7.3). With this technique, occiput-C1 translation from maximum flexion to maximum extension should be no more than 1 mm in normal adults. However, norms for children have not been established for either of these techniques.

Pseudosubluxation

The C2–3 and, to a lesser extent, the C3–4 interspaces in children have a normal physiologic displacement (4). In a study of 161 children (15), significant anterior displacement of C2 on C3 was observed in 9% of children between 1 and 7 years old. In some children, the anterior physiologic displacement of C2 on C3 is so pronounced that it appears pathologic (pseudosubluxation). To differentiate this from pathologic

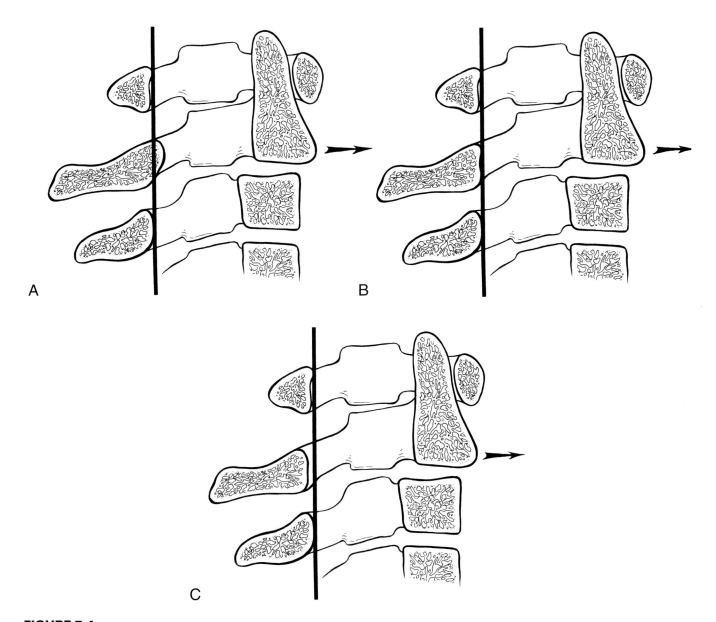

FIGURE 7.4.

The posterior line of Swischuk, showing the normal limits. **A.** Passing through or just behind the anterior cortex of C2. **B.** Touching the anterior aspect of the cortex C2. **C.** Coming within 1 mm of the anterior aspect of the cortex of C2. Reprinted with permission from Swischuk LE. Anterior displacement of C2 in children: physiologic or pathologic? A helpful differentiating line. Radiology 1977;122:759–763.

subluxation, Swischuk has used the posterior cervical line (Fig. 7.4) drawn from the anterior cortex of the posterior arch of C1 to the anterior cortex of the posterior arch of C3 (112). In physiologic displacement of C2 on C3, the posterior cervical line may pass through the cortex of the posterior arch of C2, touch the anterior aspect of the cortex of the posterior arch of C2, or come within 1 mm of the anterior cortex of the posterior arch of C2. In pathologic dislocation of C2 on C3, the posterior cervical line misses the posterior arch of C2 by 2 mm or more.

The planes of the articular facets change with growth. The lower cervical spine facets change from 55 to 70°, whereas the upper facets (i.e., C2–C4) may have initial angles as low as 30°, which gradually change to 60 to 70°. This variation in facet angulation, along with normal looseness of the soft tissues, intervetebral discs, and the relative increase in size and weight of the skull compared with the trunk, are the major factors responsible for this pseudosubluxation. Because this pseudosubluxation is a normal physiologic condition, no "treatment" is needed.

Normal Lower Cervical Spine Motion

Generally, the interspinous distances increase with age, being the smallest at C4–5 and the largest at C6–7, until 15 years of age, when it is the largest at C5–6 (90). The anteroposterior displacement from hyperflexion to hyperextension decreases from C2–3 to C6–7. The angular displacement is highest (15°) at C3–4 and C4–5 for those children 3 to 8 years of age, highest (17°) at C4–5 for those aged 9 to 11 years of age, and highest (15°) at C5–6 for those aged 12 to 15 years of age.

Congenital Problems

Torticollis

Torticollis is a combined rotatory and head tilt deformity, and indicates a problem at C1–2 (because 50% of the cervical spine rotation occurs at this joint). A head tilt alone indicates a more generalized problem in the cervical spine. The differential diagnosis of torticollis is large (2), and can be either osseous (e.g., basilar impression) or nonosseous (e.g., congenital muscular torticollis). This chapter discusses only those that have a "congenital" basis.

Congenital Muscular Torticollis (Congenital Wryneck)

Congenital muscular torticollis is the most common cause of torticollis in the infant and young child. A disproportionate number of these children have a history of a primiparous birth, or of having a breech or difficult delivery. It has, however, been reported in children with normal births, and even in children born by cesarean section (56, 62). Rarely is there a familial tendency (115).

There are several theories regarding the etiology of this disorder. The most common one is in-utero crowding because three of four children have the lesion on the right side (57) and 20% have developmental hip dysplasia (46, 75, 121). Another theory is primarily neurogenic (101), supported by histopathologic evidence of denervation and reinnervation. The primary myopathy may be initially caused by trauma, ischemia, or both, and involves the two heads of the sternocleidomastoid muscle unequally. The most recent theory states that a compartment syndrome occurs as a result of venous outflow blockage from compression to the soft tissues of the neck at the time of delivery (22). This is manifested by edema, degeneration of muscle fibers, and fibrosis of the muscle body. Histology of resected surgical specimens suggests that the lesion is caused by occlusion of the venous outflow of the sternocleidomastoid muscle (11, 123). The muscle fibrosis is variable, ranging from small amounts to the entire muscle. It has been suggested that the clinical deformity is related to the ratio of fibrosis to remaining functional muscle. If ample muscle remains, the sternocleidomastoid will probably stretch with growth and the child will not develop torticollis; if fibrosis predominates, there is little elastic potential, and torticollis will develop. With the passage of time, the fibrosis of the sternal head may entrap the branch of the spinal accessory nerve to the clavicular head of the muscle, which can then lead to a later progressive deformity (101). The fact that it can occur in children with normal birth histories or in children born by cesarean section disputes the perinatal compartment syndrome theory, and supports the in-utero crowding theory. The fact that it can occur in families (supporting a genetic predisposition) also disputes the compartment syndrome theory. The sternocleidomastoid muscle exhibited an abnormal MRI signal in 10 patients who had congenital muscular torticollis and were studied from 4 weeks to 5 years of age. In no case was a discrete mass seen within the sternocleidomastoid muscle (22). The muscle diameter also increased two to four times that of the contralateral muscle. In older patients, the signals produced were consistent with atrophy and fibrosis, similar to those encountered in compartment syndromes of the leg and forearm.

Contracture of the sternocleidomastoid muscle tilts the head toward the involved side and rotates the chin toward the opposite shoulder. The clinical features of congenital muscular torticollis depend on the time at which the physician evaluates the child. It is often discovered in the first 6 to 8 weeks of life (75). If the child is examined during the first 4 weeks of life, a mass or "tumor" may be palpable in the neck (56). Although the mass may be palpable, it is unrecognized up to 80% of the time (18). It is characteristically a nontender, soft enlargement beneath the skin and located within the sternocleidomastoid muscle belly. This tumor reaches its maximum size within the first 4 weeks of life, and then gradually regresses. After 4 to 6 months of life, the contracture and torticollis are the only clinical findings. In some children, the deformity is not noticed until after 1 year of age, which questions the "congenital" part of the name as well as the perinatal compartment syndrome theory. Because up to 20% of children with congenital muscular torticollis have developmental dysplasia of the hip (46, 75, 121), a hip examination should be performed.

If the deformity is progressive, skull and face deformities can develop (plagiocephaly), often within the first year of life. The facial flattening occurs on the side of the contracted muscle, and is probably caused by the sleeping position of the child (9). United States children usually sleep prone, and in this position it is more comfortable for them to lie with the affected side down. The face therefore remodels to conform to the bed. If the child sleeps supine, reverse modeling of the contralateral skull occurs. In the child untreated for many years, the level of the eyes and ears becomes unequal and can result in considerable cosmetic deformity.

Cervical spine radiographs should be obtained to differentiate a muscular torticollis from congenital vertebral malformations. Plain radiographs of the cervical spine in children with muscular torticollis are always normal, aside from the head tilt and rotation. If any suspicion exists about the status of the hips, appropriate imaging should be done (ultrasound/radiographs), depending on the age of the child and expertise of the ultrasonographer.

Treatment is initially conservative (7, 14, 18, 56, 62, 75). Up to 90% good results can be expected with stretching exercises alone (7). The exercises, performed by the caregivers, are guided by the physiotherapist. The ear opposite the contracted muscle should be positioned to the shoulder and the chin should be positioned to touch the shoulder on the same side as the contracted muscle. When adequate stretching has occurred in the neutral position, the exercises should be graduated to the extended position, which will achieve maximum stretching and prevent residual contractures. Treatment measures to be used along with stretching consist of modifying the child's toys and crib so that the neck will be stretched when the infant is reaching for or looking at objects of interest. The efficacy of these stretching measures versus a natural history of spontaneous resolution is not known; there are many anecdotal cases of spontaneous resolution.

Surgery is recommended for persistent deformity after 1 year of age because stretching is usually unsuccessful after this age (14, 33). The child's neck and anatomic structures are also larger after 1 year of age, making surgery easier, and the best time for surgical release is between the ages of 1 and 4 years (56, 118). Established facial deformity or a limitation of more than 30° of motion usually precludes a good result, and surgery will be required to prevent further facial flattening and cosmetic deterioration (14). Asymmetry of the face and skull can improve as long as adequate growth potential remains after the deforming pull of the sternocleidomastoid is removed; good (but not excellent) results can be obtained as late as 12 years of life (18).

Surgical alternatives are a unipolar release (either at the sternoclavicular or mastoid poles), a bipolar release, or a complete resection. The bipolar release combined with a z-plasty of the sternal attachment has yielded 92% satisfactory results in one series, whereas only 15% satisfactory results were obtained with other procedures (33). The z-plasty lengthening maintains the v-contour of the neck and cosmesis. Structures that can potentially be injured from surgery are the spinal accessory nerve, the anterior and external jugular veins, carotid vessels and sheath, and facial nerve. Skin incisions should never be located directly over the clavicle because of cosmetically unacceptable scar spreading, but rather proximal to the medial end of the clavicle and sternal notch, in line with the cervical skin creases. The postoperative protocol can vary from simple stretching exercises to cast immobilization. An orthosis to maintain alignment of the head and neck is probably a desirable part of the postoperative protocol.

Atlanto-occipital Anomalies

Occipitocervical synostosis, basilar impression, and odontoid anomalies are the most common malformations of the occipito-vertebral junction, with an incidence of 1.4 to 2.5 per 100 children (61). Both sexes are equally affected. These lesions arise from a malformation of the mesenchymal anlages at the occipito-vertebral junction.

These children resemble those who have the Klippel-Feil syndrome: short, broad necks, restricted neck movements, low hairline, high scapula, and torticollis (6, 69). The skull may be deformed and shaped like a "tower skull." Other associated anomalies include dwarfism, funnel chest, jaw anomalies, cleft palate, congenital ear deformities, hypospadias, genitourinary tract defects, and syndactyly. Neurologic symptoms may occur during childhood, but more often present around the age of 40 to 50 years. They progress slowly and relentlessly, and can be initiated by traumatic or inflammatory processes. Rarely do they present suddenly or dramatically, although they have been reported as a cause of sudden death. The most common signs and symptoms are neck and occipital pain, vertigo, ataxia, limb paresis, paresthesias, speech disturbances, hoarseness, diplopia, syncope, auditory malfunction, and dysphagia (39, 120).

Standard radiographs are difficult to obtain because of fixed bony deformities, overlapping shadows from the mandible, occiput, and foramen magnum, and the patient's difficulty in cooperating. An x-ray beam directed 90° perpendicular to the skull, rather than the cervical spine, usually gives a satisfactory view of the occipitocervical junction. Further studies (tomograms and/or CT scans) are usually needed. The anterior arch of C1 is commonly assimilated to the occiput, often with a hypoplastic posterior ring. The height of C1 is also variably decreased, allowing the odontoid to project upward into the foramen magnum (primary basilar impression). The position of the odontoid relative to the opening of the foramen magnum has been described by McRae, by measuring the distance from the posterior aspect of the odontoid to the posterior ring of C1 or the posterior lip of the foramen magnum, whichever is closer (68, 69). This should be determined in flexion because this position maximizes the reduction in the space available for the cord. If this distance is less than 19 mm, a neurologic deficit is usually present. Lateral flexion/extension views of the upper cervical spine often show up to 12 mm of space between the odontoid and the C1 ring anteriorly (69); associated C1–2 instability eventually develops in one-half of these patients (120). The odontoid may also be misshapen or malpositioned posteriorly. Up to 70% of these children have a congenital fusion between C2–3. Occipital vertebrae and condylar hypoplasia can also occur.

The MRI is used to image the neural structures. Posterior encroachment upon the upper spinal cord or medulla often occurs by a dural constricting band, with resultant neurologic findings. Compression from the posterior lip of the foramen magnum or dural constricting band can disturb the posterior columns with a loss of proprioception, vibration, and tactile senses. Nystagmus also commonly occurs because of posterior cerebellar compression. Vascular disturbances from vertebral artery involvement can result in brain stem ischemia, manifested by syncope, seizures, vertigo, and unsteady gait. Cerebellar tonsil herniation can also occur (6). The altered mechanics of the cervical spine may result in a dull, aching pain in the posterior occiput and neck with intermittent stiffness and torticollis. Irritation of the greater occipital nerve may cause tenderness in the posterior scalp.

The posteriorly projecting odontoid can cause anterior compression of the brain stem or upper cervical cord. This compression produces a range of findings and symptoms, depending on the location and degree of compression. Pyramidal tract signs and symptoms (spasticity, hyperreflexia, muscle weakness, gait disturbances) are most common, although cranial nerve involvement (diplopia, tinnitus, dysphagia, auditory disturbances) can be seen.

Treatment is difficult because surgical intervention carries a much higher morbidity and mortality risk than with anomalies of the odontoid (6, 80, 120). For this reason, nonoperative methods should be initially attempted. Cervical collars, braces, and traction often help for persistent reports of head and neck pain, especially after minor trauma or infection. Immobilization may only achieve temporary relief if neurologic deficits are present. Those with evidence of a compromised upper cervical area should take precautions not to expose themselves to undue trauma.

When symptoms and/or signs of an unstable C1–2 complex are present, a posterior C1–2 fusion is indicated. Preliminary traction to attempt reduction is used if necessary. If a reduction is possible and there are no neurologic signs, surgery has an improved prognosis (6, 39, 120). Posterior signs and/or symptoms may be an indication for posterior decompression depending on the evidence of dural or osseous compression. Results vary from complete resolution to increased deficits and death (6, 80). The role of concomitant posterior fusion has not yet been determined, but if the decompression (whether anterior or posterior) could potentially destabilize the spine, then concomitant posterior fusion should be strongly considered.

Basilar Impression

Basilar impression occurs when the skull floor is indented by the upper cervical spine. The tip of the dens is more cephalad and sometimes protrudes into the opening of the foramen magnum. This may encroach upon the brain stem, risking neurologic damage from direct injury, vascular compromise, or cerebrospinal fluid flow alteration (16, 113).

There are two types of basilar impression: primary and secondary. Primary basilar impression is a congenital abnormality often associated with other vertebral defects (Klippel-Feil syndrome, odontoid abnormalities, atlantooccipital fusion, atlas hypoplasia). The incidence of primary basilar impression in the general population is 1% (13).

Secondary basilar impression, the less common type, is a developmental condition attributed to softening of the osseus structures at the skull base. Any disorder of osseous softening can lead to secondary basilar impression (23). These disorders include metabolic bone diseases (Paget's disease [30, 92], renal osteodystrophy, rickets, and osteomalacia [48]), bone dysplasias and mesenchymal syndromes (osteogenesis imperfecta [43, 93, 97], achondroplasia [127] and hypochondroplasia [125], neurofibromatosis [150]) and rheumatologic disorders (rheumatoid arthritis, ankylosing spondylitis) (42, 64). The softening allows the odontoid to migrate cephalad and into the foramen magnum.

These patients typically present with a short neck (78% in one series) (23), which is an apparent, rather than real, deformity because of the basilar impression. They also show asymmetry of the skull and/or face (68%), painful cervical motion (53%), and torticollis (15%). Neurologic signs and symptoms are often present (73). Many children will have acute onset of symptoms precipitated by minor trauma (114). In cases of isolated basilar impression, the neurologic involvement is basically a pyramidal syndrome associated with proprioceptive sensory disturbances (motor weakness [85%], limb paresthesias [85%]). In cases of basilar impression associated with Arnold-Chiari malformations, the neurologic involvement is usually cerebellar (motor incoordination with ataxia, dizziness, nystagmus). In both types, the patients may complain of neck pain and headache in the distribution of the greater occipital nerve, and cranial nerve involvement, particularly those which emerge from the medulla oblongata (trigeminal [V], glossopharyngeal [IX], vagus [X], and hypoglossal [XII]). Ataxia is a very common finding in children (114). Hydrocephalus may develop because of obstruction of the cerebrospinal fluid flow by obstruction of the foramen magnum from the odontoid.

Basilar impression is difficult to assess radiographically. The most commonly used lines are Chamberlain's (16), McRae's (67), and McGregor's (65) in the lateral radiograph (Fig. 7.5). McGregor's line is a line drawn from the posterosuperior aspect of the hard palate to the lowermost point on the midline occipital curve. It is the best method for screening because the landmarks can be defined clearly at all ages on a routine lateral radiograph. Any odontoid tip greater than 4.5 mm above the line is concerning for basilar invagination. McRae's line is helpful in assessing the clinical significance of basilar impression because it defines the opening of the foramen magnum; in those who are symptomatic, the odontoid projects above this line. Chamberlain's line is drawn from the posterior lip of the foramen magnum to the dorsal margin of the hard palate. No more than one-third of the odontoid should project above this line. Computed tomography with sagittal plane reconstructions can show the osseous relationships at the occipitocervical junction more clearly, and magnetic resonance imaging shows the neural anatomy. Occasionally, vertebral angiography is needed (89).

Treatment of basilar impression is difficult and requires a multidisciplinary approach (orthopaedic, neurosurgery, and neuroradiology) (71, 126). The symptoms can rarely be helped by custom made orthoses (47); the primary treatment is surgical. If the symptoms are caused by a hypermobile odontoid, then surgical stabilization in extension at the occipitocervical junction will be needed. Anterior excision of the odontoid is needed if it cannot be reduced (72, 98), but it should be preceded by posterior stabilization and fusion. If the symptoms are from posterior impingement, suboccipital decompression and often upper cervical laminectomy is needed. The dura often needs to be opened to look for a tight posterior band (6, 69). Posterior stabilization should also be performed. These are general statements, and each case should be considered individually.

Unilateral Absence of C1

This congenital malformation of the first cervical vertebrae is in essence a hemiatlas, or a congenital scoliosis of C1. It was first described by Dubousset (27) in 1986. The problem is often associated with other anomalies common to children with congenital spine deformities

Two-thirds of the children present at birth, while the others develop a torticollis and are noticed later. A lateral translation of the head on the trunk with variable degrees of lateral tilt and rotation is a typical finding, best appreciated from the back. There may also be severe tilting of the eye line. The sternocleidomastoid muscle is not tight, although regional aplasia of the muscles in the nuchal concavity of the tilted side is noted. Neck flexibility is variable and decreases with age. The condition is not painful. Plagiocephaly can occur and increases as the deformity increases. Neurologic signs (headaches, vertigo, myelopathy) are present in approximately one-quarter of the patients. The natural history is unknown due to the recent description of this anomaly.

Standard AP and lateral radiographs rarely give the diagnosis, although the open-mouth odontoid view may suggest it. Tomograms and/or CT scans are usually needed to see the anomaly. The defect can range from a hypoplasia of the lateral mass to a com-

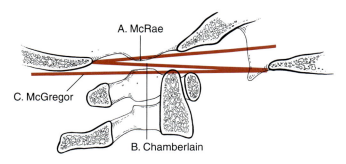

FIGURE 7.5.

McGregor line: upper surface of the posterior edge of the hard palate to the most caudad point of the skull (> 4.5 mm is abnormal). McRae line: odontoid protrusion into the foramen magnum. Chamberlain's line: from the posterior lip of foramen magnum to the dorsal margin of the hard palate.

plete hemiatlas with rotational instability and basilar impression. Occasionally the atlas is occipitalized. There are three types of this disorder. Type I is an isolated hemi-atlas. Type II is a partial or complete aplasia of one hemi-atlas, with other associated anomalies of the cervical spine (e.g., fusions of the third and fourth vertebrae, or congenital bars in the lower cervical vertebrae). Type III is a partial or complete atlanto-occipital fusion and symmetrical or asymmetrical hemiatlas aplasia with or without anomalies of the odontoid and/or lower cervical vertebrae.

Once the disorder is diagnosed, radiographs of the entire spine are needed to rule out other congenital vertebral anomalies. Vertebral angiography and MRI is needed if operative intervention is planned. Arterial anomalies are often found on the aplastic side (e.g., multiple loops, vessels smaller than normal, and abnormal routes between C1 and C2), and many of these children will have stenosis of the foramen magnum and/or an Arnold-Chiari malformation.

The deformity is observed for the presence or absence of progression. This observation is primarily clinical because radiographic measurements are difficult to obtain. Bracing does not halt deformity progression. Surgery is recommended for severe deformities. Preoperative gradual correction with a halo is used. An ambulatory method of gradual cervical spine deformity correction has been recently described using the halo-Ilizarov technique (38). A posterior fusion from the occiput to C2 or C3 is then performed. Decompression of the spinal canal is necessary when the canal size is not ample, either at that time or if it is projected that it will not be able to fully accommodate the developed spinal cord. The ideal age for posterior fusion is between the ages of 5 and 8 years, when the canal reaches adult size.

Os Odontoideum

Os odontoideum is an anomaly in which the tip of the odontoid process is divided by a wide transverse gap, leaving the apical segment without its basilar support (36, 124). It is quite rare; the exact incidence is not known. It most likely represents an unrecognized fracture at the base of the odontoid or damage to the epiphyseal plate during the first few years of life. Either of these causes can compromise the blood supply to the developing odontoid, resulting in the os odontoideum. Some authors believe that it may represent a congenital anomaly instead of occult trauma, and it is for this reason that it is included in this chapter on congenital anomalies.

These children usually present with local neck pain and, occasionally, transitory episodes of paresis, myelopathy, or cerebral-brain stem ischemia caused by vertebral artery compression from the upper cervical instability. Sudden death can also occur, although it is rare.

Radiographically, an os odontoideum is seen as an oval or round ossicle with a smooth sclerotic border, of variable size, located in the position of the normal odontoid tip. On occasion, it can be located near the basioccipital area of the foramen magnum. The base of the dens is usually hypoplastic. It is often difficult to differentiate an os odontoideum from nonunion after a fracture. The gap between the os and the hypoplastic dens is wider than in a fracture, and usually well above the level of the facets. Tomograms and CT scans are useful to further delineate the bony anatomy, and flexion/extension lateral radiographs can identify instability.

The neurologic symptoms are caused by cord compression from posterior translation of the os into the cord in extension, or the odontoid into the cord in flexion. Increased motion at the C1–2 level can lead to vertebral artery occlusion/ischemia of the brainstem and posterior fossa structures, resulting in seizures, syncope, vertigo, and visual disturbances. The long-term natural history is unknown.

Patients who have local pain or transient myelopathies can expect recovery with cervical traction and/ or immobilization. Subsequently, only nonstrenuous activities should be allowed, but the curtailment of activities in the pediatric age group can be difficult. One must weigh the risk of a small insult leading to catastrophic quadriplegia/death.

Surgery is indicated when there is 10 mm or more of instability (ADI) or a SAC of 13 mm or less (107), neurologic involvement, progressive instability, or persistent neck pain. A Gallie fusion is recommended. The surgeon must be careful when tightening the wire so that the os is not pulled back posteriorly into the canal and cord; this has disastrous consequences. In small children the wire may be eliminated. In all children a Minerva or halo cast/ vest is also used in the postoperative period.

Other Syndromes and Dysplasias

Familial Cervical Dysplasia

This recently described atlas deformity (99) has an autosomal dominant genetic pattern with complete penetrance and variable expressivity. Clinical presentation varies from an incidental finding, a passively correctable head tilt, suboccipital pain, or decreased cervical motion, to a clunking of the upper cervical spine.

Plain radiographs are difficult to interpret. Various anomalies of C1, most commonly a partial absence of the posterior ring of C1, are typically seen. Various anomalies of C2 also exist, commonly as a shallow hypoplastic left facet. Other dysplasias of the lateral masses, the facets, and the posterior elements, and occasionally the spondylolisthesis, are seen. Occiput-C1 instability is seen frequently, and C1–2 instability is seen rarely. The delineation of this complex anatomy is often best seen with a CT scan and 3-dimensional reconstruction. When symptoms of instability are present, an MRI in flexion and extension is recommended to assess the presence and magnitude of neural compression. Neural compression at the occipito-cervical junction is created by instability from the malformation(s).

Frequent observation (every 6 to 12 months) is recommended to ensure that instability does not develop either clinically (e.g., progressive weakness and fatigue, or objective signs of myelopathy), or radiographically (lateral flexion/extension views). Surgery is recommended for persistent pain, torticollis, and especially neurologic symptoms. A posterior fusion from the occiput to C2 is usually required, with gradual preoperative reduction using an adjustable halo cast (38).

Klippel-Feil Syndrome

The Klippel-Feil syndrome is a triad of a low posterior hairline, short neck, and limited neck motion (45, 53, 76, 105) resulting from congenital fusions of the cervical vertebrae. Other anomalies, both in the musculoskeletal and other organ systems, frequently occur. The congenital fusions result from abnormal embryologic formation of the cervical vertebral mesenchymal anlages. This embryologic insult, although yet unknown, is not limited to the cervical vertebrae, which explains the other associated anomalies with the Klippel-Feil syndrome. The incidence of congenital cervical fusion is approximately 0.7% (12).

Limited neck motion of varying degrees is seen. Approximately one-third of these patients have an associated Sprengel's deformity. The other anomalies associated with the syndrome are scoliosis (both congenital and idiopathic-like) (45), renal anomalies (28, 37, 70, 74, 95), deafness (66, 88, 108, 109), synkinesis (mirror movements) (5, 40), pulmonary dysfunction (3, 17, 54), and congenital heart disease (32, 81). Varying degrees of vertebral fusion, ranging from simple block vertebrae to multiple and bizarre anomalies, are seen radiographically. An associated scoliosis often makes interpretation of the radiographs difficult. Flexion and extension lateral radiographs are useful to assess any potential instability. Any segment adjacent to unfused segments may result in hypermobility and neurologic symptoms (24, 41, 55, 111). A common pattern is fusion of C1–2 and C3–4, leading to a high risk of instability at the unfused C2–3 level (31).

A thorough evaluation should be undertaken to ensure that no congenital cardiac or other neurologic abnormality exists (49, 77). Renal imaging should be done in all children; a simple renal ultrasound is usually adequate for the initial evaluation (26, 63). The neural axis is visualized most easily with an MRI. An MRI should be obtained whenever any concern for neurologic involvement exists on a clinical basis, as well as prior to any orthopaedic spinal procedure (96, 119). Also, simple flexion-extension lateral radiographs should be taken before any general anesthetic to rule out any occult instability of the cervical spine. When flexion-extension radiographs are difficult to interpret (which is not uncommon because of the multiple anomalous vertebrae), a flexion-extension CT scan can be useful, especially at the C1–2 level.

The natural history of these children primarily depends on the occurrence of severe renal or cardiac problems. Instability of the cervical spine (91) can develop with neurologic involvement, especially in the upper segments or in patients who have iniencephaly (91, 103). Degenerative joint and disc disease develops in patients who have lower segment instabilities. Because children with large fusion areas are at high risk for developing instabilities, strenuous activities should be avoided, especially contact sports. Other nonsurgical methods of treatment are cervical traction, collars, and analgesics when mechanical symptoms appear, which is usually in the adolescent or adult patient. Surgical fusion is needed when neurologic symptoms arise from instability. The real dilemma is whether prophylactic stabilization should be undertaken for asymptomatic hypermobile segments; no guide lines exist for this problem. The need for decompression at the time of stabilization depends on the exact anatomic circumstance, as does the need for combined anterior/posterior versus simple posterior fusions alone. Surgery solely for cosmesis is unwarranted and risky (8, 25).

Sandifer's Syndrome

Sandifer's syndrome is a syndrome of gastroesophageal reflux (often from a hiatal hernia) resulting in abnormal posturing of the neck and trunk, usually torticollis (78, 94). It is commonly seen in infancy or in children who have cerebral palsy. The torticollis is believed to be an attempt on the part of the child to decrease the esophagitis pain secondary to the reflux. The majority present in infancy. On occasion the diagnosis may be delayed and not discovered until childhood. The abnormal posturing may also present as opisthotonos or neural tics, and often mimics CNS disorders. The diagnosis of symptom-causing gastroesophageal reflux is frequently overlooked (10). The incidence of gastroesophageal reflux is high (up to 40% of infants) (21), with the principal symptoms being vomiting, failure to thrive, recurrent respiratory disease, dysphagia, various neural signs, torticollis, and even respiratory arrest. Upon careful examination of these infants, the tight and short sternocleidomastoid muscle or its tumor is not seen, eliminating congenital muscular torticollis. Further work-up excludes skeletal dysplasias, congenital anomalies of the cervical spine, post-infectious causes, and CNS disorders (e.g., extraocular muscle or vestibular apparatus disorders, CNS neoplasms). In these situations, the physician should consider Sandifer's syndrome in the differential diagnosis.

Plain radiographs of the cervical spine are needed to rule out congenital anomalies or skeletal dysplasias. Contrast studies of the upper gastrointestinal tract usually demonstrate the hiatal hernia and/or gastroesophageal reflux (51). Esophageal pH studies may be necessary because many children (both asymptomatic and symptomatic) show evidence of gastroesophageal reflux (52). Medical therapy is the first treatment employed. When this fails, fundoplication can be considered. In otherwise normal children, this is usually curative (51).

Other Syndromes

Fetal Alcohol Syndrome

The teratogenic fetal alcohol syndrome is characterized by CNS dysfunctions, growth deficiencies, facial anomalies, and variable major and minor malformations. The children present with developmental delay, especially in motor milestones, failure to thrive, mild to moderate retardation, mild microcephaly, distinct facies (hypoplasia of the facial bones and circumoral tissues), and congenital cardiovascular anomalies. Abnormal necks are not uncommon, and are similar to the Klippel-Feil syndrome. Fusion of two or more cervical vertebrae occurs in approximately one-half of the children, resembling the Klippel-Feil syndrome (60, 79, 117). However, fetal alcohol syndrome is distinctly different from the Klippel-Feil syndrome because the major visceral anomaly in the Klippel-Feil syndrome is the genitourinary system, whereas in the fetal alcohol syndrome it is the cardiovascular system (117).

Radiographic imaging and treatment recommendations regarding the cervical spine are the same as for the Klippel-Feil syndrome.

Craniofacial Syndromes

Cleft lip and/or palate is the most common craniofacial anomaly. It can be a solitary finding, or, more often, can be associated with other syndromes and anomalies. Children with cleft anomalies have a 13% incidence of cervical spinal anomalies, compared with the 0.8% incidence of children undergoing orthodontia care for other reasons (non-cleft) (100). This incidence is highest in those with soft palate and submucous clefts (45%). These anomalies are predominantly in the upper cervical spine, and usually are spina bifida or vertebral body hypoplasia. The potential for instability is not known, nor is the natural history. No documented information regarding treatment is available; however, the clinician should be aware of this association and make sound clinical judgements as needed.

Craniosynostosis Syndromes (Crouzon's, Pfeiffer's, Apert's, Goldenhar's)

Craniosynostosis syndromes exhibit cervical spine fusions (neural arch, facet fusions, and block vertebrae), occipito-atlanto fusions, and butterfly vertebrae (44, 59, 104). Fusions are more common in Apert's syndrome (71%) than in Crouzon's syndrome (38%) (44). Upper cervical fusions are most common in Crouzon's and Pfeiffer's syndromes (104), whereas in Apert's syndrome, the fusions are more likely to be complex and to involve C5–6 (44). However, this syndromal variation is not accurate enough for syndromic differentiation. Congenital cervico-thoracic scoliosis is frequently seen in Goldenhar's syndrome, usually from hemivertebrae (104).

The cervical fusions are "progressive" with aging; in younger children the vertebrae appear to be separated by intervertebral discs, but as the child ages, the vertebrae fuse together. Recommendations for treatment are not specifically known. The author recommends following the same principles as in the Klippel-Feil syndrome. One major problem is the potential difficulty with intubation in these children. Odontoid anomalies are rare; however, if any question exists regarding the stability of the cervical spine, lateral flexion/extension radiographs should be obtained.

Skeletal Dysplasias

Spondyloepiphyseal dysplasia, Morquio's syndrome and other mucopolysaccharidoses, achondroplasia, pseudoachondroplasia, chondrodysplasia punctata, and multiple epiphyseal dysplasia have their own unique parameters regarding epidemiology, etiology, and clinical features. This chapter discusses only the cervical spine. Overall, 48% of individuals with skeletal dysplasias show upper cervical anomalies (106).

The clinical features of upper cervical instability are often subtle and difficult to differentiate in children with skeletal dysplasias from pre-existing mechanical problems in the lower limbs associated with joint laxity and epiphyseal malformation (e.g., genu valgum, loss of endurance, tiredness). Later, sleep apnea and loss of hand-motor coordination can occur, with eventual paraparesis/quadriparesis and loss of urinary/bowel sphincter control.

Odontoid hypoplasia with instability on lateral flexion/extension views is the most frequently seen problem. Varying degrees of vertebral body dysplasia are also present. The overall proportion of children who have upper cervical anomalies and skeletal dysplasias is 100% for those with Morquio's syndrome, 75% for those with other mucopolysaccharidoses, 83% for those with SED congenita, and 57% for those with pseudoachondroplasia.

Flexion/extension CT scans and/or MRIs are often needed to better delineate the neuroanatomy. The vertebral body and odontoid hypoplasia, as well as ligamentous laxity, leads to instability and myelopathy. The incidence and natural history for irreversible neurologic damage is unknown in most of these dysplasias; however, children with Morquio's syndrome are at a very high risk.

All children with skeletal dysplasias should be screened for upper cervical instability before any surgical procedure. Those with Morquio's syndrome should be screened routinely as early as possible, regardless of whether surgery and general anesthesia is planned in the near future, because of their very high incidence of instability. When instability develops, upper cervical fusion, often from the occiput to C3–4, is needed. Halo-cast immobilization is often required; instrumentation, except for interspinous wiring, is rarely indicated.

Neurofibromatosis

Neurofibromatosis is the most common single gene disorder in humans. The proportion of patients with neurofibromatosis and cervical spine involvement is difficult to assess (30% in the series of Yong-Hing et al. [128]; 44% of those with scoliosis or kyphosis had cervical spine lesions). The children are often asymptomatic (128). Symptoms, when they do occur, are diminished or painful neck motion, torticollis, dysphagia, deformity, and neurologic signs ranging from mild pain and weakness to paraparesis/quadriparesis (19, 50). Neck masses constituted 20% of presenting symptoms in one study of neurofibromatosis patients (1).

Radiographic features of neurofibromatosis in the cervical spine are vertebral body deficiencies and dysplasia or scalloping (20, 128). This is often associated with kyphosis (lordosis being less common) and foraminal enlargement. Lateral flexion/extension radiographs are recommended for all neurofibromatosis patients before general anesthesia or surgery. MRI is helpful for assessing the involvement of neural structures and dural ectasia. CT scans are useful for evaluating the upper C-spine complex and bony definition of the neural foramen. The natural history regarding the cervical spine is unknown, but patients who have severe kyphosis often develop neurologic deterioration.

Surgical indications are cord or nerve root compression, C1–2 rotary subluxation, pain, and neurofibroma removal (19, 128). Halo-cast/vests usually are needed after fusions, with or without internal fixation, which is usually simple interspinous wiring. Kyphosis generally requires anterior and posterior fusions. If no indications for surgical treatment exist, then the patient should be observed closely. Pseudarthroses are frequent with isolated posterior fusions.

References

1. Adkins JC, Ravitch MM. The operative management of von Recklinghausen's neurofibromatosis in children, with special reference to lesions of the head and neck. Surgery 1977;82:342–348.
2. Armstrong D, Pickrell K, Fetter B, et al. Torticollis: an analysis of 271 cases. Plast Reconstr Surg 1965; 35:14–25.
3. Baga N, Chusid EL, Miller A. Pulmonary disability in the Klippel-Feil syndrome. A study of two siblings. Clin Orthop 1969;67:105–110.
4. Bailey DK. The normal cervical spine in infants and children. Radiology 1952;59:712–719.
5. Baird PA, Robinson GC, Buckler WSJ. Klippel-Feil syndrome. A study of mirror movement detected by electromyography. Am J Dis Child 1967;113:546–551.
6. Bharucha EP, Dastur HM. Craniovertebral anomalies (a report on 40 cases). Brain 1964;87:469–480.
7. Binder H, Eng GD, Gaiser JF, et al. Congenital muscular torticollis: results of conservative management with long-term follow-up in 85 cases. Arch Phys Med Rehabil 1987;68:222–225.
8. Bonola A. Surgical treatment of the Klippel-Feil syndrome. J Bone Joint Surg Br 1956;38:440–449.
9. Brackbill Y, Douthitt TC, West H. Psychophysiologic effects in the neonate of prone versus supine placement. J Pediatr 1973;81:82–84.
10. Bray PF, Herbst JJ, Johnson DG, et al. Childhood gastroesophageal reflux. JAMA 1977;237:1342–1345.
11. Brooks B. Pathologic changes in muscle as a result of disturbances in circulation. Arch Surg 1922;5:188–216.
12. Brown MW, Templeton AW, Hodges III FJ. The incidence of acquired and congenital fusions in the cervical spine. Am J Roentgenol 1964;92:1255–1259.
13. Burwood RJ, Watt I. Assimilation of the atlas and basilar impression. A review of 1, 500 skull and cervical spine radiographs. Clin Radiol 1974;25:327–333.
14. Canale ST, Griffin DW, Hubbard CN. Congenital muscular torticollis: a long-term follow-up. J Bone Joint Surg Am 1982;64:810–816.
15. Catell HS, Filtzer DL. Pseudosubluxation and other normal variations in the cervical spine in children. A study of one hundred and sixty children. J Bone Joint Surg Am 1965;47:1295–1309.
16. Chamberlain WE. Basilar impression (platybasia): bi-

zarre developmental anomaly of occipital bone and upper cervical spine with striking and misleading neurologic manifestations. Yale J Biol Med 1939; 11:487–496.
17. Chaurasia BD, Singh MP. Ectopic lungs in a human fetus with Klippel-Feil syndrome. Anat Anz 1977; 142:205–208.
18. Coventry MB, Harris LE. Congenital muscular torticollis in infancy. Some observations regarding treatment. J Bone Joint Surg Am 1959;41:815–822.
19. Craig JB, Govender S. Neurofibromatosis of the cervical spine. J Bone Joint Surg Br 1992;74:575–578.
20. Crawford Jr. AH, Bagamery N. Osseous manifestations of neurofibromatosis in childhood. J Pediatr Orthop 1986;6:72–88.
21. Darling DB, Fisher JH, Gellis SS. Hiatal hernia and gastroesophageal reflux in infants and children: analysis of the incidence in North American children. Pediatrics 1974;54:450–455.
22. Davids JR, Wenger DR, Mubarak SJ. Congenital muscular torticollis: sequela of intrauterine or perinatal compartment syndrome. J Pediatr Orthop 1993; 13:141–147.
23. de Barros MC, Farias W, Ataíde L, et al. Basilar impression and Arnold-Chiari malformation. A study of 66 cases. J Neurol Neurosurg Psychiat 1968;31:596–605.
24. de Graff R. Congenital block vertebrae C2-C3 in patients with cervical myelopathy. Acta Neurochir (Wein) 1982;61:111–126.
25. Deburge A, Briard J. Cervical hemivertebra excision. Report of a case. J Bone Joint Surg Am 1981; 63:1335–1338.
26. Drvaric DM, Ruderman RJ, Conrad RW, et al. Congenital scoliosis and urinary tract abnormalities: are intravenous pyelograms necessary? J Pediatr Orthop 1987;7:441–443.
27. Dubousset J. Torticollis in children caused by congenital anomalies of the atlas. J Bone Joint Surg Am 1986; 68:178–188.
28. Duncan PA. Embryologic pathogenesis of renal agenesis associated with cervical vertebral anomalies (Klippel-feil phenotype). Birth Defects 1993;13:91–101.
29. El-Khoury GY, Clark CR, Dietz FR, et al. Posterior atlantooccipital subluxation in Down syndrome. Radiology 1986;159:507–509.
30. Epstein BS, Epstein JA. The association of cerebellar tonsillar herniation with basilar impression incident to Paget's disease. Am J Roentgenol 1969;107:535–542.
31. Epstein NE, Epstein JA, Zilkha A. Traumatic myelopathy in a seventeen-year-old child with cervical spinal stenosis (without fracture or dislocation) and a C2–3 Klippel-Feil fusion. A case report. Spine 1984;9:344–347.
32. Falk RH, Mackinnon J. Klippel-Feil syndrome associated with aortic coarctation. Br Heart J 1976; 38:1220–1221.
33. Ferkel RD, Westin GW, Dawson ED, et al. Muscular torticollis. A modified surgical approach. J Bone Joint Surg Am 1983;65:894–900.
34. Fesmire FM, Luten RC. The pediatric cervical spine: developmental anatomy and clinical aspects. J Emerg Med 1989;7:133–142.
35. Fielding JW, Cochran GVB, Lawsing III JF, et al. Tears of the transverse ligament of the atlas. A clinical and biomechanical study. J Bone Joint Surg Am 1974; 56:1683–1691.
36. Fielding JW, Hensinger RN, Hawkins RJ. Os odontoideum. J Bone Joint Surg Am 1980;62:376–383.
37. Gehring GG, Shenasky II JH. Crossed fusion of renal pelves and Klippel-Feil syndrome. J Urol 1976; 116:103–104.
38. Graziano GP, Herzenberg JE, Hensinger RN. The halo-Ilizarov distraction cast for correction of cervical deformity. J Bone Joint Surg Am 1993;75:996–1003.
39. Greenberg AD. Atlantoaxial dislocation. Brain 1968; 91:655–684.
40. Gunderson CH, Solitare GB. Mirror movements in patients with the Klippel-Feil syndrome. Neuropathologic observations. Arch Neurol 1968;18:675–679.
41. Hall JE, Simmons ED, Danylchuk K, et al. Instability of the cervical spine and neurological involvement in Klippel-Feil syndrome. J Bone Joint Surg Am 1990; 72:460–462.
42. Hallah JT, Fallahi S, Hardin JG. Nonreducible rotational head tilt and atlantoaxial lateral mass collapse. Clinical and roentgenographic features in patients with juvenile rheumatoid arthritis and ankylosing spondylitis. Arch Intern Med 1983;143:471–474.
43. Harkey HL, Crockard HA, Stevens JM, et al. The operative management of basilar impression in osteogenesis imperfecta. Neurosurgery 1990;27:782–786.
44. Hemmer KM, McAlister WH, Marsh JL. Cervical spine anomalies in the craniosynostosis syndromes. Cleft Palate J 1987;24:328–333.
45. Hensinger RN, Lang JE, MacEwen GD. Klippel-Feil syndrome. A constellation of associated anomalies. J Bone Joint Surg Am 1974;56:1246–1253.
46. Hummer Jr. CD, MacEwen DD. The coexistence of torticollis and congenital dysplasia of the hip. J Bone Joint Surg Am 1972;54:1255–1256.
47. Hunt TE, Dekaban AS. Modified head-neck support for basilar invagination with brain-stem compression. Can Med Assoc J 1982;126:947–948.
48. Hurwitz LJ, Shepherd WHT. Basilar impression and disordered metabolism of bone. Brain 1966;89:223–234.
49. Illingsworth RS. Attacks of unconsciousness in association with fused cervical vertebrae. Arch Dis Child 1956;31:8–11.
50. Isu T, Miyasaka K, Abe H, et al. Atlantoaxial dislocation associated with neurofibromatosis. Report of three cases. J Neurosurg 1983;58:451–453.
51. Johnson DG, Herbst JJ, Oliveros MA, et al. Evaluation of gastroesophageal reflux surgery in children. Pediatrics 1977;59:62–68.
52. Jolley SG, Johnson DG, Herbst JJ, et al. An assessment of gastroesophageal reflux in children by extended pH monitoring of the distal esophagus. Surgery 1978; 84:16–24.
53. Klippel M, Feil A. Un cas d'absence des vertebres

cervicales. Nouvelle Icongographie de la Salpétriere 1912;25:223–250.
54. Kreiger AJ, Rosomoff HL, Kuperman AS, et al. Occult respiratory dysfunction in a craniovertebral anomaly. J Neurosurg 1969;31:15–20.
55. Lee CK, Weiss AB. Isolated congenital cervical block vertebrae below the axis with neurological symptoms. Spine 1981;6:118–124.
56. Ling CM. The influence of age on the results open sternomastoid tenotomy in muscular torticollis. Clin Orthop 1976;116:142–148.
57. Ling CM, Low YS. Sternomastoid tumor and muscular torticollis. Clin Orthop 1972;86:144–150.
58. Locke GR, Gardner JL, Van Epps EF. Atlas-dens interval (ADI) in children. A survey based on 200 normal cervical spines. AJR 1996;97:135–140.
59. Louis DS, Argenta LC, Seidman M. The orthopaedic manifestations of Goldenhar's syndrome. Surg Round Orthop 1987;43–46.
60. Lowry RB. The Klippel-Feil anomalad as part of the fetal alcohol syndrome. Teratology 1977;16:53–56.
61. Macalister A. Notes on the development and variations of the atlas. J Anat Physiol 1983;27:519–542.
62. MacDonald D. Sternomastoid tumour and muscular torticollis. J Bone Joint Surg Br 1969;51:432–443.
63. MacEwen DD, Winter RB, Hardy JH. Evaluation of kidney anomalies in congenital scoliosis. J Bone Joint Surg Am 1972;54:1451–1454.
64. Martel W. The occipito-atlanto-axial joints in rheumatoid arthritis and ankylosing spondylitis. Am J Roentgenol 1961;86:223–240.
65. McGregor M. Significance of certain measurements of skull in diagnosis of basilar impression. Br J Radiol 1948;21:171–181.
66. McLay K, Maran AGD. Deafness and the Klippel-Feil syndrome. J Laryngol Otol 1969;83:175–184.
67. McRae DL. Bony abnormalities in the region of the foramen magnum: correlation of the anatomic and neurologic findings. Acta Radiol 1953;40:335–354.
68. McRae DL. The significance of abnormalities of the cervical spine. Am J Roentgenol 1960;84:3–25.
69. McRae DL, Barnum AS. Occipitalization of the atlas. Am J Roentgenol 1953;70:23–46.
70. Mecklenburg RS, Krueger PM. Extensive genitourinary anomalies associated with Klippel-Feil syndrome. Am J Dis Child 1974;128:92–93.
71. Menezes AH, VanGilder JC, Graf CJ, et al. Craniocervical abnormalities: a comprehensive surgical approach. J Neurosurg 1980;53:444–454.
72. Menezes AHV. Transoral-transpharyngeal approach to the anterior craniocervical junction. J Neurosurg 1988;69:895–903.
73. Michie I, Clark M. Neurologic syndromes associated with cervical and craniocervical anomalies. Arch Neurol 1968;18:241–247.
74. Moore WB, Matthews TJ, Rabinowitz R. Genitourinary anomalies associated with Klippel-Feil syndrome. J Bone Joint Surg Am 1975;57:355–357.
75. Morrison DL, MacEwen GD. Congenital muscular torticollis: observations regarding clinical findings, associated conditions, and results of treatment. J Pediatr Orthop 1982;2:500–505.
76. Morrison SG, Perry LW, Scott III LP. Congenital brevicollis (Klippel-Feil syndrome). Am J Dis Child 1968;115:614–620.
77. Mosberg Jr. WH. The Klippel-Feil syndrome. Etiology and treatment of neurologic signs. J Nerv Ment Dis 1953;117:479–491.
78. Murphy Jr. WJ, Gellis SS. Torticollis with hiatus hernia in infancy. Sandifer syndrome. Am J Dis Child 1977;131:564–565.
79. Neidengard L, Carter TE, Smith DW. Klippel-Feil malformation complex in fetal alcohol syndrome. Am J Dis Child 1978;132:929–930.
80. Nicholson JT, Sherk HH. Anomalies of the occipitocervical articulation. J Bone Joint Surg Am 1968;50:295–304.
81. Nora JJ, Cohen M, Maxwell GM. Klippel-Feil syndrome with congenital heart disease. Am J Dis Child 1961;102:110–864.
82. Ogden JA. Radiology of postnatal skeletal development. XI. The first cervical vertebrae. Skel Radiol 1984;12:12–20.
83. Ogden JA. Radiology of postnatal skeletal development. XII. The second cervical vertebra. Skel Radiol 1984;12:169–177.
84. Ogden JA. Skeletal injury in the child. 2nd ed. Philadelphia: WB Saunders, 1990;571–577.
85. Ogden JA, Murphy MJ, Southwick WO, et al. Radiology of postnatal skeletal development. XIII. C1-C2 relationships. Skel Radiol 1986;15:433–438.
86. O'Rahilly R, Muller F, Meyer DB. The human vertebral column at the end of the embryonic period proper. 1. The column as a whole. J Anat 1980;131:565–575.
87. O'Rahilly R, Meyer DB. The timing and sequence of events in the development of the human vertebral column during the embryonic period proper. Anat Embryol 1979;157:167–176.
88. Palant DI, Carter BL. Klippel-Feil syndrome and deafness. A study with polytomography. Am J Dis Child 1972;123:218–221.
89. Pásztor E, Vajda J, Piffkó P, et al. Transoral surgery for basilar impression. Surg Neurol 1980;14:473–476.
90. Pennecot GF, Gouraud D, Hardy JR, et al. Roentgenographical study of the stability of the cervical spine in children. J Pediatr Orthop 1984;4:346–352.
91. Pizzutillo PD, Woods MW, Nicholson L. Risk factors in Klippel-Feil syndrome. Orthop Trans 1987;11:473.
92. Poppel MH, Jacobson HG, Duff BK, et al. Basilar impression and platybasia in Paget's disease. Radiology 1953;61:639–644.
93. Pozo JL, Crockard HA, Ransford AO. Basilar impression in osteogenesis imperfecta. A report of three cases in one family. J Bone Joint Surg Br 1984;66:233–238.
94. Ramenofsky ML, Buyse M, Goldberg MJ, et al. Gastroesophageal reflux and torticollis. J Bone Joint Surg Am 1978;60:1140–1141.
95. Ramsey J, Bliznak J. Klippel-Feil syndrome with renal agenesis and other anomalies. Am J Roentgenol 1971;113:460–463.
96. Ritterbusch JF, McGinty LD, Spar J, et al. Magnetic resonance imaging for stenosis and subluxation in Klippel-Feil syndrome. Spine 1991;16:539–541.

97. Rush PJ, Berbrayer D, Reilly BJ. Basilar impression and osteogenesis imperfecta in a three-year-old girl: CT and MRI. Pediatr Radiol 1989;19:142–143.
98. Sakuo T, Morizono Y, Morimoto N. Transoral atlantoaxial anterior decompression and fusion. Clin Orthop 1984;187:134–138.
99. Saltzman CL, Hensinger RN, Blane CE, et al. Familial cervical dysplasia. J Bone Joint Surg Am 1991; 73:163–171.
100. Sandham A. Cervical vertebral anomalies in cleft lip and palate. Cleft Palate Craniofac J 1986; 23:206–214.
101. Sarnat HB, Morrissy RT. Idiopathic torticollis: sternomastoid myopathy and accessory neuropathy. Muscle Nerve 1981;4:374–380.
102. Sensenig EC. The development of the occipital and cervical segments and their associated structures in human embryos. Contrib Embryol Carnegie Inst 1957;36:141–152.
103. Sherk HH, Shjut L, Chung S. Iniencephalic deformity of the cervical spine with Klippel-Feil anomalies and congenital elevation of the scapula. J Bone Joint Surg Am 1974;56:1254–1259.
104. Sherk HH, Whitaker LA, Pasquariello PS. Facial malformations and spinal anomalies. A predictable relationship. Spine 1982;7:526–531.
105. Shoul MI, Ritvo M. Clinical and roentgenological manifestations of the Klippel-Feil syndrome (congenital fusion of the cervical vertebrae, brevicollis). Report of eight additional cases and review of the literature. Am J Roentgenol 1952;68:369–385.
106. Skeletal Dysplasia Group. Instability of the upper cervical spine. Arch Dis Child 1989;64:283–288.
107. Spierings ELH, Braakman R. The management of os odontoideum. J Bone Joint Surg Br 1982;64:422–428.
108. Stark EW, Borton TE. Hearing loss and the Klippel-Feil syndrome. Am J Dis Child 1972;123:233–235.
109. Stark EW, Borton TE. Klippel-Feil syndrome and associated hearing loss. Arch Otolaryngol 1973; 97:415–419.
110. Steel HH. Anatomical and mechanical considerations of the atlanto-axial articulation. J Bone Joint Surg Am 1968;50:1481–1482.
111. Strax TE, Baran E. Traumatic quadriplegia associated with Klippel-Feil syndrome: discussion and case reports. Arch Phys Med Rehab 1975;56:363–365.
112. Swischuk LE. Anterior displacement of C2 in children: physiologic or pathologic? A helpful differentiating line. Radiology 1977;122:759–763.
113. Taylor AR, Chakravorty BC. Clinical syndromes associated with basilar impression. Arch Neurol 1964; 10:475–484.
114. Teodori JB, Painter MJ. Basilar impression in children. Pediatrics 1984;74:1097–1099.
115. Thompson T, McManus S, Colville J. Familial congenital muscular torticollis: case report and review of the literature. Clin Orthop 1986;202:193–196.
116. Tredwell SJ, Newman DE, Lockitch G. Instability of the upper cervical spine in Down syndrome. J Pediatr Orthop 1990;10:602–606.
117. Tredwell SJ, Smith DF, Macleod PJ, et al. Cervical spine anomalies in fetal alcohol syndrome. Spine 1982;7:331–334.
118. Tse P, Cheng J, Chow Y, et al. Surgery for neglected congenital torticollis. Acta Orthop Scand 1987; 58:270–272.
119. Ulmer JL, Elster AD, Ginsberg LE, et al. Klippel-Feil syndrome: CT and MR of acquired and congenital abnormalities of cervical spine and cord. J Comput Assist Tomogr 1993;17:215–224.
120. Wadia NH. Myelopathy complicating congenital atlantoaxial dislocation (a study of 28 cases). Brain 1967;90:449–472.
121. Weiner DS. Congenital dislocation of the hip associated with congenital muscular torticollis. Clin Orthop 1976;121:163–165.
122. Weisel SW, Rothman RH. Occipitoatlantal hypermobility. Spine 1979;4:187–191.
123. Whyte AM, Lufkin RB, Bredenkamp J, et al. Sternocleidomastoid fibrosis in congenital muscular torticollis: MR appearance. J Comput Asst Tomog 1989; 13:163–166.
124. Wollin DG. The os odontoideum. Separate odontoid process. J Bone Joint Surg Am 1963;47:1459–1471.
125. Wong VCN, Fung CF. Basilar impression in a child with hypochondroplasia. Pediatr Neurol 1991;7:62–64.
126. Wood DE, Good Tl, Hahn J, et al. Decompression of the brain stem and superior cervical spine for congenital/acquired craniovertebral invagination: an interdisciplinary approach. Laryngoscope 1990;100:926–931.
127. Yamada H, Nakamura S, Tajima M, et al. Neurological manifestations of pediatric achondroplasia. J Neurosurg 1981;54:49–57.
128. Yong-Hing K, Kalamchi A, MacEwen GD. Cervical spine abnormalities in neurofibromatosis. J Bone Joint Surg Am 1979;61:695–699.

CHAPTER EIGHT

Neuromuscular Scoliosis

John G. Thometz

General Principles

The early attempts at treatment of neuromuscular scoliosis involved manipulative therapy, frequently in patients with poliomyelitis. These techniques date back for hundreds of years, and a variety of rather involved manipulative techniques were employed. Spinal corsets and casts also were used in an attempt achieve some curve correction, but these early methods were unsuccessful (Fig 8.1). The first bracing system that was thought to have some effect on curve progression was developed by Dr. Walter Blount. In addition to its use in treating idiopathic scoliosis, it was also used for treatment of poliomyelitis.

Bracing systems such as the Milwaukee brace or the Boston brace are considered "active" systems that require good torso strength and control, and a satisfactory righting reflex. These are requirements not present in severely involved neuromuscular patients with scoliosis; therefore, "active" systems are contraindicated. Bracing systems that work best for these patients are considered "passive" systems, which are variations of a total contact TLSO.

Problems with the use of bracing in neuromuscular patients are numerous. The total contact circumferential brace may compromise an already diminished vital capacity. Prolonged brace wear causes pressure on the rib cage, which ultimately may lead to significant rib deformity. Patients who are marginal ambulators may have their ability to walk negatively affected by the use of the brace. Patients who have a G-tube or problems with gastroesophageal reflex may develop complications related to increased abdominal pressure. Those with a sensory deficit are prone to pressure sores.

The biggest concern regarding the use of the brace in many neuromuscular conditions revolves around whether the brace alters the natural history to any significant degree, particularly in entities such as muscular dystrophy, spinal muscular atrophy, Friedreich's ataxia, and even cerebral palsy. The brace may help those patients with very poor trunk control maintain an upright posture. Patients with severe scoliosis who unfortunately are not surgical candidates because of severe medical problems may be helped with a total contact brace or a total contact molded seating system.

The initial reports on the surgical treatment of neuromuscular scoliosis primarily relate to patients with poliomyelitis who underwent a posterior spinal fusion with cast immobilization (Fig. 8.2). Early in these series, a facet fusion was not performed. However, even when facet fusion was included, most series still reported a high pseudarthrosis rate with little improvement in the curve magnitude after fusion. Gucker (17), in 1956, reported a 60% pseudarthrosis rate, and Bonet (5), in 1965, reported a 40% pseudarthrosis rate. In both series, there was a very poor rate of curve correction.

The development of Harrington's instrumentation in the early 1960s was a significant advance. Harrington instrumentation, when combined with posterior spinal fusion, achieved an improved correction in curve magnitude and also diminished the rate of

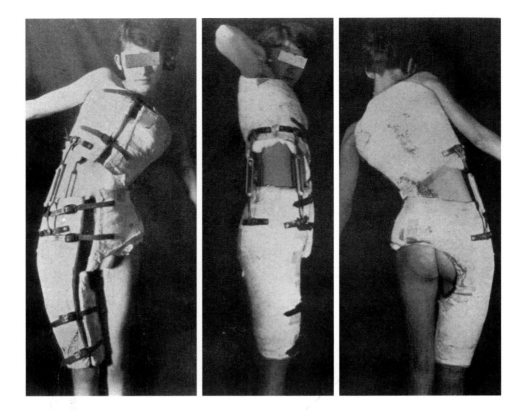

FIGURE 8.1.
Turnbuckle cast used to achieve correction of scoliosis. Reprinted with permission from Campbell W. Operative orthopaedics. St. Louis: Mosby-Year Book: 1939, reprint 1942; Figure 775, p. 1042.

pseudarthrosis significantly. Nonetheless, in the more severely involved neuromuscular patients, osteopenic bone often led to loss of fixation. Furthermore, the Harrington fusion still required a significant period of immobility.

A dramatic advance in the treatment of neuromuscular curves came with the development of the Luque segmental spinal instrumentation, which achieved stability with the use of sublaminar wires at every level to be fused (4, 6,13, 40, 50). The system was rigid and fusion rates in neuromuscular patients increased dramatically. Anterior instrumentation systems such as the Dwyer were also helpful in patients with neuromuscular scoliosis, particularly when combined with posterior instrumentation systems such as the Harrington or Luque system. Since then, multiple systems using segmental fixation have been developed and are successfully used for the treatment of neuromuscular scoliosis. Although there are multiple systems, the ultimate goal is the same: to achieve a vertical torso over the pelvis. The goal is balance of the thoracic spine over the pelvis, not maximal correction of the scoliosis.

Patients who have neuromuscular scoliosis require a careful preoperative workup. Subspecialty evaluation insures that the patient is a reasonable surgical candidate from the pulmonary and cardiac standpoint. In addition, patients who have severe neuromuscular deformities also need assessment from the standpoint of their nutritional status. Patients who are nutritionally depleted are at significantly higher risks for wound infections postoperatively.

Fusions in the neuromuscular patients are often more extensive than those in the idiopathic patients, and the blood loss may be extensive. The appropriate candidate may predonate blood. The cell saver, the use of intraoperative hypotension, and intraoperative hemodilution are important methods for diminishing blood loss. There also are systems available for retrieving blood in the postoperative period from the drain.

Hypothermia can be a problem with some patients, and heated humidified anesthesia may be helpful in maintaining body temperature along with the use of heating blankets. Spinal cord monitoring is probably useful in most cases. The usefulness of somatosensory evoked potentials varies with the type of neuromuscular disorder. With the severely disabled neuromuscular patient, the quality of the cortical evoked potentials may be poor. Methods for the use of motor evoked potentials are improving to

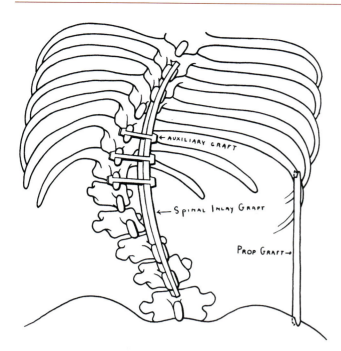

FIGURE 8.2.
For more severe cases, use of both the "spinal inlay" graft and the "prop" graft are advocated. Reprinted with permission from "The Alber Spine Fusion Operation in the Treatment of Scoliosis." Surg Gynecol Obstet 1966; April:797–803. By permission of SURGERY, Gynecology & Obstetrics, now known as the JOURNAL OF THE AMERICAN COLLEGE OF SURGEONS.

diminish the possibility of a false negative result during surgery.

Patients who need both the combined anterior and posterior procedure traditionally had this done as a two-stage procedure. If the operation is staged a week or two apart, patients should have nutritional support between the two stages. More recently, both stages have been performed during the same general anesthetic with satisfactory results. Swank (49) reported less complications with a one-stage combined anterior posterior fusion compared with the two-stage procedure. The author has experience with 16 single-stage combined anterior-posterior fusions in neuromuscular patients without significant postoperative complications.

As mentioned earlier, patients must be assessed preoperatively to make sure that they have an optimal nutritional status. Pretreatment with a gastrostomy may be required in certain cases. Urinary tract infections may be precipitated by the prolonged use of an indwelling catheter. Patients who have a diminished urine output postoperatively may have the syndrome of inappropriate antidiuretic hormone and may require assessment for this entity.

Ileus usually occurs after a major scoliosis fusion. Severe prolonged ileus may actually be a mechanical obstruction caused by the superior mesenteric artery syndrome. This obstruction generally resolves with intravenous hyperalimentation and nasogastric suction.

Atelectasis is a common postoperative problem in neuromuscular patients who often have underlying diminished pulmonary reserve. It is always important to initiate aggressive postoperative pulmonary treatment, which may require use of chest physiotherapy and the nebulizer. Patients also need to be observed for aspiration pneumonia, or severe atelectasis caused by the development of a mucous plug.

If a patient develops a superficial infection, it should resolve with intravenous antibiotics and local wound care. However, if there is a suspicion of a deep wound infection, then the wound must be opened, irrigated, and debrided, with multiple cultures taken for both aerobic and anaerobic specimens. The bone graft material is removed and irrigated and then replaced, and the instrumentation is left in place. If the wound appears clean, the wound may be closed over drains. Severe wound infections occasionally require multiple debridements and then healing by secondary intention. If a late, low grade, chronic infection develops with a presentation of a draining sinus with no systemic signs, local care may be given until the fusion is solid; at that point, the instrumentation may be removed and antibiotics given. After an infection develops, the pseudoarthrosis rate is increased.

Cerebral Palsy

The decision as to whether to treat a significant scoliosis in a patient with severe cerebral palsy requires a careful assessment of the child's mental status and functional capacity. The indications for extensive spinal surgery in the profoundly retarded patient have come into question in this area of limited health resources. If the child is a sitter, performing a scoliosis fusion to preserve the child's sitting ability is often worthwhile. Other indications for surgery may include: progression of a large thoracolumbar curve which may diminish pulmonary function, recurrent pressure sore formation in patients whose sitting balance is poor, and pain. Assessing and localizing the source of pain in these patients, however, is difficult.

Treatment decisions also must include an understanding of the curve's natural history (30). In a study of the natural history of the progression of scoliosis after skeletal maturity in adults who have cerebral palsy, Thometz and Simons (50) noted that in patients with a curve of over 50° at the time of skeletal maturity, progression was 1.4° per year (Figs.8.3 and 8.4). Patients who had an early onset of structural scoliosis had a poor prognosis. Skeletal maturity was

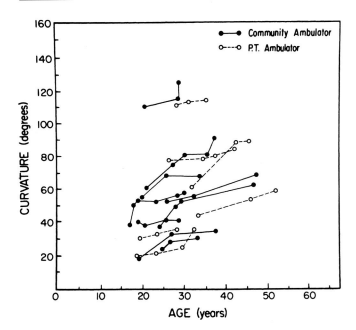

FIGURE 8.3.
Progression of scoliosis often skeletal maturing in ambulatory cerebral palsy patients. Reprinted with permission from Thometz JG, Simon SR. Progression of scoliosis after skeletal maturity in institutionalized adults who have cerebral palsy. J Bone Joint Surg Am 1988;70:1294.

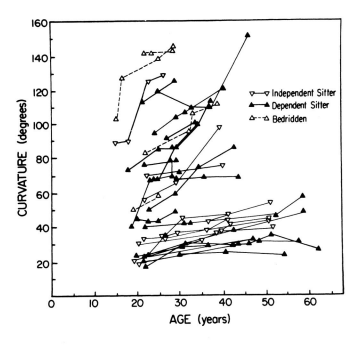

FIGURE 8.4.
Progression of scoliosis after skeletal maturity in nonambulatory cerebral palsy patients. Reprinted with permission from Thometz JG, Simon SR. Progression of scoliosis after skeletal maturity in institutionalized adults who have cerebral palsy. J Bone Joint Surg Am 1988;70:1294.

often delayed, and there were patients who were skeletally immature even in the third decade of life. Nonambulatory patients with spastic quadriplegia can show dramatic progression after skeletal maturity. Braces are not well tolerated in patients with severe cerebral palsy, and their efficacy in altering the natural history is unclear.

Lonstein and Akbarnia (28) have divided the curve patterns in cerebral palsy into two groups (Fig.8.5). The first group, the ambulatory children, develop a single or double curve typical to that seen in idiopathic scoliosis. The second group, the nonambulatory children, generally develop long thoracolumbar curves with associated pelvic obliquity. The pelvis

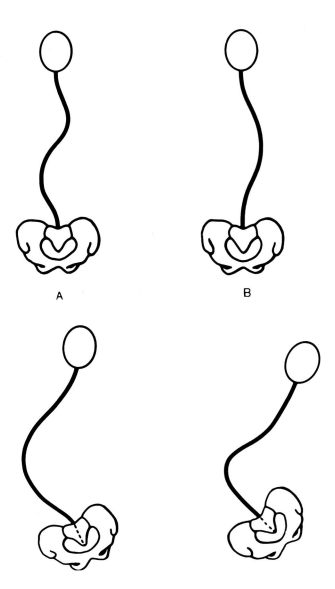

FIGURE 8.5.
Curve patterns in cerebral palsy. Top: ambulatory. Bottom: nonambulatory. Reprinted with permission from Moes textbook of scoliosis and other spinal deformities, 2nd ed. Philadelphia: WB Saunders, 1987; Figure 13.11, p. 293.

may be included in the curve in this second group, or there may be a short compensatory curve at the lumbosacral junction wherein the sacral vertebrae are not part of the larger curve.

Lonstein and Akbarnia felt that with this second group, fusion to the pelvis was mandatory to achieve a balanced spine. With the nonambulatory group, Lonstein felt that even patients with a curve similar to the ambulatory group would develop pelvic obliquity over time if fused only to the fifth lumbar vertebra. The authors concluded that all nonambulators should be fused to the sacrum. The indications for adding an anterior fusion followed evaluation of curve flexibility on the Risser Cotrel frame. If the rib cage could be balanced over the pelvis with this view, then a posterior fusion alone would be sufficient. Imbalance is unacceptable, as is pelvic obliquity greater than 10°. An anterior fusion should be performed when a large residual curvature is present even on the traction film. Patients who are significantly skeletally immature may develop the crankshaft phenomenon; this may be another relative indication for performance of an anterior fusion.

Luque instrumentation provides excellent fixation for patients with severe cerebral palsy. When using Luque spinal instrumentation with sublaminar wiring, it is important to achieve proper wire contour to avoid injury to underlying spinal cord or nerve roots (Fig. 8.6). Zindrick (56) noted that a semi-circular shape resulted in less canal penetration than the previously recommended rectangular shape, and he noted that the larger the radius of the circle, the less the penetration into the canal. Goll et al. (15) videotaped the passage of sublaminar wires and documented the depth of wire penetration in the spinal canal. They concluded that passage of the sublaminar wire must remain strictly in the midline, the bend at the tip of the sublaminar wire should not be greater than 45°, and the radius of curvature of the semi-circular wire must at least equal the width of the lamina. Once the sublaminar wire has been passed, it must be stabilized to avoid trauma to the underlying neural elements.

Yngve (55) described a useful technique for wire stabilization (Fig. 8.7). The wire is passed from a caudal to cranial direction with the tip of the wire contacting the undersurface of the lamina as the wire is advanced. Once the tip of the wire is visible at the proximal end of the lamina, the wire is grasped and gently pulled until about 6 cm of wire is exposed.

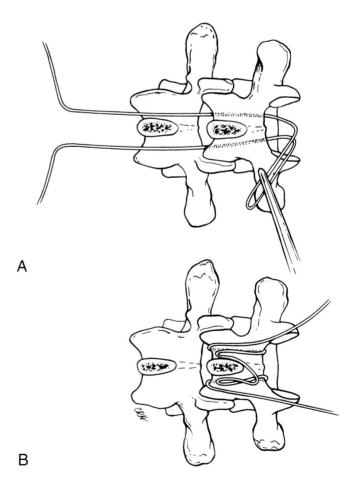

A

B

FIGURE 8.7.
A. Kocher clamp may be used to help advance sublaminar wire. **B.** The tails of the sublaminar wire are brought proximally over the lamina; the tip of the sublaminar wire is brought distally; and one strand is placed on each side of the spinous process.

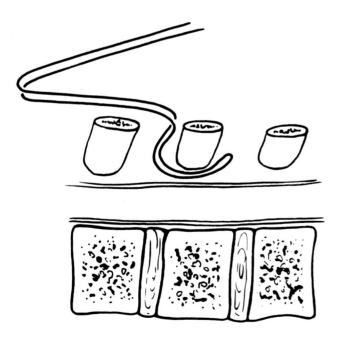

FIGURE 8.6.
The top of the sublaminar wire must remain in contact with the undersurface of the lamina during passage.

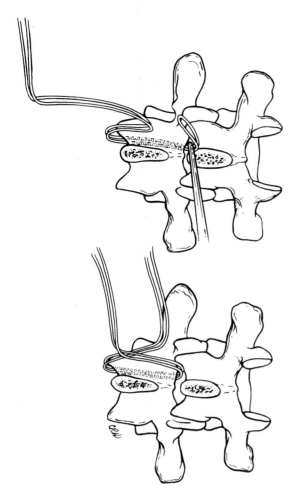

FIGURE 8.8.
Each end of the wire is bent and twisted about the lamina to prevent the wire from migrating down the canal.

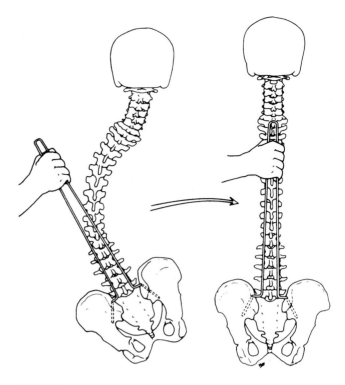

FIGURE 8.9.
Correction achieved through use of unit rod. Reprinted with permission from Rinsky L. Scoliosis management in cerebral palsy. Clin Orthop 1990;253:104.

The tip of the wire is then brought over the lamina with one strand of the wire placed on each side of the spinous process. It is contoured closely to the lamina. After this, the tails of the wire are brought proximally over the lamina in a cephalic direction and also contoured against the lamina. The tails are then bent laterally out of the wound (Fig. 8.8). The Luque rod is then modified as needed to achieve the appropriate contour, particularly in the sagittal plane. Cross links must be used when two separate rods are involved.

Broom (6) found that cerebral palsy patients had better results with instrumentation using .25 inch Luque rods rather than the smaller rods. Rinsky et al. (40), when reviewing their results with Harrington rods, unlinked Luque rods, and the unit Luque rod found far and away the best correction and least complications with the use of the unit rod (Fig. 8.9). The use of postoperative immobilization with an orthosis for 4 to 6 months postoperative is generally recommended. The most popular method for achieving pelvic fixation is the Galveston method of Allen and Ferguson (1). Stabilization of the pelvis is accomplished by driving a segment of the rod into each ilium. The amount of purchase into the ileum should be at least 6 cm.

The pelvic component of the rod is designed to fit between the cortices of the wing of the ileum. The rod is contoured to achieve the most stable fixation in a position of approximately 1 to 1.5 cm above the sciatic notch. Intraoperatively, the surgeon places his/her finger in the sciatic notch to obtain appropriate orientation. The precontoured unit rod may simplify placement of the rod for the Galveston technique, but individual patients who have a very large rigid curve or severe lumbar lordosis may require a more individualized rod configuration.

Additional techniques are available for distal fixation only to the sacrum, particularly in larger patients in whom the bone is not osteopenic. Sacral screws can be inserted into the ala laterally, into the ala directly anteriorly, or into the vertebral body and sacral promontory.

The use of segmental spinal fixation has diminished the pseudarthrosis rate. These longer fusions also need bone bank bone to obtain a satisfactory fusion. The most common areas to develop a pseudarthrosis are in the region of the thoracolumbar spine and the lumbosacral spine. If a pseudarthrosis develops and there is evidence of continued curve progression or pain, then repair is warranted.

Careful postoperative management is necessary to prevent significant respiratory complications in children with severe cerebral palsy. Severe atelectasis may develop, and pneumonia may lead to a premature death. Postoperative ileus may develop (particularly in patients who have had an anterior release), which may lead to the necessity for nutritional support.

Myelomeningocele—Kyphosis and Scoliosis

The natural history of kyphosis in myelomeningocele tends to be one of unremitting progression. This progressive kyphosis can lead to several problems, including recurrent pressure sores over the prominence, difficulty sitting, the potential risk of respiratory problems, and difficulty eating. The kyphosis limits available space for the abdominal contents, which are then pushed up against the diaphragm.

Lindseth (26) has divided kyphosis in myelomeningocele into three patterns. The first type is collapsing kyphosis. Although occasionally these curves may be stable, more often they show evidence of significant progression. Brace management may be attempted for a very mild curve at a very early age, but the brace may exacerbate the problems with diminished pulmonary reserve or cause feeding problems. Therefore, if progression is noted, early surgical treatment is warranted. Instrumentation without fusion may be attempted but often results in instrument failure. Combined anterior/posterior fusion leads to an exceedingly small spine when performed at an early age.

Therefore, Lindseth (26) developed a technique which can be used at any age, from birth on (Fig 8.10). His procedure involves decancellation of the vertebral bodies above and below the apical vertebra. The posterior elements are removed first, after which the ossific nucleus of the vertebral body is removed, but the epiphysis is left intact as is the cortical bone anteriorly. After the cortex of the vertebral bodies is removed posteriorly and laterally, the apical vertebral body is pushed anteriorly. When the kyphosis is corrected satisfactorily, it is stabilized by using a tension band wiring technique between the pedicle of the vertebral body above the apex, the apical vertebral body and the vertebral body below the apex. Satisfactory growth of the lumbar spine can provide room for the abdominal cavity.

The functioning epiphyses allow for further correction of kyphosis into lordosis. In the child older than 1 year, Lindseth recommends adding Luque in-

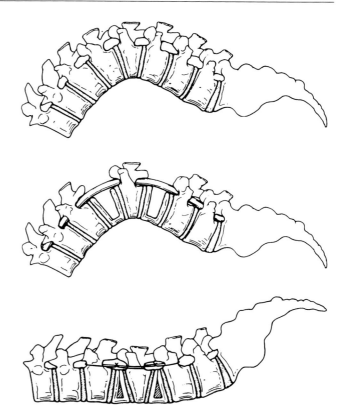

FIGURE 8.10.
Correction of C-shaped kyphosis by removal of ossific nucleus from vertebra. Reprinted with permission from Linseth R. Spine deformity in myelomeningocele. American Academy of Orthopaedic Surgeons Instruction Course Lectures, Vol XL, 1991:276.

strumentation posteriorly to stabilize the spine as part of a posterior spinal fusion.

In dealing with the surgical attempts at correcting kyphosis, one must keep in mind the anatomy of the abdominal aorta in children with a congenital lumbar kyphosis. Loder et al. (27) noted that in aortagrams of these children, the abdominal aorta bridges the lumbar kyphosis and, therefore, attempts to forcefully elongate the spine through the area of the lumbar kyphosis could result in aortic rupture. The more severe S-shaped kyphosis requires excision of vertebral bodies for correction (Fig. 8.11).

Treatment of the spinal deformity in myelomeningocele is particularly complex. Early surgical reports were notable for high infection rates, poor curve correction, and frequent pseudarthroses. Shurtleff (46) studied the progression of scoliosis in patients with myelomeningocele over time and noted that by the age of 1 year, only 3% had a curvature. In general, the less severe the neurologic involvement, the less a problem there was with scoliosis. The incidence of scoliosis increases over time (20). Eighty-eight percent of thoracic patients develop significant scoliosis.

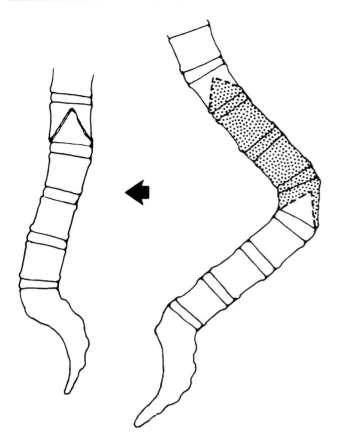

FIGURE 8.11.
Correction of rigid S-shaped kyphosis by excision of vertebrae between apex of kyphosis and the lordosis. Reprinted with permission from Morrisey RT. Lovell and Winter's pediatric orthopaedics. 3rd ed. Philadelphia: JB Lippincott, 1990;522. Bernie Kida, Illustrator.

Only 9% of the sacral level patients have a significant curve by skeletal maturity. Scoliosis is present in 90% of children with myelomeningocele over the age of 10 years.

Scoliosis in myelomeningocele is frequently progressive. With each visit, a careful neurologic examination must be performed. The patient must be assessed to ensure that no progressive motor or sensory loss exists. The gait pattern must be monitored for deterioration. The child's lower extremities should also be evaluated for evidence of spasticity, and the hips should be checked for progressive hip flexion contractures.

The patient with a progressive curvature needs a careful preoperative assessment in conjunction with the neurosurgical team to rule out lesions which are known to cause a progressive spinal curvature.

The tethered cord syndrome is a well-known cause associated with progressive spinal curvature. This may be associated with diastamyelia or lipoma. With the tethered cord syndrome, the spinal cord remains bound down to the region of the myelomeningocele. Therefore, the distal end of the spinal cord cannot migrate proximally as it normally does with age, leading to neurologic deficit and curve progression. Early recognition of the tethered cord with successful release may be successful in slowing or stopping curve progression in the milder curves.

Other entities can cause a progressive change. The development of hydromyelia may be related to a nonfunctioning shunt. The nonfunctioning shunt may not cause the usual clinical significance of hydrocephalus. If hydromyelia or syringomyelia is recognized early and treated, this may inhibit curve progression. Patients with a progressive curvature in spina bifida need assessment with the use of magnetic resonance imaging to rule out not only the possibility of tethered cord and hydromyelia, but also the possibility of malformations such as the Arnold-Chiari or the presence of dermoid cysts. Considerable judgment is required by the neurosurgeon because several of these abnormalities may be present on the magnetic resonance scan.

There are relatively few reports of brace treatment for scoliosis in myelomeningocele. The goal of the brace is to delay surgical intervention until sufficient spinal growth has developed. Patients with curvatures over 20° should be treated with a brace. Pressure sores may be a problem, and over time, deformities of the rib cage caused by compression may develop. The use of the soft Boston brace can be helpful in diminishing any tendency towards pressure sores. Muller et al. (34) confirmed that bracing works best in patients with spina bifida when initiated with a curve of less than 45°. The curves often are paralytic collapsing curves that initially show significant flexibility and good curve correction in the brace. Muller et al. found that the use of the brace did diminish the rate of scoliosis progression significantly; pressure sores were rarely a problem. The brace can be valuable as an aide in treating these milder, flexible curves.

Muller et al. noted that patients with larger curvatures tend to progress more rapidly (34). Shurtleff found that the risk for scoliosis curve progression was high in patients beyond the age of 10 years.

Patients who undergo unsuccessful brace treatment and have continued curve progression are candidates for fusion. It is better to fuse the curve at an early age rather than wait for the scoliosis to reach a huge magnitude at a later date before attempting correction. Parents of ambulatory patients should be counseled that the fusion may negatively affect the child's ambulatory capacity (31).

Patients who are nonambulatory often have their sitting balance improved with the surgical procedure. These nonambulatory patients generally require fusion to the pelvis. Pseudoarthrosis of the lumbosacral junction, however, is common because of the lack of the posterior elements. Lumbar curves must be well corrected; if the child is fused and significant pelvic obliquity remains, recurrent ischial pressure sores may be a problem. Lindseth recommends that the residual pelvic obliquity be less than 15°. McMaster (29) noted that improved fusion rates are obtained when a combined anterior-posterior arthrodesis is performed, particularly in the region where the posterior elements are missing. Anterior release and fusion followed by posterior instrumentation may be performed, or anterior instrumentation systems may be combined with posterior instrumentation to supplement the fixation.

Fixation to the pelvis is difficult in these patients because of the thin wall of the ilium. Other methods besides the Galveston techniques have been described to improve distal fixation. In Dunn's technique (12), the rods are wrapped around the sacral ala and a transverse rod connector is used to prevent migration of the rods. Until recently, Luque instrumentation has been the most common system for achieving segmental spinal stabilization. Hybrid systems which are able to use compression and distraction with the use of pedicle screws and hooks are all alternative methods for achieving segmental stabilization of the spine.

In addition to the typical collapsing neuromuscular scoliosis, patients who have myelomeningocele often have a congenital scoliosis. As in the neurologically intact child, early treatment is warranted before gross deformity develops. In the lumbar spine where the posterior elements are lacking, combined anterior/posterior fusion is the preferred treatment.

For the posterior approach, the skin must be assessed carefully. If there is significant scarring in the region of the dural sac, an inverted "Y" incision down to the sacrum can be used. Plastic surgery consultation can be helpful, and the use of a free flap to obtain satisfactory skin coverage may be necessary. As with all long fusions in neuromuscular scoliosis, both coronal and sagittal alignment must be maintained with appropriate thoracic kyphosis and lumbar lordosis.

Duchenne's Muscular Dystrophy

Duchenne's muscular dystrophy is usually evident clinically when a child is around 2 to 3 years of age, although there may be some history of mild developmental delay before this age. Genetic research has identified that the gene defect has been localized to the short arm of the tenth chromosome. This gene produces dystrophin, which is a component of the plasma membrane system in normal muscle fibers. Patients who have Duchenne's muscular dystrophy have significant deficiency of dystrophin. In patients with Duchenne's dystrophy, the dystrophin level is generally less than 3% of normal. Hip extensors are the first muscles involved, resulting in an increased pelvic tilt with ambulation along with increased lumbar lordosis. Both Gower's and Meyron's signs are helpful in demonstrating the proximal muscle weakness (53). Hip and knee flexion contractures along with equinus contractures may develop over time. At the age of 10 years, the children are generally not ambulatory. It is once the children become nonambulatory that rapidly progressive curves may develop.

Natural History of the Spinal Deformity in Duchenne's Muscular Dystrophy

Progressive scoliosis leads to significant pelvic obliquity and problems with sitting balance; the scoliosis may exaggerate their respiratory compromise or lead to problems with back or leg discomfort. In addition, seating difficulties may cause feeding problems or inhibit a child's upper extremity function. Progression of the curvature may be delayed by the use of bracing, but bracing ultimately fails to prevent curve progression.

The natural history of the scoliosis in muscular dystrophy was analyzed by Wilkins and Gibson (54). These authors thought that scoliosis in muscular dystrophy can be divided into two pathways: the "stable" pathway and the "unstable" pathway. The "stable" pathway establishes an extension posture of the lumbar spine. If this lordotic posture of the lumbar spine can be maintained, a severe scoliosis rarely develops. In the "unstable" pathway, thoracolumbar kyphosis develops and subsequently a severe curvature develops. Oda et al. (36), in a recent review of 46 patients with Duchenne's muscular dystrophy, concluded that patients who had a lumbar extension posture did not develop a significant curve and thought that these patients should not be surgically stabilized.

Other natural history studies, however, reveal that the incidence of a progressive scoliosis in Duchenne's muscular dystrophy is close to 100%. Cambridge and Drennan (9) noted that in 95% of their patients, scoliosis with an average of 75° developed during the nonambulatory phase, even in patients who used a spinal orthosis. Smith et al. (48) studied 51 patients with Duchenne's muscular dystrophy, all of whom developed scoliosis. In a review by Hsu (19) of 8 patients, all developed significant curvatures.

Patients with Duchenne's muscular dystrophy undergo a progressive deterioration in their pulmonary function. The forced vital capacity diminishes when the children become wheelchair bound. Whether operative stabilization of the spine slows the progression of the decline in the pulmonary function has been the subject of some debate. Miller et al. (32) noted no difference in the rate of decline of pulmonary function between patients who had undergone spinal stabilization and patients who did not. However, Galasko (13) found that in the surgical group, the forced vital capacity remained stable for the first 3 years after surgery, after which there was a slight deterioration. The nonoperative group had a progressive decline.

Early surgical stabilization of the scoliosis while the child's pulmonary function is satisfactory is the procedure of choice. Because of the striking incidence of progressive curves, Jenkins et al. (22) thought that it was important to operate before the forced vital force fed capacity was less than 35% of normal to minimize postoperative pulmonary problems. Brace management has been abandoned because it is effective only in delaying but not stopping the progression of the curvature.

Surgical stabilization must be done using segmental spinal instrumentation. The greatest experience has been with the use of Luque instrumentation. The Luque system achieves segmental stabilization with the use of sublaminar wiring and avoids the need for postoperative brace. The Luque technique was modified by Dr. Mosley with the creation of a unit rod, which is contoured to achieve satisfactory sagittal alignment and fixation to the pelvis. As with all neuromuscular collapsing curves, the fusion must extend proximally to the first or second thoracic vertebra. Distally, it was initially thought that all patients needed fixation to the pelvis. There was concern that patients who did not have fixation to the pelvis would over time develop significant pelvic obliquity and seating problems. Sussman (48) in 1984 analyzed a group of patients who underwent early fusion with the distal extension to the fifth lumbar vertebra. The patients had a satisfactory result, except for one patient who preoperatively had a 96° curve. This patient had increasing pelvic obliquity and curve progression. Mubarek et al. (33) reviewed 12 patients who had a fusion to the pelvis, and 10 patients who had fusion to the fifth lumbar vertebra. These patients had a minimal follow-up of 5 years. The authors found, in general, very satisfactory results with fusion to L-5 if the instrumentation was performed at a very early age (when the patient's curvature was still mild). One patient with a significant postoperative pelvic obliquity after fusion to L-5 was a patient whose preoperative curvature was 50°. Mubarek feels that if the scoliosis curvature is less than 40° and the pelvic obliquity is less than 10°, fusion to L-5 only will give satisfactory long-term results.

Spinal Muscular Atrophy

Spinal muscular atrophy is a condition of progressive flaccid paralysis that results from atrophy of the anterior horn cells throughout the spinal cord. Spinal muscular atrophy is an autosomal recessive condition. Gene studies have noted that both the acute and the chronic forms of spinal muscular atrophy are linked to regions of chromosome 5. The clinical presentation of this disorder has been subdivided into the acute infantile form (Werdnig-Hoffman) disease, and more chronic childhood forms (such as Kugelberg-Welander disease). In the infantile form, the onset begins shortly after birth, and the patients have such muscle weakness that they never develop the ability to sit or walk. Muscle weakness leads to respiratory insufficiency, recurrent pneumonia, and, ultimately, death. However, the more chronic forms have a more benign course with patients surviving to the second or third decade of life. Recently, some authors believe that some of these more benign chronic forms may in fact be nonprogressive.

The severity of this scoliosis is a relative function of the severity of the disease. The natural history studies by Philips et al. (38), Schwentker and Gibson (44), and Drennan and Russman (42) show that the vast majority of patients do develop a progressive scoliosis. As with Duchenne's muscular dystrophy, the nonambulatory patients develop the rapidly progressive curves (16, 18). The pattern of scoliosis tends to be a large, long collapsing curve. Initially, the curve is flexible; it develops more structural characteristics with time. Patients with spinal muscular atrophy may show varying degrees of structural kyphosis over time also, but this tends to be mild. If the scoliosis develops at a relatively early age, bracing is reasonable in an attempt to buy time and delay performance of the spinal fusion until there is a greater torso height. However, if that curve progression continues, it is better to perform an earlier fusion rather than wait until a gross deformity develops and perform fusion at a late date. Anterior releases have been done before the posterior fusion in spinal muscular atrophy in an attempt to gain greater correlation. In patients with severe pulmonary compromise, the risks often outweigh the benefits.

A soft TLSO may be helpful with maintaining sitting balance and, therefore, the functional status; a rigid spinal brace is often uncomfortable. Care must be taken that the brace does not worsen the patient's respiratory difficulties. If the respiratory capacity is diminished, this may necessitate discontinuation of the brace. The brace is minimally effective in preventing curve progression in the nonambulatory patient. In these patients, segmental spinal fixation is necessary to provide satisfactory fixation of the spinal curvature (45). Brown et al. (7) noted that the Luque segmental spinal instrumentation system provided superior fixation to the Harrington systemic patients undergoing spinal fusion for spinal muscular atrophy. Stabilization techniques with the Harrington system have a relatively high complication rate, and initially there was poor attention to sagittal contours to provide satisfactory seating tolerance (2).

Piasecki et al. (39) found very satisfactory results in a long-term follow-up study of spinal fusion in spinal muscular atrophy. He concluded that the procedure significantly improved the quality of life in these patients.

Spinal fusion helps maintain the patient's respiratory reserve by arresting the progression of the curvature and provides for improved seating balance. When the fusion is done early, there is a relatively low incidence of complications. These patients must have careful preoperative evaluation by pulmonary physicians and the anesthesiologist. Patients with a vital capacity of 50% or greater generally do well in the postoperative period. Great attention must be paid to the patient's respiratory care to avoid severe atelectasis or pneumonia. It is also helpful to have a physical therapist involved early in the postoperative treatment of these patients to help ensure that no degeneration in their function occurs from the standpoint of their activities of daily living.

It is controversial whether patients with spinal muscular atrophy have functional improvement after spinal fusion. Philips et al. (38) noted improved sitting balance and endurance, and Piasecki et al. (39) noted that in their group of long-term survivors, there was improved sitting balance and greater independence in the use of hands. However, Brown et al. (7) noted some decrease in functional activities, such as self-feeding, after the procedure. Postoperative physical therapy may inhibit this tendency towards the loss of some functional status.

Friedreich's Ataxia

Friedreich's ataxia is a progressive disorder characterized by spinal-cerebellar degeneration. There is a significant loss of large myelinated fibers which is very striking in the posterior columns. The cerebellum has a noticeable loss of myelinated fibers to the dentate nucleus. It is generally inherited as an autosomal recessive trait with onset between the ages of 5 and 20 years. Recent studies by Chamberlain (10) have identified the gene on chromosome nine by genetic linkage. Patients usually present with an ataxic gait, and later they develop a cavus foot (37). Friedreich's ataxia also leads to a progressive hypertrophic cardiomyopathy.

The natural history of scoliosis in Friedreich's ataxia is not as straightforward as the typical collapsing neuromuscular scoliosis. In a study of 56 patients with a mean age of 20 years, Labelle et al. (25) found a scoliosis of more of 10° in 100% of patients, and a hyperkyphosis in 66% of patients. Cady and Dubechko (8) also noted that the incidence of scoliosis in Friedreich's ataxia was extremely high. These authors noted that scoliosis in patients with Friedreich's ataxia is not always progressive; therefore, there are an appreciable number of patients who may not need treatment.

The patients who did have a progressive scoliosis generally had an onset of a curvature before the adolescent growth spurt. Labelle felt that the curvature behaved more like an idiopathic curve than a neuromuscular curvature (23, 25).

His study concluded that curves less than 40° could be observed, and curves more than 60° should be treated surgically. Those curves between 40 and 60° could be treated depending on the age of the patient at onset of the disease and progression of the curve. Cady et al. also agreed that larger progressive curves should be stabilized surgically. All authors who have discussed brace management in the treatment of scoliosis in Friedreich's ataxia note that the brace has been generally ineffective in inhibiting further curve progression. In addition, the brace often has a negative effect on the patient's gait. These considerations make the use of the brace for this condition very questionable. In Friedreich's ataxia, nonoperative management has been unsuccessful in preventing further progression of the scoliosis (21).

Labelle et al. (24) also studied the sagittal plane abnormalities in patients with Friedreich's ataxia. Increased kyphosis has been reported, but the authors confirmed that the apparent kyphosis is really a "pseudokyphosis" that is secondary to vertebral body rotation. The authors used a three-dimensional computer generated graphic representation from radiographs of patients with Friedreich's ataxia and demonstrated that on a true lateral radiograph, the lateral thoracic spine is hypokyphotic with evidence of hypokyphosis from T-1 to -T-6 (in a patient who was noted to have a right thoracic curve from T-7 to L-1). This must be taken into consideration during surgical planning so as not to exacerbate a proximal junctional kyphosis.

Good results have generally been reported using Harrington, Harrington-Luque, or Luque instrumentation. As with fusions in other ambulatory patients, instrumentation to the sacrum should be avoided because of its negative effect on those patients with marginal ambulation. However, long curves with associated pelvic obliquity must have the pelvis included in the fusion.

Rett's Syndrome

Rett's syndrome is a progressive neurologic disorder that develops in the second year of life. Early milestones are normal, but regression begins, resulting in gait apraxia, autism, and typical hand wringing movements with progressive mental and physical deterioration. Scoliosis is the most common orthopaedic problem. Scoliosis in this entity appears to occur at a higher prevalence as the child ages. By skeletal maturity, most scoliosis is present to some degree in essentially all patients. Bracing is of questionable efficacy but perhaps worth a trial in the younger child. Surgical stabilization with segmental instrumentation is best for those with relentlessly progressing curves.

Poliomyelitis

Poliomyelitis is a viral infection that results in the destruction of the motor neurons of the anterior horn cells of the spinal cord and the brain. This may result in total loss of function of the individual motor neuron. As one might expect, the more severe the involvement, the greater the likelihood of the development of the scoliotic curve. In addition, contractures about the hip may lead to pelvic obliquity, which may induce a curvature. Irwin held that the iliotibial band contracture was an important cause of creating pelvic obliquity associated with a scoliotic curve. Also, muscle imbalance and hip flexion contractures may also result in distortion of the spine. With flexible curves, judicious release of these contractures may help with spinal balance.

Continued curve progression may result in the need for spinal instrumentation and fusion. The initial descriptions of the attempts at scoliosis fusion were in patients with poliomyelitis. These were often fusions with postoperative immobilization with a cast only, resulting in a very high pseudoarthrosis rate with loss of correction. These curves generally require segmental fixation with attention to correction of the pelvic obliquity.

Arthrogryposis

Scoliosis is also a common problem in arthrogryposis. Arthrogryposis is a generic term for a broad group of disorders that are characterized by multiple joint contractures. The most common form of arthrogryposis is amyoplasia. Amyoplasia is characterized by multiple contractures of the shoulders, elbows, and upper extremities, resulting in internal rotation and adduction of the shoulder, flexion or extension or the elbow, and wrist flexion and forearm pronation. The hips are abducted and externally rotated; the knees may be either flexed for extended. Frequently, the feet are severely equinovarus. Scoliosis may develop over time, but curves may be present in infancy because of contracture of the muscles of the trunk. Contractures about the hip also may aggravate pelvic obliquity, but releasing contractures generally fails to halt curve progression. Progressive curve progression may require early combined anterior posterior fusion.

Charcot-Marie-Tooth

Scoliosis may also occur in patients with Charcot-Marie-Tooth disease. Charcot-Marie-Tooth disease is divided into two subtypes. The hereditary motor and sensory neuropathy type I, or the axonal form, more commonly has spinal involvement. There also is a neuronal form of hereditary motor and sensory neuropathy (type II). Initially, it was thought that the incidence of scoliosis in this entity is low. A more recent study by Walker et al. has shown that the incidence may approach 50%. Nonetheless, the number of curves that require treatment is low.

References

1. Allen BL, Ferguson RL. L-rod instrumentation for scoliosis in cerebral palsy. J Pediatr Orthop 1982;2:87–96.
2. Aprin H, Bowen JR, MacEwen Gd, et al. Spine fusion in patients with spinal muscular atrophy. J Bone Joint Surg Am 1982;64:1179–1187.
3. Bassett GS, Tolo VT. The incidence and natural history of scoliosis in Rett syndrome. Dev Med Child Neur 1990;32:963–966.
4. Boachie-Adgei O, Lonstein JE, Winter RB, et al. Management of neuromuscular spinal deformities with Luque segmental instrumentation. J Bone Joint Surg Am 1989;71:548.
5. Bonnett C, Brown J, Perry J, et al. The evolution of treatment of paralytic scoliosis at Rancho Los Amigos Hospital. J Bone Joint Surg Am 1975;57:206–215.
6. Broom MJ, Banta JV, Renshaw TS. Spinal fusion augmented by Luque rod segmental instrumentation for neuromuscular scoliosis. J Bone Joint Surg Am 1989; 71:32.
7. Brown JC, Zeller JL, Swank SM, et al. Surgical and functional results of spine fusion in spinal muscular atrophy. Spine 1989;14:763–770.
8. Cady RB, Bobechko WP. Incidence, natural history, and treatment of scoliosis in Friedreich's ataxia. J Pediatr Orthop 1984;4:673–676.
9. Cambridge W, Drennan JC. Scoliosis associated with Duchenne muscular dystrophy. J Pediatr Orthop 1987; 7:436.
10. Chamberlain S, Shaw J, Rowland A, et al. Mapping of mutation causing Friedreich's ataxia to human chromosome 9. Nature 1988;334:248–250.
11. Daher YH, Lonstein JE, Winter RB, et al. Spinal deformities in patients with Friedreich's ataxia: a review of 19 patients. J Pediatr Orthop 1985;5:553–557.
12. Dunn HK. Kyphosis of myelodysplasia—operative treatment based on pathophysiology. Orthop Trans 1983;7:19.
13. Galasko CSB, Delaney C, Morris P. Spinal stabilization in Duchenne muscular dystrophy. J Bone Joint Surg Br 1992;74:210.
14. Gerhsoff WF, Renshaw TS. The treatment of scoliosis in cerebral palsy by posterior spinal fusion with Luque rod segmental instrumentation. J Bone Joint Surg Am 1988;70:41.
15. Goll S, Balderston R, Stambough J, et al. Depth of intraspinal wire penetration during passage of sublaminar wires. Spine 1988;13:503.
16. Granata C, Merlini L, Magni E, et al. Spinal muscular atrophy: natural history and orthopaedic treatment of scoliosis. Spine 1989;14:760–762.
17. Gucker T III. Experiences with poliomyelitic scoliosis

after fusion and correction. J Bone Joint Surg Am 1956; 38:1281–1300.
18. Hensinger RN, MacEwen GD. Spinal deformity associated with heritable neurological conditions: spinal muscular atrophy, Friedreich's ataxia, familial dysautonomia, and Charcot-Marie-Tooth disease. J Bone Joint Surg Am 1976;58:13–23.
19. Hsu JD. The natural history of spine curvature progression in the non-ambulatory Duchenne muscular dystrophy patient. Spine 1983;8:771.
20. Hull WJ, Moe JN, Winter RB. Spinal deformity in myelomeningocele: natural history, evaluation, and treatment. J Bone Joint Surg Am 1974;56:1767.
21. Irwin CE. The iliotibial band. Its role in producing deformity in poliomyelitis. J Bone Joint Surg Am 1949; 31:141–146.
22. Jenkins J, Bohn D, Edmonds J, et al. Evaluation of pulmonary function in muscular dystrophy patients requiring spinal surgery. Crit Care Med 1982;10:645.
23. Labelle H, Beauchamp M, Lapierre L, et al. Pattern of muscle weakness and its relation to loss of ambulatory function in Friedreich's ataxia. J Pediatr Orthop 1987; 7:496.
24. LaBelle H. Duhaime M, Allard P. Kyphosis and scoliosis in 3-D in Friedreich's ataxia. Orthop Trans 1987; 11:214.
25. Labelle H, Tohmé S, Duhaime M, et al. The natural history of scoliosis in Friedreich's ataxia. J Bone Joint Surg Am 1986;68:564–572.
26. Lindseth RE. Spine deformity in myelomeningocele. Instr Course Lect 1991;40:276.
27. Loder RT, Shapiro P, Towbin R, et al. Aortic anatomy in children with myelomeningocele and congenital lumbar kyphosis. J Pediatr Orthop 1991;11:31–35.
28. Lonstein JE, Adbarnia BA. Operative treatment of spinal deformities in patients with cerebral palsy or mental retardation. J Bone Joint Surg Am 1983;65:43–55.
29. McMaster MJ. Anterior and posterior instrumentation and fusion of thoracolumbar scoliosis due to myelomeningocele. J Bone Joint Surg Br 1987;69:20.
30. Madigan R, Wallace L. Scoliosis in the institutionalized cerebral palsy population. Spine 1981;6:583.
31. Mazur J, Menelaus MB, Dicksen DR, et al. Efficacy of surgical management for scoliosis in myelomeningocele: correction of deformity and alteration of functional status. J Pediatr Orthop 1986;6:568.
32. Miller F, Moseley CF, Koreska P, et al. Pulmonary function and scoliosis in Dechenne dystrophy. J Pediatr Orthop 1988;8:133.
33. Mubarak S, Morin W, Leach J. Spinal fusion in Duchenne muscular dystrophy—fixation and fusion to the sacrum? Orthop Trans 1989;13:169.
34. Muller EB, Nordwall A. Brace treatment of scoliosis in children with myelomeningocele. Spine 1994;19:151–155.
35. Muller EB, Nordwall A, Oden A. Progression of scoliosis in children with myelomeningocele. Spine 1994; 19:147–150.
36. Oda T, Shimizu N, Yonenobu K, et al. Longitudinal study of spinal deformity in Duchenne muscular dystrophy. J Pediatr Orthop 1993;13:478–488.
37. Pelosi L, Fels A, Petrillo A, et al. Friedreich's ataxia: clinical involvement and evoked potentials. Acta Neurol Scand 1984;70:360–368.
38. Philips DP, Roye DP Jr, Farcy JPC, et al. Surgical treatment of scoliosis in a spinal muscular atrophy population. Spine 1990;9:942–945.
39. Piasecki JO, Mahinpour S, Levine DB. Long-term follow-up of spinal fusion in spinal muscular atrophy. Clin Orthop 1986;207:44–54.
40. Rinsky LA. Surgery of spinal deformity in cerebral palsy. Clin Orthop 1990;253:100–109.
41. Rivard CH, Duhaime M, Poitras B, et al. Spinal segmental instrumentation for the treatment of all types of paralytic scoliosis. J Bone Joint Surg Br 1984;66: 299.
42. Russman BS, Melchreit R, Drennan JC. Spinal muscular atrophy: the natural course of disease. Muscle Nerve 1983;6:179–181.
43. Sarwark JF, MacEwen GD, Scott CI. Current concepts review—Amyoplasia (a common form of arthrogryposis). J Bone Joint Surg Am 1990;72:465–469.
44. Schwentker EP, Gibson DA. The orthopaedic aspects of spinal muscular atrophy. J Bone Joint Surg Am 1976; 58:32–38.
45. Shapiro F, Bresnan MJ. Orthopaedic management of childhood neuromuscular disease. Part I. Spinal muscular atrophy. J Bone Joint Surg Am 1982;64–785–789.
46. Shurleff DB, Bourney R, Gordon LH, et al. Myelodysplasia: the natural history of kyphosis and scoliosis. A preliminary report. Dev Med Child Neurol 1976;18 (Suppl 37):126.
47. Smith AD, Koreska P, Moseley CF. Progression of scoliosis in Duchenne muscular dystrophy. J Bone Joint Surg Am 1989;71:1066.
48. Sussman MD. Advantage of early spinal stabilization and fusion in patients with Duchenne muscular dystrophy. J Pediatr Orthop 1984;4:532.
49. Swank S, Lonstein JE, Moe JM, et al. Surgical treatment of adult scoliosis. J Bone Joint Surg Am 1981;63:268–287.
50. Thometz JG, Simon S. Progression of scoliosis after skeletal maturity in institutionalized adults who have cerebral palsy. J Bone Joint Surg Am 1988;70:1290.
51. Thometz JG, An HS. Luque Instrumentation with sublaminar wiring In: An HS, Colter JM, eds. Spinal instrumentation. Baltimore: Williams & Wilkins, 1992;93–103 .
52. Walker JL, Nelson KR, Stevens DB, et al. Spinal deformity in Charcot-Marie-Tooth disease. Spine 1994; 19:1044–1047.
53. Walton JN, Nattrass FJ. On the classification, natural history, and treatment of the myopathies. Brain 1954; 77:169–231.
54. Wilkins KE, Gibson DA. The patterns of spine deformity in Duchenne muscular dystrophy. J Bone Joint Surg Am 1976;58:24–32.
55. Yngve D, Burke S, Price C, et al. Sublaminar wiring. J Pediatr Orthop 1986;6:605–608.
56. Zindrick MR, Knight GW, Bunch WH, et al. Factors influencing the penetration of wires into the neural canal during segmental wiring. J Bone Joint Surg Am 1989; 71:742–750.

CHAPTER NINE

Surgical Treatment of Pediatric Idiopathic Scoliosis

Keith H. Bridwell

Clinical Evaluation

The clinician/surgeon should examine the standing patient from the front and from the back. Standing from the back, the surgeon gets a perception of the patient's translatory deformity and trunk shift. Also, the clinician should look at which shoulder is higher. By looking at the patient from the front, the clinician often gets a better idea of shoulder asymmetry because patient hair often covers up the spine from behind. When the patient flexes forward, then the clinician gets a perception of the axial plane deformity. Having the patient side bend to the right or left then affords a perception of the flexibility of the patient's curves. Also, by putting the patient prone on an examining table and pushing on the apices of the appropriate curves, the clinician best assesses the flexibility of the deformity.

Radiographic Evaluation

Radiographic evaluation includes standing long cassette coronal and sagittal radiographs. Also, long cassette right and left side benders are necessary. A long cassette coronal supine film shows the surgeon just how the patient will look on the table. This author also finds the so-called long cassette push-prone radiograph to be helpful. This radiograph is taken by putting the patient prone and then pushing on the apex of the principal curve that is going to be instrumented. If the surgeon is thinking of instrumenting just the thoracic curve and not the lumbar curve, then this film is valuable because it reveals how much correction is likely in the thoracic spine and shows how the correction will affect patient balance and the lumbar curve below it. The push-prone radiograph is a substitute for the Moe traction film on a Risser table. It is easy and quick to do in the office. For those patients who have a significantly kyphotic component to their deformity, a long cassette supine hyperextension film with a soft bump over the apex of the deformity shows the flexibility of the deformity in the sagittal plane.

Decision-Making Regarding Indications for Surgical Treatment

The principal considerations when deciding on surgical treatment are the magnitude of the deformity and the patient's proximity to skeletal maturity. As Lonstein clearly showed (52), the likelihood of progression of the deformity is related to the size of the curve and to the amount of growth left at presentation.

Usually, surgeons consider surgery on curves that have a Cobb measurement between 40 and 50°. This measurement is considered a "grey zone," in that

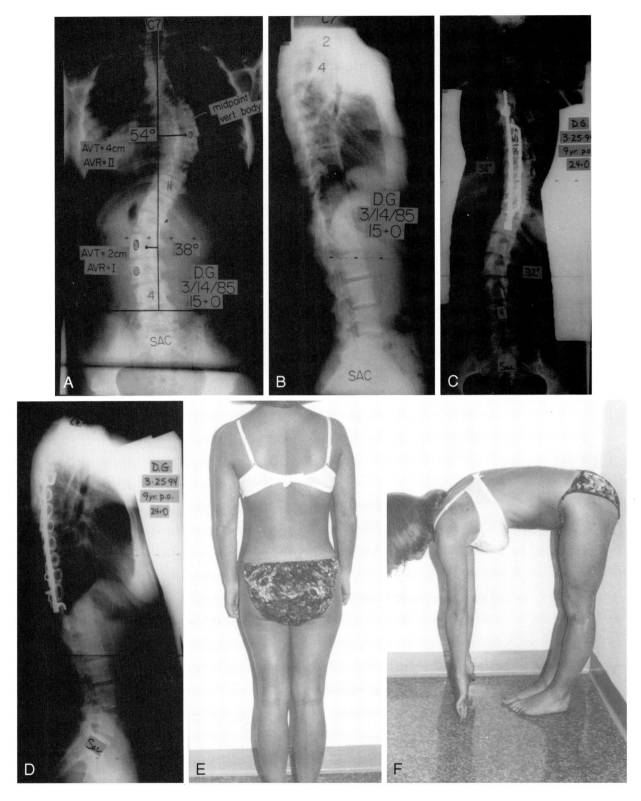

FIGURE 9.1.

A and **B.** Long cassette coronal and sagittal radiographs preoperatively showing a Type II curve pattern. The spine is in lordosis from T12 to L2. There is no thoracolumbar kyphosis. The thoracic curve is bigger than the lumbar curve in terms of Cobb measurement, apical vertebral deviation, and apical vertebral rotation. **C** and **D.** Long cassette coronal and sagittal radiographs upright at ultimate follow-up. **E** and **F.** The patient's clinical appearance at ultimate follow-up. Note her flexibility.

some curves with measurements in the 40s need operative treatment and some do not. As a general rule, however, all curves that are 50° and higher are surgical candidates.

More than just the Cobb measurement has to be considered. The amount of trunk shift, the size of the rib hump, and the curve type all are factors. If the patient has a 43° right thoracic curve, has a significant trunk shift, and is decompensated to the right, then it makes sense to instrument and fuse that curve. However, if the patient has a well-balanced double major curve pattern with both curves measuring 42° that would require a T4 to L4 instrumentation and fusion, then it might be better not to treat that patient surgically, especially if the patient has reached skeletal maturity.

Curve Classification

The curves that are discussed in this chapter are as follows: false double major, single thoracic, long thoracic, double thoracic, double major, lumbar/thoracolumbar, and left thoracic.

False Double Major Curve

This curve pattern generally is referred to as a Type II curve. It was initially described by King et al. (42). Subsequent to that, there have been numerous reports debating how to define this particular curve pattern (16, 45, 46, 75, 82, 87). This type of curve is a pattern in which both a thoracic and a lumbar curve exist. The lumbar curve crosses the midline and does have some structural component to it, but the structural component to the thoracic curve exceeds that of the lumbar curve. In most cases, it is possible to selectively instrument the thoracic curve without having to include the lumbar curve (Fig. 9.1).

The patients who are the best candidates for selective thoracic fusions are those who are skeletally mature. On examination, the principal area of clinical deformity should be in the thoracic spine. If there is a significant lumbar "hump" or waistline asymmetry, the surgeon is probably dealing with a double major curve and not a false double major curve.

Some debate exists among authors as to whether it is more important to look at the standing radiographs or the flexibility radiographs. Most feel that the thoracic curve should be somewhat bigger than the lumbar curve on the standing film. Certain authors have attempted to define what "bigger" is. Certainly the lumbar curve should be much more flexible than the thoracic curve. The flexibility index was described by King (41, 42), who stated that the percent flexibility of the lumbar curve should be greater than that of the thoracic curve. However, this index can be misleading because with true double major curves, the lumbar curve often is more flexible.

If there is no thoracolumbar kyphosis preoperatively, it is often possible to instrument posteriorly to T12 or L1, whichever is the stable vertebra. If there is any thoracolumbar kyphosis (T12 to L2 sagittal Cobb in kyphosis), then it is better to instrument and fuse down to L2 or, more commonly, L3. It is reasonable to stop at L3 if that segment is neutral in rotation.

One group thought that the best indicator of a Type II curve pattern was judged on standing films, where the apical deviation of the thoracic curve should be one and a half times greater than the lumbar curve (46). Also, the lumbar curve should be under 60°, and there should be no thoracolumbar kyphosis.

Exactly where the fine line is drawn between a Type II curve and a true double major curve is still a matter of conjecture and dispute. However, without question, there are Type II curves and it is, at times, possible to selectively instrument only the thoracic curve even though the lumbar curve does cross the midline and has some structural component to it.

Single Thoracic Curve

Single thoracic curves usually are referred to as King Type III curves (42). The apex is usually at T9 or T10. The stable vertebra is usually L2. Usually, instrumentation and fusion posteriorly is performed from T4 to L1 or L2. The lumbar segments below have no rotation to them and they do not cross the midline. Single thoracic curves are the most straightforward type of idiopathic curve to treat (Fig. 9.2).

Long Thoracic Curve

This curve is a King Type IV curve (42), which has an apex at T10, is longer, and extends all the way down to L4. L4 is the first stable vertebra, and instrumentation and fusion is usually necessary down to L4. If the curve is particularly flexible and L3 is neutrally rotated, then it is possible to stop a level higher at L3 (15, 47) (Fig. 9.3).

Double Thoracic Curve

A double thoracic curve is a curve pattern in which there are two thoracic curves. In most cases, there is a high left thoracic curve and a low right thoracic curve. Usually, the low right thoracic curve creates the trunk shift deformity and translation. It also has the bigger rib hump. However, the upper thoracic curve determines shoulder height. Therefore, if a patient with a large right thoracic curve has a high left shoulder, that is a clinical tip-off to a double thoracic curve pattern. Radiographically, if the upper thoracic curve does not correct to less than 20° in the left side

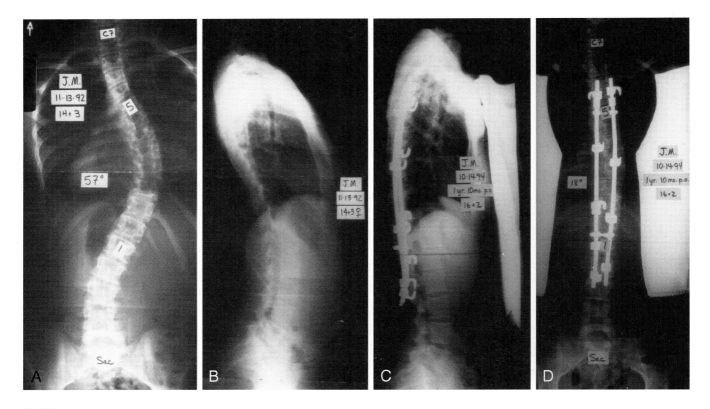

FIGURE 9.2.

A and **B.** Upright coronal and sagittal radiographs preoperatively. A Type III curve pattern. **C** and **D.** Upright coronal and sagittal radiographs at ultimate follow-up.

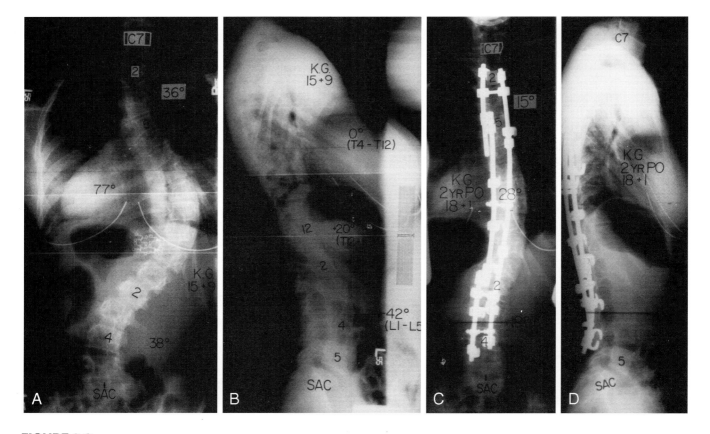

FIGURE 9.3.

A and **B.** A long Type IV thoracic curve. The apex is T10. Coronal and sagittal radiographs preoperatively demonstrate the deformity. **C** and **D.** Upright coronal and sagittal radiographs in the patient at ultimate follow-up. Selective segmental forces and rod rotation maneuvers were performed to address the coronal and sagittal deformities. The patient's upper thoracic spine was kyphotic. The lower thoracic spine was hypokyphotic, and the lumbar spine was hypolordotic.

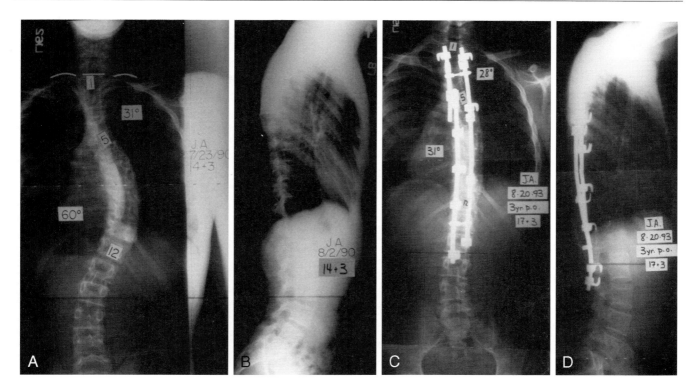

FIGURE 9.4.
A and **B.** Upright coronal and sagittal radiographs preoperatively. Note the structural characteristics of the high left thoracic curve. This is a double thoracic curve pattern. **C** and **D.** Upright coronal and sagittal radiographs on the patient postoperatively. On the left side, a rod rotation maneuver was performed, then a domino was added, and then compression forces were applied to the convexity of the upper curve. In most instances with a double thoracic curve, the lower curve will be hypokyphotic and the upper curve will be somewhat kyphotic. Therefore, the convexity of the upper curve is approached with compression forces first. If the spine was hypokyphotic all the way up to T2, then it would make more sense to approach the concavity of that upper curve first. More often than not, however, the upper curve is relatively hyperkyphotic.

bender, it probably should be included in the instrumentation and fusion. The push-prone radiograph can be beneficial here also. If pushing on the lower right thoracic curve does not change the balance of the shoulders over the pelvis, then the surgeon is probably dealing with a single thoracic curve. However, if it pushes up the left shoulder, then the surgeon is probably dealing with a double thoracic curve (43, 51) (Fig. 9.4).

Double Major Curve

This type of curve usually follows a right thoracic/left lumbar curve pattern. Clinically, the surgeon finds that the rib hump of the thoracic curve and the hump of the lumbar curve are about equal with significant waistline asymmetry. With a double major curve, the thoracic and lumbar curve usually have roughly equal apical deviation from the plumb line, roughly equal apical rotation, and roughly equal Cobb measurements. Often, with posterior fusion for this curve pattern, instrumentation and fusion is needed from T4 to L4. At times, it is possible to stop at L3 if the lumbar curve is very flexible and if L3 is relatively neutral in rotation (15, 47) (Fig. 9.5). At times, a high left thoracic curve may exist with double major curves. Therefore, it is necessary at times to instrument and fuse from T2 to L4.

Lumbar/Thoracolumbar Curves

These curves have an apex at T12 or below. Usually, a thoracolumbar curve is considered one with an apex at T11, T12, or L1, and a lumbar curve has an apex below that. With most thoracic curves, an element of hypokyphosis exists. With most thoracolumbar and lumbar curves, there is an element of hypolordosis. There are differing opinions as to whether it is better to treat lumbar curves anteriorly or posteriorly.

Usually with hook constructs, it is necessary to fuse longer posteriorly than it is anteriorly with screw constructs. Posterior pedicle screw only constructs are being investigated, but the results of this treatment are not clearly known at this time. It is generally believed that anterior instrumentation of lumbar curves allows the surgeon to fuse fewer segments and to get better correction and derotation (18, 25,

29, 32, 54, 60, 63, 67, 68, 77). However, the established literature states that anterior instrumentation is somewhat kyphogenic and is associated with a somewhat higher pseudarthrosis rate (39, 54, 64). Also, if anterior instrumentation is stopped short of the neutral and transitional vertebra distally, then the surgeon may see a "jacked up" appearance to the disc below.

The author found that by using structural grafts or cages anteriorly, the problem of Zielke instrumentation kyphosing the spine can be negated (19). For structural grafts, fresh frozen tricortical iliac wedges are used. They are then wedged into the anterior disc space after the disc has been removed. The disc space is opened up initially with a with a laminar spreader, and then that graft is put in before instrumenting the vertebral bodies with screws placed in the posterior third of the vertebral bodies. Another alternative is to use a construct of a solid rod anteriorly and to perform a 90° rod rotation maneuver (71). The rod rotation maneuver applies to lumbar and thoracolumbar curves that are under 60°. For curves over 60°, it is not always feasible to perform 90° rod rotation maneuvers anteriorly with a solid rod (Fig. 9.6).

Left Thoracic Curve

Left thoracic curves are uncommon. They are, at times, associated with syringomyelia (22, 65). Any patient with a left thoracic curve should have a very careful neurologic examination. All patients with left thoracic curves coming to surgery should probably have an MRI study preoperatively to rule out a syrinx. If, in fact, there is no associated syrinx or other spinal cord anomaly, then these curves are generally different from right thoracic curves. They tend to be hyperkyphotic rather than hypokyphotic. Therefore, they are probably best treated with compression to the convexity before distraction to the concavity. The left thoracic curves also seem to be associated with a greater degree of axial plane rotation (Fig. 9.7).

Principles of Where to Start and Stop the Fusion

The stable vertebra is the vertebra bisected by a line which bisects the sacrum and is perpendicular to the sacrum and the ilium. The stable zone should be bi-

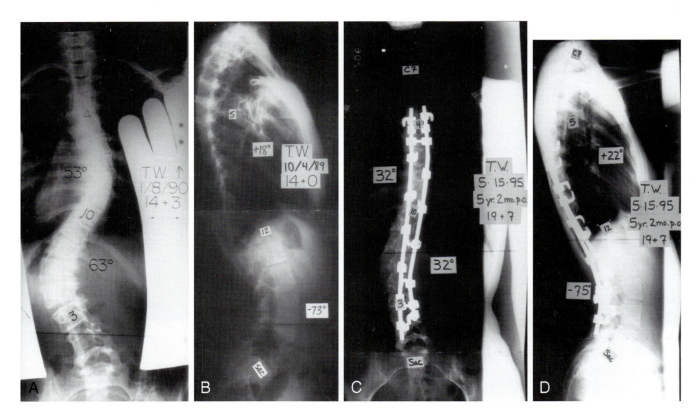

FIGURE 9.5.

A and **B.** Coronal and sagittal long cassette standing radiographs preoperatively. Note that the thoracic and lumbar curves have roughly equal Cobb measurements, apical vertebral deviation, and apical vertebral rotation. L3 is still rotated significantly. L4 is the first neutral vertebra. **C** and **D.** Coronal and sagittal standing radiographs at ultimate follow-up. Maintenance of lumbar lordosis.

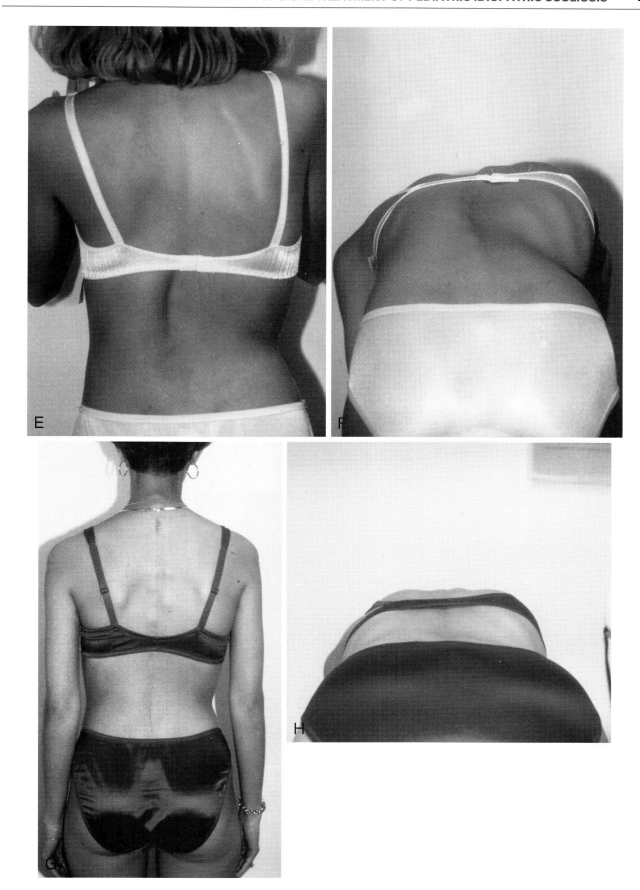

FIGURE 9.5—*continued*
E and F. Clinical photos of the patient preoperatively. G and H. Clinical photos of the patient postoperatively.

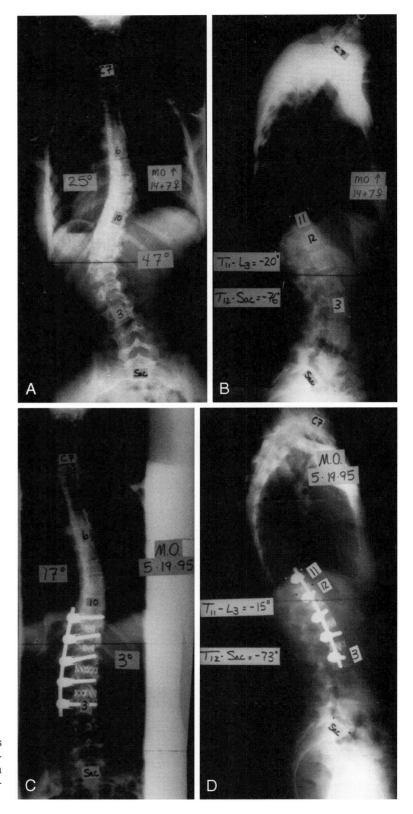

FIGURE 9.6.
A and B. Upright coronal and sagittal radiographs preoperatively. C and D. Upright coronal and sagittal radiographs postoperatively. Solid rod system and cages were used to maintain her lumbar lordosis.

sected by the center sacral line. The stable zone refers to the zone within two vertical lines drawn up from the S1 pedicles and perpendicular to the sacrum (10). Ideally, the distal end of a fusion should be within the stable zone, and the last instrumented vertebra should be bisected by the center sacral line and, therefore, be "stable."

A neutral vertebra is one with neutral rotation. If a spine fusion is carried below L2, it is ideal for that segment to be not only stable but also neutrally ro-

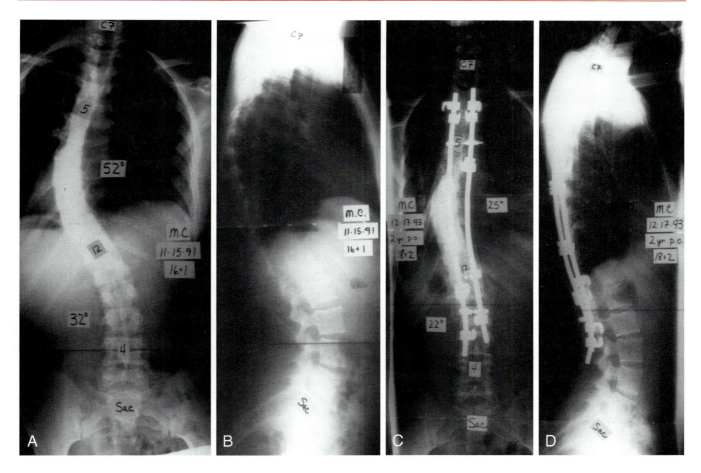

FIGURE 9.7.
A and **B.** Upright coronal and sagittal radiographs preoperatively. Note that this is a left thoracic curve and that it is hyperkyphotic rather than hypokyphotic. **C** and **D.** Upright coronal and sagittal radiographs at ultimate follow-up. Compression forces were applied to the convexity first to correct the kyphotic component of the deformity. A thoracoplasty was also performed.

tated. Rotation can be judged by the Nash-Moe method or by the use of a Perdriolle template (74). The Perdriolle template gives finer measurements, but the Nash-Moe method is more reproducible and less influenced by inter-observer error.

Sagittal Considerations

High Thoracic Kyphosis

With double thoracic curve patterns, the lower thoracic curve usually tends to be lordotic and the upper thoracic curve to be kyphotic. Therefore, it usually makes sense to correct the upper thoracic curve by compression from the left side and the lower thoracic curve by distraction and rod rotation from the left side (78).

Mid-Thoracic Hypokyphosis

Most right thoracic curves are hypokyphotic. If they are treated posteriorly, it makes sense to perform a rod rotation maneuver on the concavity to deliver additional kyphosis to the spine. Another option is using Luque rods or square Harrington rods contoured with kyphosis and sublaminar wires. The other alternative is to treat the curves anteriorly with anterior compression instrumentation, which tends to naturally kyphose the spine (8).

Thoracolumbar Kyphosis

Most thoracolumbar curves are, at the least, hypolordotic. Therefore, if they are treated posteriorly, it makes the most sense to perform a rod rotation maneuver on the convexity. If they are treated anteriorly, then the derotation achieved can negate some of the thoracolumbar kyphosis.

Lumbar Hypolordosis

Most lumbar curves are somewhat hypolordotic. If they are treated from the posterior approach, it is necessary to compress and instrument the convexity first. A surgeon should never apply a distraction force across the lumbar spine concavity until the spine is fixed on the convexity. If the surgeon is treating a lumbar curve anteriorly, then it is necessary to increase segmental lordosis. This increase can be accomplished to some extent with a rod rotation maneuver with a solid rod anteriorly, and also by the use of structural bone graft or cages.

Concomitant L5/S1 Spondylolisthesis

Some patients present with Type IV curves or double major curves and a concomitant L5/S1 isthmic spondylolisthesis. In most cases, the spondylolisthesis is low grade and should be left alone. If possible, the surgeon should fuse higher than L4. Often it is necessary to fuse down to L4. The long-term prognosis in a patient with spinal fusion to L4 and an L5/S1 isthmic spondylolisthesis has never been defined in the literature. However, it is particularly important for such a patient to have the last instrumented vertebra be perfectly parallel to the sacrum, centered on the sacrum, and with physiologic segmental lumbar lordosis.

Thoracic Hyperkyphosis

Thoracic hyperkyphosis often exists in conjunction with a left thoracic curve. Therefore, for this curve pattern, compression forces should be applied on the left side of the curve first (Fig. 9.7).

Indications and Techniques of the Posterior Approach

Rod Rotation Maneuver

With a rod rotation maneuver, translational correction is achieved, and some change in the sagittal orientation is possible (11, 12, 14, 48). The actual degree of axial correction is limited (44).

For a right thoracic curve that is hypolordotic, the rod rotation maneuver is performed on the left side. For a double major curve that is a right thoracic/left lumbar curve, the rod rotation maneuver is also performed on the left side. This approach has the effect of kyphosing the thoracic spine and lordosing the lumbar spine. If the lumbar spine alone is being instrumented, it is important to perform the rod rotation maneuver from the convex left side first to lordose the spine. These maneuvers all apply to curves that are relatively flexible.

Three Rod Technique

This method is useful for large, stiff thoracic curves, or a curve that is over 75° and corrects to no more than 40 to 50°. The three rod technique consists of initially applying a distraction rod across the apical three to four segments and then a longer distraction rod over the whole length of the curve. This author has found that it usually is helpful to have a two segment compression claw on the top and bottom segments to prevent overdistraction. Selective distraction of both rods and then translation of the small rod to the long rod with a device for traction achieves the correction. A third rod is applied to the convexity. The rod on the convexity is principally a holding and stabilizing rod (Fig. 9.8).

Translation with Segmental Wiring

By fixing a solid rod to the top and bottom of the curve and then using either sublaminar wires or intraspinous wires to pull the spine to the rod, a translational correction can be achieved. This can be accomplished with Harrington instrumentation with a square-ended Moe rod that is contoured appropriately, combined with sublaminar wires or Wisconsin wires, or this can be performed with the Texas Scottish Rite or Isola systems (1). Some correction of sagittal deformity can be achieved. The hypokyphotic spine can be given some additional kyphosis with this technique.

Orientation of the Hooks

Using purely a rod/hook construct such as CD or Texas Scottish Rite, it is necessary to change the orientation of the hooks as the discs reverse (2, 11, 12, 20, 81). Therefore, for a Type III curve, if we are to assume that the instrumentation is being carried out from T5 to L2, then the orientation of the hooks usually will be as follows: the hook at T5 on the left side will be in a distraction mode with a claw to prevent medial displacement; the hook at T7 will be an upgoing hook; the hook at T10 will be downgoing hook; the hook at T12 will be a downgoing hook; and finally, the hook at L2 will be an upgoing hook. Usually between T12 and L1, the disc spaces will start to change their orientation in the coronal plane. In the sagittal plane, they will change their orientation from kyphosis to lordosis. Hence, hooks should change their orientation as the discs change their orientation in both the coronal and sagittal planes. On the convexity, the orientation of the hooks should be the reverse of what it is on the concavity.

The Role of Pedicle Fixation

The surgeon has the choice of using either pedicle screws or hooks in the lumbar spine. Some surgeons prefer pedicle screws, thinking that better derotation and control of the sagittal plane can be achieved in this manner. Before using pedicle screws on the con-

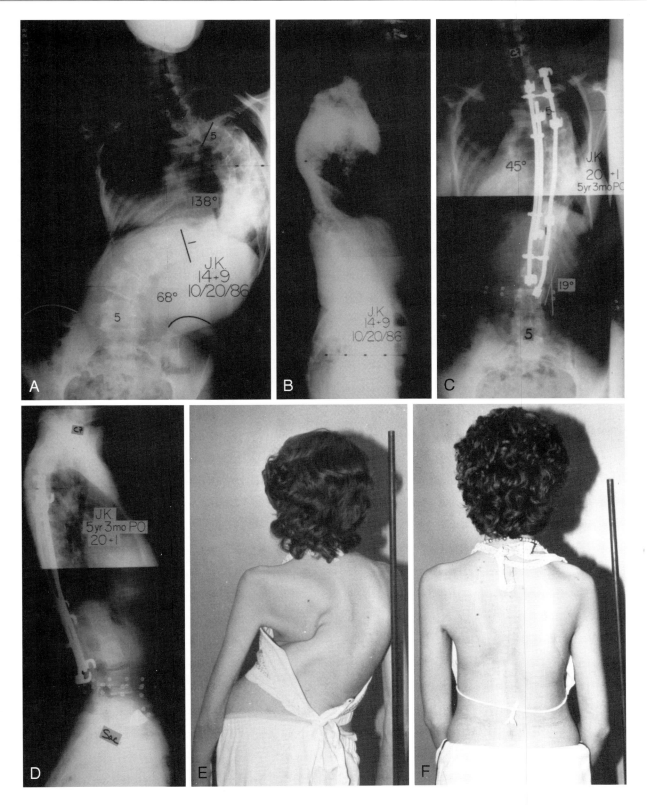

FIGURE 9.8.

A and **B.** Upright coronal and sagittal radiographs preoperatively. **C** and **D.** Upright coronal and sagittal radiographs at ultimate follow-up. Thoracic releases, followed by halo traction, followed by posterior fusion and three rod technique, were employed. **E.** The patient's clinical appearance preoperatively. **F.** The patient's clinical appearance at ultimate postop follow-up.

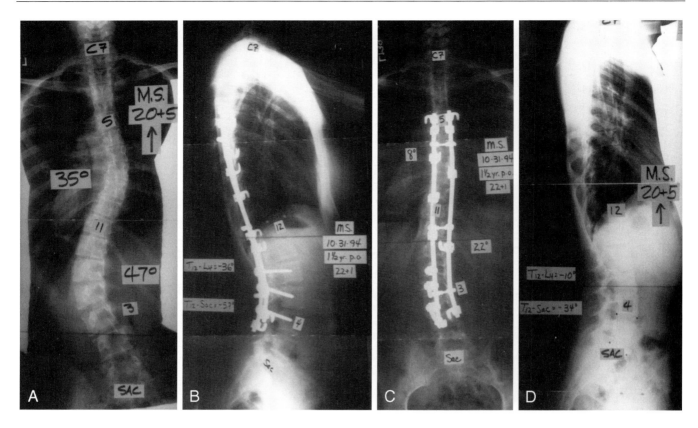

FIGURE 9.9.
A and **B.** Upright long cassette coronal and sagittal radiographs preoperatively. Note that the lumbar curve is hypolordotic. **C** and **D.** Upright long cassette coronal and sagittal radiographs at ultimate follow-up. Instrumentation was carried to the first neutral vertebra. Note that a significant amount of lumbar lordosis has been added.

vexity of a lumbar curve, the surgeon should be sure that the pedicles are big enough to accept screws. The pedicles may be dysplastic, especially on the concavity. At least theoretically, the use of pedicle fixation offers the surgeon an opportunity for better control of the sagittal plane and better rotational correction than can be achieved with posterior hook constructs (34, 59) (Fig. 9.9).

Very, Very Short Anterior Instrumentation

For most thoracolumbar and lumbar curves, the instrumented levels should be the levels that are tilted within the curve. The most cephalad and most caudad vertebrae instrumented should be the ones that are most tilted into the curves. The top and bottom vertebrae included should be of roughly neutral rotation. At times, for very flexible thoracolumbar curves, it is possible to instrument even shorter. This technique has been popularized by Hall, Millis, and Emans (32, 60) in Boston. Shorter can mean one disc space above and one disc space below if the apical segment is a vertebra. If an apical segment is a disc, then this means including that apical disc plus one disc above and one disc below. It is necessary to actually overcorrect the apical segments to achieve this very short instrumentation and fusion, which applies more to thoracolumbar curves than to lumbar curves. There is a bit of kyphosing tendency with this technique, so it is more applicable at the thoracolumbar junction than at the mid or distal lumbar spine (Fig. 9.10).

Instrumentation Without Fusion

This technique applies to curves that are not amenable to bracing or that have exceeded the capacity of bracing in skeletally immature patients. The concept is to instrument the spine and then lengthen the instrumentation every 6 to 12 months until the patient is big enough and skeletally mature enough to perform a fusion (43, 57, 62). It is easiest to perform instrumentation without fusion on single curves without much sagittal deformity. There is a tendency to see increasing kyphosis at the end segments with additional lengthenings. Also, stable fixation at the top and the bottom often is problematic because these patients are young and generally do not have good bone stock. This technique applies more to tho-

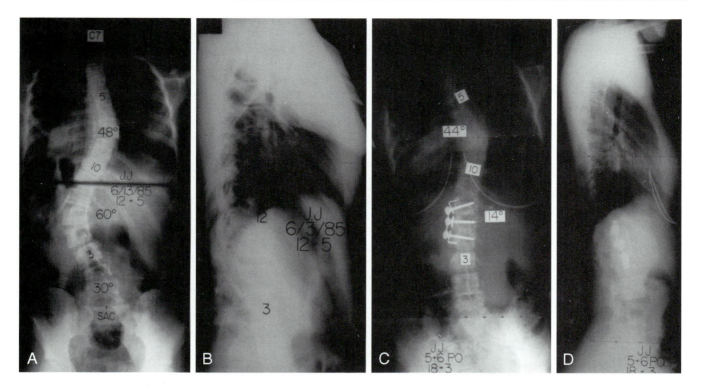

FIGURE 9.10.
A and **B.** Upright coronal and sagittal radiographs preoperatively. The thoracolumbar curve is bigger than the thoracic curve. Both have structural components. If treated posteriorly, one would probably do a T4 to L4 Harrington instrumentation and perhaps stop with TSR or CD instrumentation at L3. The patient's left thoracolumbar curve was extremely flexible on the left side bender. **C** and **D.** Upright coronal and sagittal radiographs at ultimate follow-up after instrumentation and fusion from just T12 to L2. The Hall-Millis technique was used. The patient has excellent clinical balance. Although her thoracic curve measures 40°, the thoracic deformity is imperceptible.

racic curves than it does lumbar curves or double major curves and works better in a spine that is somewhat lordotic or hypokyphotic than it does in a spine that is relatively kyphotic. If some type of two segment claw could be achieved on the top and bottom of the construct, its stability would be greater than simply one hook on the top, one hook on the bottom, and distraction in between.

Indications for Anterior Approach and Anterior Instrumentation

Determining the Fusion Levels

This technique has some application in both the thoracic spine and the lumbar spine. One of the potential advantages of anterior instrumentation is that levels usually can be saved over what is needed posteriorly. The levels that should usually be instrumented are simply the levels that are within the curve. Therefore, instrumentation from transitional vertebra to transitional vertebra is usually appropriate. The transitional vertebra is defined as the one on the top and the bottom of the curve that is the most tilted into the curve. Also, the last disc space tilted into the curve occurs at the transitional vertebra, and then the disc spaces just above proximally and just below distally will start to turn the other way.

Anterior Instrumentation Alternatives for Thoracic Curves

A small rod and compression forces with either Harms or Zielke instrumentation has been advocated (8). So far, solid rod systems have not gained popularity for the thoracic spine. There is some natural kyphosing of the hypokyphotic spine by shortening the anterior column (Fig. 9.11).

Anterior Instrumentation Alternatives for Thoracolumbar/ Lumbar Curves

In the lumbar spine, either Dwyer or Zielke instrumentation can be used. Dwyer instrumentation is now obsolete. Zielke instrumentation, if used, should be combined with structural grafting anteriorly so that the spine is not kyphosed. Traditional Zielke instrumentation is now contraindicated in the lumbar spine because it takes away segmental lordosis. Ei-

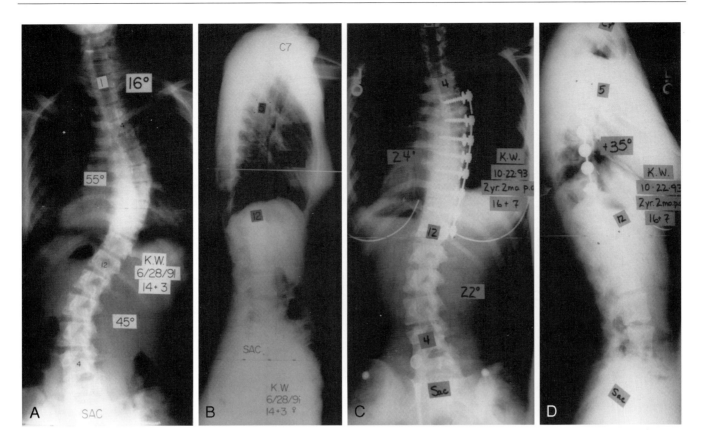

FIGURE 9.11.
A and **B.** Upright coronal and sagittal radiographs preoperatively. **C** and **D.** Upright coronal and sagittal radiographs at ultimate follow-up. Note the broken Zielke rod. However, there has been no loss of correction since this occurred, and the patient has been asymptomatic.

ther structural grafting or placement of cages before instrumentation can segmentally lordose the spine with anterior instrumentation. Another option is a solid rod/screw system. What has most commonly been used is Texas Scottish Rite screws with a Texas Scottish Rite rod. Another option, however, is to use CCD screws with a 6-mm CCD rod. A third option is to use Texas Scottish Rite variable angle screws with a 6-mm CCD rod. With all of these techniques, correction is achieved with a 90° rod rotation maneuver which converts kyphosis to lordosis and scoliosis to no scoliosis. The solid rod systems are most applicable to curves under 60° (Fig. 9.6).

Use of Structural Grafts or Cages

The authors found that with anterior instrumentation of the lumbar spine, we can actually lordose those segments. First, take out the discs back to the posterior longitudinal ligament. Then, open up the interval with a laminar spreader and place either a large fresh frozen tricortical iliac graft or cages into the anterior concave portion of the disc spaces. It is important to place the vertebral screws in the posterior third of the vertebral bodies. This has the effect of compressing the posterior disc space but distracting the anterior disc space. The overall effect is that of opening up the anterior disc space, closing down the posterior disc space, and also locking the grafts and/or cages into place with the anterior instrumentation (Fig. 9.12).

Thoracic Curves

Certainly, double thoracic curves are not ideal candidates for anterior instrumentation. Anterior instrumentation of one of the double thoracic curves worsens shoulder asymmetry. However, anterior instrumentation may afford better coronal, axial, and sagittal correction. The pseudarthrosis rate with this technique is not well known at this point. It may have a role in Type III curves, Type IV curves, and also some Type II curves—namely those Type II curves without much thoracolumbar kyphosis.

Thoracolumbar and Lumbar Curves

Thoracolumbar and lumbar curves are best instrumented and fused from transitional vertebra to transitional vertebra, fusing the entire curve and not beyond. It is possible to stop at L3 instead of L4 if L3 is rotated neutrally. However, if L3 still has signifi-

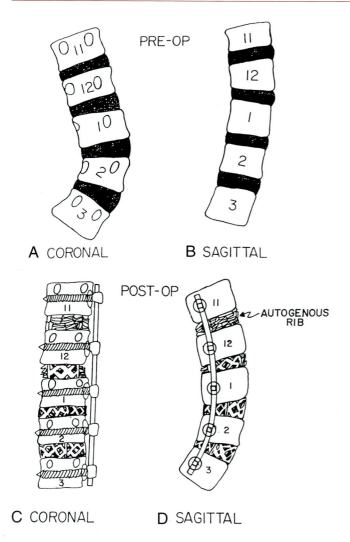

FIGURE 9.12.
Structural grafts to enhance lordosis. **A** and **B.** Coronal and sagittal depiction preoperatively. **C** and **D.** Coronal and sagittal depiction postoperatively. The posterior disc height is shortened but the anterior disc height is lengthened.

cant rotation, then it is better to instrument down to L4 either anteriorly or posteriorly. Most commonly, the principal graft used is autogenous rib graft. This can be supplemented with either fresh frozen allograft or cages to enhance lordosis. If the surgeon tries to fuse short of the transitional and neutrally rotated vertebra, there is potential to see a "jacked up" effect on the disc below.

Indications and Techniques of Anterior and Posterior Approach

Crankshaft

The Texas Scottish Rite group has defined an open triradiate cartilage as the principal risk factor for continued progression of deformity in spite of a solid posterior fusion (76). This occurs as a result of crankshaft, which refers to continued anterior vertebral body growth in spite of a solid posterior fusion (23). In a study done in St. Louis, the authors found that idiopathics between the age of 10 and 12 do not seem to crankshaft even though their triradiate cartilage is open (33). A very young idiopathic scoliosis patient (age 10 or younger) whose triradiate cartilage is open and who has a large deformity may be at risk for crankshaft. The precise set of factors that place an immature idiopathic patient at risk for crankshaft still requires further definement. Relatively few adolescent idiopathics should have anterior fusions to prevent crankshaft. Juvenile/infantile scoliosis patients who require spinal fusions are almost all at risk for crankshaft. Almost all of them who require fusions should have anterior fusions to prevent crankshaft (Fig. 9.13).

Thoracic Curves Requiring Anterior Releases

The literature varies as to when it is advisable to do an anterior thoracic release before a posterior fusion for thoracic scoliosis. If the curve exceeds 100°, this is advisable. Between 75 and 100° is somewhat of a grey zone. Whether an anterior release is needed in this range depends on how flexible that particular curve is.

Fixed Thoracic Lordosis

Both Bradford (9) and Winter (90) have shown that patients with a fixed thoracic lordosis often suffer from significantly reduced pulmonary functions. For those patients, a two-stage procedure is recommended. The first stage involves performing kyphosing vertebral body wedge resections through the disc spaces. This stage is followed by contouring a solid rod and using sublaminar wires at each level posteriorly. With this technique, the spine is gradually translated to the kyphotic rod (9). For stiff and fixed thoracic lordosis, this technique provides a greater reconstitution of normal kyphosis than simply a rod rotation maneuver performed posteriorly (Fig. 9.14).

Fixed Thoracic Hyperkyphosis

Left thoracic curves often are hyperkyphotic. Usually, they are flexible enough that the sagittal deformity can be corrected with a posterior-only procedure. Doing a supine long cassette lateral hyperextension film over a bump provides the surgeon with information regarding whether the kyphosis is flexible. If it is inflexible, it may be advisable to perform anterior releases before the posterior instrumentation and fusion. The principles are the same as those with Scheuermann's kyphosis. This is only

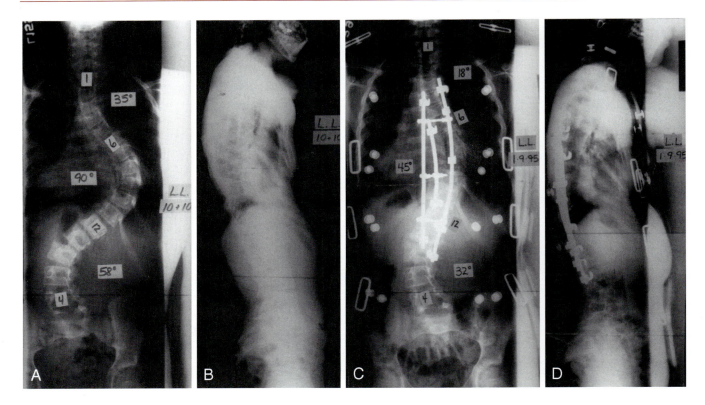

FIGURE 9.13.
A and **B.** A skeletally immature, small patient with a progressive right thoracic curve. Her triradiate cartilage is open. The size of the thoracic curve plus concern regarding potential crankshaft made concomitant anterior releases and fusion advisable. **C** and **D.** Upright coronal and sagittal radiographs postoperatively on the patient. She had anterior discectomies and fusion in the thoracic spine, and then posterior instrumentation and fusion as appropriate.

necessary if the thoracic kyphosis exceeds 75° and does not correct to 40° on the supine hyperextension lateral.

Fixed Lumbar Kyphosis T12 to the Sacrum

Most patients have between 45 and 65° of lordosis (T12 to the sacrum) (7). The normal range is wide. The amount of lumbar lordosis needed depends on how much thoracic kyphosis the patient has. With less thoracic kyphosis, the patient does not need as much lumbar lordosis. However, every lumbar segment from T12 to the sacrum should be in some lordosis. The majority of lumbar lordosis resides within the disc spaces (83).

If a patient does not have segmental lumbar lordosis, then it behooves the surgeon to surgically create physiologic segmental lordosis. In most cases, this can be accomplished with a one-stage approach. The long cassette hyperextension lateral radiograph over a soft bump indicates whether restoration of segmental sagittal lordosis can be accomplished in a single-stage procedure. If that film suggests that the sagittal deformity is not flexible, this may be an indication for an anterior release before posterior instrumentation and fusion. If the segmental sagittal Cobb angle from T12 to L3 or T12 to L4 exceeds 30° of kyphosis, then an anterior release procedure should be done, followed by a posterior instrumentation and fusion to accomplish physiologic lordosis. If the sagittal plane is off the norm by this great a degree, adequate lordization cannot be achieved with a posterior-only or an anterior-only surgery even with a rod rotation maneuver and placement of structural grafts.

Bone Grafting Techniques

Three possibilities for bone grafting include allograft, autogenous iliac bone, and autogenous rib bone obtained with a thoracoplasty.

Most surgeons would not suggest using allograft in idiopathic adolescent scoliosis patients. Allograft seems reasonable for certain paralytic patients in whom it is difficult to obtain adequate autogenous harvesting in a safe fashion because of either reduction of pulmonary functions or because of limited bone stock. In the idiopathic population, the pseudarthrosis rate should be under 5% and perhaps as low as 1%. The morbidity associated with autogenous harvesting in this patient population is low.

Posterior autogenous iliac harvesting is the gold standard for bone graft in idiopathic scoliosis pa-

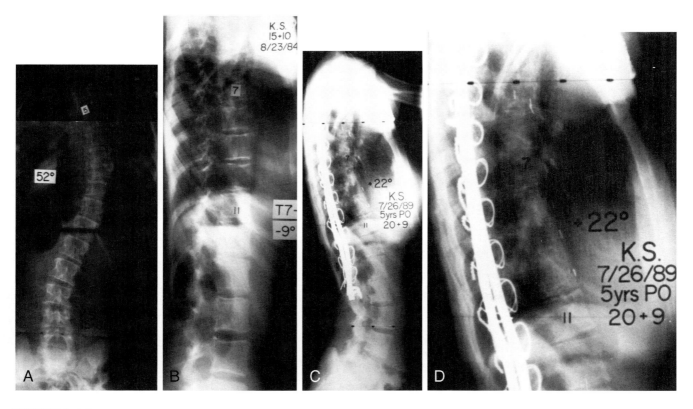

FIGURE 9.14.
A and **B.** Upright coronal and sagittal radiographs preoperatively showing a frankly lordotic thoracic curve. This did not correct significantly on sagittal flexibility radiographs. **C.** Ultimate upright sagittal radiograph showing the correction of the sagittal deformity. The patient had wedges taken through her disc spaces anteriorly and then had correction posteriorly with sublaminar wires and precontoured square Harrington rods. **D.** The postoperative coned-down sagittal view of her spine.

tients. Usually, if the posterior fusion is to L2 or above, the surgeon harvests the iliac bone graft through a separate vertical incision over the posterior ilium. If the instrumentation and fusion is to L3 or L4, the surgeon usually extends the skin incision a bit further and then raises a skin flap above the fascia over to the right ilium. The iliac fascia always should be closed over hemovacs to prevent hematomas and to reduce the incidence of wound infection. Persistent complaints regarding the bone graft site in adolescents are, in the author's experience, rare.

For patients who have significant thoracic deformity and thoracic axial rotation, thoracoplasty is a reasonable alternative (79, 80). Usually with harvesting six to eight ribs posteriorly, thoracoplasty provides an adequate bone graft supply for the fusion.

We usually perform the thoracoplasty after the definitive instrumentation and fusion are done. A flap is raised under the thoracolumbar fascia and under the latissimus dorsi muscle over to the rib cage. Next, several pieces of rib are taken, starting at the apex and working proximally and distally. A longer piece of rib usually is taken at the apex than at the end segments. It is necessary to osteotomize the rib all the way to the transverse process medially. Failure to get to the transverse process creates an unsightly medial ridge. The author used to go somewhat beyond the apex of the rib and center the rib osteotomy on the apex. Now, however, it often is sufficient to osteotomize the rib at the level of the apex. Since doing this, the author sees fewer pulmonary complications, and the cosmetic result is satisfactory (Fig. 9.15).

When we first started doing thoracoplasties, the patient's pulmonary functions were studied preoperatively, immediately postoperatively, and at intervals postoperatively (49). Frequently, a chest tube would be placed because many of the patients seemed to develop either sympathetic effusions or retropleural intrathoracic hematomas. In the idiopathic population, it is rare to violate the pleura when taking the ribs. The periosteal envelope is thick and, therefore, this complication is rare.

At present, we do not do as extensive a thoracoplasty, and chest tubes are seldom used. The study of pulmonary function tests is continued. We found that with most idiopathics in our initial series, pulmonary functions were reduced immediately postoperatively and took about one year to return to normal (49). The effect of the less extensive thoracoplasty is yet to be determined. After harvesting the ribs, we do repair the rib beds. We also advance the latissimus muscle medially to help push the ribs

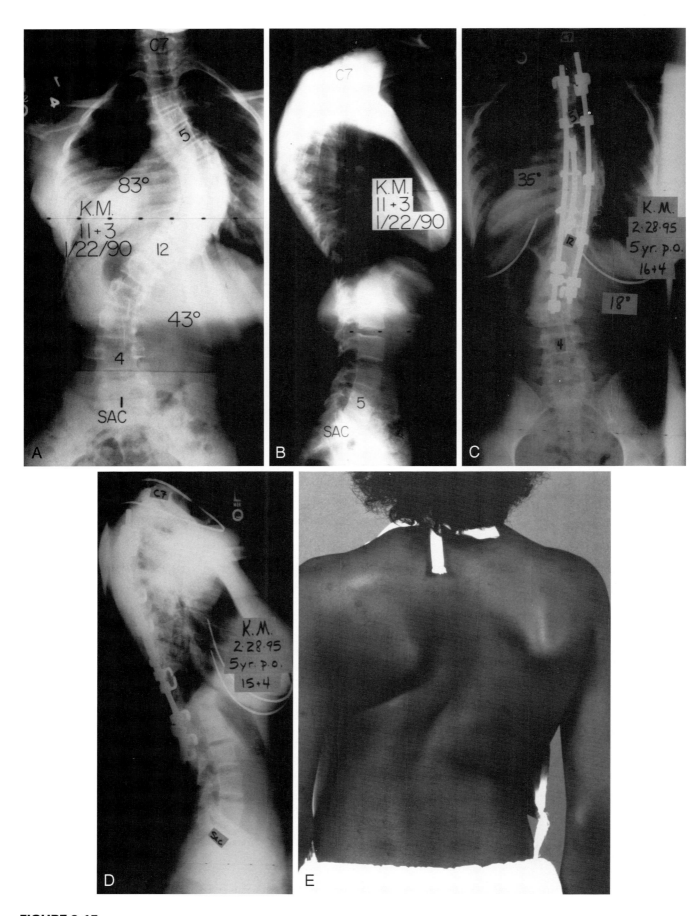

FIGURE 9.15.

A and **B.** Coronal and sagittal radiographs in the patient preoperatively. **C** and **D.** Coronal and sagittal radiographs in the patient postoperatively. Three rod technique and a thoracoplasty was performed.

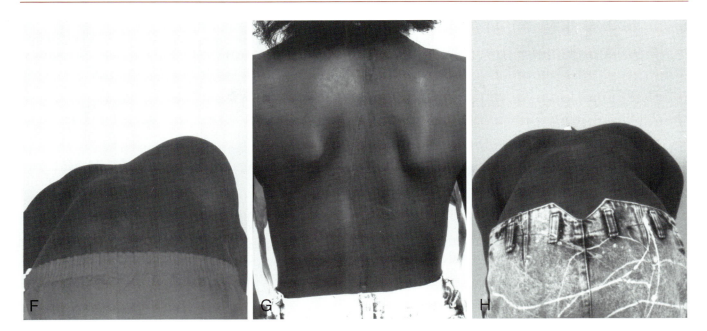

FIGURE 9.15—*continued*

E and F. The patient's coronal and axial clinical appearance preoperatively. G and H. The patient's coronal and axial appearance postoperatively. The improvement in the axial plane is a result of the thoracoplasty. The improvement in the coronal plane is caused by the instrumentation of the spine.

down, and we approximate them to the transverse processes so that such large segments of ribs do not have to be taken.

Usually, the supply of rib bone that we obtain is adequate for a fusion from T4 to L2. Sometimes it is not an adequate supply for a T4 to L4 fusion. Remember also that rib bone is almost all cortical. The osteogenic potential of rib bone may not be as good as iliac bone because there is not as much trabecular bone. However, in the pediatric idiopathic population, we have yet to see a pseudarthrosis in which rib bone was used exclusively. We do have at least one case of a pseudarthrosis in a young adult patient who was treated with rib bone only that was harvested by thoracoplasty.

As has been shown by Geissele et al., the cosmetic result and patient satisfaction from thoracoplasty is high (28). To date, no anterior or posterior instrumentation has been conclusively shown to significantly improve axial rotation in the thoracic spine. However, the axial deformity can be improved with the thoracoplasty procedure.

Postoperative Management

Immediate Postop

With most idiopathic adolescent patients who are treated with present-day posterior segmental spinal instrumentation systems (Cotrel-Dubousset, Texas Scottish Rite, Isola, Moss-Miami), it is possible to quickly mobilize the patient postoperatively without the need for a brace. Often, the patient is stood at the bedside for the first postoperative day. For an idiopathic adolescent, the time in the hospital usually is a total of 5 days. For the first 3 days, the patients usually are managed with a patient controlled analgesia system (PCA). Most commonly, a morphine PCA is used. Side effects from this include nausea, abdominal distention, and itching. If these side effects become marked, the patients are at times switched over to Toradol in an effort to reduce the amount of morphine that they need. However, we generally have been hesitant to use Toradol too extensively because of its effect on platelets. Usually, for the first 3 days after the surgery, the patient retains her Foley catheter and hemovac drains. We usually give the patient one dose of Ancef right before the surgery and then continue that until the hemovacs are removed. Usually, by the time the Foley catheter is removed, the patient is passing gas and is eating and drinking fairly well. Most patients retain fluid for 48 hours and then diurese spontaneously. This act represents a transient inappropriate ADH syndrome (6). The temptation to treat marginal urine output in a healthy idiopathic patient with fluid boluses should be resisted. Usually, blood replacement is not needed intraoperatively (especially if controlled hypotensive anesthesia [58, 70] is used), but it may be advisable within 48 hours of the surgery. Hence, preoperative autologous blood donation should always be encouraged (3).

Usually, on the third or fourth postoperative day, the intravenous narcotics are stopped and the patient is switched to oral narcotics. Upon discharge, the patient is usually sent home with an ample supply of Darvocet and a moderate supply of either Tylenol with codeine or Percodan. We find that teenagers are usually able to go back to school within 2 to 4 weeks after surgery.

Post-Hospitalization and Beyond

Patients frequently want to know how quickly they can return to their preoperative activities. This is all arbitrary, but we usually suggest that bicycling on level surfaces, stationary bicycling, and swimming are okay at approximately 3 to 4 months postoperative. At 7 months postoperative, we allow a "friendly game" of tennis. Usually, by 1 year postoperative, we allow patients to go back to water skiing or snow skiing. Finally, at 2 years postoperative, we generally allow the patients return to most everything that they were doing before the surgery. There are some exceptions to this guideline, however. We are more conservative with the long fusions (T4 to L4) than we are with the shorter fusions (T4 to L2). Usually with the longer fusions, we tend to discourage contact sports, high level gymnastics, or competitive diving sports, which all put increased loads on the segments below the fusion. We encourage general physical fitness and encourage aerobic activities.

We believe that it is mandatory to observe patients closely for at least 5 years postoperatively. We expect detection of pseudarthrosis to be later in this patient population now that more stable forms of segmental spinal instrumentation are being used. At 5 years follow-up, we then recommend that patients continue to see us every 5 years thereafter.

Complications

Wound

Recent reports suggest that the incidence of wound infection is higher with present-day systems. Dubousset, Shufflebarger, and Wenger (24) reported a 1% incidence of late infections. The Texas Scottish Rite institution recently reported a 10% incidence of deep wound infection (73). In our series of adolescent idiopathic scoliosis cases done since 1985, we have had only one case of a delayed deep wound infection in a primary idiopathic scoliosis surgery. However, concerns that present-day systems are too bulky and represent too much of a nidus for hematogenous seeding are reasonable.

Our cases of deep wound infections with reconstructive spinal surgery have been in the adult and revision population. If a deep wound infection does occur, the appropriate treatment is to debride the wound and close the tissues over tubes. We find that Jackson Pratt drains stay in longer than do standard hemovac drains. Therefore, with deep wound infections, we tend to use the Jackson Pratt drains and leave them in for 7 to 10 days. After this step, IV antibiotics for 4 to 6 weeks are advisable. Then, when the sedimentation rate is returned to normal, oral antibiotic suppression is advisable. It is important to leave the instrumentation in place for at least 1 year, if not 2 years, postoperatively until the surgeon is relatively sure that the spine fusion is solid. In most cases in which a deep wound infection does occur, it is possible to preserve the implants for 1 to 2 years. In most instances, it is eventually necessary to remove the implant to "cure" the patient of the infection. Removing the implant at an early stage is not advisable and is fraught with disastrous complications.

Pseudarthrosis

In our first 100 cases of Cotrel-Dubousset instrumentation, we did not have any pseudarthroses (48). Subsequent to that, we have had a few. One patient was associated with a deep wound infection. Another patient was associated with instrumentation pull-out proximally. Our incidence of pseudarthrosis with Zielke instrumentation alone anteriorly was high (19)—in excess of 15%. We do not have enough follow-up with the solid rod systems anteriorly to be able to comment on the incidence there. Our incidence of pseudarthrosis with combined anterior Zielke instrumentation and fusion with posterior segmental instrumentation over the same levels has been 0% (19).

With posterior segmental instrumentation, the areas of pseudarthrosis usually occur most commonly at the thoracolumbar junction, then at the very top or bottom of the construct. Pseudarthrosis at the very top of the construct may not result in much progression of deformity. However, a pseudarthrosis at the end of the construct or at the thoracolumbar junction is more likely to lead to progression of deformity and should be treated with repair, reinstrumentation, and re-bone grafting.

Decompensation

The main risk in decompensation comes in the Type II curves in which one is selectively fusing the thoracic curve and not including the lumbar curve (4, 13, 87). Whenever the surgeon selectively instruments the thoracic curve in this curve pattern, he/she should inform the parents that there is a risk that the lumbar curve will need to be added at a later date. That risk is higher if the patient is skeletally immature. That risk is also higher if the lumbar curve has a significant amount of rotation or a significant amount of apical vertebral deviation from the plumb line. When managing a Type II curve, one should either stop at the stable vertebra, stay completely out of the lumbar curve, or instrument and fuse the entire lumbar curve. It is a mistake to instrument to the apex of the structural lumbar curve.

If a thoracolumbar kyphosis exists in a Type II curve, this curve pattern is better treated as though it were a true double major curve pattern. If a thoracolumbar kyphosis exists and an instrumentation and fusion is stopped at L1, then very often a junctional kyphosis will ensue at L1/L2. Therefore, a junctional kyphosis seems to be an indicator and predictor of the structural nature of the lumbar portion of the deformity.

We therefore only selectively instrument a thoracic curve if the lumbar curve is under 60°, if there is no kyphosis between T12 and L4, and if the ratios of thoracic to lumbar Cobb measurements, apical vertebral rotation, and apical vertebral deviation all exceed 1.5 (46).

If a decompensation problem does occur, then treatment consists of extending the instrumentation and fusion into the lumbar curve to address both the coronal and sagittal imbalances. Whether this should be done all posteriorly or anteriorly and posteriorly with anterior instrumentation depends on the specific circumstances of the case involved (Fig. 9.16).

The incidence of sagittal decompensation has been reduced significantly with the use of present-day posterior segmental spinal instrumentation systems. It is important to always compress the convexity of a lumbar curve before applying any distraction to the concave side. Any rod rotation maneuver should be performed on the convex side of the lumbar curve. Failure to do so may cause a reduction in the patient's lumbar lordosis. Most lumbar curves are somewhat hypolordotic, and it is important to preserve or enhance lordosis.

Using Zielke or Dwyer instrumentation in the traditional sense almost always reduces segmental lordosis. In the future, this could be every bit as disabling as iatrogenic flatback caused by posterior Harrington instrumentation. Hence, any Zielke instrumentation anteriorly should be used in conjunction with either fresh frozen structural tricortical iliac allografts or cages to effectively increase anterior column height. Using a solid rod system and a rod rotation maneuver anteriorly without placement of structural graft anteriorly may be another option. Our preference is to always place something structural anteriorly. Either fresh frozen tricortical iliac grafts or cages work well. They provide a biomechanically stable construct that ensures that anterior column height is lengthened, not shortened.

Neurologic

The incidence of neurologic deficits after surgical treatment of idiopathic adolescent scoliosis is relatively low. However, the incidence is not zero. The standard of care throughout North America is to provide some form of spinal cord monitoring during surgeries. One option is a Stagnara wake-up test (31). With this wake-up test, the patient is lightened several minutes after the instrumentation has been applied. The patient is then asked to move his/her lower extremities. This works well if the anesthesiologist is experienced and if the patient is emotionally stable. However, many patients are not cooperative enough to perform such a test. At this point, the value of somatosensory evoked potentials and motor evoked potentials comes into play (17, 26, 27, 69).

To have an effective spinal cord monitoring team, it is necessary to monitor cases on a weekly, if not a daily, basis. In this way only can a service work effectively. It is necessary to have ongoing communication between the spinal cord monitoring technicians and the anesthesia team. Trying to monitor only a handful of cases per year will simply not work. It is necessary to monitor several cases every week to maintain the expertise of the technicians and to facilitate ongoing communication between them and the anesthesiologists so that anesthetic agents that interfere with the monitoring potentials are not being given.

For any kind of spinal deformity surgery, both Stagnara wake-up tests and somatosensory and motor evoked potentials should be employed and considered. We rehearse the Stagnara wake-up test with the patients preoperatively. If the electrical monitoring potentials are totally stable throughout the surgery (both the somatosensory and the motor potentials) then we will not perform a Stagnara wake-up test, but we always rehearse it with the patient preoperatively. In our years of using evoked potential monitoring, we have never had a false negative if both somatosensory and motor evoked potentials have been reproducible.

Over the last 10 years, we have had one case of iatrogenic neurologic deficit in a patient who was truly an idiopathic scoliotic. We have had others in the non-idiopathic population. This patient was a girl with a thoracic curve over 100°. The neurologic deficit was identified immediately with the spinal cord monitoring. It was confirmed with the Stagnara wake-up test. As a consequence, the incomplete neurologic deficit did resolve by a few weeks postoperatively because the instrumentation was removed immediately. Sublaminar wire techniques remain more popular for neuromuscular deformities than for idiopathic scoliosis because of the inherent neuro-

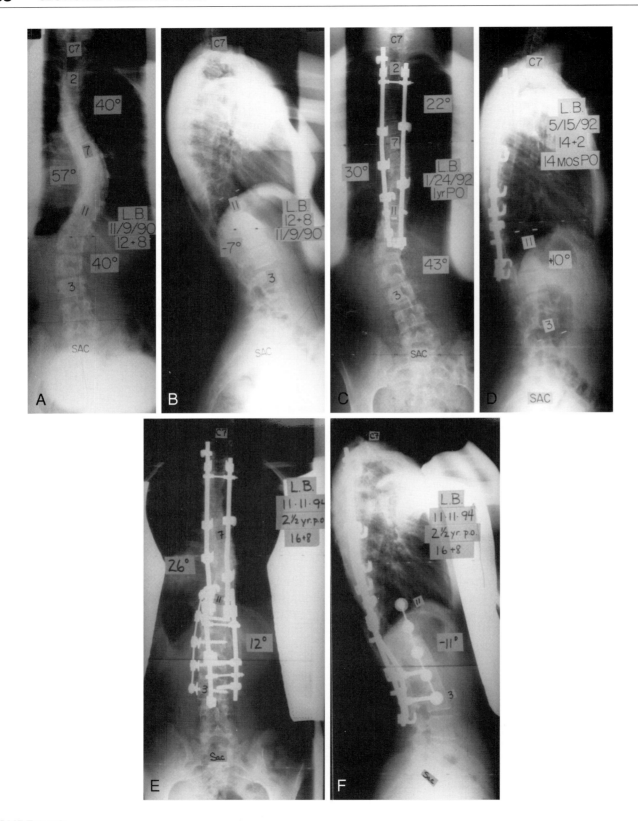

FIGURE 9.16.

A and **B.** Coronal and sagittal radiographs before treatment. **C** and **D.** Upright coronal and sagittal radiographs after initial treatment. The patient was decompensated to the left. This did not resolve 1 year after treatment. **E** and **F.** Revision was performed with anterior instrumentation and fusion and also concomitant extension of the posterior instrumentation. This all was done easily in one anesthesia. Fresh frozen tricortical iliac grafts were used anteriorly to enhance her lumbar lordosis.

logic risks (40, 88). However, sublaminar wire techniques do have a role for certain severe thoracic deformities.

Instrumentation Prominence

In thin patients, the instrumentation is often prominent and somewhat unsightly. The crosslinks or DTTs are usually the most prominent portion of the instrumentation. After that, the next most prominent portion of the instrumentation usually is the hooks in the proximal thoracic spine. It is unusual for hooks or pedicle screws in the lumbar spine to be prominent. As a consequence, most manufacturers are working on developing lower profile systems, and it was one of the driving forces to the development of the Moss-Miami system. This system is similar to the Cotrel-Dubousset system, but it has a lower profile and is easier to remove.

Summary

The first evolutionary step for surgical treatment of idiopathic scoliosis was the actual fusion technique (38, 61). Next came the concept of correction with instrumentation (35, 36, 37, 72). Subsequently, several evolutionary steps have been made to improve the capabilities of the implant. Present-day systems, such as CDI, TSR, Isola, and Moss-Miami, do allow for high patient satisfaction with their scoliosis surgery (50).

Although we now know more about the etiology of idiopathic scoliosis (5, 56), its natural history (85, 86), and nonoperative techniques (53, 89), a role for surgical treatment still exists. The effects of various surgical techniques are appreciated better in the coronal and sagittal planes than in the axial plane (84, 91). Further investigation on long-term results (≥ 20 years) is still sorely needed, especially for patients having long fusions (21, 30; 55). Before surgically treating a patient, it is very important to exclude any spinal cord anomalies (66) and to perform a "safe" surgery with low neurologic risk.

References

1. Asher M. An improved technique for the correction of adolescent idiopathic scoliosis: for thoracolumbar and lumbar deformities. Paper #61, presented at the Annual Meeting of the Scoliosis Research Society, Minneapolis, MN, 1991.
2. Ashman RB, Herring JA, Johnston CE. Texas Scottish Rite Hospital (TSRH) instrumentation system. In: Bridwell KH, DeWald RL, eds. The textbook of spinal surgery. Philadelphia: JB Lippincott, 1991;219–248.
3. Bailey TE Jr, Mahoney OM. The use of banked autologous blood in patients undergoing surgery for spinal deformity. J Bone Joint Surg Am 1987;69:329–332.
4. Banks GM, Transfeldt EE, Garvey TA, et al. Prognostic significance of decompensation occurring after Cotrel-Dubousset instrumentation. Paper #60, presented at the Annual Meeting of the Scoliosis Research Society, Minneapolis, MN, 1991.
5. Barrack RL, Whitecloud TS III, Burke SW, et al. Proprioception in idiopathic scoliosis. Spine 1984;9(7):681–685.
6. Bell GR, Gurd AR, Orlowski JP, et al. The syndrome of inappropriate antidiuretic-hormone secretion following spinal fusion. J Bone Joint Surg Am 1986;68:720–724.
7. Bernhardt M, Bridwell KH. Segmental analysis of the sagittal plane alignment of the normal thoracic and lumbar spines and thoracolumbar junction. Spine 1989;14(7):717–721.
8. Betz RR, Clements DH III, Harms J, et al. Flexible anterior instrumentation for thoracic idiopathic scoliosis. Poster Exhibit #S83, American Academy of Orthopaedic Surgeons, Orlando, Florida, 1995.
9. Bradford DS, Blatt JM, Rasp FL. Surgical management of severe thoracic lordosis. A new technique to restore normal kyphosis. Spine 1983;8:420–428.
10. Bradford DS, Lonstein JE, Moe JH, et al. Moe's textbook of scoliosis and other spinal deformities. 2nd ed. Philadelphia: WB Saunders, 1987.
11. Bridwell KH. Adolescent idiopathic scoliosis: surgical treatment. In: Weinstein SL, ed. The pediatric spine: principles and practice. New York: Raven Press, 1994, 511–555.
12. Bridwell KH. Idiopathic scoliosis. In: Bridwell KH, DeWald RL. ed. The textbook of spinal surgery. Philadelphia: JB Lippincott, 1991;97–162.
13. Bridwell KH. Surgical treatment of adolescent idiopathic scoliosis: the basics and the controversies. Spine 1994;19(9):1095–1100.
14. Bridwell KH, Betz RR, Capelli AM, et al. Sagittal plane analysis in idiopathic scoliosis patients treated with Cotrel-Dubousset instrumentation. Spine 1990;15(7):644–649 and 15(9):921–926.
15. Bridwell KH, Lenke LG. Prevention and treatment of decompensation. When can levels be saved and selective fusion be performed in idiopathic scoliosis? In: Farcy J-PC, ed. Complex spinal deformities; Spine: State of the Art Reviews, Vol. 8, No. 3. Philadelphia: Hanley and Belfus, 1994;643–657.
16. Bridwell KH, McAllister JW, Betz RR, et al. Coronal decompensation produced by Cotrel-Dubousset "derotation" maneuver for idiopathic right thoracic scoliosis. Spine 1991;16(7):769–777.
17. Brown RH, Nash CL, Berilla JA, et al. Cortical evoked potential monitoring: a system for intraoperative monitoring of spinal cord function. Spine 1984;9:256–261.
18. Chan DPK. Zielke instrumentation. Instr Course Lect 1983;32:208–209.
19. Chapman MP, Hamill CL, Bridwell KH, et al. Can we lordose the spine with Zielke instrumentation anteriorly? Paper presented at the annual meetings of North

American Spine Society, Washington, D.C., October 1995, and the American Academy of Orthopaedic Surgeons, Atlanta, GA, February 1996.
20. Chopin D, Morin C. Cotrel-Dubousset instrumentation (CDI) for adolescent and pediatric scoliosis. In: Bridwell KH, DeWald RL, ed. The textbook of spinal surgery. Philadelphia: JB Lippincott, 1991:183–217.
21. Cochran T, Irstam L, Nachemson A. Long-term anatomic and functional changes in patients with adolescent idiopathic scoliosis treated by Harrington rod fusion. Spine 1983;8:576–584.
22. Coonrad RW, Richardson WJ, Oakes WJ. Left thoracic curves can be different. Orthop Trans 1985;9:126–127.
23. Dubousset J, Herring JA, Shufflebarger H. Inevitable progression of scoliosis following posterior fusion alone in the immature spine. The crankshaft phenomenon. J Pediatr Orthop 1989;9:541.
24. Dubousset J, Shufflebarger HL, Wenger D. Late "infection" with CD instrumentation. Orthop Trans 1994; 18:121.
25. Dwyer AF, Schafer MF. Anterior approach to scoliosis: results of treatment in fifty-one cases. J Bone Joint Surg Am 1974;56:218–224.
26. Engler GL. Preoperative and intraoperative considerations in adolescent idiopathic scoliosis. Instr Course Lect 1989;38:137–141.
27. Engler GL, Spielholz NI, Bernhard WN, et al. Somatosensory evoked potentials during Harrington instrumentation for scoliosis. J Bone Joint Surg Am 1978; 60:528–532.
28. Geissele AE, Ogilvie JW, Cohen M, et al. Thoracoplasty for the treatment of rib prominence in thoracic scoliosis. Spine 1994;19(14):1636–1642.
29. Giehl JP, Zielke K. Zielke procedures in scoliosis correction. In: Bridwell KH, DeWald RL, eds. The textbook of spinal surgery. Philadelphia: JB Lippincott, 1991; 163–182.
30. Haher TR, Merola A, Zipnick RI, et al. Meta-analysis of surgical outcome in adolescent idiopathic scoliosis: a 35-year English literature review of 11,000 patients. Spine 1995;20(14):1575–1584.
31. Hall JE, Levine CR, Sudhir KG. Intraoperative awakening to monitor spinal cord function during Harrington instrumentation and fusion. Description of procedure and report of three cases. J Bone Joint Surg Am 1978;60:533–536.
32. Hall JE, Millis MB. Short segment anterior instrumentation for thoracolumbar scoliosis. In: Bridwell KH, DeWald RL, eds. The textbook of spinal surgery, 2nd ed. Philadelphia: Lippincott Raven Publishers, 1997: 665–674.
33. Hamill CL, Bridwell KH, Lenke LG, et al. Posterior arthrodesis in the skeletally immature patient. Assessing the risk for crankshaft. Is an open triradiate cartilage the answer? Spine (in press).
34. Hamill CL, Lenke LG, Bridwell KH, et al. The use of pedicle screw fixation to improve correction in the lumbar spine of patients with idiopathic scoliosis. Is it warranted? Spine 1996;21(10):1241–1249.
35. Harrington PR. Surgical instrumentation for management of scoliosis. J Bone Joint Surg Am 1960;42:1448.
36. Harrington PR. Treatment of scoliosis: correction and internal fixation by spine instrumentation. J Bone Joint Surg Am 1962;44:591–610.
37. Harrington PR, Dickson JH. An eleven-year clinical investigation of Harrington instrumentation. A preliminary report on 578 cases. Clin Orthop 1973;93:113–130.
38. Hibbs RA. A report of 59 cases of scoliosis treated by the fusion operation. J Bone Joint Surg 1924;6:3–37.
39. Horton WC, Holt RT, Johnson JR, et al. Zielke instrumentation in idiopathic scoliosis: late effects and minimizing complications. Spine 1988;13:1145–1149.
40. Johnston CE, Happel LT, Norris R, et al. Delayed paraplegia complicating sublaminar segmental spinal instrumentation. J Bone Joint Surg Am 1986;68:556–563.
41. King HA. Selection of fusion levels for posterior instrumentation and fusion in idiopathic scoliosis. Orthop Clin North Am 1988;19:247–255.
42. King HA, Moe JH, Bradford DS, et al. The selection of fusion levels in thoracic idiopathic scoliosis. J Bone Joint Surg Am 1983;65:1302–1313.
43. Klemme WR, Denis F, Koop SE, et al. Spinal instrumentation without fusion for progressive scoliosis in young children. Paper #38, presented at the annual meeting of the Scoliosis Research Society, Portland, OR, September 1994.
44. Lenke LG, Bridwell KH, Baldus C, et al. Analysis of pulmonary function and axis rotation in adolescent and young adult idiopathic scoliosis patients treated with Cotrel-Dubousset instrumentation. J Spinal Disord 1992;5(1):16–25.
45. Lenke LG, Bridwell KH, Baldus C, et al. Preventing decompensation in King type II and III curves treated with Cotrel-Dubousset instrumentation (CDI): 24–64 months' follow-up. Paper #59, presented at the annual meeting of the Scoliosis Research Society, Minneapolis, MN, 1991.
46. Lenke LG, Bridwell KH, Baldus C, et al. Preventing decompensation in King type II curves treated with Cotrel-Dubousset instrumentation. Strict guidelines for selective thoracic fusion. Spine 1992;17(8S):S274–281.
47. Lenke LG, Bridwell KH, Baldus C, et al. Ability of Cotrel-Dubousset instrumentation to preserve distal lumbar motion segments in adolescent idiopathic scoliosis. J Spinal Disord 1993;6(4):339–350.
48. Lenke LG, Bridwell KH, Baldus C, et al. Cotrel-Dubousset instrumentation for adolescent idiopathic scoliosis. J Bone Joint Surg Am 1992;74(7):1056–1067.
49. Lenke LG, Bridwell KH, Blanke K, et al. Analysis of pulmonary function and chest cage dimension changes after thoracoplasty in idiopathic scoliosis. Spine 1995; 20(12):1343–1350.
50. Lenke LG, Bridwell KH, Blanke K, et al. Radiographic and clinical assessment of Cotrel-Dubousset instrumentation in adolescent idiopathic scoliosis: 5 to 10-year follow-up. Paper presented at the Scoliosis Research Society annual meeting, Asheville, NC, September 1995.
51. Lenke LG, Bridwell KH, O'Brien MF, et al. Recognition and treatment of the proximal thoracic curve in adolescent idiopathic scoliosis treated with Cotrel-Dubousset instrumentation. Spine 1994;19(14):1589–1597.

52. Lonstein JE, Carlson JM. The prediction of curve progression in untreated idiopathic scoliosis during growth. J Bone Joint Surg Am 1984;66(7):1061–1071.
53. Lonstein JE, Winter RB. The Milwaukee brace for the treatment of adolescent idiopathic scoliosis: a review of one thousand and twenty patients. J Bone Joint Surg Am 1994;76(8):1207–1221.
54. Lowe TG, Peters JD. Anterior spinal fusion with Zielke instrumentation for idiopathic scoliosis: a frontal and sagittal curve analysis in 36 patients. Spine 1993;18(4):423–426.
55. Luk KDK, Lee FB, Leong JCY, et al. The effect on the lumbosacral spine of long spinal fusion for idiopathic scoliosis. A minimum of 10-year follow-up. Spine 1987;12:996–1000.
56. Machida M, Dubousset J, Imamura Y, et al. Pathogenesis of idiopathic scoliosis: SEPs in chickens with experimentally induced scoliosis and in patients with idiopathic scoliosis. J Pediatr Orthop 1994;14(3):329–335.
57. McCarthy RE, McCullough FL. Growing instrumentation for scoliosis. Paper #35, presented at the annual meeting of the Scoliosis Research Society, Dublin, Ireland, September 1993.
58. McNeill TW, DeWald RL, Kuo KN, et al. Controlled hypotensive anesthesia in scoliosis surgery. J Bone Joint Surg Am 1974;56:1167–1172.
59. McNulty PS, Ashman R. Biomechanical comparison of scoliosis correction with vertebral body screws and pedicle screws. Paper #262, presented at the annual meeting of the American Academy of Orthopaedic Surgeons, Orlando, FL, February 1995.
60. Millis MB, Hall JE, Emans JB. Short (3 segment) anterior instrumentation and fusion for progressive thoracolumbar scoliosis. Orthop Trans 1985;9:438–439.
61. Moe JH. A critical analysis of methods of fusion for scoliosis: an evaluation in two hundred and sixty-six patients. J Bone Joint Surg Am 1958;40:529–554.
62. Moe JH, Kharrat K, Winter RB, et al. Harrington instrumentation without fusion plus external orthotic support for the treatment of difficult curvature problems in young children. Clin Orthop 1984;185:35–45.
63. Moe JH, Purcell GA, Bradford DS. Zielke instrumentation (VDS) for the correction of spinal curvature. Analysis of results in 66 patients. Clin Orthop 1983;180:133–153.
64. Moskowitz A, Trommanhauser S. Surgical and clinical results of scoliosis surgery using Zielke instrumentation. Paper #46, presented at the Scoliosis Research Society annual meeting, Minneapolis, MN, 1991.
65. Noordeen MHH, Taylor BA, Edgar MA. Syringomyelia: a potential risk factor in scoliosis surgery. Spine 1994;19(12):1406–1409.
66. O'Brien MF, Lenke LG, Bridwell KH, et al. Preoperative spinal canal investigation in adolescent idiopathic scoliosis (AIS) curves ≥70°. Spine 1994;19(14):1606–1610.
67. Ogiela DM, Chan DPK. Ventral derotation spondylodesis. A review of 22 cases. Spine 1986;11:18–22.
68. Ogilvie JW. Anterior spine fusion with Zielke instrumentation for idiopathic scoliosis in adolescents. Orthop Clin North Am 1988;19:313–317.
69. Owen JH, Laschinger J, Bridwell KH, et al. Sensitivity and specificity of somatosensory of neurogenic motor evoked potentials in animals and humans. Spine 1988;13(10):1111–1118.
70. Patel NJ, Patel BS, Paskin S, et al. Induced moderate hypotensive anesthesia for spinal fusion and Harrington rod instrumentation. J Bone Joint Surg Am 1985;67:1384–1387.
71. Regan JJ, Shelokov AP. Correction of lumbar scoliosis in adults using the Texas Scottish Rite Hospital System anteriorly. Paper #74, presented at the Scoliosis Research Society annual meeting, Minneapolis, MN, 1991.
72. Renshaw TS. The role of Harrington instrumentation and posterior spine fusion in the management of adolescent idiopathic scoliosis. Orthop Clin North Am 1988;19:257–267.
73. Richards BS. Delayed infections following posterior spinal instrumentation for the treatment of idiopathic scoliosis. J Bone Joint Surg Am 1995;77(4):524–529.
74. Richards BS. Measurement error in radiographic assessment of vertebral rotation using the Pedriolle torsionometer. Orthop Trans 1990;14:560.
75. Richards BS, Birch JG, Herring JA, et al. Frontal plane and sagittal plane balance following Cotrel-Dubousset instrumentation for idiopathic scoliosis. Spine 1989;14:733–737.
76. Sanders JO, Herring JA, Browne RH. Posterior arthrodesis and instrumentation in the immature (Risser-grade-0) spine in idiopathic scoliosis. J Bone Joint Surg Am 1995;77(1):39–45.
77. Schafer MF. Dwyer instrumentation of the spine. Orthop Clin North Am 1978;9:115–122.
78. Shufflebarger HL, Ellis RD, Clark CE. Cotrel-Dubousset instrumentation (CDI) in adolescent idiopathic scoliosis: minimum 2-year follow-up. Orthop Trans 1989;13:79–80.
79. Shufflebarger HL, Smiley K, Roth HJ. Internal thoracoplasty: a new procedure. Spine 1994;19(7):840–842.
80. Steel HH. Rib resection and spine fusion in correction of convex deformity in scoliosis. J Bone Joint Surg 1983;65:920–925.
81. Stephens BS, Herring JA, Johnston CA, et al. Treatment of adolescent scoliosis using Texas Scottish Rite Hospital instrumentation. Spine 1994;19(14):1598–1605.
82. Thomson JD, Transfeldt EE, Bradford DS, et al. Decompensation after Cotrel-Dubousset instrumentation of idiopathic scoliosis. Spine 1990;15:927–931.
83. Wambolt A, Spencer DL. A segmental analysis of the distribution of lumbar lordosis in the normal spine. Orthop Trans 1987;11:92–93.
84. Weatherley CR, Draycott V, O'Brien JF, et al. The rib deformity in adolescent idiopathic scoliosis. A prospective study to evaluate changes after Harrington distraction and posterior fusion. J Bone Joint Surg Br 1987;69:179–182.
85. Weinstein SL. Idiopathic scoliosis: natural history. Spine 1986;11:780–783.
86. Weinstein SL, Ponseti IV. Curve progression in idiopathic scoliosis. J Bone Joint Surg Am 1983;65:447–455.
87. West JL, Boachie-Adjei O, Bradford DS, et al. Decom-

pensation following CD instrumentation: a worrisome complication. Orthop Trans 1989;13:78–79.
88. Wilber RG, Thompson GH, Shaffer JW, et al. Postoperative neurological deficits in segmental spinal instrumentation. A study using spinal cord monitoring. J Bone Joint Surg Am 1984;66:1178–1187.
89. Willers U, Normelli H, Aaro S, et al. Long-term results of Boston brace treatment on vertebral rotation in idiopathic scoliosis. Spine 1993;18(4):432–435.
90. Winter RB, Lovell WW, Moe JH. Excessive thoracic lordosis and loss of pulmonary function in patients with idiopathic scoliosis. J Bone Joint Surg Am 1975;57:972–977.
91. Wood KB, Transfeldt EE, Ogilvie JW, et al. Rotational changes of the vertebral-pelvic axis following Cotrel-Dubousset instrumentation. Spine 1991;16S:S404–408.

CHAPTER TEN

Congenital Spine Deformities

John E. Lonstein

Introduction

Spine deformities caused by anomalous vertebral development are defined as congenital. Although the anomaly is always present at birth, the deformity may not be. In general, children with congenital spine deformity tend to have a curvature noted much earlier in life than the typical patient with idiopathic scoliosis.

This early development of the deformity has resulted in a tendency for the young child with congenital scoliosis to receive less than optimum care. Congenital curves tend to be rigid and resistant to correction. The curves are frequently allowed to progress and, because of all the years of growth remaining, large deformities can result. These curves must not be allowed to progress. In many cases, early fusion is necessary, which is preferable to allowing severe curves to develop. Early fusion does not stunt the potential vertical growth because the area of the anomalies and the area that needs to be fused cannot grow in a normal vertical manner because of the defective growth potential.

Classification

Congenital deformities are classified in a number of ways, including: 1) the specific type of malformation, 2) the pattern of deformity (scoliosis, kyphosis, kyphoscoliosis, lordoscoliosis and lordosis), and 3) the area of the spine involved (cervical, cervicothoracic, thoracic, thoracolumbar, lumbar, and lumbosacral).

The vertebral anomaly is classified as abnormalities of segmentation, abnormalities of formation, or a mixture of problems that can occur at any part in the vertebral ring (anterior, anterolateral, lateral, posterolateral, or posterior). The vertebral anatomy is laid down in a mesenchymal anlage during the first 6 weeks of intrauterine development, and this is the time in which the vertebral anomalies occur. Once the mesenchymal anlage (either normal or abnormal) is established, the cartilaginous and bony stages are passive, being formed on the mesenchymal mold. Depending on where the growth potential in the vertebral ring is lost, the resulting deformity can be pure scoliosis, kyphosis or lordosis, or a combination of scoliosis plus kyphosis or lordosis.

Defects in the segmentation of the mesenchymal tissue are either a failure of segmentation or an error of segmentation. The failure can involve the whole vertebra (block vertebra) or be localized to a part of the vertebral ring (unsegmented bar). A lateral defect of segmentation causes scoliosis; a posterolateral defect causes lordoscoliosis; an anterior defect causes kyphosis; and a posterior defect causes lordosis (see Fig. 10.10). A block vertebra or an unsegmented bar causing scoliosis or lordoscoliosis are the most common failures of segmentation seen. An error of segmentation involves the failure of the two hemimetameres to pair and form a vertebra over a number of

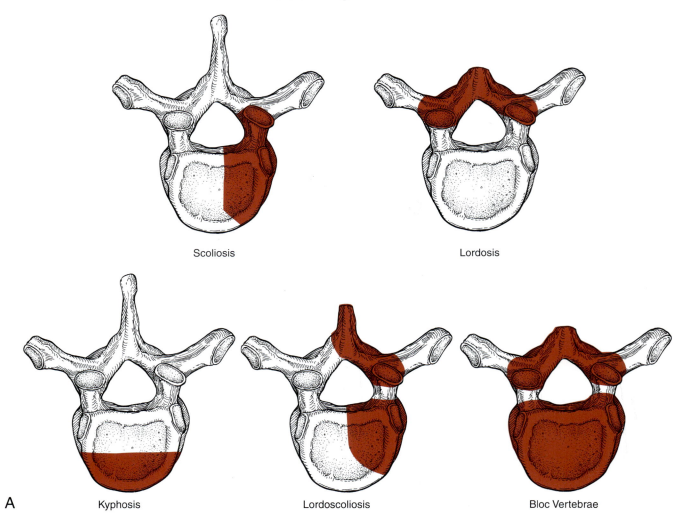
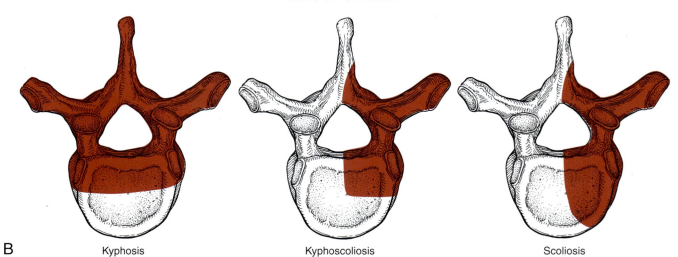

FIGURE 10.1.
Diagrams showing the vertebral ring, the site of the congenital abnormality, and the relation to the deformity that results. **A.** Failure of segmentation. The area of the vertebral ring that is unsegmented is shaded. **B.** Failure of formation. The portion of the vertebra that is formed is shaded.

segments; this error gives paired contralateral hemivertebrae—the so-called hemimetameric shift or hemimetameric segmental displacement.

Failure of formation occurs when a portion of the vertebral ring does not develop normally, giving a wedge vertebra or a hemivertebra. Remember that a hemivertebra is not an extra vertebra, but rather the remainder of an incompletely developed vertebra, and it is this absent bone and growth potential that gives the deformity. If the absent vertebral tissue is lateral, scoliosis results. If the vertebral body is completely or partially absent with normally developed posterior elements, kyphosis results. If the formation defect is lateral and anterior leaving only a posterolateral quadrant of vertebra, this produces true kyphoscoliosis caused by the posterior quadrant hemivertebra (Fig. 10.1).

Hemivertebrae are classified as segmented, semisegmented, and nonsegmented depending on their relationship to the adjacent vertebrae, as determined by the presence or absence of an intervening disc (and thus growth potential). A fully segmented hemivertebra has a disc on either side of the hemivertebra; a semisegmented hemivertebra has a disc on only one side, which is being fused on the opposite side to the adjacent vertebra; and a nonsegmented hemivertebra is fused to both of the adjacent vertebrae. In addition, in scoliosis, the hemivertebra is classified as incarcerated or nonincarcerated, depending on its relation to the spine. An incarcerated hemivertebra is "tucked into" the spine, its pedicle falling in line with the adjacent pedicles, whereas a nonincarcerated hemivertebra (generally fully segmented) protrudes from the spine with its pedicle lying out of the line of the adjacent pedicles. The latter scenario has the worse prognosis.

There can be one or more hemivertebrae, and the prognosis is poorer when they are on the same side of the spine than when they are on opposite sides. They can be adjacent to each other or separated. In addition, they can be combined with a segmentation defect on the opposite side—this is the most malignant anomaly.

The mixed group of anomalies consists of failures of formation and segmentation occurring in the same area of the spine. The anomaly and thus the anatomy can be clear cut with a clear cut prognosis, as in the case of a unilateral unsegmented bar with a hemivertebra on the opposite side. In general, the anomaly is not as clearly seen with a prognosis that is unknown, and thus the case has to be followed to see whether it is progressive.

The vertebral anomaly thus results in a spine deformity caused by the growth disturbance that occurs. The combination of the absent growth potential in the area of the anomaly and the growth in the remainder of the vertebral ring causes the deformity. The magnitude of the deformity, its behavior, and its rate of progression depend on the type of anomaly and the growth potential of the vertebrae in the area.

Genetics

The possible genetic origin of congenital spine deformities is intriguing. Wynne-Davies, in a study of 337 patients with congenital spinal anomalies, found that an isolated hemivertebra or similar localized defect were sporadic with no risk to subsequent siblings or offspring (46). Patients with multiple anomalies, however, carried a 5 to 10% risk to subsequent siblings. These findings could not be confirmed at our center in over 1200 congenital deformities, in which only about 1% of patients with congenital spinal deformities have a known relative with the problem (36). Most studies of identical twins show one with the congenital defect and the other without (11, 26). There are rare reports of both twins with congenital anomalies (1).

There is only one type of congenital spine anomaly that has a positive family history. This syndrome consists of multiple levels of bilateral failures of segmentation, with multiple fused ribs and often missing segments, and goes under many names: spondylothoracic dysplasia, spondylocostal dysplasia, spondylovertebral dysplasia, and Jarcho-Levin syndrome (5, 15, 29). Some of the children with this syndrome die early because of respiratory failure. Both recessive and dominant forms of inheritance have been reported.

Patient Evaluation

Patients with congenital spine anomalies frequently have congenital anomalies involving other organs or systems (3). It is thus extremely important that these patients receive a complete evaluation, not one restricted to the spine alone.

Genitourinary

The most common associated congenital anomaly is found in the genitourinary tract (3). Studies by MacEwen and colleagues of patients with congenital scoliosis revealed a 20% incidence of urinary tract anomalies on routine intravenous pyelography (21), whereas Hennsinger's study on cervical anomalies found a higher rate of 33% (12). This finding is not surprising from an embryologic point of view because the same undifferentiated mesenchyme will differentiate into the vertebra medially and the mesonephros ventrolaterally, the latter forming the kidney and the urinary tract. Many of the anomalies noted do not demand urologic treatment (e.g., unilateral kidney, cross-fused ectopia) because they are anatomic variations with normal renal function. However, 6% of the patients in the study by Mac-

Ewen and associates were noted to have a life-threatening urologic problem—usually an obstructive uropathy. Thus, all patients diagnosed as having a congenital spine anomaly must have a renal tract evaluation. Historically, this evaluation has been done using an intravenous pyelogram (IVP), but recently renal ultrasound or an MRI scan is used, the latter used primarily to evaluate the spinal canal in these patients. If an obstructive uropathy is detected during this screening, an IVP follows with appropriate urologic procedures performed before instituting orthopaedic treatment of the spinal deformity.

Cardiac

A second area of great concern is cardiac anomalies (3). As many as 10 to 15% of patients with congenital scoliosis have congenital heart defects (12, 28). These defects may have previously been undetected. Murmurs should never be attributed to the scoliosis and must be evaluated thoroughly. It is tempting to blame murmurs on distortion of the thorax caused by the scoliosis, but in actuality, scoliosis does not produce murmurs.

Neurologic

Neurologic problems can accompany the congenital spine deformity. Congenital kyphosis caused by failure of vertebral formation can in itself result in paraplegia. In fact, this is the most common noninfectious spinal deformity that can result in paraplegia caused by the deformity alone. In addition, there may be abnormal development of the neural elements with neurologic findings. A complete neurologic examination is thus an integral part of the assessment of anyone with a congenital spine deformity.

Spinal Dysraphism

The development of the spinal cord and vertebrae are closely associated, and therefore malformations often coexist. The spine deformity is recognized easily, but the intraspinal anomaly is difficult to recognize. These abnormalities of the spinal cord often restrict the normal mobility of the neural elements. With surgery and correction of the deformity, stretch can be placed on the tethered neural elements with resultant neurologic complications. Examination of the back and extremities for evidence of a hidden neurologic disorder is important.

The term spinal dysraphism is used to refer to these intraspinal anomalies. The prevalence of dysraphism in patients with congenital scoliosis was low in previous studies (10, 14, 23, 37), but with the use of routine MRI scans, it has shown an incidence of intraspinal lesions of 40% (4, 6,39). Diastematomyelia is the most common anomaly. This is a sagittal split in the spinal cord with a bony, fibrocartilaginous, or fibrous spur extending from the vertebral body through the split (Fig. 10.2). This spur restricts the motion of the spinal cord. Other anomalies can tether the spinal cord or cauda equina; these include a tight filum terminale, fibrous bands, and ectopic nerve roots. Other intraspinal anomalies are found alone or in combination with the previous ones; these include degrees of hindbrain herniation through the foramen magnum (Chiari malformations), fluid filled cavities within the spinal cord (syringomyelia), lipomas, epidermoid, or dermoid cysts and teratomas.

These neural canal abnormalities are associated frequently with cutaneous changes (hair patches, dimples, skin pigmentation, or hemangiomata), and various abnormalities on the examination of the lower extremities. These abnormalities include flatfeet, cavus feet, vertical tali, clubfeet, and more subtle changes, such as slight atrophy of one calf, a slightly smaller foot on one side, or asymmetrical reflexes. However, it is possible for a patient to have

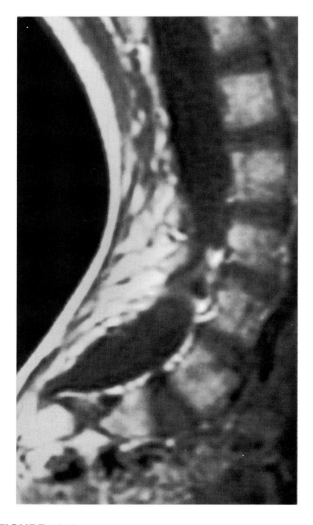

FIGURE 10.2.

An MRI scan in a severe congenital scoliosis showing the midline bony spur of the diastematomyelia. (Additional scans on the same patient are seen in Figure 10.11.)

one of these intraspinal anomalies and no associated findings. The physician must carefully evaluate the radiographs for any interpediculate widening or midline bony spicules. The use of MRI scans has greatly aided the evaluation of dysraphism. This imaging should be obtained in any patient having neurologic findings, foot deformities, bladder or bowel malfunction, cutaneous changes overlying the spine, or in patients in whom corrective spinal surgery is being planned. In larger spinal deformities, it is sometimes difficult on the MRI scan to adequately assess the whole spinal canal. In these cases, a myelogram is performed to adequately image the spinal canal.

Respiratory

Patients with congenital spine deformities must be evaluated for respiratory problems, which may present as a history of pneumonia or dyspnea. These problems can be caused by rib fusions with abnormal pulmonary mechanics and restrictive disease, severe thoracic or thoracolumbar deformities with torso distortion and a raised diaphragm, and reduced lung space, or severe thoracic lordosis with reduced lung space and abnormal rib mechanics. In some cases of congenital deformities, the pulmonary problem may be fatal (e.g., spondylocostal dysplasia or posterior failure of segmentation with resultant lordosis.)

Miscellaneous

Other congenital anomalies can occur and must be sought. Klippel-Feil syndrome refers today to any congenital fusion in the cervical spine, without the other originally described clinically features of a short neck, low hairline, and restricted range of motion. This occurs in 25% of cases (12, 42) and a strong correlation exists between Klippel-Feil syndrome, cervicothoracic congenital scoliosis, and Sprengel's deformity. Other anomalies include preauricular ear tags, mandibular hypoplasia, cleft lip, cleft palate, anal atresia, absent uterus or vagina, and Sprengel's deformity (congenital elevation of the scapula).

Radiographic Evaluation

An accurate radiologic evaluation is essential. Supine radiographs should be obtained on all children who are unable to sit or stand unaided. In addition, this view is obtained in older children to accurately visualize the vertebral anatomy, with the upright views showing the maximal deformity. The convex growth is important as mentioned previously, and thus the quality of the bone and disc spaces on the convexity must be clearly visualized and inspected. If the disc spaces are present and clearly defined and the convex pedicles are clearly formed, there is a possibility of convex growth, and the prognosis is poor. However, if the convex discs are not clearly formed, and the convex pedicles are poorly demarcated, there is less convex growth potential, and the prognosis is improved. It must be remembered that in the first year to two of life, cartilage forms a significant part of the vertebra, and thus prognostication is not as accurate as in the older child.

Routine coronal and sagittal views are initially obtained to appreciate the deformity in both planes, subsequent examinations depending on the deformity that exists. It is important to visualize the whole spine on both views because multiple anomalies are common, and they may be on opposite ends of the spine (e.g., one cervical and one lumbosacral). In addition, both views are necessary to appreciate where the anomaly is situated in the vertebral ring. A common example is an obvious unsegmented bar causing scoliosis. The lateral radiograph shows a localized area of slight lordosis in the area of the bar. This indicates that the failure of segmentation is not only lateral but extends posteriorly.

Coned down views or special projections are sometimes necessary to clearly define the vertebral anatomy. In the lumbosacral area, a Ferguson view demonstrates the area in an anteroposterior projection. A Ferguson view is a coronal radiograph with the patient supine and the x-ray beam directed parallel to the L5-S1 disc, usually with the tube tilted 35° cranially. When significant rotation is present at the apex of the scoliosis, it is impossible to delineate the vertebral anatomy clearly. A true anteroposterior projection of this apex is obtained with the derotated view of Stagnara (32).

Once the anomalies of the vertebrae and ribs have been identified, the curves are now measured. Accurate vertebral landmarks need to be selected on the end vertebrae of the curves measured, this varying from upper or lower end plate of the vertebra to the upper or lower margins of the pedicle. Exactly the same landmarks on the same vertebrae are used for subsequent measurements, ensuring the reliability of this evaluation. In addition, the vertebral anatomy is scrutinized; the size of the disc spaces and the clarity of the pedicle need evaluation because both give an indication of the possible growth potential of the concavity versus the convexity of the curve.

The radiologic evaluation thus clearly delineates the vertebral anomaly, its location in the vertebral ring, the quality of the convex growth potential, and the type and magnitude of the spinal deformity produced. This, combined with a knowledge of the natural history, determines the treatment plan.

Scoliosis

Natural History

The natural history of congenital scoliosis is well described in the literature. The earliest article is that of

Kuhns and Hormell in 1952 who reviewed 85 children and found that only 13 (15%) did not progress, with 32 (38%) progressing significantly. The most progressive cases were those with thoracic curves and multiple unbalanced anomalies (17). Later studies (20, 27, 41, 34, 25, 33, 24) give similar figures, 10% being nonprogressive, 15% being slightly progressive, and 75% progressing significantly. The best review is that of McMaster and Ohtsuka who reviewed 202 patients that were observed past the age of 10 years without treatment. They found that the final severity depended on a number of factors: 1) the type of vertebral anomaly; 2) the site of the anomaly; and 3) the age of the patient at diagnosis (24) (Table 10.1).

1) The type of vertebral anomaly. As noted previously, the growth discrepancy produced by the anomaly and the health of the opposite growth plates are important. An unsegmented bar (failure of segmentation) has no growth, and with healthy growth, plates opposite produce a predictably progressive curve, progressing at 5° per year. Additional growth on the convexity with the addition of a hemivertebra adds to the growth discrepancy, giving the most progressive anomaly. Thus, the worst anomaly is an unsegmented bar with a convex hemivertebra, followed by a unilateral unsegmented bar, double convex hemivertebrae, a single fully segmented hemivertebra, a wedge vertebra, with the least progressive being a bloc vertebra (24). Congenital scoliosis produced by mixed anomalies is difficult to predict and the patient needs to be observed for progression.

Congenital scoliosis caused by failure of formation is difficult to predict; some are nonprogressive and others progress at a rate of up to 5° per year. The prognosis depends on the presence of healthy growth centers adjacent to the hemivertebra, i.e., whether it is fully segmented, semisegmented, or unsegmented. Often, this is not clearly evident, and the child must be observed for progression. Contralateral hemivertebrae (hemimetameric segmental displacement or hemimetameric shift) when balanced often may not progress and thus do not require treatment. When separated by several segments, a double curve is produced, and both curves may progress and require fusion.

2) The site of the anomaly. For any anomaly, the rate of deterioration is worse in the thoracic and thoracolumbar regions, and is less severe in the upper thoracic or lumbar regions. However, small curves in the cervicothoracic or lumbosacral areas result in more significant clinical deformity (head tilt, shoulder elevation, decompensation) because there is less ability of the adjacent spine to compensate for the anomaly.

3) The age of the patient at diagnosis. In general, the earlier the age at diagnosis, the worse the prognosis, because this indicates marked growth imbalance. This excludes the cases detected on a neonatal radiograph taken for another reason. It must be remembered that the times of rapid growth in the child are the first two years and the adolescent growth spurt. During these times, curves progress more rapidly, with severe curves progressing even after skeletal maturity.

Although it is possible to associate a certain prognosis with a certain anomaly, this is not always feasible. It is best to consider the curve in its general character and to see what problem it produces and whether it is progressive, regardless of the specific type of anomaly. Thus, careful documentation of the deformity and the magnitude of the curve by high-quality radiographs and photographs is necessary on the first examination. Subsequent serial photography

TABLE 10.1.
Median Yearly Rate of Deterioration (in degrees) Without Treatment For Each Type of Single Congenital Scoliosis in Each Region of the Spine (187 Patients)

Site of curvature	Type of congenital anomaly					
	Block vertebra	Wedge vertebra	Hemivertebra		Unilateral unsegmented bar	Unilateral unsegmented bar and contralateral hemivertebrae
			Single	Double		
Upper thoracic	<1°–1°	★–2°	1°–2°	2°–2.5°	2°–4°	5°–6°
Lower thoracic	<1°–1°	2°–2°	2°–2.5°	2°–3°	5°–6.5°	6°–7°
Thoracolumbar	<1°–1°	1.5°–2°	2°–3.5°	5°–★	6°–9°	>10°–★
Lumbar	<1°–★	<1°–★	<1°–1°	★	>5°–★	★
Lumbosacral	★	★	<1°–1.5°	★	★	★

☐ No treatment requested ■ May require spinal surgery ☐ Require spinal fusion ★ Too few or no curves
Ranges represent the degree of deterioration before and after 10 years of age.
Modified from McMaster MJ, Ohtsuka K. The natural history of congenital scoliosis. J Bone Joint Surg Am 1982;64:1144. (Reproduced with permission.)

and radiology are important. Children should be observed at 6-month intervals and must be observed until the end of their growth. Many patients have mild curves that are stable for many years and then suddenly become severe when the adolescent growth spurt begins. Some curves never progress at all and, after being observed for many years, do not result in any significant deformity. These patients, of course, do not require any treatment, and it is foolish to apply an orthosis or perform a fusion for a condition that is not progressive and not disabling.

Nonoperative Treatment

Observation

The objective in the treatment of congenital scoliosis is to obtain a spine as straight as possible in balance over the sacrum at the end of growth. Because generally the anomaly has absent or diminished growth on the concavity of the curve and it is not possible to create growth on this side, the treatment for progressive curves is surgical. Early diagnosis with prompt identification of progression and early surgical intervention is the treatment of choice. The aim of surgery is to balance the growth by eliminating the deforming growth potential on the convexity of the curve. This elimination results in a shorter, straighter spine, which is preferable to a slightly longer but markedly crooked spine.

In the majority of cases, the prognosis is not well defined and these children need to be observed for progression. Supine radiographs are obtained until the child can easily stand unaided; all films should show the whole spine. To fully appreciate the anomaly and deformity in three dimensions, routine coronal and sagittal views are always obtained on the first visit with repeal lateral views in the presence of abnormal sagittal contours (kyphosis or lordosis). Once the anomaly has been identified and the growth plates assessed, the child is observed for progression. Radiographs are repeated every 4 months during the early growth spurt in the first 2 years of life. After this stage, films every 6 to 12 months are appropriate once no progression is seen. Careful measurement of the same landmarks on the same vertebrae is essential for accuracy and consistency. In addition, the current radiograph must always be compared to the earliest radiograph available, and also the film of the previous visit. Because the curve may progress slowly and unpredictably, it is easy to not detect progression, attributing small differences to measurement error rather than detecting the real change from the original radiograph.

Orthotic Treatment

Because the primary deformity in congenital scoliosis occurs in the bones rather than in the soft tissues, the curves tend to be rigid and thus not as amenable to orthotic treatment as idiopathic or paralytic curves. Nevertheless, there are definite, but few, indications for orthotic treatment of congenital spine deformities. The orthosis of choice is the Milwaukee brace. Underarm braces, although they provide effective curve control, do so at the expense of thoracic compression and a reduction of vital capacity—undesirable side effects.

A study by Winter and colleagues indicated that certain patients did well in the Milwaukee brace for many years, and a few could even be treated permanently in an orthosis, avoiding surgery (44). The best results were found in patients who had mixed anomalies that were flexible, and who had a progressive secondary curve. The patients who did well had flexible curves with the anomalous vertebrae making up only a part of the curve. The vertebral anomalies were in the cranial, center, or caudal portion of the curve, with the curve much longer than the anomalous area and the other vertebrae being normal. The brace is thus effective with a flexible deformity, and has no role in a rigid deformity. Progressive secondary curves need to be controlled, and the Milwaukee brace is the best method to achieve this.

The other role for orthotic treatment in congenital scoliosis is for the treatment of coronal imbalance, which may be coronal decompensation or head tilt. With coronal decompensation with single or multiple anomalies, the Milwaukee brace can be effective in correcting the malalignment, allowing the spine to become balanced with growth. With head tilt in the young child with cervicothoracic or upper thoracic anomalies, the Milwaukee brace with a posterior auricular occipital pad can correct the head tilt.

The physician must recognize the role of the orthosis when it is used, and must monitor its use to ensure that it accomplishes its goal. The orthosis must control the curve with acceptable spine alignment. Careful monitoring, both clinically and radiographically, is necessary. The area of the anomaly and the overall curve in some cases need to be measured separately. If the patient's curve progresses despite the orthosis, fusion must be performed without further delay. The orthosis should only be continued if it successfully controls the curve.

The most common error in the treatment of congenital scoliosis with a Milwaukee brace is the attempt to treat a curve that requires surgery. The second most common mistake is the failure to recognize that the orthosis is not doing an adequate job of controlling the curve, thus allowing curve progression to occur. The current radiograph must always be compared to the radiograph of the last visit as well as with the earliest radiograph available. Because curve progression is slow, if the current radiograph is only compared to the radiograph of the last visit, any slight difference can be ascribed to measurement error, and progression will be missed.

Surgical Principles

Surgery is the most common treatment of severe or progressive congenital spine deformities. It is impossible to insert growth potential where it is absent. It is only possible by surgery to stop the abnormal growth potential, thus balancing the growth in the area of the anomaly. This balance is achieved with a fusion, combined in some cases with removal the deforming growth potential on the convexity of the curve. In some young patients with smaller curves, the remaining concave growth is sufficient to achieve curve correction—an epiphysiodesis effect. In addition, in larger curves with a decompensated spine, the deformity must be corrected and the correction maintained with a spinal fusion to achieve the ultimate goal: a stable balanced spine.

Several types of operative procedures are available in the treatment of congenital deformities. Two fundamental questions emerge: What is the best procedure? and What is the best age for surgery? These questions are addressed under each subsequent deformity.

Surgical Treatment of Congenital Scoliosis

In congenital scoliosis, there is no simple answer to these two questions. The operative treatment chosen must be tailored to that specific patient. The treatment plan depends on the age of the patient; the type of deformity (scoliosis, kyphosis, lordosis, or a combination); the severity of the deformity; the area of the deformity; the rigidity of the deformity; the curve pattern; the natural history of the deformity; and the presence of other congenital anomalies. The ideal plan chooses the right procedure for the child instituted at the right age.

The indications for surgery are, first, an anomaly on presentation that has a guaranteed poor prognosis—a unilateral unsegmented bar with healthy convex growth, especially in the presence of a convex hemivertebra. In addition, double convex unsegmented hemivertebrae show severe progression. These anomalies should usually be treated fairly promptly without waiting for progression. The exception is the child under 9 to 12 months. In this case, surgery is planned for 12 to 18 months of age because surgery is easier at this age; the vertebrae are larger and less cartilaginous.

In the majority of cases, the anomaly is mixed in type, a combination of failure of segmentation and formation. A decision for surgery is made once progression occurs. This rule applies especially to the very young in whom the anomaly may be unclear because the vertebra is mainly cartilage. In these cases, the crispness of the pedicle outlines gives an indication of the vertebral anatomy and growth potential. Any progressive curves should be treated surgically, especially if they do not respond to orthotic treatment. If a 25-degree curve in a 3-year-old child progresses to 35° by age 6 years, the curve requires surgical treatment. The tendency is to avoid surgery at this age for fear of "stunting the child's growth". In reality, the child will grow taller if the curve is fused, rather than allowing the deformity to progress because the area of the anomaly is devoid of normal vertical growth potential.

There are four basic procedures for the surgical treatment of congenital scoliosis: posterior fusion, anterior and posterior fusion, convex growth arrest (anterior epiphysiodesis and posterior hemiarthrodesis), and hemivertebra or wedge excision. The fusion (posterior or combined) can be in-situ or with correction by traction, casting, bracing, or instrumentation. The aim of surgery in these cases must be kept in mind—to prevent further progression of the curve and to achieve a spine and torso balanced on a level pelvis with a non-tilted head and level shoulders. With small curves, correction is usually unnecessary to achieve these aims, and thus any correction depends on the flexibility of the curve. With larger curves and an unbalanced torso, correction is essential to achieve the surgical aims. Because fusion in congenital scoliosis is performed at a much earlier age than in other types of scoliosis, instrumentation becomes an adjunct to the procedure rather than an integral part of the fusion, playing a role in maintaining any correction rather than obtaining the correction. In addition, in cases of fusion of the young having congenital scoliosis, the patient must be observed closely until the end of growth because further surgery may be necessary to keep the spine balanced.

Posterior Fusion

The aim of posterior fusion is not curve correction, but rather curve stabilization with the prevention of further curve increase (43). Generally, congenital curves tend to be rigid and thus there is little chance of significant correction unless extensive anterior and posterior releases are performed. The fusion must cover the entire measured curve and extend to the "central gravity line." Abundant autologous iliac bone graft should be added because a wide, thick fusion mass is necessary to avoid possible bending of the fusion by the intact anterior growth plates. Where autologous and local bone is of insufficient quantity, cancellous allograft is added. Correction and immobilization are best obtained with a carefully molded Risser cast or with a well fitting Milwaukee brace.

In the past, bracing of the young child with a fusion was continued for many years to protect this fusion. There is no scientific evidence for this approach. It is a fact that the fusion is solid in the young after 4 to 6 months. Although solid, however, the fusion is immature and weak because it is biologically plastic. The best results come with protection of the fusion in a Milwaukee brace for 12 to 18 months. Thus, if the postoperative immobilization is a cast, it is removed after 4 to 6 months and a Milwaukee brace is fitted, or the postoperative bracing is continued. The immobilization is continued until the child outgrows the brace—usually after 12 to 18 months. At this point the fusion is mature enough to resist bending forces.

This procedure historically was the most common method of treatment of congenital scoliosis. The reported results are good (40, 43) with curve stabilization; the failures are caused by curve increase, which in turn is caused by bending of the fusion mass (the "crankshaft effect") in 14% of cases or by curve lengthening. Curve bending (crankshaft) is a result of continued anterior growth in the presence of a solid posterior fusion with the anterior growth resulting in rotation of the vertebral bodies around the solid posterior fusion. Curve increase is treated by a subsequent anterior fusion with ablation of the anterior growth potential, or prevented with the use of the combined anterior and posterior approach initially. Lengthening of the curve is treated by an extension of the fusion.

Today, a posterior fusion alone is reserved for an older child with a moderate deformity that is still relatively flexible or is well balanced on presentation. The child must be old enough, usually over 10 years, so that the crankshaft effect is not a possibility (Fig 10.3). In these cases, correction is obtained and maintained with instrumentation, with external immobilization in a cast or brace being added when the fixation of the instrumentation is less than optimal. A posterior fusion alone is also used in cases of progressive mixed anomalies in which the anterior growth potential on the convexity of the curve is poor. A thick wide posterior fusion stabilizes the curve and prevents subsequent anterior growth and bending of the fusion. In some of these cases a reinforcement of the fusion is performed at 6 months to increase the size of the fusion mass. If the convex anterior growth potential is good, especially in a younger child, it is better to stabilize the curve with the combined anterior and posterior approach.

The other role of a posterior fusion alone is in the case of cervicothoracic anomalies, which are usually mixed in type and result in shoulder elevation on the convexity of the curve, and head tilt. These anomalies tend to present in the young, or during the adolescent growth spurt. In the young, there is head tilt and facial asymmetry. The deformity is still flexible and the head tilt can be corrected as seen clinically by the use of gentle head traction in the supine child.

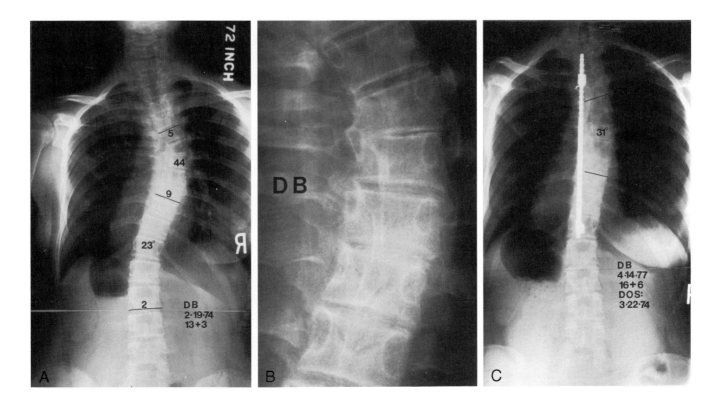

FIGURE 10.3.

A. D.B. presented at the age of 13 years and 3 months with a right thoracic curve of 44°. **B.** Coned down view of the apex of the curve shows the unilateral unsegmented bar at one level. The patient underwent a posterior fusion and instrumentation using a Harrington distraction rod. **C.** Three years later the fusion is solid and the postoperative correction is maintained.

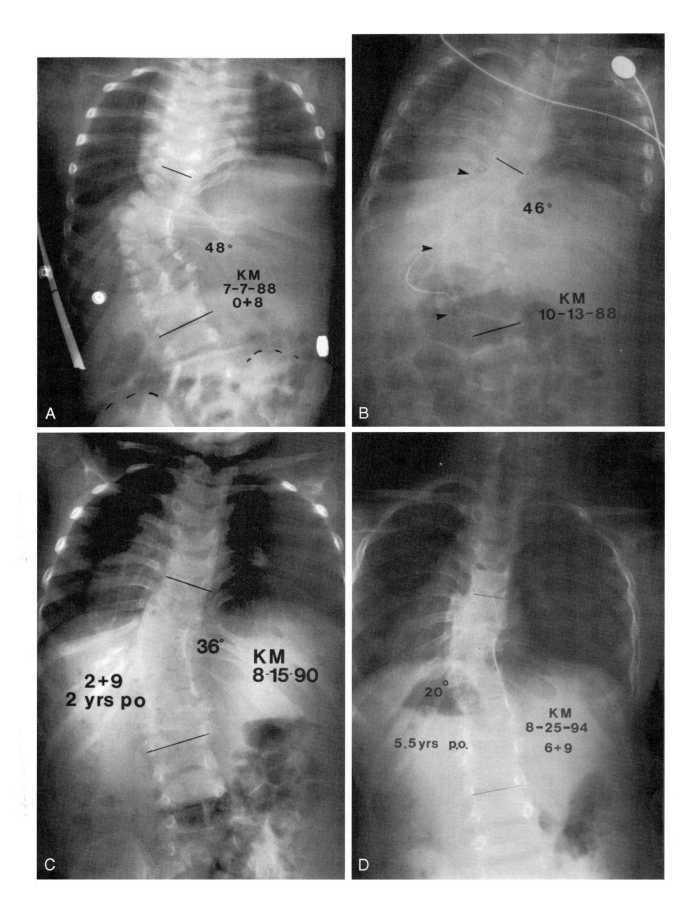

In these cases posterior fusion of cervicothoracic curve is followed by immobilization in a Milwaukee brace with a head support behind the ear to correct the head tilt. The brace is worn until the head tilt corrects and the correction is stable—usually a number of years. In these children, it is advantageous to fit the brace preoperatively and to allow the child and family to adapt to the brace before surgery, usually a period of 2 to 4 weeks. This makes the surgical procedure easier because the child is immediately placed in the brace to which he/she has already adapted. In the older child, the head tilt may be rigid. In these cases the fusion is performed, with a halo being applied under the same anesthetic. Postoperatively, the halo is placed in traction with a lateral force to correct the head tilt. Once the head tilt is corrected, the head position is maintained with the incorporation of the halo in a halo cast, which is used for 4 to 6 months until the fusion is solid.

The use of traction to gain correction is reserved for curves in which it is desired to slowly correct the curve with the patient awake, allowing careful and constant neurologic monitoring, rather than to get more rapid correction with instrumentation. It is used after preliminary removal of a tethering structure like a tight filum terminale or a diastematomyelia, or after osteotomy of an unsegmented bar. The traction is either halo-gravity or with the use of a femoral pin with pelvic obliquity, with the pin used on the side of the high pelvis. Once the correction has been obtained, it is held with a cast and the patient is kept nonambulatory for the first 3 to 4 months postoperatively, or the correction is maintained with instrumentation if the child is old enough and the vertebrae are of sufficient size. The use of traction with a posterior fusion alone used to be the most common method for achieving correction in congenital scoliosis, but in the past 10 years the combined anterior and posterior approach has been more commonly used (43).

Instrumentation is an adjunct to the posterior fusion, used to obtain or maintain correction. Correction with instrumentation is appropriate for curves in which it is safe to obtain correction in one procedure with the patient under anesthesia. There must be no evidence of spinal dysraphism, and the curve must be small enough and the child old enough that an additional anterior approach is not necessary to improve the correction or to ablate the anterior growth plates with the disc excision. Because there are many types of instrumentation available today, the surgeon should choose the system that best fits the child, the deformity, the safety factors, and the surgeon's experience.

A preoperative MRI scan is necessary when any correction is planned or the use of instrumentation is anticipated. This rules out any tethering problems and any localized spinal stenosis (39). In addition, spinal cord monitoring with the wake-up test is mandatory with the use of instrumentation in congenital spine deformities. Electronic monitoring can be used, but it augments rather than replaces the wake-up test.

Combined Anterior and Posterior Fusion

This has become an increasingly performed procedure for congenital scoliosis. It is used for thoracic, thoracolumbar, or lumbar curves with a poor prognosis, i.e., good convex growth potential. The multiple discectomies and fusion give an anterior growth arrest which reduces or eliminates any bending of the fusion ("crankshaft effect"). In addition, correction is improved because the multiple disc excisions are actually multiple convex wedge excisions. Because of the combined anterior and posterior fusion, the pseudarthrosis rate is lower. This approach obviously adds the risks of an anterior procedure, even though these risks are small.

In recent times, the two procedures usually are performed sequentially under the same anesthetic. The anterior fusion is performed first with a thoracotomy or thoraco-abdominal approach, and the approach is from the side of the convexity of the curve. The discs are excised, including the cartilage end plates, and care is taken during the excision to preserve the bony end plate because this reduces the blood loss. The disc spaces are then fused by decortication of the bony end plates (usually with a curette) and packing of the spaces with rib bone cut into small chips. If this graft is of insufficient quantity, it is augmented with cancellous allograft, with the cubes of bone being crushed into smaller pieces for the disc spaces. After closure of the anterior exposure the child is repositioned, and the posterior fusion of the whole measured curve is now performed (Fig. 10.4).

As with a posterior fusion alone, the correction

FIGURE 10.4.

This girl was first seen at the age of 8 days with a congenital scoliosis of 63°. She was placed in a Kallabis splint. **A.** At 8 months of age, a supine radiograph shows the bony anomalies consisting of concave rib synostoses associated with a concave unilateral unsegmented bar, and multiple convex hemivertebrae. There is interpediculate widening in the lumbar spine and the midline bony spur of the diastematomyelia is well seen. **B.** At the age of 11 months she underwent neurosurgical excision of the diastematomyelia, followed 2 weeks later by an anterior and posterior fusion at the apex of the curve and a cranial and caudal convex anterior and posterior hemiepiphysiodesis from T7 to L3. A Milwaukee brace was used postoperatively to achieve correction and immobilization. C. Two years later the fusion was solid with correction to 38°. **D.** Five years postoperatively, due to the convex fusion at the ends of the curve, there was curve improvement to 20°. (See previous page) can be obtained externally with traction, a cast or brace, or internally with instrumentation. The choice depends on the nature, magnitude, and flexibility of the deformity, the alignment of the spine (decompensation, head tilt), and the size and age of the child. In more severe deformities, a combination of these methods is applicable, e.g., multiple discectomies to increase flexibility, halo gravity traction to safely obtain correction with the patient awake and to achieve a balanced spine, and a cast to maintain this correction. The young child is kept nonambulatory for 3 to 4 months to eliminate the greatest deforming force on the spine: gravity. At this time, the cast and halo are removed, a Milwaukee brace is fitted, and the child is ambulatory, with brace wearing continuing for 12 to 18 months as mentioned earlier.

Convex Growth Arrest (Anterior Epiphysiodesis and Posterior Hemiarthrodesis)

Convex growth arrest is not new, first being described by MacLennan in 1922 (22), and subsequently by Roaf and others (2, 30, 35, 38). It is achieved by anterior and posterior convex fusion (anterior hemiepiphysiodesis and posterior hemiarthrodesis), and was designed to arrest excessive convex growth and allow the concave growth to occur and hopefully correct the deformity. It is thus indicated in cases with a progressive scoliosis, or moderate scoliosis on presentation with single or adjacent convex hemivertebrae and a chance for concave growth with normal or near normal concave growth plates. To be successful, the surgery must be performed when there are a sufficient number of years of growth remaining (i.e., under age 5) and is contraindicated if there is any kyphosis in the area of the anomaly. Another indication for convex growth arrest is in cases with a marked potential for bending of the fusion (i.e., a young patient with healthy convex growth). In these cases, removal of the convex growth forces is essential to achieve the best result.

The anterior and posterior procedures are performed under the same anesthetic. It is essential to address the whole measured curve, sometimes adding a normal level to the convex fusion to increase the possibility of curve improvement by concave growth. Anteriorly, the convex half of the disc is excised with hemiepiphysiodesis and is done with interbody fusions using small chips of rib bone with or

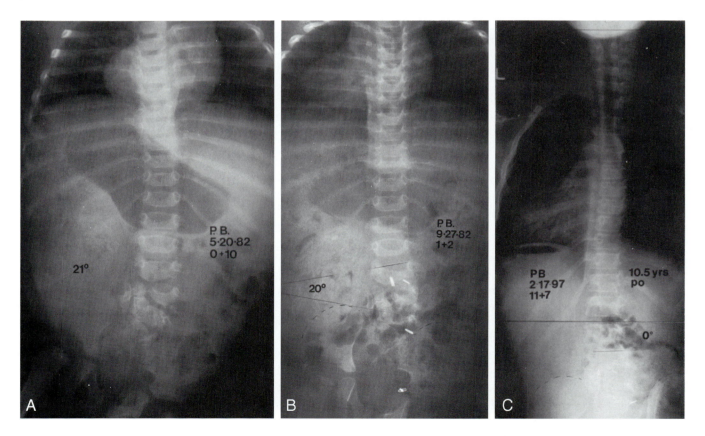

FIGURE 10.5.
A. This 10-month-old girl had a L4 hemivertebra with a 21-degree curve and marked pelvic obliquity. She underwent an anterior and posterior convex growth arrest with postoperative immobilization in a body cast with bilateral leg extensions. **B.** Four months later the convex fusion is solid with correction of the curve and pelvic obliquity. **C.** Ten years later the curve is 0° with correction of the pelvic obliquity. Note that no overcorrection has occurred.

without the addition of an inlay rib strut graft. The posterior hemiarthrodesis is done opposite the area of the anterior surgery, care being taken to only expose the area of the proposed fusion because any additional exposure in a child cranially or caudally, or exposure of the concave side, may in itself result in arthrodesis (Fig. 10.5).

The child is placed in a postoperative body cast (with leg extensions added with lumbar curves) because correction can usually be obtained in the segments adjacent to the hemivertebra. The cast is trimmed appropriately so that the chest tube (inserted more anteriorly than normal) can be removed from under the cast. The child is kept nonambulatory for 3 to 4 months, the cast is removed, and the child is placed in a well fitting Milwaukee brace which is worn full-time for 12 to 18 months. This use of an orthosis after fusion in a young child is necessary because at 4 month postoperatively the fusion mass is continuous but immature, and continued support is necessary to achieve a strong mature solid fusion. This protection is actually necessary in all cases of fusion in the young child.

Convex growth arrest surgery can give two possible results. Gradual improvement of the curve over a number of years can result because of the concave growth. The surgery can give a fusion effect, which occurs where the concave growth potential is misjudged; poor concave growth actually is present with no possibility of concave growth with curve improvement. The addition of an obviously healthy disc to the fusion area cranially and caudally increases the chance of a true epiphysiodesis effect. In some cases, the curve may increase, either immediately or years later. This is caused by residual convex growth and indicates a pseudarthrosis, which must be treated with repeat arthrodesis.

Hemivertebra or Wedge Excision

Hemivertebra excision is essentially an anterior and posterior wedge osteotomy that is combined with correction and fusion. It is used for rigid angulated scoliosis in which compensation cannot be achieved with other methods (18). It is usually applied in the lumbosacral area for a lumbosacral hemivertebra, which causes decompensation because there is no mobile spine below the hemivertebrae to allow compensation (9, 13, 16, 31). There is no way to achieve a balanced spine other than by a wedge excision. The procedure is best performed before age 5, before the secondary curve above has developed structural changes. The hemivertebra and the adjacent discs are excised using a lumbotomy approach, and a corresponding wedge of the hemivertebra and the pedicle are removed posteriorly with a fusion of the adjacent vertebrae (Fig. 10.6). Depending on the age of the child and the size of the vertebrae, the correction is maintained with a body cast with a leg extension or with the use of internal fixation, usually a compression system on the convexity of the excised segment, with the use of hooks and/or pedicle screws. The use of internal fixation is preferable (Fig. 10.7). Postoperatively, the child is immobilized in a body cast, usually with a leg extension, and is nonambulatory for 3 to 4 months.

In rare cases, there are dysplastic changes at the level of the hemivertebra with insufficient bone stock for compression instrumentation. In this case, a preliminary convex hemifusion is performed posteriorly, followed by excision of the wedge 9 to 12 months after the hemifusion is solid and can support the instrumentation.

Hemivertebra excision or a wedge excision are also used in more severe and rigid deformities or in reconstructive surgery in which discectomies alone would be inadequate to achieve a balanced spine. The approach is from the convexity of the curve as above, followed by discectomies. Correction is obtained with excision of a wedge of the adjacent end plates converting the discectomy into a wedge osteotomy. In addition, any significantly deforming hemivertebra is excised, and in reconstructive cases a wedge of bone is excised, the line of bone removal being marked with clips. The posterior procedure is now performed under the same anesthetic. With wide discectomies, the facets and adjacent laminar edges are excised to allow correction. With a hemivertebral or wedge excision, a wedge of bone is removed posteriorly, which matches the anterior excision using the anterior clips as a guide. Multiple wedges are preferable to a single wedge for correction because this allows a little correction at multiple levels rather than all the correction occurring at one level. Multiple wedges are safer neurologically, and in addition, a single large wedge makes the spine more unstable, thus increasing the chance of neurologic problems.

At the completion of the posterior releases, there are two choices. Either the spine can be fused with decortication and the addition of abundant autologous iliac bone graft, or the wound can be closed with a planned return after traction to fuse the spine with possible stabilization with instrumentation. The patient is now placed in halo gravity or halo femoral traction to obtain slow traction with the patient awake, allowing careful neurologic monitoring while correction occurs. Traction continues until the correction is obtained with restoration of spinal balance, usually after 2 to 3 weeks. At this stage, reoperation with fusion and possible insertion of instrumentation occurs. It must be remembered that the instrumentation is used to maintain the correction obtained in traction, and *not* to obtain any additional correction.

This treatment plan usually is performed in small

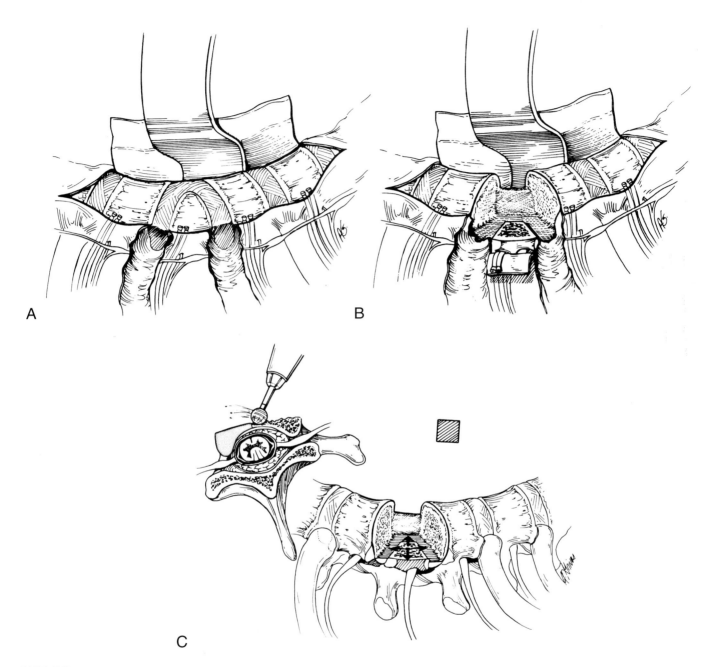

FIGURE 10.6.
Technique of hemivertebra excision. The procedure involves two stages, an anterior and posterior removal, under the same anesthesia. An anterior approach is performed on the convexity of the curvature (thoracotomy, thoraco-abdominal, or lumbotomy) and the hemivertebra is identified by direct visualization, by subperiosteal exposure of the curvature and hemivertebra area, or with an intraoperative radiograph. In the thoracic spine, the rib head at the level of the hemivertebra is removed. Using subperiosteal dissection the hemivertebra and adjacent discs are visualized (**A**). The discs are excised back to the posterior annulus and across the spine to the opposite side, leaving only the opposite lateral annulus as a stabilizing structure. After removal of the discs, the hemivertebra is removed to the posterior cortex with rongeurs and curettes, the latter used in a transverse rotating manner so that the hard posterior cortex of the vertebra is exposed but not penetrated (**B**). The spinal canal must now be entered. This is done best through the posterior cortex of the hemivertebra rather than through the posterior annulus. A diamond-tipped burr or fine gouges and curettes are used to make this opening, which is enlarged gradually with curettes and/or rongeurs (**C**). The dissection is carried cranially and caudally to

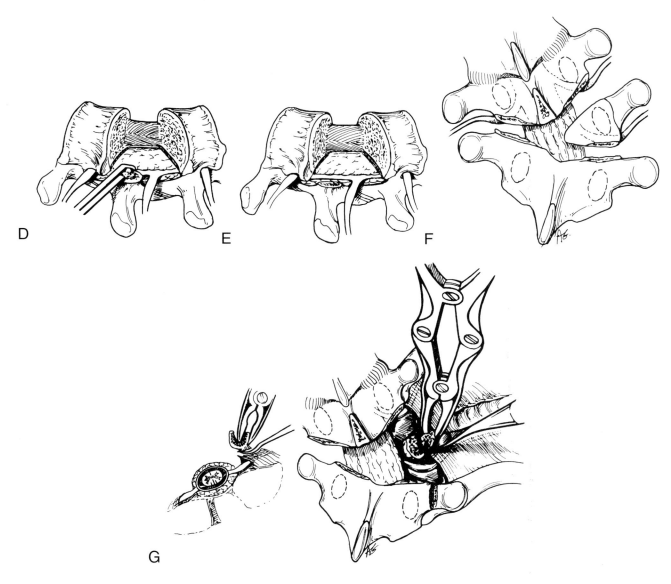

remove the annular tissue. This is best done in the midline first, and carried across to the far side, leaving the near side bone to be removed last. The lower portion of the near bone is removed in the area of the foramen so that the exiting nerve root is seen. The pedicle is now removed. The posterior cortex is gradually nibbled upwards from the foramen and laterally from the midline until just the pedicle remains (**D**). The base of the pedicle is now nibbled off, proceeding posteriorly to the waist of the pedicle, with the remainder of the pedicle to be removed from the posterior approach (**E**). Bone chips from the removed hemivertebra are placed in the space over thrombin-soaked Gelfoam or a fat graft against the dura. With the patient prone, the spine is exposed in the area to be fused, and the levels are identified with a radiograph in the operating room. The ligamentum flavum is removed above and below the hemivertebra, extending the removal laterally and removing the superior and inferior facets so that the nerve roots can be seen exiting at the foramina (**F**). In the lumbar spine the transverse process can be transected at its base and the lateral portion left in place, and in the thoracic spine the whole transverse process is excised. The remaining laminar bone is now removed with a Kerrison rongeur so that only the pedicle remains (**G**). The stump of the pedicle can now be removed by grasping it with a fine tipped rongeur with one jaw inside and the other jaw outside the pedicle. The pedicle is gently twisted and rotated with careful dissection of the periosteum on its outer surface so that it comes out as a single piece. If this does not occur, it can be removed with bites of a fine tipped rongeur and a curette. The wedge is closed with cast correction in the very young, or when the bone size is sufficient, with instrumentation (the pediatric hooks, two pedicle screws, or a hook and a screw). Reprinted with permission from Winter RB, Lonstein JE, Denis F, et al. Atlas of spinal surgery. Philadelphia: WB Saunders, 1995.

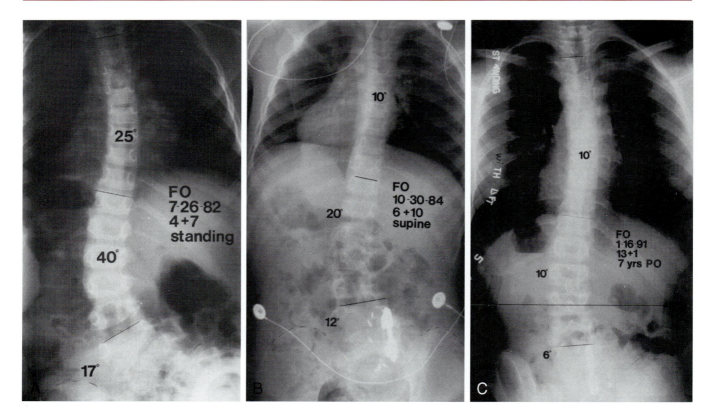

FIGURE 10.7.
A. This girl presented at the age of 4 years and 7 months with a right L5 hemivertebra with trunk translation to the left and a compensatory 40-degree left lumbar curve. This curve progressed and, at the age of 6 years and 10 months, she was referred to Dr. Winter who performed an anterior and posterior hemivertebra excision with fixation using hooks and a small Harrington compression rod. **B.** Postoperatively the curves were improved with correction of the torso shift. **C.** Seven years postoperatively the fusion is solid, the torso is in balance, and the curve correction is maintained.

children in whom the instrumentation would not add anything and allow ambulation; thus decortication and fusion is usually performed as part of the original posterior procedure. The patient is now placed in a halo cast or a Risser body cast with leg extensions. The immobilization used depends on the age of the child and the site of the curve. The patient is kept nonambulatory for 3 to 4 months, at which time the halo and cast are removed. A Milwaukee brace is now fitted, the patient is ambulatory, and bracing continues for 12 to 18 months as mentioned previously.

Kyphosis

Natural History

Kyphotic deformities are less common than scoliosis, but they can have serious consequences if left untreated, like causing paraplegia. Paraplegia is more common with failure of formation, which gives a sharp angular kyphosis. It also is more common with kyphosis in the upper thoracic area because this is the part of the spinal cord with the poorest collateral circulation—the so-called watershed area of the blood supply of the spinal cord. The paraplegia may occur early, but is more common during the adolescent growth spurt with rapid increase in the untreated kyphosis, and may occur after minor trauma (7, 19, 45).

Congenital kyphosis can be caused by a failure of formation or a failure of segmentation, the former being more common. The failure of formation can be purely anterior resulting in kyphosis (Fig.10.8), or anterolateral with a posterior corner hemivertebra resulting in kyphoscoliosis. In addition, the failure can involve more than one level, and there may be a sagittal translation in these cases—the so-called congenital spondylolisthesis. In addition, in rare cases, there may be a congenital narrowing of the spinal, termed segmental spinal dysgenesis (8). In general, kyphosis caused by failure of formation is universally progressive and can lead to paraplegia if untreated, as noted previously. The progression is caused by the growth imbalance and the mechanical effect of kyphosis.

Kyphosis with any hemivertebra is thus important because it gives a different prognosis with progression and the danger of paralysis. The possibility of a hemivertebra seen on a coronal view that is posterolateral and not only lateral must always be consid-

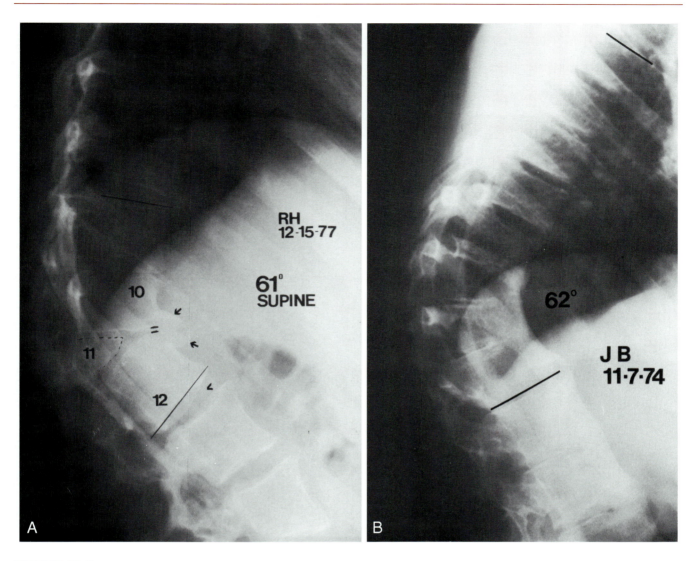

FIGURE 10.8.
Examples of congenital kyphosis. **A.** Failure of anterior formation of T11 with a posterior hemivertebra causing an angular kyphosis. **B.** Failure of anterior segmentation with an anterior bar and a rounded kyphosis.

ered. This emphasizes the need to obtain coronal and sagittal views on all congenital deformities to appreciate the anomaly and deformity in three dimensions.

Defects of anterior segmentation causing kyphosis are less common. They may involve single or multiple levels, and may result in a rounded kyphosis with little risk of paraplegia. Commonly, the kyphosis caused by the defect of segmentation starts in the late juvenile years with progressive ossification of the disc space anteriorly (Fig.10.8B). In the very early stages differentiation from Scheuermann's disease can be difficult, but with time the progressive anterior ossification becomes obvious. With the anterior bar and continued posterior growth, progressive kyphosis results. The rate of progression is less than that with a formation failure because the bar forms in the late juvenile years and the growth discrepancy is not as great.

Nonoperative Treatment

There is no role for nonoperative treatment of congenital kyphosis. The natural history indicates a universally poor prognosis and thus the treatment is surgical.

Surgical Treatment

In congenital kyphosis, the choices are between a posterior approach and a combined anterior and posterior approach. Because the defect is defined clearly, it is easier to discuss the treatment with respect to the vertebral anomaly.

Defects of Segmentation

The choice of treatment depends on the magnitude of the deformity and whether correction is desired.

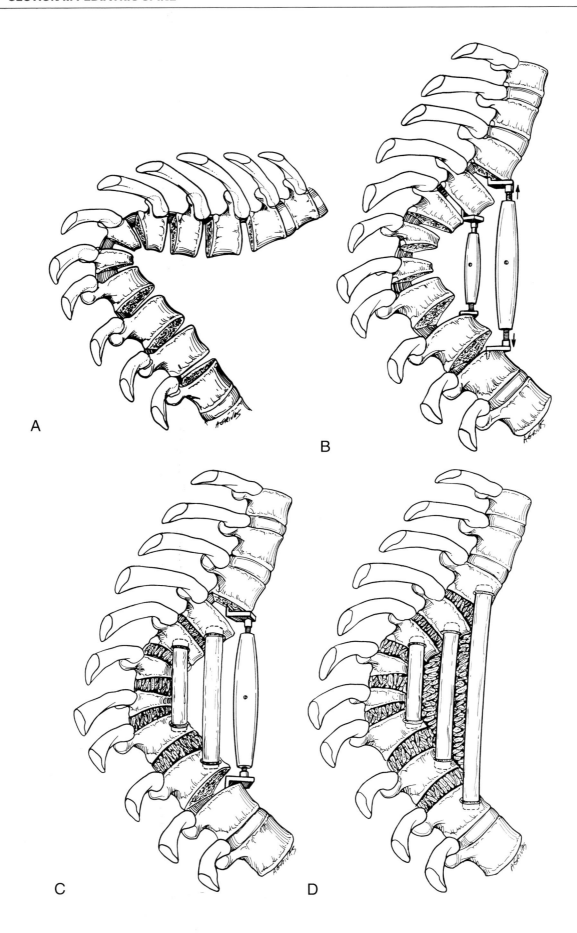

POSTERIOR FUSION

If the defect is detected early with an acceptable kyphosis with no need for correction, a posterior fusion extending at least one vertebra cranial and one caudal to the segmentation defect is ideal. The fusion must include the whole of the abnormal sagittal curve. Abundant autologous iliac bone graft is added to achieve as thick a fusion as possible. Because the deformity is rigid, instrumentation is not used unless the congenital kyphosis is part of a longer kyphosis that requires treatment and fusion. This posterior fusion removes the posterior deforming growth forces.

ANTERIOR OSTEOTOMY AND FUSION AND POSTERIOR FUSION

When the kyphosis presents later with a significant deformity that needs correction, the combined approach is best. Anteriorly, the unsegmented areas are osteotomized with section of the anterior longitudinal ligament and removal of any residual disc posteriorly. The posterior annulus is left intact and the spinal canal is not entered. An anterior fusion is now performed by packing the disc spaces with small chips of rib bone, extending the fusion to include any additional levels that need to be included in the fusion area. A sequential posterior fusion is now performed under the same anesthetic, thus ensuring that the full extent of the kyphosis is addressed. Instrumentation and bone graft are added. The choice of instrumentation depends on the curve and the experience and preference of the surgeon.

Failure of Formation

The treatment plan depends on whether the kyphosis is detected early or late, and if late, whether neurological loss, such as paraparesis or paraplegia, exists.

POSTERIOR FUSION (EPIPHYSIODESIS)

The best procedure is an early posterior fusion that extends one normal level cranial and caudal to the anomalous area. This procedure is best done on patients under age 3 years and with kyphoses under 55 to 60°. Postoperatively, the child is placed in a hyperextension cast and the child is kept nonambulatory for 4 to months. In the very young (under 18 months) or in whom a pseudoarthrosis is detected, a repeat posterior procedure is performed to reinforce the fusion and/or repair the pseudarthrosis. It is generally recommended that routine exploration and graft augmentation be performed at 6 months to obtain a thick fusion. The child is immobilized in a brace or cast and ambulated, the total time of additional immobilization being 18 months until the fusion is solid and mature.

The early posterior fusion allows anterior growth with a slow steady improvement in the angle of the kyphosis—a true epiphysiodesis effect. In their review of 17 cases of congenital kyphosis fused posteriorly alone before the age of 5, Winter and Moe found improvement in the kyphosis in 12 patients (71%) with an average 9-year follow-up (40).

In children older than 5 with less severe kyphosis, under 50 to 55°, a posterior fusion alone can be successful in controlling the kyphosis and stabilizing the curve. Many of these cases are kyphoscoliosis, and instrumentation is added where possible to obtain any correction allowed by the flexibility of the deformity, and to stabilize the curve during the fusion process.

ANTERIOR AND POSTERIOR FUSION

For kyphosis greater than 55 to 60°, an anterior and posterior fusion is necessary. It is important to include the whole extent of the kyphosis in the fusion, not limiting one's approach to the area of the anomaly. Anteriorly the tether is the abnormal cartilage in the area of the hemivertebra, the anterior longitudinal ligament, and the annulus fibrosis. They all need to be removed. The discs are excised completely over the whole extent of the kyphosis back to the posterior annulus and to the opposite side. At the apex of the kyphosis in the area of the anomaly, care is taken to excise all the anterior cartilage and fibrocartilage, and any disc between the hemivertebra and the adjacent vertebrae (Fig.10.9A).

After the anterior release, correction can now be obtained by gentle distraction on the head by the anesthesia staff to stabilize the spine while the surgeon

FIGURE 10.9.
Technique of anterior fusion in congenital kyphosis caused by a failure of anterior formation, i.e., hemivertebra. **A.** The extent of the whole kyphosis is visualized with subperiosteal exposure of the vertebrae. The discs are excised over the area of the proposed fusion with removal of the anterior tether: the anterior longitudinal ligament, the anterior annulus, and the fibrocartilage in the area of the hemivertebrae. In kyphoses of moderate degree correction is obtained with longitudinal traction combined with pressure applied by the surgeon over the apex of the kyphosis. In an angular kyphosis, an anterior distractor (Santa Casa) is inserted to gradually elongate the concavity with correction of the kyphosis. This correction is obtained slowly and patiently, with spinal cord monitoring or a wake-up test being done during or after the distraction (**B**). **C.** After obtaining maximal correction, posterior fibular struts are inserted into slots in the vertebral bodies. **D.** The anterior distractor is removed, followed by insertion of an anterior fibular strut bridging the anterior extent of the kyphosis. The disc spaces and all the area between the fibular struts is filled with bone—autologous rib, iliac crest augmented with allograft cancellous bone when necessary. Reprinted with permission from Winter RB, Lonstein JE, Denis F, and Smith MD. Atlas of spinal surgery. Philadelphia: WB Saunders, 1995. (See previous page)

corrects the kyphosis with posterior pressure. In older children and adults with larger vertebrae, an anterior distractor can be used (Santa Casa or Slot) to obtain this correction (Fig.10.9B). Correction is maintained with an anterior fusion with chips of bone inserted in the disc spaces. In addition, rib struts are added, bridging the kyphosis anteriorly and restoring the anterior support. In larger kyphoses with bone of adequate size, an anterior graft of autogenous fibula is inserted to maintain the correction. The anterior strut is inserted in slots curetted in the vertebral bodies, with the anterior strut being inserted while correction is being obtained with pressure over the apex of the kyphosis. The principle is to build an anterior bridge, filling the concavity of the kyphosis with bone (Fig.10. 9C and D).

A posterior fusion is now performed, usually sequentially under the same anesthetic. Compression instrumentation is added, which stabilizes the kyphosis and allows any possible correction at the ends of the curve. This is the safest force for the neural structures in these cases because it actually relaxes the spinal cord. Historically, the Harrington compression system was used for kyphosis, or combined with a distraction rod for kyphoscoliosis. This has been replaced by the third generation multiple hook rod systems, but the principles are unchanged. The choice of instrumentation depends on the experience and choice of the surgeon (Fig. 10.10).

With the use of instrumentation and secure fixation, the child is ambulatory without immobilization. If the fixation is not secure or is in question, additional external protection in a cast or brace is best. In the young patient in whom instrumentation is impossible or would not add sufficient stabilization, the child is placed in a hyperextension cast and kept nonambulatory for 3 to 4 months. At this time, a brace is fitted and worn for 12 to 18 months until the fusion is mature.

It is tempting in these cases to obtain correction in traction, either halo-gravity or halo-femoral. This can be obtained either preoperatively or between the anterior and posterior procedures. The use of traction in these cases carries a high incidence of paraplegia. The apex of the kyphosis is rigid with the spinal cord stretched over the apical vertebral bodies. Traction corrects the ends of the curve, pulling the cord against the apical bone with resultant neurologic

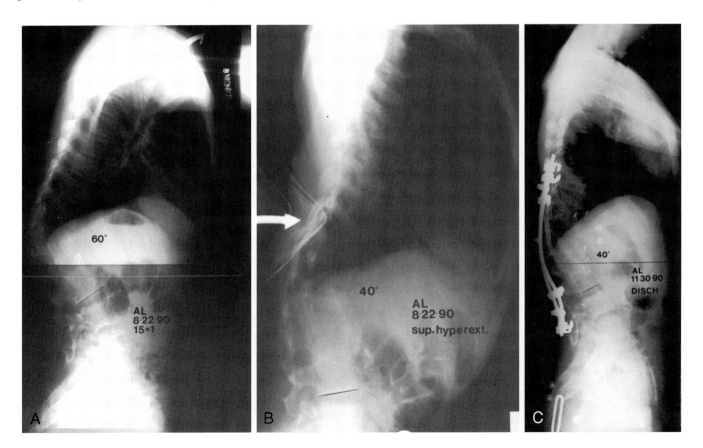

FIGURE 10.10.
A. This 14-year, 1-month-old male presented with a congenital kyphosis of 60°. **B.** On hyperextension, it corrected to 40°. The anomaly caused by a hemivertebra combined with an anterior unsegmented bar—a mixed deformity. **C.** This deformity was treated with an anterior fusion with rib strut grafts followed by posterior fusion Cotrel-Dubousset instrumentation, with correction to 40°.

loss. Traction thus plays no role in the treatment of congenital kyphosis (45).

Treatment of Congenital Kyphosis and Neurological Loss (19)

As mentioned previously, congenital kyphosis caused by failure of formation can be complicated by paraparesis or paraplegia due to the deformity alone. The spinal cord is stretched over the anterior bone at the apex of the deformity. With growth, especially the adolescent growth spurt, the kyphosis increases, worsening this stretch. Interference with cord function and neurologic loss can result caused by growth alone or combined with minor trauma. This result is more common with kyphosis in the area of poor cord blood supply, the upper thoracic area, which is the watershed area of cord blood supply.

The neurologic loss can range from mild, with minor weakness, reflex change, and bladder symptoms, to frank paraparesis or paraplegia. All these patients should have imaging of the spinal canal. Historically, this imaging has been done using large volume myelography, but today the MRI scan is used most often because of the excellent visualization of the spinal canal and its contents. Large volume myelography with CT is still used in cases of severe deformity where it is impossible to visualize the spinal canal and cord adequately with an MRI scan. In cases with minor loss, the bladder function is best evaluated with a cystometrogram and a bladder neck EMG so that any neurologic effects of the cord compression on the bladder can be detected.

In patients who present with minor neurologic deficits with congenital kyphosis, the kyphosis is treated with a combined anterior and posterior fusion as described previously. In these cases, the straightening of the apex during the anterior procedure has the effect of releasing the compression of the apical bone against the spinal cord. In cases of mild paraparesis with a flexible apex as shown on a hyperextension film, the patient is placed on bed rest. In some cases this bed rest with the apex in hyperextension results in improvement in the paraparesis. The bed rest is continued as long as there is neurologic improvement—usually a number of weeks. If the recovery is normal or to a residual minor loss, the improved position is stabilized with a combined anterior and posterior fusion as mentioned previously.

In cases with more marked neurologic loss or in which the bed rest does not result in neurologic improvement in mild paraparesis, an anterior spinal cord decompression is performed. The anterior approach and releases are performed as described previously. The anterior bone compressing the spinal cord is now removed, ensuring that the removal covers the whole area of compression that was identified on the preoperative imaging study. After removal of the anterior compressing bone, the dural sac and cord move anteriorly into decompressed area. An anterior fusion is now done with interbody fusion and the insertion of rib and fibula strut grafts as described previously.

A posterior fusion with or without instrumentation is now performed. It can be under the same anesthetic, or in cases in which there is excessive blood loss with the decompression, the posterior fusion is staged and performed 1 to 2 weeks later. The patient is kept nonambulatory for 2 to 4 weeks to allow maximal cord recovery and allow the postoperative edema in and around the cord to subside. Further treatment as regards external immobilization and an addition period nonambulatory depends on the use of posterior instrumentation, and the security of its fixation as discussed before.

Lordosis

Congenital lordosis is the least common of the congenital spine deformities and is caused by a failure of posterior segmentation. The cases with failure of posterior formation are extremely rare. The unsegmented bar can be only posterior, causing pure lordosis, or posterolateral, resulting in lordoscoliosis. Its position in the vertebral ring determines whether scoliosis or lordosis is the prominent feature. The predominantly scoliosis cases are discussed in previous text, while those with lordosis as the major deformity are discussed here. The area of segmentation loss usually extends over multiple levels, and the deforming force is the anterior growth. With increasing lordosis there is reduction of the spine-sternal distance and alteration in the rib mechanics in respiration with resultant respiratory restriction, respiratory failure, and even early death.

Nonoperative Treatment

There is no role for any nonoperative treatment in congenital lordosis because the natural history is progressive. The treatment in all cases is thus surgical.

Surgical Treatment

The deforming force in these cases is anterior growth; therefore. all cases need an anterior approach. The only method to correct the congenital lordosis is osteotomy of the unsegmented bar; thus, any case requiring correction needs a combined anterior and posterior approach. As these patients have pulmonary restrictive disease, an anterior approach has greater risks. If there is already an element of pulmonary failure, these risks increase. If pulmonary artery hypertension is already present, surgery is probably contraindicated due to the high mortality in these cases.

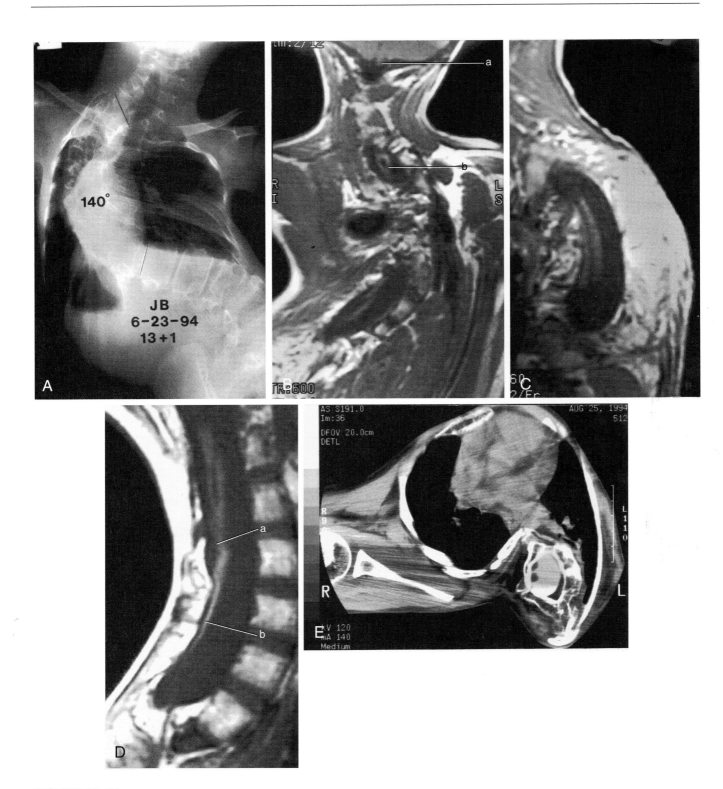

FIGURE 10.11.

A. This 13-year, 1-month-old girl presented with 140° congenital scoliosis, and as a routine preoperative evaluation, an MRI scan was done to exclude spinal dysraphism. **B.** This sagittal MRI cut shows a Chiari I abnormality (a) and a syrinx in the cervico-thoracic cord (b). **C.** A split spinal cord is seen in the thoracic area, with the diastematomyelia shown in Figure 10.2.**D.** This sagittal cut in the lumbar area shows a low lying conus (a) and a tight filum terminale (b). Because of the severe scoliosis, numerous MRI cuts are necessary to visualize the whole spinal canal. Because of this, and to confirm the anatomy, a myelogram was also performed on this patient. A sample CT cut of the myelogram shows better visualization of the split spinal cord and the marked vertebral rotation (**E**).

Anterior Fusion

In early cases in which correction is not necessary, an anterior fusion is performed with disc excisions, removal of the cartilage end plates, and packing of the disc spaces with bone chips. This removes the anterior growth potential and gives an anterior fusion opposite the unsegmented bar. This is the ideal procedure, but is rarely performed because of the rarity of this anomaly and the usual presentation with a larger lordosis.

Anterior and Posterior Procedure

Generally the cases present later where correction is necessary, involving anterior closing wedges and osteotomy of the bar posteriorly. Anteriorly, the discs are excised over the whole area of the lordosis, and thin wedges of the adjacent vertebral end plates are excised, converting the disc excision into an osteotomy that is wider anteriorly. The disc spaces are not packed with bone chips because the wedges need to lose anteriorly.

Posteriorly, the bar is exposed and multiple osteotomies are performed, with exposure extending to all the vertebrae to be fused considering the coronal and sagittal curves. The best method for correction is with the passage of sublaminar wires and approximation of the spine with these wires to a kyphotically contoured rod: Harrington, Luque, or one of the third generation multiple hook rod systems. In addition, it may be necessary to perform rib resections bilaterally to prevent the spine correction from being hampered by the ribs. This is performed in two stages: an internal thoracoplasty with rib resections performed during the anterior approach; and the opposite side resections performed during the posterior procedure. In some in which the lordosis is not too great, the same effect can be achieved with bilateral transverse process osteotomies during the posterior procedure. This process allows some spinal correction without the restriction imposed by the ribs.

Treatment of Spinal Dysraphism

The common feature in spinal dysraphism is tethering of the spinal cord to some degree by the intraspinal anomaly. This tethering results in neurologic sequelae, e.g., small foot, cavus foot, calf atrophy, alteration in bladder function, and, rarely, pain. The diagnosis of dysraphism may be confirmed by investigating one of these signs or symptoms in a spine or foot clinic. In addition, the lesion may be detected during an evaluation of a congenital scoliosis with or without external (skin dimple, hair patch) or radiographic findings (bony spur, widened interpediculate distance). A high index of suspicion is necessary in all cases of congenital spine deformities to exclude these intraspinal anomalies (Fig. 10.11).

Surgical treatment consists of releasing the cord tethering, and the exact procedure is tailored for the specific anomaly. A tight filum terminale is sectioned, a diastematomyelia is removed, a Chiari malformation is treated with fourth ventricle decompression, syringomyelia is shunted, and lipomas and teratomas are excised. This treatment should be performed by a neurosurgeon who is skilled and experienced in this area. The procedure includes the use of microscopes, bipolar cautery, and electronic neurologic monitoring. The most complex problem to treat is a lipoma in which the nerve rootlets are intertwined with the lipomatous tissue, often making safe and complete removal of the lipoma difficult, if not impossible. Neurologic deterioration can follow the neurosurgical procedure, and this must be kept in mind while planning and counseling regarding surgery.

The question is whether all these lesions should be removed surgically once detected. A considerable amount of controversy still exists in this regard. There is no argument in the case of a lesion with obvious signs and/or symptoms. The discussion involves the lesion detected during routine screening of a congenital spine deformity. Some neurosurgeons advocate removal of all lesions once detected, while others advocate a more conservative approach, the latter being the author's preferred treatment plan. If any correction of the spinal deformity by any method (releases, traction, instrumentation) is planned, the dysraphic lesion is treated. The neurosurgical procedure is best performed first as a separate surgery, and then the spinal fusion is performed 2 or more weeks later using careful neurologic monitoring. The safest way to achieve correction in these cases is with traction, bracing, or serial casts. These methods allow careful neurologic monitoring with the patient awake during the correction.

In cases in which no neurologic deficit exists and no correction with stretching of the spine is planned, the dysraphic lesion does not need to be treated before the spinal fusion. Continued neurologic monitoring continues in these cases and in cases with a dysraphic lesion, no neurological deficit, and no surgery. This monitoring continues past the end of growth into adulthood because symptoms have been seen presenting later at any age from 20 to 60 years.

Summary

All patients with a congenital spine deformity need a complete evaluation to exclude other congenital anomalies, especially those involving the spinal canal and its contents. Complete and accurate radiographic assessment in the coronal and sagittal planes is essential so that the type of vertebral anomaly and its anatomic position in the vertebral ring is established as well as the associated deformity and its magnitude. What is important is the growth disturbance produced by the anomaly, and the growth potential of the remainder of the vertebral ring; this imbalance results in the deformity and determines its rate of progression. As the natural history of congenital deformities is well established, this assessment points to the prognosis and determines the treatment plan.

In general principle, the treatment is fairly straightforward. Observation for curve progression is used for those deformities and anomalies in which the natural history and prognosis is not clear. Nonoperative treatment by bracing plays a limited role; it is reserved for congenital scoliosis to improve spinal balance (including head tilt) and to control compensatory curves. It has no role in the treatment of rigid curves, congenital kyphosis, or congenital lordosis.

The principle of surgery is to balance growth, thus preventing curve progression. It is impossible to insert growth. Therefore, the only thing that can be done is to remove the growth in the vertebral ring opposite the anomaly with an appropriate fusion. In some cases, it is possible to perform a convex fusion where there is concave growth potential and sufficient growth remaining so that the concave growth corrects the curve (the epiphysiodesis effect). In other cases, curve improvement is obtained with releases and correction, with the safest correction obtained in traction. It is also safer to shorten the convexity of a curve than to lengthen the concavity. Many surgical procedures are available—there is no ideal or correct procedure for a specific anomaly or deformity. The procedure and treatment plan chosen is tailored for the patient and depends on the anomaly, the deformity produced, its natural history, the patient's age, and the presence of other congenital anomalies, especially neurologic.

References

1. Akbarnia BA, Heydarian K, Ganjavian MS. Concordant congenital spine deformity in monozygotic twins. J Pediatr Orthop 1983;3(4):502.
2. Andrew T, Piggott H. Growth arrest for progressive scoliosis: combined anterior and posterior fusion of the convexity. J Bone Joint Surg Am 1985;67:193.
3. Beals RK, Robbins JR, Rolfe B. Anomalies associated with vertebral malformations. Spine 1993;18:1329.
4. Bradford DS, Heithoff KB, Cohen M. Intraspinal abnormalities and congenital spine deformities. J Pediatr Orthop 1991;11:36.
5. Cantu JM, Urrusti J, Rosales G, et al. Evidence for autosomal recessive inheritance of costovertebral dysplasia. Clin Genet 1971;2:149.
6. Dowling FE, Lynch AF, Blake NS. Spinal cord abnormalities in congenital scoliosis—clinical and radiographic evaluation. Orthop Trans 1987;11:103.
7. Dubousset J, Gonon EP. Cyphoses et cypho-scolioses angulaires. Rev Chir Orthop 1983; Suppl II:69.
8. Faciszewski T, Winter RB, Lonstein JE, et al. Segmental spinal dysgenesis. A disorder different from spinal agenesis. J Bone Joint Surg Am 1995;77:530.
9. Freedman LS, Leong JCY, Luk KDK, et al. One stage combined anterior and posterior excision of hemivertebrae in the lower lumbar spine. J Bone Joint Surg Br 1987;69:854.
10. Goldberg C, Fenton G, Blake NS. Diastematomyelia: a critical review of natural history and treatment. Spine 1984;9:367.
11. Hattaway GL. Congenital scoliosis in one of monozygotic twins: a case report. J Bone Joint Surg Am 1977; 59(6):837.
12. Hensinger R, Lang JE, MacEwen GD. Klippel-Feil syndrome: a constellation of associated anomalies. J Bone Joint Surg Am 1974;56:1246.
13. Holte D, Winter RB, Lonstein JE, et al. Hemivertebra excision and wedge resection in the surgical treatment of patients with congenital scoliosis. J Bone Joint Surg Am 1995;77:159.
14. Hood RW, Riseborough E, Nehme A, et al. Diastematomyelia and structural spinal deformities. J Bone Joint Surg Am 1980;62:520.
15. Jarco S, Levin PM. Hereditary malformations of the vertebral bodies. Bull Johns Hopkins Hosp 1938;62:215.
16. King JD, Lowery GL. Results of lumbar hemivertebral excision for congenital scoliosis. Spine 1991;16(7):778.
17. Kuhns JE, Hormell RS. Management of congenital scoliosis. Arch Surg 1952;65:250.
18. Leatherman KD, Dickson RA. Two-stage corrective surgery for congenital deformities of the spine. J Bone Joint Surg Br 1979;1979:324.
19. Lonstein JE, Winter RB, Moe JH, et al. Neurological deficits secondary to spinal deformity: a review of the literature and report of 43 cases. Spine 1980;5:331.
20. MacEwen GD, Conway JJ, Miller WT. Congenital scoliosis with a unilateral bar. Radiology 1968;90(4):711.
21. MacEwen GD, Winter RB, Hardy JH. Evaluation of kidney anomalies in congenital scoliosis. J Bone Joint Surg Am 1972;54(7):1451.
22. MacLennan GD. Scoliosis. Br Med J 1922;2:864.
23. McMaster MJ. Occult intraspinal anomalies and congenital scoliosis. J Bone Joint Surg Am 1984;66(4):588.
24. McMaster MJ, Ohtsuka K. The natural history of congenital scoliosis. A study of two hundred and fifty-one patients. J Bone Joint Surg Am 1982;64(8):1128.
25. Nasca RJ, Stelling F, Steel HH. Progression of congenital scoliosis due to hemivertebrae and hemivertebrae with bars. J Bone Joint Surg Am 1975;57(4):456.
26. Peterson HA, Peterson LF. Hemivertebrae in identical twins with dissimilar spinal columns. J Bone Joint Surg Am 1967;49(5):938.
27. Rathke WF, Sun HY. Untersuchungen uber Missbildungsskoliosen. Z Orthop Ihre Grenzgeb 1963;97:173.
28. Reckles LH, Peterson HA, Bianco AJ, et al. The association of scoliosis and congenital heart disease. J Bone Joint Surg Am 1975;57:449.

29. Rimoin DL, Fletcher BD, McKusick VA. Spondylocostal dysplasia. A dominantly inherited form of short trunked dwarfism. Am J Med 1968;45:948.
30. Roaf R. The treatment of progressive scoliosis by unilateral growth arrest. J Bone Joint Surg Br 1963;45:637.
31. Slabaugh PB, Winter RB, Lonstein JE, et al. Lumbosacral hemivertebrae. A review of twenty-four patients, with excision in eight. Spine 1980;5:234.
32. Stagnara P. Les deformations due Rachis. Paris: Masson, 1985:344.
33. Touzet P, Rigault P, Padovani JP. Les hemivertebrales: classification, histirie naturelle et elements de prognostic. Rev Chir Orthop 1979;65:173.
34. Tsou P, Yau A, Hodgson A. Congenital spinal deformities: natural history, classification, and the role of anterior surgery. J Bone Joint Surg Am 1974;56:1767.
35. Winter RB. Convex anterior and posterior hemiarthrodesis and hemiepiphysiodesis in young children with progressive congenital scoliosis. J Pediatr Orthop 1981;1(4):361.
36. Winter RB. Congenital deformities of the spine. New York: Thieme-Stratton, 1983.
37. Winter RB, Haven JJ, Moe JH, et al. Diastematomyelia and congenital spine deformities. J Bone Joint Surg Am 1974;56:27.
38. Winter RB, Lonstein JE, Denis F, et al. Convex growth arrest for progressive congenital scoliosis due to hemivertebrae. J Pediatr Orthop 1988;8:633.
39. Winter RB, Lonstein JE, Denis F, et al. The prevalence of spinal canal or cord abnormalities in idiopathic, congenital and neuromuscular scoliosis. Orthop Trans 1992;16:135.
40. Winter RB, Moe JH. The results of spinal arthrodesis for congenital spine deformities in patients younger than 5 years old. J Bone Joint Surg Am 1982;64:419.
41. Winter RB, Moe JH, Eilers VS. Congenital scoliosis: a study of 234 patients treated and untreated. J Bone Joint Surg Am 1968;50:1.
42. Winter RB, Moe JH, Lonstein JE. The incidence of Klippel-Feil syndrome in patients with congenital scoliosis and kyphosis. Spine 1984;9(4):363.
43. Winter RB, Moe JH, Lonstein JE. Posterior spinal arthrodesis for congenital scoliosis. J Bone Joint Surg Am 1984;66:1188.
44. Winter RB, Moe JH, MacEwen GD, et al. The Milwaukee brace in the nonoperative treatment of congenital scoliosis. Spine 1976;1:85.
45. Winter RB, Moe JH, Wang JF. Congenital kyphosis. J Bone Joint Surg Am 1973;55:223.
46. Wynne-Davies R. Congenital vertebral anomalies: etiology and relationship to spin bifida cystica. J Med Genet 1975;12:280.

CHAPTER ELEVEN

Juvenile Kyphosis

Serena S. Hu and David S. Bradford

Introduction

Juvenile kyphosis was first defined in 1920 by Scheuermann, who described radiologic findings of wedging of the vertebral bodies and endplate irregularities (38). These radiologic changes suggested disturbances of the vertebral epiphyses that were similar to Legg-Calve-Perthes disease of the hip (38). Others have noted the herniations of disc material into the endplates, and suggested refining the definition of juvenile kyphosis, including wedging of 5° or more of three adjacent vertebra (4, 40, 42).

The incidence of Scheuermann's disease in the general population is reported to be 0.4 to 8% (2, 14, 42). One study from New Zealand, examining 500 students aged 17 to 18 years, found an incidence of radiographic changes typical of Scheuermann's disease (mild to severe endplate changes, with or without Schmorl's nodes) in 56% of the males surveyed and 30% of the females (17). Data on the incidence in males versus females varies, with some studies reporting a higher incidence in males, others reporting a higher incidence in females, and still others reporting an equal distribution among males and females (15, 17, 38). Familial incidence implies autosomal dominance in at least some of the cases (16, 21, 28).

Pathogenesis

A number of factors have been implicated in the pathogenesis of juvenile kyphosis. Several researchers have noted that such patients have lower bone densities than their unaffected peers (8, 24). It has been unclear from these studies, however, whether the osteoporosis was the primary condition or an associated factor that may predispose to increased kyphosis, Schmorl's nodes, and vertebral wedging. Histology obtained during anterior fusion in young patients with Scheuermann's has demonstrated irregular endplates and endplate disruption, along with herniation of disc material into the vertebral body, which is thought to suggest vertebral osteoporosis (10).

An anterior extension of the affected vertebral bodies in cadaver specimens has also been observed; these findings are consistent with Scheuermann's (14, 39). The authors of this study suggested that the anterior extension implied an abnormality of endochondral ossification similar to that seen in patients with Blount's disease. Histologic studies have revealed abnormal and loose-appearing cartilage in the vertebral endplates as well as irregular mineralization and ossification (19, 20). Faulty ossification, with resultant wedging and irregular vertebral bodies, resulted. Also, Schmorl's nodes formed at the failed junction between the weakened cartilage plate and the nucleus pulposus. Another hypothesis is that the primary etiology is an abnormality in collagen aggregation because autopsy specimens of patients with juvenile kyphosis appear to have regions within the endplate that are devoid of collagen (3).

Diagnosis

Patients with juvenile kyphosis often present because of concerns about poor posture on the part of parents or health care professionals. Patients generally develop the condition in preadolescence, although they may present somewhat later. It is important to differentiate Scheuermann's disease from postural roundback. Patients with postural roundback demonstrate a gently rounded thoracic kyphosis that is flexible clinically. They do not have the radiographic findings described for patients with Scheuermann's. Patients with Scheuermann's kyphosis, when viewed from the side or on a lateral radiograph, have a more abrupt curve that is relatively rigid upon hyperextension (Fig. 11.1)

Increased thoracic kyphosis generally is accompanied by hyperlordosis of the lumbar spine. The resultant increased stress on the pars interarticularis may account for the increased incidence of spondylolysis reported in these patients (33). In a number of studies, varying degrees of scoliosis have also been found in 39% to 70% of patients observed for Scheuermann's kyphosis (7, 11, 12, 29, 38). Pain is uncommon as a presenting problem in adolescents and preadolescents with kyphosis; it appears to be more common with thoracolumbar involvement and in skeletally mature patients (1, 5, 47). One large survey reported a significant association between back pain lasting more than 1 week and radiographic changes associated with Scheuermann's disease (17).

The diagnosis of Scheuermann's disease is made if there is radiographic evidence of: 1) vertebral body endplate irregularity; 2) disc space narrowing; 3) one or more vertebral bodies with wedging of at least 5°; and 4) increased thoracic kyphosis (normal is defined as 25° to 40°) (Fig. 11.2) (2, 42). Scheuermann's disease can also affect the thoracolumbar and lumbar spine. Clearly, any degree of kyphosis in these

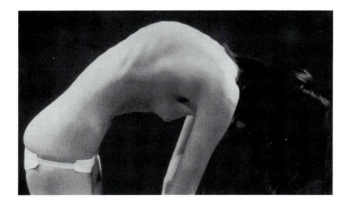

FIGURE 11.1.
Lateral photograph of patient with juvenile (Scheuermann's) kyphosis during forward bending. Note the sharp, angular curve.

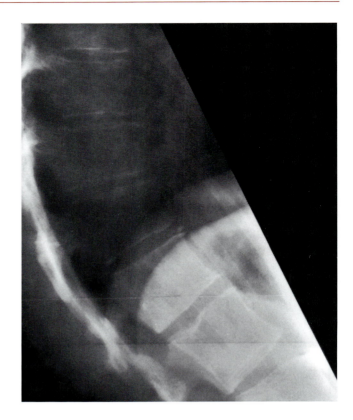

FIGURE 11.2.
Radiographic changes include vertebral body wedging, endplate irregularity and Schmorl's nodes.

regions is considered abnormal and is a possible indication of Scheuermann's disease. Severe Scheuermann's kyphosis can result in cosmetic deformity, back pain, or neurologic deficit (6). Kyphosis greater than 65 to 70° is usually noticeable and may progress after skeletal maturity (6, 9, 11).

Neurologic deficits are rare, although several case reports in the literature describe gradual and progressive lower extremity weakness with long tract signs developing in patients who have had radiographic findings consistent with juvenile kyphosis (9, 22, 44, 48). The deficit is generally secondary to thoracic disc herniation but can also occur because of tenting of the spinal cord over the curve apex or by the presence of extradural spinal cysts.

Limited data exists on the natural history of Scheuermann's kyphosis. Murray et al. recently reviewed patients a minimum of 10 years after diagnosis (average follow-up, 32 years), comparing them with an age-matched control group (31). In their series, kyphosis patients tended to have more intense back pain, less strenuous jobs, decreased range of motion of the trunk, and different pain from the controls. The subjects demonstrated no significant differences from controls with respect to self-consciousness, self-esteem, pain interference with activities of daily living, use of pain medication, or participation in recreational activities. Patients with kyphosis greater than 100° had restrictive lung disease. The effect of pain on activities correlated highly with severity of the kyphosis and a more cephalad level of the apex. Only 57% of the patients diagnosed during the period in question participated in this study.

Nonoperative Treatment

Skeletally immature patients who have kyphosis measuring greater than 45 or 50° and radiographic evidence of Scheuermann's kyphosis (endplate changes and vertebral body wedging) may be candidates for brace treatment. Historically, many patients have been treated initially with Risser antigravity casts or even traction. Such treatments are not used frequently at the present time, however. Bracing for thoracic kyphosis requires use of a Milwaukee brace. Pads are placed over the apex of the kyphosis paraspinally and corrective forces are applied, countered by the pelvic mold and neck piece (Fig. 11.3). Full-time brace wear is preferred. Many orthopedic surgeons recommend an exercise regime designed to decrease lumbar lordosis and correct the thoracic kyphosis through stretching of the pectorals and hyperextension exercises. Patients are observed at four-month intervals, lateral radiographs are taken in the brace at each follow-up visit, and the brace is adjusted as needed. Weaning from brace wear, begun as the patient nears skeletal maturity, proceeds gradually and may be slowed if correction is lost.

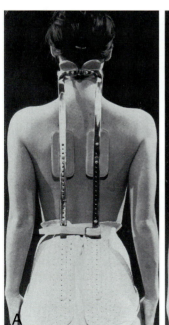 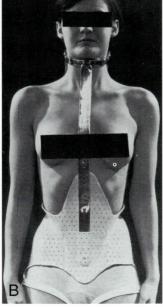

FIGURE 11.3.

Back (**A**) and front (**B**) views of Milwaukee brace with apical pads for correcting Scheuermann's kyphosis.

Milwaukee brace treatment has been effective in decreasing overall kyphosis in patients who have significant growth remaining. In general, brace correction was similar to that seen on hyperextension radiographs obtained at the beginning of treatment. Approximately 50% correction can be expected initially in these patients. After brace wear is discontinued, some loss of correction can also be expected. In the majority of patients, however, the kyphosis is improved and/or the correction is maintained at follow-up as compared to the deformity when treatment was initiated (29, 37). Vertebral body wedging can also be improved, perhaps secondary to the unloading of the anterior endplates achieved with bracing (29, 37). Also, patients with poor brace compliance and those with curves greater than 75° were more likely to have deformity progression requiring surgical correction (37).

Sachs et al. reviewed the results of 120 patients who were treated using the Milwaukee brace for their kyphosis (37). Patients began brace treatment at an average age of 12 years and completed treatment at an average age of 16 years. They were observed for at least 5 years after completion of treatment. Seventy-six of the patients who were compliant with brace wear demonstrated improvement of their kyphosis at follow-up, relative to their deformity at presentation, whereas 24 were worse despite brace wear. Seven of these patients went on to surgical correction for increasing deformity greater than 60°. (The majority of these had initial curves measuring greater than 74°.) Of the 10 patients who were noncompliant with brace wear, 8 had increased kyphosis.

The Milwaukee brace was also used to treat a series of 62 patients with Scheuermann's kyphosis reported on by Montgomery and Erwin (29). Average initial curve was 62° and the corrected curvature averaged 41°. The authors' patients were treated for an average of 18 months, beginning at a mean age of 14 years. Follow-up for at least 18 months after brace discontinuation showed an average 15° loss of correction.

Surgical Treatment

Patients may be considered for surgical intervention if their kyphosis progresses despite brace treatment or if they are skeletally mature and their deformity is substantial. Severe pain localized just distal to the apex of the kyphosis or kyphosis greater than 70° may be other indications for surgery. Mild to moderate degrees of pain accompanied by moderately severe, nonprogressive kyphosis can be treated conservatively with such measures as physical therapy and antiinflammatories.

Posterior spinal fusion using compression instrumentation with Harrington rods has been described by several authors (11, 34, 43, 45, 46). The technique involves bilateral placement of Harrington compression rods, with at least three hooks on each side above the deformity and three on each side below the apex. Upper hooks are placed over the lamina or transverse processes, while distal hooks are placed under the lamina. Compression is applied across the apex to correct the curve. Standard bone grafting and fusion is performed.

The largest of these series was that of Speck and Chopin, who reported on 59 patients with an average age of 17 years, and follow-up over four years (43). The average preoperative kyphosis was 77°, which had improved to 41° at final follow-up. Seven of 12 skeletally mature patients had an anterior fusion as well, generally 2 to 4 weeks after the posterior fusion. Loss of correction of 10° or more occurred in 9 patients, presumably because the fusions were performed over too short a segment in most cases. The authors noted that among skeletally mature patients, those who had had a combined anterior and posterior fusion lost only 1° of correction, whereas skeletally mature patients who had had a posterior fusion alone lost an average 14° of correction. Clinical appearance improved significantly for all of their patients. Twenty-eight reported significant thoracic or lumbar pain preoperatively. Only 10 patients had back pain at follow-up; four of these noted only mild pain that did not interfere with work.

Bradford et al. reviewed a series of 22 patients treated with Harrington instrumentation (11). The presenting complaints were cosmetic deformity in all patients and pain in 10 patients. One patient presented with spastic paraparesis secondary to cord compression at the curve apex. Mean age at surgery was 17 years. Risser antigravity casts were worn for 5 to 18 months after surgery. Average kyphosis was 70° at the time of surgery and corrected to an average 26° in patients whose curves averaged less than 70° preoperatively; at follow-up the average kyphosis was 38°. In patients whose preoperative curve was greater than 70°, the average kyphosis was 36° postoperatively and 55° at follow-up. All patients in the latter group lost at least 5° of correction during the follow-up period, whereas only half of those in the former group lost correction. All patients felt that their deformity had been improved by the procedure, although their surgeons felt that four of these patients had an unsatisfactory cosmetic result. The 10 patients who had presented with pain experienced relief of this symptom after the surgery.

Taylor's series of 27 patients produced similar results (46). His group included patients whose average age was 17 years and whose mean preoperative curve was 72°. Their average loss of correction was 6° at a mean follow-up of over 2 years. These patients were kept on a Stryker frame for 2 weeks after surgery and then wore body jackets.

Use of larger diameter Harrington compression rods in flexible but significant curves greater than 65° is preferred by some surgeons (34, 45). For the 10 young patients studied by Otsuka et al., successful pain relief and deformity correction from 71° to 38° was accompanied by an average loss of correction of 8° at follow-up. Sturm et al., whose patients ranged from 12 to 37 years of age, reported similar results (34, 45). They thought that the technique was useful in adults as long as anterior bony bridging was not present.

The frequently observed loss of correction, as well as the presence of increasing curve stiffness when patients are treated during adulthood, has prompted increased use of combined surgical approaches for the treatment of Scheuermann's kyphosis. It was hoped that the addition of an anterior release and fusion would permit better curve correction in stiff or severe curves and that an anterior fusion would decrease the posterior tensile forces and thus decrease the loss of correction often found. Bradford et al. reviewed a series of 24 skeletally mature patients who underwent anterior release and fusion followed by posterior fusion with Harrington compression instrumentation (7). Sixteen of their patients were placed in traction between stages and all were placed in Risser casts postoperatively for 9 to 12 months. Their patients averaged 21 years of age and follow-up ranged from 2 to 5 years. Deformity and pain were the presenting problems in nearly all their patients. Average kyphosis measured 77° preoperatively and 41° postoperatively. The average loss of correction was 6°; those who experienced the greatest loss of correction did so below the fusion; it was thought that this was secondary to a too-short posterior fusion. All patients with operative pain reported significant pain relief. It was concluded that despite a significant complication rate, a combined approach should be considered for skeletally mature, symptomatic patients whose curves are greater than 70°.

Similar results were noted by Herndon et al. in their series of 13 patients (18). Traction between surgery stages did not preserve the correction achieved. Their analysis also suggested that failure to fuse all the involved levels was the most common reason for loss of correction exceeding 6°. Nerubay and Katznelson, reviewing their results in 14 patients, including 10 patients who were in traction between surgeries, found that traction did not improve the overall correction (32). Lowe used double Luque rods for the posterior stage for those who underwent a combined procedure (25). He used traction between stages but no regimen of postoperative immobilization. Despite a somewhat increased average initial kyphosis (84°) as compared to the other studies, correction was comparable and was maintained at follow-up.

The surgical technique for anterior fusion includes a thoracotomy, ligation of the segmental vessels on the side being exposed, and exposure of the disc spaces at the apex and stiffest portion of the curve. The surgeon can perform the thoracotomy on either side. If there is a coexisting scoliosis, however, the approach is generally easier on the side of the convexity. The exposure must be adequate to permit complete discectomy and removal of the anterior longitudinal ligament. This ligament becomes contracted and thickened in severe Scheuermann's kyphosis and, if not completely released, it will act as a tether preventing correction. Osteophytes can completely bridge the interspace, preventing correction, and must be resected during the anterior release. Certainly, if thoracic discs or bony canal compression exist and are associated with neurologic compromise, anterior decompression can be done at this time (23). After complete discectomy, bone graft from the rib harvested from the thoracotomy, supplemented by local bone, should be placed loosely into the disc spaces. Many surgeons have found it helpful to place a portion of the rib graft as a structural graft within the disc space, notching the vertebral endplates slightly to permit opening of the space and secure placement. The structural graft helps to maintain distraction across the disc space and facilitates correction.

More recent use of the Cotrel-Dubousset instrumentation has shown good results (26). Thirty-two patients with initial deformities measuring greater than 75° underwent anterior release and fusion, followed by posterior fusion with CD instrumentation. Their average kyphosis was 85° preoperatively and 43° at follow-up. Average loss of correction was only 4° at a minimum follow-up of 2 years. Proximal junctional kyphosis was seen in 10 patients; this was associated with greater than 50% correction of the kyphotic deformity. Distal junctional kyphosis was seen in nine of the patients and was thought to be secondary to failure to include the first lordotic disc. Nearly all the patients were satisfied with their postoperative appearance. Of the majority of patients who preoperatively reported back pain as interfering with daily activities, 65% noted mild postoperative pain with vigorous activity. For variable hook-rod systems such as CD instrumentation, the basic configuration is two or more claw constructs above the apex of the curvature and at least one and one-half

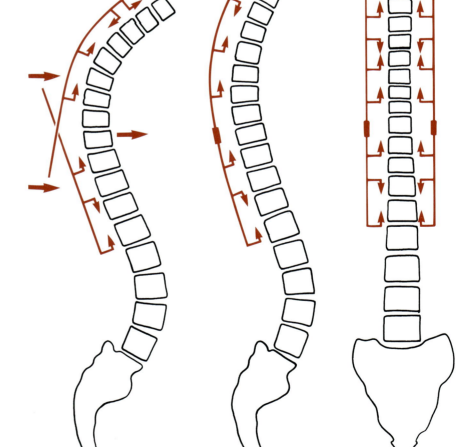

FIGURE 11.4.
Diagram of Double domino—instrumentation construct, used with variable hook systems in the surgical correction of juvenile kyphosis. **A.** Compression and cantilever bending forces on the two rods. **B.** The two rods are linked together by the double domino devices. **C.** Claw constructs on both rods are shown.

claws below the apex. The proximal claw construct is a down-going laminar or transverse process hook placed over the transverse process at the most proximal vertebra to be fused; it is clawed with an up-going pedicle hook at the adjacent level. If fixation or osteoporotic bone is a concern, a sublaminar hook may be used for the top hook instead. At least one additional claw consisting of a down-going hook over the transverse process of the vertebra one to two levels below the first claw, and an up-going pedicle hook at the level below is necessary above the apex of the curve. Distal to the apex, an up-going hook should be placed one or two levels below the apex of the kyphosis, followed by a claw construct one to two levels below this hook. The two end claws should have closed hooks. The authors, as well as others, have found that pedicle screws can improve the fixation distally when fusing into the lumbar spine (26). The rod is contoured to the desired kyphosis and maneuvered into place, levering against the apex of the kyphosis to facilitate correction and permit seating of the rod into the hooks. Compression is applied

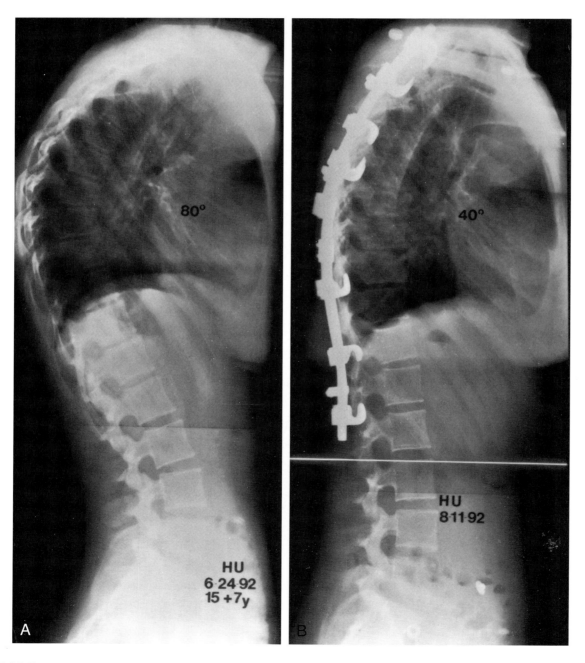

FIGURE 11.5.
Preoperative (**A**) and postoperative (**B**) lateral radiographs show correction of this 16-year-old female's Scheuermann's kyphosis. Because of her skeletal immaturity and flexible curve, isolated posterior instrumentation and fusion was sufficient.

across each claw and the entire construct is placed in compression (13). Alternatively, a temporary contralateral rod can be used as a lever as one maneuvers the first rod into place (41). We have found that using two shorter overlapping rods on each side of the spine facilitates rod placement and permits better control of the amount of correction (Fig. 11.4). The shorter rods are linked using the CD domino; additional compression can be placed across the apex at this time. We have found this double domino—technique to be technically easier and to produce results equivalent to those achieved via single-rod techniques (Fig. 11.5). The bulkiness created by the two dominos, which tend to lie at or near the apex, can be problematic in thin patients, however. Also, the bulk of the implant can jeopardize the grafting procedure and, hence, the posterior spinal fusion. This should be taken into account when selecting an implant. The presence of significant coexisting scoliosis affects the sequence of rod application and hook seating. In some instances, the hook configuration may need to be altered to account for the application of corrective forces to the kyphosis and how this would affect the coronal deformity.

Surgical Complications

The complications inherent to spinal deformity surgery are no less frequent when the deformity is in the sagittal plane than when it is in the coronal plane. Because of the forces placed at the ends of the instrumentation, hook pullout is common, either at the time of surgery or later. Many smaller studies report occasional hook pullouts; larger series have documented hook pullout in 11 to 18% of these kyphosis cases (11, 43, 45). The majority of the pullouts were proximal, and they frequently occurred, and were corrected, during surgery. Hook pullouts can occur either secondary to osteoporotic bone or with inadequate hook placement. This complication occurred more often with posterior fusion alone; it has been reported only sporadically in series studying combined surgery. Hardware failure can occur either in the presence of a pseudarthrosis or because of additional trauma. The reported incidence of hardware failure varies; meta-analysis produces an overall rate of 4 to 5% for all patients, and slightly less for combined procedures (7, 11, 25, 36, 46, 43, 45). The length of follow-up for these reports ranged from 1 year to more than 5 years. The reported incidence of pseudarthrosis in patients who have undergone surgical correction of their Scheuermann's kyphosis varies widely among different studies. It has been reported to occur in 2 to 18% of cases (7, 10, 32, 45, 46). However, some studies noted hardware failure but did not always operate or describe exploration of the fusion at the time of hardware removal (43, 45).

Others, as noted previously, noted loss of correction but did not document whether addition investigation was undertaken to determine the presence of a pseudarthrosis. Given the rate of late hardware failure and high incidence of loss of correction, the true pseudarthrosis rate seems higher than specified in the literature. In Bradford et al.'s series of posterior fusion patients, all patients who had hardware failure were surgically explored specifically for pseudoarthrosis; they reported an 18% incidence (11).

Wound infections may be either superficial or deep. Superficial infections often can be cared for locally, using appropriate antibiotics. Deep infections, however, require complete irrigation and debridement as well as appropriate intravenous antibiotics. The wound infection rate in the literature varies from 0% to 9% (7, 11, 25, 46, 43, 45). Instrumentation may need to be removed if the infection becomes chronic or is diagnosed after a delay.

The risk of neurologic compromise with kyphosis surgery may be greater than that experienced with scoliosis surgery because of the risk to the anterior spinal artery and therefore the blood supply to the spinal cord. However, cord injuries have only rarely been reported in the literature. When anterior fusion is necessary to treat a rigid deformity or a mature patient, care must be taken to not divide the segmental arteries bilaterally as well as to avoid coagulation of bleeders within the foramen. With posterior fusion and instrumentation, introduction of the rod can lengthen the anterior column and place stretch on the spinal cord and its blood supply. Traditional spinal cord monitoring, which monitors somatosensory tracts, does not monitor anterior columns and therefore may provide false negatives because loss of motor function can occur before the somatosensory tracts are affected. Wake-up tests, although they do not produce false negatives, are not continuous and are an all-or-none test. Motor-evoked potentials may eventually provide reliable and continuous monitoring of anterior column integrity.

Speck and Chopin had one patient out of a series of 65 who developed Brown-Sequard syndrome 4 hours after his posterior fusion for Scheuermann's kyphosis (43). His instrumentation was promptly removed and he had complete neurologic recovery. Lowe reported 4 of 24 patients who noted painful paresthesias after sublaminar wire instrumentation and fusion (25). Nerubay had one patient develop paraparesis and numbness after staged combined anterior and posterior fusion (32). She was still able to walk and her motor power returned to normal after six months, although she noted continued bilateral numbness. Her 84° kyphosis had been corrected to 60°. Herndon et al. reported one patient, out of a series of 13, who developed temporary weakness of the right ankle and toe extensors after her anterior fusion (18). The 1993 Morbidity and Mortality report of the Scoliosis Research Society noted 15 cases of cord injury in a cohort of 8000 spinal reconstructive surgeries of all types (30). All but one of these were partial cord injuries with partial recovery. Five of these cord injuries were in kyphosis cases, three among them in patients with Scheuermann's kyphosis. Only three were in scoliosis patients, despite the fact that there were more than seven times as many scoliosis cases as kyphosis cases.

Other reported complications include painful bursae over prominent hardware, treated either with partial hardware removal or extension of fusion, pressure sores under casts, deep vein thrombosis (11), pulmonary embolism, psychiatric problems, pneumothorax or hemothorax, coagulopathy with resultant death, and other cardiopulmonary problems (7, 11, 18, 25, 34, 45, 46). Gastrointestinal problems, such as duodenal compression, can occur secondary to secondary stretch or superior mesenteric artery compression, as seen with scoliosis patients. This problem can be treated with nasogastric aspiration or even hyperalimentation. On rare occasions, duodenojejunostomy may be required (7, 11, 46).

Thoracoscopy

Thoracoscopy is a promising new technique in the correction of kyphosis. An endoscope, such as that used by thoracic surgeons to perform lung and other resections, is used for visualizing the thoracic spine. Early reports show a significant learning curve with this technique but decreased pain and perioperative morbidity compared with open thoracotomy in anterior release (27, 35). Most spine surgeons have preferred to work, at least initially, with a general surgeon experienced in thoracoscopy. These authors have reported on 27 thoracic discectomies, 27 anterior releases for scoliosis, and 2 anterior releases for Scheuermann's kyphosis. After discectomy and resection of the anterior longitudinal ligament, morselized rib graft can be placed in the disc space. These two series included three cases of paraparesis, all of which resolved. Intercostal neuralgia was a common complication, but it resolved in the majority of cases. The authors reported shorter hospital stays and fewer intensive care days, compared with open thoracotomy procedures. Follow-up time was short, however; as of yet there are no available data evaluating fusion rates or comparing curve correction or loss of correction in deformity patients.

Thoracoscopy appears particularly promising for patients with Scheuermann's kyphosis when the anatomy is relatively undistorted and the cleaned disc spaces are small and easy to bone graft. It may be a viable and useful technique if adequate curve correction and fusion rates can be achieved in these patients. Although we have had little experience thus far with this technique as applied to kyphosis, review of others' cases leads us to question the adequacy of the anterior fusion that can be achieved using this technique.

Pulmonary Function

The effect of severe idiopathic kyphosis on pulmonary function, if any, is unclear. In a 1975 study of 22 patients by Bradford et al., half had had pulmonary function tests prior to surgical intervention (11). Only 2 of those 11 had abnormal pulmonary function. One 16-year-old had a 128° kyphosis, a vital capacity of 50% of predicted, and a maximum breathing capacity of 43%. Studies were not repeated after surgical correction in this patient. A 23 year old had a 62° deformity and a vital capacity of 65% of predicted, with a maximum breathing capacity of 56%. After surgical correction, his vital capacity increased by 400 milliliters, to 75% of predicted. Surgery did not adversely affect patients whose pulmonary function was normal preoperatively. Herndon et al. performed pulmonary function testing in 11 of their 13 patients, all of whom had normal parameters preoperatively (18). Eight of their patients were re-evaluated after surgery. Average preoperative values were 103% of predicted vital capacity and 105% of predicted total lung capacity; these figures decreased to 94% and 96% respectively after surgery, which was statistically significant. The interval of time that elapsed before postoperative pulmonary testing was not specified, however. One patient had impaired pulmonary function postoperatively, with 68% of predicted vital capacity and 75% of predicted total lung capacity. Unfortunately, this patient had not had preoperative studies. An analysis of pulmonary function in 52 patients with Scheuermann's kyphosis was performed by Murray et al. (31). The majority of patients had measurements at or above predicted values. After adjusting for age, lower inspiratory capacity was found to be related to a kyphotic curve of greater magnitude. Patients who had kyphotic curves greater than 85° had a significantly lower inspiratory capacity than did those with lesser degrees of kyphosis. The former group of patients still had scores greater than 75% of predicted, however. Murray noted in a study of the natural history that patients with kyphosis greater than 100° tended to have restrictive lung disease (31).

Conclusions

Juvenile kyphosis is a relatively common condition that responds to conservative measures in many cases. Milwaukee bracing is effective at improving the deformity in skeletally immature patients with flexible curves, although some loss of correction may be seen over time. Braces are less likely to be successful when the patient's initial curve is greater than 74° or when the patient is noncompliant with brace wear.

Surgical correction may be indicated for progressive kyphosis unresponsive to bracing in a growing child or symptomatic kyphosis measuring greater than 70°. If surgery is indicated, posterior fusion with instrumentation is generally satisfactory for skeletally immature patients, the majority of whom have flexible spines. Anterior fusion, combined with posterior fusion with instrumentation, is preferred for skeletally mature patients or for patients with stiff curves. Although Harrington compression rod instrumentation has been satisfactory in the past, newer variable hook-rod systems have good early follow-up and appear to permit greater correction. Any surgical plan must include fusion and instrumentation of all kyphotic segments. Without this, curve progression in the unfused region is likely. Complications can be significant. Back pain and clinical appearance can be improved, however, in the majority of patients symptomatic for this condition.

References

1. Ascani E, Montanaro A. Scheuermann's disease: In: Bradford DS, Hensinger RN, eds. Pediatric spine. New York: Thieme, 1985.
2. Ascani E, Salsano V, Giglio G. The incidence and early detection of spinal deformities. Ital J Orthop Traumatol 1977;3:111–117.
3. Aufdermaur M. Juvenile kyphosis (Scheuermann's disease): radiology, histology and pathogenesis. Clin Orthop 1981;154:166–174.
4. Beadle OA. The intervertebral disc. Medical Research Council, Special Report series 1931:161.
5. Blumenthal SL, Roach J, Herring JA. Lumbar Scheuermann's: a clinical series and classification. Spine 1987;12:929–932.
6. Bradford DS. Vertebral osteochondrosis (Scheuermann's kyphosis). Clin Orthop 1981;158:83–90.
7. Bradford DS, Ahmed KB, Moe JH, et al. The surgical management of patients with Scheuermann's disease. J Bone Joint Surg Am 1980;62:705–712.
8. Bradford DS, Brown DM, Moe JH, et al. Scheuermann's kyphosis: A form of osteoporosis? Clin Orthop 1976;118:10–15.
9. Bradford DS, Garcia A. Neurologic complications in Scheuermann's disease. J Bone Joint Surg Am 1969;51:567–572.
10. Bradford DS, Moe JH. Scheuermann's juvenile kyphosis: a histologic study. Clin Orthop 1975;110:45–53.
11. Bradford DS, Moe JH, Motalvo FJ, et al. Scheuermann's kyphosis: results of treatment by posterior spine arthrodesis in twenty-two patients. J Bone Joint Surg Am 1975;57:439–449.
12. Deacon P, Berkin CR, Dickson RA. Combined idiopathic kyphosis and scoliosis. J Bone Joint Surg Br 1985;67:189–192.
13. Denis F. Cotrel-Dubousset system and Scheuermann's kyphosis. Presented at the G.I.C.D. Update Course, Los Angeles, CA, December 1990.
14. DiGiovanni BF, Scoles PV, Latimer BM. Anterior extension of the thoracic vertebral bodies in Scheuermann's kyphosis. Spine 1989;14:712–16.
15. Dommisse GF. The vulnerable, rapidly growing thoracic spine of the adolescent. S Afr Med J 1990;77:211–213.
16. Findlay A, Conner AN, Connor M. Dominant inheritance of Scheuermann's juvenile kyphosis. J Med Genet 1989;26:400–402.
17. Fisk JW, Baigent ML, Hill PD. Scheuermann's disease: clinical and radiologic survey of 17 and 18 year olds. Am J Phys Med 1984;63:18–30.
18. Herndon WA, Emans JB, Micheli LJ, et al. Combined anterior and posterior fusion for Scheuermann's kyphosis. Spine 1981;6:125–130.
19. Ippolito E, Bellocci M, Montanaro A, et al. Juvenile kyphosis: An ultrastructural study. J Ped Orthop 1985;5:315–322.
20. Ippolito E, Ponseti IV. Juvenile Kyphosis. J Bone Joint Surg Am 1981;63:175–182.
21. Kemp FH, Wilson DC. Some factors in the aetiology of the osteochondritis of the spine. Br J Radiol 1947;20:410–417.
22. Klein DM, Weiss RL, Allen JE. Scheuermann's dorsal kyphosis and spinal cord compression: case report. Neurosurgery 1986;18:628–631.
23. Lonstein JE, Winter RB, Bradford DS, et al. Neurologic deficits secondary to spinal deformity. Spine 1980;5:331–355.
24. Lopez R, Burke SW, Levine DB, et al. Osteoporosis in Scheuermann's disease. Spine 1988;13:1099–1103.
25. Lowe TG. Double L-rod instrumentation in the treatment of severe kyphosis secondary to Scheuermann's disease. Spine 1987;12:336–341.
26. Lowe TG, Kasten MD. An analysis of sagittal curves and balance after Cotrel-Dubousset instrumentation for Scheuermann's disease. Spine 1994;19:1680–1685.
27. McAfee PC, Regan J, Picetti G. The incidence of complications in endoscopic anterior thoracic spinal reconstructive surgery: a prospective multicenter study comprising the first 50 consecutive cases. Presented at the 9th Annual Meeting of the North American Spine Society, Minneapolis, MN, October 1994:19–22.
28. McKenzie L, Sillence K. Familial Scheuermann's disease: a genetic and linkage study. J Med Genet 1992;29:41–45.
29. Montgomery SP, Erwin WE. Scheuermann's kyphosis! Long-term results of Milwaukee brace treatment. Spine 1981;6:5–8.
30. Morbidity and Mortality Report, Scoliosis Research Society, Dublin, Ireland. September, 1993.
31. Murray PM, Weinstein SL, Spratt KF. The natural history and long-term follow-up of Scheuermann's kyphosis. J Bone Joint Surg 1993;75(2):236–248.
32. Nerubay J, Katznelson A. Dual approach in the surgical

treatment of juvenile kyphosis. Spine 1986;11:101–102.
33. Ogilvie JW, Sherman J. Spondylosis in Scheuermann's disease. Spine 1987;12:251–253.
34. Otsuka NY, Hall JE, Mah JY. Posterior fusion for Scheuermann's kyphosis. Clin Orthop 1990;251:134–139.
35. Regan JJ, Ben-Yishay A, Crawford AH. Spinal thoracoscopy: technique evaluation. Anterior procedures for adult spinal deformity. Presented at the 9th Annual Meeting of the North American Spine Society, Minneapolis, MN, Oct. 19–22, 1994.
36. Reinhardt P, Bassett GS. Short segmental kyphosis following fusion for Scheuermann's disease. J Spinal Disord 1990;3:162–168.
37. Sachs B, Bradford D, Winter R, et al. Scheuermann's kyphosis: follow-up of Milwaukee brace treatment. J Bone Joint Surg Am 1987;69:50–58.
38. Scheuermann HW. Kyfosis dorsalis juvenilis. Ugeskr. Laeger, 1920;82:385.
39. Scoles PV, Latimer BM, DiGiovanni BD, et al. Vertebral alterations in Scheuermann's kyphosis. Spine 1991;16:509–515.
40. Schmorl G. Die Pathogenese der juvenilen Kyphose. Fortschr geb Rontgen 1930;41:359–383.
41. Shufflebarger HL, Clark C. Treatment of kyphosis using CDI. Presented at the G.I.C.D. U.S.A. Update Course on Cotrel-Dubousset instrumentation. Los Angeles, CA, December, 1990.
42. Sorensen KH. Scheuermann's juvenile kyphosis. Copenhagen: Munksgaard, 1964.
43. Speck GR, Chopin DC. The surgical treatment of Scheuermann's kyphosis. J Bone Joint Surg Br 1986;68:189–193.
44. Stambough JL, VanLoveren HR, Cheeks ML. Spinal cord compression in Scheuermann's kyphosis: case report. Neurosurgery 1992;30:127–130.
45. Sturm PF, Dobson JC, Armstrong WGD. The surgical management of Scheuermann's disease. Spine 1993;18:685–691.
46. Taylor TC, Wenger DR, Stephen J, et al. Surgical management of thoracic kyphosis in adolescents. J Bone Joint Surg Am 1979;61:496–503.
47. Wilcox PG, Spencer CW. Dorsolumbar kyphosis or Scheuermann's disease. Clin Sports Med 1986;5:343–351.
48. Yablon JS, Kasdon DL, Levine H. Thoracic cord compression in Scheuermann's disease. Spine 1988;13:896–898.

CHAPTER TWELVE

Lumbar Spondylolisthesis

Chun-sing Yu and Steven R. Garfin

Introduction

Spondylolisthesis is the forward displacement of a vertebral body on the one below it. It is derived from the Greek word "olisthanein," which means "to slip." The diagnosis of lumbar spondylolisthesis usually is made on plain radiography in the course of evaluating a patient with low back pain and/or leg pain. Subsequent management depends on the age of the patient, the severity of symptoms, the pathogenesis and natural history of the slip, and assessing the risk:benefit ratio of the available treatment modalities.

Classification

The widely used classification described here, originally proposed by Wiltse et al., is based on etiology and anatomy. It is clinically useful as a guide to treatment and prognosis (135).

Congenital Spondylolisthesis

Congenital spondylolisthesis is defined as spondylolisthesis that occurs at the level of a congenital vertebral abnormality. Wiltse and Rothman distinguish 3 subtypes (136):

Subtype A

In this subtype, the L5-S1 facet joints are dysplastic and axially (horizontally) oriented (Fig. 12.1). Hence, they are unable to resist forward translation of L5 on S1 when the lumbosacral spine is subject to the loads of an erect posture.

Subtype B

In this subtype, the facet joints are malorientated in the sagittal plane so that they are almost parallel to each other (facet tropism) (Fig. 12.2). Again, the ability of the facet joints to resist forward translational forces is diminished.

Subtype C

In this subtype, other congenital anomalies of the spine, such as a hemivertebra and/or congenital kyphosis, predispose to spondylolisthesis (107, 139).

Isthmic Spondylolisthesis

In isthmic spondylolisthesis, bilateral defects of the pars interarticularis effectively "disconnect" the inferior articular processes from the superior articular processes and pedicles, thus allowing the latter vertebral elements and the attached vertebral body to translate forward. Three subtypes are distinguished, based on the pathogenesis and nature of the pars defect:

Subtype A

In this subtype, a break exists in the pars interarticularis (spondylolysis) (Fig. 12.3) that is caused by

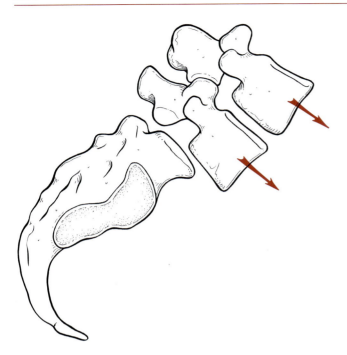

FIGURE 12.1.
Congenital spondylolisthesis. Axially oriented facet joints.

repeated episodes of relatively minor trauma (fatigue fracture) (137). An inherited weakness in the pars is suggested by the high incidence of spondylolysis seen in some families. This subtype represents the most common form of spondylolisthesis.

Subtype B

In this subtype, repeated occurrence and healing of spondylolysis, in association with gradual forward slippage of the vertebral body, results in the formation of an elongated, but intact, pars.

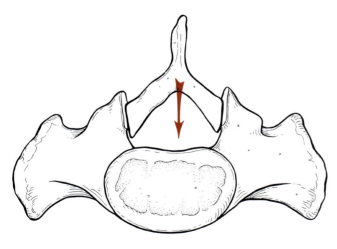

FIGURE 12.2.
Congenital spondylolisthesis. Sagittally maloriented facet joints.

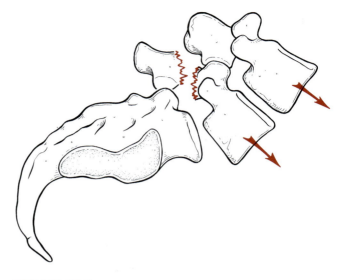

FIGURE 12.3.
Isthmic spondylolisthesis.

Subtype C

Rarely, severe trauma can cause an isolated acute fracture of the pars (25).

Degenerative Spondylolisthesis

Degenerative changes in the facet joints and intervertebral disc allow mild forward slippage of the superior vertebra to occur. The pars interarticularis is intact. The extent of slippage usually does not exceed 30%.

Traumatic Spondylolisthesis

Severe trauma can cause fractures of parts of the vertebra other than the pars, notably the articular processes and the pedicles (135). Forward slippage of the affected vertebra occurs gradually. This type is to be distinguished from an acute fracture-dislocation, although the structural defects may be almost the same.

Pathologic Spondylolisthesis

Disorders of bone and/or soft tissue weaken the stabilizing structures of the spine and predispose to spondylolisthesis. Generalized disorders that may lead to spondylolisthesis include arthrogryposis, osteopetrosis, Marfan's syndrome, and osteogenesis imperfecta (119, 140). Localized disorders include varying types and degrees of infection and tumor.

Post-surgical Spondylolisthesis

During posterior decompressive surgery of the spine, excessive resection of the facet joints may destabilize the corresponding vertebral segment and allow gradual forward slippage to occur, unless fusion of the affected segment is concomitantly performed.

Natural History

Congenital Spondylolisthesis

Congenital spondylolisthesis is uncommon and accounts for 14 to 21% of spondylolisthesis cases (14, 80). The female:male ratio is approximately 2:1 (135). The presence, or absence, of an intact neural arch can determine the natural history and clinical presentation of congenital spondylolisthesis. If there is no spina bifida, or just a narrow spina bifida in the presence of a normal pars, slip progression beyond 25 to 35% can cause significant cauda equina compression (135, 136). Severe hamstring tightness and altered gait are then likely to result, as well as bowel and/or bladder dysfunction. If there is a wide spina bifida and/or an associated pars defect, slippage tends to occur earlier and to become more severe, but with relatively less hamstring spasm and neurologic disturbance.

Subtype A

This subtype is associated frequently with a wide spina bifida. The slip occurs in childhood and can become severe during the adolescent growth spurt, the period in which the patient usually presents (136).

Subtype B

The slip is usually mild and symptoms occur in adulthood (136).

Isthmic Spondylolisthesis

Isthmic spondylolisthesis is the most common form of spondylolisthesis. Approximately 50 to 70% of patients with spondylolysis develop spondylolisthesis (34, 137). The female:male ratio is about 1:2, which is reversed from the congenital type (34, 122).

Fredrickson et al. prospectively studied 500 randomly selected first grade students for 20 to 25 years (34). They found a 4.4% incidence of spondylolysis at age 6 years. By adulthood, this incidence had increased to 6%, although only 34% of the original 500 patients were available for follow-up at age 18. No patient with a pars defect was lost to follow-up once the defect was discovered. The male:female ratio was 2:1 at age 6 and remained the same into adulthood. The vast majority of cases involved the fifth lumbar vertebra. Most pars defects occurred bilaterally. Two patients with unilateral defects subsequently developed bilateral defects. Healing of the spondylolysis was demonstrated in only one patient, a 6-year-old girl with a unilateral defect at L5, which healed sometime between the ages of 12 and 28. Spondylolisthesis occurred in 13 of the 19 patients whose pars defects were detected at age 6, and in 20 of the 27 adults with pars defects. It did not develop in patients with a unilateral defect.

In most patients, the slip was detected at about the same time that the pars defect was demonstrated. The overall amount of slip did not exceed 30% in any of the young patients. Progression of slip was uncommon, with the largest change occurring during the early teenage years. The average increase was 16% in males and 14% in females. Only 4 of the 27 patients with spondylolysis had low back pain during follow-up. Subsequently, one patient underwent laminectomy and discectomy for a herniated disc. Spina bifida occulta occurred more frequently in patients with a pars defect than in those without a defect.

In an ancillary study, the radiographs of 500 normal neonates were reviewed. Because the pars interarticularis is cartilaginous in the neonate, only a spondylolisthesis, if present, could be demonstrated. However, no such cases were found.

Genetic Factors

Inheritance plays a significant role in the development of spondylolysis, but the specific mode of inheritance is unknown. Wynne-Davies and Scott radiographically surveyed the first-degree relatives of 35 patients with pars defects and found that 15% were affected similarly (142). Interestingly, the incidence was even higher (33%) among first-degree relatives of 12 patients with congenital spondylolisthesis. Albanese and Pizzutillo made similar findings in 222 first-degree relatives of 70 index patients with pars defects (1). They also found a high incidence (61%) of spina bifida occulta in the index patients.

There are variations in the incidence of spondylolysis and spondylolisthesis among different races. Stewart reported a 50 to 60% incidence in Eskimos (117). Rowe and Roche found an incidence of 6.4% in white American men, 2.8% in black men, 2.3% in white women, and 1.1% in black women (94).

Enviromental Factors

The development of spondylolysis and spondylolisthesis in a genetically predisposed individual appears to occur only in the presence of the appropriate environmental influences. A pars defect at birth has never been found on gross and histologic examination of stillborn infants (6, 94). Rarely, spondylolisthesis has been reported in infants (12). Pars defects almost invariably occur only after walking begins, suggesting that an erect posture increases stress on the pars.

Spondylolysis is more common in gymnasts, football players, and other athletes (9, 55, 74). Activities that require repeated hyperextension of the spine likely place excessive stress on the pars.

Patients who have excessive lumbar lordosis caused by disorders such as spastic diplegia and Scheuermann's kyphosis are also at increased risk of spondylolysis (44, 84). Nonambulatory patients, however, do not develop the lesion (93).

Slip Progression

It is presently not possible to reliably predict future slip progression based on clinical and radiologic parameters (27, 105). In most cases, the amount of displacement initially detected remains relatively static (27, 96, 105). The factors that predispose to the severe slips seen in some patients are unknown.

Progression, if it does occur, usually takes place during the growth spurt of early puberty (ages 9 to 12 in girls, 11 to 14 in boys) (8, 34, 77, 105). Patients with higher slips (greater than 20 to 30%) at initial diagnosis have been reported to have a higher risk of slip progression (8, 77, 105, 133). Although female gender and spina bifida are associated more frequently with severe slips, they are of no statistical value in predicting slip progression (8, 14, 27, 105, 106).

Pregnancy does not increase significantly the risk of slip progression, nor do severe slips significantly increase the risk of complications during pregnancy (97).

Saraste et al. found the lumbar index (a measure of L5 vertebral body wedging) to be valuable in predicting slip progression, but other authors have disagreed (34, 96, 105).

Risk of Symptoms

Most patients with spondylolysis or mild spondylolisthesis are asymptomatic (34). Saraste found that the risk of low back pain and sciatica was higher in patients with at least 15 mm of slippage than in those with less than 15 mm of slippage (98). Additionally, patients with L4 spondylolysis had significantly greater intensity and frequency of low back pain compared with patients with L5 spondylolysis (95). Other authors have found that the risk of back pain does not increase with higher grades of spondylolisthesis (40, 122).

Clinical Evaluation

Complete evaluation involves obtaining a thorough history and physical examination followed by radiographic and other studies, if indicated. Because most patients present with back pain and/or leg pain, the initial part of the evaluation should be as for any patient who presents with these symptoms. Characteristic clinical features of patients with spondylolisthesis are described below.

Presenting Complaints

Back Pain

Back pain is the most common presenting symptom (122). It is typically mechanical in nature, i.e., it is intermittent, aggravated by strenuous activity and relieved with rest. If this symptom persists for more than 1 to 2 weeks in a child, an organic cause should be excluded. Hensinger, in a study of 100 skeletally immature patients who had back pain for at least 2 months, found that 18 had an infection or a tumor (52). In addition, 66 patients had evidence of occult fracture, spondylolysis, spondylolisthesis, kyphosis, or scoliosis.

Leg Pain

Leg pain is uncommon (in children and adolescents), and is usually referred from the back (122). The pain occurs in the buttocks and posterior thighs, but does not go below the knees. Occasionally, adolescents may report pain only in the greater trochanteric area (131). In adults, however, leg pain is a frequent complaint and may be sciatic or claudicant in nature (26).

Neurologic Symptoms

Radicular symptoms (pain, numbness, and/or paraesthesia in a dermatomal distribution) are more common in the adult patient. Rarely, severe spondylolisthesis can give rise to significant leg weakness and sphincter disturbances secondary to cauda equina compression (81).

Abnormal Posture/Gait

Some patients are first brought to medical attention because of postural and/or gait abnormalities.

Physical Findings

Local Signs

Tenderness may be elicited by deep palpation of the spinous process above the level of slip (typically the L4 spinous process in a lumbosacral slip). A spinous process step-off can often be felt immediately above the level of higher grade slips (grade 2 or higher). Paravertebral muscle spasm can accompany symptomatic spondylolisthesis and limit forward flexion of the trunk.

Hamstring Tightness

Hamstring tightness can develop regardless of the grade of slip but is more commonly associated with severe slips (5, 81). It is manifested as diminished straight leg raising and limited forward flexion of the trunk. This finding is believed to represent either an attempt by the body to control the unstable spondylolisthetic level (typically L5-S1), or an attempt to rotate the pelvis into a more vertical position to help restore the patient's center of gravity (5, 81). A herniated disc in association with spondylolisthesis may also give rise to similar symptoms (positive straight leg raising interpreted as hamstring tightness).

Lumbosacral Kyphosis

Bony remodeling at the L5-S1 junction frequently occurs in severe slips (grade III or higher) that have been present for a while. The L5 body becomes wedge-shaped and the superior part of the S1 body becomes dome-shaped. This allows L5 to rotate antero-inferiorly over S1, producing a kyphotic deformity at the lumbosacral junction (Fig. 12.4). This deformity pushes the body's center of gravity anterior to the hip joints. To stand upright, the patient has to rely on several compensatory mechanisms. These mechanisms include contracting the hamstrings to rotate the pelvis into a more vertical position, increasing the lordosis of the upper lumbar spine, and flexing the hips and knees.

Lumbosacral kyphosis also makes the iliac wings appear wider and the buttocks appear flat, producing the characteristic heart-shaped pelvis when viewed posteriorly.

Trunk Shortening

Trunk shortening is caused by the combination of L5 slipping antero-inferiorly, lumbosacral kyphosis, and compensatory lumbar hyperlordosis. It is associated with loss of the waist line and the appearance of anterior and flank creases in the abdominal wall. In very high grade slips, the lower rib cage may even abut the iliac crests.

Gait Abnormalities

An abnormal gait may be observed (in patients with severe slips), characterized by flexed hips and knees, a shortened stride, and a wide base of support (5, 81).

Neurologic Deficits

The nerve roots exiting adjacent to a pars defect (typically the L5 roots in L5-S1 spondylolisthesis) can be compressed by three pathologic structures: 1) the hypertrophic fibrocartilage that fills the defect; 2) osteophytes arising adjacent to the defect; and 3) degenerative hypertrophic facets caudal to the defect (32, 40, 133). In addition, the sacral roots can be stretched as they pass over the postero-superior corner of the sacrum in L5-S1 spondylolisthesis. In severe slips, this stretching can potentially give rise to bladder and bowel dysfunction.

Imaging Studies

The initial films for evaluating a patient with suspected spinal pathology include anteroposterior (AP) and lateral radiographs of the lumbosacral spine. The upper lumbar spine should also be included in the radiographic evaluation (69). Because most cases of spondylolysis occur in the lower two lumbar segments, there is a tendency to miss lesions in the upper lumbar spine.

Although a significant hereditary component is present in congenital and isthmic spondylolisthesis, routine radiographic screening of asymptomatic family members is not recommended.

Anteroposterior Radiograph

In severe slips, the L5 vertebra can be viewed end-on through the sacrum, giving the so-called "upside-down Napoleon's hat" sign (Fig. 12.5). Other associated findings include spina bifida occulta, scoliosis, and lumbarization or sacralization.

Lateral Radiograph

The severity of spondylolisthesis is measured on the lateral radiograph. To reliably measure the radiographic parameters of spondylolisthesis, it is neces-

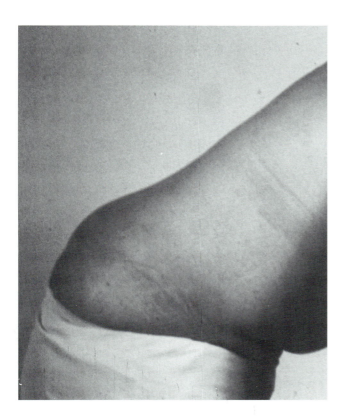

FIGURE 12.4.
Severe spondylolisthesis. Prominent lumbosacral kyphosis on forward flexion of the trunk.

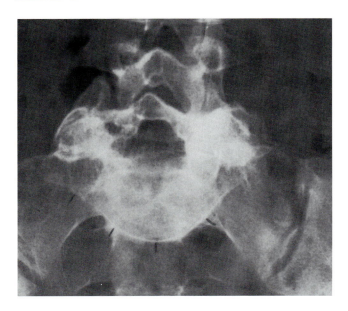

FIGURE 12.5.
Severe spondylolisthesis. Anteroposterior radiograph demonstrating upside-down Napoleon's hat sign.

sary to obtain a standing lateral radiograph focused at the level of the slip (Fig. 12.6). Lowe et al. have found that 26% of their 50 patients with spondylolisthesis or bilateral spondylolysis demonstrated more than a 2-mm increase in displacement when standing radiographs were compared with supine radiographs (68).

Displacement and angulation are the two most widely used radiographic parameters for describing the severity of spondylolisthesis.

Displacement

Meyerding's method of measuring displacement divides the antero-posterior diameter of the upper surface of the inferior vertebral body into four quarters (Fig. 12.7) (78). Slippage of the superior vertebral body is then graded as I, II, III, or IV for anterior displacements of one, two, three, or four quarters, respectively. Taillard's method is more precise (120). It measures anterior displacement of the superior vertebral body as a percentage of the AP diameter of the upper surface of the inferior vertebral body (Fig. 12.7). Other authors have proposed various methods to overcome measurement difficulties caused by bony remodeling and osteophyte formation (14, 138). Displacement is considered severe if it is grade III or higher (50% or more).

Angulation

Angulation refers to the angular relationship between the L5 and S1 vertebrae, and it quantifies lumbosacral kyphosis. It is also referred to as slip angle or sagittal rotation. Amundson et al. have described a modification of the method proposed by Speck et

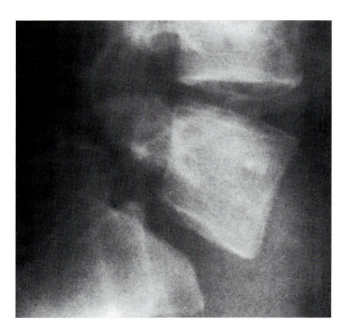

FIGURE 12.6.
Isthmic spondylolisthesis. Lateral standing radiograph focused at L5-S1. Arrows indicate spondylolytic defect.

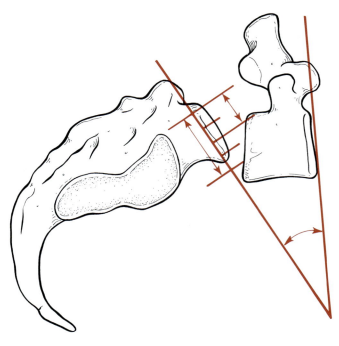

FIGURE 12.7.
Displacement: Meyerding's method of measuring anteroposterior displacement. Displacement: Taillard's method of measuring anteroposterior displacement. Angulation: Amundson's method of measuring lumbosacral kyphosis.

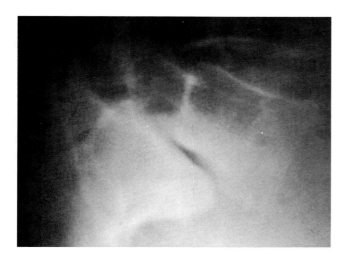

FIGURE 12.8.
Longstanding spondylolisthesis. Disc space narrowing at L5-S1 and osteophyte formation at the posteroinferior corner of the L5 body.

al. (3, 111). It involves measuring the angle formed between a line drawn along the superior endplate of L5 and the perpendicular of a line drawn along the posterior cortex of the S1 and S2 vertebral bodies (Fig. 12.7). A high slip angle (especially if greater than 40 to 50°) is associated with potentially greater instability, greater risk of slip progression, and lower chances of successful surgery (obtaining a solid fusion and good functional results) (14).

Adaptive Changes

In severe L5-S1 spondylolisthesis, bony remodeling results in a trapezoidal L5 body and a dome-shaped cranial surface of S1. In long-standing spondylolisthesis, disc degeneration leads to disc space narrowing at the involved segment (Fig. 12.8). Some slip progression usually occurs as the disc space narrows, but ultimately this process, with its associated osteophyte formation, has the effect of stabilizing the spine.

Oblique Radiographs

If spondylolysis is suspected, but the lateral radiograph is equivocal, oblique views can be obtained. These views classically demonstrate the pars defect as a break in the "neck" of the "Scottie dog" (Fig. 12.9). Technical expertise is required for producing good oblique views.

Dynamic Radiographs

The role of dynamic radiographs in the evaluation of spondylolisthesis has not been established. Traction-compression radiographs, as described by Friberg,

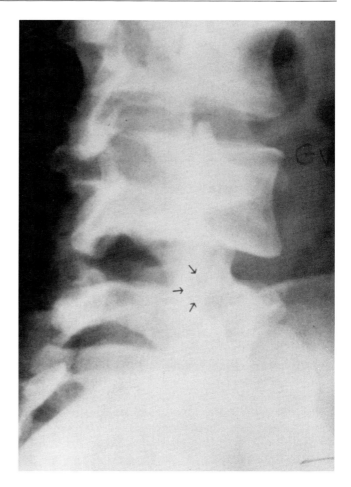

FIGURE 12.9.
Spondylolysis. Oblique radiograph demonstrating break in the "Scottie dog's neck" (arrows).

were shown to be more sensitive than flexion-extension radiographs or standing-recumbent radiographs in detecting translatory motion in spondylolisthesis (35, 59). Patients with symptomatic spondylolisthesis have greater amounts of translatory motion (6.7 ± 3.7 mm) than those with asymptomatic spondylolisthesis (1.9 ± 2 mm) (36). Roentgen stereophotogrammetry is highly accurate and sensitive in the detection of intervertebral motion but has practical limitations in a clinical setting.

Radionuclide Scanning

Some patients with back pain and spondylolysis demonstrate increased activity at the pars defect on technetium bone scanning (124). This finding is believed to indicate ongoing healing of the pars defect and suggests that such patients may benefit from a period of immobilization. However, there is a lack of evidence to support this proposed role for radionuclide scanning.

Single photon emission computerized tomographic (SPECT) scanning has been compared with plain bone scanning and found to be more sensitive in detecting increased activity in symptomatic patients with spondylolysis and/or spondylolisthesis (24). It permits more accurate localization of the area of increased activity. However, the activity on SPECT scanning varies with the duration of spondylolysis and the grade of spondylolisthesis (70).

Myelography

Myelography has become less popular because of its invasive nature and the availability of more informative imaging modalities, such as CT and MRI.

Computerized Tomography (CT)

Computerized tomography has been useful in the diagnosis and evaluation of spondylolysis and spondylolisthesis (Fig. 12.10). Teplick et al. have described a number of characteristic CT features of spondylolysis that permit its recognition, even though this lesion can sometimes be difficult to distinguish from the adjacent facet joint (121). The most helpful feature is the location of the pars defect on the CT slice just cephalad to the neural foramina. Normally, this slice shows the pedicles and lamina forming an intact ring.

CT can demonstrate specific sites of neural compression in patients with neurologic problems (73). Although the neural elements are better defined if CT scanning is combined with myelography, this has the disadvantage of being invasive.

CT can also demonstrate other co-existing pathology (e.g., herniated disc, degenerative stenosis) at the same or another level.

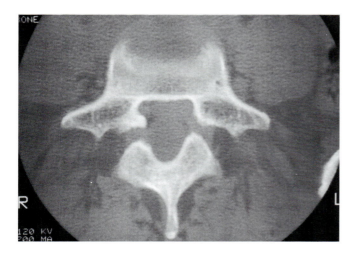

FIGURE 12.10.
Spondylolysis. Axial CT scan demonstrating breaks in the pars interarticularis (arrows).

Magnetic Resonance Imaging (MRI)

With the increasing availability and capabilities of MRI, as well as greater experience in its use and interpretation, this modality may replace CT for the indications listed previously.

Sagittal T1-weighted images can best demonstrate spondylolysis, spondylolisthesis, and any associated nerve root impingement within the neural foramina (57). Axial images, however, can be indeterminate or misleading.

Nonoperative Treatment

For the asymptomatic patient with spondylolysis or mild spondylolisthesis, no activity restriction or treatment is recommended (134). For the asymptomatic patient with spondylolisthesis of grade III or higher, activity restriction and even surgical treatment has been recommended, although no general agreement exists.

Symptomatic patients should initially be treated nonoperatively if the following criteria are met: 1) slip is less than 50 percent; 2) slip is not progressive; and 3) neurologic deficits are absent.

Rest, activity restriction, and short-term pain or anti-inflammatory medication form the mainstays of nonoperative treatment. Normal activities can be resumed when symptoms have resolved. If symptoms are severe, the use of a corset, brace, or body cast may be beneficial (7, 116). Physical therapy is recommended to improve the flexibility of tight hamstrings and, more importantly, the strength of deconditioned back muscles. Sinaki et al. found that flexion back strengthening exercises were more effective than extension exercises in relieving symptoms related to spondylolisthesis (109).

Nonoperative treatment is successful in the vast majority of patients with symptomatic spondylolysis or mild spondylolisthesis (9, 89).

Operative Treatment

The goals of operative treatment for spondylolysis and/or spondylolisthesis should include: 1) relief of back pain and leg pain; 2) restoration of spinal stability; 3) recovery of neurologic deficit; and 4) improvement of posture and gait.

Indications

Operative treatment can be considered in the following situations:

1. Failure of nonoperative treatment to provide significant long-term relief of the patient's symptoms
2. Significant or progressive neurologic deficit
3. Slip of 50% or greater

4. Documented slip progression beyond 25 to 50%
5. Associated development and progression of a scoliosis that is typical for spondylolisthesis (long "C"-shaped curve originating at L5)

With the exception of significant or progressive neurologic deficit, none of the other indications should be considered as absolute. Selection of surgical candidates should also take into account the age of the patient and the risk-benefit ratio of surgery. In adult patients especially, it can be difficult to attribute chronic low back pain to spondylolysis or spondylolisthesis.

Classification of Operative Techniques

The various operations that have been described for spondylolysis and/or spondylolisthesis can be classified into the following broad categories: 1) pars defect repair; 2) decompression without fusion; 3) fusion in situ; 4) closed reduction; and 5) open reduction.

Pars Defect Repair

Repair of the pars defect has been proposed for spondylolysis and Grade I isthmic spondylolisthesis to avoid fusing the involved intervertebral motion segment. It consists of local bone grafting of the pars defect and the use of a screw or wires to achieve reduction and fixation of the defect. Buck's technique involves the insertion of a screw across the pars defect (18). Morscher et al. developed a hook-screw device (79). Scott proposed wire fixation of the transverse processes to the spinous process of the same vertebra (17, 82). So far, the reported series have been retrospective and contain relatively small numbers of patients (17, 42, 79, 82, 86, 92, 141). They suggest that pars defect repair benefits relatively young patients who have not yet developed disc degeneration. Patients with degenerated discs are believed to be at risk for persistent back pain despite successful pars fusion (17).

Decompression Without Fusion

Laminectomy was the first operation reported for spondylolisthesis (64). Later, Gill et al. described excision of the loose lamina and decompression of the nerve roots by removal of the hypertrophic fibrocartilage in the pars defect (40). They performed this operation in 18 adult patients in whom the most common mechanism of pain was believed to be L5 nerve root compression. After long-term follow-up of 43 patients, it was concluded that in adults, postoperative slip progression occurred in relatively few patients, was limited, and did not necessarily cause symptoms (39, 41). Despite having only two children in their series, Gill and White thought that their procedure did not contribute to postoperative slip progression in younger patients.

Davis and Bailey found that patients with minimal or no arthritic changes (disc space narrowing, endplate sclerosis, hypertrophic bone formation) at the level of the spondylolysis or spondylolisthesis had better postoperative results than patients with moderate to severe arthritic changes (28).

Osterman et al. performed decompression without fusion in patients less than 20 years old only if they had neurologic symptoms and total slippage (they believed that the totally olisthetic vertebra was usually stable) (87). They recommended that surgical treatment for patients less than 30 years old should consist of posterior or posterolateral fusion, with concomitant decompression only if neurologic symptoms or signs were present. Decompression without fusion was mainly indicated for patients over 40 years old with nerve root symptoms. The authors noted a deterioration in their initial results when 75 patients were reevaluated 5 or more years after surgery. Slip progression was noted in 27% of the patients, although this did not affect the clinical results of surgery. Poorer outcomes occurred mostly in patients who demonstrated increasing disc degeneration.

Vestad and Naes also found that the extent of postoperative slip progression did not correlate with symptom relief (128). In their series, there was a 30% failure rate in patients who underwent decompression alone compared with 6% in patients who had concomitant fusion.

Fusion In Situ

POSTEROLATERAL FUSION

Posterolateral fusion is the most widely used surgical treatment for spondylolisthesis. It refers to fusion of the "lateral gutters," which consist of the transverse processes, articular processes, and/or sacral ala (130). In children and adolescents, a high rate of success in achieving solid fusion (80 to 100%) and symptomatic relief (80 to 100%) has been reported in many studies, even for patients with severe slips (45, 66, 90, 134).

In adults, however, the results of posterolateral fusion in situ are less satisfactory. The reported fusion rate in adults varies between 67 and 100%, and is lower than that for adolescents with the same degree of slip (62, 88, 112, 123). Haraldsson and Willner found that only 57% of their adult patients, as opposed to 95% of their teen-aged patients, were completely free of symptoms postoperatively (45). All their patients had radiographically solid fusions. Hanley and Levy (43) analyzed variables affecting results in the surgical treatment of 50 patients with grade I to III spondylolisthesis. The factors associated with an unsatisfactory outcome included compensation cases, pseudarthrosis, middle age, male gender, smoking, and radicular symptoms.

In general, for L5-S1 spondylolisthesis, a single level fusion is adequate. However, for 50% or greater slippage, an L4-S1 fusion is recommended because it offers a better mechanical advantage when healed, and the L5 transverse processes are technically difficult to access in high grade slips (134).

Postoperative slip progression can occur despite radiographically solid fusion, especially in patients with severe slips. The amount of progression is usually small (up to 1 Meyerding grade) and ceases after the second postoperatve year (14, 26, 49, 58, 104).

Concomitant decompression of the cauda equina and affected nerve roots has been recommended for patients who show evidence of neurologic compromise, including motor, reflex and sensory changes, tight hamstrings, and gait abnormalities (87, 122, 126). However, other authors believe that decompression is seldom indicated and that solid fusion of the unstable segment is sufficient for neural recovery (13, 14, 134). It is thought that stabilization eliminates abnormal stretching and irritation of the nerve roots. It has also been suggested that the fibrocartilage mass at the pars defect decreases in size after successful fusion (134). Despite the controversy, it is generally agreed that neural deompression is indicated in patients with bladder and bowel dysfunction or with a motor deficit that affects normal walking (14). It is also strongly indicated in patients with congenital spondylolisthesis who have an intact neural arch. In such a situation, the L5 lamina slides forward and compresses the cauda equina against the posterosuperior aspect of the body of S1. These patients can have severe hamstring tightness that may not resolve after in situ fusion alone. They are also at risk of developing a cauda equina syndrome.

Decompression may increase the risk of slip progression during the healing period of the fusion mass, particularly in patients with severe slips (13, 134). In such cases, it is necessary to consider prolonged bed rest, cast or brace immobilization, and/or internal fixation.

Although neurologic complications are rare with fusion in situ and/or decompression by the posterior approach, there are reports of cauda equina deficits after these procedures in patients with severe spondylolisthesis (72, 102). The cause is believed to be related to the transmission of forces exerted during decortication with mallet and osteotome (72).

The use of various pedicular screw fixation devices has been advocated to improve the clinical results and union rate after posterolateral fusion in situ for spondylolysis and spondylolisthesis (11, 67, 114). However, in a prospective randomized study by McGuire and Amundson, no statistically significant increase in the fusion rate was demonstrated when plate and pedicle screw fixation was added to decompression and posterolateral fusion for patients with grade I and II spondylolisthesis (75).

POSTERIOR FUSION

Posterior fusion essentially consists of fusion of the laminae and/or spinous processes by a variety of techniques (2, 13, 53). The facet joints may be fused as well (53). Symptomatic relief is reported in 65 to 95% of patients, with solid fusion obtained in 60 to 100% (49, 58, 65, 118, 122). Despite these results, the procedure is presently not popular because it necessitates extending the fusion to include the vertebra above the spondylolisthetic vertebra. This occurs because fusing to the loose posterior element of the spondylolytic vertebra will not afford fixation of the anterior elements.

POSTERIOR INTERBODY FUSION

Cloward described the use of posterior lumbar interbody fusion (PLIF) in the treatment of spondylolisthesis (23). The technique involved complete removal of the neural arch and intervertebral disc at the spondylolisthetic level, distraction of the disc space by means of a "vertebra spreader," and insertion of multiple corticocancellous bone grafts into the disc space. Of 93 patients surveyed, 89% were completely free of back and leg pain at 4 to 30 years postoperatively. However, solid bony fusion was radiographically demonstrated in only 71% of 97 patients. Despite the biomechanical advantages, this technique has not been popular because of its relative difficulty (101). An attempt to simplify the procedure by using only two tricortical bone grafts and no disc space distraction produced dismal results (127).

For patients with severe L5-S1 spondylolisthesis and spondyloptosis, Bohlman has described the insertion of a fibular dowel graft from the posterior aspect of the sacrum, across the L5-S1 disc space, into the L5 body (10). A bilateral posterolateral fusion is performed at the same time. This method provides stable fixation without instrumentation and also avoids the need to fuse to L4 in such cases. The potential complications include graft dislodgement, sacral fracture, and neurovascular injury.

ANTERIOR FUSION

In 1932, Capener suggested that the ideal operation for the prevention of slipping in spondylolisthesis would be an anterior interbody fusion but thought that the operation would be technically impossible (21). In the following year, however, Burns recorded the first anterior interbody fusion for spondylolisthesis (20).

Anterior interbody fusion for spondylolisthesis can be done either with strut grafts inserted into the decorticated disc space, or with a fibular dowel graft inserted through the L5 vertebral body, across the disc space, and into the body of S1. Anterior lumbosacral console fusion, as described by Verbiest, consists essentially of placing tibial cortical grafts and cancellous bone between the inferior surface of a severely slipped L5 body and the anterior surface of the sacrum (126).

Many studies on the use of anterior interbody fusion in spondylolisthesis have included patients with different types and grades of spondylolisthesis and some who have had previous posterior surgery (38, 61, 125, 132). These studies report a fusion rate of 86 to 96% and a clinical success rate of 69 to 100%. Cheng et al. however, studied 20 adult patients with spondylolysis or mild isthmic spondylolisthesis and no previous surgery. They reported a solid fusion rate of 75%, with 95% having excellent or satisfactory clinical results (22).

Using anterior lumbosacral fusion in 11 patients with severe spondylolisthesis, Verbiest was able to achieve solid fusion in 10 patients and freedom from symptoms and signs in 9 (126).

Reduction of Spondylolisthesis

Reduction of severe spondylolisthesis and spondyloptosis is an attractive concept in terms of anatomy, biomechanics, and cosmesis. The potential advantages of reducing the spondylolisthetic deformity include: 1) preservation of adjacent uninvolved motion segments by reducing the need to fuse to these levels in severe slips; 2) prevention of slip progression and enhancement of graft union by reducing the tensile and bending forces working against the fusion mass; 3) restoration of body posture and mechanics by correcting lumbosacral kyphosis and height loss; 4) improvement of appearance and self-image; and 5) decompression of neural structures by relieving stretch over the postero-superior aspect of the caudal vertebral body.

Because of these substantial advantages, much attention has been focused on the development of techniques to achieve reduction safely and to maintain the resultant correction with the least possible morbidity.

Bradford has suggested the following criteria for the selection of candidates for reduction of spondylolisthesis: 1) slippage of greater than 60%; 2) slip angle greater than 50°; 3) symptoms uncontrollable by nonoperative means; and 4) between 12 and 30 years of age (16). He did not consider previously failed posterior surgery to be a contraindication to reduction.

Closed Reduction

Closed reduction refers to the use of primarily external devices to achieve reduction. The procedure can be initiated either before or after the fusion operation.

Scherb, in 1921, was the first to report the reduction of spondylolisthesis. He managed to achieve intraoperative reduction by manually repositioning a very mobile L5 in a 14-year-old girl (100). Unilateral posterior fusion with a unicortical tibial autograft was then performed and reduction was reported to be maintained at one year.

Jenkins, in 1936, described the use of longitudinal traction and a pelvic sling to achieve partial reduction (56). An anterior interbody fusion with a tibial dowel was subsequently performed.

Harris, in 1951, reported the use of longitudinal femoral pin traction combined with anterior traction through anterior iliac crest tongs to flex and translate the sacrum (50). Traction was applied both before and after posterolateral fusion. The iliac crest tongs were subsequently incorporated in a pantaloon cast for 3 months. Lance later used Steinmann pins instead of tongs for improved iliac fixation (63). He also described neural decompression by removing the posterior prominence of the body of the first sacral vertebra.

Scaglietti et al. used serial plaster casts to achieve and maintain reduction. Reduction was achieved by: 1) applying longitudinal traction to the spinal column; 2) hyperextending the hips to rotate the pelvis and thus correcting lumbosacral kyphosis; and 3) pushing the sacrum anteriorly by direct pressure (99). In 6 patients below 20 years of age, serial plaster casting was applied for at least 4 months before posterior fusion by the Hibbs' method. In 14 patients older than 20 years, preoperative serial casting was applied for 3 to 4 weeks. The authors believed that progressive reduction over a prolonged period was necessary to allow the lumbosacral neurovascular structures to adapt themselves to their new anatomic relationships. The authors subsequently found that posterior fusion without instrumentation resulted in loss of reduction of up to 50% despite 10 months of postoperative cast protection. Hence, internal fixation was added to help achieve and maintain reduction.

Snijder et al. believed that preoperative reduction was unnecessary and described the use of a traction apparatus using wires through the spinous processes to achieve reduction (110). This apparatus was spring-loaded and mounted on a modified Milwaukee brace. The patient remained in bed until an anterior interbody fusion was considered solid.

McPhee and O'Brien described the use of halofemoral traction after laminectomy and alar-transverse fusion (76). This was followed by an anterior interbody fusion. O'Brien et al. later reviewed the long-term results of this technique in 22 patients and reported that 20 patients were asymptomatic and only 2 had lost their reduction (83).

Ohki et al. combined halo-pelvic or halo-femoral traction with spinous process traction wiring and an anterior interbody fusion (85). They achieved sound fusion with complete remission of symptoms in all five of their patients.

Bradford reviewed the use of various closed reduction techniques with posterolateral fusion in 22 patients (15). He was able to obtain a two-thirds reduction in average slip angle but could not change appreciably the slip percentage.

Burkus et al. compared the results of in situ posterolateral fusion with those of posterolateral fusion followed by closed reduction using the technique of Scaglietti et al. (19, 99). They found that reduction did not result in increased functional capability, improved cosmetic appearance, or neurologic improvement. However, patients who were reduced had a decreased rate of late progression of the lumbosacral deformity. They also had a lower rate of pseudarthrosis, although this finding was not statistically significant.

Closed reduction techniques have the disadvantages of prolonged bed rest and immobilization, frequent failure to achieve or maintain satisfactory correction, and significant risk of neurologic injury. In general, reduction is maintained more reliably by anterior fusion than by posterolateral fusion.

Open Reduction

Open reduction refers to the use of an intraoperative device to achieve reduction. The reduction device may or may not be a part of an instrumentation system used for internal fixation.

Operations involving open reduction can be classified into: 1) posterior procedures; and 2) combined anterior-posterior procedures.

Posterior Procedures

Harrington and Tullos, in 1969, were probably the first to report the open reduction of spondylolisthesis (47). In two teen-aged patients with severe spondylolisthesis, they placed distraction rods and hooks between the L1 laminae and a transiliac sacral bar. Reduction occurred spontaneously upon the application of distraction. The rods were then wired to pedicle screws inserted into L5. Their technique was able to achieve nearly complete correction of slippage but caused transient cauda equina syndrome in one patient. Later modifications to their original technique included placement of the sacral bar anterior to the spinal canal, omission of the pedicle screws, and addition of posterior interbody fusion (46, 48). In their series of 24 patients with severe spondylolisthesis, Harrington and Dickson reported "a very desirable amount of reduction," improvement in symptoms and signs, and successful fusion in all patients (46).

Scaglietti et al. supplemented their closed reduction technique with open reduction and internal fixation by distraction rods and hooks (99). They designed "rider" hooks for fixation to the sacral ala, and cup-shaped hooks for fixation to the inferior articular processes of the second or third lumbar vertebra. After early failure of their instrumentation in one patient, they recommended a second-stage anterior interbody fusion to prevent loss of reduction in cases in which the shape of the S1 body provided inadequate support anteriorly.

Vidal et al. combined Harrington rod distraction with posterior interbody fusion in 16 patients (129). Although they were able to achieve average slip reduction of 75 to 80%, they encountered appreciable difficulties with maintaining sagittal alignment. These difficulties included horizontalization of the sacrum and loss of normal lumbosacral angulation.

Kaneda et al. reviewed 53 patients with isthmic spondylolisthesis treated by distraction rod instrumentation and posterolateral fusion (60). They obtained solid fusion in 91% and excellent or good clinical results in 93% of patients. However, they were only able to correct the average slip from $26 \pm 11\%$ to $21 \pm 10\%$ at follow-up. The average slip angle actually worsened from $4 \pm 7\%$ to $-3 \pm 7\%$.

The development of more rigid pedicle screw instrumentation systems provided new possibilities for spondylolisthesis reduction.

Schollner developed a one-stage posterior procedure which consisted of: 1) discectomy with or without sacral dome resection; 2) insertion of a Cobb elevator into the L5-S1 disc space to lever L5 superiorly; 3) insertion of dual-threaded pedicle screws into L5; 4) pulling L5 posteriorly by tightening a nut on the pedicle screws against a slotted plate; 5) posterior interbody fusion combined with posterolateral fusion; and 6) pedicle screw-plate fixation (71). Matthiass and Heine later reported on the use of this procedure in 51 patients (71). Complete slip reduction was achieved in 18 patients and partial slip reduction in 17 patients. Steffee and Sitkowski treated 14 patients with severe slips using a similar technique and were able to maintain complete reduction in 11 patients (115). Three patients who did not have an interbody fusion lost reduction.

Sijbrandji suggested that bone grafting was unnecessary after reduction and that interbody fusion could occur by bony contact between the decorticated surfaces of the L5 and S1 vertebral bodies (108). In his series of nine patients with severe slips, he achieved and maintained complete reduction in seven patients. In the two remaining patients, the slip percentages after operation were 15 and 25%, respectively, with no loss of correction at follow-up. Lumbosacral kyphosis could also be corrected, although follow-up values were not reported.

Edwards and his associates in the Spinal Fixation Study Group developed the concept of gradual instrumented reduction of spondylolisthesis without the need for extensive release procedures (3). Using rods, pedicle screws, and a special reduction device, they were able to simultaneously apply the corrective forces of distraction, posterior translation, and sacral flexion. These forces were applied over several hours to obtain viscoelastic stress-relaxation of contracted soft tissues without the need for disc excision or anterior release. Posterolateral fusion was then performed and routine interbody fusion avoided. Sacral screw fixation at both S1 and S2 enabled greater rotational forces to be applied to restore lumbosacral lordosis, and also provided more secure maintenance of reduction. Edwards, in a prospective study of 25 patients treated with this technique (Fig. 12.11), reported an average slip correction of 91%, an average lumbosacral kyphosis correction of 88%, and an average trunk height increase of 32 mm (33). Similar results have been reported for 180 patients with L5-S1 spondylolisthesis treated by other members of the Spinal Fixation Study Group (3). Complications included transient radiculopathy in 3%, permanent neurologic deficit in 1%, infection in 1%, and S2 screw pull-out in 2% of patients. Solid fusion was achieved in 88% of patients at 1 year.

Schwend et al. used sublaminar wires and a rectangular rod to obtain reduction and fixation in 20 children with severe lumbosacral spondylolisthesis (103). Eight patients also had preoperative hyperextension casting because of limited L5-S1 motion on extension radiographs. Four of these patients also had anterior lumbosacral release because the L5-S1 junction was assessed to be particularly rigid. The average slip percentage improved from 76% preoperatively to 55% postoperatively, and the average slip angle improved from 25° to 5°. Patients could ambulate within the first postoperative week and solid fusion without slip progression was attained in all patients. Seven patients had transient neurologic complications.

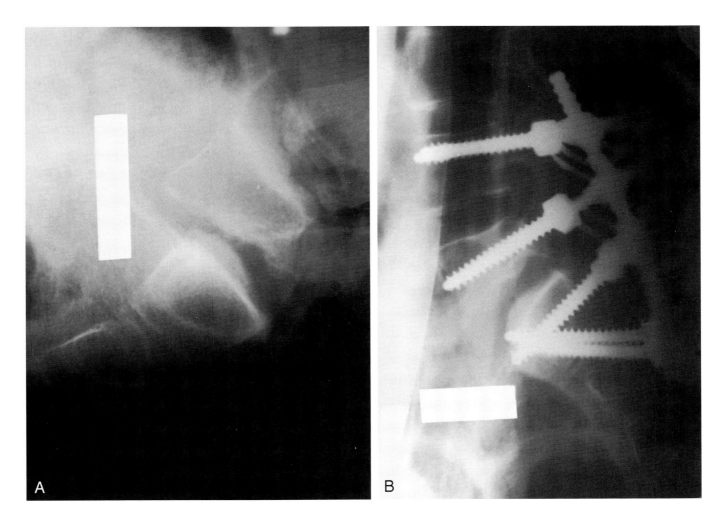

FIGURE 12.11.

A and **B.** Severe spondylolisthesis: Preoperative (A) and postoperative (B) radiographs of an adolescent male who underwent internal reduction and fixation with Edwards instrumentation.

Combined Anterior-Posterior Procedures

A variety of surgical regimes have been described which employ both the anterior and posterior approaches to achieve reduction, fixation, and fusion. In general, these major reconstructions have been performed only in adolescents with severe spondylolisthesis or spondyloptosis.

Denecke, in 1956, described the use of both the posterior and trans-coccygeal approaches to obtain reduction and fixation (29). After laminectomy, the trans-coccygeal approach was used to resect the inferior aspect of the L5 vertebral body. The posterior route was used again to resect the sacral dome and insert reduction devices bilaterally into the disc space. Finally, the trans-coccygeal route was used to insert a pin or screws axially from the sacrum to L5 or L4, and to perform interbody fusion.

DeWald et al. used the posterior approach to perform laminectomy, sacral dome resection, reduction with Harrington distraction rods, and posterolateral fusion (30). The anterior approach was then used for discectomy, further reduction, and interbody fusion. Postoperatively, patients wore a pantaloon cast and stayed in bed for 3 months. The distraction rods were removed after 6 to 12 months. At follow-up, complete reduction was maintained in 8 of 14 patients, and partial reduction in 5. Cauda equina syndrome developed in one patient and reduction was lost after removal of instrumentation.

Dick and Schnebel first performed anterior release and interbody fusion with bone paste harvested from the posterior iliac crest using an acetabular reamer (31). Reduction was then performed with pedicle screws and rods. No bone grafting was carried out posteriorly. In 2 of their 15 patients, they also used percutaneous pedicle screws and external fixation for initial distraction and kyphosis correction before the procedures previously described. They reported an average slip improvement of 46% and an average kyphosis improvement of 20°. Despite permanent neurologic complications in three patients, complete relief of pain and significant improvement in function was achieved in all patients.

Poussa et al. compared the results of reduction and in situ fusion in 22 adolescents who had severe spondylolisthesis (91). Reduction was accomplished in 11 patients using pedicle screws and rods in combination with an external fixator. Fusion was then carried out posterolaterally and anteriorly. In situ fusion was performed in 11 patients using a variety of techniques, including posterolateral fusion alone, posterolateral fusion combined with anterior fusion, and anterior fusion alone. The authors found no differences between the two groups of patients in terms of pain relief and functional status. However, four patients in the reduction group were dissatisfied with the final appearance of their backs as compared to none in the group that had in situ fusion. Reduction procedures were also associated with more complications and re-operations. No neurologic complications, however, occurred in the reduction group, whereas one patient who was fused in situ posterolaterally and anteriorly developed unilateral L5 root paralysis.

Gaines and Nichols described performing a complete L5 vertebrectomy in two patients with spondyloptosis (37). This was followed by posterior instrumented reduction of L4 onto the sacrum. Shortening the spine allowed relaxation of the soft tissues and cauda equina so that reduction was facilitated and the risk of neurologic injury minimized. Postoperatively, bed rest in a spica cast lasted from 3 to 7 months. Published reports indicate that this technique is able to significantly improve the slip percentage and lumbosacral kyphosis in the majority of patients (4, 37, 54). Trunk height also can be increased despite complete vertebrectomy.

Combined anterior-posterior reduction procedures have a high complication rate with neurologic injury reported in up to 30% of patients. Hardware failure and pseudarthrosis have occurred in 10 to 20% of patients.

Conclusion

Spondylolysis and spondylolisthesis are frequent findings in children and adolescents who present with back pain and/or leg pain. When it is reasonably certain that this abnormality is responsible for the patient's symptoms, nonoperative measures are successful for most low-grade slips. When indicated, surgical treatment for grade I and II slips is relatively straightforward and predictable. For higher grade slips, surgery is more complex and less rewarding. The development of safer and more effective reduction and fixation techniques will, hopefully, improve the surgical results for patients with severe slips.

References

1. Albanese M, Pizzutillo PD. Family study of spondylolysis and spondylolisthesis. J Pediatr Orthop 1982; 2:496–499.
2. Albee FH. Transplantation of a portion of the tibia into the spine for Pott's disease. A preliminary report. JAMA 1911;57:885–886.
3. Amundson G, Edwards CC, Garfin SR. Spondylolisthesis. In: Rothman RH, Simeone FA, eds. The spine. 3rd ed. Philadelphia: WB Saunders, 1992:913–969.
4. Ani N, Keppler L, Biscup RS, et al. Reduction of high-grade slips (grades III–V) with VSP instrumentation. Report of a series of 41 cases. Spine 1991;16:S302–S310.

5. Barash HL, Galante JO, Lambert CN, et al. Spondylolisthesis and tight hamstrings. J Bone Joint Surg Am 1970;52:1319–1328.
6. Batts M Jr. The etiology of spondylolisthesis. J Bone Joint Surg 1939;21:879–884.
7. Bell DF, Ehrlich MG, Zaleske DJ. Brace treatment for symptomatic spondylolisthesis. Clin Orthop 1988; 236:192–198.
8. Blackburne JS, Velikas EP. Spondylolisthesis in children and adolescents. J Bone Joint Surg Br 1977; 59:490–494.
9. Blanda J, Bethem D, Moats W, et al. Defects of pars interarticularis in athletes: a protocol for nonoperative treatment. J Spinal Disord 1993;6:406–411.
10. Bohlman HH, Cook SS. One-stage decompression and posterolateral and interbody fusion for lumbosacral spondyloptosis through a posterior approach. Report of two cases. J Bone Joint Surg Am 1982;64:415–418.
11. Boos N, Marchesi D, Aebi M. Treatment of spondylolysis and spondylolisthesis with Cotrel-Dubousset instrumentation: a preliminary report. J Spinal Disord 1991;4:472–479.
12. Borkow SE, Kleiger B. Spondylolisthesis in the newborn. A case report. Clin Orthop 1971;81:73–76.
13. Bosworth DM, Fielding JW, Demarest L, et al. Spondylolisthesis: a critical review of a consecutive series of cases treated by arthrodesis. J Bone Joint Surg Am 1955;37:767–786.
14. Boxall D, Bradford DS, Winter RB, et al. Management of severe spondylolisthesis in children and adolescents. J Bone Joint Surg Am 1979;61:479–495.
15. Bradford DS. Closed reduction of spondylolisthesis. An experience in 22 patients. Spine 1988;13:580–587.
16. Bradford DS. Treatment of severe spondylolisthesis. A combined approach for reduction and stabilization. Spine 1979;4:423–429.
17. Bradford DS, Iza J. Repair of the defect in spondylolysis or minimal degrees of spondylolisthesis by segmental wire fixation and bone grafting. Spine 1985; 10:673–679.
18. Buck JE. Direct repair of the defect in spondylolisthesis. Preliminary report. J Bone Joint Surg Br 1970; 52:432–437.
19. Burkus JK, Lonstein JE, Winter RB, et al. Long-term evaluation of adolescents treated operatively for spondylolisthesis. A comparison of in situ arthrodesis only with in situ arthrodesis and reduction followed by immobilization in a cast. J Bone Joint Surg Am 1992; 74:693–704.
20. Burns BH. An operation for spondylolisthesis. Lancet 1933;1:1233.
21. Capener N. Spondylolisthesis. Br J Surg 1932;19:374–386.
22. Cheng CL, Fang D, Lee PC, et al. Anterior spinal fusion for spondylolysis and isthmic spondylolisthesis. Long term results in adults. J Bone Joint Surg Br 1989; 71:264–267.
23. Cloward RB. Spondylolisthesis: treatment by laminectomy and posterior interbody fusion. Clin Orthop 1981;154:74–82.
24. Collier BD, Johnson RP, Carrera GF, et al. Painful spondylolysis or spondylolisthesis studied by radiography and single-photon emission computed tomography. Radiology 1985;154:207–211.
25. Cope R. Acute traumatic spondylolysis. Report of a case and review of the literature. Clin Orthop 1988; 230:162–165.
26. Dandy DJ, Shannon MJ. Lumbosacral subluxation (group I spondylolisthesis). J Bone Joint Surg Br 1971; 53:578–595.
27. Danielson BI, Frennered AK, Irstam LK. Radiologic progression of isthmic lumbar spondylolisthesis in young patients. Spine 1991;16:422–425.
28. Davis IS, Bailey RW. Spondylolisthesis. Long-term follow-up study of treatment with total laminectomy. Clin Orthop 1972;88:46–49.
29. Denecke H. Reposition der luxierten Wirelsaule bei Spondylolisthese. Ver Deutsch Orthop 1956;44:404–410.
30. DeWald RL, Faut MM, Taddonio RF, et al. Severe lumbosacral spondylolisthesis in adolescents and children. Reduction and staged circumferential fusion. J Bone Joint Surg Am 1981;63:619–626.
31. Dick WT, Schnebel B. Severe spondylolisthesis. Reduction and internal fixation. Clin Orthop 1988; 232:70–79.
32. Edelson JG, Nathan H. Nerve root compression in spondylolysis and spondylolisthesis. J Bone Joint Surg Br 1986;68:596–599.
33. Edwards CC. Prospective evaluation of a new method for complete reduction of L5-S1 spondylolisthesis using corrective forces alone. Orthop Trans 1990;14:549.
34. Fredrickson BE, Baker D, McHolick WJ, et al. The natural history of spondylolysis and spondylolisthesis. J Bone Joint Surg Am 1984;66:699–707.
35. Friberg O. Lumbar instability: a dynamic approach by traction-compression radiography. Spine 1987; 12:119–129.
36. Friberg O. Functional radiography of the lumbar spine. Ann Med 1989;21:341–346.
37. Gaines RW, Nichols WK. Treatment of spondyloptosis by two stage L5 vertebrectomy and reduction of L4 onto S1. Spine 1985;107:680–686.
38. Ghosez JP, Himmer O, Devyver B, et al. Operative treatment of spondylolisthesis. Comparison of 3 arthrodesis techniques. Rev Chir Orthop 1992;78:515–528.
39. Gill GG. Long-term follow-up evaluation of a few patients with spondylolisthesis treated by excision of the loose lamina with decompression of the nerve roots without spinal fusion. Clin Orthop 1984;182:215–219.
40. Gill GG, Manning JG, White HL. Surgical treatment of spondylolisthesis without spine fusion. J Bone Joint Surg Am 1955;37:493–518.
41. Gill GG, White HL. Surgical treatment of spondylolisthesis without spine fusion. A long term follow-up of operated cases. Acta Orthop Scand 1965;85 Suppl:5–99.
42. Hambly M, Lee CK, Gutteling E, et al. Tension band wiring-bone grafting for spondylolysis and spondylolisthesis. A clinical and biomechanical study. Spine 1989;14:455–460.

43. Hanley EN Jr, Levy JA. Surgical treatment of isthmic lumbosacral spondylolisthesis. Analysis of variables influencing results. Spine 1989;14:48–50.
44. Harada T, Ebara S, Anwar MM, et al. The lumbar spine in spastic diplegia. A radiographic study. J Bone Joint Surg Br 1993;75:534–537.
45. Haraldsson S, Willner S. A comparative study of spondylolisthesis in operations on adolescents and adults. Arch Orth Traum Surg 1983;101:101–105.
46. Harrington PR, Dickson JH. Spinal instrumentation in the treatment of severe progressive spondylolisthesis. Clin Orthop 1976;117:157–163.
47. Harrington PR, Tullos HS. Reduction of severe spondylolisthesis in children. South Med J 1969;62:1–7.
48. Harrington PR, Tullos HS. Spondylolisthesis in children. Observations and surgical treatment. Clin Orthop 1971;79:75–84.
49. Harris IE, Weinstein SL. Long-term follow-up of patients with grade-III and IV spondylolisthesis. Treatment with and without posterior fusion. J Bone Joint Surg Am 1987;69:960–969.
50. Harris RI. Spondylolisthesis. Ann R Coll Surg Engl 1951;8:259–297.
51. Hendersen ED. Results of the surgical treatment of spondylolisthesis. J Bone Joint Surg Am 1966;48:619–642.
52. Hensinger RN. Back pain in children. In: Bradford DS, Hensinger RN, eds. The pediatric spine. New York: Thieme, 1985:41–60.
53. Hibbs RA. A report of fifty-nine cases of scoliosis treated by the fusion operation. J Bone Joint Surg 1924;6:3–37.
54. Huizenga BA. Reduction of spondyloptosis with 2-stage vertebrectomy. Orthop Trans 1983;7:21.
55. Jackson DW, Wiltse LL, Cirincoine RJ. Spondylolysis in the female gymnast. Clin Orthop 1976;117:68–73.
56. Jenkins JA. Spondylolisthesis. Br J Surg 1936;34:80–85.
57. Jinkins JR, Matthes JC, Sener RN, et al. Spondylolysis, spondylolisthesis, and associated nerve root entrapment in the lumbosacral spine: MR evaluation. Am J Roent 1992;159:799–803.
58. Johnson JR, Kirwan EO. The long-term results of fusion in situ for severe spondylolisthesis. J Bone Joint Surg Br 1983;65:43–46.
59. Kalebo P, Kadziolka R, Sward L, et al. Stress views in the comparative assessment of spondylolytic spondylolisthesis. Skel Radiol 1989;17:570–575.
60. Kaneda K, Satoh S, Nohara Y, et al. Distraction rod instrumentation with posterolateral fusion in isthmic spondylolisthesis. 53 cases followed for 18–89 months. Spine 1985;10:383–389.
61. Kim NH, Kim DJ. Anterior interbody fusion for spondylolisthesis. Orthopedics 1991;14:1069–1076.
62. Kim SS, Denis F, Lonstein JE, et al. Factors affecting fusion rate in adult spondylolisthesis. Spine 1990;15:979–984.
63. Lance EM. Treatment of severe spondylolisthesis with neural involvement. A report of two cases. J Bone Joint Surg Am 1966;48:883–891.
64. Lane WA. Case of spondylolisthesis with progressive paraplegia: laminectomy. Lancet 1893;1:991.
65. Laurent LE, Osterman K. Operative treatment of spondylolisthesis in young patients. Clin Orthop 1976;117:85–91.
66. Lenke LG, Bridwell KH, Bullis D, et al. Results of in situ fusion for isthmic spondylolisthesis. J Spinal Disord 1992;5:433–442.
67. Louis R. Fusion of the lumbar and sacral spine by internal fixation with screw plates. Clin Orthop 1986;203:18–33.
68. Lowe R, Hayes D, Kaye J, et al. Standing roentgenograms in spondylolisthesis. Clin Orthop 1976;117:80–84.
69. Lowe J, Libson E, Ziv I, et al. Spondylolysis in the upper lumbar spine. A study of 32 patients. J Bone Joint Surg Br 1987;69:582–586.
70. Lusins JO, Elting JJ, Cicoria AD, et al. SPECT evaluation of lumbar spondylolysis and spondylolisthesis. Spine 1994;19:608–612.
71. Matthiass HH, Heine J. The surgical reduction of spondylolisthesis. Clin Orthop 1986;203:34–44.
72. Maurice HD, Morley TR. Cauda equina lesions following fusion in situ and decompressive laminectomy for severe spondylolisthesis. Four case reports. Spine 1989;14:214–226.
73. McAfee PC, Yuan HA. Computed tomography in spondylolisthesis. Clin Orthop 1982;166:62–71.
74. McCarroll JR, Miller JM, Ritter MA. Lumbar spondylolysis and spondylolisthesis in college football players. A prospective study. Am J Sports Med 1986;14:404–406.
75. McGuire RA, Amundson GM. The use of primary internal fixation in spondylolisthesis. Spine 1993;18:1662–1672.
76. McPhee IB, O'Brien JP. Reduction of severe spondylolisthesis. A preliminary report. Spine 1979;4:430–434.
77. McPhee IB, O'Brien JP, McCall IW, et al. Progression of lumbosacral spondylolisthesis. Australas Radiol 1981;25:91–95.
78. Meyerding H. Spondylolisthesis: surgical treatment and results. Surg Gynecol Obstet 1932;54:371–377.
79. Morscher E, Gerber B, Fasel J. Surgical treatment of spondylolisthesis by bone grafting and direct stabilization of spondylolysis by means of a hook screw. Archiv Orthop Traum Surg 1984;103:175–178.
80. Newman PH. Stenosis of the lumbar spine in spondylolisthesis. Clin Orthop 1976;115:116–121.
81. Newman PH. A clinical syndrome associated with severe lumbosacral subluxation. J Bone Joint Surg Br 1965;47:472–481.
82. Nicol RO, Scott JH. Lytic spondylolysis. Repair by wiring. Spine 1986;11:1027–1030.
83. O'Brien JP, Mehdian H, Jaffray D. Reduction of severe lumbosacral spondylolisthesis. A report of 22 cases with a ten-year follow-up period. Clin Orthop 1994;300:64–69.
84. Ogilvie JW, Sherman J. Spondylolysis in Scheuermann's disease. Spine 1987;12:251–253.
85. Ohki I, Inoue S, Murata T, et al. Reduction and fusion of severe spondylolisthesis using halo-pelvic traction with a wire reduction device. Int Orthop 1980;4:107–113.

86. Ohmori K, Suzuki K, Ishida Y. Translamino-pedicular screw fixation with bone grafting for symptomatic isthmic lumbar spondylolysis. Neurosurg 1992; 30:379–384.
87. Osterman K, Lindholm TS, Laurent LE. Late results of removal of the loose posterior element (Gill's operation) in the treatment of lytic lumbar spondylolisthesis. Clin Orthop 1976;117:121–128.
88. Peek RD, Wiltse LL, Reynolds JB, et al. In situ arthrodesis without decompression for Grade-III or IV isthmic spondylolisthesis in adults who have severe sciatica. J Bone Joint Surg Am 1989;71:62–68.
89. Pizzutillo PD, Hummer CD 3d. Nonoperative treatment for painful adolescent spondylolysis or spondylolisthesis. J Pediatr Orthop 1989;9:538–540.
90. Pizzutillo PD, Mirenda W, MacEwen GD. Posterolateral fusion for spondylolisthesis in adolescence. J Pediatr Orthop 1986;6:311–316.
91. Poussa M, Schlenzka D, Seitsalo S, et al. Surgical treatment of severe isthmic spondylolisthesis in adolescents. Reduction or fusion in situ. Spine 1993;18:894–901.
92. Roca J, Moretta D, Fuster S, et al. Direct repair of spondylolysis. Clin Orthop 1989;246:86–91.
93. Rosenberg NJ, Bargar WL, Friedman B. The incidence of spondylolysis and spondylolisthesis in nonambulatory patients. Spine 1981;6:35–38.
94. Rowe GG, Roche MB. The etiology of separate neural arch. J Bone Joint Surg Am 1953;35:102–109.
95. Saraste H. Symptoms in relation to the level of spondylolysis. Int Orthop 1986;10:183–185.
96. Saraste H, Brostrom LA, Aparisi T. Prognostic radiologic aspects of spondylolisthesis. Acta Radiol Diagn 1984;25:427–432.
97. Saraste H. Spondylolysis and pregnancy—a risk analysis. Acta Obst Gyn Scand 1986;65:727–729.
98. Saraste H. Long-term clinical and radiological follow-up of spondylolysis and spondylolisthesis. J Pediatr Orthop 1987;7:631–638.
99. Scaglietti O, Frontino G, Bartolozzi P. Technique of anatomical reduction of lumbar spondylolisthesis and its surgical stabilization. Clin Orthop 1976;117:165–175.
100. Scherb R. Zur indikation und technik der Albee-de Quervainschen operation. Schweiz Med Wochen 1921;2:763–765.
101. Schlegel KF, Pon A. The biomechanics of posterior lumbar interbody fusion (PLIF) in spondylolisthesis. Clin Orthop 1985;193:115–119.
102. Schoenecker PL, Cole HO, Herring JA, et al. Cauda equina syndrome after in situ arthrodesis for severe spondylolisthesis at the lumbosacral junction. J Bone Joint Surg Am 1990;72:369–377.
103. Schwend RM, Waters PM, Hey LA, et al. Treatment of severe spondylolisthesis in children by reduction and L4-S4 posterior segmental hyperextension fixation. J Pediatr Orthop 1992;12:703–711.
104. Seitsalo S. Operative and conservative treatment of moderate spondylolisthesis in young patients. J Bone Joint Surg Br 1990;72:908–913.
105. Seitsalo S, Osterman K, Hyvarinen H, et al. Progression of spondylolisthesis in children and adolescents. A long-term follow-up of 272 patients. Spine 1991; 16:417–421.
106. Seitsalo S, Osterman K, Poussa M, et al. Spondylolisthesis in children under 12 years of age: long-term results of 56 patients treated conservatively or operatively. J Pediatr Orthop 1988;8:516–521.
107. Shapiro J, Herring J. Congenital vertebral displacement. J Bone Joint Surg Am 1993;75:656–662.
108. Sijbrandij S. A new technique for the reduction and stabilisation of severe spondylolisthesis. A report of nine cases. Int Orthop 1985;9:247–253.
109. Sinaki M, Lutness MP, Ilstrup DM, et al. Lumbar spondylolisthesis: retrospective comparison and three-year follow-up of two conservative treatment programs. Arch Phys Med Rehab 1989;70:594–598.
110. Snijder JG, Seroo JM, Snijder CJ, et al. Therapy of spondylolisthesis by repositioning and fixation of the olisthetic vertebra. Clin Orthop 1976;117:149–156.
111. Speck GR, McCall IW, O'Brien JP. Spondylolisthesis: the angle of kyphosis. Spine 1984;9:659–660.
112. Stauffer RN, Coventry MB. Posterior lateral lumbar spine fusion. J Bone Joint Surg Am 1972;54:1195–1204.
113. Stears JC. Radiculopathy in spondylosis/spondylolisthesis. The laminar/ligamentum flavum process. Acta Radiol Suppl Stockh 1986;369:723–726.
114. Steffee AD, Brantigan JW. The variable screw placement spinal fixation system. Report of a prospective study of 250 patients enrolled in Food and Drug Administration clinical trials. Spine 1993;18:1160–1172.
115. Steffee AD, Sitkowski DJ. Reduction and stabilization of grade IV spondylolisthesis. Clin Orthop 1988; 227:82–89.
116. Steiner ME, Micheli LJ. Treatment of symptomatic spondylolysis and spondylolisthesis with the modified Boston brace. Spine 1985;10:937–943.
117. Stewart TD. The age incidence of neural arch defects in Alaskan natives, considered from the standpoint of etiology. J Bone Joint Surg Am 1953;35:937–950.
118. Suezawa Y, Bernoski FP, Jacob HA. A comparison of the long term results of three types of posterior fusion of the lumbar spine for spondylolisthesis. Int Orthop 1981;5:291–297.
119. Szappanos L, Szepesi K, Thomazy V. Spondylolysis in osteopetrosis. J Bone Joint Surg Br 1988;70:428–430.
120. Taillard W. Etiology of spondylolisthesis. Clin Orthop 1976;117:30–39.
121. Teplick JG, Laffey PA, Berman A, et al. Diagnosis and evaluation of spondylolisthesis and/or spondylolysis on axial CT. Am J Neuroradiol 1986;7:479–491.
122. Turner RH, Bianco AJ. Spondylolysis and spondylolisthesis in children and teenagers. J Bone Joint Surg Am 1971;53:1298–1306.
123. Van den Berghe L, Maes G, Fabry G, et al. In situ posterolateral fusion for spondylolisthesis. Acta Orthop Belg 1991;57(Suppl I):214–218.
124. Van den Oever M, Merrick MV, Scott JH. Bone scintigraphy in symptomatic spondylolysis. J Bone Joint Surg Br 1987;69:453–456.
125. Van Rens TJ, van Horn JR. Long-term results in lum-

bosacral interbody fusion for spondylolisthesis. Acta Orthop Scand 1982;53:383–392.
126. Verbiest H. Impending lumbar spondyloptosis. Problems with posterior decompression and foraminotomy: treatment by anterior lumbosacral console fusion. Clin Neurosurg 1973;20:197–203.
127. Verlooy J, De Smedt K, Selosse P. Failure of a modified posterior lumbar interbody fusion technique to produce adequate pain relief in isthmic spondylolytic grade 1 spondylolisthesis patients. A prospective study of 20 patients. Spine 1993;18:1491–1495.
128. Vestad E, Naes B. Spondylolisthesis. Treatment by excision of the loose lamina and resection of the pedicle. Acta Orthop Scand 1977;48:472–478.
129. Vidal J, Fassio B, Buscayret C, et al. Surgical reduction of spondylolisthesis using a posterior approach. Clin Orthop 1981;154:156–165.
130. Watkins MB. Posterolateral fusion of the lumbar and lumbosacral spine. J Bone Joint Surg Am 1953;35:1014–1018.
131. Wenger DR, Lee CS. Spondylolisthesis in children and adolescents. Semin Spine Surg 1993;5:308–319.
132. Whitecloud TS 3d, Butler JC. Anterior lumbar fusion utilizing transvertebral fibular graft. Spine 1988;13:370–374.
133. Wiltse LL. The etiology of spondylolisthesis. J Bone Joint Surg Am 1962;44:539–560.
134. Wiltse LL, Jackson DW. Treatment of spondylolisthesis and spondylolysis in children. Clin Orthop 1976;117:92–100.
135. Wiltse LL, Newman PH, Macnab I. Classification of spondylolysis and spondylolisthesis. Clin Orthop 1976;117:23–29.
136. Wiltse LL, Rothman SLG. Spondylolisthesis: classification, diagnosis and natural history. Semin Spine Surg 1993;5:264–280.
137. Wiltse LL, Widell EH Jr, Jackson DW. Fatigue fracture: the basic lesion in isthmic spondylolisthesis. J Bone Joint Surg Am 1975;57:17–22.
138. Wiltse LL, Winter RB. Terminology and measurement of spondylolisthesis. J Bone Joint Surg Am 1983;65:768–772.
139. Winter RB. Congenital kyphosis. J Bone Joint Surg Am 1973;55:253–256.
140. Winter RB. Severe spondylolisthesis in Marfan's syndrome: report of two cases. J Pediatr Orthop 1982;2:51–55.
141. Winter M, Jani L. Results of screw osteosynthesis in spondylolysis and low-grade spondylolisthesis. Archiv Orthop Traum Surg 1989;108:96–99.
142. Wynne-Davies R, Scott JHS. Inheritance and spondylolisthesis. A radiographic family survey. J Bone Joint Surg Br 1979;61:301–305.

CHAPTER THIRTEEN

Pediatric Spine Injuries

Roger M. Lyon

Introduction

The care of spinal injuries in the pediatric age group is very challenging even for the most well-trained spine surgeon. Fortunately, spinal injuries in children are much less common than in adults. In fact, even if patients up to 18 years old are included, most major trauma centers only care for a few of these injuries per year. Reasons for this include anatomic differences in the spine of children and behavioral differences. Of the few large published series on pediatric spine injuries, most of the patients are in the 12 to 18-year-old age group (13, 16, 38, 43, 70, 85, 100). Because the older child (>12 years old) has spinal characteristics that more closely resemble the adult spine, to make generalizations about the care of spine injuries in children less than 10 or 12 years old based on most of these studies would be misleading.

Unlike the adult spine, the child's spine is constantly changing in terms of anatomic features, size, and composition. As it is growing larger, its proportion of cartilage to bone is decreasing, its growth plates are closing, and its mechanical properties are changing. These continual anatomic changes make evaluation of the child's spine an especially difficult task, particularly in the cervical spine. Most of the anatomy has to be understood as it relates to radiographic anatomy and specifically with the presence of multiple radiolucent lines representing cartilaginous plates (physeal plates). The dates of epiphyseal appearances and disappearances may vary with age, and are often expressed as an age range. It is therefore essential to have a thorough understanding of the radiographic features of a child's spine to accurately identify abnormalities.

For most purposes, the pediatric age group is defined as newborn to 18 or 20-years-old. In the case of spinal development, different aspects of the spine reach their adult form at different ages. For instance, the level of the conus medullaris achieves its adult relationship with the vertebral bodies just a few months after birth. However, the ring apophyses may not fuse with the primary ossification centers (especially in males) until age 20 to 22 (12). However, for practical purposes, the child's spine takes on most of the adult characteristics by age 10 or 12.

For purposes of this chapter, the discussion of pediatric spine injuries will be limited, except where stated, to the below 12 year old age group.

Etiology

The causes of pediatric spinal injuries reflect the activities in which children are often involved. The majority of these injuries result from motor vehicle accidents (especially in patients older than 16 years), a somewhat lesser amount from falls, and a small percentage (10%) from sports (9, 24, 43, 60, 74).

Other less common mechanisms of injury include penetrating trauma (including gun shot wounds and knife wounds), birth injuries, and child abuse (3, 4, 111). Spinal injuries account for less than 2 to 3% of all injuries to children. Most injuries involve the thoracic spine, with the lumbar, cervical, and sacral areas being involved less often and in that order. Isolated sacral injuries are rare. They are associated more commonly with pelvic fractures.

Spinal injuries tend to occur mainly in two different age groups: 5 years old or younger and older than 10 years. Approximately 50% of these patients have associated injuries, and 20% have an associated neurologic injury (6, 9). Overall spine injuries increase in frequency around the time of adolescence and into early adulthood (70). In terms of injuries unique to the child, most of these occur in children from birth to age 10. Injuries in children over age 10 are similar in mechanism and fracture patterns to those in the adult, and for the most part have no significant differences in their management.

Anatomy

The first two cervical vertebrae are unique in their development and the remaining five cervical vertebrae all develop similarly (91). The atlas at birth is composed of three ossification centers, one for the body and one for each of the two neural arches (Fig. 13.1). The center for the body is usually not present at birth. It may appear during the first year of life, but may remain entirely absent throughout life. The neural arch usually closes by the third year, although it can remain open into adulthood. The posterior ring of the atlas may develop partially, or remain completely absent. The synchondroses between the body of the atlas and the neural arches are best seen on the open mouth view. The synchondroses usually close by the seventh year of life, and they are occasionally mistaken for fractures.

Failure of segmentation of the atlas from the skull can occasionally lead to narrowing of the foramen magnum and signs of neurologic dysfunction that may not appear until the second or third decades of life. This anomaly may put the child at risk for spinal cord injury, even with minor trauma, by narrowing of the foramen magnum, which results in excessive motion or instability in the upper cervical spine.

The second cervical vertebrae (the axis) has four ossification centers at birth: one for each neural arch, one for the body, and a fourth for the odontoid process (Fig. 13.2). In an open mouth view, the odontoid process is sandwiched between the neural arches (Fig. 13.3). Its ossification center is present at birth and sits on top of the ossification center of the body of the axis, and it is separated from it by a synchondrosis. Below this are the synchondroses between the body and the neural arches. The epiphysis and synchondroses combine to form a letter "H" shape. The epiphysis of the odontoid runs across the apparent base of the odontoid, but at a level well below that of

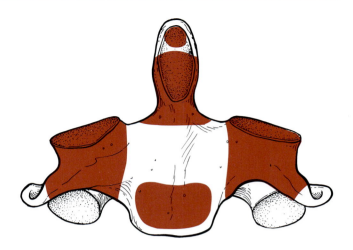

FIGURE 13.2.
Four ossification centers of the axis.

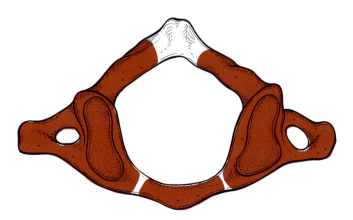

FIGURE 13.1.
Three ossification centers of the atlas.

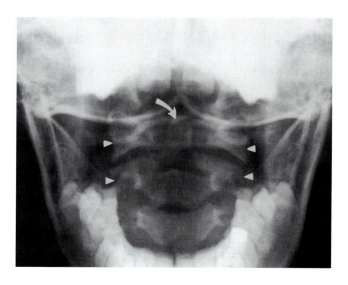

FIGURE 13.3.
An open mouth view showing the odontoid process (arrow) between C1 and C2 neural arches (arrowheads).

the level of the articular processes of the axis. This line is occasionally mistaken for a fracture of the odontoid in both children and adults. However, most odontoid fractures occur at the level of the articular facets.

The odontoid fuses with the neural arches and the body of the axis between three and six years of age, essentially the same time the body joins the neural arches. Occasionally, this synchondrosis is present in the axis on the open mouth view in a child up to age 11.

The cartilage anlage of the odontoid process ossifies from two independent centers, one on either side of the midline during the fifth fetal month. These are usually fused in the midline at birth. Persistence of this vertical line is sometimes confused with a fracture. The tip of the odontoid is not ossified at birth. The small ossification center at the tip of the odontoid (os terminale) appears between 3 and 6 years of age and fuses with the main portion of the odontoid by 12 years of age. When it persists, it is occasionally confused with a fracture. The third to the seventh cervical vertebrae each ossify from three centers: one from the body and one from each neural arch (Fig. 13.3). The neural arches close between the second and third year. The neural central synchondroses between the neural arches and the body fuse between the third and the sixth year of life. On lateral radiographs, the ossified part of the vertebral bodies in young children are wedge shaped until they become more square at about age 7.

The joints of Luschka (uncovertebral articulations) usually seen on the AP radiograph in the adult cervical spine are not present in the developing spine under 8 to 10 years of age. The apophyseal rings in the upper and lower surface of the vertebral body ossify late in childhood and fuse to the vertebral body by age 25. These ring apophyses are secondary ossification centers and as such they do not contribute significantly to vertebral body height. The thoracic and lumbar vertebrae have a common ossification pattern (Fig. 13.4). One ossification center develops in each of the two neural arches, from which one ossification center forms in the vertebral centrum. The cartilage separating the ossification center from the neural central synchondrosis is slightly anterior to the anatomic base of the pedicles and ossifies between the age of three and six years.

Secondary ossification centers develop at the tips of the spinous, transverse, and mammillary processes during puberty and represent apophyses. The lateral and anterior portions of the central epiphysis remain thicker than the rest of the epiphyses and appear radiographically and histologically as a groove extending around the developing vertebral body. Between 7 and 8 years of age, small linear foci of ossification develop in the end plates. By 12 to 15 years of age, these foci coalesce to form the ring apophysis, which can be seen on radiographs. The ring does not extend around the entire circumference of the vertebral body, but only around the centrum (11).

The longitudinal growth of the vertebral body is by endochondral ossification with the vertebral end plate similar to that of other physes in the body (12).

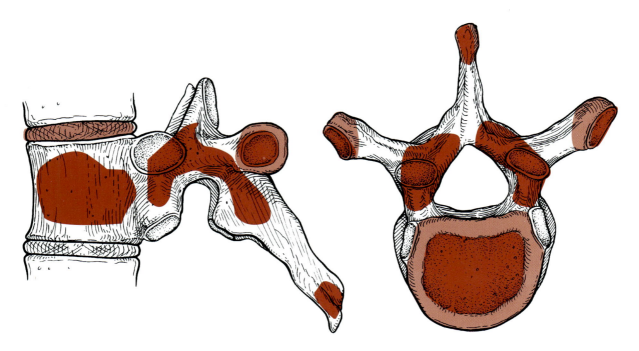

FIGURE 13.4.
Three ossification centers of the thoracic and lumbar vertebrae.

As the child gets older, these ossification centers enlarge and the cartilage:bone ratio gradually decreases (14). Adult proportions are reached by age 10. The bodies enlarge radially by perichondrial and periosteal bone apposition, with the lumbar vertebrae growing to a greater degree in width after age 2 years. The neural arches and pedicles enlarge by the same mechanism. Radiographically, the intervertebral spaces widen in relation to the vertebral bodies.

In the infant, the lateral radiograph usually demonstrates a horizontal conical shadow of decreased density extending inward from the anterior and posterior walls of the vertebral bodies, which occasionally can be confused with a fracture. The posterior notch results from indentation of the posterior vertebral wall at the point of entrance and emergence of the posterior arteries and veins. The indentation is present in all vertebrae and all ages. In the infant, the anterior conical shadow is more obvious than the posterior shadow, and results from the presence in this area of large sinusoidal space within the vertebrae. The anterior notch is not permanent and disappears with ossification of the anterior lateral walls of the body, usually within the first year of life. The vertebral disc in children consists of three main components: the annulus fibrosis, the nucleus pulposus and the vertebral cartilaginous end plate.

The nucleus pulposus in children has a water content of 88%, which is higher than in adults. This high percentage allows the disc to be much more deformable and less susceptible to injury. In infants and children under age 7 and 8, trauma often can lead to end plate fractures instead of disc ruptures. Schmorl's nodes are often noted. As the nucleus pulposus matures, the incidence of both osseous and disc injuries increases. In the fetal period, the spinal cord initially ends at the sacral level. At birth, the level of termination of the spinal cord is L3 and achieves the adult level of L1 to 2 at about 2 months after birth.

The sacral segments do not fuse to form a single bone until the fourth decade of life. The five sacral vertebrae are separated initially by four atypical intervertebral discs. The middle two discs ossify first, then the fourth disc, and the first disc is the last to ossify. Thus, in a child, fractures of the sacrum may occur through an intervertebral disc.

Biomechanics

Bone Properties

Fractures that are significant in adults may be less so in children who have more elastic soft tissue, the potential for remodeling, and normal mineralization of their bones. Certain injuries are unique to children, including periosteal sleeve injuries, most cases of spinal cord injury without radiographic abnormalities (SCIWORA), and child abuse. The cervical region is the most flexible area of the spine, and is more so in children. This flexibility makes separating out normal from abnormal motion especially difficult. To date, most of the biomechanical studies done on the spine have been done on the adult spine, and may only have limited application in the child less than 10 years of age. Throughout the child's growth, there are continual changes in the ability of the spine to sustain loads. By age 10, the biomechanical differences between the spine in the child and the adult are probably minimal.

The child's spinal column is quite flexible and can reportedly stretch approximately 2 cm prior to any significant injury of the structure itself. Unfortunately, the spinal cord itself is less extensible than the child's spinal column, and only can stretch approximately 5 to 6 mm before it sustains significant injury (80).

The relatively large size of the head in the younger children (less than 8 years old) along with a relatively poorly developed cervical musculature allows the cervical spine to be at risk for significant injury. This situation is extreme in the case of the newborn; at this stage the child is incapable of even supporting the head and therefore is unable to protect the spine from external forces. There has been little work on the biomechanics of different motion segments in the spine of children.

A biomechanical study done to examine the sagittal plane motion of C1 on C2 found that anterior/posterior force caused displacement, namely, anterior displacement of the atlas on the axis up to 3 mm prior to rupture of the transverse ligament. Once the transverse ligament was ruptured, there was between 3 and 5 mm of translation. Translation over 5 mm between C1 and C2 is an indication of gross instability with all the ligamentous structures having failed. Because of the larger cartilaginous spaces in children, the actual measurement between the front of the odontoid and the anterior ring of C1 (posterior cortex) may be slightly larger.

Pathomechanics

Mechanisms of Injury

To understand many spine injuries it is helpful to understand the column concept of the spine as described by Holdsworth (two columns) and by Denis (three columns) (67, 32). This concept was developed for the adult thoracic and lumbar spine, although it has been extrapolated to children and adolescents with adjustments for anatomic and biomechanical differences.

The column system permits injuries to be divided

into four major types: 1) the compression fracture, which is a failure of the anterior column with an intact middle column; 2) a burst fracture, which is failure under compression (usually axially) of both the anterior and middle columns; 3) a seat belt fracture, which is a compression injury of the anterior column, with distraction of the middle and posterior columns through either bony or ligamentous elements; and 4) a fracture dislocation, in which all three columns fail (Fig. 13.5).

Spinal stability has many different definitions, but Denis (33) groups instability into three main types: 1) first degree instability, which is a mechanical instability with risk of kyphosis; 2) second degree instability, which is a neurologic instability such as collapsing "stable" burst fracture; and 3) third degree instability, which is both mechanical and neurologic instability, such as an unstable burst fracture or a fracture dislocation. Because of the unique anatomic features of the upper cervical spine, the column concept does not apply in that area.

Harris et al. classified cervical spine injuries according to their mechanism of injury which has been attributed to predominant force vectors acting on the spine (63). The predominant vectors include flexion, extension, vertical compression, or combinations of these.

A flexion force can result in anterior subluxation, bilateral facet dislocation, simple wedge compression fractures, clay shoveler fractures, and flexion tear drop fractures. Flexion rotation injuries can result in unilateral facet dislocations. Extension rotation injuries can result in pillar fractures. Vertical compression force can result in Jefferson burst type fracture of the atlas, or the classic burst fracture.

A primary hyperextension force can result in hyperextension/dislocation, avulsion fracture of the anterior arch of the atlas, extension tear drop fracture of the atlas, fracture of the posterior arch of the atlas, a laminar fracture, traumatic spondylolisthesis, or hyperextension fracture/dislocation. A lateral flexion force can result in an uncinate process fracture (not usually seen in the child less than 10 years old). Nonspecific mechanisms can result in atlanto-occipital disassociations, as well as odontoid fractures.

These classification systems seek to establish a mechanism of injury based on the appearance of the fracture pattern on plain radiographs and computerized tomography. What is not evident from these mechanisms and from the classification schemes is the amount of soft tissue injury in the area, including ligaments, tendons, muscles, and the spinal cord and neural elements. One main goal of classification systems is to establish a particular injury as stable or unstable.

There are minor spinal fractures that are not covered by the usual classifications schemes; these are fractures of spinous and transverse processes very often encountered with blunt trauma. At times the associated injuries can be severe, but the fractures themselves are relatively minor and usually do not need any specific treatment. Transverse process fractures in the thoracic region may be associated with significant chest trauma; those in the thoracolumbar region may be associated with significant renal injury; and those in the lower lumbar spine may be associated with unstable pelvic fractures.

Diagnosis

Significant force is necessary to cause spinal injuries and fractures. Therefore, most patients with pediatric spine injuries are true multi-trauma patients. They may have significant head, chest, abdomen, pelvis, and extremity injuries in addition to their spinal injury. Any initial evaluation should involve a thorough history.

Establishing a mechanism of injury is extremely important because it allows determination of the energy involved. High energy injuries, such as most automobile accidents, usually involve more significant injury than low energy injuries, such as falls. If the history does not correlate with what the findings are in the child, child abuse must be considered and appropriate steps must be taken.

Many times the child cannot provide specific details surrounding the incident. These details should

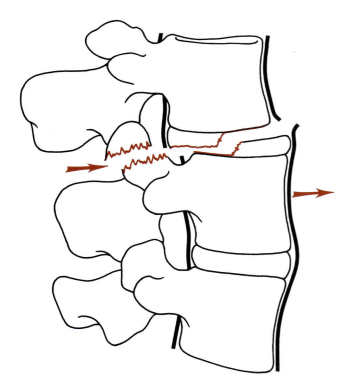

FIGURE 13.5.
A fracture-dislocation with failure of all three columns.

be sought from other individuals who may have been involved in, or witnessed, the incident to try to arrive at some judgement about risk for spinal injury. A high level of suspicion for a significant spinal injury would include anyone with a significant head injury, any high energy injury with multiple fractures, or any altered or loss of consciousness.

It is also important to elicit any history of transient neurologic deficit even in children who appear neurologically normal. They may have occult instability, which has to be investigated thoroughly before "clearing" the spine.

The importance of the physical examination cannot be overemphasized. As with any multiple trauma patient, the initial evaluation should be directed to the usual ABCs of trauma management. Once this is done and the patient is thought to be stable, evaluation of the spine should be performed. Before the examination, any trauma patient should be assumed to have a spine injury until proven otherwise.

In a cooperative, verbal child, any area of pain should be identified first. Usually the patient is supine on a back board and the back is not readily accessible. If there is a high suspicion of a spine fracture, a cursory neurologic exam should be performed to make sure the patient is moving all four extremities appropriately and that the sensation is intact on all four extremities to at least light touch and pinprick. If the patient can lift each of the limbs off of the bed on his or her own, at least a certain level of baseline neurologic function has been established. With an uncooperative or comatose child, one must proceed as though an unstable spine injury is present.

It may be wise to get an initial lateral radiograph of the cervical spine before any moving of the patient if there is a high degree of suspicion of cervical spine injury. The neck should be examined first because it is the most accessible in the supine position. While someone is stabilizing the neck and head, the neck can be palpated anteriorly, posteriorly, and on both sides without motion of the neck. If the palpation does not reveal any significant areas of pain and the patient is alert, the patient may be instructed to raise his head or her off of the bed and rotate the head to either side; if this is done without pain, the patient can then be log-rolled into the decubitus position for visual inspection and thorough palpation of the entire spine from the occiput down to the sacrum.

In the comatose or uncooperative patient with a high degree of suspicion for spinal injury, a complete set of spine radiographs should usually proceed moving the patient. The skin over the back and abdomen should be evaluated carefully for any skin breaks, ecchymosis, or swelling. Any deformity should be noted, including localized swelling and widening of spinous processes. Localized areas of tenderness should be radiographed with extra suspicion for injuries. A more thorough neurologic evaluation can be done at this time—testing reflexes (bulbocavernosus reflex if other reflexes absent), sensation (including perianal sensation), and strength of the major muscle groups (including rectal exam for sphincter tone).

Every attempt should be made to perform a complete neurologic examination, even though this can be very challenging in the very young patient with other painful injuries. A rectal examination should be performed in all patients. Patients with apparent complete cord injury, either paraplegia or quadriplegia, should have the bulbocavernosus reflex tested to determine whether they are in a period of spinal areflexia or "spinal shock." This test aids in the overall prognosis for potential return of neurologic function to the areas of neurologic compromise.

Determining the extent of neurologic injury in the infant is difficult at best. Even in the presence of paralysis, the child may have a reflex mass flexion withdrawal which may be indistinguishable from the response in an otherwise normal child. The lack of voluntary motor function and sensory loss confirms the diagnosis of spinal cord injury. Any patient with a compromised clinical assessment (i.e., comatose, altered consciousness, combative, uncooperative, or unable to communicate) needs continued spine precautions and repeat examinations until adequate assessment can be assured. With added attention to detail and very thorough precautions in the injured child, missed or delayed diagnosis of spinal injury can be minimized.

The entire patient should be examined carefully for any other associated injuries, particularly abdominal injuries if the patient was involved in a motor vehicle accident as a restrained passenger using a lap belt. Children have a high incidence of abdominal injury, visceral rupture, and flexion distraction injures of the lumbar spine.

All patients with significant spinal injuries should have bladder catheterization initially. A more thorough evaluation of bladder function is made on a more delayed basis. Associated injuries, such as cardiac contusion, pneumothorax, hemothorax, aortic injury, abdominal visceral ruptures, and renal and bladder injuries are life-threatening injuries that can accompany significant spinal injuries. These injuries may not manifest themselves in initial trauma evaluation, but may present on a slightly delayed basis. Appropriate evaluation to rule out these injuries is important in the initial and subsequent care of these patients.

Imaging of Spinal Fractures

Accurate diagnosis in the case of spinal injuries relies heavily on the use of appropriate spinal imaging modalities. The major imaging studies to evaluate spinal injuries are plain radiography, tomography, computerized tomography, MRI, myelography, and technetium bone scintigraphy. These modalities, when used appropriately, identify the location and severity of the injuries, including assessment of spinal alignment, stability, and the extent of any canal comprise.

Plain radiography remains the initial imaging study of choice for any spinal injury. Initial evaluation of the cervical spine should include a lateral x-ray of the cervical spine from the occiput down to and including the top of the T1 body. When assessed appropriately, this study is highly sensitive for cervical spine injuries. In addition to the lateral, an AP of the cervical spine and open mouth odontoid view should be obtained. Oblique views of the cervical spine can aid with diagnosis although they are not needed on every patient.

If the initial screening radiographs are normal and the patient still has significant neck pain, flexion extension views can be helpful in ruling out cervical spine instability. The lateral cervical spine radiographs should be examined closely for occipital C1 alignment by determining Powers ratio. Despite "normal" radiographs, a significant spinal injury is possible. No spine can be "cleared" on radiographs alone. The spine must be cleared on both a radiographic and clinical basis before discontinuing spine precautions. For the spine to be cleared clinically, the patient must not have significant pain in the area and must have a full range of motion.

Careful assessment of the C1–2 articulation is important, checking the atlantodens interval, which measures up to 5 mm in children, and also checking the space available for the cord in using the rule of thirds (10). The open mouth view visualizes the odontoid and the lateral masses of C1 to further check the articulation of C1 and C2 for any potential injury. The distance between the lateral masses of the C1 should be checked, fracture of the odontoid should be ruled out, and any significant rotational deformity should be identifiable (95).

Initially, the soft tissues in the anterior aspect of the vertebral column should be checked. In a resting non-crying child, the soft tissues on the anterior aspect of C2 should not measure more than 7 mm, or two-thirds the width of C2 vertebral body. On the lower cervical spine, anterior to approximately C6, the soft tissues can measure as much as 14 mm in width without being pathologic (49). Any significant alterations in thickness of the soft tissues anterior of the spine should raise suspicion of significant spinal injury.

Next, the bony articulations from C2 down through the top of T1 should be inspected carefully, noting the bone quality itself, the alignment of the anterior portion of the vertebral bodies, the shape of the vertebral bodies, the height of each disc space, posterior vertebral line, the facet joints, the posterior laminar line, and posterior elements. These should all be checked for alignment and for evidence of fractures.

The normal spine in young children differs considerably from that in adults, especially in the cervical region. Lack of awareness of the normal radiographic appearances may lead to misdiagnosis. Common transient developmental features and more unusual normal variants may be mistaken for spinal trauma in children as listed previously. The multiple primary and secondary ossification centers and their intervening synchondroses are often mistaken for evidence of fracture or avulsion fragmentation.

In young children, the lateral radiographs of the thoracic and lumbar spine may occasionally show a vertically oriented radiolucent cleft. This cleft may represent a more anteriorly positioned neurocentral synchondroses. A similar cleft may also represent a bifid vertebrae. Morphologic variations in the lumbosacral region are common. Lumbarization of the first sacral segment to form a sixth lumbar vertebrae or bilateral or unilateral fusion of the L5 to the sacrum is often seen.

Incomplete osseous fusion of the neural arch of L5 or S1 is present in up to 50% of some populations. A gradual decrease in this percentage occurs throughout childhood, but remains high even in adolescence.

Variations caused by displacement of vertebrae may resemble subluxation and can be a major area of concern. Significant anterior displacement of the second or third cervical vertebrae resembling a true subluxation is common in children between 1 and 7 years of age. This probably occurs in a frequency of approximately 20%. Less frequently similar displacement would even be seen between the third and fourth cervical vertebrae. This localized area of increased spinal motion can only be correctly called pseudosubluxation in the asymptomatic child or a child in whom other studies of significant spinal column injury are negative.

On lateral radiograph, an increased atlantodens interval occurs in about 20% of normal children. There may be no lordosis in the cervical spine in approximately 50% of children. The absence of uniform angulation, absence of cervical lordosis, and absence of flexion curves have been reported in high percentage normal asymptomatic children. All of these appear to suggest, but do not necessarily indicate, ligamentous injury. Normal anterior wedging of the immature vertebral bodies may appear like a compression fracture. Spinous process, secondary ossification centers may be confused with avulsion fractures.

In the young child, radiographic diagnosis is complicated further by the relative elasticity of the cartilaginous spine and supporting ligamentous structures, which may allow severe cord damage in the absence of significant radiographic findings (64, 65). Burke studied 7 children 13 months to 12 years of age and noted that 5 of the younger children sustained flexion rotation injuries with a preponderance of thoracic spine involvement in extensive longitudinal traction injuries extending over several levels (24). Even in the three children in whom the vertebral injury could be radiographically demonstrated, actual cord involvement extended several segments above the osseus involvement (8, 25, 29).

Hyperextension injuries may reduce spontaneously, causing radiographs to look benign. Soft tissue swelling of the perivertebral fat stripes may be the only indication of this type of injury. Another indication of such an injury may be a small piece of bone pulled away from the anterior inferior edge of the ossifying vertebral column at the point of separation of the end plate, anterior longitudinal ligament, and annulus. Difficulties in measuring the sagittal and interpedicular diameters of the cervical spine canal on plain radiographs in children is a known problem.

Naik's values can be consulted for the interpretation of spinal canal's sagittal diameters (88). Additional imaging modalities may be helpful in both cases of established spine injury as well as high suspicion injuries with normal plain radiographs.

Normal Variance

The following normal radiographic findings have been misinterpreted as injury:

1. The apical ossification center of the odontoid.
2. The secondary ossification center at the tips of the transverse and spinous processes.
3. Incomplete ossification, especially of the odontoid process with apparent superior subluxation of the anterior arch of C1.
4. Persistence of the synchondrosis at the base of the odontoid.
5. Anterior wedging of a young child's vertebrae misinterpreted as a compression fracture.
6. Findings associated with hypermobility, pseudo subluxation, especially at C2–3.
7. Increase in the atlanto-dense interval of >4 mm.
8. Absence of the ossification center of the anterior arch of C1 in the first year of life suggesting posterior displacement of C1 on the odontoid.
9. Physiologic variations in soft tissue width anterior to the cervical spine.
10. Overlying anatomy, such as ear, braided hair, teeth, or hyoid bone.
11. Angulation of the odontoid seen in 4% of all children.
12. Horizontally placed facets in the younger child creating the illusion of Pillar fracture.
13. Congenital anomalies, such as osteoid odontoideum, spina bifida, and non-segmentation.

Plain Tomography

Good quality plain tomography can help define certain injuries. Injuries in the transverse plane usually can be seen quite readily with good quality plain tomography. Plain tomography may be the modality of choice for flexion distraction (seat belt) injuries. With the wide availability of CT scans and sagittal reconstructions, however, plain tomography is used less and less, although it still can provide extremely useful information.

CT Scanning

Computerized tomography is one of the main stays for evaluating spine injuries. It is an important adjunct to the plain radiographies in all but the most simple of spine fractures. The CT scan should be used when bony injuries are suspected or known to exist to help determine the extent of bony injury, canal comprise, and to assess overall spinal stability. Vertebral end plate fractures are imaged better by this modality than any other. Occasionally the addition of contrast intravenously or myelographically can enhance the imaging of the canal or neuroforamen.

The use of three-dimensional reconstructions in the CT images can help conceptualize these injuries in a more straight forward three-dimensional image. This is extremely helpful in planning of both surgical and nonsurgical treatment of these injuries.

Magnetic Resonance Imaging

The MRI is also an adjunct to the plain radiographs for imaging of spinal injuries. It is rapidly becoming an indispensable part of evaluating severe spinal injuries. Its main indications are for evaluation of the soft tissue injuries associated with spinal fractures, including herniated discs, neuroforaminal encroachment, hematomas, spinal cord edema, post-traumatic spinal cord cysts, and extent of damage to ligaments and other soft tissue that surrounds in the spinal column. Any child with a neurologic deficit should have an MRI of the spine in addition to any other imaging modality.

Myelography

Myelography has a very limited role in children's thoracic and lumbar fractures and is not used unless MRI is either unavailable or contraindicated.

Bone Scintigraphy

Radionuclide imaging using technetium-99 phosphate can be helpful in diagnosing more occult injuries of the spine and establishing an approximate location. This is especially true in spondylolysis of the pars intra articularis. It is helpful when combined with laboratory studies in differentiating trauma from other etiologies that might present as back pain, such as infection or tumor. It is also useful in evaluating children who are the victims of non-accidental trauma. The single photon emission computed tomography (SPECT) scan is an important adjunct to the diagnose of stress fractures, especially of the pars intra articularis, because it may be positive even in the presence of normal bone scans.

A clinical examination and knowledge of the pathophysiology of spine trauma determine which imaging modality is used. Because of the inherent elasticity of the soft tissues in childrens' spines, trauma can cause damage that will not be evident on plain radiography.

Other factors, such as the need for anesthesia for MRIs in young children, exposure to radiation, and the cost of these studies, must also be considered when imaging spine injuries. The determination of spinal alignment, displacement, and extent of canal comprise is the goal of these imaging modalities and should occur with a judicious use of tests.

Differential Diagnosis

Whenever a child is being evaluated for a spinal injury, one must keep in mind that there is a long list of diagnoses that tend to look as though they are the result of acute trauma, but actually represent an underlying condition. Congenital spine abnormalities are not common but certainly can confuse the issue when the patient has been involved in trauma. Although congenital hemi-vertebrae would not be painful, generalized back pain with a wedge-shaped vertebra on spine radiographs could be confused with an acute traumatic injury. Congenital spine abnormalities do have a typical appearance and would not be associated with pain either by history or by physical examination. If doubt about the abnormality still exists, a bone scan would be normal and would confirm the diagnosis of a congenital problem.

Klippel-Feil syndrome may also be confusing in interpretation of the C-spine radiograph after trauma. Fused vertebrae can also lead to some minor spinal alignment variations that can be mistaken for traumatic instability.

Infection

A spinal infection can occasionally be misinterpreted as a fracture. As in a fracture, a spinal infection can result in acute onset of back pain. Typically, there will be no history of significant trauma. (Occasionally a pathologic fracture can occur through an infected vertebral body.) In cases of infection, wedging can also occur in adjacent vertebrae due to diskitis (116). Plain radiographs often demonstrate narrowing of the intervertebral discs.

Patients with vertebral osteomyelitis are typically very ill, but this is not always the case. There is often fever, leukocytosis, and an increased erythrocyte sedimentation rate. A blood culture is often positive. A bone scan may not differentiate among the fracture, tumor, or infection. MRI may show replacement or edema of the marrow elements. Occasionally a biopsy is needed to obtain the correct diagnosis.

Neoplasm

Primary tumors, both benign and malignant, involve the spine. As the marrow and cancellous bone become replaced by tumor, the vertebral body is widened and pathologic fractures can occur. These fractures can be differentiated by history and radiographic features. Usually there is only minimal, if any, history of trauma. Radiographically, the bony elements of tumor will be abnormal with evidence of prior bone destruction, formation, or abnormal fracture pattern. Often, other imaging modalities, including an MRI or CT scan, are used to support the diagnosis (62). Biopsy is often necessary to confirm the diagnosis.

Metabolic Disease

Any of the metabolic diseases that lead to osteopenia can significantly weaken the vertebrae so that minor trauma can lead to a pathologic fracture. Osteogenesis imperfecta patients often have spinal fractures at different levels. The mucopolysaccharidosis often involve the spine and can result in vertebral body fractures. Morquio syndrome is characterized by involvement of all the vertebrae.

The radiographic appearance is similar to spondyloepiphyseal dysplasia with platyspondylisis. A careful history and physical examination as well as laboratory investigation usually help make the diagnose of metabolic bone disease.

Spondyloepiphyseal Dysplasia

Occasionally the abnormalities in spondyloepiphyseal dysplasia which include flattening of the vertebral bodies relative to the normal height can mimic fractures. Radiographic findings of epiphyseal and vertebral body dysplasia along with the usual family history and short stature can confirm the diagnosis of spondyloepiphyseal dysplasia.

Scheuermann's Disease

Scheuermann's disease is characterized by wedging of multiple thoracic vertebrae. These patients have characteristic round back deformity with chronic thoracic back pain and ridged kyphosis. The radiographic picture is one of narrow disc space increased anterior posterior diameter of the apical thoracic vertebrae, loss of normal height of the involved vertebrae, and end plate irregularity (30). Schmorl's nodes may be present but are not necessary to make the diagnosis. Classically, the wedging is described as three consecutive vertebrae with wedging of at least 5°. The clinical and radiographic presentation of Scheuermann's disease usually eliminates trauma as etiology for the wedging of the vertebral body.

Early Management

Whenever a spine injury is suspected, the patient must be handled appropriately. Immediate immobilization to allow transportation is key to avoid further neurologic injury to the patient. Spinal injuries should be considered whenever a patient is unconscious after trauma or reports numbness, weakness, and neck or back pain. Even transient neurologic symptoms after trauma warrant immobilization until instability can be ruled out. Spinal immobilization usually requires use of a back board combined with devices designed specifically to immobilize the head and neck. Combinations of tape and sandbags provide much more effective immobilization of the head and neck than can be achieved with a hard collar alone. Positioning of children less than 10 years old on a standard backboard tends to force the cervical spine into relative kyphosis because young children have large heads in comparison to the rest of their body (Fig. 13.6). Therefore, the use of a mattress to raise the torso relative to the head or a recess to accommodate the occiput is recommended (66). This discrepancy between the circumference of the head and the circumference of the chest attains 50% of its adult size.

Athletic injuries are a common cause of cervical spine injuries in older pediatric patients. A spine board should always be present in playing fields and gymnasiums where high risk sports like football and gymnastics take place.

In helmeted sports, the patient should be transported with the helmet in place, but the face mask should be cut away, allowing access to the airway. A high spinal cord injury commonly has compromised respiratory function that requires endotracheal intubation. The helmet is then removed in the emergency room while the head is stabilized manually. Attention must be directed to the ABCs: airway, breathing, and circulation.

The recommended technique to establish an airway in a spinal cord injury patient is controversial, and no studies have specifically addressed this issue in the pediatric patient. Cervical collars do not adequately immobilize the spine during orotracheal intubation. In line traction does tend to minimize spinal motion during intubation, but has some theoretical danger of overdistracting the rare case of highly unstable cervical spine injuries (7, 84).

Clinical studies of cervical spine fractures that underwent oral intubation compared to those patients intubated nasally found no patients with neurologic deterioration attributed to intubation technique (68,

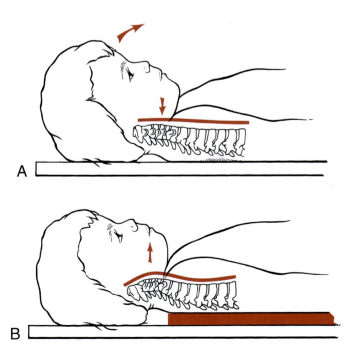

FIGURE 13.6.
A. Positioning of a child on a standard backboard produces the cervical spine into a kyphotic position. **B.** The use of a mattress to raise the torso accommodates the child's large head to provide safer lordotic cervical spine alignment.

110). Fiberoptic guided intubation tends to minimize spine motion during intubation.

Children with spinal injuries should remain on a backboard during initial transport and assessment. It is reasonable after the initial physical examination and radiographic assessment to remove the patient from the spine board with the usual precautions to an appropriate hospital bed to accommodate the specific injuries. The patient should be removed from the backboard as soon as it can be done safely because it only takes 1 or 2 hours to produce a full thickness skin breakdown in a neurocompromised patient from pressure necrosis.

Children with an unstable cervical spine injury should be immobilized initially using a Gardner-Wells tong and traction, or a sufficiently rigid brace.

Cervical Spine Injuries

Cervical spine injuries are uncommon in children. When they do occur, they occur in the child less than age 8, most often in the upper cervical spine (above C4). In the child greater than age 8, they usually occur below C4.

Obstetrical Trauma

Obstetrical trauma has been reported as the cause of serious and occasionally fatal cervical spine injuries. Atlanto-occipital and atlanto-axial dislocations, odontoid fractures, and cord transections have all been reported (104a), and most of these injuries occur in forceful breech extractions. Forceful breech extractions appears to be the most common cause of cervical spine injuries in newborns, but can also be seen in cephalic presentations.

Hyperextension of the neck in utero with the fetus in breech position will result in an estimated 25% incidence of spinal cord transection if the child is delivered vaginally (1, 19). Obviously, cesarean section is recommended in these cases.

Spinal cords removed from newborns who have died from obstetrical trauma demonstrate injury over long segments, suggesting that longitudinal traction is the major injuring factor (103a). However, in adults, spinal cord injury is usually well localized to a short segment of the cord. The large percentage of cartilage in the skeletal elements of neonates is difficult to evaluate radiographically, and significant injury may be missed easily because it may involve the cartilaginous portion of the vertebral body and spare the bony elements. (Radiographs can remain normal despite significant spinal cord injury in newborns.) Any newborn suspected of having a spinal injury or neurologic deficit should be evaluated with plain radiographs and a MRI of the spine. Cast immobilization using a Minerva type cast should be used until adequate healing can be seen radiographically—usually 6 to 8 weeks. Operative treatment is rarely, if ever, indicated.

Occipoatlantal Dislocations

Traumatic dislocation of the occiput from the atlas occurs commonly in fatal cranial spinal injuries. Few children survive this injury because of the neurologic deficit that results from injury to the upper cervical cord, brain stem, and cranial nerves. Dislocation is usually the result of high energy trauma commonly involving a motor vehicle (Fig. 13.7) (21). Severe associated injury is common. Survival with this injury is being reported with increasing frequency, in part, because of better emergency care results in early cardiopulmonary resuscitation and ventilatory support for these patients, who previously would not have survived.

Bucholz and Burkhead reported an incidence of 8% in victims of fatal traffic accidents, making it the single most common injury encountered (20). The injury was more than twice as frequent in the pediatric age group—15%, compared with 6% in adults. This finding is consistent with a higher incidence of upper cervical spine injuries in children as compared to adults.

The degree of neurologic injury in patients who survive occipito atlanto dislocation varies. Patients rarely present with normal neurologic examinations or with minimal deficit. In a series of Montane et al., two patients presented with minor weakness and hyper-reflexia, and one patient had a more severe neurologic injury, only retaining anti-gravity strength in her extremities unilaterally (86). The latter patient also sustained several episodes of heart block and respiratory arrest, suggesting injury to the cardiorespiratory centers in the brain stem. A fourth patient who did not survive suffered a complete cord transection at C1 and a severe head injury.

A patient presented by Zigler et al. survived with a complete paralysis at the C1 level, as well as palsy of the spinal accessory nerve (121). This resulted in a flail neck, which necessitated fusion from the occiput to the thoracic spine to avoid the need for external support. The patient also required tracheostomy because he was ventilatory dependent.

Ogden described an 8-year-old girl with irregular pulse and respiration, which resolved on extension of the neck (92). Page et al. described a patient with a C5 quadriplegia and palsy of the tenth and twelfth cranial nerves on initial presentation, with assent to a C2 level (93). Evarts described a patient with left hemiparesis and palsies of the sixth, ninth, tenth, and twelfth cranial nerves (44).

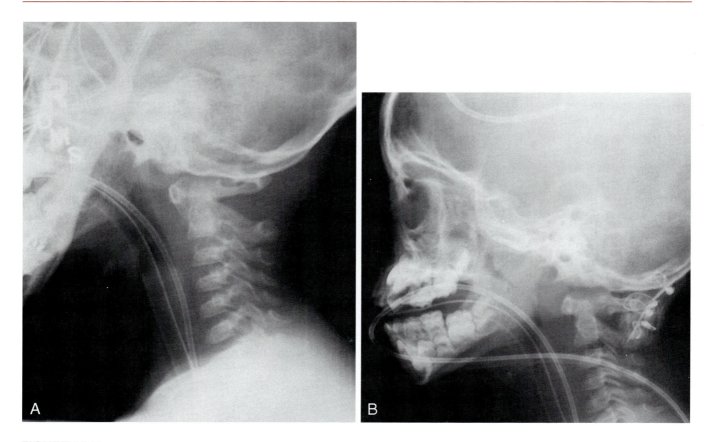

FIGURE 13.7.

A. A child with an atlanto-occipital instability following a motor vehicle accident. **B.** This patient underwent occiput-C2 fusion with wiring.

Radiographic diagnosis of occipito atlanto dislocation may not be apparent until traction is applied to the skull. It is important to check lateral radiographic and cervical spine immediately after applying traction to avoid overdistraction of this or other ligamentous injuries.

Several radiographic parameters are helpful in determining the extent of injury in the occipito atlanto articulation. The distance between the basion and the dens should not exceed 5 mm in adults and 10 mm in children (117). The greater distance in children has been attributed to incomplete ossification of the dens.

The Powers ratio should also be evaluated (97). This ratio is the distance between the basion and the posterior arch of the atlas divided by the distance between the opisthion and the anterior arch of the atlas (Fig. 13.8). Values greater than 1.0 are definitely abnormal, and values less than 0.9 are definitely normal. The advantage of this ratio is that it is dimensionless, and thus unaffected by magnification on the radiograph.

If the landmarks are not identified easily on a lateral cervical spine radiograph, they can be measured on a midline sagittal reconstruction of a CT scan. The ratio is sensitive to anterior occipito atlanto dislocation because one line (BC) parallels the direction of the dislocation, while the second (OA) is almost perpendicular to it. The Powers ratio may be insensitive to posterior occipito atlanto dislocation, as described by Eismont and Bohlman (39). It is invalid if there is

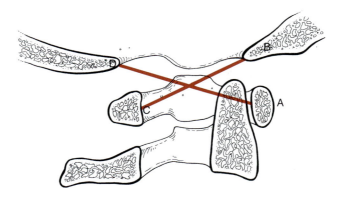

FIGURE 13.8.

The Power's ratio (BC/OA) >1 is abnormal: The distance between the basion and the posterior arch of the atlas divided by the distance between the opisthion and the anterior arch of the atlas.

a fracture of the atlas or congenital abnormality of the foramen magnum.

Another measurement that can be used to evaluate the stability of the occipitoatlanto joint is horizontal translation on flexion/extension. The basion should not translate more than 1 mm relative to the odontoid (102, 118). This value has only been established for adults and has not been validated in children. However, flexion/extension radiographs should never be done on an unresponsive patient or if evidence of spinal instability exists on routine radiographs.

Treatment of occipitoatlanto dislocation is controversial. Immobilization in a halo or Minerva cast has been advocated by some authors (92). Most recent authors advocate operative treatment with posterior occipitocervical fusion (55). Because traction can distract the occipitocervical junction, traction is contraindicated. Halo immobilization is recommended as soon as the injury is identified. It provides the most secure stabilization available, and should be placed preoperatively. Nontraumatic instability has also been described in children at the occipitoatlanto junction. Most often it is associated with congenital fusions of the upper cervical spine or other anomalies of the cervical spine. If severe instability is documented and neurologic findings are present, posterior occipitocervical fusion from the occiput to C1 is indicated (55).

Gilles et al. proposed that occipitoatlanto instability may be a factor in infant sudden death syndrome (56). In a cadaver study, Gilles demonstrated that during extension of the head, the atlas invaginates into the foramen magnum, resulting in bilateral vertebral artery compression and cerebral ischemia.

Atlas Fractures

Burst fractures of the C1 ring are uncommon in children. The mechanism of injury is thought to be a blow to the head. This blow transmits a compressive force to the occipital condyles, which displaces the lateral masses of the atlas laterally. If the force is severe enough, the transverse ligament ruptures or is avulsed at its point of attachment. In the child under age 7, the fracture may occur through the neurocentral synchondroses. The child usually will have a severe headache and limitation of neck rotation. The CT scan is usually diagnostic. It is important not to confuse the normal appearing synchondroses or anomalous ossification centers of the anterior arch with fractures. Neurologic deficits are uncommon.

Treatment of C1 fractures should include immobilization for 3 to 6 months with either a Minerva cast or halo, followed by a brace. Healing can be followed using serial CT scans. Stability of the atlanto axial articulation should be confirmed on flexion/extension radiographs before discontinuing treatment. Allen and Ferguson advocate an initial 4- to 6-week period of traction if more than 4 mm lateral displacement of the lateral mass is seen (5). Generally these fractures heal without complications, and surgery is rarely indicated.

Atlanto Axial Segment

Lesions occurring at the atlanto axial interval in children can be separated into traumatic and atraumatic instabilities. These lesions are then further divided as being either rotational or translational. Stability at this joint is almost entirely dependent on ligaments that must simultaneously protect the articulation and allow for extensive mobility. Although the primary motion is rotation, small amounts of flexion/extension, vertical translation, and lateral slide also occur.

Approximately 50% of cervical rotation takes place between the first and second segments around the anterior odontoid process. Therefore, the lateral wall of the vertebral foramen of C1 rotates to a considerable extent, across the canal at C2, physiologically decreasing the opening of the spinal canal between the two segments. The spinal canal of C1 is large compared with the other cervical segments and safely accommodates this degree of rotation and some degree of pathologic displacement without cord pressure. According to Steel, the cord moves into this free space when there is a displacement of C1 on C2 (109). The canal at C1 is occupied equally by the cord, the odontoid, and free space. This is commonly known as Steel's rule of thirds. Anterior displacement of the atlas exceeding the thickness of the odontoid may place the adjacent segment of the cord in jeopardy.

The significance of trauma in this highly mobile articulation lies in the fact that it houses the vulnerable cervical medullary portion of the spinal cord that can be damaged by C1 on C2 displacement. The vertebral arteries which supply a significant amount of blood to the upper cord and cerebellum are fixed in the foramen transversarium of C1 and C2, and can be carried forward and compressed by an atlanto axial shift with subsequent ischemia to neuro tissue.

Atlanto Axial Instability (Translational Instabilities)

Traumatic atlanto axial subluxation/dislocation in children secondary to transverse ligament rupture is an extremely uncommon injury. A dislocation of the atlanto-axial joint without a fracture occurs when the transverse ligament of the atlas is torn. This allows the spinal cord to be compressed between the intact odontoid and the posterior arch of the atlas. Usually it is a lethal injury.

Fielding recommends 8 to 12 weeks of immobilization for treatment of acute traumatic rupture of the transverse ligament, but no clinical series in children has been reported to evaluate the efficacy of nonoperative treatment (48). Treatment can be done in a halo or Minerva cast with the head in slight extension. Any nonoperative treatment should be followed by stress films of the cervical spine. If the displacement persists, posterior C1-C2 fusion is recommended.

Nontraumatic instability is associated with a variety of developmental disorders, including Down syndrome, Klippel-Feil syndrome, and many of the skeletal dysplasias. This association may be caused by the laxity of the transverse ligament or hypoplasia of the odontoid. In Down syndrome, the incidence of instability has been reported to be as high as 20%. These patients are at risk for catastrophic injury after trivial trauma, and they should be screened routinely for instability, even if asymptomatic, at age 5 and on a yearly basis thereafter. If the atlanto dens interval (ADI) is greater than 5 mm, they should avoid high risk activities and should undergo repeat C-spine radiographs on a yearly basis. C1-2 fusion is indicated if ADI is greater than 10 mm or if signs of myelopathy are present. A small number of patients have no obvious predisposing factors.

The normal ADI is 3 mm in children. If an ADI greater than 5 mm is encountered, the patient should avoid contact sports and other activities that carry a high risk of flexion injury. If ADI is greater than 10 mm, or if the patient has any symptoms or signs of spinal cord compression, C1-C2 posterior spinal fusion is recommended. A C1-C2 fusion in Down syndrome is fraught with complications, and this should not be taken lightly.

Atlanto Axial Rotatory Subluxation

Rotatory instability of the atlanto axial joint is common in the pediatric population. Although it can occur as a result of minor or major trauma, its etiology is commonly atraumatic.

Grisel described this condition in 1930, which resulted in the term Grisel's syndrome (57). Various causes include upper respiratory and throat infections, tuberculosis, and rheumatoid disease. A small number of patients have no obvious predisposing factors. Grisel's syndrome is thought to develop when infectious agents are carried to the area of the ligaments that support the atlanto axial complex via the venous plexus, which drains the posterior superior nasal pharynx resulting in inflammation and secondary ligamentous laxity. If ligamentous laxity exists, rotation of the neck can result in subluxation of the atlanto axial joints.

A combination of muscle spasm, swollen capsular, and synovial tissue are believed to be responsible for blocking the subluxation from reducing spontaneously. Patients present with torticollis and neck pain which varies from mild discomfort to severe pain. The torticollis can be differentiated from congenital muscular torticollis by the position of the head with the chin pointing to the side of the muscle spasm. Neurologic deficit is uncommon, but quadriparesis has been caused by this condition.

Standard radiographs can be used to confirm the diagnosis, but interpretation is difficult because of rotation of the head and neck. Dynamic CT with the head turned maximally to the right and left is the best way to confirm a diagnosis, by showing a loss of normal rotation between C1 and C2. Once other injuries have been ruled out, treatment protocols are the same regardless whether the onset was traumatic or atraumatic. Treatment should be tailored to the degree of severity in each case. If symptoms have been present for a week or less, cervical collar immobilization, bed rest, and analgesic medication may be adequate to allow resolution of the muscle spasm and torticollis. If symptoms persist for more than a week, cervical traction with a head halter or Gardner-Wells tongs should be used until spasm resolves and subluxation is reduced. Fielding recommends an arbitrary maximum weight of 6.8 kilograms in children (48). A Minerva type brace/cast or halo should be used for 6 or 9 more weeks to allow adequate healing of inflamed tissues. It is thought that after reduction and immobilization for this period of time, the lesion will heal without instability even if the cause of the original inflammation continues.

If symptoms have been present for more than a month, reduction with traction is unlikely. This is referred to as rotatory fixation by Fielding and Hawkins (50). In their patients, there was an average delay of diagnosis of over 11 months. They recommend an initial period of traction, followed by posterior cervical fusion of C1 on C2. If reduction is not achieved, fusion should be in situ, rather than risk neurologic deficit by attempting a reduction under general anesthesia.

Odontoid Fractures

In children below age 11, C1 on C2 displacement almost always results from a fracture of the odontoid at the level of the growth plate between the odontoid and the axis body. This fracture tends to "decompress" the cord and result in less cord injuries than the true atlantoaxial dislocation. The lateral C-spine radiograph usually demonstrates the anteriorly displaced odontoid process with a normal ADI but reduced SAC.

Treatment for fracture of the dens at its base depends on the displacement. Traction on the cervical spine in slight extension usually results in reduction of the displaced or angulated odontoid. The fracture usually heals promptly when stabilized in a Minerva cast or halo for 8 to 12 weeks. Post-treatment stability should be checked with flexion, extension, and lateral radiograph of the cervical spine. Failure to recognize this injury may lead to resorption of the basilar portion of the odontoid. This resorption produces the appearance of the absent odontoid or an os odontoid. In the case of C1-C2 instability, a posterior C1-C2 fusion is indicated.

Fractures of the odontoid in young children almost always occur as an epiphyseal separation of the growth plate at the base of the dens. Most cases result from severe falls or motor vehicle accidents, but separation of the growth plate can occur with minor trauma as well. Usually the dens is displaced forward with the atlas and does not compress the spinal cord. The atlanto dens interval is not increased on a lateral radiograph; however, the space available for the cord is reduced depending on the degree of displacement. Neurologic deficit is uncommon.

In a series by Sherk et al., only patients with associated head injury had a neurologic deficit (103). Fracture displacement of at least 50% was universal in Sherk's reported cases, but if displacement is not present, identification of the fracture on radiographs may be difficult. Tomograms may show widening of the growth plate. Anterior angulation of the odontoid fragment is an almost constant finding and may help identify the minimally displaced fracture. As in other cervical spine injuries, occipital pain, muscle spasm, and limited neck motion are common findings.

Reduction and casts or Halo immobilization are appropriate treatment for this injury. Six to eight weeks of immobilization are required. When appropriately immobilized nonunion is rare, so is avascular necrosis or growth disturbance of the odontoid fragment. Fracture of the odontoid occurring in older children at the base of the dens after closure of the growth plate is extremely uncommon. When it occurs, it follows the same pattern seen in adults. It is important not to confuse epiphyseal scar at the base of the odontoid with a fracture.

Failure to recognize odontoid fracture in childhood may be responsible for the clinical syndrome of os odontoideum. Previously, it was believed that os odontoideum was a congenital abnormality caused by failed fusion of the odontoid process to the vertebral centrum. Several case reports in the literature document the os odontoideum or the absence of the odontoid process occurring after trauma to the cervical spine. There are nine reported cases of development of an os odontoideum after injury with preinjury documentation of normal radiographs.

Fielding believes that injury to the blood supply combined with retraction of the dens by the alar ligaments contributes to creating a nonunion of the odontoid (48). Os odontoideum leads to atlanto axial instability because the odontoid is no longer attached to C2.

In a symptomatic or asymptomatic patient with documented instability, treatment is by C1-C2 posterior cervical fusion (83). Controversy exists regarding the asymptomatic patient without radiographic instability. Some authors advocate observation and repeated examination, while others recommend fusion to prevent neurologic injury with minor trauma.

C2 Pedicle Fracture

The so-called "hangman's fracture" has been reported in an infant as young as 7 weeks old. No data exists regarding the mechanism of injury in children, but it is believed to be similar to that in adult hangman's fractures. In most reported series, there has been no neurologic deficit. Weiss and Kaufman reported the case of a hangman's fracture in a 12-month-old child with central cord syndrome, and Pizzutillo et al. had only one of five patients with a neurologic deficit (96, 115).

Radiographic evaluation of this injury is complicated by two factors. The neural central synchondroses can mimic a fracture on oblique radiographic views and can persist beyond the age of 7 years, at which time it is usually closed. The more difficult problem in radiographic evaluation is differentiating the physiologic subluxation at C2-3 from pathologic subluxations, secondary to horizontal orientation of the pedicles and facet joints of C2. Pseudosubluxation of C2-3 is present in 50% of children up to age 8. It is secondary to physiologic ligamentous laxity and horizontally oriented facet joints in this age group.

Swischuk's posterior cervical line is useful in evaluating hypermobility at this level (112). The posterior laminar line is identified at the base of the spinous process at C1, 2, and 3 in a line drawn connecting this landmark at C1 and C3. The posterior laminar line of C2 should lie within 1 mm of this line. If it lies more than 1.5 mm posterior to Swischuk's line, one should become suspicious of a fracture separating the anterior body and posterior lamina (112). If the distance is more than 2 mm, a fracture is almost certainly present.

If the lateral radiograph view is normal, the same criteria should be applied to the flexion radiograph. A true lateral radiograph view is essential for this technique to be used reliably. Treatment of Hangman's fractures in an infant is similar to treatment in an adult. If the body of C2 is not displaced significantly on C3, immobilization in a rigid collar or custom fabricated splint (SOMI or Minerva type) should be adequate. If there is more than 3 mm anterior displacement of C2 on C3, a more rigid immobilization is indicated. A Minerva cast or halo is most appropriate (78). Surgery is rarely indicated on an acute basis.

Subaxial Injuries

Subaxial injuries are distinctly different in children below age 8 and those over age 8. In the younger group, injuries are visually above C4. In the older group, the injuries are usually below C4 and result in injury patterns similar to those seen in adults. Flexion injuries predominate. Complete dislocations appear to be uncommon until late adolescence. Compression fractures are the most common injury. Residual kyphosis, following flexion injury, may be less well tolerated in the growing child than in adults. Some authors advocate posterior fusion to prevent late disability.

Most commonly, posterior interspinous wiring and fusion of the involved levels is sufficient. They should be accompanied by a brace for 2 to 3 months postoperatively. Subaxial injuries in infants and young children may have normal radiographic appearance in the face of serious cervical instability and neurologic deficit.

One important type of subaxillary injury in young children is separation of the vertebral end plate from the vertebral body. This usually occurs through the epiphysis, similar to a physeal injury in a long bone. Salter Harris Type I injuries occur in infants and young children, and Type III injuries occur in older adolescence, as the physis begins to close. It usually results from flexion injuries causing subluxation or dislocation of the facet joints. It does not result in rupture of the intervertebral disc as it does in adults with this injury. True incidence of this injury is not known because it is difficult to identify on radiographs. This injury is most common at the C2-3 level. The fracture may recoil after injury and return to normal alignment, making radiographic identification impossible. The most likely radiographic finding is widening of the intervertebral disc space.

Physeal separation may play an important rule in injuries where neurologic deficit has occurred but no radiographic abnormality is seen. In the cervical spine, this usually involves the inferior end plate. Salter Harris Type I injuries are extremely unstable. If these injuries are identified in a child, Ogden advocates operative stabilization (92). A single level posterior instrumentation and fusion is adequate. Posterior intraspinous wiring can be used for fixation. Postoperative bracing or casting for 2 to 3 months is recommended. In contrast, Type III injuries do not completely separate the physes from the vertebra. Therefore, if stability is maintained, these injuries will heal quickly if immobilized in a Minerva cast or halo brace.

Ogden states that surgical treatment is rarely necessary in young children with C spine compression fractures even with ligamentous instability. He advocates reduction and traction, followed by rigid immobilization. Treatment of fractures or dislocations of the lower cervical spine should consist of reduction of the fracture or dislocation with skeletal traction and then stabilization of the spine in a halo or Minerva cast.

Surgical stabilization is indicated in children only if there is a progressive neurologic deficit, severe unreducible deformity, and delayed spinal instability (108). If canal decompression is indicated, an anterior approach is needed. Posterior decompression is usually suboptimal, and laminectomy may result in increased instability (107). Multiple level laminectomies (more than 4 or 5) in children result in progressive late kyphotic deformity and require prophylactic fusion. If posterior fusion is required, autogenous bone graft should be used because the use of allograft is associated with an unacceptably high rate of pseudoarthrosis.

Thoracic and Lumbar Spine Injuries

In a three column system, injuries of the thoracic and lumbar spine can be divided into four major types: compression fracture, which is failure of the anterior column with an intact middle column; a burst fracture, which is failure under compression of both anterior middle columns; a seat belt fracture, which is a compression injury of the anterior column with distraction of the middle and posterior columns to either bony or ligamentous elements (flexion distraction); and a fracture/dislocation with all three columns failing compression, rotation shear of the anterior column distraction, shear of the middle column, and distraction with rotation shear of the posterior column.

Flexion (Compression) Fractures

The normal kyphotic alignment of the thoracic spine predisposes it to compressive (flexion) injuries. Compression fractures of the thoracic spine are relatively common and those involving the lumbar spine are uncommon. The vertebral bodies typically have a wedge shape on lateral radiographs with the posterior cortical height maintained. Anterior vertebral bony compression is usually 20% or less, and commonly occurs at several levels. Fortunately, most compressive fractures of the thoracic spine are stable injuries with additional support from the rib cage, which prevents excessive translational movements during trauma.

The anterior column is compromised with the middle and posterior columns intact. The end plates may be involved in the fractures. The superior end plate sustains injury twice as often as the inferior end plate. Even in those fractures with 50% compression, posterior elements are often not involved. Although there may be pain and tenderness in the posterior spine, there is usually no palpable widening of the interspinous distance. Neurologic findings are rare.

Vertebral body wedging in the sagittal plane usually remodels with reconstitution of the vertebral height, especially in children less than 10 years old (69). Frontal (coronal) plane wedging does not correct as well. If the end plates are fractured, there is usually no correction with growth, presumably because of disruption of the growth centers and partial growth arrest. Slight axial deviations (less than 10°) can be corrected by asymmetric growth of adjacent vertebral bodies.

Compression fractures that do not have posterior involvement or apophyseal ring fractures are usually stable, both mechanically and neurologically. If there is any middle or posterior column involvement, there is potential for instability. A CT scan is usually indicated in compression fractures with more than 30% loss of anterior vertebral body height or any loss of posterior vertebral body height to rule out a burst fracture with middle column instability.

Nonoperative Treatment

Most compression fractures, except for some severe compressions and multiple fractures in the thoracic spine, are stable injuries and can be treated nonoperatively in an extension thoracolumbosacral orthosis (TLSO). Compression fractures heal in 6 to 8 weeks, and they do not tend to progress (46). If the compression is mild, the patient can be treated symptomatically with rest, with or without external support. Children are usually asymptomatic in 1 to 2 weeks. Posterior tenderness at the level of the fracture may continue for several weeks, but it responds to symptomatic treatment. In an end plate fracture or disc herniation, symptoms may persist a little longer. The outcome of nonoperative treatment with casting and bed rest has been satisfactory. Compression fractures less than 50% loss of anterior body height are good candidates for nonoperative treatment.

Acute fractures with significant angular kyphosis or significant pain should be treated in an extension type TLSO for 6 to 8 weeks or until pain is gone.

Severe Compression Fractures

Compression fractures rarely require surgery. When there is more than 50% loss of anterior height or if there are multiple compression fractures leading to increased kyphosis, posterior instrumentation is necessary. Contoured Harrington rods or any of the newer multiple hook rod systems may be used. Instrumentation should be long enough in the thoracic spine to encompass the kyphosis and apply compressive forces. Patients who have multiple compression fractures should be watched closely because further deformity in both coronal and sagittal planes can develop.

Burst Fractures

When a vertical (axial) compression force is applied, the vertebral end plate fractures, and the nucleus of the disc is forced into the vertebral body, which explodes and shatters. Burst fractures usually occur in the lower thoracic region, thoracolumbar junction, and lumbar region, where axial loading is possible.

By definition, these injuries are unstable in that they involve the anterior and middle columns simultaneously. These burst fractures are mechanically unstable with collapse and painful kyphosis; they also are neurologically unstable both acutely and chronically with a retropulsed bone into the spinal canal (36). The extent of bursting cannot always be appreciated on plain radiography. CT scanning has proved invaluable in the evaluation of burst fractures, both as an aid to diagnosis and as a guide to further treatment.

If the fracture involves the end plates, progressive deformity may result. Compensation for this deformity by asymmetric growth of neighboring vertebra seldom cancels out the deformity completely. Children should be observed carefully for this complication. Spontaneous, interbody fusion seldom occurs, and should not be relied on to provide long-term stability. Satisfactory results in burst fracture with or without neurologic deficit have been reported following nonoperative treatment.

For a burst fracture of the thoracic spine, the length of instrumentation may be similar to that for compression fractures, without compressive force. Contouring of the rods and achieving three point fixation helps reduce the deformity and restore the spinal alignment. In the lumbar region, instrumentation can be short one level above and one level below the fractured vertebra using pedicle fixation. After reduction, if loss of anterior body height is greater than 60%, anterior grafting from either posterior/anterior approach may be required.

It may be possible to use one pedicle screw at the fracture level. This will aid in the strength of the construct. If the patient requires decompression, especially in the lower lumbar spine, this can be accomplished through the other pedicle. Occasionally, limited anterior body bone grafting can be accomplished posteriorly through the pedicle. Harrington instrumentation can be used for longer instrumentation levels with contoured rods and application of three-point fixation, distraction, and short fusion.

Thoracolumbar junction fractures with severe anterior angulation of the vertebral body require instrumentation with a Kanada device or other similar instrumentation, which allows reconstitution of

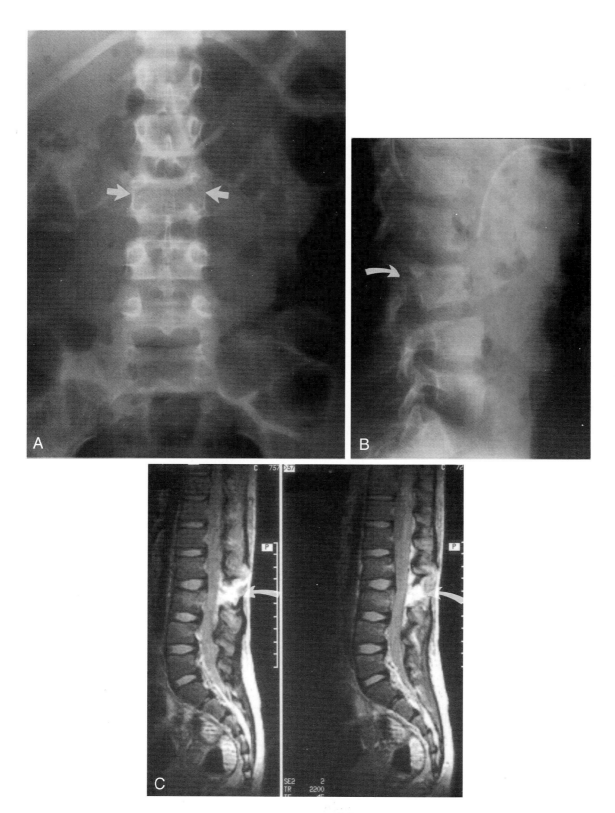

FIGURE 13.9.
Flexion-distraction injury through L3. **A.** An anteroposterior radiograph showing the fracture through the pedicles (arrows). **B.** A lateral radiograph shows the angulation and fracture through the posterior arch and the pedicle (arrow). **C.** A sagittal MRI shows soft tissue disruption through L2-L3 interspinous ligaments (arrow).

vertebral height or short fusion, one vertebrae above and one vertebrae below. In a case of neurologic deficit, the anterior decompression is possible at the same time.

Flexion Distraction Injuries

Chance described three fractures of the lumbar spine in which the fracture goes through the neural arches and pedicles and exits through the vertebral body anteriorly (Fig. 13.9) (27). He thought that the fracture was secondary to a flexion injury. It is now accepted that a combination of flexion and distraction are the cause of this type of fracture (98, 105).

Gumley suggested a classification based on location of the fracture of the posterior elements of the vertebra (58). Type I extends through the spinous process and travels symmetrically forward through all the posterior bony elements to emerge in a variable position in the vertebral body. Type II is identical except that the fracture line transverses the posterior elements between the spinous processes. Type III is asymmetric, involving the posterior elements more on one side than the other, which is possibly associated with a rotational force occurring around the seat belt strap.

Children are particularly susceptible to the seat belt flexion distraction injury because of their high center of gravity and poorly fitting seat belts for their body size (2, 23) (Fig. 13.16). Bony chance fractures are best treated with an extension cast or rigid TLSO for 2 to 3-month full-time wear. If acceptable sagittal alignment cannot be achieved by closed means, operative reduction by a posterior approach is indicated (72).

If reduction is not achieved by nonoperative methods of postural reduction and casting, operative reduction and fixation may be indicated. Posterior compression force is required to reduce the fracture. This can be achieved by interspinous wiring in small children, or by standard hook rod systems in patients over age 6 or 7. Instrumentation and fusion is usually extended one level above and one level below the injury. A postoperative brace (TLSO) is highly recommended.

Soft tissue chance injuries can occasionally be treated nonoperatively in children. A periosteal sleeve injury can heel well and result in long-term spinal stability (13).

Fracture Dislocation Injuries

These fractures usually occur at the thoracolumbar junction. They are often associated neurologic injuries of either the conus medullaris or nerve roots. This injury is always unstable, requiring operative stabilization (17, 18). Injuries that have bony stability may only require posterior instrumentation and fusion. Significant bony instability usually necessitates anterior and posterior spinal instrumentation and fusion.

Fracture dislocation injuries are very unstable, and they require rigid fixation with long instrumentation levels and multiple anchors starting close to the fracture level (26). Long instrumentation assures increased stability. In addition, if the patient has complete neurologic deficit, longer fusion and instrumentation may be needed to prevent subsequent paralytic spine deformity. If short segmental instrumentation is used, it should be extended at least two levels above and two levels below with the addition of postoperative bracing. A rigid TLSO is optimal.

Decompression is dictated by the individual patient's clinical presentation. Decompression is indicated in patients with significant canal compromise who have incomplete cord or cauda quina injuries (37).

Minor Spinal Fractures

Fractures of the spinous and transverse processes are often encountered with blunt trauma to the back; although the fractures themselves may be minor, the associated injuries may be severe. Transverse process fractures of the thoracic region may be associated with significant pleural cavity trauma; those in the thoracolumbar region may be associated with renal damage; and those in the lower lumbar region may accompany unstable pelvic fractures. These associated injuries must be investigated thoroughly before these minor injuries are treated symptomatically.

Sacral Fractures

Isolated sacral fractures are rare in children. They usually occur along with significant pelvic injuries which are themselves uncommon in children. They also occur in association with more obvious thoracolumbar spine fractures.

Fractures of the sacrum may involve the sacral nerve roots and cause neurologic deficit (14). High level sacral injuries S1 to S2 or S2 to S3 are more likely to cause bladder problems than lower injuries such as S4 to S5. Foraminal entrapment of S3 and S4 is less likely than that of S1 or S2 because of the size of the nerve root relative to the foramina at these levels. If sacral fractures are undiagnosed and untreated, they may result in neurologic symptoms and deficits in the lower extremities and lead to urinary, rectal, and sexual dysfunction, as well as perianal and genital sensory loss. Neurologic problems often remain the major chronic sequelae after the more obvious pelvic trauma is healed.

Denis et al. studied 263 patients with sacral fractures and a series of 776 patients with pelvic injuries and introduced a new classification scheme (34). He divides sacral fractures into three zones (Fig. 13.10): Zone I, alar zone, involves a fracture through the ala

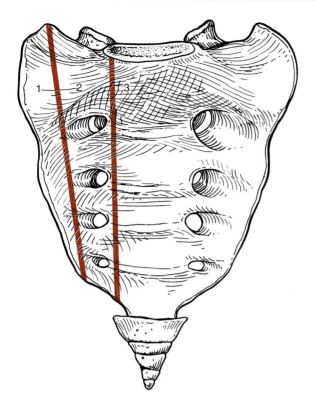

FIGURE 13.10.
Sacral fracture zones by Denis.

without any damage to either the foramen or the central sacral canal. Zone II, foraminal zone fractures, involves one or several foramina. It also goes through the ala without impinging on the central sacral canal. Zone III, central zone, involves primarily the central sacral canal. The fracture line may involve two zones, or in the case of transverse fractures, all three zones. Any fracture involving multiple zones and the central canal is considered a Zone III fracture because the central canal is the most significant component of the injury. The majority of sacral fractures are not associated with neurologic deficit. More serious sequelae result from fracture dislocation of the sacrum before synostosis of the sacrum has occurred.

Zone I fractures are rarely associated with neurologic deficit, although they may occasionally involve L5 nerve root or the sciatic nerve. Vertical shear type fractures may compress the L5 root between the ala and the transverse process of L5. Initial traction may help reduce the compression, but if displacement and neurologic deficit continue, open reduction may be necessary. If the sacral fracture has been displaced vertically 2 cm or more for more than 72 hours, reduction is difficult because the paravertebral musculature will have contracted.

Zone II fractures may involve one or several foramina. Neurologic injuries are found in 28% of these fractures; they may include bowel or bladder dysfunction and L5, S1, S2, and nerve injuries. If the CT scan shows reduction of sacral foramen size of at least 50%, early surgical decompression may be indicated. In a case of unstable fractures, open reduction posteriorly in conjunction with anterior pelvic external fixation may be required.

Zone III fractures involve primarily the sacral canal. Neurologic damage results in more than 50% of these cases and involves the bowel and bladder in the majority of the cases. It may also involve L5 and S1 nerve roots independently or in combination. Transverse sacral fractures may be associated with thoracolumbar burst fractures. Treatment of Zone III fractures without neurologic deficit is aimed at pelvic stabilization. Neurologically involved patients require careful evaluation, including CT scan with thin cuts, tilted gantry, and sagittal reconstruction. Postvoid bladder residuals are also helpful in determining bladder function pre- and postoperatively.

Decompression of sacral roots in the acute phase may be necessary to improve neurologic function. Delayed decompressions are often difficult, and they may not lead to significant recovery.

Vertebral Apophysis Fractures

Fractures involving the vertebral apophyseal end plate are unique injuries to the developing spine (13, 106). The strength of the intervertebral disc and its attachments in children and adolescents allow excessive forces involved in spinal trauma to be transmitted to the relatively weak cartilaginous vertebral apophysis end plate. Severe trauma to the spine in the younger child (less than 10 years old) frequently results in a complete separation of the vertebral apophysis from the primary spongiosa of the vertebral body without failure of the intervertebral disc or annulus fibrosis (Fig. 13.11). The actual fracture is through the hypertrophic zone of the growth plate. The inferior growth plate is involved twice as often as the superior growth plate. This type of fracture may spontaneously reduce and may not be seen on plain radiographs. If the injury was severe enough to cause a spinal cord injury, the SCIWORA syndrome will be present.

The injury to the posterior elements in this type of fracture is usually through soft tissue attachments to bone, creating a periosteal sleeve type fracture. These fractures heal readily with closed reduction as needed and cast immobilization. Post-treatment stability should be documented with flexion extension films.

If open reduction is required, it can usually be accomplished using a posterior approach. Fracture reduction is then usually maintained with a cast or brace until adequate healing has been achieved. Unstable spine injuries in children can heal and become sufficiently stable to justify not using internal fixation and fusion.

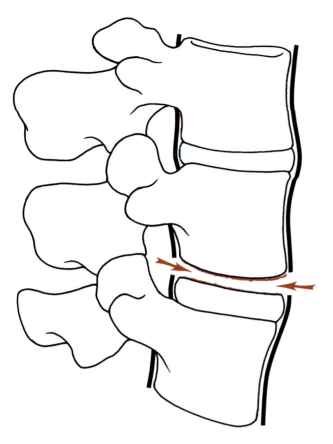

FIGURE 13.11.
Separation of the vertebral apophysis from the vertebral primary spongiosa.

An uncommon cause of back pain in adolescents is a fracture of the vertebral ring apophysis, usually referred to as a vertebral limbus fracture or slipped vertebral apophysis (Fig. 13.12) (82). This fracture usually involves the lumbar vertebra and occurs most often as a result of sports activity, such as gymnastics or weight lifting (61, 81, 82). Usually it is not associated with high energy trauma. The overriding complaint is back pain—sensory or motor loss is rare. Several distinct types occur (Fig. 13.13) (113). The inferior end plate is usually involved. Plain films may be normal. CT scan is usually diagnostic. Surgical excision through a posterior approach is recommended (41, 42). MRI may be helpful to rule out other causes of back pain prior to surgery.

Fractures Resulting from Child Abuse

The true incidence of spinal injuries as a result of child abuse is not known, but the range is from 0 to 3% in large series (51). One of the reasons for this discrepancy may be from a lack of consistency in obtaining a skeletal survey in child abuse victims among different institutions. Most radiology departments include an anterior, posterior radiograph of the entire spine and skeletal series, but the lateral radiograph is often not included. Furthermore, in abused children, spinal injuries occasionally show mild kyphosis, but most patients do not have significant clinical findings referable to their spines. It is not unusual that many of these injuries go unrecognized, and they may be more common than what is reported in the literature.

Because these injuries are likely to be associated with extremely violent assaults, routine evaluation of the spine is mandatory. In a study of child abuse by Kleinman, in 45 children with 85 spinal fractures, the average age of injury was 22 months (75). Most of the spinal fractures resulting from child abuse involve the vertebral bodies. Posterior elements are involved only occasionally. Varying degrees of anterior compression are seen. There may be anterior notching of the vertebral body near the superior end plate. There may be decreased disc space caused by disc herniation.

Severe injuries, such as fracture dislocations with or without neurologic deficit, have also been reported. Spinal cord hematoma may be seen without bony involvement. Significant fracture dislocations, especially those not associated with neurologic deficit, may go unrecognized and result in significant spinal deformity later in life. Fracture dislocations in most cases result from hyperflexion, extension, or a combination of the two. Multiple compression fractures are not unusual findings.

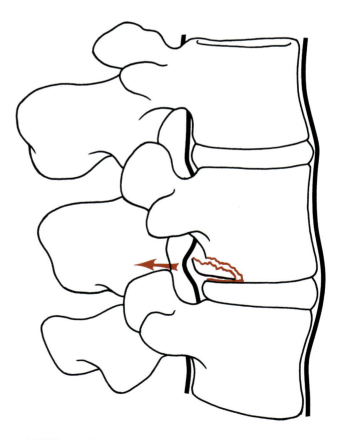

FIGURE 13.12.
A vertebral limbus fracture.

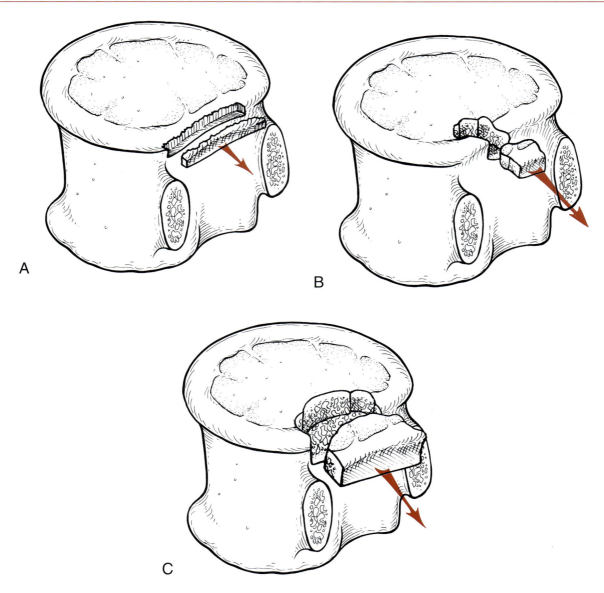

FIGURE 13.13.

Types of vertebral limbus fracture. **A.** A thin margin of the apophysis is separated. **B.** A small fragment of the apophysis is separated. **C.** A large piece consisting of the apophysis and vertebral body is separated.

Fractures of the upper extremities may be seen associated with spine fractures. For example, if a child is held above a table or counter and his/her buttocks are slammed down, he/she can use his/her outstretched arms to break the impact, causing fractures of the upper extremities. Most fractures are in the region of the thoracolumbar and lumbar spine. Fractures and fracture dislocations of the cervical region are also seen.

In evaluating the changes in the vertebral bodies and the disc spaces in child abuse, one should consider developmental changes or infection. Disc space narrowing caused by infection is usually more severe than that caused by trauma and disc herniation. The value of the bone scan in detecting spinal injuries in cases of child abuse is not clear. Standard radiographic studies generally are the primary method of detecting spinal trauma in child abuse.

According to Kleinman, vertebral body fractures and subluxations are fractures with moderate specificity for child abuse, but if the history of trauma is absent or inconsistent with injuries, they become high specificity lesions (75). Once child abuse is detected, the principles of diagnosis and treatment of child abuse victims should be followed.

Treatment of Pediatric Spinal Fractures

Management of thoracic and lumbar spine fractures in children have similar goals: namely, a stable spine without significant deformity which accommodates the neural elements, is function and free of pain (31). There are some factors that lead to more severe deformities than would be seen in an adult with the similar injury. An asymmetric injury to the vertebral end plate in a child can result in progressive angulatory deformity typical of partial growth arrests. If a kyphotic deformity is allowed to remain after treatment of spine fractures, it may spontaneously progress. This progression occurs more often when there has been a crushed vertebral body and end plate.

On the positive side, the continued growth of a vertebral body may help in remodeling of the deformity and reconstitution of the vertebral body. This is often seen in compression fractures. The spinal canal compromise seen in burst fractures has more potential for remodeling in a child than in an adult. Fragments that have not caused neurologic deficit may be left alone. Further remodeling can be expected if the spine is otherwise stable.

Operative Treatment

Operative treatment is indicated most often in unstable spine injuries. The alternatives in surgical management of spine fractures in children are reduction, fusion, decompression, and instrumentation. The assessment of a child's spine should include evaluation of spinal alignment, stability, and degree of canal compromise. If the initial imaging studies show that the alignment of the spine is satisfactory, there is no displacement of the fracture site, and the spinal canal has not been violated by bony or disc fragments, no reduction is necessary.

The need for surgical stabilization depends on the degree of stability. In the case of a neurologic deficit, the spinal canal should be evaluated by imaging, such as MRI or CT contrast studies. A patient with complete neurologic deficit who has no apparent spinal fracture or whose spine is aligned and stable does not require surgical intervention. Patients with incomplete neurologic deficit and spinal canal compromise and patients who are worsening neurologically are candidates for spinal canal decompression.

Thoracic and Lumbar Spine Fractures

The goal of operative treatment of spine fractures is threefold: To provide an environment for maximal neurologic recovery, preserve maximal spinal mobility, and provide long-term stability and a balanced spine. In the thoracic spine, arthrodesis and instrumentation can be extended a few levels above and below the fracture. A longer posterior instrumentation may be necessary to correct an angular kyphosis in this region. In addition, mobility of the thoracic spine is not significantly affected by longer instrumentation and fusion.

In the lumbar spine, shorter instrumentation is desirable to preserve maximal mobility and lessen long-term degenerative changes. Pedicle screws may be beneficial for the lumbar spine in the adolescent patient. However, in the younger child, the pedicles may not be of sufficient size.

Thoracolumbar fractures, especially those associated with increased kyphosis and neurologic deficit, may be approached with an anterior decompression, grafting, and instrumentation or posteriorly by a posterolateral decompression, posterior interbody grafting, and posterior instrumentation. If the loss of anterior vertebral height is significant, anterior strut grafting is preferable to posterolateral interbody fusion. In the case of a burst fracture, decompression can be done anteriorly, posteriorly, or laterally.

The surgical approach and the choice of instrumentation depend on the type of fracture, location, neurologic deficit, and surgeon's experience.

Decompression

The indications for decompression in patients with spinal fractures who are neurologically intact are controversial. There is significant potential for remodeling of the spinal canal in children. Therefore, decompression in neurologically intact patients who have spinal canal compromise may not always be necessary. If patients require anterior grafting for correction of kyphosis, decompression should be done at the same time. Children who have neurologically incomplete lesions and who have plateaued or are getting worse neurologically are candidates for decompression.

There is evidence that early anterior decompression may lead to improved neurologic recovery. There are several methods that allow anterior decompression of the spinal cord. Posterolateral decompression includes removal of the entire pedicle at the fracture level and the disc superior to the level of the fracture, as well as an eggshell procedure of the vertebral body to allow room for the fragments to reduce. Special instruments are necessary to accomplish this goal. Anterior decompression through an anterior approach involves removal of the entire vertebral body at the offending level and usually necessitates the use of an anterior strut graft. Most often this is then followed by posterior surgery for stabilization.

With the exception of birth fractures, in which anterior surgery is required to remove bone fragments compressing the spinal cord, anterior fusion is generally avoided in the growing child. Anterior fusion destroys the anterior growth potential if posterior growth continues and a kyphotic deformity can result. If posterior fusion is required, autologous bone graft should be used. Use of allograft bone is associated with a high rate of pseudoarthrosis. In posterior fusions, iliac crest bone graft is routinely used, taking care to minimize injury to the cartilaginous iliac apophysis.

Traumatic Spondylolysis

It was once thought that spondylolysis at the L5 level was secondary to congenital anomaly of the spine. However, there is significant evidence to suggest that the trauma is the actual etiology. Spondylolysis is rare before the age of five, and it is often first seen in children who are 8 to 9 years old. A review of the history of these patients and all the studies demonstrate that there is no one major severe trauma, but rather multiple minor insults to the back. The etiology of spondylolysis is unknown. Wiltse suggests that there is a stress fracture of the pars interarticularis (119). Rowe and Roche believe that normal hip flexion contractures may accentuate lumbar lordosis and allow increased force through the pars interarticularis leading to fracture (99).

Jackson et al. found an incidence of spondylolysis in female gymnasts that was four times higher than that of the normal population (71). Interior football linemen also experienced an increased incidence of spondylolysis.

Although the preponderance of evidence favors a traumatic origin, there are several studies that demonstrate a familial tendency towards spondylolysis and spondylolisthesis. An increased incidence of spondylolisthesis in patients with spina bifida occulta may result from lack of development of the proximal sacrum.

The clinical presentation of traumatic spondylolisthesis is usually pain localized to the lower back that is aggravated by strenuous activities such as gymnastics or weight lifting. The child may have hamstring tightness, although there is usually no other evidence of nerve root irritation. The pain may be exacerbated by twisting movement. Occasionally, tenderness may be elicited at the level of the L5, S1 region posteriorly.

Radiographs, including anterior, posterior, lateral, and oblique views, are often very specific in the diagnosis of spondylolisthesis. However, because of the overlying bone structures involved, no fractures may be noted. In these cases, technetium bone scans or SPECT scans may be necessary to fully evaluate the child with low back pain. A CT scan through the area can also be helpful in demonstrating these injuries.

Sherman et al. described 11 patients who had reactive sclerosis and hypertrophy of a single pedicle of the lumbar vertebra with a contralateral spondylolysis in the same vertebral segment (104). They believe that this was a physiologic response to stress on the opposite neural arch. The sclerotic pedicle can be confused with the sclerosis of an osteoid osteoma.

Therefore, further studies should be undertaken before an excision of this lesion is performed because the spine could be rendered unstable with spondylolysis of the opposite side.

The treatment of spondylolysis is usually nonoperative because the defect heals in most children. The back should be mobilized with either a corset or lumbosacral orthosis. The child should be restricted from vigorous activities, and therapy should be instituted for stretching of the abdominal and hamstring muscles. If nonoperative treatment fails to relieve symptoms within 6 to 9 months, surgical treatment may be indicated. This treatment can consist of bilateral lateral column fusion from L4 or L5 to S1. Direct bone repair with a screw or wiring of the defect with bone grafting with repair with a pedicle screw and wire above the spinous process has been described with some success (22).

The Gill procedure or laminectomy should never be performed in children without fusion because removal of the posterior elements may lead to increased instability.

Halo Application

The halo-brace (cast) has been used successfully in children and infants as young as 7 months of age (89). Custom-made components usually will be needed depending on the size of the patient. The steps for fitting the halo-brace are as outlined in Mubarak et al. (87). A preapplication CT scan of the skull can

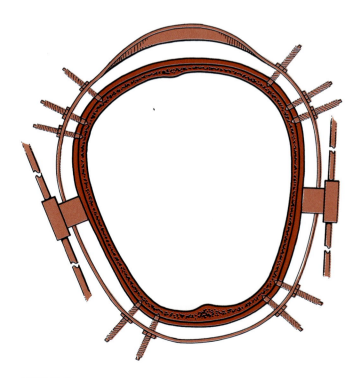

FIGURE 13.14.

Halo application in the child: up to 10 to 12 pins can be applied with 2 inch/lbs.

help locate the halo pins in areas of thicker bone. The ring is usually placed under a general anesthetic just below the equator of the skull. Ten to twelve standard halo pins can be used and tightened to 2 in/1bs circumferentially (Fig. 13.14). The vest and suprastructure are then applied (53).

Routine daily pin care is needed. If pin sites become infected, oral or intravenous antibiotics may be needed. Persistent infections in the face of aggressive treatment may require pin removal (45, 52, 87). Extra care must be taken in the use of the halo-brace in patients under 2 years of age. Incomplete fusion of cranial sutures, open fontanels, and deformable cranial bones can be significant problems. These difficulties are minimized by short periods of halo use, custom fitted rings, and a high number of low tongue pins (76, 87).

Disc Herniation

Although not as common as in adults, lumbar disc herniation does occur in children and adolescents. Presenting complaints are similar to adults with leg pain in a typical sciatic distribution (15, 35). The straight leg raise test is highly sensitive and specific for the presence of a herniated lumbar disc in children (15, 35, 40, 54, 73, 77, 101). Nonoperative treatment with bed rest, activity restriction, and analgesics are usually sufficient treatment. Trauma is a significant factor in causing disc herniation in children. Associated structural abnormalities that may predispose to herniated discs include spina bifida occulta, sacralization of L5 and 6, and lumbar vertebra (15, 35, 40). MRI is helpful in establishing the diagnosis and level of compression. The results of surgical management of lumbar disc herniation in children is excellent. Discectomy using a laminectomy without fusion is the procedure of choice (15, 35, 40, 54, 73, 77, 101). Recurrence rate at the operative level is 6% and twice that at another level (35).

SCIWORA

Spinal cord injury without radiographic abnormality (SCIWORA) occurs almost exclusively in children and is common in younger children, infants, and newborns (28). It occurs most commonly in the cervical spine, specifically the cervicothoracic junction, but also occurs in the thoracic and lumbar spine. A higher percentage of these injures are complete injuries. Children less than 8 years old have a lower incidence of neurologic recovery. Onset of symptoms can be delayed up to 4 days post injury (94). A MRI is indicated in all these cases to define the specific lesion. Causes include physeal end plate fracture with instability, stretch injuries, infolding of the ligamentum flavum, infarction of the cord (most common at the T4-L1 level), acute thoracic disc herniation, and protrusion of cartilaginous end plate into the canal. Nonoperative immobilization for 1 to 3 weeks is the treatment of choice. Operative decompression is not effective unless progressive neurologic deterioration occurs and a specific lesion can be identified (120).

Return to Activities (Sports)

The physician who is treating the child with spinal injuries is concerned about the child's injury and when treatment can be finished. However, usually the child is more concerned over when he/she can return to regular activities. This is always a challenge for any physician but especially for those dealing with children. Often times, the child who is nearing the end of treatment will be active despite the presence of a halo brace, Minerva cast, or body jacket. Once these devices are removed, an element of protection against reinjury is eliminated. At the same time, the child feels unleashed. This is not a good time to let the child go. The child and parent need to be counseled as to the need for restraint and the possibility of reinjury. The child should not be allowed to return to normal activities (i.e., sports) for 6 to 12 weeks after discontinuing treatment. Rarely is formal physical therapy needed unless there is a persistent limitation of motion or weakness. The child should not return to unrestricted activity until the injury has healed, the spine is stable, and there is no significant pain or loss of motion. Return to activities should be done on a graduated basis.

Injury Prevention

Prevention of spinal injuries in children is everyone's responsibility. Although not all of these injuries are preventable, there are many ways to decrease their incidence. Children are unaware of their decisions that put them at risk of having a spine injury. It is the responsibility of adults and ultimately parents to minimize the risk of spinal injury in their children. The physician can and should be an advocate for child safety, usually through education of the parents and children. Parents should be informed as to what activities are high risk for spinal injuries and what active role they can take to protect their child while not overreacting.

Complications

Late Deformity

Significant long-term posttraumatic deformities of the spine do occur in children and should be treated aggressively. Growth of adjacent vertebra rarely correct the primary deformity completely. The amount of reconstitution of height in fractured vertebral bodies is not predictable.

Severe deformity always results in compensation by adjacent parts of the spine, which leads to a secondary deformity. This process can lead to overload symptoms in the spine, which are very difficult to resolve.

Paraplegia or Quadriplegia

Fortunately, severe spinal cord injury is not common in young children. Complete cord lesions in children carry a prognosis similar to those in adults with no real chance of recovery. For incomplete lesions seen, the return of neurologic function is quite variable and a complete return is possible. For those patients unfortunate enough to have a complete cord lesion as a child (preadolescent), nearly 100% will develop a significant progressive spinal deformity. Most, if not all, of these patients will require operative spinal fusion with instrumentation. The young child (less than 10 years old and Risser 0) will need a combined anterior discectomy and fusion and posterior instrumentation and fusion to the pelvis to obtain a stable, balanced spine.

References

1. Abroms IF, Bresnan MJ, Zuckerman JE. Cervical cord injury secondary to hyperextension of the head in breech presentation. Obstet Gynecol 1973;41:369–378.
2. Agran PF, Dunkle DE, Winn DG. Injuries to a sample of seatbelted children evaluated and treated in a hospital emergency room. J Trauma 1987;27:58–64.
3. Akbarnia BA. The role of the orthopaedic surgeon in child abuse. In: Morrissy RT, ed. Pediatric orthopaedics. 3rd ed. Philadelphia: JB Lippincott, 1990.
4. Akbarnia BA, Torg JS, Kirkpatrick RT, et al. Manifestations of the battered-child syndrome. J Bone Joint Surg Am 1974;56:1159.
5. Allen BL, Ferguson RL. Cervical spine trauma in children. In Bradford DS, Hensinger RN, eds. The pediatric spine. New York: Thieme, 1985.
6. Anderson MJ, Schutt AH. Spinal injury in children: a review of 156 cases seen from 1950–1978. Mayo Clin Proc 1980;55:499–504.
7. Aprahamian C, Thompson BM, Finger WA, et al. Experimental cervical spine injury model: evaluation of airway management and splinting techniques. Am Emerg Med 1984;13:584–587.
8. Aufdermaur M. Spinal injuries in juveniles: Necropsy findings in 12 cases. J Bone Joint Surg Br 1974;56:513–519.
9. Babcock JL. Spinal injuries in children. Pediatr Clin North Am 1975;22:487–500.
10. Bailey DK. Normal spine in infants and child radiology. 1952;59:712.
11. Bick EM, Copel JW. Longitudinal growth of the human vertebra. J Bone Joint Surg Am 1950;32:803–814.
12. Bick EM, Copel JW. The ring apophysis of the human vertebra. J Bone Joint Surg Am 1951;33:783–787.
13. Black BE, O'Brien E, Sponseller PD. Thoracic and lumbar spine injuries in children: different then in adults. Contemp Ortho Oct 1994:253–260.
14. Bonnin JG. Sacral fractures and injuries of the cauda equina. J Bone Joint Surg 1945;27:113–122.
15. Bradford DS, Garcia A. Lumbar intervertebral disk herniation in children and adolescents. Orthop Clin North Am 1971;2:583–592.
16. Bradford DS, Iza J. Repair of the defect in spondylolysis or minimal degrees of spondylolisthesis by segmental wire fixation and bone grafting. Spine 1985;10:673–679.
17. Bradford DS, Akbarnia BA, Winter RB, et al. Surgical treatment of fracture and fracture dislocations of the thoracic spine. Orthop Trans 1977;1:99.
18. Brenner B, Moiel R, Dickson J, et al. Instrumentation of the spine from fracture-dislocations in children. Childs Brain 1977;3:249–255.
19. Bresnan MJ, Abroms IF. Neonatal spinal cord transection secondary to intrauterine hyperextension of the neck in breech presentation. J Pediatr 1974;5:734–737.
20. Bucholz RW, Burkhead WZ. The pathological anatomy of fatal atlanto occipital dislocations. J Bone Joint Surg Am 1979;1:248–250.
21. Bucholz RW, Burkhead WZ, Graham W, et al. Occult cervical spine injuries in fatal traffic accidents. J Trauma 1979;19:768–771.
22. Bucks JE. Direct repair of the defect in spondylolisthesis. J Bone Joint Surg Br 1970;52:432–437.
23. Burdi AR, Huelke DF. Infant and children in the adult world of automobile safety design: pediatric and anatomic considerations for design of child restraints. Biomechanics 1969;2:267–280.
24. Burke DC. Traumatic spinal paralysis in children. Paraplegia 1974;11:268–276.
25. Campbell J, Bonnett C. Spinal cord injury in children. Clin Orthop 1975;112:114–123.
26. Chambers HG, Akbarnia BA. Thoracic, lumbar and sacral spine fractures and dislocations. Weinstein SL, ed. New York: Raven Press, 1994:743–766.
27. Chance GQ. Note on a type of flexion fracture of the spine. Br J Radiol 1948;21:452–453.
28. Cheshire DJD. The pediatric syndrome of traumatic myelopathy without demonstrable vertebral injury. Paraplegia 1977–1978;15:74–85.
29. Choi JU, Hoffman HJ, Hendrick EB, et al. Traumatic infarction of the spinal cord in children. J Neurosurg 1986;65:608–610.
30. Cohn SL, Akbarnia BA, Luisiri A, et al. Disc space infection versus Scheuermann's disease. Orthopaedics 1988;2:330–335.
31. Crawford AH. Operative treatment of spine fractures in children. Orthop Clin North Am 1990;21:325–339.
32. Denis F. The three column spine and its significance in the classification of acute thoracolumbar spinal injuries. Spine 1983;8:817–831.
33. Denis F. Spinal instability as defined by the three column spine concept in acute spinal trauma. Clin Orthop 1984;189:65–76.
34. Denis F, Davis S, Comfort T. Sacral fractures: an im-

portant problem. Retrospective analysis of 236 cases. Clin Orthop 1988;227:67–81.
35. DeOrio J, Bianco A. Lumbar disc excision in children and adolescents. J. Bone Joint Surg. Am 1982;64:991.
36. Dewald RL. Burst fractures of the thoracic and lumbar spine. Clin Orthop 1984;189:150–161.
37. Dickman CA, Rekate HL, Sonntag VKH, et al. Pediatric spinal trauma: vertebral column and spinal cord injuries in children. Pediatr Neurosci 1989;15:237–256.
38. Dietrich AM, Ginn-Pease ME, Bartkowski HM, et al. Pediatric cervical spine fractures: predominately subtle presentation. J Pediatr Surg 1991;26(18):995–1000.
39. Eismont EJ, Bohlman HH. Posterior atlanto-occipital dislocation with fractures of the atlas and odontoid process. J Bone Joint Surg Am 1978;60:397–399.
40. Epstein JA, Epstein N, Marc J. Lumbar intervertebral disk herniation in teenage children: recognition and management of associated anomalies. Spine 1984;9:427–431.
41. Epstein NE, Epstein JA. Limbus lumbar vertebral fractures in 27 adolescents and adults. Spine 1991;16:962–966.
42. Epstein NE, Epstein JA, Mauri T. Treatment of fractures of the vertebral limbus and spinal stenosis in five adolescents and five adults. Neurosurgery 1989;24:595–604.
43. Evans DL, Bethem D. Cervical spine injuries in children. J Pediatr Orthop 1989;9:563–568.
44. Evarts CM. Traumatic occipito-atlantal dislocation. Report of a case with survival. J Bone Joint Surg Am 1970;52:1653–1660.
45. Ewald FC. Fracture of the odontoid process in a seventeen month old infant treated with a halo. J Bone Joint Surg Am 1982;53:1636.
46. Ferguson RL. Thoracic and lumbar spinal trauma of the immature spine. In: Rothman RH, Simeone FA, eds. The spine. Philadelphia: WB Saunders, 1992:501–512.
47. Reference deleted.
48. Ferguson JW. Cervical spine injuries in children. In: Sherle HH et al., eds. The cervical spine: the cervical spine research society editorial committee. Philadelphia: JB Lippincott, 1989.
49. Fielding JW, Hawkins RJ. Roentgenographic diagnosis of the injured neck: Instructional course lecture XXV. American Academy of Orthopedic Surgeons 1976:149–170.
50. Fielding JW, Hawkins RJ. Atlanto-axial rotatory fixations. J Bone Joint Surg Am 1977;59:37.
51. Galleno H, Oppenheim WL. The battered child syndrome revisited. Clin Orthop 1982;162:11.
52. Garfin SR, Botte MJ, Nickel VL, et al. Complications in the use of the halofixation device. J Bone Joint Surg Am 1986;68:320–325.
53. Garfin SR, Roux R, Botte MJ, et al. Skull osteology as it affects halo pin placement in children. J Pediatr Orthop 1986;6:434.
54. Garrido E, Humphreys RP, Hendrick EB, et al. Lumbar disc disease in children. Neurosurgery 1978;2:22–26.
55. Georgopoulos G, Pizzutillo PD, Lee MS. Occipito-atlanto instability in children. J Bone Joint Surg Am 1987;69(3):429–436.
56. Giles FH, Biha M, Sotrel A. Infantile atlanto-occipital instability: the potential danger of extreme extension. Am J Child 1979;133:30–37.
57. Grisel PO. Enucleation de l'athas et torticollis nasopharyngren. Presse Med 1930;38:50.
58. Gumley G, Taylor TKF, Ryan MD. Distraction fractures of the lumbar spine. JBJS British 1982;64:520–525.
59. Reference deleted.
60. Hadley MN, Zabramski JM, Browner CM, et al. Pediatric spinal trauma: review of 122 cases of spinal cord and vertebral column injuries. J Neurosurg 1988;68:18–24.
61. Handel SF, Twiford TW, Reigel DH, et al. Posterior lumbar apophyseal fractures. Radiology 1979;130:629–633.
62. Hann IN, Gupta S, Palmer MK, et al. The prognostic significance of radiological and symptomatic bone involvement in childhood acute lymphocytic leukemia. Med Pediatr Oncol 1979;6:51–55.
63. Harris JH, Edeiken-Monroe B, Kopaniky DR. A practical classification of acute cervical spine injuries. Orthop Clin North Am 1986;17:15–30.
64. Hazel WA, Jones RA, Morrey BF, et al. Vertebral fractures without neurological deficit. A long-term follow-up study. J Bone Joint Surg Am 1988;70:1319–1321.
65. Hegenbarth R, Ebel K-D. Roentgen findings in fractures of the vertebral column in childhood: examination of 35 patients and its results. Pediatr Radiol 1976;5:34–39.
66. Herzenberg JE, et al. Emergency transport and positioning of young children who have an injury of the cervical spine. J Bone Joint Surg Am 1989;71:15–22.
67. Holdsworth F. Fractures, dislocations, and fracture dislocations of the spine. J Bone Joint Surg 1970;52:1534–1551.
68. Holley J, Jordan R. Airway management in patients with unstable cervical spine fractures. Am Emerg Med 1989;18:1237–1239.
69. Horal J, Nachemson A, Scheiler S. Clinical and radiological long term follow-up of vertebral fractures in children. Acta Orthop Scand 1972;43:491–503.
70. Hubbard DD. Injuries of the spine in children and adults. Clin Orthop 1974;100:56–65.
71. Jackson DW, Wiltse LL, Cirincione RJ. Spondylolysis in the female gymnast. Clin Orthop 1976;117:68–73.
72. Johnson DL, Falci S. The diagnosis and treatment of pediatric lumbar spine injuries caused by rear seat lap belts. Neurosurgery 1990;26:434–441.
73. Kamel M, Rosman M. Disc protrusion in the growing child. Clin Orthop 1984;185:46–52.
74. Kewalramani LS, Tori JA. Spinal cord trauma in children: neurological patterns, radiologic features, and pathomechanics of injury. Spine 1980;5:11–18.
75. Kleinman PK, ed. Diagnostic imaging of child abuse. Baltimore: Williams & Wilkins, 1987.
76. Kopits S, Stelngass M. Experience with halo-cast in small children. Surg Clin North Am 1970;50:935.
77. Kurihara A, Kataoka O. Lumbar disc herniation in children and adolescents. Spine 1989;5:443–451, 1989.
78. Lavernia CL, Botte MJ, Garfin SR. The spine. In: Rothman, Simeone, eds. Spinal orthoses for traumatic and degenerative disease in the spine. 3rd ed. Philadelphia: WB Saunders, 1992:1197–1224.

79. Lebbuchl NH, Eismont FJ. Cervical spine injuries in children; in The Pediatric Spine. Principles and Practice. Weinstein SL, ed. New York: Raven Press, 1994:725–741.
80. Leventhall HR. Birth injuries of the spinal cord. J Pediatr 1960;56:447–453.
81. Lippitt AD. Fracture of a vertebral body endplate and disc protrusion causing subarachnoid block in an adolescent. Clin Orthop 1976;116:112–115.
82. Lowrey JJ. Dislocated lumbar vertebral epiphysis in adolescent children: report of three cases. J Neurosurg 1973;38:232–234.
83. Mah JY, Thometz J, Emans J, et al. Threaded K-wire spinous process fixation of the axis for modified Gallie fusion in children and adolescents. JPO 1989;9:675–679.
84. Majernick TG, Brenick R, Houston JB, et al. Cervical spine movement during orotracheal intubation. Am Emerg Med 1986;15:417–420.
85. McPhee IB. Spinal fractures and dislocations in children and adolescents. Spine 1981;6:533–537.
86. Montane I, Eismont FJ, Green BA. Traumatic occipitoatlantal dislocation. Spine 1991;16:112–116.
87. Mubarak SJ, Camp JF, Vvletich W, et al. Halo application in the infant. J Pediatr Orthop 1989;9:612–614.
88. Naik DR. Cervical spinal canal in normal infants. Clin Radiol 1970;21:323–326.
89. Nickel VL, Perry J, Garrett A, et al. The halo. A spinal skeletal traction fixation device. J Bone Joint Surg Am 1968;50:1400.
90. Nykamp PW, Levy JM, Christensen F, et al. Computed tomography for a bursting fracture of the lumbar spine. J Bone Joint Surg Am 1978;60:1108–1109.
91. O'Rahilly RS, Benson DR. The development of the vertebral column. In: Bradford DS, Hensinger RM, eds. The pediatric spine. New York: Thieme, 1985:3–17.
92. Ogden JA. Spine. In: Skeletal injury in the child. 2nd ed. Philadelphia: WB Saunders, 1990:571–626.
93. Page CP, Story JL, Wissinger JP, et al. Traumatic atlantooccipital dislocation: Case report. J Neurosurg 1973;39:394–397.
94. Pang D, Wilberger JE. Spinal cord injury without radiographic abnormalities in children. J Neurosurg 1982;57:114–129.
95. Pennecot GF, Gouraud D, Hardy JR, et al. Roentgenographical study of the stability of the cervical spine in children. J Pediat Orthop 1984;4:346–352.
96. Pizzutillo PD, Rocha EF, D'Astors J, et al. Bilateral fracture of the pedicle of the second cervical vertebra in the young child. J Bone Joint Surg Am 1986;68:892–896.
97. Powers B, Miller MD, Kramer RS, et al. Traumatic anterior atlanto-occipital dislocation. Neurosurgery 1979;4:12–17.
98. Rennie W, Mitchell N. Flexion distraction fractures of the thoracolumbar spine. J Bone Joint Surg Am 1973;55:386–390.
99. Rowe GG, Roche MB. The etiology of separate neural arch. J. Bone Joint Surg Am 1953;35:102–110.
100. Ruge JR, Sinson GP, McLone DG, et al. Pediatric spinal injury: The very young. J Neurosurg 1988;68:25–30.
101. Russwurm H, Bjerkreim I. Lumbar intervertebral disc herniation in the young. Acta Orthop Scand 1978;40:148–163.
102. Shapiro R, Youngberg AS, Rothman SLG. The differential diagnosis of traumatic lesions of the occipito-atlanto-axial segment.
103. Sherk HH, Nicholson JT, Chung SMK. Fractures of the odontoid process in young children. J Bone Joint Surg Am 1978;60:921–924.
103a. Sherk HH, Schul L, Lane J. Fractures and dislocations of the cervical spine in children. Orthop Clin North Am 1976;7:593–604.
104. Sherman FC, Wilkinson RH, Hall JE. Ractive sclerosis of a pedicle in spondylolysis in the lumbar spine. J Bone Joint Surg Am 1977;59:49–54.
104a. Shulman ST, Madden JD, Esterly JR, et al. Transsection of spinal cord. A rare obstetrical complication of cephalic delivery. Arch Dis Child 1971;46:291–294.
105. Smith WS, Kaufer H. Patterns in mechanisms of lumbar injury associated with lap seatbelts. J Bone Joint Surg Am 1969;51:239–254.
106. Sovio OM, Bell HM, Beauchamp RD, et al. Fracture of the lumbar vertebral apophysis. J Pediatr Orthop 1985;550–552.
107. Stabler CL, Eismont FJ, Brown MD, et al. Failure of posterior cervical fusions using cadaveric bone graft in children. J Bone Joint Surg Am 1985;67:370–375.
108. Stauffer ES, Mazur JM. Cervical spine injuries in children. Pediatr Ann 1982;11:502–511.
109. Steel HH. Anatomical and mechanical consideration of the atlanto-axial articulation. In Proceedings of the American Orthopedic Association. J Bone Joint Surg Am 1968;56:1481–1482.
110. Suderman VS, Crosby ET, Lui A. Elective oral tracheal intubation in spine injured adults. Am J Anaesth 1991;38:785–789.
111. Swischuk LE. Spine and spinal cord trauma in the battered child syndrome. Radiology 1969;92:733–738.
112. Swischuk LE. Anterior displacement of C2 in children physiologic or pathologic? helpful differentiating line. Pediatr Radiol 1977;122:759–763.
113. Takata K, Inove S, Takahashi K, et al. Fracture of the posterior margin of a lumbar vertebral body. J Bone Joint Surg Am 1988;70(4):589–594.
114. Taylor JR. Growth of human intervertebral discs and vertebral bodies. J Anat 1975;120:49–68.
115. Weiss MH, Kaufman B. Hangman's fracture in an infant. Am J Dis Child 1973;126:268–269.
116. Wenger DR, Bobechko WP, Gilday DL. The spectrum of intervertebral disc space infection in children. J Bone Joint Surg Am 1978;60:100–108.
117. Wholey MH, Bruwer AJ, Baker HL. The lateral roentgenogram of the neck. Radiology 1958;71:350–356.
118. Wiesel SW, Rothman RH. Occipitoatlantal hypermobility. Spine 1979;4:187–191.
119. Wiltse LL. Spondylolisthesis in children. Clin Orthop 1961;21:156–163.
120. Yngve DA, Harris WP, Herndon WA, et al. Spinal cord injury without osseous spine fracture. J Pediatr Orthop 1988;8:153–159.
121. Zigler ZE, Waters RL, Nelson RW, et al. Occipito–cervical thoracic spine fusion in a patient with occipito–cervical dislocation with survival. Spine 1986;11:645–646.

SECTION 3
Spinal Trauma

CHAPTER FOURTEEN

Spinal Cord Injury and Lower Cervical Spine Injuries

Paul A. Anderson

Introduction

Recent advances in research, patient assessment, early resuscitation, and rehabilitation have greatly improved the outcome of many patients with spinal and spinal cord injuries. Unfortunately, the means to achieve reversal of complete spinal cord injury still remains enigmatic. Preventive efforts aimed at public education, the use of safety restraints, and elimination of drunk driving has resulted in decreased rates of injuries from sports activities and vehicular trauma. Unfortunately, the incidence of spinal cord injury in the population has not changed due to increases in spinal cord injuries related to firearms. Newer surgical techniques to allow decompression and stabilization of the cervical spine have increased the interest of surgeons in the care of patients with spinal trauma. In this chapter, the principles of patient assessment and the classification of injury as well as the treatment of cervical spine and spinal cord injuries are discussed.

Evaluation of the Spinal Injured Patient

The initial assessment of traumatized patients focuses on maintenance of their airway, breathing, and circulation. If required, intubation can be performed while an assistant holds the head straight with gentle traction. Spinal cord injured patients will have a paradoxical diaphragmatic breathing pattern, and patients with higher neurologic levels of injury may deteriorate over the first 24 to 48 hours and require mechanical ventilation. Cervical cord injured patients frequently have neurogenic shock caused by loss of sympathetic tone. Hemodynamically, they present with hypotension and bradycardia. Although blood loss from other causes should be excluded, neurogenic shock is best treated with vasopressors and atropine. Because the autoregulation of spinal cord blood flow is lost after trauma, it is important to maintain systolic pressure to at least 90 mm Hg. After the primary assessment, the secondary examination to exclude other life-threatening injury is performed. During the secondary examinations, the spinal column and neurologic status of the patient is assessed carefully.

Physical Examination

A history of the mechanism of injury is important to identify the magnitude and direction of forces that may have caused skeletal injury. Additionally, potential associated injuries, such as bowel injury in seat belt related trauma or facial fracture in patients with cervical extension injures, can then be identified. Inspection of the patient for contusions and lac-

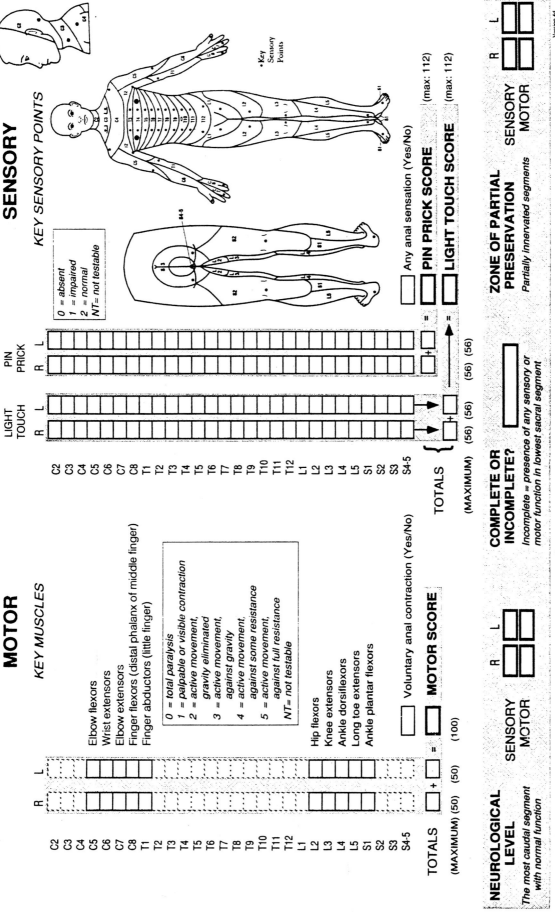

FIGURE 14.1.
American Spine Injury Association (ASIA) Spinal Cord Injury Assessment Form. Reproduced with permission from the American Spine Injury Association: Standards for Neurological and functional Classification of Spinal Cord Injury, revised. Chicago, IL. American Spine Injury Association, 1992.

eration of the head or neck or abdominal abrasion from seat belts helps to identify forces imparted to the spinal column. To complete inspection, the patient should be log-rolled with the help of an assistant and the collar removed so that the entire spinal column can be visualized. Contusions about the spine, dorsal swelling, or gibbus deformities are likely indications of significant spinal injuries. While the patient is in the log-rolled position, the spine from the occiput to the sacrum is palpated, checking for tenderness, swelling, and gaps between spinous processes. Reproducible focal spinous process tenderness is a sensitive indication of spinal column injury even when radiographs are negative. In polytraumatized patients, we have discovered occult fractures in 40% of patients with focal tenderness but negative radiographs. Palpable gaps between spinous processes indicate distractive injuries to the posterior elements and in most cases represents an unstable spine that is best treated surgically.

After palpation, the patient is placed supine and a complete neurologic examination is done (7). The neurologic examination includes testing of the motor and sensory and reflex functions of the patient. Each dermatome is tested for pin prick, light touch, and position sensation. This is best done by starting at the head and neck and proceeding caudally. Grading of sensation is normal, impaired, or absent. The motor system is assessed by manual muscle grading from 0 to 5 of each muscle group in both the upper and lower extremities. Because sacral sparing may be the only retained function indicating an incomplete spinal cord lesion, perineal function must be assessed carefully. A digital rectal exam is performed, noting the anal tone and the ability to voluntarily contract. Testing is performed for the bulbocavernosus reflex and perianal pinprick sensation. Deep tendon reflexes and pathologic reflexes, such as clonus, Babinski, and Hoffman's sign, are tested. Prompt recording of the neurologic exam in the medical record is essential to allow accurate determination of the patient's progress.

The American Spinal Injury Association (ASIA) has developed standards for assessing and classifying spinal cord injuries (7). An assessment form (Fig. 14.1) allows detailed recording of a complete neurologic examination. Functionally, patients may be assessed by the ASIA Impairment Scale, which is modified from Frankel (Table 14.1). The level of neurologic function is defined by ASIA as the most caudal level with at least Grade 3 motor function. The overall motor function of the patient can be quantified using the motor score. The motor score ranges from 0 to 100 and is determined by the summation of bilateral manual muscle test score for ten key muscle groups. These muscle groups include: elbow flexors (C5), wrist extensors (C6), elbow extensors (C7), finger flexors (C8), hand intrinsics (T1), hip flexors (L2), knee extensors (L3), ankle dorsiflexors (L4), long toe extensors (L5), and ankle plantar flexors (S1).

TABLE 14.1.
Modified Frankel Impairment Scale

A. Complete. No motor or sensory function below the level of injury including sacral segments
B. Incomplete. Some sensation but no motor function.
C. Incomplete. Preserved motor function. The key muscle groups are less than grade 3.
D. Incomplete. Preserved motor function. The key muscle groups are greater than or equal to grade 3.
E. Normal.

Radiographic Examination

All traumatized patients require antero-posterior chest, pelvic, and lateral cervical radiographs as part of initial assessment. To properly clear the cervical spine, antero-posterior cervical and open mouth odontoid radiographs are also obtained. The entire cervical spine from the occiput to T1 should be visualized. Commonly missed fractures are odontoid fractures, facet fractures, and injuries at the cervicothoracic junction (24). If the entire cervical spine cannot be well visualized with routine radiographic views, then additional special techniques, such as lateral "swimmers" and trauma oblique radiographs, can be obtained. In some cases, CT scans may be required to adequately assess the cervical spine. If a spinal fracture is found, then a complete spinal series, including the cervical, thoracic, and lumbar spine, is obtained; 10 to 15% of patients will have noncontiguous spinal injuries (67).

A CT scan is recommended in the majority of patients with identifiable fractures or dislocations on plain radiographs, although fractures in a transverse plane may be seen poorly (i.e., Type II odontoid fractures or horizontal fractures through facets). Magnetic resonance imaging may have increased benefits because of its ability to determine the soft tissue component of the injury and predict the prognosis of neurologic recovery in some patients (36, 85). Early diagnosis of soft tissue injuries, such as traumatic disc herniations, may allow surgeons to treat patients more appropriately and achieve complete neural decompression (47). The presence of ligamentous injuries can be determined accurately using fat suppression MRI techniques (T2 weight or STIR sequences).

Pathophysiology of Spinal Cord Injury

Early treatment in the first few hours after injury may lead to significant neural recovery and improved long-term function. Therefore, patients with spinal cord injuries should be evaluated rapidly to allow early institution of treatment. To better understand the importance of initial therapy, the pathophysiology of spinal cord injury and experimental treatment methods are reviewed here.

Experimental and clinical observation have identified two phases of spinal cord injury. The primary insult is the initial trauma directed to the cord that causes irreversible nerve cell and axonal loss. The severity of the initial trauma is directly related to the kinetic energy transferred to the neural tissue (15, 44). In most cases, the forces are directed to the ventral surface of the cord due to crushing from retropulsed bone and disc fragments or from excessive traction forces due to vertebral column lengthening from distraction on kyphotic angulation. Assenmacher and Ducker found that in primates, a 300 gm/cm force resulted in incomplete neural injuries, whereas a 500 gm/cm force was associated with complete neural deficits (15). Clinically, the magnitude of the forces in humans cannot be determined accurately to aid physicians caring for patients. Also, radiographs poorly correlate with displacement that occurs transiently during injury (32).

Histologic studies have demonstrated that immediately after experimental injury, the structure of the cord is intact (44). Later within the first 24 hours, a progressive disruption and necrosis of the neural tissue occurs. This progressive destruction has been termed the secondary injury, and the mechanism and method to mitigate its effects are the subject of extensive research.

Immediately after injury, a failure of axonal repolarization caused by potassium leakage blocks spinal cord conduction (11). Ischemia caused by disruption or compression of intramedullary vessels and the loss of autoregulation of spinal cord blood flow exacerbates this condition (44). Histologic examination immediately after injury shows minimal changes. Within 3 to 5 minutes, petechial hemorrhage appears in the central grey matter with minimal changes in the white axonal matter. Throughout this process, the grey matter is always affected more severely than the white matter. Within 30 minutes, the petechial hemorrhage coalescences into hemorrhages, and neuronal necrosis appears. The axons are swollen but still intact. Within 4 hours, significant changes are apparent in the white matter consisting of oligodendritic necrosis and axonal swelling although structurally they are still intact. At 8 hours following injury, axonal necrosis and maximal swelling are observed. The pathophysiologic mechanism responsible for this progressive neuronal destruction, especially of the white matter, is the subject of investigation (62, 64).

Previously, the secondary injury was thought to be secondary to vascular ischemia (12). However, more significant biochemical alterations have been identified. After injury, there is a rapid depletion of adenosine triphosphate (ATP) that results in failure of calcium dependent membrane transport systems and enzymes (64, 102, 103). This allows the accumulation of intracellular and intramitochondrial calcium, thereby uncoupling oxidative phosphorylation further depleting ATP. Enzymes such as phospholipase A2 are activated, which cause lysis of membranes and myelinated tissues. Arachidonic acid is released and metabolized to various prostaglandins and thromboxane structures, which have adverse effects such as vasoconstriction, platelet thrombosis, and lyosomal enzyme release. Significantly, lipid peroxide free radicals are formed, causing chain reactions and breakdown of membranes and myelin. A circular cascade is created, which leads to progressive destruction (Fig. 14.2).

Attempts to limit the abnormal biochemical processes of secondary injury has led to pharmacologic management of spinal cord injury (10, 27). The two agents with proven clinical efficacy in humans are corticosteroids and gangliosides. Methylprednisolone is a corticosteroid with a preferential ability to limit lipid peroxidation in traumatized central nervous systems (27). Bracken et al. reported the results of the National Spinal Cord Injury Study 2 (NSCIS 2) (26). Three drugs—a placebo, naloxone, and high dose methylprednisolone—were compared in a multicenter, randomized, double-blinded study of 476 patients. No differences in neurologic outcomes were observed between the placebo and naloxone groups. The group that was administered methylprednisolone had statistically significantly increased motor and sensory scores although clinically the results were only modest. Only patients who had the drug given within 8 hours of injury benefited. Both incomplete and complete patients showed improvement when given methylprednisolone.

Other steroid molecules have been investigated and show activity at altering abnormal biochemical processes (59). An aminosteroid, trilazoid, without any glucocorticoid activity has been shown to promote neural recovery in head injury models. This agent is currently undergoing testing in the NSCIS 3 study.

Gangliosides are naturally occurring large glycoprotein molecules with high density in neural tissues (81). They appear to aid in membrane transport function and maintenance of structure. In cell cultures they have cytogenic and trophic effects. Animal studies demonstrated efficacy of gangliosides in head injury models. Geissler et al. compared ganglioside GM1 to placebo in a randomized double-blind study of spinal cord injury patients (52). Statistically significant increased functional recovery was seen in

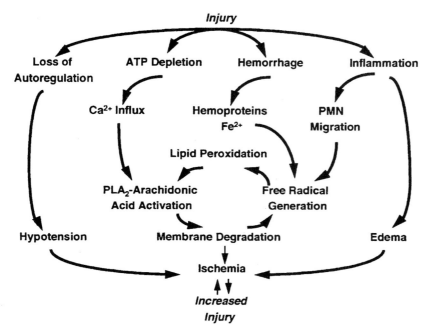

FIGURE 14.2.
Biochemical changes that occur in central nervous system after traumatic injury. ATP = adenosine triphosphate, PMN = polymorphonuclear leukocyte, PLA2 = phospholipase A2. Reprinted with permission from Slucky AV, Eismont FJ. Treatment of acute injury of the cervical spine. Instructional Course Lectures 1995;44:67–80.

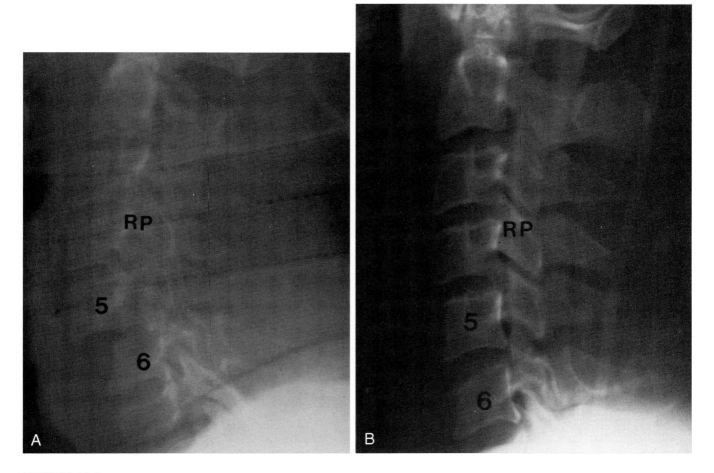

FIGURE 14.3.
A. A thirty-five-year-old male construction worker sustained the C5-6 bilateral facet dislocation shown on the lateral cervical radiograph. On examination forty-five minutes after injury, he was a C5 complete quadriplegic. Reduction was achieved 30 minutes later. He noted an immediate return of sensation in his extremities and within 1 hour he had regained motor function. **B.** Lateral radiograph after reduction. Seventy-two hours later, the patient was neurologically intact and underwent a Bohlman triple wire arthrodesis.

the group given GM1 ganglioside. To be effective, the drug can be administered up to 72 hours after injury. Presently, gangliosides are also undergoing clinical testing in a multicenter study.

Mechanical factors have received less attention but are of great interest to physicians caring for spinal cord injuries. Trauma renders the spine unstable whereby the spinal cord becomes injured. Because of persistent instability, the potential for recurrent neural injury exists. Ducker et al. convincingly demonstrated the value of skeletal stabilization when they evaluated a variety of pharmacologic agents and their effect on neural recovery (45). They found simple immobilization of the injured spine more important than any of the experimental drugs. Breig has shown that residual kyphosis or anterior cord compression creates increased tension on axonal tracts and decreased cord perfusion (28). Additionally, compression of nerve roots may decrease segmented radicular blood flow, increasing cord ischemia. The abnormal tensile forces can be corrected by fracture reduction and complete decompression.

In many cases, viable nerve tissues remain following injury but have limited recovery because of persistent cord compression. Bohlman and Anderson have documented recovery of these tissues up to 12 months from injury (11, 22). Other studies show an inverse relationship between time from injury to neurologic recovery (42, 78). Additionally, a short window of opportunity may exist in some patients in whom an immediate decompression may reverse the spinal cord injury and prevent any secondary insults. Delamarter et al. created spinal cord injuries in beagles using a constricting band, creating 50% occlusion of the spinal cord (39). Animals who had the band immediately released or after 1 hour made full clinical recovery. Animals in which the band was left in place for 6 or 24 hours developed complete paraplegia. In humans, we have observed four cases of immediate reversal of quadriplegia by fracture reduction within two hours of injury (Fig. 14.3).

Early treatment of spinal cord injuries is not without risks. Marshall et al. reported a multicenter study of 283 patients of whom 14 developed neurologic deterioration (71). Four patients were in the surgically treated group, all of whom had surgery within the first 5 days. No patients having surgery after 5 days experienced deterioration. However, a slightly higher percentage of patients deteriorated within the first 5 days during nonoperative treatment. Early surgery has been associated with decreased morbidity and hospitalization costs (63, 86).

Classification

Many classification systems have been described to assess cervical injuries, but none have been universally acceptable. An accurate classification system is important to identify common fracture patterns, determine prognosis, assist in planning reduction maneuvers that reverse injury vectors, and help determine proper treatment methods. The basic concept of stability was emphasized by Nicoll (75). He evaluated 152 miners who sustained fractures of the thoraco-lumbar spine. Stable fractures included anterior or lateral wedge fractures and fractures of the neural arch above L4. These fractures were characterized by having intact intraspinous ligaments. The patients with stable fractures did not develop progressive deformity or neurologic deficits and were able to return to mining. Unstable fractures were associated with injury to the posterior osseous-ligamentous structure and were associated with increasing deformity and disability. Such fractures included fracture subluxation with post-element damage, all fracture dislocations, and posterior element fractures at L4 or L5. Holdsworth confirmed the observations of Nicoll (61). He furthered the understanding of fractures by dividing the spinal column into two columns: the anterior and posterior columns. Stable fractures had injuries associated to only one column, whereas unstable injuries had two column injuries. He emphasized the importance of evaluation of the posterior osseous-ligamentous complex by both physical examination and careful review of radiographs. Today, MRI with fat suppression techniques can accurately determine the presence of occult posterior ligamentous injury in the sub-axial cervical spine.

White and Punjabi used cadaveric testing to determine parameters that could be used to determine clinical instability (99). They define instability as a "loss of ability of the spine under physiologic loads to maintain relationships in such a way that there is neither damage nor subsequent irritation to the spinal cord or nerve roots and, in addition, there is no development of incapacitating deformity or pain." In the cadaveric specimens, they progressively sectioned ligaments from anterior to posterior and from posterior to anterior. After each sectioning, the spine was loaded and deformations were measured. They found significant motion occurred when all posterior ligaments and a single anterior ligamentous structure or all anterior ligamentous and a single posterior ligamentous structure were sectioned. The deformation measured was 3.5 mm of antero-posterior translation and 11° of kyphotic angulation. To aid in the clinical evaluation of stability, White has recommended use of a checklist (Table 14.2) (99). Each element of the checklist is assessed and the total positive values are summated. If the value is greater than five, then the spine is probably unstable. This checklist is to be used primarily for the evaluation of acute trauma. Patients with values greater than five do not necessarily require surgery but usually, at a minimum, are

TABLE 14.2.
Checklist for the Diagnosis of Clinical Instability

Element	Point Value
Anterior elements destroyed or unable to function	2
Posterior elements destroyed or unable to function	2
Relative sagittal plane translation >3.5 mm	2
Relative sagittal plane rotation >11°	2
Posterior stretch test	2
Cord injury	2
Root injury	1
Abnormal disc narrowing	1
Congenital spinal stenosis	1
Dangerous loading anticipated	1
	>5 = Clinical Instability

TABLE 14.4.
Classification of Cervical Injuries

1. **Hyperflexion Injuries**
   Posterior ligamentous injuries
   Unilateral facet dislocation
   Bilateral facet dislocation
2. **Axial Loading**
   Compression fracture
   Burst fracture
3. **Axial Loading Flexion**
   Tear drop fractures
4. **Extension Injuries**
   Isolated fractures of posterior ligaments
   Anterior longitudinal ligament rupture
   Central cord syndrome
   Traumatic retrolisthesis

treated with a halo-vest. Although not uniformly accepted, this checklist provides an objective framework to assess clinical instability.

Allen and Ferguson and their colleagues developed a comprehensive classification system based on six different fracture mechanisms that were determined from analysis of radiographs (Table 14.3) (6). Each fracture type is associated with subtypes which vary according to the severity of the injury. This system is excellent for use in in-vitro studies, but has limited clinical applications. The system is cumbersome and in many patients it is difficult to reliably determine its fracture phylogeny. Denis expanded the ideas of Holdsworth by introducing the three column concept (41). The third column is the middle column consisting of the posterior vertebral body wall, the posterior longitudinal ligament, and the posterior third of the disc and annulus. Although artificially created, the middle column is clearly important because it is most often the site of neural impaction. McAfee et al. emphasized the importance of the middle column and described six thoracolumbar fracture types based on forces directed to the middle column (72). Although useful in the classification of thoracolumbar fractures, the three column theory has little applicability in cervical injuries.

The AO group has developed a classification system based on primary force vectors (53). Type A injuries are compression injuries, Type B are distractive injuries, and Type C are multiplanar instabilities caused by rotation or shear. Subtypes in each group represent a continuum of progressive severity. This classification system strongly correlates with stability and the incidence of neurologic deficits as one progresses from Type A to Type C. However, at the present time, this system has not been used in the United States for cervical injuries.

Because of the lack of an accepted classification system, we will define fractures in broad groups based on fracture mechanism and then in sub-groups using common names associated with fracture morphology (24) (Table 14.4). To properly classify a spinal injury, the physician must carefully examine the patient for tenderness, swelling, and gaps between the spinous processes. A meticulous neurologic examination must be performed. The plain radiographs are assessed for anterior and posterior column injuries, fractures, and subluxations. Posterior ligamentous injury is often subtle and radiographs should be scrutinized for interspinous widening. In the majority of cases, a CT and/or MRI should be obtained. The MRI is especially useful in identifying disc herniation and ligamentous injuries.

Hyperflexion Injuries

Ligamentous Injuries

Hyperflexion and distractive forces created in the posterior osseous ligamentous complex during rapid head acceleration or deceleration can result in tensile failure of these structures (79). A progressive ligamentous injury occurs from posterior to anterior. Clinically, a variable degree of soft tissue injury is present. Initially, it is often difficult to differentiate minor from severe injuries. Minor sprains may be painful but present little long-term significance. Major ligamentous disruptions are highly unstable and require aggressive treatment to diminish risk of long-term pain and neurologic deficits.

TABLE 14.3.
Allen and Ferguson Mechanistic Classification of Cervical Injuries

	Stages
Compressive flexion	1–5
Vertebral flexion	1–3
Distractive flexion	1–4
Compressive extension	1–5
Distractive extension	1–2
Lateral flexion	1–2

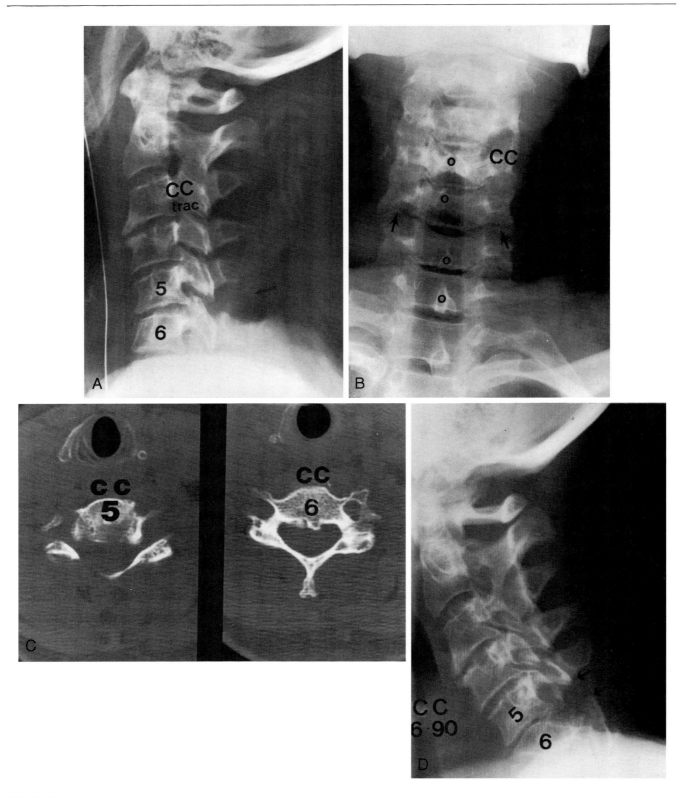

FIGURE 14.4.
A. Lateral radiograph of 73-year-old female who reported neck pain after a motor vehicle accident. Wide separation of C5-6 spinous processes is present but was overlooked. **B.** Interspinous widening is seen on anteroposterior radiograph. **C.** A CT scan was performed and was interpreted as negative for fracture. **D.** This flexion-extension radiograph performed by the patient without assistance demonstrates a complete C5-6 dislocation. Initially, the patient was neurologically intact. After flexion-extension, she developed a central cord syndrome. She was treated with methylprednisolone, immediate reduction, and delayed posterior fusion. After reduction, she rapidly recovered the lost neurologic function.

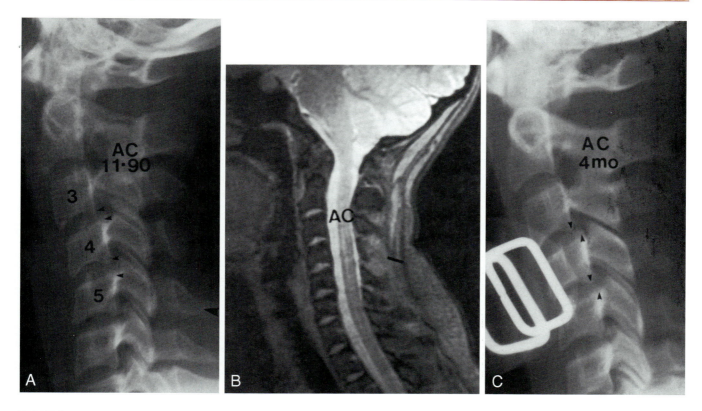

FIGURE 14.5.
A. Lateral radiograph of sixteen-year-old female after a vehicular crash. She reported neck pain and was tender focally at C3-C4. Subluxation and interspinous widening is seen at C3-4 and C4-5. **B.** MRI demonstrates increased signal in soft tissues indicative of ligamentous injury. **C.** The patient was treated with hard collar immobilization. Twelve weeks after the injury, she had increasing neck pain, recurrent subluxation, and kyphosis and was treated by a posterior cervical arthrodesis.

Patients with ligamentous injuries present with pain and difficulty moving their head and neck. The pain is often not present immediately after the trauma but is noted several days later after an inflammatory response ensues. The diagnosis is delayed frequently because the initial radiographs are interpreted as negative. A consistent physical finding in acute cases is repeatable focal tenderness in the absence of radiographic change. A palpable gap between spinous processes is rarely identifiable in the cervical spine compared to the thoracolumbar spine.

Plain radiographs may show only subtle abnormalities (Fig. 14.4A,B). Local kyphosis, angulation of the adjacent endplates at a single disc level, or interspinous widening may be present. Occasionally, abnormalities will not be present because patients are positioned supine with their necks in extension, thus reducing any deformity. Interspinous widening is often more obvious on the antero-posterior image. Flexion-extension radiographs are recommended frequently to assess the severity of injury and stability but can cause dislocations and spinal cord injury. We have observed two such cases done under controlled conditions in which the patients flexed their own necks; we have, therefore, abandoned this study (Fig.14.4C,D). CT with sagittal reconstruction, especially at the cervico-thoracic junction, can be useful when the posterior elements may not be visualized. Facet joint diastasis on axial images and interspinous widening or facet joint subluxations are indicative of posterior ligamentous injuries. MRI with fat suppression techniques is useful in identifying posterior ligamentous injuries. Findings include high intensity signals in the interspinous spaces or facet joints and discontinuity of hypointense vertical lines that represent ligamentous structures (Fig. 14.5). The White criteria is used to quantify the overall severity of injury. If the point value is less than five, then the injury is treated as a minor sprain, and if greater than five, it is treated as a major ligamentous disruption.

Unilateral Facet Dislocation

Unilateral facet dislocations arise typically from a hyperflexion-rotation force (79). Although many authors believe that these are stable injuries, a significant ligamentous injury occurs biomechanically, resulting in unilateral facet dislocations. In cadaver, unilateral facet dislocations were associated with in-

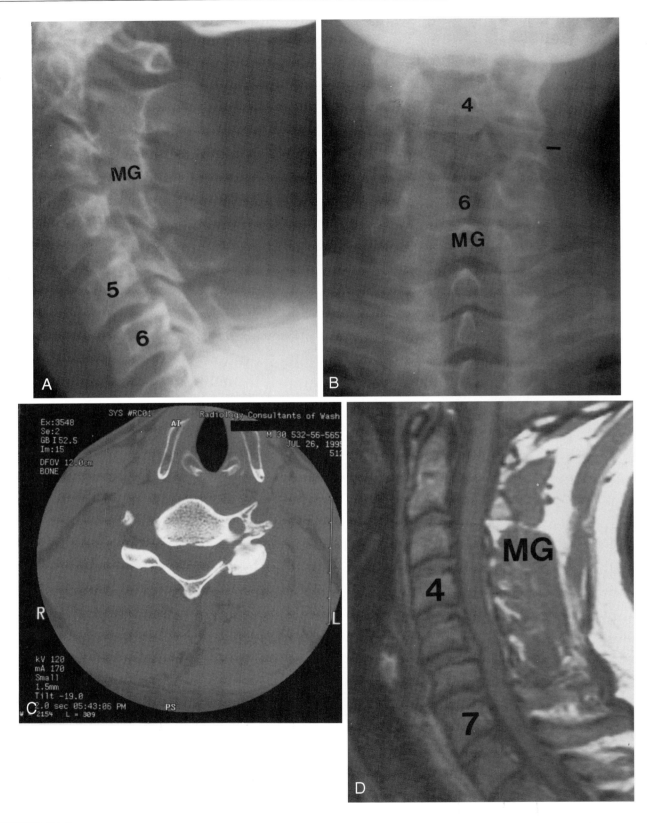

FIGURE 14.6.

A. Three weeks after a motor vehicular crash, a twenty-eight-year-old presented with a lateral radiograph showing a C5-6 subluxation. Neurologically, the patient had weakness in left arm and leg. **B.** Anteroposterior views, which demonstrate rotational deformity of the C5 lateral mass. Both the C4-5 and C5-6 facet joints are visualized because they are rotated into the plane of the x-ray beam. **C.** Fractures of both the pedicle and lamina are present, rendering the lateral mass free to rotate. Roy-Camille has termed this injury fracture separation of the lateral mass. **D.** A traumatic C5-6 disc herniation with spinal cord compression is seen on MRI. He was treated by anterior discectomy and fusion with Morscher plate.

jury to the supra- and interspinous ligaments, disc annulus, ipsilateral joint capsule, and ligamentum flava. Thus, these injuries have the potential for significant instability.

Unilateral facet dislocations can be classified into three types: pure unilateral facet dislocation, unilateral fracture dislocation, and fracture separation of the lateral mass (70). The radiographic hallmark is a 25% anterior vertebral body subluxation. On lateral radiographs, local kyphosis or interspinous widening may be seen but is often absent. The anteroposterior radiograph demonstrates rotation of the spinous process towards the side of dislocated facet. Also, the articulation may become abnormally visible as the radiographic beam is now abnormally in the plane of the facet. In unilateral facet fracture dislocations, articular fractures may be seen but often require CT for visualization. Fracture separation of the lateral mass results from fracturing of the pedicle and lamina on one side, which creates a free-floating lateral mass (Fig. 14.6). On the lateral view, the involved lateral masses appears malrotated compared to its contralateral pair and the adjacent levels. On the antero-posterior view, a fracture of the pedicle is present along with the very obvious malrotated lateral mass. Because the lateral mass has two articulations, this injury involves two motion segments. MRI imaging demonstrates a 10 to 20% incidence of disc herniation in patients with unilateral facet dislocations (Fig. 14.6D).

Clinically, patients present with minimal neurologic findings, although in patients with congenital spinal stenosis, significant cord injuries may be present. Isolated radiculopathies of the root passing out the neuroforamena of the level involved are overlooked frequently but present in greater than 50% of cases. Pure unilateral facet dislocations are the most stable and may be difficult to reduce. After reduction, the upward slope of the facets prevents redislocation. In fracture dislocations and fracture separation of this lateral mass redisplacement, frequently occurs despite closed reduction and halo-vest immobilization.

Bilateral Facet Dislocations

Bilateral facet dislocations result from tensile failure of the posterior osseo-ligamentous complex during hyperflexion often combined with small amounts of rotation (79). In more severe cases, distraction of all ligamentous structures may result in complete separation of the motion segment except for the neural and vascular tissue. Bilateral facet dislocation is highly unstable and is associated with ligamentous injury to all posterior structures, the posterior longitudinal ligament, and the disc annulus. Often the only intact structure is the anterior longitudinal ligament, which helps to realign the dislocation during traction reduction. The soft tissue injury is extensive and is associated with traumatic disc herniation in 30 to 50% of cases (43, 47). Spinal cord injury is present in the majority of cases secondary to tension created in the neural tissues and to crushing between the caudal vertebral body and the cranial lamina. Patients occasionally present neurologically intact because of the fracturing of the lamina or the presence of large spinal canals. Radiographically, a minimum of 50% anterior vertebral body translation is present, although this is occasionally overlooked at the cervico-thoracic junction. Local kyphosis or interspinous widening are variably seen. Abnormal disc narrowing may indicate the presence of associated traumatic disc herniation behind the cranial vertebral body. Fractures of the posterior elements, including bilateral laminar spinous process and facet fracture, are seen in greater than 50 percent of cases. Vertebral artery occlusion has been documented by angiography in 50 to 60% of patients with facet dislocation but is of unknown clinical significance (101). When translation is greater than 50% or when distraction is present, the patients often have higher levels of spinal cord than skeletal injury or are at risk for ascension of their neurologic deficits.

Axial Loading Injuries

Pure axial loading injuries result in fracturing of the vertebral body. With smaller amounts of compression or hyperflexion, a wedge compression fracture is created, and with larger amounts, a burst fracture is created. Radiographically burst fractures have retropulsed bone fragments that are similar morphologically to those at the thoraco-lumbar junction. Stability of these injuries is determined by the associated injury to the posterior elements.

In the tear-drop fracture, flexion axially loading forces cause fracture of the vertebral body, shearing across the intervertebral disc, and retrolisthesis of the vertebral body into the spinal canal (Fig. 14.7) (87). Tensile failure of the posterior osseous ligamentous complex creates interspinous separation and fracturing of the lamina and spinous processes in the majority of cases. These are highly unstable injuries and are associated frequently with spinal cord injuries. The posterior longitudinal ligament usually is preserved and guides realignment during fracture reduction. They should be differentiated from an avulsion fracture of the anterior inferior corner of the vertebral body caused by hyperextension, usually a more benign fracture. This "avulsion teardrop" fracture at first glance can be confused with the flexion compression teardrop fracture. This could result in inappropriately treating an unstable flexion teardrop for the more stable avulsion type.

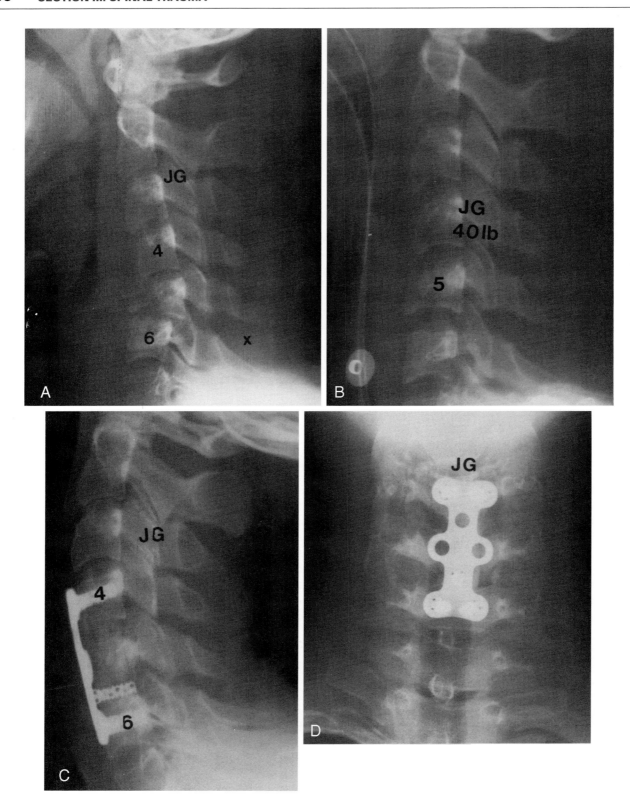

FIGURE 14.7.

A. A teardrop fracture of Schneider is seen on the lateral radiograph. This 19-year-old male was an incomplete quadriplegic. The teardrop fragment from the anterior inferior corner of the C6 vertebra is seen. More importantly, the posterior aspect of vertebral body is rotated into the cord and osseous ligamentous injury is present in the posterior elements denoted by (x). **B.** Cervical tong traction of forty pounds resulted in successful reduction. **C.** The patient was treated with anterior decompression iliac strut fusion and placement of Morscher plate. **D.** Postoperative antero-posterior radiograph.

Extension Injuries

Forced hyperextension is a common mechanism of injury in patients who impact their heads forward into windshields or in elderly patients who fall. These injuries may be missed on plain radiographs and result in long-term pain and disability. Minor fractures from a stability standpoint include ruptures of the anterior longitudinal ligament and isolated fractures without facet or vertebral body subluxation, such as spinous process lateral mass and laminar fractures. Jönsson et al. examined 22 consecutive victims of traffic accidents who had sustained skull fractures using a cryoplane technique (66). Twenty of the

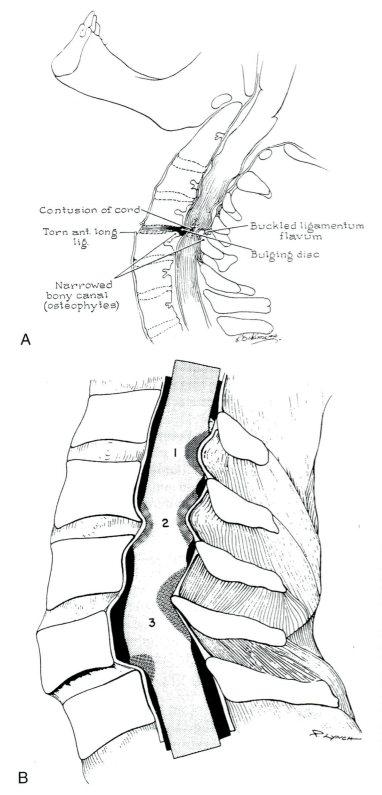

FIGURE 14.8.

A. During forced hyperextension in patients with narrow spinal canals, the cord can become pinched between the bulging disc and infolded ligamentous flava. Reprinted with permission from Bohlman HH, Ducker JB, Lucas JT. Spine and spinal cord injuries. In: Rotherman RH, Simeone FA, eds. The spine, 2nd ed. Philadelphia: WB Saunders:682. **B.** Anatomic factors that are associated with central cord injuries caused by hyperextension. (1) Infolding of the ligamentum flava. (2) Bulging of the intervertebral disc. Also frequently seen is 1 to 3 mm of retrolisthesis. (3) Compression of the spinal cord between lamina and posterior margin of the vertebral body occurs. Reprinted with permission from White AA III, Panjabi MM. Practical biomechanics of spinal trauma. In: White AA, Panjabi MM, eds. Clinical biomechanics of the spine. 2nd ed. Philadelphia: JB Lippincott, 1990:239.

twenty-two had trauma directed to the face or frontal bone. Radiographs were negative but multiple occult findings were present. Findings included prevertebral hematoma (4 cases), paravertebral hematoma (4 cases), ligamentum flava disruption (8 cases), facet joint injuries (69 cases), longus colli disruption (2 cases), uncovertebral hematoma (77 cases), disc disruption (36 cases), cartilaginous endplate avulsion (2 cases), and occult fractures (4 cases). They concluded that current routine plain radiographic evaluation of patients subjected to trauma greatly underestimates the musculoskeletal injury especially, in hyperextension injuries.

Hyperextension in a patient with congenital spinal canal stenosis or cervical spondylosis can result in shortening of the spinal column and infolding of the posterior disc annulus and ligamentum flava (Fig. 14.8A) (88). The spinal cord is thus pinched, resulting in central cord necrosis and a central cord syndrome. The major axonal tracts within the spinal cord are laminated with cervical tracts located centrally and lumbo-sacral tracts located laterally. In a central cord syndrome caused by an extension injury, the grey matter and cervical anterior horn cells are damaged, creating the neurologic picture of relative sparing of the lower extremities and more severe involvement of the upper extremities. Prognostically, patients with central cord syndromes generally recover the ability to ambulate but have poor return of hand function.

Radiographically spinal canal size can be assessed by the Pavlov method, which is determining the ratio of the midsagittal diameter of the spinal canal to antero-posterior diameter of the vertebral body (94). If the ratio is less than 0.8 then the spinal canal is probably stenotic. A more accurate determination can be made on CT or MRI. In patients with central cord syndromes, radiographs usually demonstrate spondylosis, osteophyte formation, and disc space narrowing. Small amounts of retrolisthesis is seen at the site of cord trauma and is often thought to be preexisting (Figure 14.8B). However, in many cases, this retrolisthesis is traumatically induced by the hyperextension. Small amounts of residual retrolisthesis can greatly narrow the spinal canal, creating persistent cord compression. This observation has been confirmed by MRI in which acute disco-ligamentous disruptions can be documented in patients with extension injuries. Tong traction is effective in reducing these subluxations as well as stabilizing the spine and should be used in all cases.

General Treatment

History

Ancient civilizations recognized the poor prognosis of spinal cord injuries and recommended no treatment because patients would all inevitably die. Hippocrates described closed reduction techniques for thoracolumbar fracture (2). He applied traction to the prone patient using arm and leg straps attached to turnbuckles. Once spinal column length was restored, manual reduction was performed by the surgeon or by levers. He assailed others whom he called charlatans who made public spectacles when they strapped patients to ladders and literally hung them upside down in the town center. In the second century, Galen proposed the idea of removal of the neural arch to decompress the marrow. Paul of Aegina in the seventh century may have been the first to actually perform the laminectomy. Ambrose Paré, a 15th-century Parisian surgeon, performed an unsuccessful laminectomy on a spinal-injured patient. Hadra is thought to be the first to apply internal fixation when in 1891 he circlaged the spinous process with a silver wire loop in an open wound. Harvey Cushing, the father of neurosurgery in the United States, recommended decompression of the spinal cord via laminectomy. This practice unfortunately continued until very recent times. Davies and Böhler astutely realized that fracture reduction rather than laminectomy achieved decompression of the spinal cord (20, 38). Rogers in 1942 reported a simple safe technique of fusion using interspinous wires, which resulted in a high rate of success (82). Modifications of the technique have been developed, although interspinous wire fixation and bone graft remains the standard technique for posterior fusion today (25). Smith and Robinson developed an anterior technique to decompress the neural surface of the spinal cord (90). Bailey, Cloward, and Verbiest applied the anterior approach to patients with fractures (16, 33, 98). New techniques using anterior and posterior titanium plates have been developed to achieve increased rigidity for traumatic applications.

Controversies and Current Trends

Controversies regarding the role of surgery have existed until recently. Guttmann and Bedbrook found that the surgically treated patients had less neurologic recovery and were more likely to have ascension of their lesion (17, 50, 58). At the time, laminectomy was the procedure of choice, but today it is condemned and rarely indicated. Current treatment is to decompress the neural elements in patients with neurologic deficits and to stabilize the spine with as few as possible motion segments permanently stiffened. The philosophy is based on several important principles and confirmed by animal studies. However, clinical data to support this aggressive philosophy are lacking. Another controversy is the effect of timing and its relation to neurologic recovery.

The choice of treatment of cervical spine injuries is based on many factors. Most importantly is the fracture type and stability. Once properly classified, a patient can be treated according to an algorithm based on fracture type as described later. The treatment choice should counteract the abnormal biomechanics of injury. An important secondary factor is the presence of residual cord or root compression in patients with neurologic deficits. Decompression appears to increase recovery if performed within twelve months (11, 22). Whether the injury is primarily bony or ligamentous is of primary importance. In general, bony injuries treated nonoperatively often heal, whereas ligamentous injuries have a poor capacity for healing and are best treated surgically. Other factors determining treatment include patient age, bone density associated injuries, and postoperative bracing limitations. In patients who are neurologically intact, the surgeon must remember that the final outcome cannot be any better than a neurologically intact patient. The choice of treatment methods of lower cervical injuries includes nonoperative treatment with orthosis or halo-vest and operative treatment with either anterior or posterior decompression and fusion with instrumentation.

The goals of treatment of cervical spine fractures and dislocation are to protect the neurologic structures, reduce and stabilize fractures and dislocations, and provide a long-term stable painless spinal column. Initial treatment in most cases is stabilization and, if required, reduction by tong traction. Once physical and radiologic examinations are complete, definitive treatment can be planned. In some cases, the degree of instability may not be initially apparent and therefore definite treatment may be changed over time. This treatment is not necessarily poor or inadequate, but it is appropriate and prevents unnecessary overtreatment. In this section, treatment algorithms will be described for the fracture types previously described. The initial management of spinal cord injuries is also reviewed.

Nonoperative Treatment

The soft collar provides little stabilizing effect on intersegmental forces but does limit overall range of motion and gives comfort. This method may be appropriate in stable injuries, especially in older patient populations. The hard collar, when properly fitted and worn, gives sufficient immobilization to treat many injuries. However, patients poorly tolerate the Philadelphia collar because of sweating and skin maceration. Also, achieving a good fit is often difficult. We have found the Miami J collar to have improved patient tolerance because it has a Gortex lining and is more easily adjustable to patients. This orthosis is excellent for patients who have stable fractures or postoperative management.

Cervico-thoracic braces, such as the Minerva, Yale, or Guillford braces, achieve fixation from upright bars that attach to anterior and posterior thoracic pads. The pads are stabilized by straps that pass under the arm and over the shoulders. Some orthoses have exchangeable pads so that patients may shower while wearing the brace. These braces offer enough comfort and sufficient immobilization so that they can be used successfully for many fracture patterns.

The halo-vest provides the greatest degree of cervical immobilization. Satisfactory results have been achieved in patients with upper cervical injuries, except those with type II odontoid fractures. The halo-vest appears to be less suited for patients with unstable lower cervical injuries. Whitehill reported five patients with bilateral facet dislocation who lost reduction in a halo-vest (100). Similarly, Glaser and Bucholz and their colleagues documented loss of reduction in 10% of all patients and 37% of patients with facet subluxations (30, 55). Although often minor, up to a 57% complication rate has been reported (51). These complications are primarily related to the skull pins and include loosening, infection loss of fixation, skull penetration and brain abscess. Less well known is the lack of stability of intersegmental motion afforded by the halo-vest. Anderson et al. obtained supine and upright lateral radiographs in patients with unstable cervical injuries (14). They found that an average of 1.7 mm translation and 7° of angulation occurred at the fracture site during the position change. Additionally, the halo-vest is poorly tolerated because of its restriction of activities of daily living.

Biomechanic and kinematic studies have compared the immobilization effect of various orthoses. Johnson et al. found that little reduction in overall cervical range of motion occurred from the soft cervical collar (65). The Philadelphia collar results in 71% restriction of range of motion in flexion-extension but only 54% in rotation. The cervico-thoracic braces resulted in 88% diminished flexion-extension motion and 82% in rotation. The halo-vest restricted flexion-extension by 96% and rotation by 99%. Intersegmental motion was not as affected in all braces because of the snaking effect in which one segment would flex while the next would compensate with extension.

Treatment of Spinal Cord Injury

Patients who have spinal cord injuries caused by fractures and dislocation of the cervical spine require rapid evaluation and treatment. The first goal is to protect the spine from further injury. This goal is accomplished by the use of extraction collars, placement of patients on backboards, and the use of tape and sandbags. Once a spinal injury is documented, tong traction is applied to maintain alignment, thus preventing further trauma. Supplemental oxygen is given via nasal cannula and the blood pressure is maintained to at least 90 mm Hg. High dose methylprednisolone is administered for acute spinal cord injuries within 8 hours of trauma. A loading dose of 30 mg/kg and a maintenance dose of 5.4 mg/kg/hr for 23 hours is administered.

Fractures and dislocations are reduced as rapidly as possible. Although some authors recommend obtaining imaging studies before fracture reduction, this can result in delays that can be harmful to the remaining viable neural tissue. Fracture reduction has been recognized as the simplest method to "decompress" the spinal canal. Delays, especially in the first hours after injury, may result in permanence of neurologic injury. Many controversies exist, including how traction should be applied, the timing of reduction, and the maximum amount of weight that can be used safely. Recent studies document the safety and efficacy of even very large traction weights when used in a rigid protocol (35, 56, 91). The application of cranial tongs, such as Gardner-Wells, is simple and relatively free of complication. Skull fractures or craniotomy defects are relative contraindications to tong placement. The tongs are placed 1 cm above the pinna in line with the external auditory meatus. Shaving is not required. The skin is prepared with antiseptic solution and local anesthetic down to the periosteum. The skull pins are tightened symmetrically until the skull pin tensionometer indicates that sufficient tension has been applied when the plunger backs out 1 mm. Initially, 5 to 10 lbs. of traction weight are applied with the head in a neutral position. A lateral radiograph is checked and a repeat neurologic examination is performed. If the fracture has not reduced, then 10 to 15 lbs. are added and a repeat neurologic check is performed and a radiograph obtained. The radiograph is scrutinized for fracture alignment and signs of overdistraction, including disc space or facet joint diastasis. If these signs are present, the process is stopped. Addition of traction weight continues until the fracture is reduced or there is an adverse change in neurologic status or signs of overdistraction. Traction weights equal to 70% of body weight have been used safely and efficaciously (35, 91). Once the fracture has been reduced, the weight can be decreased except in bursting type fracture. The use of MRI compatible tongs is recommended, although they do not withstand as high traction weights as well as do stainless steel tongs. Once the fracture is reduced, the patient can undergo neural imaging.

If the fractures cannot be reduced, strong consideration should be given to performing an open reduction and internal fixation (89). The surgical approach depends on fracture type and direction of neural compression. Although not based on any scientific studies, early surgery is recommended in these cases.

The next component of treatment is stabilization. In patients with unstable fractures and neurologic deficits, this usually will be performed surgically. The choice of treatment depends on fracture type as described later in the chapter. The timing of surgery is controversial. Early surgery within the first 5 days may be associated with increased chance of neurologic deficit (71). However, early surgery allows rapid patient mobilization and has decreased the overall morbidity, hospital stay, and cost of treatment (63, 69, 86).

A major goal of the surgical procedure is to achieve adequate neural decompression and stabilization. Preoperatively, patients are imaged with MRI. If compression is anterior, then an anterior approach is recommended. For the rare posterior compressive lesion, laminectomy with or without foraminotomy is performed. Sufficient internal fixation should be used to allow rapid mobilization and avoidance of the halo-vest in quadriplegics, if at all possible.

Treatment of Specific Fracture Types

Minor Fractures

Stable injuries, such as spinous process fractures, laminar fractures, lateral mass fractures without subluxation, vertebral body compression fractures, and avulsion fracture of the anterior longitudinal ligament, can be considered minor fractures. These injuries are isolated to one side of the spine and are not associated with any narrowing of the spinal canal. In questionable cases, patients are evaluated by the White Criteria (Table 14.2). Treatment of these minor fractures includes simple immobilization in a hard collar or cervico-thoracic brace for 6 to 8 weeks. After placement of the orthosis, upright lateral radiographs are obtained to assure that the injury is stable before the patient is discharged from the hospital. The patient is then assessed biweekly with repeat radiographs. Increasing pain or neurologic symptoms indicate fracture site motion. The treating physician must always be ready to alter his/her initial diagnosis of a stable injury and change treatment as required. After the period of immobilization, flexion-extension radiographs are obtained to assess healing. Other surgeons initially recommend flexion-extension radiographs to assess stability. We believe that these may be hazardous and therefore prefer to treat the patient and provide serial follow-up to assess healing and alignment.

Hyperflexion Injuries

Ligamentous Injuries

Hyperflexion ligamentous injuries can be classified as minor or severe. The minor injuries have a White criteria of less than five and are not associated with vertebral body subluxation or intradiscal disruption. These mild ligamentous injuries may be expected to heal with immobilization as described previously for minor fractures. The severe hyperflexion ligamentous injury represents an unstable injury with poor healing capacity. Additionally, during closed treatment, loss of reduction has been reported frequently (30, 55, 100). Therefore, the treatment for the severe ligamentous injury is a posterior fusion with a Bohlman triple wire technique. If a spinous process or lamina fracture is present, fixation using lateral mass plates or an anterior plate can be performed. When the severity of ligamentous injury is uncertain, we recommend initial conservative treatment with frequent follow-up.

Unilateral Facet Dislocations

The treatment of unilateral facet dislocations is controversial. Although a significant ligamentous injury is present, many authorities believe that these injuries are stable after reduction. However, during nonoperative treatment, these rotationally unstable injuries have frequently lost reduction, especially in the presence of a facet fracture. Factors that may influence the treatment include difficulty of reduction, presence of a fracture, and extent of reduction. Long-term outcome has demonstrated that the best function is achieved when an anatomic alignment is present at the end of treatment, regardless of treatment (18, 83).

The following treatment algorithm for patients with unilateral facet fracture dislocation is recommended. Patients with pure dislocations and difficult reductions are treated in a halo-vest for 8 to 12 weeks. During follow-up, the alignment is monitored carefully. Patients who redislocate are reduced and treated by a posterior fusion. Patients with unilateral facet fracture dislocation or who are reduced easily are treated primarily by a single level posterior fusion. Because of the facet fracture with loss of rotational control, interspinous wire fixation is frequently inadequate. Supplementation with an oblique facet wire as described by Anderson, Edwards, Levine, and their colleagues, or by lateral mass plates is recommended (9, 46). Before surgery, an MRI or CT-myelogram is assessed for presence of a disc herniation or displaced facet fractures that narrow the neuroforamina. If they are present, decompression by anterior approach or a foraminotomy should be performed if warranted by the patient's neurologic state. Anterior interbody fusion with plate fixation appears to be an adequate method of treatment for patients with unilateral facet dislocation who have been reduced by closed means (3, 13). In the rare case of failure of closed reduction, an open reduction by levering the facets, manipulating the spinous processes, or removing a small amount of the superior articular facet can be done. After arthrodesis, the patient is immobilized in a hard collar for 6 to 8 weeks.

Bilateral Facet Dislocations

Bilateral facet dislocations are highly unstable and are best treated by closed reduction and surgical arthrodesis. Attempts at halo-vest management results in greater than 50% incidence of loss of reduction (100). Also, these patients are usually quadriplegic, and avoidance of the halo vest can speed their rehabilitation and lessen the risk of pulmonary complications.

The controversy in the management of bilateral facet dislocations relates to the associated intervertebral disc herniation and the timing of reduction (47, 96). MRI studies have demonstrated a 10 to 42% incidence of disc herniation in patients with bilateral facet dislocations. Theoretically, during reduction the intervertebral disc can remain posterior to the cranial vertebral body, causing further neurologic injury. Eismont et al. reported six cases of associated disc herniation, three of which worsened after reduction (47). In these three cases, reduction occurred during surgery after an unsuccessful closed attempt. Tribus reported a similar case of traumatic disc herniation associated with bilateral facet dislocation treated successfully by an anterior discectomy and fusion. Risk factors for this catastrophic complication include abnormal disc narrowing, irreducibility or difficult reduction, worsening of the neurologic state during reduction, and operative versus closed reduction. Eismont et al. and Tribus recommend MRI studies in patients who are neurologically intact or who have incomplete deficits before reduction (47, 96). If an anterior disc herniation is present, an anterior discectomy should be performed before any attempt at reduction. The disadvantage of this approach is the difficulty in obtaining an emergent MRI on trauma patients resulting in a delay in fracture reduction. The management of patients with bilateral facet dislocation thus depends on the neurologic status and availability of MRI.

Patients who have complete or significant incomplete neurologic deficits should have immediate attempt at closed reduction aimed to rapidly and indirectly decompress the neural tissues. After reduction, an MRI is obtained. If spinal cord compression secondary to a disc herniation is present, an anterior discectomy and interbody fusion with autogenous bone graft and plate is performed. Patients without associated disc herniation are treated by posterior fusion with interspinous wire or plate techniques.

Patients with minimal deficits should have MRI before attempts at reduction are made. The patient is kept on the back board with the extraction collar and placed in the scanner. For patients who have disc herniation, an anterior discectomy is done before reduction. After disc removal and distraction, a reduction can be attempted by the closed technique aided by fluoroscopy or with the use of disc distractor. If reduction is achieved, anterior fusion with plate fixation can be performed. If the reduction is unsuccessful, a bone graft is placed in the disc space and an open reduction and posterior fusion is performed. The interbody graft may migrate and require replacement after the posterior procedure.

Axial Loading Injuries

The hallmark of axial loading injuries is the comminution of the vertebral body and retropulsion of bone into the spinal canal. Stable axial loading injuries include burst fractures without significant posterior column involvement. These injuries usually occur at C6 or C7 levels. These fractures are reduced easily with tong traction and can be treated in a halo-vest. For patients with associated neurologic deficits, a surgical approach is recommended to facilitate rehabilitation and decrease the likelihood of recurrent injury. Because the pathology is located anteriorly, an anterior corpectomy and reconstruction with iliac crest strut graft and anterior plate is recommended. If flexion or extension is combined with axial loading, then the posterior osseo-ligamentous structures are injured, resulting in an unstable pattern. The teardrop fracture of Schneider is a usual example. These fractures can be reduced with traction, although large weights may be required. Optimal definitive treatment is anterior corpectomy and reconstruction with iliac crest strut graft and an anterior plate. Burst fractures associated with facet dislocation may require combined anterior and posterior arthrodesis.

Extension Injuries

Classically, extension injuries causing central cord syndromes were thought to occur from degenerative or congenital stenosis and were not associated with instability. Careful review of radiographs, however, show that these patients often have 2 to 3 mm of retrolisthesis in the mid-cervical spine (22). Small amounts of retrolisthesis in narrow canals can be associated with significant cord compression. Recently, MRI has documented the presence of acute annular disruption and increased signal in the intervertebral discs, suggesting that the subluxation is acute and not from spondylosis. Although these extension injuries stabilize over time, the initial treatment of all extension injuries with cord injury is tong traction. The goal of traction is to stabilize the spine, indirectly reduce the luxations, and lengthen the spinal column, pulling the bulging disc and infolded ligamentum flavum out of the spinal canal.

Definitive treatment of patients with central cord syndrome is controversial (22). Many patients are treated successfully by a short (3 to 5 day) period of traction and then immobilization in a collar. Patients are then assessed regularly and those not improving neurologically are evaluated by MRI or CT-myelogram. If cord compression is present, then a decompression is performed. Although recovery can occur for up to 1 year, we prefer to perform decompression within 3 to 4 weeks. The choice of anterior versus posterior decompression depends on the number of levels involved, site of compression, and overall alignment of the cervical spine. In most cases of one to three level involvement from anterior disc disease, an anterior decompression and fusion can be performed. In patients with multilevel disease and lordotic cervical spines, a posterior laminaplasty or laminectomy may be indicated. In trauma cases, we always perform an adjunctive posterior fusion with lateral mass plates and screws. Occasionally, for combined anterior-posterior compression, a two stage anterior-posterior approach is needed. A rare type of extension injury is the traumatic retrolisthesis in which vertebral body subluxation is 50% or greater. These injuries are difficult to reduce and are best treated by an anterior vertebrectomy and plate stabilization.

Surgical Treatment

Anesthesia Considerations

Patients who have unstable cervical spinal columns must be managed carefully to avoid iatrogenic neural injury during intubation and positioning. To avoid neck motion, an awake nasotracheal technique aided by fiberoptic scope is done while the patient is maintained in skeletal traction. Immediately after intubation, the neurologic function is tested and the patient is transferred to a turning frame. If a posterior approach is to be used, the patient is turned prone on the turning frame and the neurologic function is again tested. At this time, general anesthesia is induced and a lateral radiograph is obtained to check alignment. Visualization is aided by pulling downward on the shoulder with tape. Alignment corrections are made by adjusting the position of the face piece before skin incision. After positioning, the brachial plexus is palpated to assess whether excessive traction is present. The face is checked for excessive pressure points. No pressure should be applied to the orbits.

The anesthesiologist should avoid succinylcholine in patients with acute neurologic deficits because this is associated with massive leakage of potassium from muscle cells and cardiac arrest. Somatosensory evoked potentials are used only in cases in which an intraoperative reduction is to be performed and when decompression of a high grade stenotic lesion is to be decompressed.

Anterior Decompression and Fusion

Residual spinal cord compression may impair function of viable neural tissue, preventing maximal recovery (21). Because the majority of patients have ventral compression, decompression of retropulsed bone or disc fragments theoretically offers the best chance for neurologic recovery. Other advantages of anterior decompression include ease of positioning of patients with unstable cervical spines and a simple splitting approach using tissue planes, which avoids the more extensive soft tissue stripping of the posterior paraspinal musculature. Occasionally, in cases of fractures of the posterior elements, fewer segments can be arthrodesed by choosing an anterior approach.

Disadvantages primarily relate to stability and soft tissue swelling in the anterior neck. In acute traumatic cases, an anterior cervical plate can be applied to achieve sufficient stability to allow mobilization of the patient. For late cases, anterior decompression and arthrodesis without fixation appears satisfactory unless there is persistent posterior ligamentous instability or laminectomy. Complete quadriplegic patients have limited respiratory capacity and often cannot overcome the retropharyngeal soft tissue swelling that occurs after anterior decompression. Complications such as aspiration pneumonia and respiratory arrest can be minimized by keeping patients intubated for 2 to 3 days after surgery.

Bohlman and Anderson reviewed the results of late anterior decompression in 109 patients with spinal cord injuries who had reached a neurologic plateau in recovery (11, 22). All patients had residual cord and/or root compression. The average time from injury to surgery was a mean of 14 months. The follow-up averaged 5.6 years with a range of 2 to 14 years. The patients were divided into two groups based on neurologic function at the time of surgery. Fifty-eight patients had incomplete motor quadriplegia (Frankel Grade C and D) and 51 had complete motor quadriplegia (Frankel A and B). Twenty-nine of the 58 patients with incomplete motor quadriplegia became ambulators, and another 6 improved significantly on their preoperative ambulation ability. Noteworthy improvement in upper extremity function was seen in 39 of the 58 patients. In the group with complete motor quadriplegia, only one patient regained the ability to ambulate. However, upper extremity root recovery and improvement in activity of daily living as measured by the Bartel Index occurred in 31 of the 58 patients. Predictors of success were age of patient less than 50 years, greater degree of preoperative neural function, and surgery within 12 months of injury. Thus far, no study had addressed adequately the efficacy of acute anterior decompression within the first few days.

Anterior decompression and fusion is indicated in patients with residual ventral cord or root compression and persistent neurologic deficits. The timing of treatment is controversial, although most surgeons now recommend early treatment rather than the older approach of waiting for patients to achieve neurologic plateau. Patients who are neurologically intact do not require "prophylactic" decompression, although if they have an unstable injury that requires surgical stabilization, an anterior approach may be warranted. Similarly, patients who have a burst of teardrop fractures that have been reduced may be treated by an anterior approach. In most cases of acute trauma, adjunctive anterior plate fixation is recommended.

Surgical Technique—Anterior Decompression and Fusion

Preoperatively, patients have had attempted reduction with cranial tong traction and are evaluated with MRI or CT myelography. They are brought to the operating room in traction and have an awake naso-tracheal intubation. After a neurologic check, the patient is transferred to the operating table in traction and placed under general anesthesia. A small roll is placed under the shoulders and the arms are taped downwards. A lateral radiograph is obtained to check alignment.

A left-sided Smith-Robinson approach is used (90). A transverse incision extending from the midline to the anterior border of the sternocleidomastoid muscle is made at an appropriate level above the clavicle. The platysma and superficial layer of the deep cervical fascia are divided transversely. The sternocleidomastoid is dissected free from the middle layers of the deep cervical fascia. By blunt dissection between the trachea and carotid sheath, a plane is developed through the alar to the prevertebral fascia. This membranous structure is divided, exposing the ventral bodies and disc spaces. Localization of the level is confirmed radiographically. Complete disc removal back to the posterior longitudinal ligament of the cranial and caudal disc is performed (Fig. 14.9A). An operating microscope or loupes and a head lamp can facilitate visualization. The vertebral body is removed from an anterior to posterior direction using rongeurs and an air driven burr (Fig. 14.9B). Bony decompression continues until only a thin shell of posterior cortex remains,

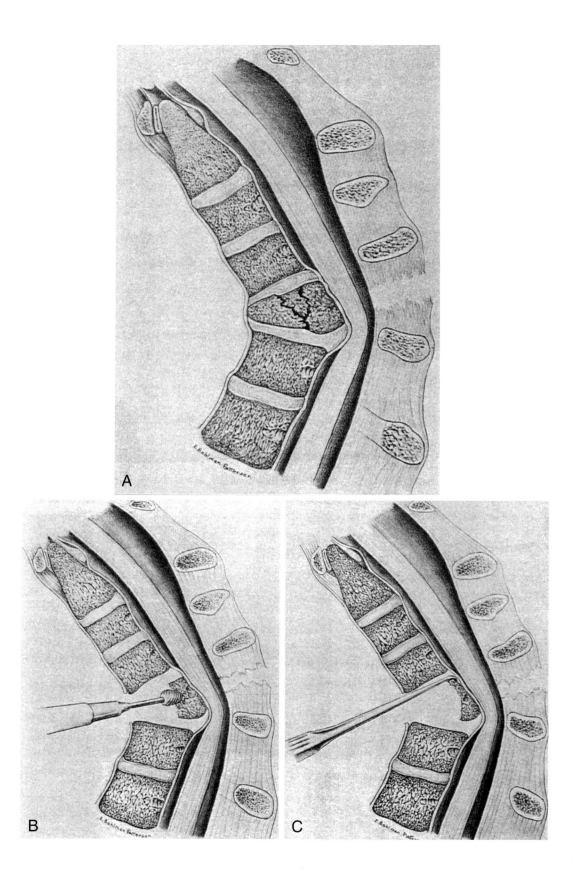

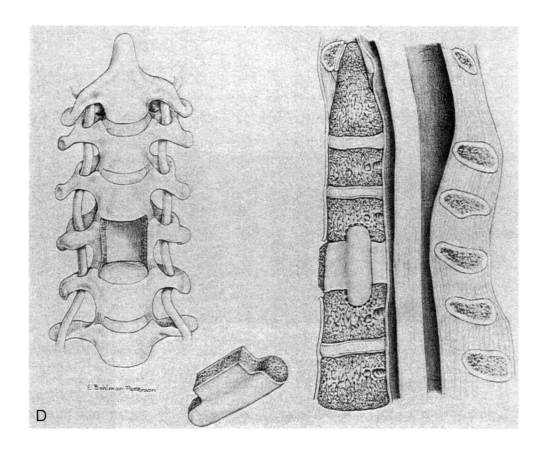

FIGURE 14.9.
A. Lateral view of burst type fracture with retropulsion of bone and disc into spinal canal. Reprinted with permission from Bohlman HH. Acute fracture and dislocation of the cervical spine: an analysis of 300 hospitalized patients and review of the literature. J Bone Joint Surg Am 1979;61:123. **B.** In an anterior decompression, the disc and vertebral body are removed back to the posterior longitudinal ligament. The vertebral body is resected with rongeurs and an air driven burr. Reprinted with permission from Bohlman HH, Eismont FJ. Surgical techniques of anterior decompression and fusion for spinal cord injuries. Clin Orthop Related Res 1981;154:60. **C.** Vertebral body resection continues until only a thin posterior wall remains. This wall can be removed easily with curettes. Reprinted with permission from Bohlman HH, Eismont FJ. Surgical techniques of anterior decompression and fusion for spinal cord injuries. Clin Orthop Related Res 1981;154:60. **D.** Realignment is achieved with traction or use of distraction pins. Mortices are made in the endplate. An appropriate length iliac crest graft is harvested and made into a T-shape creating tenons. The tenons are seated into the mortices. Reprinted with permission from Bohlman HH. Acute fracture and dislocation of the cervical spine: an analysis of 300 hospitalized patients and review of the literature. J Bone Joint Surg Am 1979;61:123.

which can then be removed with curettes (Fig. 14.9C). In patients with associated disc herniation, the posterior longitudinal ligament is removed to assure adequate cord decompression. Decompression is carried out laterally until the dura or posterior longitudinal ligament appears convex—this is usually 12 to 15 mm in width. Care must be taken to maintain orientation to the midline, thus avoiding extending the decompression laterally into the vertebral artery. In patients with kyphosis, traction or the use of a Caspar disc distraction can allow correction by increasing anterior column length.

The endplanes of the remaining cranial and caudal vertebrae are removed. Mortices in endplates are created with a burr or curette and measurements for the length and depth of bone graft are taken (Fig. 14.9D). A tricortical autogenous iliac crest graft is harvested with an ossicating saw and machined into a T-shape creating tenons to fit in the previously prepared mortices. Under traction, the graft is keyed into the mortices caudally and gently tapped downward cranially until the tenons lock into the mortices. In the majority of trauma cases, supplemental fixation as described later are added. The traction is released and the graft is tested for fit. A lateral radiograph is obtained before wound closures. A small Penrose drain is placed and the platysma and skin are closed in layers. Patients with neurologic deficits are monitored in the intensive care unit overnight. Postoperatively, patients are immobilized in a cervico-thoracic brace for 8 to 12 weeks.

Anterior Cervical Plate Fixation

Anterior decompression and fusion decreases overall spinal stabilization by removal of the anterior longitudinal ligament and intervertebral discs (49, 92). In trauma cases, this can be associated with loss of reduction or graft dislodgment, especially in the presence of posterior osseo-ligamentous damage (11, 22, 92). Also, pseudarthrosis rates after discectomy and fusions have been reported to occur from 10 to 50%. To decrease failures and increase the chance of bony union, the anterior cervical plate was developed. Numerous biomechanical studies have shown the inferiority of anterior fixation compared with posterior fixation (34, 73, 93, 97). Abitbol et al. determined that the anterior cervical plate was only 25 to 50% as stiff in resisting flexing (1). Anterior fixation was significantly better in resting extensions than posterior fixation. However, clinical studies of patients treated with anterior cervical plates are in disagreement with these in vitro biomechanical studies (3, 13).

Bohler first used an anterior cervical plate and reported his results in 1967 (19). Orozco developed an AO/ASIF cloverleaf or H-plate that is affixed with 3.5-mm screws (Fig. 14.10) (76). This technique proved to be simple, effective, and low-cost . Ripa et al. reported the outcome of 92 patients with spinal injuries treated by the anterior decompression with the Orozco plate (77). All but one patient healed the fusion. Twelve patients had less than ideal hardware placement, including disc penetration, plate malposition, and adjacent disc and poor graft technique. Four patients had screw loosening, one of which required removal for dysphagia. Caspar et al. improved the instrumentation and popularized his trapezoidal plate (31). The screws in the Orozco and Caspar systems are not fixed to the plate and, therefore, have a tendency to loosen. Under load, the screws are subject to cantilever bending and can toggle and back out. To minimize this complication, most investigators recommend screw engagement of the posterior cortex. However, this step has been associated with iatrogenic neural injury and has decreased the enthusiasm for this technique. Rigidly locked screw-plate systems have been developed to allow unicortical screw purchase without risk of loosening. Morscher et al. used Thorpe screws (developed for maxillo-facial surgery) placed into a cloverleaf titanium plate (74). The screw has a special hollow head that, after insertion in the vertebral body, is expanded against the edge of the plate hole by an expansion set screw. Biomechanically, the unicortical Morscher plate has equal stiffness to the Caspar plate with bicortical screw purchase (95). Anderson et al. examined the efficacy of the cervical spine locking plate in patients with combined anterior and posterior injury (13). Thirty seven patients were treated who had a follow-up of 1.5 years. Thirty four patients had uneventful healing, one patient was found to have an asymptomatic fibrous union, and one patient with plate fracture had a symptomatic non-union. The remaining patient had early failure when the screws pulled out of the caudal vertebral body. This patient was treated successfully by revision and a posterior cervical fusion. This and other studies demonstrate clinically that anterior cervical plating is efficacious in over 90% of patients, despite the adverse in-vitro biomechanical results.

Surgical Technique—Orozco Plate Fixation

Anterior decompression and fusion with autogenous iliac crest graft is performed as described previously. The cranial and caudal vertebral bodies are subperiosteally exposed. Any osteophytes that would interfere with plate placement are resected. Orozco plates are available in several plate lengths with different hole spacings. The best fitting plate is chosen and positioned over the spine. Lateral C-arm fluoroscopy is used to check plate position to avoid positioning over unfused intervertebral discs. The plate holes

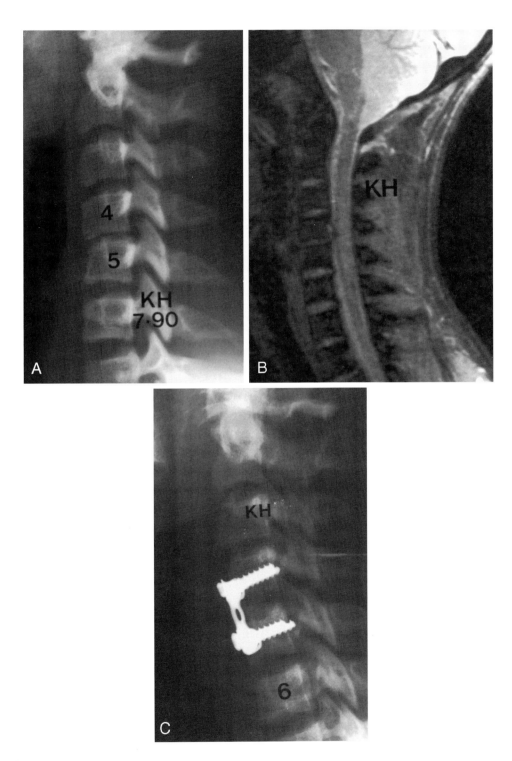

FIGURE 14.10.
A. A fifteen-year-old wrestler was dropped onto his head and sustained a unilateral facet fracture dislocation seen on lateral radiograph. Note the abnormal disc narrowing indicating possible herniation into the spinal canal. Neurologically, the patient was an incomplete quadriplegic. **B.** MRI demonstrates a herniated disc with cord compromise. The patient was treated by an anterior discectomy and application of Orozco plate. **C.** Postoperative lateral radiograph.

318 SECTION III: SPINAL TRAUMA

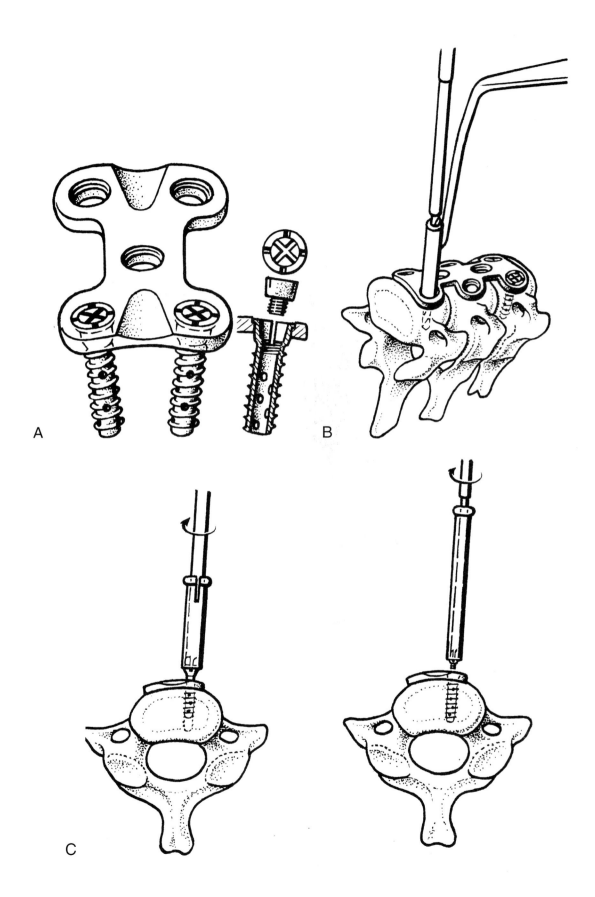

should be positioned so that they are located near the middle of the vertebral body. For longer constructs, the plate is contoured to match cervical lordosis. Proper drilling and screw placement are critical to avoid iatrogenic complications. To diminish the chance of loosening and increase construct rigidity, screws should engage to posterior vertebral cortex. Initial screw length is selected by measuring the midsagittal antero-posterior height of the body before graft placement. A 2.0-mm drill or K wire with an adjustable drill guide is advanced, angling slightly upward and medially. C-arm fluoroscopy is used to check drilling depth. Using the adjustable drill guide allows the drill to be advanced by small increments until the posterior cortex has been reached. Once the posterior cortex has been perforated, the screw length is checked from the adjustable drill guide. The near cortex is tapped and cortical 3.5 mm AO/ASIF screws are inserted again using fluoroscopy. Screws are not placed in the bone graft. After all screws are inserted, they are tightened sequentially. Postoperatively, patients wear a Miami J or cervico-thoracic brace for 8 to 10 weeks.

Surgical Technique—Cervical Spine Locking Plate (Fig. 14.11)

The cervical spine locking plate has plate length available in sizes ranging from 16 to 55 mm. Longer plates are available but must be used with caution because large forces are concentrated at the points of caudal fixation and may be subject to failure. Screw sizes are 4.0 and 4.35 mm in 14-mm lengths. The screw heads are hollow so that a second expansion screw can be inserted into the head, causing it to expand. When inserted in vivo, the screw rigidly locks to the plate.

Anterior decompression, grafting, and preparation are as described before. The selected plate is placed on the spine and checked for position and length radiographically. The plate holes should lie in the mid position of the vertebral bodies and the plate should not overlie an unfused disc. The plate is held firmly and a hoe is drilled with a stopped 3.0 mm drill and drill guide. The drill is angled medially and 12° cranially in the superior vertebra and medially and straight downward in the inferior vertebrae. The drill automatically stops at a depth of 14 mm. The near cortex is tapped and screws are inserted loosely. The process is repeated at the other holes. Once all screws are inserted, they are tightened sequentially. The small set screws are inserted into the head of the vertebral body screws and tightened. A lateral radiograph is taken and the wound is closed. No screws are inserted into the strut graft. Postoperatively, patients are immobilized in a Miami J brace for 8 to 10 weeks.

Posterior Decompression

Posterior decompression via laminectomy is rarely indicated except in cases of depressed lamina fractures or for multilevel spondylosis in patients with extension injuries and central cord syndrome. Biomechanically, laminectomy has little decompressive effect on a ventral lesion, whereas it significantly increases spinal instability (5). In trauma cases, laminectomy should always be combined with arthrodesis with facet wiring or the lateral mass plate technique. In the spondylitic spine, a multilevel laminectomy can allow some posterior displacement of the cervical cord as long as the spinal alignment remains lordotic (48). Unfortunately, C5 or C6 radiculopathies can occur secondary to increased root tension as the cord displaces posteriorly.

Before any surgery, the assessment of patients with traumatic injuries should include the patency of the neuroforamina. Patients with facet injuries may have displaced fractures or disc herniations that create foraminal stenosis. Foraminectomy may be warranted and can be performed at the time of posterior fusion.

Surgical Technique—Laminectomy

The patient is positioned prone and the lamina is exposed as described later for posterior fusion. A laminectomy is performed by bilateral vertical osteotomy at the junction of the lamina and lateral mass using a 3- to 4-mm high speed burr. As the inner cortex and canal is approached the cutting burr is changed to a diamond-tipped burr to avoid dural laceration. Care

FIGURE 14.11.

A. The Morscher AO/ASIF system consists of a plate with specially designed screws and screw holes that allow rigid connection between plate and screw. The screws angle medially to give a triangulation effect that resists plate disengagement. After other screws are inserted, a small locking screw is inserted into the screw head, which expands the head and creates a rigid interlock. Reprinted with permission from Aebi M, Webb JK. The spine. In: Allgower, ed. Manual of internal fixation, 3rd ed. Berlin: Springer Verlag, 1991:627–682. **B.** Drilling using a 3-mm stopped drill allowing 14 mm of depth. Only tapping of the near cortex is required. Reprinted with permission from Aebi M, Webb JK. The spine. In: Allgower, ed. Manual of internal fixation, 3rd ed. Berlin: Springer Verlag, 1991:655. **C.** This drawing shows screw insertion and application of locking screw.

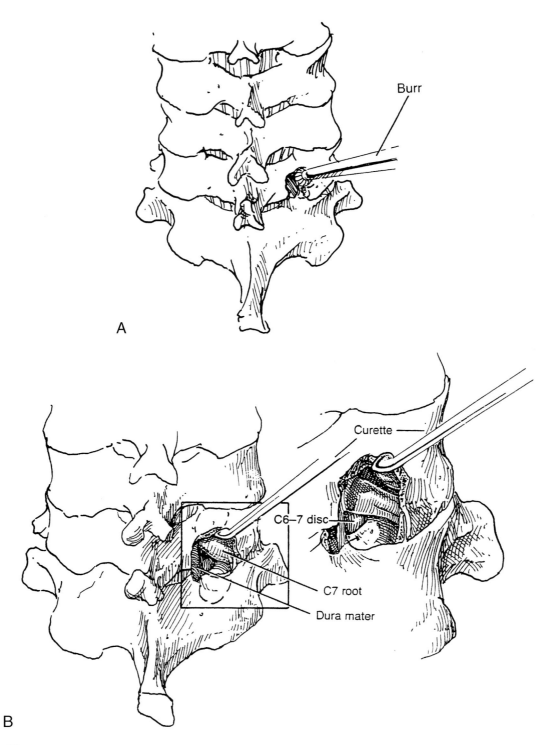

FIGURE 14.12.

A. A foraminotomy is performed with a 3 to 4 mm high speed burr. Drilling starts along the inferior surface of the cranial lamina at the facet joint. Only one-third to one-half of the facet joint can be sacrificed. **B.** The exiting nerve root is located deep and slightly cranial to the facet joint. If necessary, the root can be retracted upward exposing the disc. The foramen is checked for patency with small nerve hooks. Reprinted with permission from Cusick JF, Larson SJ. Foramenotomy. In: The Cervical Spine Research Society, ed. The cervical spine: an atlas of surgical procedures. Philadelphia: JP Lippincott, 1994:217.

is taken not to disrupt joint capsules or resect any portion of the facets. Once the lamina are divided, the interspinous ligaments and ligamentum are divided while pulling upward on the spinous processes until the entire lamina is freed. Care is taken to release any dural adhesions. After laminectomy, a posterior fusion with lateral mass plates is performed.

Surgical Technique—Foraminotomy **(Fig. 14.12)**

Biomechanical studies have shown that up to 50% of the facet joints can be removed without development of instability (104). In traumatic situations, the possibility of instability is greatly increased and therefore an arthrodesis is always performed. From the dorsal approach, the lower cervical spine foramen are located directly below and slightly cranially to the facet joint. A foraminotomy is performed primarily with a burr and curettes. Kerisone rongeurs are avoided because their foot can traumatize the nerve roots. The burr is used to remove bone along the caudal edge of the superior vertebra at the junction of the lateral mass with the lamina going outwards to the midpoint of the facet. Drilling proceeds downward until the edge of the dura and the take off of the nerve root is visualized. This visualization is facilitated by using the diamond burr and curettes. The neuroforamina is decompressed laterally until small nerve hooks or probes can be passed outward. After foraminotomy, a posterior fusion is performed.

Posterior Cervical Fusion

The posterior cervical fusion is the utilitarian surgical procedure in the management of cervical spine injuries. The procedure is highly effective and safe with excellent long-term outcome. In the majority of cases of cervical instability, a simple posterior fusion technique should be used. Newer techniques using rigid fixation can potentially overcome inherent biomechanical weaknesses of standard interspinous wire techniques but are associated with increased complications and cost.

Biomechanical studies have helped to clarify the roles of various posterior cervical fixation techniques (1, 34, 73, 93). The interspinous wire and the Bohlman triple wire technique provide sufficient stability in hyperflexion injuries. To be stable, these techniques require an intact neural arch and facet articulations. Halifax clamps perform poorly in cyclical loading secondary to screw loosening or hook dislodgment and should be avoided. There is little role for sublaminar wire fixation because it provides stability only equal to interspinous wire techniques and it unnecessarily invades the spinal canal. Fixation with plates and screws to the lateral masses or pedicles is gaining popularity. Biomechanically, lateral mass plates are associated with increased resistance to rotational and axial loading forces and overall provide the stiffest cervical constructs (9). In a comprehensive biomechanical study, Abitbol et al. evaluated four posterior biomechanical plates (AO plates, Modular Fixation System, Haid plates, Harms plate), an interspinous wire technique and two anterior plates (Cervical Spine Locking plate and Caspar plate) (1). In torsion and axial loading, the lateral mass plates were significantly stiffer compared with the wire or anterior plate. In flexion, the AO plate, Mod-Fix, and interspinous wire were equal and had a significantly greater flexural stiffness. In extension, the anterior plate constructs were significantly stiffer.

The choice of which technique depends on the pathoanatomy, surgeon's expertise, and biomechanic requirements. In the majority of cases, simple techniques using interspinous wires and autogenous bone grafts will suffice. Indications for posterior cervical fusion include unstable fractures that do not require anterior decompression and have significant posterior column injury. These fractures include most hyperflexion injuries and some axial loading injuries. Posterior fusion can be used as an adjunct to anterior decompression or for the treatment of anterior pseudarthrosis. The following surgical techniques will be reviewed: Bohlman triple wire, facet wire, and lateral mass fixation with AO reconstruction plates.

Interspinous Wire Technique

Rogers initially described a technique by passing wires through drill holes in the base of the spinous process (82). Autogenous bone grafts were wedged under the wires. He reported excellent long-term outcome in 37 patients. Two patients developed nonunion and one patient had a loss of reduction. To increase construct rigidity, Bohlman et al. added a second and third wire passed through holes in the spinous processes, which affixed cortico-cancellous plates of bone graft (23). Biomechanically, the Bohlman triple wire technique greatly increases flexural and rotational rigidity (34).

Surgical Technique—Bohlman Triple Wire **(Fig. 14.13)**

After prone positioning, the spine is exposed via a midline incision. A cuff of interspinous ligament and ligamentum nuchae is protected during dissection to decrease the risk of iatrogenic extension of the fusion or instability. Drill holes are placed with a 3-mm air driver burr at the base of the spinous processes. The hole is enlarged with a towel clip or Leween clamp. A 20-gauge wire is passed through the holes and looped around the spinous process and passed back through the hole. The free ends are tightened and the

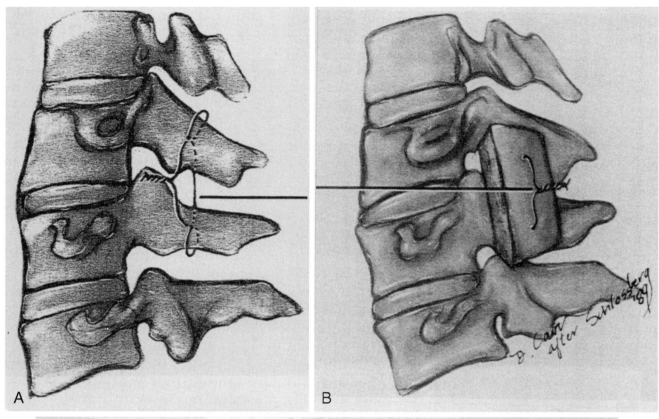
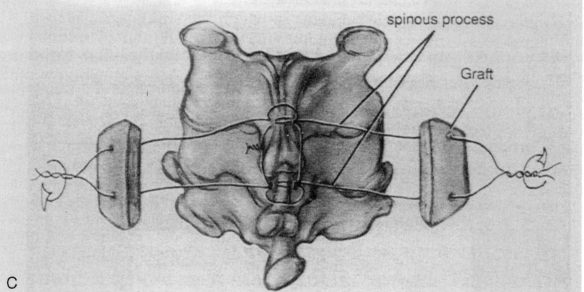

FIGURE 14.13.
A. Bohlman triple wire technique. Three millimeter drill holes are placed in the base of the spinous processes with an air driven burr. A 20-gauge wire is double looped around both spinous processes and tightened. **B.** Second and third 22-gauge wires are passed through corticocancellous bone grafts and through the holes previously placed in the spinous process. **C.** The wires are twisted, compressing the bone grafts against the spinous processes. Reprinted with permission from Delamarter R. Wire fixation of the lower cervical spine. Tech in Ortho 1994;9:68–74.

alignment is checked radiographically. Plates of cortico-cancellous bone grafts are harvested and drill holes are placed to accept wires. Twenty-two gauge wires are passed through the bone grafts and the hole in the spinous process and are tightened, affixing the grafts to the spinous processes. Postoperatively, patients are immobilized in a cervico-thoracic brace for 6 to 8 weeks.

Facet Wire Technique

When lamina and spinous processes are deficient or missing, the interspinous wire techniques cannot be used. In such cases, the Robinson Southwick facet wire technique may be used to achieve posterior fixation (80). Wires passed through the facets and out the facet joint are tightened over bone graft struts. In cases of facet fracture and subluxation, greater rotational stability may be required than provided by the interspinous wire technique. Edwards, Matz, and Levine described the oblique wire, which is passed through the cranial facet and around the caudal spinous process (46). They reported successful fixation in 26 of 27 patients with unilateral facet dislocations. These techniques can be applied at multiple segments.

Surgical Technique—Facet Wire (Fig. 14.14)

The dissection is carried out to the far edge of the facets to be arthrodesed. All joint capsules are removed. Drill holes are made with a 3- to 4-mm burr, which starts at the center of the lateral mass and is directed slightly downward, exiting into the facet joint. The articular cartilage is denuded to facilitate wire passage. Twenty or 22-gauge wire is passed downward through the drill hole and the end is brought out through the joint. This step is facilitated by gently opening the joint using an osteotome as a lever. The use of double or triple-stranded wire or cable eases bending of the wire around corners, which is necessary for this technique. After all wires have been passed, the wires are looped and tightened around the ribs or iliac crest corticocancellous plates of bone graft. Postoperatively, patients are managed in the halo-vest or cervico-thoracic brace for 10 to 12 weeks depending on stability.

In the oblique wire technique, to stabilize a unilateral facet dislocation, a facet wire is placed as described previously in the cranial lateral mass. The wire is then looped around the caudal spinous process and tightened. An interspinous wire is added for additional stability.

Lateral Plate Mass Fixation

Roy-Camille developed the technique of lateral mass fixation using plates with 13 mm hole spacing (84).

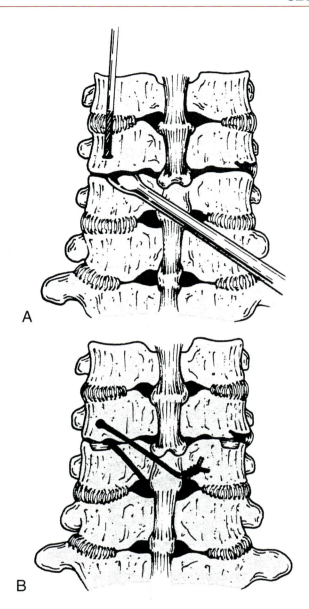

FIGURE 14.14.
A. Oblique wire technique. A drill or burr is used to make a hole passing from the lateral mass into the facet joint. To aid in drilling, the joint is gently distracted and a freer is placed into the joint to act as a back stop. **B.** A 20–22 gauge wire is passed around the caudal spinal process and tightened. Reprinted with permission from Bucholz RW. Lower cervical spine injuries in skeletal trauma. In: Browner BD, Levine AM, Jupiter JB, Trafton PG, eds. Fracture dislocation and ligamentous injuries. Philadelphia: WB Saunders, 1992:699–728.

The plates are affixed to the lateral masses with 14 or 16-mm screws. The lateral mass plates are easy to apply, can be used over multiple segments, and have had excellent results. Magerl modified the technique using the AO/ASIF hook plate (57). Fixation is obtained from a hook that is placed around the inferior edge of the caudal lamina and through a hole in the plate in which a screw is placed into the cranial lateral mass. To give three point fixation, an H-graft is placed between the spinous processes. Anderson modified these techniques using AO/ASIF reconstruction plates and reported successful outcomes in 30 of 30 patients (9). Although interspinous wire techniques can be used for the majority of patients, plate fixation has several advantages. Because it is stiffer, patients require less postoperative bracing and fracture reduction is maintained, especially in patients with rotational or axial instability. Plates can be applied extensilely, including across the craniocervical and cervicothoracic junction. Plates are now available in titanium, which allows postoperative MRI imaging. In patients with laminar or spinous process fractures, plate fixation can shorten the overall length of fixation or can be applied more easily than facet wire fixation. Specific indications for lateral mass fixation include deficiency or absence of lamina and spinous processes, rotational or axial instabilities, multilevel instabilities, pathologic fracture, extension to craniocervical junction or cervicothoracic junction, and requirement for decreased bracing.

Lateral mass screw placement is critical to the safety and efficacy of this technique. Two basic techniques have been described and evaluated (Fig. 14.15). Roy-Camille et al. start the screw at the summit or center of the lateral mass and direct the screw straight forward and 10° outward (84). Magerl screws start 1 to 2 mm medially and cranially to the center of the lateral mass (57). The screws are oriented 25 to 35° cranially and 25° outward. Heller et al. performed an anatomic study to determine the safety of the Roy-Camille and Magerl techniques (60).They found that experienced surgeons had a 3.6% chance of root injury with the Magerl technique compared with 0% with the Roy-Camille technique. However,

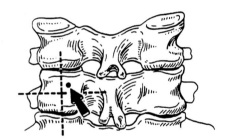

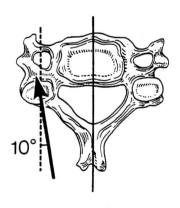 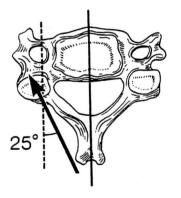

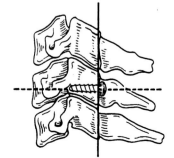 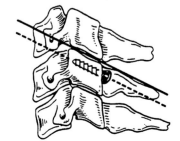

FIGURE 14.15.
Roy-Camille and Magerl techniques for lateral mass screw placement. Reprinted with permission from Heller JG, Carlson GD, Abitbol JJ, et al. Anatomic comparison of the Roy-Camille and Magerl techniques for screw placement in the lower cervical spine. Spine 1991;16:S552-S557.

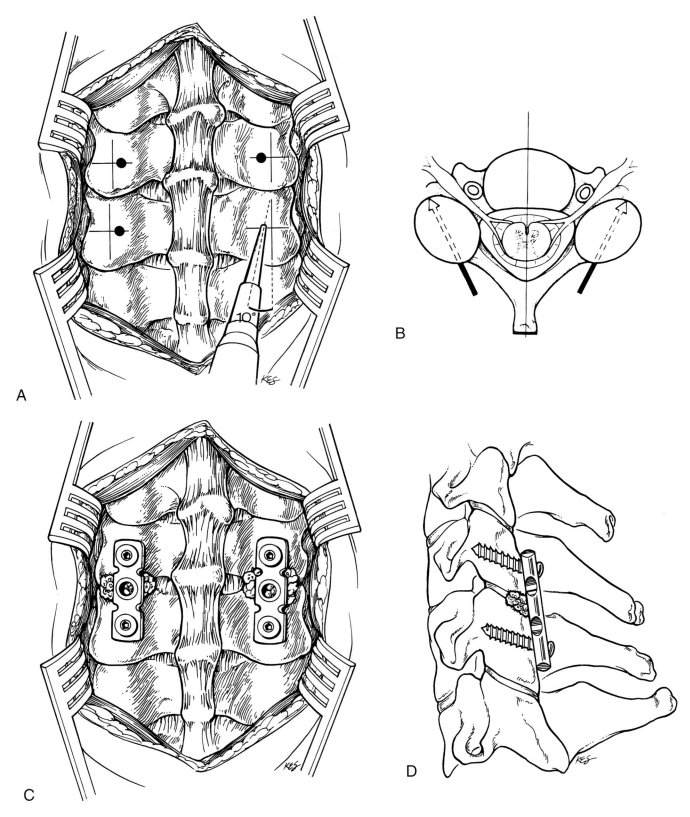

FIGURE 14.16.

A. Dorsal view of the cervical spine. The starting point for lateral mass screw placement is 1 to 2 mm medial to the center of the lateral mass. The screw is directed cranially 20 to 30° and outward 10 to 20°. **B.** Axial view of the cervical spine. Note the important landmark of the valley at the junction of the lamina and lateral mass. The vertebral artery and most dorsal extent of the nerve root are located directly anterior to this point. Screws must start lateral and angle outward to avoid neurovascular injury. Reprinted with permission from Aebi M, Webb JK. The spine. In: Allgower M, ed. Manual of internal fixation, 3rd ed. Berlin: Springer Verlag, 1991:627–682. **C.** Lateral view after plate fixation with AO reconstruction plates. **D.** Dorsal view after lateral mass fixation. A, C, and D reprinted with permission from Anderson PA, Henley MB, Grady MS, et al. Posterior cervical arthrodesis using AO reconstruction plates. Spine: Symposium on Internal Fixation 1991; 16:S72-S79.

the Roy-Camille technique was associated with a 13% incidence of facet joint violation. Based on an anatomic study, An et al. recommended a starting point similar to Magerl and a direction of 15° cephalad and 30° lateral (8). To accommodate this angulation, An recognized that new plates will need to be designed. Montesano et al. biomechanically compared the Roy-Camille and Magerl techniques and found that Magerl screws had significantly better pullout strength (73). Additionally, they noted that longer screws could be placed safely using the Roy-Camille technique. Gill et al. found that bicortical screw purchase greatly increased pullout strength (54). Anderson et al. reported the use of lateral mass fixation with AO reconstruction plates (9). These plates have the advantage of being sized properly and are available in different lengths to accommodate many applications. They are now available in titanium. Plates with hole spacings of 8 and 12 mm are available to accommodate individual variations in distances between lateral masses. We have reviewed 102 consecutive cases and found that all patients went on to fusion with minimal loss of position after surgery. Two patients had a transient isolated C7 radiculopathy caused by screw placement. It may have been secondary to anatomic variations that occur at C7. As described by An et al., the C7 lateral mass is transitional and may be absent or truncated, making identification of starting points difficult (8). Recently placement of C7 pedicle screws has been advocated (68).

Surgical Technique—Cervical Lateral Mass Fixation with AO Reconstruction Plates *(Fig. 14.16)*

The patient is positioned and exposure of the dorsal elements is performed as described previously. For proper screw placement, the borders of the lateral mass are exactly determined. This determination requires exposure out to the far lateral edge. The medial border is the junction of the lamina and lateral mass. A valley is usually present to aid in identification of this important landmark. Directly forward of this valley is the most dorsal extent of the exiting nerve root and the vertebral artery. Thus, all lateral mass screws must be placed lateral to this valley and angled outward. The lateral border is the far edge of the facet. The superior and inferior borders are the cranial and caudal facet joint, respectively. Once the square or rectangularly shaped lateral mass has been identified, the starting point for screw insertion is selected. This point is 1 to 2 mm medial to the center of the lateral mass.

A 2-mm K-wire or drill is placed in an adjustable drill guide set to allow only 15 mm of advancement. The drill is advanced from the starting point, angling upward 20 to 30° (parallel to the facet joints) and outward 15°. After drilling is complete, the hole is checked for perforation of the far cortex with a smaller blunt K-wire. If the far cortex is not perforated, then the drill guide is adjusted to allow 1 to 2 mm more of advancement, and the process is repeated. Drilling continues until a depth of 20 mm or perforation has occurred. The length of drill to achieve perforation is noted to aid in screw length selection. The hole is tapped with a 3.5 mm cancellous tap.

The drilling process proceeds free-hand rather than through the plate. This allows accurate screw placement needed to avoid neurovascular injuries. In multilevel constructs, only the most cranial and caudal levels are drilled initially. Malleable templates are used to determine plate choice, length, and contour. If necessary, plates can be contoured with bending pliers. In longer constructs, the plate is affixed cranially and caudal and then the intervening lateral masses are drilled through the plate holes. The screws are initially inserted with light torque and at the end of the procedure are tightened sequentially. The dorsal third of the facet joints are decorticated and packed with autogenous bone graft. If desired, an interspinous wire can be added to increase stability. The lamina and spinous processes medial to the plates are decorticated with a burr and covered with cancellous bone graft. The paraspinal muscles and nuchal ligaments are closed in two layers. Postoperatively, patients wear a Miami J or Minerva brace for 8 weeks (Fig. 14.17).

Conclusion

Cervical spine injuries require prompt recognition and early treatment to maximize recovery. The use of newer imaging techniques has greatly aided our understanding of these injuries, but has not led to a comprehensive classification system. Treatment is determined primarily from fracture morphology (stability) and neurologic status. The goal of treatment as outlined by Rogers: 1) Protect the neural tissue; 2) Reduce fractures and dislocations; and 3) Stabilize the spine to provide a stable, painless spine long term (82). Pharmacologic treatment in cases of spinal cord injuries appears to improve chances of neurologic injury. The standard surgical techniques—anterior decompression and fusion, and interspinous wire fixation—have excellent reported results and low complication rates. However, patients require immobilization, and these techniques are less effective in more unstable cases. Newer surgical techniques involving plate fixation either anteriorly or posteriorly have reported excellent outcomes with low complication rates.

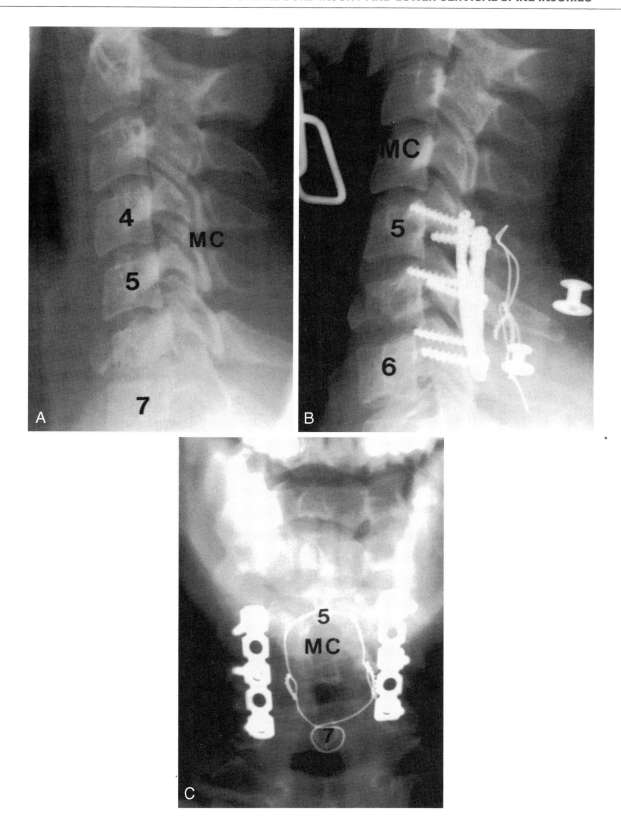

FIGURE 14.17.

A. Lateral radiograph of an eighteen-year-old female in vehicular trauma sustaining unstable tear drop type fracture. After reduction, she returned to normal neurologic function. **B.** She was treated by posterior arthrodesis with AO reconstruction plates. Lateral radiograph demonstrates excellent screw placement and fracture reduction. **C.** Postoperative anteroposterior radiograph.

References

1. Abitbol JJ, Zdeblick T, Kunz D, et al. A biomechanical analysis of modern anterior and posterior cervical stabilization techniques. Twentieth Annual Meeting of the Cervical Spine Research Society, December 2–4, 1992, Palm Springs, CA.
2. Adams F. The genuine works of Hippocrates. Baltimore: Williams & Wilkins, 1939:231–243.
3. Aebi M, Mohler J, Zäch GA, et al. Indication, surgical technique, and results of 100 surgically-treated fractures and fracture-dislocations of the cervical spine. Clin Orthop 1986;203:244–257.
4. Aebi M, Webb JK. The spine. In: Allgower M, ed. Manual of internal fixation, 3rd ed. Berlin: Springer Verlag, 1991:627–682.
5. Allen BL Jr, Tencer AF, Ferguson RL. The biomechanics of decompressive laminectomy. Spine 1987;12:803–808.
6. Allen BL, Ferguson RL, Lehmann R, et al. Mechanistic classification of closed indirect fractures and dislocations of the lower cervical spine. Spine 1982;7:1–27.
7. American Spinal Injury Association, ed. Standards for neurologic and functional classification of spinal cord injury, revised. Chicago: American Spinal Injury Association, 1992.
8. An HS, Gordin R, Renner K. Anatomic considerations for plate-screw fixation of the cervical spine. Spine 1991;16:S548–S551.
9. Anderson PA, Henley MB, Grady MS, et al. Posterior cervical arthrodesis using AO reconstruction plates. Spine. Symposium on Internal Fixation 1991;16:S72–S79.
10. Anderson DK, Braughler JM, Hall ED, et al. Effects of treatment with U-74006F on neurological outcome following experimental spinal cord injury. J Neurosurg 1988;69:562–567.
11. Anderson PA, Bohlman HH. Anterior decompression and arthrodesis in patients with traumatic, complete motor cervical spine cord injury. Long term neurologic recovery in 52 patients: part II. J Bone Joint Surg Am 1992;74:683–691.
12. Anderson TE. Spinal cord contusion injury: experimental dissociation of hemorrhagic necrosis and subacute loss of axonal conduction. J Neurosurg 1985;62:115–119.
13. Anderson PA, Newell D, Armengaro M, et al. Stabilization of combined anterior and posterior instability with the cervical locking plate. Orthop Trans 1995;19–1:195–196.
14. Anderson PA, Budorick TE, Easton KB, et al. Failure of halo-vest to prevent in-vivo motion in patients with injured cervical spines. Spine 1991;16:S501–S505.
15. Assenmacher DR, Ducker TB. Experimental traumatic paraplegia. J Bone Joint Surg Am 1971;53:671–680.
16. Bailey RW, Badgley CE. Stabilization of the cervical spine anterior fusion. J Bone Joint Surg Am 1960;42:565–594.
17. Bedbrook G. Spinal injuries with tetraplegia and paraplegia. J Bone Joint Surg Br 1979;61:267–284.
18. Beyer CA, Cabanela ME, Benquist TH. Unilateral facet dislocations and fracture dislocation of the cervical spine. J Bone Joint Surg Br 1991;73:977–981.
19. Bohler J, Gaudernak T. Anterior plate stabilization of fracture-dislocations of the lower cervical spine. J Trauma 1980;20:203–205.
20. Böhler L. The treatment of fractures. 4th ed. (English). Baltimore: W Wood & Co., 1935.
21. Bohlman HH, Bahniuk E, Raskulinecz C, et al. Mechanical factors affecting recovery from incomplete cervical spinal cord injury: a preliminary report. Johns Hopkins Med J 1979;145:115–125.
22. Bohlman HH, Anderson PA. Anterior decompression and arthrodesis in patients with incomplete motor cervical spinal cord injury: long term results of neurologic recovery in 58 patients: part I. J Bone Joint Surg Am 1992;74:671–682.
23. Bohlman HH, Ducker JB, Lucas JT. Spine and spinal cord injuries. In: Rothman RH, Simeone FA, eds. The Spine, 2nd ed. Philadelphia: WB Saunders:682.
24. Bohlman HH. Acute fracture and dislocation of the cervical spine: an analysis of 300 hospitalized patients and review of the literature. J Bone Joint Surg Am 1979;61:123.
25. Bohlman HH. The triple-wire technique for posterior stabilization of fractures and dislocations of the lower cervical spine. The cervical spine: an atlas of surgical procedures 1994;9:145–150.
26. Bracken MB, Shepard MJ, Collins WF, et al. A randomized controlled trial of methylprednisolone or Naloxone in the treatment of acute spinal cord injury: results of the Second National Acute Spinal Cord Injury Study. New Eng J Med 1990;322:1405–1411.
27. Bracken MB, Collins WF, Freeman DF, et al. Efficacy of methylprednisolone in acute spinal cord injury. JAMA 1984;251:45–51.
28. Breig A. The therapeutic possibilities of surgical bioengineering in incomplete spinal cord lesions. Paraplegia 1972;9:173–182.
29. Bucholz RW. Lower cervical spine injuries in skeletal trauma. In: Browner BD, Levine AM, Jupiter JB, Trafton PG, eds. Fracture dislocation and ligamentous injuries. Philadelphia: WB Saunders, 1992:699–728.
30. Bucholz RD, Cheung KC. Halo vest versus spinal fusion for cervical injury: evidence from an outcome study. J Neurosurg 1989;70:884–892.
31. Caspar W, Barbier DD, Klara PM. Anterior cervical fusion and Caspar plate stabilization for cervical trauma. Neurosurg 1989;25:491–502.
32. Chang DG, Tencer AF, Ching RP, et al. Geometric changes in the cervical spinal canal during impact. Spine 1994;18:973–980.
33. Cloward RB. Treatment of acute fractures and fracture dislocations of the cervical spine by vertebral body fusion: a report of eleven cases. J Neurosurg 1961;18:201–209.
34. Coe JD, Warden KE, Sutterlin CE, et al. Biomechanical evaluation of cervical spine stabilization methods in a human cadaveric model. Spine 1989;14:1122–1131.
35. Cotler HB, Herbison GJ, Nasuti JF, et al. Closed reduction of traumatic cervical spine dislocation using traction weights up to 140 pounds. Spine 1993;18:386–390.

36. Cotler HB, Kulkarni MV, Bondurant FJ. Magnetic resonance imaging of acute spinal cord trauma: preliminary report. J Orthop Trauma 1988;2(1):1–4.
37. Cusick JF, Larson SJ. Foramenotomy. In: The Cervical Spine Research Society, ed. The cervical spine: an atlas of surgical procedures. Philadelphia: JB Lippincott, 1994:217.
38. Davis AG. Fractures of the spine. J Bone Joint Surg 1929;11:133–156.
39. Delamarter RB, Sherman J, Carr JB. Spinal cord injury: the pathophysiology of spinal cord damage and subsequent recovery following immediate or delayed decompression. Twenty-first Annual Meeting Cervical Spine Research Society, New York, NY, Dec 1–4, 1993.
40. Delamarter R. Wire fixation of the lower cervical spine. Tech in Ortho 1994;9:68–74.
41. Denis F. Spinal instability as defined by the three-column spine concept in acute spinal trauma. Clin Orthop 1984;189:65–76.
42. Dolan EJ, Tator CH, Endrenyi L. The value of decompression for acute experimental spinal cord compression injury. J Neurosurg 1980;53:749–755.
43. Doran SE, Papadopoulos SM, Ducker TB, et al. Magnetic resonance imaging documentation of coexistent traumatic locked facets of the cervical spine and disk herniation. J Neurosurg 1993;79:341–345.
44. Ducker T, Kindt G, Kempe L. Pathological findings in acute experimental spinal cord trauma. J Neurosurg 1971;35:700–708.
45. Ducker TB, Saleman M, Daniell HB. Experimental spinal cord trauma, III; therapeutic effect of immobilization and pharmacologic agents. Surg Neurol 1978;10:71–76.
46. Edwards CC, Matz SO, Levine AM. The oblique wiring technique for rotational injuries of the cervical spine. Orthop Trans 1986;10:455.
47. Eismont FJ, Arena MJ, Green BA. Extrusion of an intervertebral disc associated with traumatic subluxation or dislocation of cervical facets. J Bone Joint Surg Am 1991;73:1555–1560.
48. Epstein JA, Epstein ME. The surgical management of cervical spine stenosis, spondylosis and myeloradiculopathy by means of the posterior approach. In: The Cervical Spine Research Society, ed. The cervical spine, 2nd ed. Philadelphia: JB Lippincott, 1989:625–643.
49. Flynn TB. Neurologic complications of anterior cervical interbody fusion. Spine 1982;7:536–539.
50. Frankel H, Hancock DO, Hyslop G, et al. The value of postural reduction in the initial management of closed injuries of the spine with paraplegia and tetraplegia. Part I. Paraplegia 1969;7:179–192.
51. Garfin SR, Botte MJ, Waters RL, et al. Complications in the use of the halo fixation device. J Bone Joint Surg Am 1986;68:320–325.
52. Geisler FH, Dorsey FC, Coleman WP. Recovery of motor function after spinal-cord injury: a randomized, placebo-controlled trial with GM-1 ganglioside. New Eng J Med 1991;324:1829–1838.
53. Gertzbein SD, ed. Classification of thoracic and lumbar fractures. In: Fractures of the thoracic and lumbar spine. Baltimore: Williams & Wilkins, 1992:25–57.
54. Gill K, Paschal S, Corin J, et al. Posterior plating of the cervical spine. A biochemical comparison of different posterior fusion techniques. Spine 1988;13:813–816.
55. Glaser JA, Whitehill R, Stamp WG, et al. Complications associated with the halo vest. J Neurosurg 1986;65:762–769.
56. Grady MS, Anderson PA. Cervical spine injuries: management. Contemp Neurosurg 1991;13:1–6.
57. Grob D, Magerl F. Dorsal spondylodesis of the cervical spine using a hooked plate. Orthopade 1987;16:55–61.
58. Guttman LI. Organization of spinal units: history of the national spinal injuries centre, Stoke Mandeville Hospital, Aylesbury. Paraplegia 1967;5:115–126.
59. Hall ED. Effects of the 21-aminosteroid U74006F on posttraumatic spinal cord ischemia in cats. J Neurosurg 1988;68:462–465.
60. Heller JG, Carlson GD, Abitol JJ, et al. Anatomic comparison of the Roy-Camille and Magerl techniques for screw placement in the lower cervical spine. Spine 1991;16:S552–S557.
61. Holdsworth F. Fractures, dislocations, and fracture-dislocations of the spine. J Bone Joint Surg Am 1970;52:1534–1551.
62. Ikata T, Iwasa K, Morimoto K, et al. Clinical considerations and biochemical basis of prognosis of cervical spinal cord injury. Spine 1989;14:1096–1101.
63. Jacobs RR, Asher MA, Snider RK. Thoracolumbar spinal injuries. A comparative study of recumbent and operative treatment in 100 patients. Spine 1980;5:463–477.
64. Janssen L, Hansebout RR. Pathogenesis of spinal cord injury and newer treatments. A review. Spine 1989;14:23–32.
65. Johnson RM, Hart DL, Simmons EF, et al. Cervical orthoses: a study comparing their effectiveness in restricting cervical motion in normal subjects. J Bone Joint Surg Am 1977;59:332–339.
66. Jönsson H Jr, Bring G, Rauschning W, et al. Hidden cervical spine injuries in traffic accident victims with skull fractures. J Spinal Disord 1991;4:251–263.
67. Keenen TL, Anthony J, Benson DR. Noncontiguous spinal fractures. J Trauma 1990;30:489–501.
68. Kotani Y, Cunningham BW, Abumi K, et al. Biomechanical analysis of cervical stabilization systems: an assessment of transpedicular screw fixation in the cervical spine. Spine 1994;19:2529–2539.
69. Krengel WF, Anderson PA, Henley MB. Early stabilization and decompression for incomplete paraplegia due to a thoracic-level spinal cord injury. Spine 1993;18:2080–2087.
70. Levine AM. Facet injuries in the cervical spine. In: Camins MB, O'Leary PF, eds. Disorders of the cervical spine. Baltimore: Williams & Wilkins, 1992:298–302.
71. Marshall LF, Knowlton S, Garfin SR. Deterioration following spinal cord injury: a multicenter study. J Neurosurg 1987;66:400–404.
72. McAfee PC, Yuan HA, Fredrickson BE, et al. Value of computed tomography in thoracolumbar fractures: an analysis of one-hundred consecutive cases and a new classification. J Bone Joint Surg Am 1983;65:461–473.

73. Montesano PX, Juach EC, Anderson PA, et al. Biomechanics of the cervical spine internal fixation. Spine: Symposium on Internal Fixation 1991;16:S10–S16.
74. Morscher E, Sutter F, Jennis M, et al. Die Vordere Verplattung der Halswirbelsaule mit dem Hohlschrauben-plattensystem. Chirurg 1986;57:702–707.
75. Nicoll EA. Fractures of the dorso-lumbar spine. J Bone Joint Surg Br 1949;31:376–394.
76. Orozco D, Llovet-Tapies J. Osteosintesis en las fractures de raquis cervical. Rev Ortop Traumatol 1970; 14:285–288.
77. Ripa DR, Kowall MG, Meyer PR, et al. Series of ninety-two traumatic cervical spine injuries stabilized with anterior ASIF plate fusion techniques. Spine 1991; 16S:46–53.
78. Rivlin AS, Tator CH. Effect of duration of acute spinal cord compression in a new acute cord injury model in the rat. Surg Neurol 1978;10:39–43.
79. Roaf R. A study of the mechanics of spinal injury. J Bone Joint Surg Br 1960;42:810–823.
80. Robinson RA, Southwick WO. Indications and techniques for early stabilization of the neck in some fracture dislocations for the cervical spine. South Med J 1960;53:565.
81. Rodden FA, Wiegandt H, Bauer BL. Gangliosides: the relevance of current research to neurosurgery. J Neurosurg 1991;74:606–619.
82. Rogers WA. Fracture and dislocations of the cervical spine. An end result study. J Bone Joint Surg Am 1957; 39:341–376.
83. Rorabeck CH, Rock MG, Hambin RJ, et al. Unilateral facet dislocation of the cervical spine: an analysis of the results of treatment in 26 patients. Spine 1987; 12:23–27.
84. Roy-Camille R, Saillant G, Mazel C. Internal fixation of the unstable cervical spine by a posterior osteosynthesis with plates and screws. The cervical spine. Philadelphia: JB Lippincott, 1989:390–403.
85. Schaefer DM, Flanders A, Northrup BE, et al. Magnetic resonance imaging of acute cervical spine trauma: correlation with severity of neurologic injury. Spine 1989;14:1090–1095.
86. Schlegel J, Yuan H, Frederickson B, et al. Timing of operative intervention in the management of acute spinal injuries. Proceedings of the 6th Annual Meeting, Orthopaedic Trauma Association, Toronto, Canada, 1990:38.
87. Schneider RC, Crosby EC, Russo RH, et al. Traumatic spinal cord syndromes and their management. Clin Neurosurg 1973;20:24–492.
88. Schneider RC, Knighton R. Chronic neurological sequelae of acute trauma to the spine and spinal cord; the syndrome of chronic injury to the cervical spinal cord in the region of the central canal. J Bone Joint Surg Am 1959;41:905–919.
89. Slucky AV, Eismont FJ. Treatment of acute injury of the cervical spine. Instructional Course Lectures 1995; 44:67–80.
90. Smith GW, Robinson RA. The treatment of certain cervical spine disorders by anterior removal of the intervertebral disc and interbody fusion. J Bone Joint Surg Am 1958;40:607–623.
91. Star AM, Jones A, Cotler JM, et al. Immediate closed reduction of cervical spine dislocations using traction. Spine 1990;15:1068–1072.
92. Stauffer ES, Kelly EF. Fracture-dislocation of the cervical spine: instability and recurrent deformity following treatment by anterior interbody fusion. J Bone Joint Surg Am 1977;59:45–48.
93. Sutterlin CE III, McAfee PC, Warden KE, et al. A biomechanical evaluation of cervical spinal stabilization methods in a bovine model. Spine 1988;13:795–802.
94. Torg JS, Pavlov H, Genuario SE, et al. Neuropraxia of the cervical spinal cord with transient quadriplegia. J Bone Joint Surg 1986;68:1354–1370.
95. Traynelis VC, Donaher PA, Roach RM, et al. Biomechanical comparison of anterior Caspar plate and three-level posterior fixation techniques in a human cadaveric model. J Neurosurg 1993;79:96–103.
96. Tribus CB. Cervical disk herniation in association with traumatic facet dislocation. Techniques in Orthopaedics 1994;9:5–7.
97. Ulrich C, Wörsdörfer O, Claes L, et al. Comparative study of the stability of anterior and posterior cervical spine fixation procedures. Arch Orthop Trauma Surg 1987;106:226–231.
98. Verbiest H. Anterior operative approach in cases of spinal cord compression by old irreducible displacement or fresh fractures of the cervical spine. J Neurosurg 1962;19:389–400.
99. White AA III, Panjabi MM. The problem of clinical instability in the human spine: A systematic approach. In: White AA, Panjabi MM, eds. Clinical biomechanics of the spine, 2nd ed. Philadelphia: JB Lippincott, 1990:277–378.
100. Whitehill R, Richman JA, Glaser JA. Failure of immobilization of the cervical spine by halo-vest. J Bone Joint Surg 1986;68:326–332.
101. Willis BK, Greiner F, Orrison WW, et al. The incidence of vertebral injury after midcervical spine fracture or subluxation. Neurosurg 1994;34(3):435–441.
102. Yashon D. Pathogenesis of spinal cord injury. Orthop Clin 1978;9:247–261.
103. Young W. Secondary injury mechanisms in acute spinal cord injury. J Emerg Med 1993;11:13–22.
104. Zdeblick TA, Zou D, Warden KE, et al. Cervical stability after foraminotomy: a biomechanical in vitro analysis. J Bone Joint Surg 1992;74:22–27.

CHAPTER FIFTEEN

Upper Cervical Spine Injuries in the Adult

Alexander R. Vaccaro and Jerome M. Cotler

Introduction

Traumatic disorders of the cervicocranium represent a unique subset of cervical spine injuries that differ from those of the subaxial cervical spine through their pathoanatomy, clinical presentation, and treatment. Clinicians treating patients with injuries to the upper cervical spine need to be well versed in the static and dynamic anatomy of this region to diagnose subtle instability patterns which require specialized treatment. Although the majority of lethal traumatic injuries to the spine involve the upper cranial region, patients that survive transport to a regional trauma center tend to have minimal, if any, neurologic deficit as a result of the capacious spinal canal volume in this region and the relatively small ratio of cord size to canal area. Because of the paucity of neurologic dysfunction seen after trauma to this area, injuries to the upper cervical region are frequently overlooked, especially in the multiple injured patient or patients with altered mental status unable to localize discomfort to the upper cervical region. Therefore, the evaluating team should be diligent in ruling out pathology in this region, especially in patients with obvious soft tissue or bony injuries above the level of the clavicle. In addition, injuries to the upper cervical spine are associated frequently with contiguous and noncontiguous spinal fractures that complicate management. This chapter discusses the anatomy, pathogenesis, diagnosis, classification, and nonoperative and operative treatment of traumatic injuries to the adult upper cervical spine.

Occipital Condyle

Occipital condyle fractures are rare and are missed frequently unless the treating physician has a high index of suspicion for its presence. This fracture may occur alone or in combination with injuries of the atlanto-occipital complex, odontoid, or subaxial spine (68, 75, 107).

Mechanism of Injury

This injury has been reported in patients between 18 and 82 years of age and is usually the result of a high-speed deceleration accident associated with axial compression, with or without rotation, and an anterior, posterior, or lateral shear force (17, 52).

Clinical Diagnosis

The severity of neurologic deficit after injury to the occipital condyles may range from none to complete tetraparesis with respiratory compromise. Patients without neurologic deficit tend to report significant upper neck discomfort with limitation or range of motion. Injuries to cranial nerve VI (abducens), XI (glossopharyngeal), and XII (hypoglossal) may be caused by direct nerve injury or involvement of the anterior brain stem (16, 30) have been reported. Patients may also present with symptoms of vertebrobasilar artery insufficiency.

Radiographic Evaluation

Visualization of the basiocciput is extremely difficult with plain roentgenographs because of the overlying facial anatomy. If clinical suspicion is high for injury to this region, i.e., unexplained prevertebral swelling or lower cranial nerve dysfunction, then a frontal AP radiograph of the atlanto-occipital joint projected through the maxillary sinus allows reasonable visualization of this region. More sensitive imaging tools include biplanar tomography, high resolution CT scanning with reformatting in the axial, sagittal and coronal planes with or without intravenous or intrathecal contrast, and, if necessary, cervical myelography or MR imaging (17, 30, 52).

Injury Classification

The classification scheme used by the authors is a three-part system described by Anderson in 1988 (Fig. 15.1) (11). Type 1 injuries include impacted

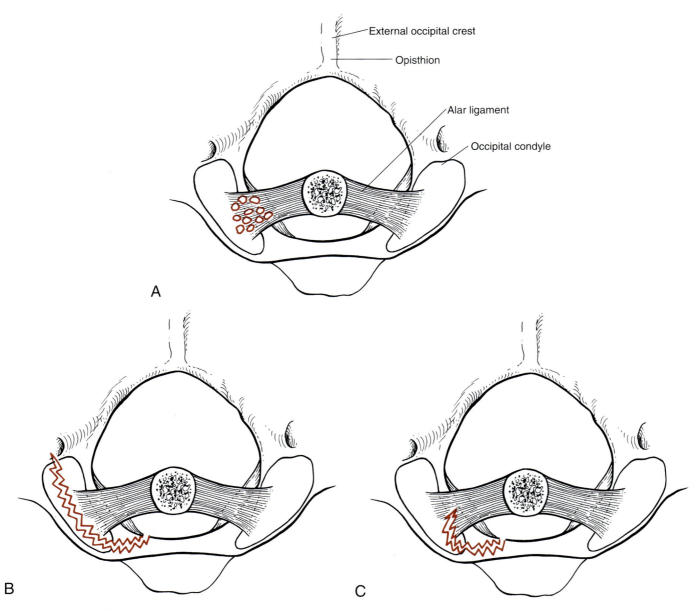

FIGURE 15.1.
The Anderson classification of occipital condyle fractures. **A.** Type I—an impacted comminuted fracture of the occipital condyle with minimal or no displacement. **B.** Type II— a fracture of the occipital condyle with propagation into the foramen magnum, also known as a basilar skull fracture. **C.** Type III—an alar ligament avulsion fracture of the occipital condyle.

comminuted condyle fractures with minimal or no displacement, usually resulting from an axial load. Type II injuries are caused by a direct load to the cervicocranium, resulting in a basilar skull fracture with extension of the fracture line through the occipital condyle into the foramen magnum, rarely resulting in any significant ligamentous disruption. Type III injuries result from a significant shear, lateral bending, or rotatory force, resulting in a bony avulsion injury of the occipital condyle through pull of the alar ligament. These injuries are highly unstable.

Treatment

Type I and Type II occipital condyle fractures are stable injuries and may be treated with a rigid cervical orthosis for approximately 2 to 3 months, at which time dynamic flexion and extension plain radiographs are taken to determine the presence of any soft tissue ligamentous instability. Type III injuries result in compromise to the alar ligament, the primary ligamentous constraint to occipitoatlantal rotation, and lateral bending, and are therefore unstable injuries. This injury should be treated in a halo vest and followed closely in the post-injury period for any evidence of occipital cervical displacement. Surgery is rarely indicated for fractures of this region, especially in the absence of symptomatic brain stem compression or gross instability. The first reported case of surgical treatment of an occipital condyle fracture was in 1992 in a 34-year-old patient with symptomatic brain stem and vertebral artery compression who underwent a unilateral suboccipital craniectomy and C1 laminectomy for brain stem compression (17).

Occipitoatlantal Injuries

As of 1993, only approximately 34 survivors of occipitoatlantal subluxation or dislocation, mostly children, have been reported in the literature (31, 68, 72, 78, 113). The majority of these patients remained significantly neurologically impaired at their latest follow-up (19). The true incidence of this injury is difficult to discern because the majority of patients do not survive transport to a hospital setting (3, 19). Approximately one-third of reported surviving patients had their injury overlooked, most likely secondary to significant paraspinal spasm that maintained the appearance of radiographic alignment (61). The primary bony and ligamentous stabilizing elements of this region include the capsule of the atlanto-occipital joint and the bony articulation of the occipital condyle with the superior lateral mass of the atlas. The paired alar ligaments stabilize the occiput to the upper cervical spine through their attachment to the dens, along with the apical ligament that attaches the dens to the basion. This ligament serves as a stabilizing element during lateral bending and axial rotation (9, 25).

Mechanism of Injury

At the completion of postmortem examinations on 313 victims of multiple trauma, of which 19 had fatal atlanto-occipital dislocations, Alker postulated that the primary mechanism of injury resulting in atlanto-occipital disruption was hyperflexion (3). Bucholz and Burkhead performed similar postmortem studies on 112 victims of multiple trauma, of which 9 cases succumbed to atlanto-occipital dislocations. They believed that the mechanism of injury consisted primarily of hyperextension and longitudinal distraction (19). Other authors, citing the limited degree of intrinsic rotation that occurs at the occipitoatlantal junction, have supported forced rotation with or without lateral flexion as the primary etiology of this injury (73, 78, 111).

Clinical Diagnosis

The spectrum of neurologic deficits in patients who incur injury to this level is similar to that seen in patients with occipital condyle fractures, i.e., little if any neurologic loss to high tetraplegia with respiratory compromise (68). Damage to the caudal ten pairs of cranial nerves, the brain stem, upper cervical spinal cord, and first three cervical nerves have been reported in survivors of this injury (35, 36, 68, 78). Unilateral injury to the vertebral basilar system secondary to cervical hyperextension, longitudinal distraction, and excessive rotation has been reported. This injury may result in a complex of neurologic impairments referred to as Wallenberg's syndrome, which consists of cerebellar ataxia, a deficit to the ipsilateral cranial nerves of V, IX, X, and XI, contralateral loss of pain and temperature, and an ipsilateral Horner's syndrome.

A high index of suspicion must be afforded to a patient with a suspected upper cervical spine injury with significant suboccipital neck pain and evidence of ecchymosis in the suboccipital region, especially if loss of consciousness or possible symptoms of brain stem compression have been reported (61).

Radiographic Evaluation

Several static and dynamic plain radiographic relationships have been defined in both the rheumatoid and nonrheumatoid upper cervical spine to determine the presence of instability or injury to the level of the cervicocranium (33, 88, 117). The presence of abnormal vertebral soft tissue swelling at the level of C2 (greater than 7 mm) may indicate the presence of injury at the occipitoatlantal level (21). In addition, the presence of free air in the retropharyngeal space may indicate a posterior pharyngeal wall disruption, a finding noted at autopsy in patients who succumb to this injury (7). Normally, on a lateral plain radiograph, the anterior superior tip of the odontoid should be in line with the apex of the basion (117). The average distance between these two structures is approximately 9 to 10 mm in the adult and 4 to 5 mm in the child (53). This measurement is referred to as the Wholey dens-basion method or distance (117). A distance greater than 15 mm in an adult and 12 mm in a child is considered abnormal. In the sagittal plane, the relationship between the basion and dens should change less than 1 mm in flexion or extension (68, 78). The basilar line of Wackenstein describes the normal relationship between the clivus and the odontoid on a lateral radiograph and is drawn tangentially along the posterior surface of the clivus in continuity with the posterior cortex of the dens (Fig. 15.2) (112). The Powers ratio consists of four points, BC and OA, that defines two separate lines, one drawn from the basion to the anterior border of the posterior arch of the atlas (BC) and the other from the opisthion to the posterior border of the anterior atlas arch (OA) (Fig. 15.3) (88). The distance of BC divided by OA should be approximately 0.77 mm, with 1 mm being the upper limit of normal. Values greater than 1 mm imply significant anterior occipitoatlantal subluxation or dislocation. This ratio does not apply to children and may provide false negative values in cases of longitudinal distraction or posterior subluxation (31). Plain roentgenographs are sensitive 50 to 75% of the time in determining occipitoatlantal injuries. AP and lateral tomography and high resolution CT scanning with reconstruction, especially in the sagittal plane, better discern bony landmarks necessary to perform precise measurements.

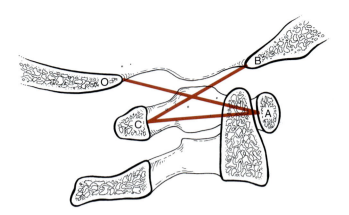

FIGURE 15.3.

An illustration of the Powers ratio describing the relationship of the occiput to the atlas on a lateral plain roentgenograph. The ratio BC/OA should be approximately 0.77. A ratio of 1 or greater suggests anterior subluxation of the occipitoatlantal joint.

Injury Classification

Traynelis divided injuries to the occipitoatlantal complex into three groups. Group I injuries have radiographic evidence of longitudinal distraction; Group II injuries consist of anterior subluxation or dislocation; and Group III injuries consist of posterior subluxation or dislocation (111).

Treatment

Any injury to the occipitoatlantal complex is considered extremely unstable and requires immediate halo application during all phases of patient evaluation. If reduction is necessary to improve alignment or decompress vital neurologic structures, light traction of 2 to 3 pounds, rarely exceeding 5 pounds, is applied with the appropriate vector forces to accomplish accurate alignment. Careful radiographic follow-up and serial neurologic examinations must be done, especially when paracervical muscle spasms subside and result in further instability at this level. Long-term halo immobilization cannot be relied on to insure stability at this level, and primary occipitocervical fusion is necessary to insure long-term spinal stabilization.

Atlas Fractures

Fractures of the atlas represent approximately 3 to 13% of injuries to the cervical spine (46, 58, 64, 65). Interestingly, associated cervical spine injuries, especially involving the odontoid, occur as much as 5% of the time in association with atlas injuries (35, 63, 66).

Disruption of the transverse ligament, the primary stabilizer to the C1, C2 level in flexion, may occur

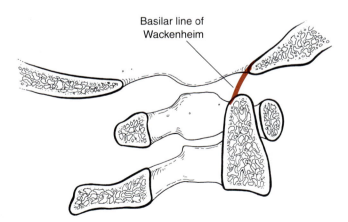

FIGURE 15.2.

A sagittal illustration with applied measurements describing the spatial relationship of the occiput to the upper cervical spine.

with certain atlas fractures. This ligament, which traverses between the medial tubercles of the lateral masses of the atlas within a posterior groove on the odontoid process, is part of the cruciform ligamentous complex. This complex has a superior extension that extends to the basion of the occiput and an inferior extension that terminates along the posteroinferior surface of the dens, referred to respectively as the upper and lower cruciform bands. Besides stabilizing the odontoid to the anterior ring of C1, the transverse ligament allows the odontoid to act as a stable pivot point for C1, C2 rotation. In close proximity to the transverse ligament are the accessory ligaments. These ligaments originate from the C1 lateral masses in conjunction with or anterior to the transverse ligament and assist in stabilizing the atlas to the odontoid peg in flexion, extension, and lateral deviation.

Mechanism of Injury

Activities associated most frequently with fractures to the atlas include motor vehicle accidents followed by falls and miscellaneous trauma. The primary vector force reported most frequently is an axial load to the vertex of the skull that causes compressive approximation of the occipital condyles, C1 superior facets, and C1, C2 articular processes. This may be followed by hyperextension, lateral bending, or rotation (74, 75). The presence of an associated spinal injury further delineates the probable force mechanics involved. In the setting for compressive load, the ring of C1 fails in tension, resulting in body disruption at the narrowest point along the C1 ring. This point most commonly is at the junction of the anterior and posterior ring arch with the lateral masses, resulting in spreading of the articular processes. If hyperextension is the primary force, the posterior C1 arch may be compressed between the occiput and C2 posterior element. This results in bony failure, usually at the arches' narrowest point in the superior groove that bilaterally contains the vertebral vessels (77).

Clinical Diagnosis

Fortunately, neurologic injury associated with atlas fractures is rare because of the large vertebral canal in this region and the tendency of this fracture to displace in a centrifugal manner (99). Patients with associated upper cervical spine fractures, especially posterior displaced odontoid fractures, report the highest incidence of neurologic deficit (66). Lateral displacement of the lateral masses may compress the glossopharyngeal (XI), vagus (X), and hypoglossal (XII) nerves between the C1 transverse process and the styloid process (75). Injuries to the abducent nerve (VI) and spinal accessory nerve (XI) have also been reported. Peripheral nerves at risk to injury include the suboccipital nerve (C1) as it crosses over the ring of C1 and the greater occipital nerve (C2) as it transverses the atlantoaxial membrane. Symptoms of posterior fossa ischemia may rarely result from injury to the vertebral vessels as they cross over the posterior arch of the atlas (64). Injuries to the brain stem caused by cranial settling due to C1 lateral mass displacement may result in symptoms of basilar impression (29). The majority of patients report significant suboccipital discomfort in the setting of upper paracervical muscle spasm. Patients may report a subjective sense of instability and manifest a significant restriction of cervical motion (101).

Radiographic Evaluation

Standard plain lateral and open mouth odontoid radiographs are the usual screening imaging modalities used to diagnose C1 ring fractures. Stable arch fractures, especially the posterior arch, present with no obvious soft tissue swelling on a lateral roentgenograph and may be missed with plain roentgenographic surveys. A method to improve the sensitivity of a plain lateral roentgenograph is to position the x-ray tube over the body of C3 which, because of the obliquity of image acquisition, offsets the posterior arches of C1, thereby allowing them to be more clearly visualized (100). The most sensitive means of visualizing the ring of C1 is by transaxial CT scanning with the CT gantry aligned parallel to the C1 ring. This mode of imaging does not detect transverse fractures of the odontoid, which are the same plane of the imaging cut. AP and lateral tomograms further delineate fracture patterns whose configuration lies in the transverse plane of the ring of C1, such as an anterior arch avulsion injury. This form of imaging is also useful when an associated odontoid fracture is suspected.

Injury to the transverse ligament may be inferred by excessive spreading of the C1 lateral masses on an open mouth odontoid view or, most commonly, through direct visualization of a medial tubercle avulsion via a transverse CT image. An increase in the atlantodens interval greater than 3.5 to 4 mm on a lateral plain roentgenograph is also a possible indicator of transverse ligament incompetency or laxity. Spence discovered through biomechanical cadaveric experimentation that the transverse ligament was incompetent when divergent spreading of the lateral masses occurred greater than 6.9 mm, with an intact ligament usually present with spread less than 5.7 mm (106).

Injury Classification

Since the time of Sir Geoffrey Jefferson, who reviewed 46 atlas fractures in 1920, several authors have described various classification schemes of atlas injuries to prognosticate outcome and guide treatment (Fig. 15.4) (58, 63, 74, 77, 81). Levine described three types of atlas injuries (66, 70). Type I fractures consisted of bilateral fractures to the posterior C1 arch. Type II fractures consisted of a free floating lateral mass with a fracture of the adjacent anterior and posterior arch with a contralateral posterior arch frac-

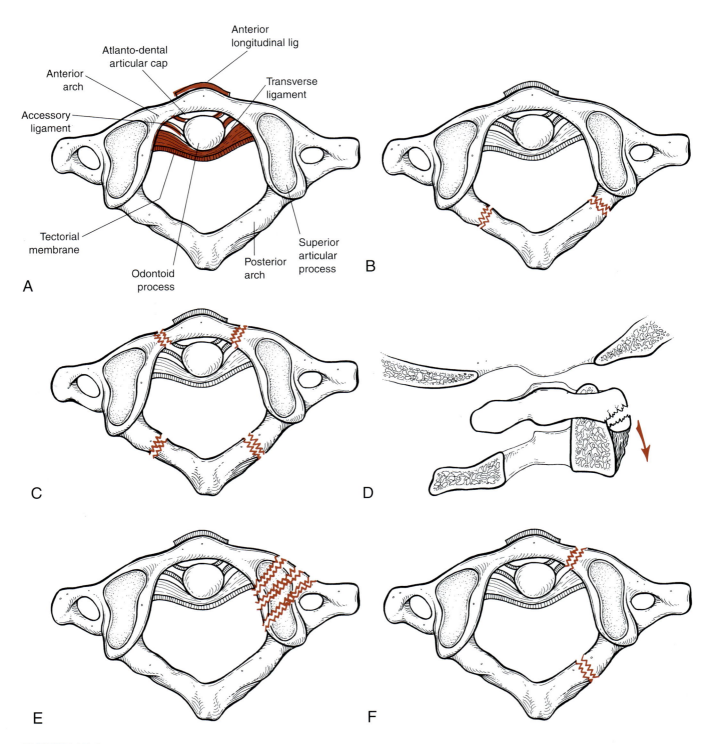

FIGURE 15.4.
A. An illustration of the bony and ligamentous anatomy of the atlas as well as fracture patterns described in various classification systems. **B.** Bilateral posterior arch fracture. **C.** Four-part burst fracture. **D.** Hyperextension avulsion fracture of the anterior inferior C1 arch. **E.** Comminuted lateral mass fracture. **F.** Ipsilateral anterior and posterior arch fracture. **G.** Unilateral anterior arch fracture. **H.** Unilateral C1 mass fracture. **I.** Transverse process fracture.

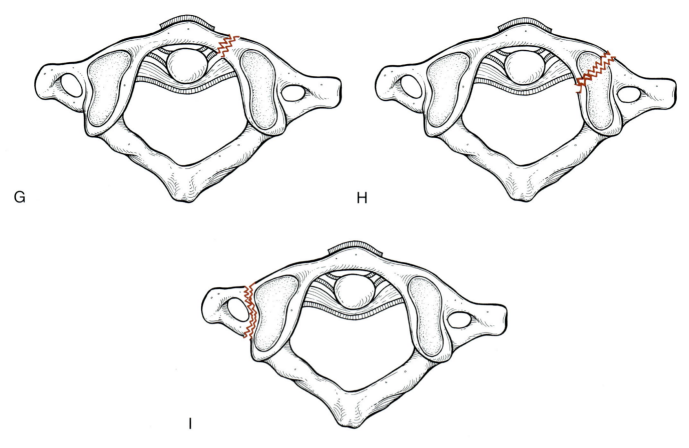

FIGURE 15.4.—continued

ture. Type III fractures included a 3 or 4 part burst fracture. Segal and Stauffer modified Gehweiler's 5 part atlas classification system (99). The original system consisted of Type 1 fractures, which included anterior arch fractures. Type II fractures included fractures of the posterior arch, and Type III fractures included injuries to the lateral masses. Type IV fractures described four part burst fractures, and Type V fractures included fractures of the transverse process. Segal and Stauffer described a comminuted type, which included an isolated comminuted lateral mass fracture with a fracture line anterior and posterior to a unilateral lateral mass similar to Levine's Type II fracture. They reported four patients with this fracture type. At follow-up, two patients unsuccessfully healed their injury, with one having a poor result and the other having a fair functional result. Stewart reported a hyperextension avulsion fracture of the anterior arch of C1 caused by traction at the insertion of the longus colli and anterior longitudinal ligament (110). Landells retrospectively correlated fracture type with long-term symptoms in his three-part classification system (65). Type I fractures consisted of injuries to a single arch, Type II consisted of fractures to both arches, and Type III included lateral mass fractures with extension into either the anterior or posterior arch. Late symptoms were reported in 50% of patients with Type I injuries, 70% with Type II fractures, and 33% with Type III fractures.

Treatment

There is disagreement in the literature over the optimum method of treatment of atlas fractures; especially those fractures with disruption of the transverse ligament. The benefits of fracture reduction and articular congruity, the hallmark of peripheral appendicular joint management, has not been shown in retrospective studies to alter symptomatic outcome of patients with these injuries at follow-up.

Fractures with transverse ligament competency may be treated with a cervical or cervicothoracic orthosis for approximately 6 to 12 weeks until fracture healing is documented (58, 64, 74). If one believes fracture reduction is necessary, axial tong traction with weights in the range of 10 to 30 pounds may be used to improve fracture alignment. Traction is maintained for approximately 5 to 8 weeks until the fracture fragments become sticky, at which time transfer to halo immobilization can begin. At the conclusion of immobilization, dynamic flexion extension lateral roentgenographs may be done to evaluate for evidence of residual instability and therefore the need for surgical stabilization.

A review of patient outcomes in large retrospective services cite various results regardless of fracture types. Many patients report consistent suboccipital discomfort and decreased cervical range of motion. Two-thirds of patients with burst fractures reported by Siegel and Stauffer had fair or poor cervical motion to follow-up, although the majority of patients reported no significant alterations of their normal activities of daily living (99). The majority of patients in Levine's series (80%) complained of neck discomfort that did not require surgical intervention and follow-up (66). Siegel and Stauffer suggested that residual fractional displacement may correlate with a poor result at follow-up (99). Three of eighteen patients in their series had significant spreading of the C1 lateral masses with compromise of the transverse ligament. All three of these patients went onto nonunion with eventually poor clinical results. This result contrasts with Sherk and Nicholson's and Hinchey and Bickel's observations that patients found to have fibrous nonunions at follow-up reported good to excellent eventual outcomes (15, 59, 102). Landells reported 35 patients with atlas fractures—5 of 6 patients with significant spreading of their C1 lateral masses treated nonoperatively had no evidence of clinical instability at follow-up (65). However, four of the five patients reported significant suboccipital discomfort. Levine noted no evidence of atlantoaxial instability or evidence of degenerative changes at follow-up (4.5 years) in six patients treated with 7 days of skeletal traction with an initial mean lateral mass displacement of 7.6 mm regardless of an incongruous reduction. Hadley also found no evidence of instability in five patients with lateral mass displacement greater than 6.9 mm at an average follow-up of 2.5 years (58). The primary causative factor that relates to degenerative changes may be the initial articular damage to the occipital C1, C2 articulations at the time of injury rather than the resulting incongruity (66, 68). The ability to achieve an anatomic reduction has not been reported consistently in clinical review series. Levine reported residual lateral displacement of 3.9 mm from an original displacement of 12.3 mm with skeletal traction (66). Fowler, in a series of 48 patients, was only able to reduce 3 of 13 patients treated with traction (46).

Injuries to the midsubstance of the transverse ligament without an associated osteoperiosteal avulsion fracture are potentially ominous injuries that many believe require immediate surgical stabilization because of the potential for significant atlantoaxial instability with resultant neurologic compromise. Fielding reported on 11 patients with rupture of the atlantoaxial ligaments after trauma (39). Nine of these patients eventually underwent a posterior atlantoaxial fusion. In addition, Fielding performed biomechanical cadaveric studies on 20 cervical spine specimens to elucidate the stability of the C1, C2 complex. He noted that in 15 of his specimens that were tested to failure, the transverse ligament failed in its midsubstance, whereas in the other five specimens, failure occurred at the junction of the transverse ligament and medial tubercle of the C1 lateral mass. He noted that with midsubstance failure of the transverse ligament, the auxiliary ligaments of stability (i.e., alar, apical) were inadequate to prevent further significant C1 displacement. As a result of these findings, Fielding advocated primary C1, C2 surgical stabilization in patients with midsubstance transverse ligament injuries (39). Spence noted midsubstance failure of the transverse ligament in 6 of 10 cadaveric specimens tested to failure (106). He also suggested aggressive surgical stabilization in cases of transverse ligament disruption. Many authors believe that in cases of osteoperiosteal avulsion fractures of the transverse ligament, the auxiliary ligaments (apical, tectorial, alar) and capsular structures are intact and impart adequate stability until fracture healing occurs. Panjabi and associates created atlas fractures experimentally in 10 fresh frozen cadaveric spines (83). They noted that in eight specimens with transverse ligament disruption secondary to axial loading, all specimens had intact alar, tectorial membrane and C1, C2 capsular ligaments. Fowler found no evidence of instability in three of four patients with transverse ligament avulsion injuries at follow-up (46). Hadley found no evidence of atlantoaxial instability at follow-up of five patients with displacement of the lateral masses greater than 6.9 mm (58). Similar results were reported by Landells (92).

In summary, patients with evidence of transverse ligament avulsion injuries may be treated conservatively with or without traction reduction. Evidence of instability may be ascertained at follow-up with dynamic flexion extension plain radiographic films. Consideration for primary surgical stabilization should be given for midsubstance transverse ligament injuries and evidence of instability on imaging studies. The optimum treatment of displaced atlas fractures (lateral mass displacement greater than 6.9mm) can only be determined with well-controlled prospective studies that evaluate the efficacy of traction versus immediate brace treatment.

Rotatory Subluxation of the Atlantoaxial Joint

The primary ligamentous stabilizer of the atlantoaxial joint is the transverse ligament, which prevents pathologic anterior displacement of the ring of C1 on C2, as well as allows the ring of C1 to pivot around the odontoid peg. The secondary, or auxiliary, stabilizing ligaments to C1, C2 rotation include the alar ligaments and the facet capsules. The superior and inferior articular facets of C2 are located in different vertical planes with the superior articular surface more anterior and inclined less vertical than the inferior articular surface. The horizontal orientation of the C1, C2 articular facets facilitates rotation at this level (22). Dislocation of the C1, C2 articulation begins to occur at around 63 to 65° degrees of rotation. At this point, the upper cervical canal may be narrowed up to 7 mm (42). If anterior subluxation of C1 on C2 of approximately 5 mm is present because of transverse ligamentous insufficiency, a C1, C2 unilateral facet dislocation may occur at around 45° of rotation, resulting in canal narrowing of about 12 mm (42). Further rotation may lead to a decrease in the space available for the spinal cord with resultant neurologic compromise (114). Vertebral vessel compromise is rare within the extremes of normal cervical rotation because of its lateral position within the lateral masses. Pathologic or extreme rotation may disrupt or compress these vessels, resulting in brain stem or cerebellar ischemia (42).

Mechanism of Injury

Pathologic processes which weaken or disrupt the C1, C2 ligamentous structures (trauma, inflammation), cause bony deformity (metabolic bone disease, genetic disorders of collagen formation and bone growth), or impart abnormal rotatory forces to the upper cervical spine (ocular, vestibular dysfunction), may result in pathologic rotatory subluxation or dislocation of the C1, C2 vertebral bodies (68).

This disorder is reported most frequently in the pediatric population after an upper respiratory inflammatory illness or trivial trauma, although significant deformity may be seen in the adult patient after trauma, or in cases of tumor or infection (60). Inflammatory processes, such as an upper respiratory infection, tonsillitis, mastoiditis, rheumatoid arthritis, or ankylosing spondylitis with involvement of the upper retropharyngeal space, may lead to significant synovial capsular effusion of the C1, C2 joint and attenuation of the surrounding ligamentous structures, resulting in rotatory or anteroposterior subluxation of the atlantoaxial joint (21, 89). An example of this is Grisel's syndrome, seen primarily in the pediatric population, in which inflammatory products from the posterior nasopharynx drain through pharyngeal lymphovenous channels into the venous plexus, surrounding the atlantoaxial joint capsule.

Abnormal rotatory forces to the C1, C2 process also may be caused by tumorous involvement of the sternocleidomastoid muscle or abnormal voluntary posturing resulting from ocular or vestibular dysfunction (40). Posterior dislocation of C1 and C2 with an intact odontoid may be the result of severe hyperextension in the setting of trauma, especially if the paracervical muscles are relaxed (118). As of 1991, only four survivors of this injury have been reported, all without significant neurologic deficit (118).

There has been conjecture as to the etiology of C1, C2 rotatory fixation after longstanding subluxation. With prolonged stretching and attenuation of the capsular ligamentous complex, gradual soft tissue contracture with scarring on this complex may prevent future articular realignment. Persistent subluxation leading to fixation may result from longstanding sternocleidomastoid contracture, traumatic injuries with incongruity or displacement of the atlantoaxial joint, or hyperemic decalcification of the surrounding ligamentous complex (21, 40). In addition, with capsular effusions seen in the previous inflammatory conditions, synovial fringes or attenuated and disrupted ligamentous structures, i.e., alar ligaments, may become entrapped within the joint cavity, preventing normal alignment. This pathologic finding has been confirmed on autopsy examination in infants and in small children; meniscus-like synovial folds have been identified in both the occipitoatlantal and atlanto-occipital joints (89).

Clinical Diagnosis

Patients with pathologic rotatory subluxation of the C1, C2 joint usually report a pertinent history suggestive of the pathogenesis of this disorder. A history of trauma or a recent upper respiratory infection may precede the characteristic clinical presentation of the cock robin-appearance in which the skull is rotated in one direction approximately 20° and tilted to the opposite direction approximately 20° with minimal cervical flexion. Rarely, the clinical deformity may be less apparent if compensatory occipitoatlantal rotation occurs in the opposite direction of atlantoaxial subluxation.

This compensatory rotation may result from significant paracervical spasm or a primary injury to the occipital-C1 joint (6). Compensatory rotation may also exist in the lower cervical spine, decreasing any apparent clinical deformity (21).

Commonly, patients report significant suboccipital discomfort associated with marked restriction in range of motion. Neurologic dysfunction may manifest after traumatic C1, C2 instability with an atlantodens interval of 7.5 mm or greater. Symptoms of weakness usually manifest before the subjective complaint of pain, especially if pathologic rotation is not present (39). On physical examination, one may palpate a prominence in the retropharyngeal space caused by asymmetry of the C1, C2 articulation (101).

With longstanding rotatory deformities, patients may develop flattening or plagiocephaly on the involved side. This has been shown to correct spontaneously at long-term follow-up with appropriate treatment (40, 42).

Radiographic Evaluation

Interpretation of plain roentgenographs in a patient with a rotatory abnormality of the C1, C2 joint in the peritrauma period is difficult because of problems with patient cooperation, patient positioning, and superimposition of soft tissue on bony landmarks that obscures subtle bony abnormalities. These difficulties may lead to a significant delay in diagnosis. Fielding reported an average delay in diagnosis of 11.6 months in his report on fixed deformities of the atlantoaxial joint (42). Anatomically, the occiput and C1 tend to rotate together in unison, although subtle physiologic rotation does exist between these two structures. With rotation greater than 50° between C1 and C2, midline deviation of the C2 spinous process may occur with the C2 spinous process and the chin, in the presence of head tilt, both lying on the same side of the midline (86).

In instances of pathologic compensatory occipitoatlantal rotation opposite C1, C2 rotatory subluxation, the lateral plain roentgenograph may reveal decreased skull rotation in relationship to C1, with the skull appearing in profile with the C2 vertebral body. On an AP roentgenograph, the skull and C2 vertebral body may appear in line with each other in reference to C2 spinous process with obvious rotation of the ring of C1 (6). In the coronal view with head rotation to the right, the left C1 lateral mass appears broader as it moves superiorly and closer to the odontoid process (Fig. 15.5). The right C1 lateral mass appears further from the midline and has its inferior border partially obscured by the ipsilateral C2 superior articular process, illustrating the so-called wink-sign (8, 21). When significant C1, C2 rotatory subluxation exists with lateral tilting of the head, the cranium overlaps the ring of C1, giving the appearance of an occipital-C1 ring assimilation on a plain lateral roentgenograph with loss of the normal superimposition of the anterior and posterior C1 arches (8). The lateral roentgenograph is also useful in determining transverse ligament integrity and pathologic soft tissue swelling. With C1, C2 rotation, the lateral mass of C1 may appear as a wedge-shaped mass anterior to the odontoid process.

AP and lateral tomography and axial CT scanning allow excellent visualization of the C1, C2 articulation and illustrate not only the presence of rotation, but also subluxation between these two vertebral bodies (Fig. 15.6). Physiologic rotation at the C1, C2 joint noted on any imaging studies is not pathognomonic for pathology unless fixation is confirmed on dynamic studies. Dynamic studies of choice include the open mouth plain roentgenograph or axial CT scanning in the plane of the C1 ring, with head rotation 15 to 20° in one direction and then in the opposite direction to determine the presence of a fixed deformity (19, 75). Cineradiographic and dynamic MRI evaluation is also useful but less frequently used in the diagnosis of this disorder.

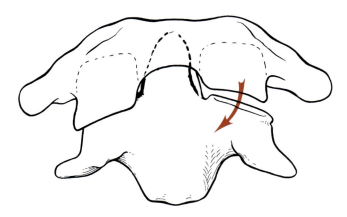

FIGURE 15.5.
A coronal schematic illustration of C1, C2 rotation. The occiput is rotating to the left, resulting in forward translation of the right C1 lateral mass, making it appear broader, more cephalad, and closer to the odontoid process. The left lateral mass, which is moving posteriorly, appears narrower and appears further from the odontoid with its inferior border obscured by the C2 superior articular mass.

Injury Classification

Rotatory subluxation is usually described in terms of its mechanism or etiology, i.e., traumatic atlantoaxial rotatory subluxation. In longstanding cases in which fixed deformity develops, Fielding classified this disorder into four groups depending on its severity (Fig. 15.7) (42). Type I fixation, the most common type, is seen most frequently in children and describes pathologic atlantoaxial rotatory fixation within the range of physiologic C1, C2 rotation without evidence of soft tissue damage. The lateral atlantodens interval is usually 3 mm or less. Type II fixation describes an incompetent transverse ligament with unilateral anterior C1 lateral mass displacement of approximately 3 to 5 mm with rotation centered around the nondisplaced contralateral C1, C2 articular process. Type III fixation describes bilateral C1, C2 lateral mass subluxation of greater than 5 mm with one lateral mass complex subluxed greater than the other side. Both primary and secondary soft tissue restraints are deficient in this subtype. Type IV fixation describes posterior subluxation of the ring of C1 or C2, usually occurring in situations of odontoid deficiency, as in the severely affected rheumatoid pop-

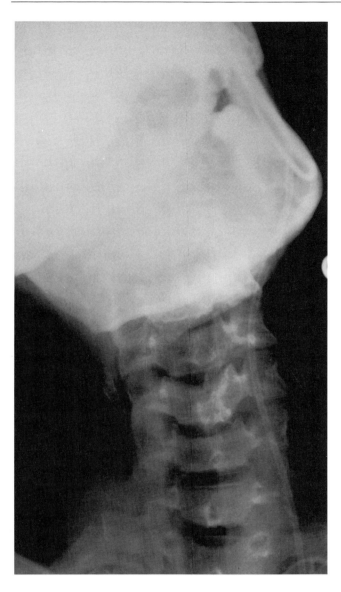

FIGURE 15.6.

An AP plain roentgenograph reveals rotation of the occiput to the left with the head tilted to the right.

ulation. Again, one lateral mass usually is subluxed more than the other, resulting in relative C1, C2 rotation.

Treatment

Treatment of rotatory disorders of the C1, C2 articulation is predicated on its etiology, the presence or absence of neurologic injury, the age of the patient, and the duration of symptomatology. Fortunately, the majority of the patients may be treated successfully with observation, bed rest, or a soft cervical collar for comfort. If a patient is seen within the first week of symptoms, head halter traction with low weights, (i.e. 3 to 5 pounds depending on the age and weight of the patient) can be used with appropriate analgesics and sedation (89). Symptoms that are present for longer than 1 week and less than 1 month, or those unresponsive to the previous modalities, generally respond to hospital admission and skeletal traction with weights determined by the age and size of the patient. Axial traction, useful for flexion or extension deformities of the cervical spine, is less efficient in reducing rotatory deformities. The physician must be aware of the presence of compensatory occipital-C1 rotatory deformity, which may inadvertently worsen with incorrectly applied traction (26).

Children usually require traction weights up to approximately 7 pounds and adults up to 15 pounds. Weights may be increased to approximately 15 pounds in a child and 20 to 30 pounds in an adult. Once occipital cervical alignment is found to be neutral, i.e., reduction is obtained, traction may be continued for 1 to 2 weeks until cervical rotation is symmetrical. If symptoms are of short duration, reduction can usually be obtained within 24 hours with many patients reporting the sensation of a pop and then immediate relief of symptoms at the time of reduction (75). After this, the patient may be immobilized in a cervical orthosis or halo brace until capsular healing has occurred (40). The duration of brace treatment depends on the length of prereduction symptomatology. In general, brace immobilization is continued for approximately 6 weeks until dynamic studies are performed to confirm capsular stability. Some surgeons advocate closed reduction of atlantoaxial rotatory deformities under general anesthesia or through open mouth direct palpation of the anterior ring of C1 through the posterior oral pharynx with local anesthesia. These methods, although effective, carry greater risk of neurologic injury because of lack of volitional neurologic monitoring and the speed of reduction (42). If subluxation is associated with pathologic rotation, i.e., atlantodens interval greater than 5 mm in children and greater than 3 mm in adults, surgical stabilization is recommended because of the presence of significant soft tissue compromise. In patients who present with a traumatic posterior dislocation of C1 and C2 with an intact odontoid, Moskovich recommends a three-stage maneuver to accomplish reduction with the least risk to the spinal cord (79). Initially, light traction is applied in an axial direction with slight flexion to create an anterior vector force, causing the anterior ring of C1 to maintain contact with the posterior border of the odontoid until reduction is accomplished. Stage two begins once reduction has occurred and consists of light weight traction in extension to maintain contact between the posterior border of the anterior C1 ring and the anterior border of the odontoid. Stage three is the final phase before a posterior C1, C2 fusion and consists of light weight traction of approximately 5 pounds to maintain appropriate alignment.

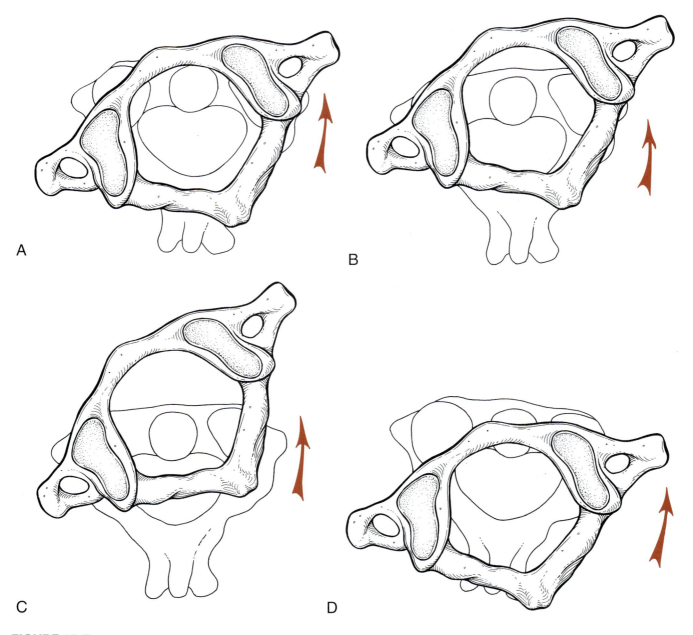

FIGURE 15.7.
The Fielding classification of atlantoaxial rotatory fixation. **A.** Type I—atlantoaxial rotatory fixation without evidence of subluxation. Rotation is within the normal physiologic range of motion. **B.** Type II—atlantoaxial rotatory fixation with evidence of unilateral C1 lateral mass displacement of 3–5 mm. **C.** Type III—atlantoaxial rotatory fixation with evidence of bilateral C1 lateral mass subluxation greater than 5 mm. **D.** Type IV—atlantoaxial rotatory fixation with evidence of bilateral posterior C1 lateral mass subluxation on C2.

If symptoms associated with deformity are present for longer than 1 month, closed reduction and immobilization is rarely successful. Many therefore advocate attempted skeletal reduction followed, if successful or not in reducing deformity, with a posterior C1, C2 fusion. In general, a posterior C1, C2 fusion is an acceptable treatment option in patients with deformity present for longer than 3 months, patients who have evidence of instability, after failure of closed treatment, and in those whose deformities recur after successful closed reduction. If an in situ fusion is done without instrumentation, one should consider continuation of light weight skeletal traction for 1 to 2 weeks to prevent early recurrence of deformity. Clark has recommended an in situ occipital-C2 fusion in patients with associated evidence of pathologic occipital-C1 rotation after a period of light weight skeletal traction (26). Fielding believed that occipital-C1 rotatory abnormalities usually correct after fusion of the atlantoaxial joint and, therefore, excluded the occiput from the fusion to preserve occipital cervical flexion (6).

Odontoid Fractures

Odontoid fractures represent approximately 5 to 15% of all cervical spine fractures (1, 7,9). The incidence of this fracture has increased slightly over the last two decades because of increased survival resulting from improvements in in-field medical treatment and triage to tertiary trauma centers specializing in spinal cord injury (84). These fractures are reported three times more frequently in males than in females, with the average patient age being in the mid-forties (10, 84).

Because of the high incidence of nonunion reported after treatment of these injuries, many investigators have looked into risk factors that may predispose to nonhealing. Initially, many physicians believed that the odontoid process was served by an end vessel vascular network which was divided at the time of fracture, thereby resulting in an avascular proximal fragment. Both cadaveric and in vivo animal injection studies have refuted this hypothesis and revealed that the odontoid is served by an extensive intra- and extra-osseous anastomotic vascular network (9, 96). Schiff and Park, Althoff and Goldie, and Schatzker and associates demonstrated, through injection studies, the existence of bilateral anterior and posterior ascending vessels that branch off from the vertebral arteries at the level of the C3 vertebral body and supply penetrating branches to the base of the dens with eventual anastomosis in an apical arcade (5, 94, 96). Additionally, arterial branches supplying the dens body and the apical arcade with contributions to both the apical and accessory ligaments were identified from both internal carotid arteries, ascending pharyngeal vessels, and several vessels of the occipital artery. The existence of central odontoid ascending vessels was confirmed in both cadaveric and in vivo animal studies (95).

Schatzker found in a dog model that fractures occurring below the level of the accessory ligament tended to heal as opposed to fractures above this ligament; these fractures tended to displace because of traction by the apical and alar ligaments (94). This finding was supported by his analysis of 37 patients with odontoid fractures and favored the hypothesis that fracture healing may be related more to fracture displacement than to arterial ischemia.

Mechanism of Injury

Anteriorly displaced odontoid fractures are reported approximately seven times more frequently than posteriorly displaced fractures, although this ratio reverses in the elderly population in which posteriorly displaced fractures are more common (9, 12, 28, 48, 85). The majority of these fractures in the middle-aged population result from high impact axial load injuries with an associated shear force—usually the result of a motor vehicle accident. This injury mechanism is also responsible for the commonly associated fracture of the C1 vertebral body. An axial load may result in a C1 burst fracture, whereas isolated C1 arch or lateral mass fractures result from associated flexion, extension, or laterally applied forces. Odontoid fractures in the elderly may occur simply after a minor fall from the standing position because of the degree of osteoporosis present within their axial spine. The taut transverse ligament assists in displacing the odontoid anteriorly with a flexion force while the bony ring of C1 acts to posteriorly displace the odontoid with an extension force (3, 9, 28). The level of the odontoid fracture depends on the forces applied to the upper cervical spine and on the position of the ring of C1 in relationship to the odontoid at the time of trauma. After performing biomechanical studies on 34 cadaveric specimens, Mouradian postulated that laterally applied forces through head rotation or oblique impact loading were necessary to produce odontoid fractures (80). Unfortunately, a reproducible cadaveric model has not been created to elucidate the exact mechanism of this injury (77).

There is debate in the literature as to the mechanism of odontoid tip avulsion fractures. Many authors believe that these fractures are actually primary injuries to the occipitoatlantal region resulting from an alar ligament avulsion rather than primary injuries to the odontoid. In a review of the literature up to 1990, Scott (98) found only six cases of odontoid tip fractures reported. These injuries usually are associated with a rotational mechanism that necessitates evaluation of the occipitoatlantal axial ligamentous complex, such as the alar and apical ligaments and the tectorial membrane.

Clinical Diagnosis

Patients who present with a fracture of the odontoid usually report poorly localized nonspecific suboccipital discomfort associated with posterior neck tenderness, paravertebral muscle spasm, and significant decreased range of motion (28). Because of the capacious nature of the upper cervical canal, a neurologic deficit is rare, reported in approximately 15 to 25% of all cases. Although unusual, neural impairment may range from irritation of the greater occipital nerve to tetraplegia with brain stem dysfunction (9). Neurologic embarrassment, when present, is usually more frequent in patients over age 60 (91).

As a result of the mechanism of injury (i.e., motor vehicle accidents) in the middle-aged population, odontoid fractures may be associated with other musculoskeletal injuries in up to 50% of patients (62, 84). Although it is difficult to determine the etiology of death in fatal accidents due to a multitude of factors, it is postulated that the incidence of mortality related to odontoid injuries ranges from 3.3 to 18% of cases (7, 9, 10, 104, 105).

Radiographic Evaluation

Initial radiographic evaluation at the odontoid process should include a lateral and open mouth odontoid view. These views may be supplemented with AP and lateral plain tomography or axial CT evaluation with sagittal or three-dimensional reformation. A poorly aligned CT gantry or imaging in the plane of a transverse odontoid fracture may completely miss this injury (9, 38).

Classification

Numerous authors have recommended various classification systems for describing injuries to the odontoid process (4, 10, 13, 56, 85, 87, 94). Recent systems have attempted to correlate fracture displacement with treatment recommendations and eventual prognosis. The most widely used system from which many of the other classification schemes base their description is the three-part system of Anderson and D'Alonzo (Fig. 15.8) (10). In this classification system, a Type I fracture is an oblique avulsion fracture caused by pull of one alar ligament and possibly the apical ligament of the tip of the dens. To date, only six cases have been reported, of which four clearly represent injuries to the occipitoatlantal or occipitoatlantoaxial junction, thereby making this a secondary injury to the odontoid process (10, 32, 35, 77). This fracture should not be confused with the secondary center of ossification, i.e., the ossiculum terminale, which is present in a minority of patients. Rarely, an avulsion fracture at this level may displace superiorly into the foramen magnum, resulting in compression of the pontomedullary junction of the brain stem. A Type II fracture, the most common, is located at the base or waist of the dens and should not be confused in the skeletally immature patient with injuries to the neurocentral synchondrosis, which is located more inferiorly in the centrum of the C2 body (25, 73). An occult injury to this level after minor trauma may be the predisposing incident to the development of an unfused proximal dens fragment, referred to as the os odontoideum (43, 44). This entity is differentiated from a true fracture because of its obvious axial separation from the base of the odontoid and its smooth cortical borders.

Comminution at the base of the dens associated with a Type II fracture makes closed reduction with skeletal traction more difficult and portends a worse prognosis with closed treatment. This fracture pattern may be associated with additional soft tissue injury to the alar and transverse ligamentous complex (56). A Type III fracture extends within the body of C2 and may course through both C2 superior articular facets.

Treatment

Patients with an identified fracture to the odontoid should be immobilized immediately to prevent further fracture displacement and the potential for neurologic compromise. We recommend initial light weight skeletal traction of approximately 5 to 10 pounds in all patients. Careful neurologic and radiographic monitoring is necessary, especially in patients with Type I injuries, which may represent a marker for significant occipitoatlantal dissociation or instability. Fractures with significant displacement are reduced with light weight skeletal traction with the institution of appropriate vector forces. We use a bivector apparatus that enables the placement of two simultaneous vector forces along a 180° axis. This in turn allows for fracture disimpaction in the superior or axial direction with simultaneous anterior displacement of the proximal fracture fragment in posteriorly displaced fractures with an anterior vector force. These steps ensure a more simplified, safe, and efficient means of closed reduction using weights less than approximately 25 pounds superiorly and 20 pounds anteriorly. Factors that have been reported to affect outcome include the patient's age, fracture type, neurologic status, direction of displacement and degree of angulation, delay in treatment, and stability of reduction. These factors must all be considered when choosing between nonoperative and operative treatment methods in the acute fracture period.

Type I Injuries

Injuries to the odontoid tip should be studied carefully for the presence of occipitoatlantoaxial instability. If an injury to this complex is not present, this fracture should then be immobilized in a cervical orthosis for approximately 3 months until dynamic studies illustrate fracture stability.

Type II Injuries

There is no clear consensus as to the optimum treatment methods for fractures of the odontoid base. Many authors recommend immediate surgical stabilization (10), while others prefer closed reduction and brace immobilization until fracture healing or the expression of delayed or nonunion occurs (7, 10, 15, 23). The nonunion rate reported in some studies

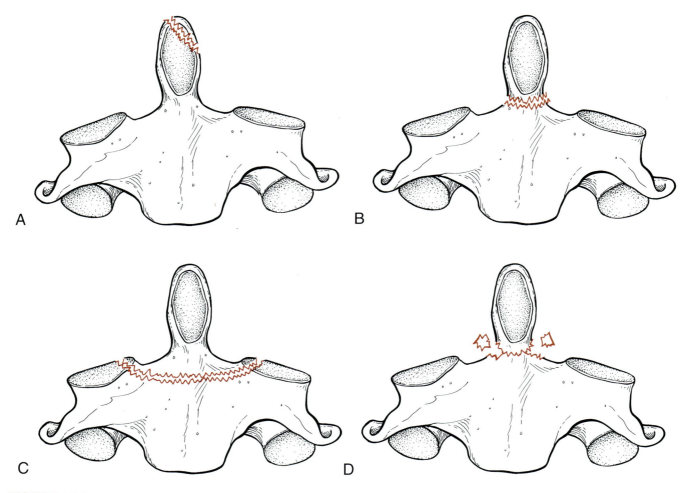

FIGURE 15.8.
The Anderson and D'Alonzo three-part odontoid fracture classification, including the Type IIA fracture described by Hadley. **A.** Type I—an oblique ligamentous avulsion fracture of the tip of the dens. **B.** Type II—a fracture at the base or waist of the dens. **C.** Type III—a fracture with extension into the body of C2. **D.** Type IIA—a Type II fracture with anterior and posterior cortical comminution.

for this fracture type is as high as 88% (average 33%), thereby motivating many surgeons to recommend initial surgical stabilization (9, 34, 109). Ekong noted a 41% nonunion rate in Type II fractures in patients over the age of 55 or fractures displaced greater than 4 to 6 mm (37). Ryan suggested that adequate fracture overlap of at least 60% was necessary for bony healing to occur with these fractures (90). Clark and White performed a multicenter retrospective review of 144 odontoid fractures, of which 96 were considered Type II fractures (27). They found that halo immobilization resulted in eventual fracture stability in 70% of patients, i.e., lack of fracture fragment movement on follow-up flexion extension films, whereas fractures stabilized with a posterior cervical fusion resulted in fracture stability in 96% of cases. A statistically increased incidence of nonunion and malunion was noted in fractures with significant displacement (greater than 5 mm) and angulation (greater than 10°). They therefore recommended consideration of primary cervical fusion for significantly displaced or angulated Type II fractures.

Hadley reported on 68 patients with acute Type II fractures who were treated with extended immobilization regardless of their alignment status on postinjury traction films (56, 57). He noted a 78% incidence of nonunion in fractures displaced greater than 6 mm, as opposed to a 10% nonunion rate in fractures displaced less than 6 mm. He found no correlation between fracture healing and the patient's age, neurologic status, or direction of fracture displacement. Dunn advocated initial halo reduction in all patients with Type II fractures in a series of 128 patients (30). He recommended a primary posterior cervical fusion in certain high risk groups, including patients with greater than 3 mm of posterior fracture displacement (100% union), patients greater than 65 years of age (78% nonunion rate), after initial delay in diagnosis and treatment (greater than seven days), or unstable fractures that are poorly aligned with closed reduction (100% union rate).

Bell and Myers reported a 97% union rate in their series of Type II fractures treated with initial skeletal traction for 6 weeks followed by SOMI brace immobilization for 3 months (14). Donovan reported on 28 patients treated with halo immobilization for Type II and Type III odontoid fractures and noted a 75% union rate at follow-up (32). He noted no correlation between fracture union and the patient's age or degree of fracture displacement and recommended primary posterior cervical fusion for all Type II odontoid fractures.

At the Regional Spine Cord Injury Center of Delaware Valley (RSCICDV) at Thomas Jefferson University Hospital, 70 consecutive patients with odontoid injuries admitted between 1980 and 1990 were evaluated retrospectively (28). Seventy-five percent of patients with Type II fractures treated by halo immobilization eventually went on to nonunion, compared with a 100% union rate for patients treated with a primary posterior cervical fusion. Patients with greater than 5 mm of displacement, age over 60, or loss of a previous reduction also had an increased incidence of nonhealing. We therefore concluded that halo immobilization may be effective in nondisplaced or minimally displaced Type II odontoid fractures with consideration made for surgical stabilization in certain high-risk groups outlined in our study.

Type III Fractures

Type III odontoid fractures generally have a high healing success rate because of greater cancellous bony overlap and the rarity of fragment distraction. Paradis and Jones recommended treating these fractures with 4 or 5 weeks of traction followed by a total of 4 to 5 months of immobilization (84). They reported a union rate of 84% in 13 patients treated in this manner at the Mayo Clinic. Husby and Sorensen reported only a 14% nonunion rate in 21 fractures treated nonoperatively (62). These results, however, have not been substantiated universally in various retrospective reviews. Clark and White reported four cases of malunion and one case of nonunion in 10 patients treated in a cervical orthosis (27). Of a total of 48 Type III fractures in their series, 13% went onto a nonunion while 15% went onto a malunion. For fractures displaced greater than 5 mm, 40% failed to unite at follow-up.

Apuzzo and associates recommended primary posterior cervical fusion in elderly patients with fracture displacement greater than 4 mm after reporting a 54% nonunion rate in 13 patients (12). At Thomas Jefferson University Hospital, we reported a 22% incidence of nonunion in 60 patients treated with skeletal tong traction followed by halo immobilization (28). Three of the four nonunions in our series had significant posterior fracture displacement at initial evaluation.

In fractures that show evidence of impaction, consideration for treatment with a cervical orthosis may be given because of the fracture's inherent stability (25, 51). In general, these injuries should be reduced with light skeletal traction, followed by halo immobilization for a minimum of 3 months. If evidence of delayed union or nonunion occurs at follow-up, consideration for surgical stabilization should be given.

Combination C1 and odontoid fractures are common. Primary treatment in this situation usually is predicated on the type of odontoid fracture present. More recently, many surgeons have recommended primary anterior odontoid screw stabilization to preserve C1, C2 rotation and to avoid the morbidity of prolonged halo immobilization, especially if the odontoid fails to unite after 3 months of brace treatment. Meyer and Cotler, as well as Hadley, suggest that a primary C1, C2 fusion may be done if adequate sublaminar wire purchase can be obtained with the remaining nonfractured posterior C1 ring (58, 74).

The majority of treating physicians consider fracture healing to be the only acceptable endpoint to this fracture. Stable nonunions have the potential to displace with minor trauma or to cause anterior thecal sac compression and subsequent myelopathic symptoms caused by callus hypertrophy with subtle fracture fragment movement. This result has motivated many surgeons to recommended surgical stabilization in all cases of nonunion. Ryan and associates recently followed nine odontoid nonunions in the elderly for 21 months and reported no evidence of adverse neurologic consequences (91). They therefore suggested that vigorous treatment to obtain union may not be necessary in this patient subgroup.

Axis Fractures

Traumatic spondylolisthesis of the axis is disruption of the pars interarticularis of the C2 vertebra. The morphology of the articular facets of the axis differs from the remaining subaxial cervical spine in that the superior articular process is anteriorly offset from the inferior articular process rather than in the same sagittal plane. A common location for fractures of the C2 vertebra is between the superior and inferior articular processes, i.e., the pars interarticularis and not through the pedicle, which anatomically does not exist at the C2 level. A fracture of the pars interarticularis of the axis is commonly called a hangman's fracture. Fortunately, fractures of this structure usually result in fracture fragment separation with actual widening of the space available for the cord at this level.

The incidence of traumatic fractures to the axis is

approximately 12 to 18% of all acute cervical spine fractures (51, 75). As with fractures to this region of the upper cervical spine, fractures of the axis are commonly associated with other cervical spine injuries (14 to 33%), such as the posterior arch of C1, the odontoid process, or the subaxial cervical vertebral bodies (41, 47, 48, 74). In addition to associated spinal injuries, trauma to other regions of the body is common, including injuries to the thoracic cage, cranium, trachea, and facial and scalp lacerations (47). Although survivors of traumatic fractures of the axis report a paucity of neurologic deficits (3 to 10%), approximately 25 to 40% of these injuries result in immediate death at the scene of the accident caused by the combination of spinal cord injury and associated musculoskeletal and viscus injuries (19, 20, 36, 41).

Mechanism of Injury

Fractures of the axis are usually the result of an acceleration/deceleration injury caused by motor vehicle accidents, falls, or diving accidents (41, 97). The etiology and biomechanics of a lethal C2 fracture dislocation through hanging was illustrated by Wood-Jones in 1912–1913 (21, 119). They analyzed specific knot placements during hanging when a severe hyperextension distraction force was applied. Fortunately, as mentioned, these injuries generally result from acceleration/deceleration forces without distraction and, therefore, significant spinal cord stretching or transection does not occur.

Cadaveric and clinical studies have confirmed that hyperextension is a major force vector in fracture production (69). Hyperextension with an associated axial load to the cervical cranium results in compression to the posterior facet joints with accentuation of shear forces concentrated on the pars interarticularis and adjacent articular masses and foramen transversarium (21, 50, 69, 74). The pars interarticularis is a focus of force application because of its transverse orientation, elongated shape, and location midway between C2 inferior and superior articular processes, both of which are located in different transverse and vertical planes (41, 69). The pars interarticularis is usually fractured bilaterally but asymmetrically, implying a combination of force vectors probably related to the presence of cervical rotation.

Diagnosis

The signs and symptoms of fractures of the axis are similar to other injuries at this level of the spine and tend to be nonspecific. Discomfort in the distribution of the greater occipital nerve (C2) along with other stigmata of trauma to the head and neck region are usually present.

Radiographic Evaluation

Aside from plain radiographs, an axial CT image illustrates well the fracture lines involving the pars interarticularis. Lateral plain tomography is also useful in illustrating a fracture to this region in the sagittal plane.

Injury Classification

The preferred classification system to date is the modification of the three-part classification system of Effendi by Levine and Edwards (Fig. 15.9) (36, 67). This system describes a sequence of injuries to the second cervical vertebra and surrounding soft tissue, implying not only the mechanism of injury, but also an anatomic description of compromised structures and preferred treatment. A Type I fracture is a fracture through both pars and/or adjacent superior or inferior articular processes with less than 3 mm of fracture displacement. No evidence of fracture angulation or excessive translation on flexion extension plain roentgenographs are noted. This fracture results from a hyperextension axial loading force with injury to only the bony elements without compromise of the contiguous soft tissues.

A Type II fracture has more than 3 mm of displacement at the fracture site and evidence of significant fracture angulation on the lateral plain roentgenograph. There also may be an associated compression fracture to the anterior superior body of C3 or an avulsion fracture to the posteroinferior body of C2 because of the pull of the posterior longitudinal ligament. This injury results from an extension, axial loading force similar to a Type I injury. In addition, before any significant injury to the anterior disc or anterior longitudinal ligament, a rebound flexion, axial compression force occurs, resulting in disruption of the posterior longitudinal ligament and the C2-C1 disc space from posterior to anterior, with subsequent subperiosteal elevation of the anterior longitudinal ligament off the body of C3. This results in significant fracture site angulation and a compression injury to the anterosuperior body of C3.

A Type IIA fracture has slight or no translation but significant fracture angulation because of a predominant flexion distraction force. The pathoanatomy of this fracture is not well understood, but it is thought that as a result of a flexion and distraction force, the posterior longitudinal ligament and disc space between the C2 and C3 vertebral bodies are disrupted with subperiosteal elevation of the anterior longitudinal ligament off the C3 vertebral body.

Although the pathoanatomy of Type II and IIA fractures are poorly understood, it is important to recognize their appearance on a static lateral plain roentgenograph; Type IIA fractures may significantly displace at the fracture site with axial traction. In ad-

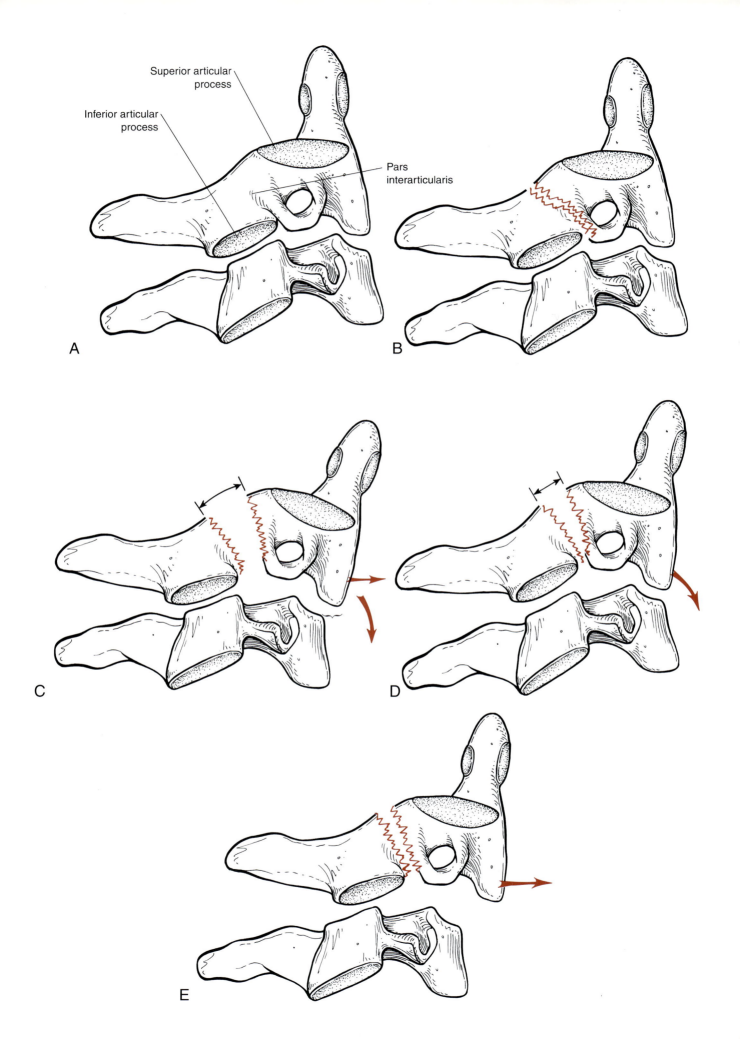

dition to horizontal displacement, the fracture orientation of a Type II injury is usually oriented in a vertical direction at the junction of the anterior pars and C2 body, whereas the fracture line in the Type IIA fracture is more oblique.

A Type III fracture usually results from a pure flexion force that results in either a unilateral or bilateral dislocation or fracture dislocation of the C2, C3 facet joint, followed by a fracture of the midportion of the pars interarticularis or posterior elements. The fracture of the posterior elements is usually a lamina fracture in an oblique orientation extending from anterior superior to posterior inferior, exiting posterior to the inferior facet joint. This injury usually signifies disruption of both the anterior and posterior longitudinal ligaments.

Burke, in 1989, and later Star and Eismont in 1993, described an atypical variant to the hangman's fracture in which the fracture line extended unilaterally or bilaterally through the posterior body and cortex of the axis (22, 108). With anterior translation of the C2 body and cephalad cervicocranium, the canal area at the level of fracture actually narrows rather than increases, causing potential spinal cord compression between the posterior cortical margin of the nondisplaced C2 body and the neural arch. Star and Eismont reported on six patients with this fracture configuration of which one-third (2/6) presented with a neurologic deficit (108).

Many hangman variants have been described in the literature. It is important to recognize the character of each individual fracture to infer the correct pathoanatomy and allow safe and effective treatment.

C2 Lateral Mass Fractures

Isolated fractures of the lateral mass of the axis result from axial compression and lateral flexion. These fractures are considered stable injuries and are rarely associated with any neurologic deficit, buy may result in considerable symptomatic arthritic changes at long-term follow-up.

C2 Body Fractures

Isolated C2 body fractures may result from either a compressive or distraction force, resulting in considerable fracture instability depending on its type. A typical distraction injury seen on the lateral plain roentgenograph is the appearance of an anterior inferior C2 body fracture. This fracture may either represent a benign hyperextension tear drop avulsion injury by the anterior longitudinal ligament (seen commonly in the elderly osteoporotic spine) or a hyperextension body fracture dislocation resulting from an avulsion injury through the insertion of Sharpey's fibers of the anterior annulus of the C2, C3 disc space. Burke found that in a hyperextension tear drop fracture, the vertical height of the body fracture fragment is equal to or greater than the horizontal length of the fracture fragment. He also found that there is minimal soft tissue swelling noted on the lateral plain roentgenograph (22). In a hyperextension body fracture dislocation, the transverse fracture width is greater than the vertical fracture height. There is also significant prevertebral swelling noted on a lateral plain roentgenograph.

C2 Lamina Fractures

Isolated fractures of the C2 lamina usually result from hyperextension or compressive forces and are usually associated with other fractures or ligamentous injuries to the cervicocranium.

Treatment

The vast majority of injuries to the axis may be treated nonoperatively with or without cervical traction. Fortunately, a majority of injuries at this level are not associated with neurologic embarrassment and associated spinal cord compression that necessitates surgical decompression. The usefulness of Levine and Edwards' fracture classification is that the pathoanatomy of each fracture type and each mechanism of injury is described, assisting in fracture management (67). Type I hangman fractures are minimally displaced and are considered stable injuries. They may be treated with a rigid cervicothoracic orthosis or halo for approximately 2 to 3 months. At the completion of immobilization, dynamic films should be obtained to assess the presence of ligamentous instability. At follow-up, approximately 30% of patients may be left with advanced symptomatic degenerative disc disease. Rarely does the C2, C3 disc autofuse in this fracture subtype because of the lack of significant disc disruption at the time of injury.

Type II fractures may exhibit significant translation and angulation. Published reports recommend prolonged halo or tong traction for 4 to 6 weeks in

FIGURE 15.9.
A. Effendi's three-part classification system of traumatic spondylolisthesis of the axis classification system as modified by Levine and Edwards. **B.** Type I—a bilateral fracture through the pars interarticularis with less than 3 mm of fracture displacement without evidence of angulation. **C.** Type II—a fracture of the pars interarticularis with translation greater than 3 mm with significant angulation. **D.** Type IIA—a fracture of the pars interarticularis with no or slight translation, but with significant angulation. **E.** Type III—a fracture of the pars interarticularis with evidence of a unilateral or bilateral facet dislocation of C2 on C3.

extension with low weights (10 to 20 pounds) in fractures presenting with displacement of greater than 4.5 mm or angulation greater than 15 mm (69). A cervical roll may be placed posteriorly at approximately the C4, 5 level to assist in obtaining cervical lordosis and fracture reduction. Unfortunately, no study has documented long-term disability caused by symptomatic arthrosis, fracture nonunion, or instability from residual fracture displacement in patients who are not adequately reduced on initial evaluation (41, 47). Even with attempted traction reduction for 4 to 6 weeks, many authors have reported residual fracture translation of 60% and angulation 40% of the original displacement (67). Type II fractures with less significant displacement usually can be reduced easily in slight extension with low weight axial traction and immobilized immediately in halo orthosis for 8 to 12 weeks. Closed reduction under anesthesia with fluoroscopic guidance is also a practiced means of treating Type II fractures, but it must be considered prudently in light of the success noted with other treatment methods (50). Francis, and later, Fielding, noted no difference in clinical outcome in a similar patient population treated with either immediate halo immobilization, short-term traction, or traction for 6 weeks (41, 47). Clinical instability at follow-up may be treated with an anterior C2, C3 fusion if nonhealing is noted at the par interarticularis or a posterior C1-C3 or C2-C3 fusion in cases of instability with healing present at the fracture site. Seventy percent of Type II fractures eventually go on to spontaneous fusion at the C2, C3 disc space at follow-up because of residual hematoma formation that results from disc disruption and contiguous endplate injuries at this level (20, 67).

Because of their unique pathoanatomy, Type IIA fractures should not be treated in traction due to the possibility of overdistraction at the fracture site. These injuries should be reduced gently in extension and immobilized in a halo for approximately 3 months (67, 69).

Type III fractures with a unilateral or bilateral jumped facet are extremely difficult to reduce by closed means and usually require an open reduction followed by internal fixation. If the fracture is at the level of the pars bilaterally, then spinous process wiring of C2 to C3 is adequate fixation, followed by rigid halo immobilization for reduction and stabilization of the pars interarticularis fracture. If the fracture is more posterior at the level of the C2, C3 facet, fusion may need to be extended to the C1 level to maintain alignment of the C2–3 facet joint. Alternative means of stabilization after reduction include C2 pedicle or isthmus screw fixation across the pars defect or reduction and internal fixation followed by an anterior C2, C3 fusion with or without internal fixation. In this situation, the only potential intact structure, i.e. the anterior longitudinal ligament, would be compromised.

The need for surgical treatment of a C2 hangman fracture is rare. Surgery should be considered in cases of Type III fracture-dislocations or evidence of objective instability at the C2, C3 level at follow-up on dynamic flexion extension lateral roentgenographs. The long-term outcome of this injury is favorable, with an expected nonunion rate of about 5.5% and with a residual neurologic deficit reported in approximately 6.5% of cases (47).

Surgical Treatment of Upper Cervical Spine Injuries

Technical Considerations

Posterior Cervical Exposure

Posterior surgical approaches to the cervical spine are discussed elsewhere in this book; therefore, only specific highlights will be explored. The vertebral artery exits the C1 foramen transversarium from inferior to superior and courses lateral to medial within a superior groove on the C1 posterior lamina prior to ascending into the foramen magnum. The course of this vessel must be kept in mind when performing any posterior exposure of the C1 level to avoid injury to this superficial structure. A posterior exposure of the cervical spine at this level should be extended no further than 1 cm from the midline in children and 1.5 to 2 cm in the adult to protect the vertebral artery.

The C2 spinous process anatomically is considerably larger than the remaining spinous processes in the subaxial spine, except for the C7 level. This size is due to its biomechanical role as an important insertion site for the posterior deep cervical musculature of the neck and the interspinous and supraspinous ligaments. On all exposures to the upper cervical spine, the inferior muscular attachments into the C2 spinous process should be preserved to maintain the physiologic posterior tethering structures, thereby maintaining normal cervical lordosis. If one is unable to retain these muscular attachments during exposure, compulsive attention to reattachment of these structures at the time of closure should be carried out.

Instrumentation

Sublaminar Wires

A useful method of safe C1 and C2 sublaminar wire passage is through the assistance of a free vascular aneurysmal needle threaded with a #1 silk. The pointed end of the vascular needle is removed with a wire cutter, and the eye of the needle is threaded with a #1 silk. The eye of the needle is then passed beneath the respective lamina from inferior to superior after the attached ligamentum flavum has carefully been dissected free with the use of sharp small curved curettes and right angled instruments. Once the needle with attached silk thread is passed successfully beneath the lamina, the thread is then tied to a chosen sublaminar wire, which is then pulled gently beneath the respective lamina. A right-angled instrument may be used to protect the underlying dural sac at the C1, C2 level by imparting a posterior directed force to the sublaminar wire as it passes between both lamina. Wires may also be passed through the C2 spinous process at the level of the spinolaminar line with the use of a right-angled burr. Wire may also be passed through the substance of the lamina of the C1 level to avoid sublaminar wire placement.

Wire fixation to the occiput may be accomplished in numerous ways, two of which are described here. The first is through drill holes through both cortices of the calvarium, approximately 5 mm lateral to the apex of the occipital inion. This method risks injury to the underlying epidural veins, sinuses, and dura. The second method involves developing a trough with a 4- to 5-mm burr on both sides of the inion. A right angled burr is then used to connect a passageway between both gutters for wire placement. A towel clip further enlarges the burr holes for passage of a 16- to 24-gauge wire (115). The level of wire passage should be approximately 1 to 2.5 cm about the inferior rim of the foramen magnum (82). The wire may be looped on itself for greater holding strength.

An effective means of stabilizing the C1, C2 joint posteriorly through the use of sublaminar wires is the modification of the technique described by Brooks in 1978 (18). In this technique, sublaminar wires are placed beneath the lamina of C1 midline. This technique improves the degree of rotational stability afforded by the standard Gallie fusion. The Gallie fusion technique was described originally as using a single looped wire passed underneath the lamina of C1 with both free ends of the wire passed within the loop to lasso the posterior C1 ring (49). The wires were then subsequently fixed over a bone graft between the C1, C2 lamina and then secured to themselves after being passed through the spinous process of C2 (Fig. 15.10). The Brooks fusion has increased rotational stability. More recently described techniques using screw fixation have further improved the stability obtained in posterior C1, C2 fusion techniques—this is discussed in the next section.

Screw Fixation

Screws may be used for posterior fixation of the upper cervical spine within the isthmus of C2, the C2, C1 facet complex, and the occiput.

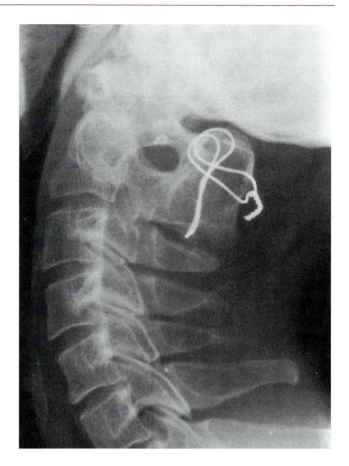

FIGURE 15.10.

Lateral plain radiograph showing C1-C2 modified Gallie wiring and solid fusion.

C2 Isthmus or Pedicle Screws

C2 isthmus fixation is an effective means of upper cervical spine fixation. Before their placement, a transaxial CT scan of the C2 vertebral body should be obtained to determine the width and angulation of the C2 isthmus (pedicle) and to identify the path of the vertebral artery. During exposure of the C2 isthmus, dissection is carried laterally along the superior border of the C2 lamina to its junction with the C2 isthmus. A Penfield #4 is then used to gently palpate the inner or medial wall of the C2 isthmus to determine appropriate screw direction and to evaluate for thread penetration within the canal at the time of screw insertion. Because of the path of the vertebral artery from inferomedially to superolaterally within the C2 foramen transversarium, the starting point for screw insertion is the upper medial quadrant of the C2 lateral mass. The direction of screw passage is approximately 15 to 20° medially and 15 to 20° superiorly, allowing passage of the screw into the dense subchondral bone of the C2 superior articular facet. A 3.5 mm cancellous screw measuring approximately 14 to 16 mm is used most frequently with in the C2 isthmus.

Posterior C1-C2 Facet Screw Fixation

An effective method of immobilizing the C2, C1 articular facet is through C1-C2 facet screw fixation as described by Magerl (71) (Fig. 15.11). This technique is biomechanically superior to both the Gallie and Brooks fusion techniques (55). In this method, a 3.5 mm cortical screw is placed obliquely in the sagittal plane, beginning at the posterior inferior C2 facet, transversing superiorly through the C2 superior articular process into the inferior C1 articular process, and finally ending within the C1 lateral mass (Fig. 15.12). Again, before screw insertion, a thinly sliced CT scan with sagittal reconstruction should be obtained to document the path of the vertebral artery as well as to determine the appropriate screw length at surgery. Before the operative procedure, the patient is placed in a halo ring, which is attached to a modified Mayfield headrest through a screw attachment. This allows clear visualization of the C1, C2 vertebral body with lateral fluoroscopy with the patient positioned prone at the time of surgery. The patient is ventilated with an extended tubing between the endotracheal tube and the respirator to allow the pa-

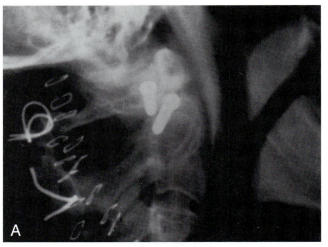

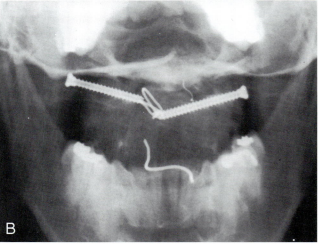

FIGURE 15.12.

A. An AP and (**B**) lateral plain roentgenograph illustrating a C1, C2 fusion with bilateral screw fixation by the lateral approach of Whitesides and Kelly.

tient's head to be opposite from the anesthesiologist, thereby allowing easy entry of the fluoroscopic unit. The C2, C1 facet joint is exposed, with careful attention to avoid injury to the greater occipital nerve which exits between the C1 and C2 lamina. A cavernous complex of veins is usually encountered overlying the C2, C1 facet joint. Excessive time should not be spent in coagulating these veins because of their lack of true endothelial boundaries. This venous complex should be packed off with a Gelfoam and paddy and then gently elevated and dissected laterally for exposure of the underlying C1, C2 facet joint. After both joints are exposed bilaterally, their articular cartilage is curetted sharply with a small 3–0 curved curette. The surgical exposure is limited to the C1, C2 level, necessitating percutaneous placement of the 3.5-mm cortical screw at approximately the C6 to T1 level to obtain the appropriate sagittal alignment for screw fixation. The appropriate

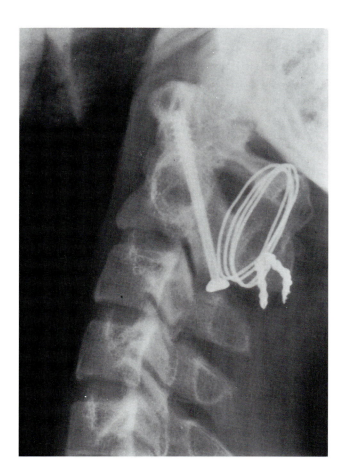

FIGURE 15.11.

Lateral plain radiograph showing Brooks wiring and fusion and Magerl's C1-C2 facet screws.

level of screw insertion is confirmed by placing a probe along the outside of the patient's neck and obtaining a lateral fluoroscopic image. The standard equipment for placement of the fixation screw includes a large outer cannular and inner blunt trochar, an inner drill cannula, a 3.5-mm cortical tap, and a long 2.5-mm drill bit. All drilling is performed under lateral fluoroscopic visualization as well as visual inspection of the medial isthmus of C2 to avoid canal intrusion. Once drilling is accomplished, an inner 3.5-mm cortical tap is placed through the cannular system, followed by the screw. Many surgeons prefer to reduce the C2,C1 facet joint temporarily with a K-wire on one side and then proceed with fixation on the other side to maintain reduction.

The starting point of screw fixation is around 2 mm lateral to the lamina lateral mass junction of C2 at the posteroinferior border of the C2 inferior facet. The path of the drill in the coronal plane is parallel to the canal to avoid canal penetration and vertebral artery injury. The sagittal plane direction is determined by fluoroscopy and is usually 50 to 60° from the horizontal. The average length of screw is approximately 40 to 45 mm in the adult patient. A Gallie or Brooks fusion is added routinely at the completion of the procedure to insure fusion of the C2, C1 articulation. Before tightening down both screws, cancellous bone graft is placed within the C2, C1 decorticated facet joints.

Posterior Occipital Screw Placement

Screw placement into the occiput is fraught with potential difficulties, depending on the choice of unilateral or bicortical screw fixation. Although bicortical screw fixation would appear to be the most stable biomechanically, this has not been proven in cadaveric studies and must be considered in light of the potential complications to the underlying dura and venous sinuses. Before attempting screw fixation, the surgeon should have a good understanding of the topographic anatomy of the occiput. Five landmarks should be identified after the exposure of the occiput. These landmarks include the superior nuchal line, the inferior nuchal line, the inion, the external occipital protuberance, and the posterior edge or rim of the foramen magnum. The thickness of the occiput increases as one moves from the foramen magnum to the superior nuchal line. This thickness also increases as one moves from lateral to medial towards the inion. The structures that should be avoided during screw application include the transverse sinus, which is located at approximately the level of the superior nuchal line or slightly above it in most people, and the confluence of the sinuses, which tends to be at the level of the external occipital protuberance or slightly above it. Penetration of the outer sinus wall may result in excessive blood loss, while penetration of the inner sinus wall may result in a fatal subdural hematoma.

The optimal occipital cervical implant should be a plate that allows screw fixation into the subaxial cervical lateral masses and isthmus of C2 and curves gently from lateral to medial over the thickest portion of the occiput. This implant should extend proximally to the level of the superior nuchal line. Because of the limitation of existing screw implants, 2.7 cortical screws are used most frequently in the occiput due to their short length. Using standard AO instrumentation, 3.5 cortical screws may be used when the screw length is 10 mm or greater. The choice of unicortical or bicortical fixation depends on the surgeon.

Anterior Dens Screw Fixation

The placement of a screw anteriorly for fixation of a Type II or shallow Type III odontoid fracture is done to preserve axial rotation at the C1, C2 facet joint. It is also done in cases of posterior element deficiency in fractures in which sublaminar wire passage at C1 is not possible. Some authors prefer screw placement in polytrauma patients or in the elderly to avoid the use of a bulky, and at times, obstructive halo vest. To date, there have been no reported cases of catastrophic neurologic events with the use of an anterior odontoid screw (54). The successful application of this technique requires a presurgical transaxial CT scan to measure the diameter of the odontoid waist, thus determining the number of screws that may be placed safely within it. The preferred implants at this time are two 3.5-mm cancellous lag screws requiring a minimum of an 8 mm wide odontoid waist. Recently, several studies have shown that a single screw, with less attendant risk, may be just as effective as two screws in obtaining a fusion (24, 54, 93). Sasso found no difference between one and two screws in loads to failure using a single 3.5-mm cortical screw, and concluded that the accuracy of reduction was more important than the number of screws used (93).

Patient selection is vital to the success of this technique. Patients who have a barrel chest or short neck make drill insertion at the appropriate angle difficult. An anatomic reduction of the odontoid should be obtained before the operative procedure because of the danger and technical difficulty of obtaining reduction intraoperatively. To facilitate screw placement, patients who present initially with a posteriorly displaced fracture should undergo reduction and then be positioned with their neck in slight extension and their head translated anteriorly. Patients who present initially with an anterior displaced odontoid fracture that is subsequently reduced should have their head positioned in slight posterior translation with their cervical spine slightly extended.

Nasotracheal intubation and a radiolucent mouthpiece can improve the visualization obtained with biplanar fluoroscopy at the time of surgery. Both shoulders may be displaced forward with the placement of a posterior transverse roll to improve ease of drill and screw placement. The standard Smith-Robinson surgical approach is done, usually centered at the C5, 6 level to allow for accurate screw placement in the sagittal plane (103). The anteroinferior endplate of the C2 vertebral body is identified, and a small recess may be made within the C2, 3 disk or anterosuperior C3 body to allow for ease of guide wire or drill placement. The drill path should be directed towards the posterosuperior tip of the odontoid. The choice of one or two 3.5-mm cancellous lag screws or a single 4.5-mm screw depends on the preference of the surgeon. The average screw length is approximately 32 to 40 mm (76). The odontoid tip may be minimally penetrated for better fixation.

Complications with this technique have been reported by several authors. Worsdofer reported 23 patients and noted six screw breakouts, three nonunions, one carotid artery injury, one fracture re-dislocation and late myelopathy, and the formation of an esophagotracheal fistula (120). Aebi reported on 15 patients and noted two screw breakouts and one case of nonunion (2). Although this technique appears theoretically promising in reducing the morbidity of a posterior cervical fusion that may decrease axial rotation, because of its infrequent use and unfamiliarity with most surgeons, a standard posterior C1, C2 fusion appears to be the operation of choice in most clinical settings.

Lateral Retropharyngeal Approach

An alternative means of fusing the C2, C1 joint when a posterior approach is not feasible is the lateral approach to the upper cervical spine, as described by Whitesides and Kelly in 1966 (116). This approach exposes the lateral aspect of the upper cervical vertebrae through posterior rather than anterior dissection to the carotid sheath. At the completion of exposure, the anterior articular facet of C2, C1 is exposed. The intertransverse membrane between the C1 and C2 transverse processes is preserved and the articular cartilage is subsequently denuded within the C2, C1 joint surface in preparation for autologous bone grafting. Once the bone grafting is completed, a 2-mm guide wire is placed at the anterior base of the C1 transverse process and directed 25° inferiorly in the coronal plane and 10° posteriorly in the sagittal plane. This placement is done bilaterally and is confirmed with intraoperative radiography. A cannulated drill is then placed over the guide wire, followed by an appropriate-length 3.5 cortical screw. The lateral C1 mass can be over drilled with a 3.5 cannulated drill to compress the facet joint at screw insertion. This technique is rarely useful, but it should be considered when other approaches may not be technically feasible.

Conclusion

The appropriate management of upper cervical spine injuries requires a high index of suspicion for associated spinal injuries as well as subtle ligamentous instabilities that may be missed on initial evaluation. A thorough knowledge of the anatomy, biomechanics, and clinical significance of the various classification systems for each injury pattern must be mastered to institute effective care to this patient population. New techniques for surgical stabilization of this region of the spine are evolving. They should be technically mastered in the cadaveric laboratory before their application in the clinical setting because of the potential for serious neurologic and vascular injury in this region of the spinal. Fortunately, the majority of injuries at this level can be treated effectively with nonoperative means.

References

1. Ackerson TT, Patzakis MJ, Moore TM, et al. Fractures of the odontoid: A ten-year retrospective study. Contemp Orthop 1982;4:54–67.
2. Aebi M, Etter C, Coscia M. Fractures of the odontoid process: treatment with anterior screw fixation. Spine 1989;14:1065–1070.
3. Alker GJ Jr, OH YS, Leslie EV. High cervical spine and craniocervical junction injuries in fatal traffic accidents. Orthop Clin North Am 1978;9:1003–1010.
4. Althoff B. Fracture of the odontoid process. An experimental and clinical study. Acta Orthop Scand Suppl 1979;177:1–95.
5. Althoff B, Goldie IF. The arterial supply of the odontoid process of the axis. Acta Orthop Scand 1977;48:622–629.
6. Altongy JF, Fielding JW. Combined atlanto-axial and occipitoatlantal rotatory subluxation. A case report. J Bone Joint Surg Am 1990;72:923–926.
7. Amyes EW, Anderson FM. Fracture of the odontoid process of the axis. Arch Surg 1956;72:377–393.
8. An HS. Posterior instrumentation of the cervical spine. In: Cotler HS, Spinal JM, eds. Instrumentation. Baltimore: Williams & Wilkins, 1992:37–47.
9. Anderson LD, Clark CR. Fractures of the odontoid process of the axis. In: Cervical Spine Research Society Editors Committee, eds. The cervical spine. 2nd ed. Philadelphia: JB Lippincott, 1989:325–343.
10. Anderson LDD, D'Alonzo RT. Fractures of the odontoid process of the axis. J Bone Joint Surg Am 1974;56:1663–1674.
11. Anderson PA, Montesano PX. Morphology and treatment of occipital condyle fractures. Spine 1988;13:731–736.

12. Apuzzo MLK, Heiden JS, Weis MH, et al. Acute fractures of the odontoid process. J Neurosurg 1978;48:85–91.
13. Barros TEP, Fielding JW. Traumatic spondylolisthesis of the axis with unusual distraction. J Bone Joint Surg Am 1990;72:124–125.
14. Bell W, Meyer P. Non halo/non-surgical management of C1-C2 fractures. Ortho Trans 1983;7:481.
15. Bohlman HH. Acute fractures and dislocations of the cervical spine. An analysis of three hundred hospitalized patients and review of the literature. J Bone Joint Surg Am 1979;61:1119–1142.
16. Bolender N, Cromwell LD, Wendling L. Fracture of the occipital condyle. Orthop Clin North Am 1978;131:729–731.
17. Bozboga M, Unal F, Hepgul K, et al. Fracture of the occipital condyle. Case report. Spine 1992;17:1119–1121.
18. Brooks AL, Jenkins EB. Atlanto-axial arthrodesis by the wedge compression method. J Bone Joint Surg Am 1978;60:279–284.
19. Bucholz RW, Burkhead WZ. The pathologic anatomy of fatal atlanto-occipital dislocation. J Bone Joint Surg Am 1979;61:248–250.
20. Bucholz RW. Unstable hangman's fractures. Clin Orthop 1981;154:119–124.
21. Bunders DA, Rechtine GR, Bohlman HH. Upper cervical spine injuries. Orthop Rev 1984;13:23–32.
22. Burke JT, Harris JH. Acute injuries of the axis vertebrae. Skeletal Radiol 1989;18:335–346.
23. Chan BPK, Morwessel RM, Leung KYK. Treatment of odontoid fractures with halo cast immobilization. Orthop Trans 1981;5:118–119.
24. Chang KW, Liu YW, Cheng PG, et al. One Herbert double-threaded compression screw fixation of displaced Type II odontoid fractures. J Spinal Disord 1994;7:62–69.
25. Clark CR. Dens fractures. Semin Spine Surg 1991;3:39–46.
26. Clark CR, Kathol MH, Walsh T, et al. Atlantoaxial rotatory fixation with compensatory counter occipitoatlantal subluxation. A case report. Spine 1986;11:1048–1050.
27. Clark CR, White AA. fractures of the dens: a multicenter study. J Bone Joint Surg Am 1985;67:1340–1348.
28. Craft DV, Cotler JM, Bauerle WB. A rational approach to the management of type II and type III odontoid fractures. Unpublished data. Presented at the AAOS annual meeting, Washington, DC, 1991.
29. Day GL, Jacoby CG, Dolan KD. Basilar invagination resulting from untreated Jefferson's fracture. Am J Roentgenol 1979;133:529–531.
30. Desai SS, Coumas JM, Danylevich A, et al. Fracture of the occipital condyle: case report and review of the literature. J Trauma 1990;30:240–241.
31. Dickman CA, Papadopoulos SM, Sonntag VKH, et al. Traumatic occipitoatlantal dislocations. J Spinal Disord 1993;6:300–313.
32. Donovan MM. Efficacy of rigid fixation of fractures of the odontoid process and retrospective analysis of fifty-four cases. Orthop Trans 1979;3:309.
33. Dublin AB, Marks WM, Weinstock D, et al. Traumatic dislocation of the atlanto-occipital articulation (AOA) with short term survival with a radiographic method of measuring the AOA. J Neurosurg 1980;52:541–546.
34. Dunn ME, Seljeskog EL. Experience in the management of odontoid process injuries. An analysis of 128 cases. J Neurosurg 1986;18:306–310.
35. Eismont FJ, Bohlman HH. Posterior atlanto-occipital dislocation with fractures of the atlas and odontoid process. Report of a case with survival. J Bone Joint Surg Am 1978;60:397–399.
36. Effendi B, Roy D, Cornish B, et al. Fracture of the ring and axis. A classification based on the analysis of 131 cases. J Bone Joint Surg Br 1981;63:319–327.
37. Ekong CEU, Schwartz ML, Tator CH, et al. Odontoid fracture: management with early mobilization using the halo device. Neurosurgery 1981;9:631–637.
38. El-Khoury GY, Kathol MH. Radiographic evaluation of cervical spine trauma. Semin Spine Surg 1991;3:3–23.
39. Fielding JW, Cochran G, Lawing JF III, et al. Tears of the transverse ligament of the atlas. A clinical and biomechanical study. J Bone Joint Surg Am 1974;56:1683–1691.
40. Fielding JW, Francis WR, Hawkins RJ, et al. Atlantoaxial rotary deformity. Semin Spine Surg 1991;3:33–38.
41. Fielding JW, Francis WR, Hawkins RJ, et al. Traumatic spondylolisthesis of the axis. Clin Orthop 1989;239:47–52.
42. Fielding JW, Hawkins RJ. Atlanto-axial rotatory fixation. J Bone Joint Surg Am 1977;59:37–44.
43. Fielding JW, Hawkins RJ. Roentgenographic diagnosis of the injured neck. American Academy of Orthopaedic Surgery Instructional Course Lectures 1976;25:149–169.
44. Fielding JW, Hensinger RN, Hawkins RJ. Os odontoideum. J Bone Joint Surg 1980;62A:376–383.
45. Fielding JW, Stillwee WT, Spyropoulos EC. Use of computed tomography for the diagnosis of atlantoaxial rotatory fixation. J Bone Joint Surg 1978;60A:1102–1104.
46. Fowler JL, Sandhu A, Fraser RD. A review of fractures of the atlas vertebra. J Spinal Disord 1990;3:19–24.
47. Francis WR, Fielding JW, Hawkins RJ, et al. Traumatic spondylolisthesis of the axis. J Bone Joint Surg Br 1981;63:313–318.
48. Gabrielsen TO, Maxwell JA. Traumatic atlanto-occipital dislocation. Am J Roentgenol 1966;97:624–629.
49. Gallie WE. Fractures and dislocations of the cervical spine. Am J Surg 1939;46:495–501.
50. Gargin SR, Rothman RH. Traumatic spondylolisthesis of the axis (Hangman's fracture). In: Cervical Spine Research Editors Committee, eds. The cervical spine. Philadelphia: JB Lippincott, 1989:344–354.
51. Gerhart TN, White AA III. An impacted dens fracture in an elderly woman. Clin Orthop 1982;167:173–175.
52. Goldstein SJ, Woodring JA, Young AB. Occipital condyle fracture associated with cervical spine injury. Surg Neurol 1982;17:350–352.
53. Grantham SA, Lipson SJ. Rheumatoid arthritis of the cervical spine. In: Cervical Spine Research Society Ed-

itors Committee, eds. The cervical spine. 2nd ed. Philadelphia: JB Lippincott, 1989:564–572.
54. Graziano G, Jaggers C, Lee M, et al. A comparative study of fixation techniques for Type II fractures of the odontoid process. Spine 1993;18:2383–2387.
55. Grob D, Crisco JJ, Panjabi MM, et al. Biomechanical evaluation of four different posterior atlantoaxial fixation techniques. Spine 1992;17:481–490.
56. Hadley MN, Browner CM, Liv SS, et al. New subtype of acute odontoid fractures (type IIA). Neurosurgery 1988;22:67–71.
57. Hadley MN, Dickman CA, Browner CM, et al. Acute axis fractures: a review of 229 cases. J Neurosurg 1989;71:642–647.
58. Hadley MN, Dickman CA, Browner CM, et al. Acute traumatic atlas fractures: management and long term outcome. Neurosurgery 1988;23:31–35.
59. Hinchey JJ, Bickel WH. Fractures of the atlas. Review and presentation of data on eight cases. Ann Surg 1945;121:826–832.
60. Holness RO, Huestis WS, Howes WJ, et al. Posterior stabilization with an interlaminar clamp in cervical injuries: technical note and review of the long term experience with the method. Neurosurgery 1984;14:318–322.
61. Hosong N, Yonenobu K, Kawagoe K, et al. Traumatic anterior atlanto-occipital dislocation. Spine 1992;18:786–790.
62. Husby J, Sorensen KH. Fracture of the odontoid process of the axis. Acta Orthop Scand 1974;45:182–192.
63. Jefferson E. Fracture of the atlas vertebra. Report of four cases and a review of those previously recorded. Br J Surg 1920;7:407–422.
64. Keterson L, Benzel E, Orrison W, et al. Evaluation and treatment of atlas burst fractures (Jefferson fractures). J Neurosurg 1991;75:213–220.
65. Landells CD, Peteghem PKV. Fractures of the atlas: classification, treatment and morbidity. Spine 1987;13:450–452.
66. Levine AM, Edwards CC. Fractures of the atlas. J Bone Joint Surg Am 1991;73:680–691.
67. Levine AM, Edwards CC. The management of traumatic spondylolisthesis of the axis. J Bone Joint Surg Am 1985;67:217–226.
68. Levine AM, Edwards CC. Traumatic lesions of the occipito-atlanto-axial complex. Clin Orthop 1989;239:53–68.
69. Levine AM, Rhyne AL. Traumatic spondylolisthesis of the axis. Semin Spine Surg 1991;3:47–60.
70. Levine AM, Edwards CC. Treatment of injuries in the C1-C2 complex. Orthop Clin North Am 1986;17:31–44.
71. Magerl F, Seeman PS. Stable posterior fusion of the atlas and axis by transarticular screw fixation. In: Kehr P, Weidner A, eds. The cervical spine. Wein-New York-Vienna: Springer-Verlag, 1987:322–327.
72. McAfee PC, Cassidy JR, Davis RF, et al. Fusion of the occiput to the upper cervical spine. A review of 37 cases. Spine 1991;16S:490–494.
73. McAfee PC. Cervical spine trauma. In: Frymoyer JW, ed. The adult spine: principles and practice. New York: Raven Press, 1991:1063–1106.
74. Meyer PR Jr, Cotler HB. Fusion techniques for traumatic injuries. In: Coster JM, Cotler HB, eds. Spinal fusion: science and techniques. New York: Springer-Verlag, 1990:189–246.
75. Meyer PR Jr, Heim S. Surgical stabilization of the cervical spine. In Meyer PR Jr, ed. Surgery of spine trauma. New York: Churchill Livingstone, 1989:397–523.
76. Meyer PR Jr, Rusin JJ, Haak MH. Anterior instrumentation of the cervical spine. In: An HS, Cotler JM, eds. Spinal instrumentation. Baltimore: Williams & Wilkins, 1992:61–66.
77. Miz G. Cervical spine instability and biomechanics of treatment. In: Errico TJ, Rauer RD, Waugh T, eds. Spinal trauma, 2nd ed. Philadelphia: JB Lippincott, 1991:123–140.
78. Montane I, Eismont FJ, Green BA. Traumatic occipitoatlantal dislocation. Spine 1991;16:112–116.
79. Moskovich R, Crocard HA. Post-traumatic atlantoaxial subluxation and myelopathy. Efficacy of anterior decompression. Spine 1990;15:442–447.
80. Mouradian WH, Fietti VG Jr, Cochran GVV, et al. Fractures of the odontoid. A laboratory and clinical study of mechanism. Orthop Clin North Am 1978;9:985–1001.
81. Murphy MJ, Wu JC, Southwick WO. Complications of halo fixation. Ortho Trans 1979;3:126.
82. Murphy MJ, Southwick WO. Surgical approaches and techniques. In: Cervical Spine Research Society Editors Committee, eds. The cervical spine, 2nd ed. Philadelphia: JB Lippincott, 1989:775–791.
83. Panjabi MM, Oda T, Crisco JJ, et al. Experimental study of atlas injuries I. Biomechanical analysis of their mechanism and fracture patterns. Spine 1991;16S:460–465.
84. Paradis GR, Jones JM. Post traumatic atlantoaxial instability: the fate of the odontoid process fracture in 46 cases. J Trauma 1973;13:359–366.
85. Pederson AK, Kostuik JP. Complete fracture-dislocation of the atlantoaxial complex: case report and recommendations for a new classification of dens fractures. J Spinal Disord 1994;7:350–355.
86. Pierce DS, Barr JS. Fractures and dislocations at the base of the skull and upper cervical spine. In: Cervical Spine Research Editors Committee, eds. The cervical spine. Philadelphia: JB Lippincott, 1989:312–324.
87. Pierce DS, Barr JS. Use of the halo in cervical spine problems. Ortho Trans 1979;3:125.
88. Powers B. Traumatic anterior-occipital dislocations. Neurosurgery 1979;4:12–17.
89. Price AE. Unique aspects of pediatric spine injuries. In: Errico TJ, Bauer RD, Waugh T, eds. Spinal trauma. Philadelphia: JB Lippincott, 1991:581–625.
90. Ryan MD, Taylor TKF. Odontoid fractures, a rational approach to treatment. J Bone Joint Surg Br 1982;64:416–421.
91. Ryan M, Taylor TKF. Odontoid fractures in the elderly. J Spinal Disord 1993;6:397–401.
92. Sassard WR, Heinig CF, Pitts WR. Posterior atlantoaxial dislocation without fracture. Case report with successful conservative treatment. J Bone Joint Surg Am 1974;56:625–628.

93. Sasso R, Doherty BJ, Crawford JM, et al. Biomechanics of odontoid fracture fixation. Spine 1993;18:1950–1953.
94. Schatzker J, Rorabeck CH, Waddell JP. Fractures of the dens (odontoid process). An analysis of thirty-seven cases. J Bone Joint Surg Br 1971;53:392–405.
95. Shatzker J, Rorabeck CH, Waddell JP. Non-union of the odontoid process: an experimental investigation. Clin Orthop 1975;108:127–137.
96. Schiff DCM, Parke WW. The arterial supply of the odontoid process. J Bone Joint Surg Am 1973;55:1450–1456.
97. Schneider RC, Livingston KE, Cave AJE, et al. Hangman's fracture of the cervical spine. J Neurosurg 1965;22:141–154.
98. Scott EW, Haid RW, Peace D. Type I fractures of the odontoid process: implications for atlanto-occipital instability. J Neurosurg 1990;72:488–492.
99. Segal LS, Grimm JO, Stauffer SE. Non-union of fractures of the atlas. J Bone Joint Surg Am 1987;69:1423–1433.
100. Sherk HH. Fractures of the atlas and odontoid process. Orthop Clin North Am 1978;9:973–983.
101. Sherk HH. Lesions of the atlas and axis. Clin Orthop 1975;109:33–41.
102. Sherk HH, Nicholson JT. Fracture of the atlas. J Bone Joint Surg Am 1970;52:1017–1024.
103. Smith GW, Robinson RA. The treatment of certain cervical spine disorders by anterior removal of the intervertebral disc and interbody fusion. J Bone Joint Surg Am 1958;40:607–624.
104. Sonntag VKH, Hadley MN, Spetzler RF. The transoral-transclival approach to the upper cervical spine. In: Sundaresan N, et al., eds. Tumors of the spine. Diagnosis and clinical management. Philadelphia: WB Saunders, 1990:319–329.
105. Southwick WO. Current concept review: management of fractures of the dens (odontoid process). J Bone Joint Surg Am 1980;62:482–486.
106. Spence KF, Decker S, Sell KW. Bursting atlantal fracture associated with rupture of the transverse ligament. J Bone Joint Surg Am 1970;52:543–549.
107. Spencer JA, Yeakley JW, Kaufman HH. Fracture of the occipital condyle. J Neurosurg 1984;15:101–103.
108. Starr JK, Eismont FJ. Atypical hangman's fractures. Spine 1993;18:1954–1957.
109. Steel HH. Anatomical and mechanical considerations of the atlanto-axial articulations. J Bone Joint Surg Am 1968;50:1481–1482.
110. Stewart G. Horizontal fracture of the anterior arch of the atlas. Radiology 1977;122:349–352.
111. Traynelis VC, Marano GD, Dunker RO, et al. Traumatic atlanto-occipital dislocation. Case report. J Neurosurg 1986;65:863–870.
112. Wackenheim A. Roentgen diagnosis of the craniovertebral region. Berlin: Springer-Verlag, 1974.
113. Washington ER. Non-traumatic atlanto-occipital and atlanto-axial dislocation. J Bone Joint Surg Am 1959;41:341–344.
114. Werne S. Studies in spontaneous atlas dislocation. Acta Orthop Scand Suppl 1957;23:1–28.
115. Wertheim SB, Bohlman HH. Occipitocervical fusion. Indications, techniques and long-term results in thirteen patients. J Bone Joint Surg Am 1987;69:833–836.
116. Whitesides TE Jr, Kelly RP. Lateral approach to the upper cervical spine for anterior fusion. South Med J 1966;59:879–883.
117. Wholey MH, Bruwer AJ, Baker HL. The lateral roentgenogram of the neck. Radiology 1958;71:350–356.
118. Wong DA, Mack RP, Craigmile TK. Traumatic atlanto-axial dislocation without fracture of the odontoid. Spine 1991;16:587–589.
119. Wood-Jones F. The ideal lesion produced by judicial hanging. Lancet 1913;1:53.
120. Worsdorfer O, Arnad M, Neugebauer R. Problems of anterior screw fixation of odontoid process fractures. Presented at the Second Common Meeting of the European and American Sections of the Cervical Spine Research Society. Marseilles, France, June 1988:12–15.

CHAPTER SIXTEEN

Thoracolumbar Spine Injuries

Geoffrey M. McCullen, Hansen A. Yuan, and Bruce E. Fredrickson

Introduction

Trauma to the thoracolumbar spine presents frequently. Such injuries, when associated with neurologic deficit, occur in approximately 50 of 1,000,000 people per year (99, 122). Most victims are males between the ages of 15 and 29 (99, 122). In a multicenter review of more than 1000 patients, 16% of injuries occurred between T1 and T10, 52% between T11 and L1, and 32% between L1 and L5 (65). Nearly half result from motor vehicle accidents, 20% from falls, 13% in sports-related events, and 11% from violence (122). Seat belts have significantly reduced the incidence of severe neurologic injury (65).

Associated injuries occur often (up to 50% of cases) depending on the type of fracture (25, 67, 72, 128, 142). These additional injuries often divert the attention of the evaluating physician and may lead to a missed or delayed diagnosis of the spine fracture. Half of those with spinal fracture resulting from a distraction force have an intra-abdominal injury, typically a ruptured viscus (72). Twenty percent have an associated pulmonary injury. Ten percent experience intra-abdominal bleeding secondary to a splenic or hepatic laceration (102). Multiple, noncontiguous spine fractures are detected in 6 to 15% of cases (94, 128). The 1-year mortality for thoracic level paraplegia is approximately 7% (40).

Isolated thoracolumbar fractures are also frequently seen in elderly women secondary to low energy trauma and pre-existing osteoporosis. These injuries may cause severe pain. Differentiation between osteoporotic fractures and pathologic fractures resulting from metabolic bone disease or osteomyelitis is often difficult. Paraplegia may occur from a slowly progressive deformity that occurs with vertebral body collapse (131).

Despite recent advances in surgical techniques and instrumentation, several issues are still contested: 1) indications for surgical intervention; 2) the optimal timing of such intervention; and 3) the best approach to decompression and fusion (anterior, posterior, and combined).

This chapter reviews the basic elements of diagnosis and treatment of thoracolumbar spine fractures. Special emphasis is placed on reviewing existing data, which may help to resolve some of the controversial issues.

Pathogenesis

Musculoskeletal Injury

Understanding how injuries affect the thoracolumbar spine requires a knowledge of spinal anatomy, biomechanics, and the common injury mechanisms. Many different classification schemes have been developed to define the injury and direct the treatment. These include anatomic, mechanistic and morphologic analyses, each emphasizing a different aspect of the injury.

The spine is faced with the difficult role of providing both stability and mobility. Anteriorly, the ver-

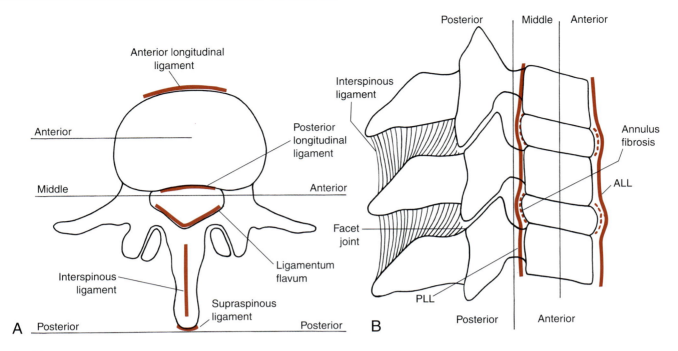

FIGURE 16.1.
Bony and ligamentous vertebral components emphasizing the columnar concepts of Holdsworth and Denis. **A**: axial plane. **B**: sagittal plane.

tebral body and disc joint face compressive loads. Posteriorly, the paired facet joints control rotation and sagittal plane translation. Ligaments providing stability between vertebrae include the anterior longitudinal ligament (ALL), the posterior longitudinal ligament (PLL), interspinous ligaments, the annulus fibrous, and the facet joint capsule.

Sagittal plane spinal contours include cervical lordosis, thoracic kyphosis, and lumbar lordosis. At the thoracic level, ribs provide an additional point of stability, making this segment less mobile than the adjacent spine. Facet joint orientation varies from a 45° angle to the coronal plane in the cervical and thoracic spine to increasing sagittal plane alignment in the lumbar spine. Transitional junctions exist between these anatomically and mechanically distinct segments at the cervicothoracic, thoracolumbar, and lumbosacral junctions. These zones are vulnerable to injury because forces tend to concentrate at the interface between mechanically different parts of the spine. Of 508 consecutive spine fractures treated at a single institution, 29% occurred at the cervicothoracic junction, and 21% occurred at the thoracolumbar junction (128).

The distance of a particular vertebrae from the center of gravity also affects its mechanical advantage. The T7 vertebral body lies at the apex of the thoracic kyphosis and therefore is the vertebrae most removed from the center of gravity. This region also coincides with the "watershed" zone, T5-T9, with decreased vascular supply to the spinal cord (37).

Thus, the junctions at either end of the thoracic spine and the mid-portion of the thoracic kyphosis are the "at risk" areas in thoracolumbar spine injury.

Anatomic Classification

Holdsworth was the first to propose a 2 "column" concept in an attempt to clinically define spinal stability (Fig. 16.1A and B) (82, 83). The anterior column transmits compressive load and consists of the vertebral body and intervertebral disc, the ALL, and the PLL. The posterior column carries tensile stress and includes the paired facet joints, the neural arch, and the interspinous ligaments.

Disruption of more than one column defines an "unstable" injury. Holdsworth emphasized the importance of the posterior ligaments, functioning as a tension band and effectively balancing the load that travels through the anterior column. For vertebral body burst fractures, a "stable" configuration implies that the posterior ligaments remain intact, whereas they are ruptured in "unstable" injuries.

Denis added to the work of Holdsworth with the development of the 3 column classification (28, 29). The anterior column consists of the anterior two-thirds of the vertebral body and the ALL. The middle column includes the posterior third of the vertebral body and disc with the PLL. The posterior column incorporates everything posterior to the PLL (Figs. 16.1A and B).

Using the Denis paradigm, disruption of more than

2 columns indicates instability. However, not all columns contribute equally to spinal stability. The middle column is actually not of great importance regarding biomechanical stability when compared with the contributing elements within the anterior or posterior columns (87, 119). Retropulsion of the middle column may cause neurologic dysfunction. The middle column therefore defines the type of intervention required.

Serial transections of cadaveric specimens have been performed to evaluate these columnar concepts (121). There is a difference in measured stability depending on whether the specimens are sectioned from anterior to posterior (AP) or posterior to anterior (PA). The PA sequence leads to failure in flexion under physiologic loads when all posterior components and one anterior component have been destroyed. The AP sequence causes failure in extension when all anterior components plus two posterior components are destroyed (121).

Mechanistic Classification

The specific spinal injury that occurs is a function of the rate, magnitude, and direction of the applied load, the position of the body at the time of applied load, and the pre-existing anatomic variations in the structure. Holdsworth described four types of forces (flexion, flexion with rotation, extension, and compression) (82, 83). Expansion of these mechanisms may reflect the six degrees of freedom of spinal motion about three axes: compression, distraction, flexion, extension, rotation, and shear (51).

Compression

With pure axial compression, the highest stresses concentrate in the middle of the end plate in the cancellous bone under the nucleus and the middle of the posterior wall cortex (132). With increasing load, the vertebral body fails, resulting in an anterior compression fracture. If load continues, the body implodes, the pedicles are driven apart, and the middle column retropulses posteriorly, resulting in a "burst." A "stable burst" implies that the posterior ligaments are intact (Fig. 16.2). Extensive damage occurs to the disc above and below the burst vertebrae (44,57).

Flexion-Compression

This is the most common mechanism of injury, representing nearly 50% of thoracolumbar fractures (25). The anterior column is compressed while posteriorly the ligamentous complex is under tension. The anterior vertebral body fails, followed by middle column retropulsion and posterior ligament disruption (119). The ALL remains intact. The PLL may be stretched depending on the severity of the posterior

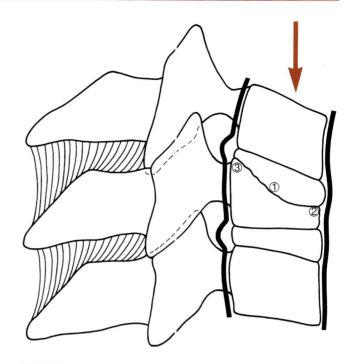

FIGURE 16.2.

Pure axial compression causes: (1) failure of the endplate under the nucleus; (2) anterior vertebral body compression or "wedge" fracture; (3) retropulsion of the middle column with intact posterior ligaments—a "stable burst" fracture.

tensile forces. "Unstable" burst fractures occur with disruption of the posterior ligaments (Fig. 16.3) (83). With the loss of the tethering effect of these posterior ligaments, late progression of kyphosis at the injured zone is possible.

Distraction

Distraction injuries occur less frequently than those caused by compression. Flexion-distraction mechanisms represent approximately 5% of thoracolumbar injuries (25). When the axis of rotation is in the anterior vertebral body (Figs 16.4 and 16.15), the result is a compression fracture of the anterior vertebral body and posterior ligament disruption with unilateral or bilateral facet joint disruption-dislocation. A concomitant burst fracture may be seen in up to 15% (67).

When the center of rotation is brought anterior to the vertebral column, an effective distraction force is applied to all three columns (Fig 16.5). In a seat-belt injury, the fulcrum is the seat-belt at the anterior abdominal wall (29). Posterior and middle columns disrupt in tension on an intact anterior hinge.

Tensile failure can occur through ligament, bone, or through a variable path that includes both. Chance first described three cases in 1948 and, as a group, such injuries continue to carry his name (23). He observed a fracture line through the spinous process,

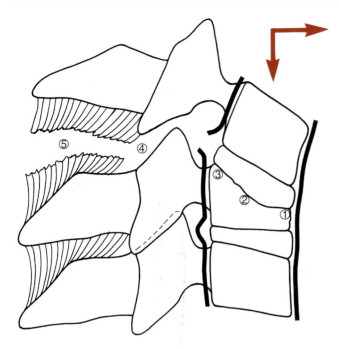

FIGURE 16.3.
Flexion-compression causes tensile stresses of the posterior ligamentous complex in addition to a vertebral body "burst": (1) failure of the endplate under the nucleus; (2) anterior vertebral body compression; (3) middle column retropulsion; (4) facet joint-capsule disruption; (5) interspinous ligament failure.

lamina, transverse processes, and pedicle, exiting on the superior surface of the vertebral body just anterior to the neural foramen (see Fig 16.14). Additional fracture patterns of the posterior elements in flexion-distraction mechanisms were later defined by Gumley (72). Type 1 enters the spinous process and travels through all bony elements and emerges in a variable position within the vertebral body (traditional Chance fracture). Type 2 enters between the spinous processes (ligamentous), and Type 3 is asymmetric, involving the posterior elements more on one side than the other because of a rotational component in the applied force. Gertzbein added a classification to describe such injuries of the anterior column (67). In group A, the injury exits through the disc, whereas in group B, the fracture passes through the vertebral body. In group C, which represents 50% of the series, extension occurs through the superior end-plate.

Fifty percent of distraction injuries suffer associated intra-abdominal injuries, including small bowel laceration, ruptures of the liver, and descending colon (67, 72). Noncontiguous spine fractures occur with greater frequency (approximately 38%), and an abnormal neurologic exam is seen in 27% (67).

Lateral distraction injuries are rare—approximately 1% of all thoracolumbar fractures (31). Multiple transverse process and rib fractures occur uni-laterally on the distracted side of the spine. Of three cases reported, all had associated life-threatening injuries (31).

Extension

This rare mechanism, which includes the lumberjack's fracture, occurs in approximately 2 to 5% of spine injuries (25, 32). It is caused by a force, such as a falling tree, striking the lower back, with relative hyperextension occurring within the upper spine. The ALL is inevitably torn, with variable injury to the anterior annulus fibrosis (Fig. 16.6) (119). The posterior compressive forces generated may fracture the posterior elements, with resulting fragments displacing ventrally into the spinal canal (119).

Rotation

The facet joint, in concert with the annulus, is the primary structure opposing rotational forces. When such forces are applied, one facet joint may fracture and dislocate anteriorly while its counterpart fails in tension with disruption of the joint capsule (112, 119). Representing 14% of all thoracolumbar spine injuries, these fractures traverse multiple ribs and transverse processes (Fig. 16.7) (25). A Holdsworth slice fracture, the result of a rotational force, proceeds anteriorly through the superior vertebral body after facet joint failure (Fig. 16.8) (83). The capability of this mechanism to destabilize the spine is manifest

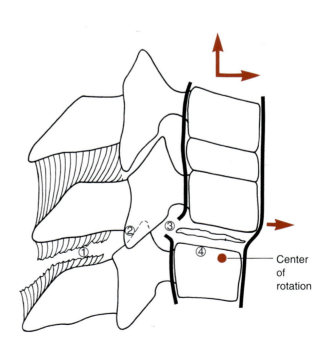

FIGURE 16.4.
Flexion-distraction with the center of rotation in the anterior vertebral body: (1–3) tensile disruption of the interspinous ligaments, facet joint and the PLL; (4) anterior vertebral body wedge with an intact ALL.

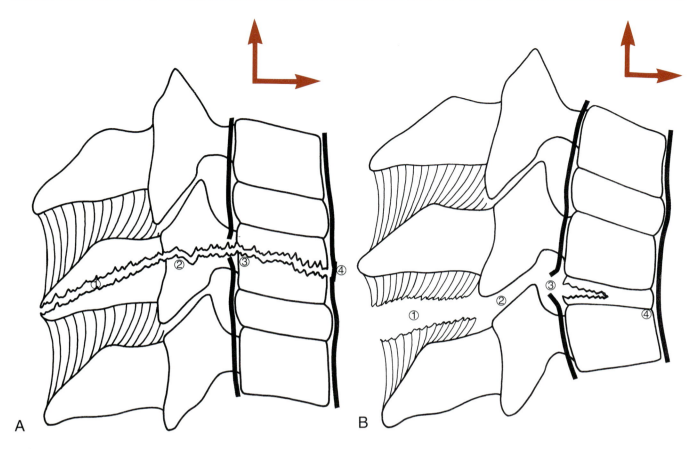

FIGURE 16.5.
Flexion-distraction with center of rotation brought further anteriorly results in an effective distraction force on all three columns: (1–3) posterior ligaments or bone sequentially fail in tension leaving an intact anterior hinge (4). **A.** Bony Chance fracture. **B.** Pure ligamentous injury.

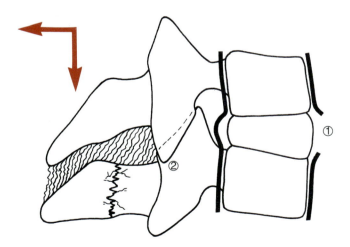

FIGURE 16.6.
Extension: (1) the anterior column fails in tension with either an avulsion fracture of the anterior-inferior vertebral body or disruption of the ALL and annulus; (2) posterior elements face compression loads leading to facet and lamina fractures. If the load continues, a posterior shear-translation between vertebra may develop.

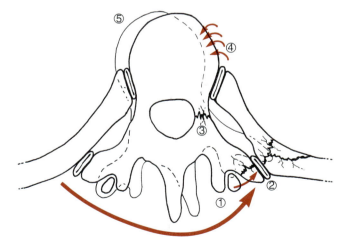

FIGURE 16.7.
Rotation: (1) one facet fails in compression, the other is disrupted in tension; (2–3) fractures occur through the compressed facet, the costotransverse joint and pedicle; (4) the annulus or the vertebral body yield to the rotational shear stresses, resulting in a fracture-dislocation (5).

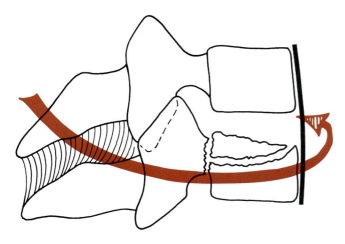

FIGURE 16.8.
The Holdsworth "slice" fracture caused by a rotational force.

in the increased risk for both neurologic injury and spinal deformity. Neurologic deterioration occurring after admission to the hospital, although a rare complication, has been associated more frequently with a torsional mechanism of injury (66). Seventy-five percent of patients with rotational fracture-dislocations and paraplegia develop late, progressive deformity if it is not stabilized (126).

Shear

The most destabilizing of all injury mechanisms is that of a shear force, occurring with a 10% relative frequency (25). Failure of all three columns results, representing the highest risk for concurrent neurologic compromise (66, 112). Fracture-dislocation may occur through the facet joints, allowing the vertebral body to translate with failure of the ALL, PLL, and anulus fibrosis. Surgical exploration often demonstrates complete ligament discontinuity (112). Multiple fractures may occur at the transverse processes and ribs (Figs. 16.9 and 16.16) (28).

Morphologic Classification

Morphologic classifications are simple, frequently used descriptions of resultant vertebral body morphology after an injury. The selected term is based on an interpretation of the static radiograph. As such, it is not meant to imply a mechanism or to define stability. These terms, such as "compression fractures," "burst fractures," and "fracture-dislocations," describe the morphology but are nonspecific.

Neurologic Injury

Injuries to the cord or cauda equina occur in approximately 10 to 38% of thoracolumbar injuries (7, 94, 128). The incidence of neurologic deficit with shear and torsional mechanisms resulting in fracture-dislocations increases to nearly 50% (112, 113). Injuries to the watershed area between T5 and T9 also have increased risk of neurologic deficit because of the tenuous vascular supply and narrow canal dimensions (37).

Neural structures are injured most commonly by a combination of compression and stretch forces. Musculoskeletal injury acutely causes hemorrhage, edema, and direct bony compression on the neural elements. Ischemia follows. Enzymes are released, which affect membrane stability and initiate a progressive, self-destructive sequence. Calcium channels fail and lead to the disruption of electrophysiologic coupling (88).

Although counter-intuitive, it has been difficult to find an association between the extent of canal compromise seen radiographically and the severity of the neurologic deficit after a burst fracture (28, 69, 89). This difficulty probably exists because static roentgenograms do not show the maximum displacement that occurs at the time of the injury. The presence of edema, hemorrhage, and disc fragments as they relate to the available spinal canal reserve (space dimensions and blood supply) may further account for the discrepancy.

Although the canal compromise is easy to estimate from a CT scan, determining the criteria for a "critical" stenosis, which indicates increased risk of late neurologic sequelae, is more difficult. Animal studies have shown that greater than 50% acute canal compromise produces significant neurologic deficits and subsequent axonal degeneration of motor roots distal

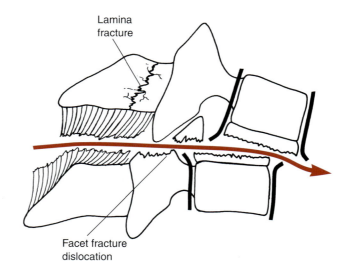

FIGURE 16.9.
Shear: the most disruptive of the injury mechanisms. Injury occurs in all three columns, including the interspinous ligaments, the facet joint, the ALL, PLL, and the annulus.

55% at L2 are at increased risk of neurologic deficit (81).

Clinically, neurologic deficits are classified as complete, incomplete or progressive, based on serial neurologic exams.

Complete

A complete injury indicates there is a definable sensory and motor level beyond which there is no functional activity (less than antigravity strength). Spinal shock may be present for approximately 24 to 48 hours, during which time all reflexes mediated through the spinal cord below the site of injury are blocked by unknown mechanism. The bulbocavernosus reflex, via the sacral roots, is used to determine the end of spinal shock. Tugging the Foley or gently squeezing the glans penis sends a monosynaptic reflex through the conus medullaris, which ends with the contraction of the peri-anal muscles. An injury may be deemed complete after spinal shock ends and the complete neurologic deficit remains. The prognosis for a functional neurologic recovery is poor (26).

Incomplete

In an incomplete injury, some of the ascending and descending spinal cord tracts are still in continuity. The terminus of the cord is usually at the L1 level and is known as the "conus medullaris." Injuries to this area may affect the lower cord, which is the site of origin for the cell bodies of the sacral nerve roots. Conus medullaris syndrome represents an isolated injury to the terminus of the cord. This type of injury results in loss of rectal tone, inability to void, and perianal dysesthesias and numbness (Fig. 16.10).

Frankel, in 1969, described a classification system that, although simplistic, is still used today (55). Five levels are defined, A through E (Figs. 16.11). Most patients within Frankel A and B will not recover. Up to 11% of these patients may show some nonfunc-

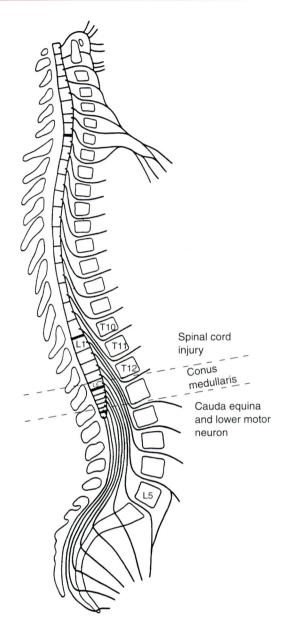

FIGURE 16.10.
The relationship between the musculoskeletal system and the nervous system. The end of the cord is usually at L1 and is known as the conus medullaris, the site of origin for the sacral nerve roots. Damage to the cauda equina represents a lower motor neuron or peripheral nervous system injury.

A	"Complete"	complete sensory and motor loss below the lesion
B	"Sensory Only"	complete motor paralysis, with some sensation present below the level of the lesion sacral sparing
C	"Motor Useless"	some motor power present below the lesion, but of not practical use
D	"Motor Useful"	useful motor power below the lesion. All can move the lower limbs and many can walk with or without aids
E	"Recovery"	the patient is free of neurologic symptoms. Abnormal reflexes may be present

FIGURE 16.11.
Frankel Classification

to the stenosis (95). Decompression improves the neurologic function. Histologically, the decompressed axons return to normal number and volume (95). Unfortunately, with one exception, human clinical studies have been unable to show an association between the extent of canal compromise and neurologic deficit, early or late (81). Hashimoto and coworkers state that burst fractures resulting in 35% or more canal compromise at T11/12, 45% at L1, or

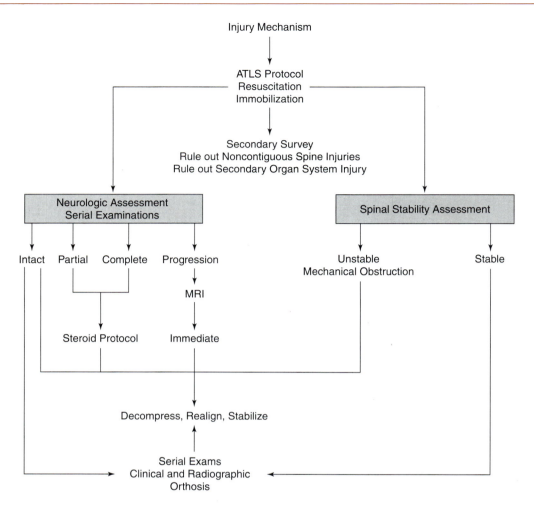

FIGURE 16.12.

Thoracolumbar spine fracture treatment algorithm. Approach and timing depend on the concurrent assessment of neurologic function and spinal stability.

tional improvement (40). Frankel C and D patients are expected to improve at least one motor grade with or without treatment (76).

Late Neurologic Change

A late neurologic change may result from gradual cord degeneration, cystic myelopathy, or syringomyelia. Those with such complications present with evolving pain, typically described as a dull ache, that may radiate into the extremities. An otherwise unexplainable progressive loss of neurologic function, usually a sensory loss involving the spinothalamic tracts and rarely motor weakness, can occur years after the original injury (9, 150, 155). Syringomyelia develops within the watershed area of the cord, between the anterior and posterior arterial blood supply, as a result of crush, liquefaction necrosis, and lysosomal autodigestion. A symptomatic syrinx affects 1.6 to 3.2% of those with spinal cord injury, with increased risk in those with persistent cord compression and impaired cerebrospinal fluid circulation (127, 138). Three forms of surgical treatment have been employed to relieve the associated pain: 1) cord transection; 2) tube syringotomy from the cyst to the subarachnoid space; and 3) tube syringotomy from the cyst to the peritoneal cavity (139). After such intervention, motor power lost resulting from the syrinx has shown the most consistent improvement. Sensory abnormalities, alternatively, are less likely to respond (139).

Diagnosis

Two systems, the musculoskeletal and the neurologic, are simultaneously evaluated (Fig 16.12). A mechanism of injury should be reconstructed using the history and reports from eye-witnesses and emergency workers at the scene. With this information, a prediction of the likely resultant injuries can be made.

Examination should include a careful palpation of the entire length of the spine. Each segment should be evaluated for interspinous widening, step-off, and tenderness, which would indicate posterior ligamentous injury. Close examination of the abdomen for abdominal wall bruising or peritoneal signs is necessary to avoid missing this frequent site of associated injury.

Neurologic exam should be repeated frequently and motor, sensory, and reflex changes should be documented to avoid missing a neurologic deterioration. Close inspection of the sacral nerve function may reveal either an isolated injury to the conus or sacral sparing in a patient otherwise thought to have a complete injury.

Radiographs

Plain radiographs of the entire spine in two planes should be performed on all high energy trauma patients to evaluate for noncontiguous injuries, especially when clinical assessment is impaired because of brain injury or drug and alcohol intoxication. AP image should be inspected in a systematic fashion, examining bone contour and alignment and soft tissue. Detectable interpedicular widening occurs in 45% of burst fractures (Fig 16.13A) (5). Widening of the distance between spinous processes indicates disruption of the posterior ligaments (Fig 16.15A).

The lateral radiographic images are inspected directly for bone injury and indirectly for soft tissue disruption. Segmental kyphosis is measured by the Cobb technique. A percentage of the loss of the anterior and posterior heights is calculated. Loss of posterior height is the most useful predicator of the presence of a burst fracture (5). Disruption of the posterior cortical line may be difficult to see because of the overlying pedicle; however, when detected, it indicates a burst fracture (Fig 16.13).

Plain radiographs may miss 25% of burst fractures, which often are misdiagnosed as stable wedge fractures (5). CT scans provide axial images and are better able to detect middle column injury, retropulsed fragments, or laminar fractures (Fig 16.14C). It is also the method used to quantify the degree of bony comminution and canal compromise. When facet joints are dislocated in a flexion-distraction injury, this is recognized on CT scan as a "naked" facet sign (118) (Fig 16.15B). Sagittal plane CT reconstructions often are more accurate in determining canal compromise in patients with bilateral facet dislocations.

The most recent addition to the evaluation scheme is the MRI. This study is best used to directly evaluate the soft tissue integrity: disc, ligament, and nerve. Disruption of the ALL, PLL, and interspinous ligaments can be determined (16). Checking for ligamentous continuity allows the surgeon another means to predict the effect of distraction instrumentation in reducing retropulsed burst fragments via ligamentotaxis. The ALL and PLL are seen as thin, linear signal voids paralleling the anterior and posterior borders of the vertebral body and discs. The ALL is best seen with T1 images because it contrasts with the surrounding, bright paraspinous fat. The PLL is best seen on T2 images against the adjacent, high-signal CSF (Fig 16.15C).

In addition, MRI can accurately evaluate the neural elements in patients who have neurologic deficit. On T2, a high signal intensity within the cord indicates a contusion. Swelling can be identified by the presence of a deformity on the surface of the cord seen on both sagittal and axial images. An epidural hematoma may be seen in spine fractures in patients with ankylosing spondylitis. Unexplained deficits or progressive neurologic change necessitate an MRI examination to search for a correctable cause within the soft tissue elements, such as a traumatically herniated disc.

Indications for Surgery

Three basic options are available to the surgeon: reduction, stabilization, and decompression. At times, performing a reduction and stabilization leads to a secondary (indirect) decompression. The indications for and methods of surgical intervention depend on the alignment and stability of the fracture, the neurologic assessment, and the status of other organ systems (61).

Neurologically Intact

Acute Instability

For the neurologically intact patient, surgery may be required to treat an acutely unstable three column injury to restore alignment and provide immediate stability. Rapid mobilization avoids the debility associated with prolonged recumbency. Fracture-dislocations (rotation and shear mechanisms), flexion-distraction injuries with displacement, and severe flexion-compression injuries with significant kyphosis and canal compromise meet these general criteria.

Reduction is accomplished by reversing the mechanism of injury. Flexion-distraction injuries reduce with a corrective force that provides extension and compression, necessitating an intact middle column. Flexion-compression injuries require distraction, extension, and an intact ALL.

Late Instability

Determining when late instability will occur is difficult because an early, multifactorial assessment must be used to predict the possibility of a delayed change. This type of stability should not be thought

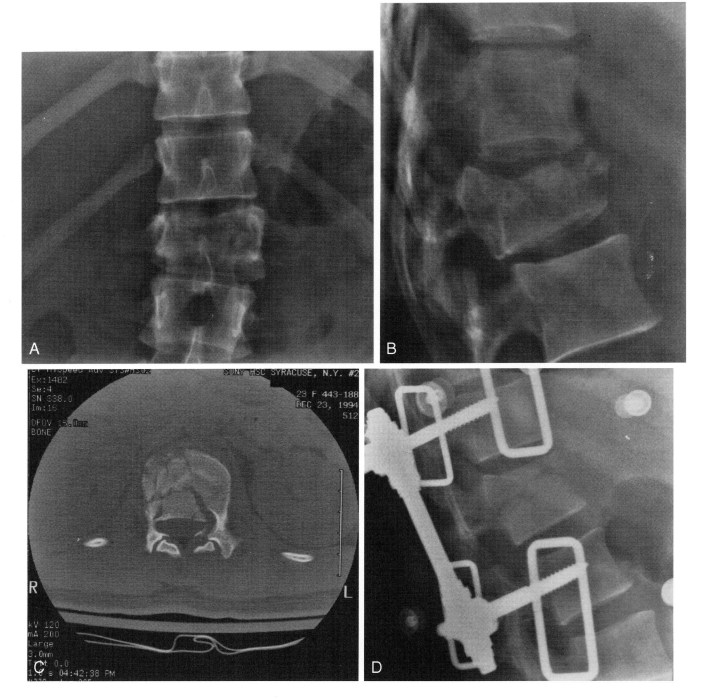

FIGURE 16.13.
40-year-old female, neurologically intact, with an L1 burst fracture caused by a motor vehicle accident. **A.** AP radiograph of the L1 burst showing a widening between the pedicles. **B.** Lateral radiograph showing anterior vertebral body height decreased by 50% when compared with adjacent vertebra. The posterior margin of the vertebral body is disrupted. The posterior-superior body is retropulsed. Segmental kyphosis from T12-L2 is 25°. **C.** Axial CT image showing the comminuted burst fracture with the retropulsed fragment causing approximately 40% canal compromise. **D.** Postoperative lateral image after short segment pedicle screw instrumentation (AO fixateur interne). Vertebral body height is restored and the retropulsed fragment is reduced. Kyphosis measures 7°.

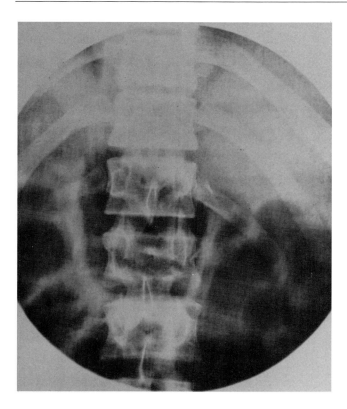

FIGURE 16.14.
Coronal image of an L1 Chance fracture. The fracture plane proceeds through the spinous process, pedicles, and into the vertebral body. Often, these fractures are difficult to detect.

of as an all-or-nothing concept. Rather, it is best conceptualized as a continuum with multiple levels of stability needs.

For flexion-compression injuries with greater than 50% loss of anterior vertebral body height and 30° of kyphosis, there is an increased likelihood of concomitant loss of stability of the posterior ligaments and an elevated risk of late progression of the deformity (10, 51). When patients are examined 2 years after the injury, those with more than 30° of initial kyphosis have an increased incidence of significant back pain (65). Hyperlordosis of the lumbar spine, a compensation for the thoracolumbar kyphotic deformity, results in facet joint overload, degeneration, and pain (106, 144).

In an attempt to quantify the risk of developing late kyphosis in burst fractures, Farcy et al. developed the sagittal index (SI) (49). SI is a measure of the kyphotic segmental deformity corrected for the normal sagittal contour at the particular level (kyphotic deformity-normal contour = SI). Those with an SI of less than 15° were treated successfully with conservative measures.

Bony comminution, osteoporosis, and consecutive vertebral injuries also add to the risk of late progression of deformity, although their respective contributions are more difficult to quantify. When such factors are present and are combined with a high grade canal compromise (greater than 50%), the surgeon may select surgical intervention because progression of kyphosis in this setting carries an increased risk of causing a neurologic deficit. Tencer et al., in studying contact pressure on the cord-meningeal complex, found that 20° of angulation was acceptable if there was less than 35% canal compromise (136). Surgical reconstruction of late kyphosis is best identified and treated early because it carries a 25% risk of major complications (125).

In flexion-distraction injuries, complete ligament disruptions tend not to heal, whereas bony disruptions heal over 3 months time. Therefore, bony "Chance" injuries are frequently treated with external immobilization, and ligamentous injuries require operative stabilization and fusion.

Complete Neurologic Deficit

The presence of a neurologic deficit implies spinal instability. The exception to this rule occurs in children who, because of ligamentous laxity and relatively horizontal facet joint alignment, may allow a mobility of the spine greater than that tolerated by its neural elements: SCIWORA (spinal cord injury without radiologic abnormality).

Complete injuries to the central nervous system very rarely show any improvement with time. Ducker et al. reported that 11% of patients with complete thoracic and thoracolumbar injuries recovered useful motor function (40). Peripheral nerve injuries at the root level, adjacent to the cord injury, may improve with or without surgical intervention. Reduction, either open or closed, should be performed on all displaced spine injuries to create an improved mechanical environment for healing of both the musculoskeletal system and the peripheral nervous system. The use of succinylcholine during anesthetic induction is contraindicated in patients with neurologic injury because of the elevated release of potassium.

When compared with nonoperative methods, internal stabilization has decreased hospitalization and rehabilitation time and improved spinal alignment with ultimately less complications (35, 54, 84, 85, 130, 146). Such stabilization, while preventing progressive deformity, does come at a cost. Spinal fusion over multiple lumbar segments has deleterious effects on spinal movement and trunk extensor strength by up to 25% (79). Open techniques also have been largely unable to demonstrate an improved neurologic recovery over postural reduction (35).

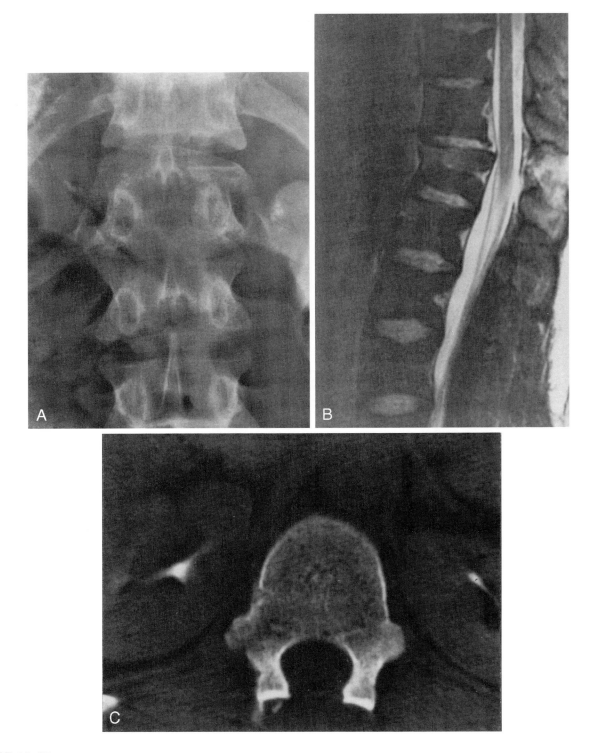

FIGURE 16.15.
35-year-old man, neurologically intact, after a motor vehicle accident. **A.** AP radiograph of a flexion-distraction injury at T12-L1. Note the widening between the spinous processes of T12 and L1. **B.** Axial CT demonstrates the naked facet sign. **C.** Sagittal plane MRI shows high signal in the interspinous region, indicating disruption of the posterior ligaments. T12 is subluxed forward on L1. The PLL is disrupted. The terminus of the cord is seen at L1.

Incomplete Neurologic Injury

Incomplete thoracic paraplegia is a relatively rare injury, representing only 1.2 to 18% of all patients with thoracic fractures and neural deficits (13, 100). If a retropulsed burst fragment or a displaced fracture-dislocation causes continuing mechanical deformation of the neural elements, removing the obstruction improves the likelihood but not the rate of neurologic recovery (66, 110). The most important factor determining the extent of a neurologic recovery is the severity of the damage sustained by the nerve tissue at the time of injury (7, 75). Deterioration of neurologic function after a partial spinal cord injury is relatively uncommon, with an overall incidence of 3 to 5% (66, 108).

While animal models of spinal cord injury have consistently shown improvement with early decompression (36, 124), this has not been the case in human clinical studies (108, 110). Some studies have shown that recovery is not enhanced by early open reduction and fixation (7, 54). In fact, a higher complication rate with neurologic worsening has been seen in association with an intervention within the first 5 days (108). Others have documented significantly improved rates of neurologic recovery with early intervention when compared with historical controls (24, 100).

Clinical studies may not be able to show the association between the promptness of the decompression and the ultimate level of neurologic function for several reasons. First, the severity of the spine and neurologic and associated injuries between study groups are difficult to quantitate and compare. Second, grading classifications for neurologic recovery may lack sensitivity and possess an inherent interobserver variability. Third, detectable recovery does occur even without intervention or when intervention is performed remotely, making statistically significant differences between early and late interventions difficult to detect.

Nonoperative Treatment

Early Medical Management

Nonoperative treatment begins in the emergency room with identification of the injury and prevention of further injury by proper immobilization and hemodynamic resuscitation. The heart rate is the primary determinate used to differentiate neurogenic shock from hemorrhagic shock. Neurogenic shock occurs as a result of cord damage with loss of autonomic (sympathetic) tone, vasodilation, and pooling of the blood in the periphery. Close monitoring of fluids and occasional use of atropine can be used to maintain satisfactory blood pressure and pulse rate.

Those with partial or complete neurologic injuries should receive intravenous methylprednisolone beginning within the first 8 hours after injury (bolus: 30 mg/kg followed by an infusion rate of 5.4 mg/kg/hr for 23 hours). If the patient first presents more than 8 hours after the spinal cord injury, methylprednisolone should not be given. This recommendation is based on a multi-center, randomized, placebo controlled study of 337 patients (18). The use of steroids did not appear to increase the risk of postoperative wound infections or GI bleeding. Criticisms regarding this study include: 1) failure to stratify patient injury characteristics; 2) the use of summed motor scores without a functional assessment; and 3) the lack of consideration of the effect of operative interventions later performed (12). Despite these shortcomings, the use of IV steroids is the standard of care at present.

Other methods have attempted to decrease cord metabolism, increase regional blood flow, enhance cellular membrane stability, suppress the processes of secondary cell destruction, and hopefully promote neural regeneration (41, 64, 88). Systemically administered medications have included GM-1 ganglioside, opiate antagonists, calcium channel blockers, mannitol, DMSO, and vitamin E (64, 88).

GM-1 ganglioside is a complex acidic glycolipid found within the cell membranes within the central nervous system. During spinal cord recovery, ganglioside promotes neurite sprouting and outgrowth and limits Wallerian degeneration (64). In a small prospective, randomized, placebo-controlled clinical study, GM-1 ganglioside enhanced the return of lost motor function (64).

Opiate antagonists, such as naloxone and thyrotropin-releasing hormone (TRH), work by decreasing the hypermetabolic state after trauma secondary to the rise of endorphins. Bracken and coworkers initially presented data indicating that naloxone did not have a beneficial effect (18). Subsequently, a revised analysis pointed out the time-dependent nature of the administration and recovery. If naloxone is given within the first 8 hours after injury, a greater recovery is seen 1 year after injury when compared with placebo-controlled patients (17).

Mannitol and DMSO serve dual functions. First, working as diuretics, local edema is diminished. Second, functioning as free-radical scavengers, toxic byproducts are deactivated. Oxygen free radicals are released by the destruction of membrane lipids. These free radicals have a secondary, injury-provoking capability.

Localized cord cooling decreases metabolic requirements and has shown some encouraging results in animal models and clinical trials (77). Unfortunately, cooling devices are cumbersome, often making clinical use impractical.

If neglected, the paraplegic patient faces complications arising within the respiratory, urinary, gastrointestinal and integument systems. These are best prevented by early and persistent attention to: 1) rapid mobilization as spinal stability allows; 2) maintenance of adequate nutrition (at least 3000 calories/day); 3) chest physiotherapy and assisted coughing; 4) intermittent catheterization of the bladder to begin at the completion of acute treatment phase at a frequency to ensure an output of no more than 400 mL; 5) GI prophylaxis with H2-blockers and antacids; and 6) protection of pressure points with periodic inspection of all skin surfaces (38).

Kinetic beds allow skin pressure redistribution and assist in pulmonary toilet. The Roto-Rest bed is extremely effective in immobilizing unstable thoracolumbar fractures, whereas the Stryker frame allows distraction at the fracture site, up to 5° of angular deformity and 25 mm of anterior-posterior displacement during turning (115).

Closed Reduction and Immobilization

The majority of thoracolumbar spine injuries can be reduced by closed techniques. Beginning in 1944 at the Stokes Mandeville Hospital, Sir Ludwig Guttman was the first to emphasize and popularize such methods (74, 75). He used postural reduction in hyperextension while the patient rested in the supine position with pillow support beneath the fracture. Frankel, who trained under Guttman, found only a 13% rate of failure of closed reduction when treating bilateral jumped facets (55). Others have reported that up to 70% of all displaced thoracolumbar spine fractures are able to be closed-reduced (7). An "acceptable" reduction may be variably defined, depending on the author and the area of analysis.

Neurologic recovery after closed reduction has been well documented. For incomplete deficits, return of at least one Frankel Grade can be expected in 65% (55, 85) to 95% (26). Failure to reduce does not exclude the possibility of a neurologic recovery (55).

After reduction, Frankel treated patients for 10 to 12 weeks in recumbency. Only 2 of 394 cases of unstable flexion-compression injuries were considered to remain unstable after the recumbent period (55).

Late progression of kyphotic deformity after flexion-compression injuries may occur after closed treatment and may lead to a late neurologic compromise. The frequency, rate, and severity of neurologic sequelae occurring with progressive kyphosis after nonoperative treatment has been variable in the literature to date (26, 30, 101, 117, 123, 142). These discrepancies are most likely caused by subtle differences in the patient populations studied, particularly the degree of posterior column disruption.

Reviewing 34 patients with a neural deficit, Davies et al. found 2 with a gibbus formation requiring excision of spinous processes, 6 with pain, and 2 with temporary neural deterioration (26). Like Frankel's study, this study rarely detected instability at follow-up. No segment exhibited more than 15° of movement between the flexed and the extended position.

Denis et al. reported on 104 intact patients with burst fractures treated conservatively. Seventeen percent developed late neurologic symptoms and 25% were unable to work (30). Krompinger et al. studied 29 patients, similarly treated, with no cases of clinically detectable neurologic deterioration. However, 21% did note periodic leg pain and 10% were unable to work secondary to back pain (101).

In contrast, Mumford et al. has shown an average increase in kyphosis of only 3°, with only 2% of 41 patients showing a neurologic deterioration (117). 90% had returned to work. Reid and coworkers have also reported good outcomes among 21 neurologically intact patients, none requiring surgery for increasing kyphosis or increasing neurologic deficit (123).

Retropulsed bone does resorb slowly with time (21, 52, 101, 117). Canal remodeling has improved the average canal compromise from 37% to 14% for Mumford (117). Krompinger documented remodeling in 11 of 14 patients whose initial canal compromise was greater than 25% (101).

Patwardhan et al. used a finite element model to predict the ability of a TLSO orthosis to restore segmental stiffness (120). Single level injuries causing up to 50% loss of segmental stiffness can be returned to normal stability with the use of a brace. Beyond 85% loss of stiffness, as occurs with three column injuries, the orthosis alone would not be expected to prevent progression of deformity. The TLSO is only effective between T7 and L4. Immobilizing cephalad to T7 requires a CTLSO incorporating the cervical spine. Stabilizing the lumbosacral junction necessitates the use of a thigh extension (53, 58). Hyperextension braces, such as the Jewett, do not control rotational forces and are best used for compression and "stable" burst fractures (21).

In summary, flexion-compression burst fractures can be treated nonoperatively in a TLSO if the posterior ligaments are intact, the loss of anterior height is less than 50%, and there is less than 30° of kyphosis. In this setting, prolonged bed rest is not required, and early ambulation can commence within an orthosis (21, 120). A slight increase in kyphosis is expected on follow-up. This increase is balanced by the body's ability to clear the canal by simultaneously resorbing the retropulsed fragment, making late neurologic changes a rare occurrence.

Surgical Treatments

Posterior Techniques

Among the first devices designed to provide an instrumented fixation were the Meurig-Williams plates and the Weiss Springs. Fastened to the spinous processes with screws, these mechanically disadvantaged devices faced high rates of failure (75, 126). The instrumentation provided no intrinsic reduction capability.

Harrington Distraction

In 1947, Harrington began to develop a spinal instrumentation for use in polio patients with scoliosis. It involved distraction applied from two posterior points. In 1958, this technique was applied to a fracture-dislocation of the spine with the initial report appearing in 1973 (35). Spanning of 2 to 3 levels, both above and below the site of injury, is required to gain the necessary mechanical advantage (85). Long instrumentation techniques provide a greater lever arm for reduction with improved correction of the deformity (57, 133).

Reduction of the retropulsed fragment in flexion-compression injuries via distraction instrumentation was initially believed to be affected by ligamentotaxis through stretching of the PLL. Biomechanical studies have subsequently shown that the PLL has relatively little influence on achieving this indirect reduction (56, 80). The true reducing ligaments are the outer layers of the annulus that originate from the superior vertebra in the midportion of the endplate and insert into the lateral margins of the intracanal fragment (56). If both the annulus, ALL, and PLL are disrupted as seen in translational injuries, posterior distraction may actually worsen the kyphosis, allowing overdistraction while failing to restore canal dimensions (4, 86, 108, 112). Distraction without reduction of the retropulsed fragment leads to tensioning of the cord over the fragment (136). A high-grade canal compromise (>67%) implies annular injury with diminished effectiveness of indirect techniques (70). There is a narrow window of opportunity for the use of posterior distraction; the best results are obtained when accomplished within 4 days from the time of injury (44, 70, 145).

Harrington instrumentation improved fracture reduction, with fewer complications and less rehabilitation time than closed techniques (54, 85, 133). The primary disadvantage of Harrington instrumentation is the length of instrumentation required (5 to 6 motion segments). This length creates problems, especially in the mid- and lower-level lumbar injuries where the caudal segments are incorporated into the fusion (3). Flat back, which is the iatrogenic loss of lumbar lordosis that occurs with distraction, can cause disabling low back pain (86). Without lumbar lordosis, the center of gravity is pushed forward, and the lower-most lumbar segments must compensate by hyperlordosis, thereby increasing facet joint load with ultimate degeneration and pain. For this reason, Harrington instrumentation should not be used to treat injuries of the lower lumbar spine (3, 129).

With only two points of fixation, high stresses are experienced at the hook-lamina junction. The incidence of hook cut-out is high—up to 10% (25, 35, 54, 108, 129, 145). The junction of the upper hook and the lamina is the most common site of failure (71, 109). Without individual vertebral segmental fixation, rotation and shear injuries are difficult to control and an orthosis is required.

Harrington Modifications

Since its introduction, many modifications of the Harrington technique have followed. In an attempt to lessen the severity of a secondary flat back deformity, Moe created square hooks that allowed a gentle contouring of the rod in the lumbar spine. Edwards added high density polyethylene sleeves threaded over the Harrington rod and used to fill the potential space between the rod and the anatomic position of the posterior elements. The sleeve is placed at the center of the pedicle of the fractured vertebrae, serving as the fulcrum for a three-point fixation to reduce the kyphotic deformity. The posterior neural arch and pedicles, at the level where the sleeves are to be placed, must be intact. Edwards found that canal area improved 32% if Harrington rods with Edwards sleeves were inserted within 2 days of the injury (44).

Jacobs introduced the rod-long, fuse-short technique in an attempt to preserve motion segments (85). Only the injured zone is fused. Instrumentation is removed at approximately 1 year. Problems with this technique include osteoarthritis of the immobilized but unfused facets and progressive kyphosis after rod removal (27, 62, 90, 91).

Kahanovitz et al. reported on 8 patients using this technique with the removal of hardware at 6 to 26 months after implantation (91). Areas of fibrillation and fissuring were identified within the cartilage of the facet joints at the instrumented but not fused levels. Histologic review confirmed erosion of the vascular tide mark, osteophyte formation and fibrillation consistent with osteoarthritis of the immobilized facets. Kahanovitz also used a dog model to show that facet osteoarthritis arose in the temporarily stabilized but not fused segments (90). Clinically, however, these changes do not appear to create detectable problems (27, 62). Examining plane radiographs, Gardner found only 2 of 75 facets had autofused, with 85% of patients reporting minimal or no pain (62).

Harrington Compression

Harrington also developed a system capable of performing compression between vertebrae. This mode of fixation provides stability for flexion-distraction injuries to reconstruct the posterior tension band. Fusion length is 1 or 2 segments. The middle column must be intact. The facets act as a fulcrum and therefore must also be intact. Compression may cause bulging of injured disc.

Despite the shortcomings, Harrington instrumentation continues to have a definite role in thoracolumbar injuries. Compared with the newer systems described later in the text, Harrington is less costly and is easier to insert, requiring half of the operating time and resulting in half the blood loss (129).

Posterior Segmental Fixation

Luque developed a segmental fixation system requiring sublaminar passage of a double stranded, 18-gauge, stainless-steel wire at multiple levels. These wires are then lashed to a rigid rod. Biomechanical studies have confirmed the ability of this construct to restore to a level that is half the rotational stiffness of the intact spine (73). The technique is less able to support axial loads (50, 111). The weakness of the Luque system when applied to thoracolumbar injuries is its inability to apply distractive or compressive forces because the position of the wire wrapped around the rod cannot be controlled or manipulated. Therefore, the system is unable to restore vertebral body height and contour and is only moderately effective at restoring lumbar lordosis (105).

Wisconsin wires, introduced by Dennis Drummond, are placed through the spinous processes and increase the torsional stability of the Harrington construct (39). The Harre-Luque technique calls for Luque segmental wiring to be added to the Harrington rod-hook construct, also improving rotational-torsional control and resistance of axial compression, thereby obviating the need for postoperative bracing (59, 60, 109, 111).

In 1985, Cotrel and Dubousset introduced a system that effectively blended Harrington with segmental fixation. Multiple hooks are placed along a rod, allowing individual compression or distraction forces to be placed at varying locations along the rod as required. Successful treatment of thoracolumbar fractures with this instrumentation has been reported (48). Second generation systems have emerged based on this concept. The system shows versatility because pedicle screws can also be added, where appropriate, to the construct.

Pedicle Screw Segmental Instrumentation

In 1982, Dick described the "fixateur interne," a modification of the Magerl external skeletal fixation system (2, 33, 34, 147). Two pairs of Schanz screws are placed in the pedicles immediately above and below the fractured vertebrae. The screws are connected to rods (Fig. 16.16). Sagittal reduction is accomplished first by using the long lever arms of the Schanz screws and squeezing them together until the desired lordosis is achieved. Next, sagittal body height and axial canal dimensions are restored by distraction. Positioning the spine in lordosis before applying distraction significantly loosens the PLL with a slight increase in canal compromise, leading to the suggestion that distraction be applied before angular correction (57, 80). Distraction, whether applied before or after the kyphosis correction, is the effective mechanism in reducing the fracture fragment (56, 57). Kyphosis correction does not contribute to canal clearance (57).

The primary benefit of pedicle screw systems is the three column purchase, allowing shorter fusion with preservation of motion segments. The most significant concern is the miss rate during screw placement, with a reported frequency between 10 to 28% (98). In addition, such devices lack sufficient mechanical support in axial rotation; therefore, an external orthosis may be required to augment fixation in cases of rotational instability (98). Farcy et al., using a bovine model, have shown that rotational instability is best controlled by a single level pedicle screw instrumentation, whereas axial instability is best controlled by a two-level construct (50).

The ability of the fixator interne to indirectly reduce retropulsed bone appears similar to that of the Harrington system. Using CT scan pre- and postoperatively, the average improvement in the percent canal compromise has been between 14 and 50% (47, 70, 134, 140).

Sagittal plane restoration through correction of kyphosis has also been successful. Lindsey et al., in reviewing 80 consecutive patients, showed an operative correction from 17.4° preoperatively to 7.9° postoperatively (103). Seventy percent of these cases had no formal fusion with the implant removed at 1 year. There was a loss of 3.5° of correction at 1 year, with 5° of additional loss after implant removal, the majority occurring through the upper disc space. The disrupted end-plates often fuse with the adjacent vertebral body (104).

Despite three column purchase, short segment fusion faces extensive loads that contribute to hardware failure (22, 116). McLain et al. reviewed 19 patients treated with short segment fusion with pedicle screws (116). Despite the use of transverse traction

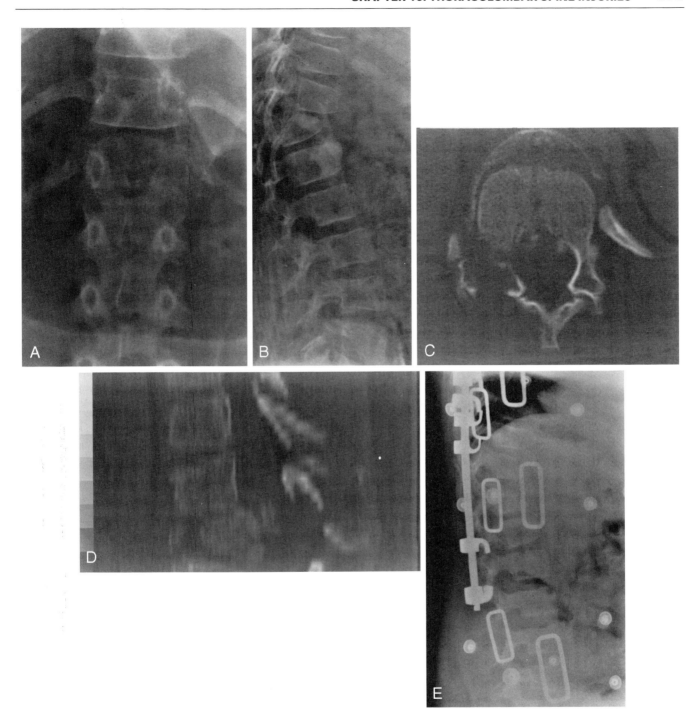

FIGURE 16.16.
9-year-old female, paraplegic after a sledding accident. **A.** The T12 pedicle on the right is not seen, indicating that a displaced fracture has occurred at the vertebral body-pedicle junction. There is widening between the spinous processes of T11–12. **B.** Lateral image shows the T11–12 fracture-dislocation. All three columns are disrupted. **C.** Axial CT demonstrates the double image, the result of capturing both T11 and T12 on the same cut. The right pedicle is comminuted and displaced. **D.** Although the canal appears capacious on the axial plane CT, significant canal compromise is appreciated on this sagittal reconstruction. **E.** After open reduction and posterior rod-hook instrumentation, sagittal alignment is restored.

devices to link the rods and the use of a custom-molded orthosis, 10 patients had vertebral collapse and translation and hardware failure in the early postoperative period. The presence of bent screws or low-grade kyphosis (less than 10°) did not always portend a pseudarthrosis or a clinical failure (22, 116).

To predict the circumstances under which short segment fusions fail, McCormack and coworkers have developed the "load sharing classification," which grades: 1) the proportion of the vertebral body that is damaged; 2) the spread of the fracture fragments; and 3) the amount of traumatic kyphosis that is corrected (114). Pedicle screw failure is likely to occur if there is greater than 30% comminution of the vertebral body detected on sagittal plane section CT; more than 2 mm spread between fracture fragments on axial image; and more than 10° of kyphosis correction required. Segmental pedicle fixation two levels above the kyphosis at the thoracolumbar junction has been suggested to avoid implant failure (22, 99).

Laminectomy

Decompressive laminectomy performed for thoracolumbar injuries is destabilizing, ineffective, and has been universally condemned as an isolated procedure (11, 13, 83, 84). In biomechanical studies, there is no neural decompression attributable to laminectomy with up to an average of 35% occlusion of the canal (135). If a laminectomy is done in the upper thoracic spine or at the thoracolumbar junction, posttraumatic kyphosis, pain, and progressive neurologic deficit results (11, 75, 106, 144). The risk of these outcomes can be diminished appropriately by combining laminectomy with a posterior instrumented stabilization (25). Laminectomy is acceptable in the setting of a lower lumbar spine injury (3).

Currently, there are only three indications for posterior laminectomy: 1) comminuted posterior elements causing direct neural compression; 2) an epidural hematoma requiring evacuation; and 3) a laminar fracture in association with a vertebral body burst and an incomplete neurologic deficit. Approximately one-third of patients with an incomplete neurologic deficit and a laminar fracture seen on CT scan have an associated dural tear, with 13% having neural elements entrapped within the fracture (20, 78, 94).

Posterolateral Decompression

Because of the inability to predict accurately the canal clearance that occurs with ligamentotaxis, some authors have recommended intraoperative assessment with either myelography or ultrasound (27, 44, 45, 140). Four percent of incomplete patients treated by Edwards and coworkers had sufficient focal impingement remaining after posterior indirect reduction to warrant immediate posterolateral or subsequent anterior decompression (Fig. 16.17) (44). Unfortunately, the large size of the ultrasound probe (1.5 cm width, 2.0 cm length) requires the surgeon to perform a generous laminotomy.

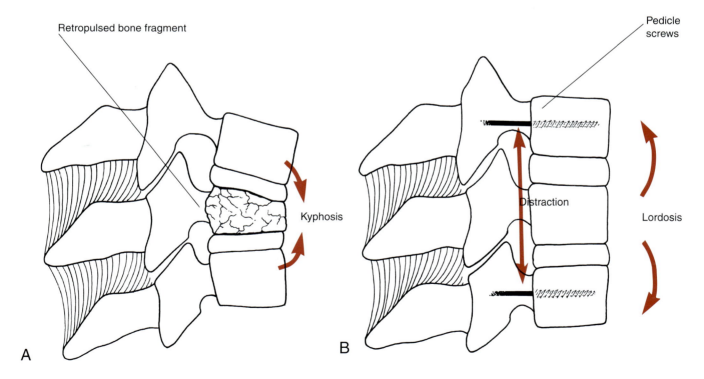

FIGURE 16.17.
Methods of indirect reduction technique: posterior distraction and lordoses forces to provide ligmentotaxis and indirect decompression of the canal. **A.** Burst fracture with kyphosis and retropulsed bone fragment. **B.** Transpedicular distraction and lordosis contouring.

Flesch and coworkers described posterolateral decompression via costotransversectomy (Fig 16.18) (54). The body of the burst fracture is entered through a transpedicular approach using a high speed drill and curette. Bone anterior to the retropulsed fragment is brided with rongeurs and curettes, effectively undermining the posteriorly displaced bone. The remaining cortical shell is then fractured and driven anteriorly. Some medial retraction of the neural elements may be required; therefore, this technique is best done in the lower lumbar spine below the conus where the canal dimensions are larger. Problems include inadequate visualization often secondary to epidural bleeding and often resulting in an inadequate decompression. Reported clinical results are generally good (63, 78, 113). Hardaker, in a review of 58 patients using a bilateral transpedicular decompression technique, reported 77% with neurologic improvement. Thirty-four of forty with incomplete deficit improved one or more Frankel grades (78).

Transpedicular bone grafting to augment healing of comminuted vertebral fractures after posterolateral decompression has been recommended by several authors (2, 33, 103). It is, however, not possible to control the position of the graft material; possible posterior extrusion can cause canal stenosis. In addition, late collapse is not prevented by such a grafting technique because kyphosis occurs secondary to a loss height of the disc space and not of the vertebral body (62).

Anterior Decompression and Fusion

Advantages

The primary indication for an anterior decompression is significant canal compromise with a partial neurologic injury in a setting that portends failure of a posterior indirect reduction. The indications include: 1) a large retropulsed fragment with significant (>50%) canal compromise; 2) anterior column comminution and marked kyphosis; and 3) a time lapse of greater than 4 days from the time of injury. The cauda equina can tolerate 85% canal occlusion, whereas the cord can tolerate only 20%, especially in the watershed area of the mid-thoracic spine (97).

The anterior technique provides a direct and therefore more predictable decompression. Whether this improved decompression leads to enhanced neurologic recovery rates depends more on the level (cord, conus, cauda equina) and the initial severity of the injury than on the estimate of the static canal compromise.

In a retrospective review of more than 1000 fractures treated by 64 Scoliosis Research Society members from 12 countries, anterior decompression was not more effective than posterior when comparing improvement in Frankel scores (66). Alternatively, after a review of 80 patients, Kostuik recommended the anterior technique after demonstrating an average recovery of 1.6 Frankel grades (96, 97). Other studies indicate that anterior decompression may also be more effective in restoring bladder function (15, 46, 110), with more than one-third returning to normal (15, 110). Fifty percent of those unable to walk regained the ability (110).

Anterior approaches are also recommended for the late treatment of symptomatic post-traumatic kyphosis that causes pain or neurologic deficit (14, 97, 106, 125, 137). Bohlman et al. obtained relief of pain in 93% of 45 patients who underwent anterior decompression an average of 4.5 years after their fracture (14). Posterior fusion to relieve pain associated with post-traumatic kyphosis is not successful for two reasons. First, it affords no improvement in the degree of canal compromise. Second, with a large bending moment, the bone graft is placed under tension, thereby predisposing to pseudarthrosis. For a large (>40 degrees), rigid kyphotic deformity, a posterior instrumented fusion should accompany an anterior procedure.

Anterior decompression may also alleviate neurogenic claudication secondary to chronic compression of the cord or cauda equina. Motor recovery has been observed when corpectomy was performed years after the injury (14, 110, 137). In one patient, this improvement took as long as 7 years after corpectomy to be realized (110).

Disadvantages

The principle disadvantages of anterior techniques are the extent of the procedure and, until recently, the lack of stable fixation devices. The approach could cause a significant deterioration of pulmonary function, especially in polytrauma patients with chest wall trauma and lung contusion. Blood loss during the approach is approximately 250 cc with 500 to 1500 cc further loss occurring during vertebrectomy secondary to bleeding from the body and from epidural veins (42, 46, 76, 92).

The ability to obtain reduction of displaced vertebrae via anterior technique can be difficult. Dislocations and translations must be approached posteriorly because the usual site of obstruction to reduction are the fractured and displaced posterior elements, which require excision.

Technique

It is best to approach the side with the greatest compromise. A right-sided approach offers the best exposure to the vertebral bodies without interference

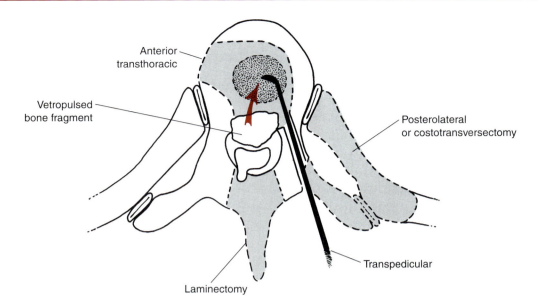

FIGURE 16.18.
Routes of direct decompression: (1) anterior transthoracic/ retroperitoneal; (2) posterolateral via a costotransversectomy; and (3) laminectomy, which is rarely indicated.

from the aorta, which overlies the upper thoracic vertebra on the left. Between T12-L4, the left sided approach is preferred. In this region, the aorta assumes a more central location on the vertebra. The thicker walled aorta is more resilient to retraction and mobilization than is the thinner vena cava. The patient is placed into the lateral decubitus position. To assist in the exposure and allow adjacent vertebra to open to receive the structural bone graft, the table is jackknifed, with the apex directed toward the fractured vertebra.

For an extensile thoracolumbar approach (required for a burst fracture at T11-L1), an incision is made along the course of the tenth rib, beginning at the posterior axillary line and extending anteriorly to the lateral border to the rectus sheath. The intercostal muscles are divided, followed by subperiosteal dissection of the rib with Alexander and Doyon elevators. The cartilaginous costal arch, at the articulation with the anterior rib, has been referred to as the keystone. Transversely splitting the keystone allows entry into the retroperitoneum beneath the diaphragm. Posteriorly, the rib is osteotomized as close as possible to the costotransverse junction. Blunt dissection of the peritoneum from the inferior surface of the diaphragm is completed. The thoracic cavity is entered through the bed of the excised rib. The diaphragm is incised, anterior to posterior, approximately 10 to 15 mm from the costal margin to the aortic hiatus. Tagging sutures placed at intervals assist in proper orientation at the time of closure. Segmental vessels, lying in the "valleys" at the mid-vertebral body, are identified and ligated as necessary.

Isolated exposure of L1-L5 or T3-T11 do not require take-down of the diaphragm. For a L1-L5 approach, a flank incision can be made, with entry into the retroperitoneum via excision of the eleventh or twelfth rib if desired. For T3-T11, excise the rib that corresponds to the level to be decompressed.

Fractured vertebrae are then removed by use of high speed burr and curettes. The opposite pedicle from the site of entry must be visualized to ensure adequate decompression. Adjacent end-plates are preserved and are decorticated to a finely bleeding surface. Tricortical grafts are keyed into vertebral cancellous bone and the table is flattened, locking it into place. The graft may face shortening and subsidence by as much as 8 mm with more expected if the endplates are disrupted iatrogenically (22).

Anterior Instrumentation

The flexion-compression injuries addressed with anterior decompression and strut graft fusion require additional stability for satisfactory healing with maintenance of position assured during bone graft incorporation. Generally, in the past, this required a staged procedure with anterior decompression with strut graft followed by posterior instrumentation (68, 106).

Improvements in anterior instrumentation now obtain a stability which approaches that obtained with posterior instrumentation. Anterior instrumentation is most effective when balanced by an intact posterior ligamentous tension band (107, 125). With complete transection of the posterior elements, biomechanical testing has shown that the fixation provided by the anterior instrumentation alone may not be adequate (107). In addition, vertebral bodies weakened by osteoporosis will not give sufficient support for anterior devices.

Like posterior spinal instrumentation, anterior instrumentation had its origins in the application of scoliosis. Zeilke was the prototype. Been et al. have reviewed 29 patients treated with anterior decompression and stabilization with the Slot-Zeilke device and followed them for 3 years (8). There was a loss of correction of 5° or more in 41%. With one solitary rod to transmit axial load, the Slot-Zeilke device is weak during compression, forward bending, and torsion.

Dual rod systems were developed to improve these shortcomings. The Dunn system was strong but bulky (42). Two rods were linked rigidly by vertebral body bridges that had been secured to each vertebra at two points. Unfortunately, its size and ventral positioning have led to fatal complications secondary to aortic erosions (19, 43). The implant has since been removed from the market.

The Kostuik-Harrington device uses either a compression or distraction Harrington rods attached to vertebral body screws (46, 96, 97). Although this system allows an intraoperative correction of kyphosis by distraction, it has been biomechanically unstable when tested in axial rotation (149, 150).

Single and double plating have been performed successfully (76). The low profile Syracuse I-plate is an AO-ASIF DC plate that serves a neutralization function. The plate was modified into an I shape with a gentle curve of the upper and lower ends so that the plate wraps around the vertebrae (6, 148). Only two 6.5-mm screws can be placed into each vertebra. Screws are not able to be placed into the bone graft.

Introduced in 1984, the Kaneda system accomplishes an instrumented reduction with rigid maintenance of fixation (92, 150). A rigid, transverse connector connects the dual vertical rods and contributes to stability in all loading modes (1). Biomechanical studies using calf spines and instrumentation after a lumbar corpectomy have shown greater torsional stiffness with Kaneda than the intact spine and are equal to the 2 above-2 below CD pedicle screw instrumentation (66, 73, 149).

Newer devices, including the Z-plate™ (Danek Inc, designed by Zdeblick) and University Plate™ (Acromed Inc, designed by An) continued to improve rigidity and provide reduction capabilities; they also are low profile. Long-term clinical results of these plates have yet to be published.

Comparative Studies

Several studies, all with relatively small numbers of patients from single institutions, have been done to compare directly the effectiveness of anterior versus posterior procedures regarding canal clearance, sagittal plane correction, and neurologic improvement (15, 46, 69). Esses and colleagues studied 40 patients in a prospective, randomized fashion using either the AO fixator interne or anterior decompression and instrumentation with the Kostuik-Harrington device (46). While the average canal compromise with use of the fixator interne changed from 44% preoperatively to 16.5% postoperatively, anterior decompression led to a decrease from 58% to 4%. There was 11.3° of kyphosis correction with posterior technique versus 9.3° with anterior technique (this was found not to be statistically significant). Their conclusion: posterior distraction can decompress the canal and correct kyphosis if done within 72 hours from the time of injury.

Bradford et al. retrospectively reviewed 87 patients with incomplete neurologic deficits (15). Motor improvement was found in 88% with anterior decompression, versus 64% with posterior indirect reduction. Similarly, bowel and bladder control returned in 69% treated anteriorly compared to 35% posteriorly.

Gertzbein et al., comparing 60 consecutive patients with neurologic deficit and greater than 20% canal compromise, found that neurologic improvement did not vary significantly between approaches (69). Using Frankel grades, there was an 83% improvement rate with a posterior procedure versus 88% with an anterior technique.

Conclusion

The last 40 years has seen great improvements in the treatment of thoracolumbar fractures. These advances are borne on an evolving understanding of spinal mechanics, injury mechanisms, and improved instrumentation. Although techniques may change, treatment will always be guided by well-founded principles. Acute surgical intervention is required to preserve or improve neurologic function, reduce bony deformity, stabilize the spine, and mobilize the patient as quickly as possible (Fig 16.19).

The future is sure to bring forth advances in the mechanical, biological, and preventative methods of spinal injury. Minimally invasive techniques, including laparoscopy and endoscopy of the chest and retroperitoneum, promise to provide an expanded application and enable decompression and stabilization with less surgically-induced trauma. Efforts will be directed toward blocking the secondary injury cascade and manipulating central nervous sys-

MECHANISTIC	MORPHOLOGIC	ANATOMIC	THERAPEUTIC
Axial Compression	I) compression	anterior and middle columns compressed	Orthosis
	II) "stable" burst	a) vertebral body shortened	Orthosis
		b) retropulsed middle column	Orthosis versus posterior distraction
		c) posterior ligaments are intact	
Flexion-compression	I) Wedge	anterior column compressed	Orthosis
	II) interspinous widening	posterior elements disrupted in tension	Posterior instrumentation distraction and extension, consider posterolateral decompression versus anterior decompression with anterior instrumentation
	III) "unstable" burst	retropulsed middle column	
Flexion-distraction	true "Chance" fracture	tensile injury through bone (center of rotation is anterior to vertebral body)	Orthosis (if anatomic)
	"ligamentous Chance"	tensile injury through ligaments	Posterior compression instrumentation
	bilateral "jumped facet"	(center of rotation is posterior to ALL)	Open reduction, posterior compression instrumentation if middle column is intact
		tensile failure of posterior ligaments disc space, interspinous widening intervertebral translation	
Extension	anterior opening of disc	tensile failure of ALL and anterior annulus	Orthosis
	"Lumberjack" shear	3 column ligamentous injury	open reduction, segmental spinal fusion
Rotation	Fracture-dislocation	fracture-dislocation of facet(s) "slice" fracture intervertebral translation	open reduction, posterior segmental spinal fusion
Shear	Fracture-dislocation	facet, pedicle, lamina fractures multiple transverse process fractures, rib fractures intervertebral translation	open reduction, posterior segmental spinal fusion

FIGURE 16.19.
Summary Table

tem plasticity and regeneration potential. The most able of the stated methods is prevention. Public awareness campaigns, auto safety, and other devices diminish the frequency and the severity of such injuries.

References

1. Abumi K, Panjabi MM, Duranceau J. Biomechanical evaluation of spinal fixation devices. Part III: stability provided by six fixation devices and interbody graft. Spine 1989;14:1249–1255.
2. Aebi M, Etter C, Kehl T, et al. The internal skeletal fixation system. Clin Orthop Rel Res 1988;227:30–43.
3. An HS, Vaccaro A, Cotler JM, et al. Low lumbar burst fractures: comparison among body cast, Harrington rod, Luque rod, and Steffee plate. Spine 1991;16:440–444.
4. Anden U, Lake A, Norswall A. The role of the anterior longitudinal ligament in Harrington rod fixation of unstable thoracolumbar spinal fractures. Spine 1980;5:23.
5. Ballock RT, Mackersie R, Abitbol J, et al. Can burst fractures be predicted from plain radiographs? J Bone Joint Surg Br 1992;74:147–150.
6. Bayley JC, Yuan HA, Fredrickson BE. The Syracuse I-Plate. Spine 1991;16(3):5120–5124.
7. Bedbrook GM. Treatment of thoracolumbar dislocation and fractures with paraplegia. Clin Orthop Rel Res 1975;112:27–43.
8. Been HD. Anterior decompression and stabilization of thoracolumbar burst fractures by the use of the Slot-Zielke device. Spine 1991;16(1):70–77.
9. Bleasel A, Clouston P, Dorsch N. Post-traumatic syringomyelia following uncomplicated spinal fracture. J Neurol Neurosurg Psychiatry 1991;54:551–553.
10. Bohlman HH. Late progressive pain following fractures of the thoracolumbar spine. J Bone Joint Surg Am 1976;58:728.
11. Bohlman HH. Current concepts review: treatment of fractures and dislocations of the thoracic and lumbar spine. J Bone Joint Surg Am 1985;67(1):165–169.
12. Bohlman HH, Ducker TB. Spine and spinal cord injuries. In: Herkowitz HN, Garfin SR, Balderston FJ, et al, eds. The spine. 3rd ed. Philadelphia: WB Saunders, 1992:973–1103.
13. Bohlman HH, Freehafer A, Dejak J. The results of treatment of acute injuries of the upper thoracic spine with paralysis. J Bone Joint Surg Am 1985;67:360–369.
14. Bohlman HH, Kirkpatrick JS, Delamarter RB, et al. Anterior decompression for late pain and paralysis after

fractures of the thoracolumbar spine. Clin Orthop Rel Res 1994;300:24–29.
15. Bradford DS, McBride GG. Surgical management of thoracolumbar spine fractures with incomplete neurologic deficits. Clin Orthop Rel Res 1987;218:201–216.
16. Brightman RP, Miller CA, Rea GL, et al. Magnetic resonance imaging of trauma to the thoracic and lumbar spine. Spine 1992;17:541–550.
17. Bracken MB, Holford TR. Effects of timing of methylprednisolone or naloxone administration on recovery of segmented and long-tract neurological function in NASCIS II. J Neurosurg 1993;79:500–507.
18. Bracken MB, Shepard MJ, Collins WF, et al. A randomized, controlled trial of methylprednisolone or naloxone in the treatment of acute spinal-cord injury. New Engl J Med 1990;322(20):1405–1411.
19. Brown LP, Bridwell KH, Holt RT. Aortic erosions and lacerations associated with the Dunn anterior spinal instrumentation. Orthop Trans 1986;10:16–17.
20. Cammisa FP, Eismont FJ, Green BA. Dural laceration occurring with burst fractures and associated laminar fractures. J Bone Joint Surg Am 1989;71:1044–1052.
21. Cantor JB, Lebwohl NH, Garvey T, et al. Nonoperative management of stable thoracolumbar burst fractures with early ambulation and bracing. Spine 1993;18:971–976.
22. Carl AL, Tjromanhauser SG, Roger DJ. Pedicle screw instrumentation for thoracolumbar burst fractures and fracture-dislocations. Spine 1992;17:317–324.
23. Chance GQ. Note on a type of flexion fracture of the spine. Br J Radiol 1948;21:452.
24. Clohisy JC, Akbarnia BA, Bucholz RD, et al. Neurologic recovery associated with anterior decompression of spine fractures at the thoracolumbar junction (T12-L1). Spine 1992;17:325–330.
25. Cotler JM, Vernace JV, Michalski JA. The use of Harrington rods in thoracolumbar fractures. Orthop Clin North Am 1986;17(1):87–103.
26. Davies WE, Morris JH, Hill V. An analysis of conservative (non-surgical) management of thoracolumbar fractures and fracture-dislocations with neural damage. J Bone Joint Surg Am 1980;62:1324–1328.
27. Dekutoski MB, Conlan ES, Salciccioli GG. Spinal mobility and deformity after Harrington rod stabilization and limited arthrodesis of thoracolumbar fractures. J Bone Joint Surg Am 1993;75(2):168–176.
28. Denis F. The three column spine and its significance in the classification of acute thoracolumbar spinal injuries. Spine 1983;8(8):817–831.
29. Denis F. Spinal instability as defined by the three-column spine concept in acute spinal trauma. Clin Orthop Rel Res 1984;189:65–76.
30. Denis F, Armstrong GWD, Searls K, et al. Acute thoracolumbar burst fractures in the absence of neurologic deficit. Clin Orthop Rel Res 1984;189:142–149.
31. Denis F, Burkus JK. Lateral distraction injuries to the thoracic and lumbar spine. J Bone Joint Surg Am 1991;73:1049–1053.
32. Denis F, Burkus JK. Shear fracture-dislocations of the thoracic and lumbar spine associated with forceful hyperextension (lumberjack paraplegia). Spine 1992;17(2):156–161.
33. Dick W. The "Fixatuer Interne" as a versatile implant for spine surgery. Spine 1987;12(9):882–899.
34. Dick W, Kluger P, Magerl F, et al. A new device for internal fixation of thoracolumbar and lumbar spine fractures: the "Fixateur Interne." Paraplegia 1985;23:225–232.
35. Dickson JH, Harrington PR, Erwin WD. Harrington instrumentation in the fractured, unstable thoracic and lumbar spine. Tex Med 1973;69:91.
36. Dolan EJ, Tator CH, Endrenyi L. The value of decompression for acute experimental spinal cord compression injury. J Neurosurg 1980;53:749–755.
37. Dommissee GF. The blood supply of the spinal cord. J Bone Joint Surg Br 1974;56:225.
38. Donovan WH, Dwyer AP. An update on the early management of traumatic paraplegia (nonoperative and operative management). Clin Orthop Rel Res 1984;189:12–21.
39. Drummond DS. Harrington instrumentation with spinous process wiring for idiopathic scoliosis. Orthop Clin North Am 1988;19:281–289.
40. Ducker TB, Russo GL, Bellegarrique R, et al. Complete sensorimotor paralysis after cord injury: mortality, recovery, and therapeutic implications. J Trauma 1979;19(11):837–840.
41. Ducker TB, Salcman M, Daniell HB. Experimental spinal cord trauma, III: therapeutic effect of immobilization and pharmacologic agents. Surg Neurol 1978;10:71–76.
42. Dunn HK. Anterior stabilization of thoracolumbar injuries. Clin Orthop Rel Res 1984;189:116–124.
43. Dunn HK. Anterior spine stabilization and decompression for thoracolumbar injuries. Orthop Clin North Am 1986;17(1):113–119.
44. Edwards CC, Levine AM. Early rod-sleeve stabilization of the injured thoracic and lumbar spine. Orthop Clin North Am 1986;17(1):121–145.
45. Eismont FJ, Green BA, Berkowitz BM, et al. The role of intraoperative ultrasonography in the treatment of thoracic and lumbar spine fractures. Spine 1984;9(8):782–787.
46. Esses SI, Botsford DJ, Kostuik JP. Evaluation of surgical treatment for burst fractures. Spine 1990;15:667–673.
47. Esses SI, Botsford DJ, Wright T, et al. Operative treatment of spinal fractures with the AO internal fixator. Spine 1991;16(3):S146–150.
48. Fabris D, Costantini S, Nena U, et al. Cotrel-Dubousset instrumentation in thoracolumbar seat belt-type and flexion-distraction injuries. J Spinal Disord 1994;7(2):146–152.
49. Farcy JC, Weidenbaum M, Glassman SD. Sagittal index in management of thoracolumbar burst fractures. Spine 1990;15:958–965.
50. Farcy J, Weidenbaum M, Michelsen CB, et al. A comparative biomechanical study of spinal fixation using Cotrel-Dubousset instrumentation. Spine 1987;12(9):877–881.
51. Ferguson RL, Allen BL. A mechanistic classification

of thoracolumbar spine fractures. Clin Orthop Rel Res 1984;189:77–88.
52. Fidler MW. Remodeling of the spinal canal after burst fracture. J Bone Joint Surg Br 1988;70(5):730–732.
53. Fidler MW, Plasmans CMT. The effect of four types of support on the segmental mobility of the lumbosacral spine. J Bone Joint Surg Am 1983;65(7):943–947.
54. Flesch JR, Leider LL, Erickson DL, et al. Harrington instrumentation and spine fusion for unstable fractures and fracture-dislocations of the thoracic and lumbar spine. J Bone Joint Surg Am 1977;59:143–153.
55. Frankel HL, Hancock DO, Hyslop G, et al. The value of postural reduction in the initial management of closed injuries of the spine with paraplegia and tetraplegia. Paraplegia 1969;7:179–192.
56. Fredrickson BE, Edwards WT, Rauschning W, et al. Vertebral burst fractures: an experimental, morphologic, and radiographic study. Spine 1992;17(9):1012–1021.
57. Fredrickson BE, Mann KA, Yuan HA, et al. Reduction of the intracanal fragment in experimental burst fractures. Spine 1988;13:267–271.
58. Fredrickson BE, Yuan H, Miller HM. Burst fractures of the fifth lumbar vertebra. J Bone Joint Surg Am 1982;64(7):1088–1093.
59. Gaines RW, Breedlove RF, Munson G. Stabilization of thoracic and thoracolumbar fracture-dislocations with Harrington rods and sublaminar wires. Clin Orthop Rel Res 1984;189:195–203.
60. Gaines RW, Carson WL, Satterlee CC, et al. Experimental evaluation of seven different spinal fracture internal fixation devices using nonfailure stability testing. Spine 1991;16(8):902–909.
61. Gaines RW, Humphreys WG. A plea for judgment in management of thoracolumbar fractures and fracture-dislocations. Clin Orthop Rel Res 1984;189:36–41.
62. Gardner VO, Armstrong GWD. Long-term lumbar facet joint changes in spinal fracture patients treated with Harrington rods. Spine 1990;15(6):479–484.
63. Garfin SR, Mowery CA, Guerra J, et al. Confirmation of the posterolateral technique to decompress and fuse thoracolumbar spine burst fractures. Spine 1985;10(3):218–223.
64. Geisler FH, Dorsey FC, Coleman WP. Recovery of motor function after spinal-cord injury: a randomized, placebo-controlled trial with GM-1 Ganglioside. New Engl J Med 1991;324(26):1829–1838.
65. Gertzbein SD. Scoliosis Research Society. Multicenter spine fracture study. Spine 1992;17:528–539.
66. Gertzbein SD. Neurologic deterioration in patients with thoracic and lumbar fractures after admission to the hospital. Spine 1994;19(15):1723–1725.
67. Gertzbein SD, Court-Brown CM. Flexion-distraction injuries of the lumbar spine. Clin Orthop Rel Res 1988;227:52–60.
68. Gertzbein SD, Court-Brown CM, Jacobs RR, et al. Decompression and circumferential stabilization of unstable spinal fractures. Spine 1988;13(8):892–895.
69. Gertzbein SD, Court-Brown CM, Marks P, et al. The neurological outcome following surgery for spinal fractures. Spine 1988;13:641–644.
70. Gertzbein SD, Crowe PJ, Fazl M, et al. Canal clearance in burst fractures using the AO internal fixator. Spine 1992;17:558–560.
71. Gertzbein SD, MacMichael D, Tile M. Harrington instrumentation as a method of fixation in fractures of the spine. J Bone Joint Surg Br 1982;64:526–529.
72. Gumley G, Taylor TKF, Ryan MD. Distraction fractures of the lumbar spine. J Bone Joint Surg Br 1982;64(5):520–525.
73. Gurr KR, McAfee PC, Shih C. Biomechanical analysis of anterior and posterior instrumentation systems after corpectomy. J Bone Joint Surg Am 1988;70:1182–1191.
74. Guttman L. History of the National Spinal Injuries Center, Stokes Mandeville Hospital. Paraplegia 1967;5:115–126.
75. Guttman L. Spinal deformity in traumatic paraplegics and tetraplegics following surgical procedures. Paraplegia 1967;7:38–49.
76. Haas N, Blauth M, Tscherne H. Anterior plating in thoracolumbar spine injuries. Spine 1991;16:100–111.
77. Hansebout RR, Tanner JA, Romero-Sierra C. Current status of spinal cord cooling in the treatment of acute spinal cord injury. Spine 1984;9(5):508–511.
78. Hardaker WT, Cook WA, Friedman AH, et al. Bilateral transpedicular decompression and Harrington Rod stabilization in the management of severe thoracolumbar burst fractures. Spine 1992;17(2):162–171.
79. Hardcastle P, Bedbrook G, Curtis K. Long-term results of conservative and operative management in complete paraplegics with spinal cord injuries between T10 and L2 with respect to function. Clin Orthop Rel Res 1987;224:88–96.
80. Harrington RM, Budorick T, Hoyt J, et al. Biomechanics of indirect reduction of bone retropulsed into the spinal canal in vertebral fracture. Spine 1993;18:692–698.
81. Hashimoto T, Kaneda K, Abumi K. Relationship between traumatic spinal canal stenosis and neurologic deficits in thoracolumbar burst fractures. Spine 1988;13:1268–1272.
82. Holdsworth FW. Fractures, dislocations, and fracture-dislocations of the spine. J Bone Joint Surg Br 1963;45(1):6–20.
83. Holdsworth FW. Fractures, dislocations, and fracture-dislocations of the spine. J Bone Joint Surg Am 1970;52(8):1534–1551.
84. Holdsworth FW, Hardy A. Early treatment of paraplegia from fractures of the thoraco-lumbar spine. J Bone Joint Surg Br 1953;35(4):540–550.
85. Jacobs RR, Asher MA, Snider RK. Thoracolumbar spinal injuries. Spine 1980;5(5):463–477.
86. Jacobs RR, Casey MP. Surgical management of thoracolumbar spinal injuries. Clin Orthop Rel Res 1984;189:22–35.
87. James KS, Wenger KH, Schlegel JA, et al. Biomechanical evaluation of the stability of thoracolumbar burst fractures. Spine 1994;19(15):1731–1740.
88. Janssen L, Hansebout RR. Pathogenesis of spinal cord injury and newer treatments: a review. Spine 1989;14(1):23–32.
89. Johnsson R, Herrlin K, Hagglund G. Spinal canal remodeling after thoracolumbar fractures with intraspi-

nal bone fragments: 17 cases followed 1–4 years. Acta Orthop Scand 1991;62:125–127.
90. Kahanovitz N, Arnoczky SP, Levine DT, et al. The effects of internal fixation of the articular cartilage of unfused canine facet joint cartilage. Spine 1984; 9(3):268–272.
91. Kahanovitz N, Bullough P, Jacobs RR. The effect of internal fixation without arthrodesis on human facet joint cartilage. Clin Orthop 1984;189:204.
92. Kaneda K, Abumi K, Fujiya M. Burst fractures with neurologic deficits of the thoracolumbar-lumbar spine. Spine 1984;9:788–795.
93. Keenen TL, Antony J, Benson DR. Dural tears associated with lumbar burst fractures. J Orthop Trauma 1990;4:243–245.
94. Keenen TL, Antony J, Benson DR. Noncontiguous spinal fractures. J Trauma 1990;30(6):489–491.
95. Kirkpatrick JS, Bolesta MJ, Bohlman HH, et al. Axon regeneration after decompression of the conus medullaris. Spine 1994;19(21):2433–2435.
96. Kostuik JP. Anterior fixation for fractures of the thoracic and lumbar spine with or without neurologic involvement. Clin Orthop 1984;189:103–115.
97. Kostuik JP. Anterior fixation for burst fractures of the thoracic and lumbar spine with or without neurologic involvement. Spine 1988;13:286–293.
98. Krag MH. Biomechanics of thoracolumbar spinal fixation: a review. Spine 1991;16(3):S84–S99.
99. Kraus JF, Franti CE, Riggins RS, et al. Incidence of traumatic spinal cord lesions. J Chron Dis 1975; 28:471–492.
100. Krengel WF, Anderson PA, Henley MB. Early stabilization and decompression for incomplete paraplegia due to a thoracic-level spinal cord injury. Spine 1993; 18(14):2080–2087.
101. Krompinger WJ, Fredrickson BE, Mino DE, et al. Conservative treatment of fractures of the thoracic and lumbar spine. Orthop Clin North Am 1986;17(1):161–170.
102. Levine AM, Bosse M, Edwards CC. Bilateral facet dislocations in the thoracolumbar spine. Spine 1988; 13(6):630–640.
103. Lindsey RW, Dick W. The fixateur interne in the reduction and stabilization of thoracolumbar spine fractures in patients with neurologic deficit. Spine 1991; 16(3S):S140–S145.
104. Lindsey RW, Dick W, Nunchuck S, et al. Residual intersegmental spinal mobility following limited pedicle fixation of thoracolumbar spine fractures with the fixateur interne. Spine 1993;18(4):474–478.
105. Luque ER, Cassis N, Ramirez-Wiella G. Segmental spinal instrumentation in the treatment of fractures of the thoracolumbar spine. Spine 1982;7(3):312–317.
106. Malcolm BW, Bradford DS, Winter RB, et al. Post-traumatic kyphosis. J Bone Joint Surg Am 1981;63:891–899.
107. Mann KA, McGowan DP, Fredrickson BE, et al. A biomechanical investigation of short segment spinal fixation for burst fractures with varying degrees of posterior disruption. Spine 1990;15(6):470–478.
108. Marshall LF, Knowlton S, Garfin SR, et al. Deterioration following spinal cord injury. J Neurosurg 1987; 66:400–404.
109. McAfee PC, Bohlman HH. Complications following Harrington instrumentation for fractures of the thoracolumbar spine. J Bone Joint Surg Am 1985;67(5):672–686.
110. McAfee PC, Bohlman HH, Yuan HA. Anterior decompression of traumatic thoracolumbar fractures with incomplete neurological deficit using a retroperitoneal approach. J Bone Joint Surg Am 1985;67:89–104.
111. McAfee PC, Werner FW, Glisson RR. A biomechanical analysis of spinal instrumentation systems in thoracolumbar fractures. Spine 1985;10(3):204–217.
112. McAfee PC, Yuan HA, Fredrickson BE, et al. The value of computed tomography in thoracolumbar fractures. J Bone Joint Surg Am 1983;65:461–473.
113. McAfee PC, Yuan HA, Lasda NA. The unstable burst fracture. Spine 1982;7(4):365–373.
114. McCormack T, Karaikovic E, Gaines RW. The load sharing classification of spine fractures. Spine 1994; 19(15):1741–1744.
115. McGuire RA, Green BA, Eismont FJ, et al. Comparison of stability provided to the unstable spine by the kinetic therapy table and the Stryker frame. Neurosurg 1988;22(5):842–845.
116. McLain RF, Sparling E, Benson DR. Early failure of short-segment pedicle instrumentation for thoracolumbar fractures. J Bone Joint Surg Am 1993; 75(2):162–167.
117. Mumford J, Weinstein JN, Spratt KF, et al. Thoracolumbar burst fractures, the clinical efficacy and outcome of nonoperative management. Spine 1993; 18:955–970.
118. O'Callaghan JP, Ullrich CG, Yuan HA. CT of facet distraction in flexion injuries of the thoracolumbar spine: The "naked" facet. AJNR 1980;1:97–102.
119. Oxland TR, Panjabi MM, Southern EP, et al. An anatomic basis for spinal instability: a porcine trauma model. J Orthop Res 1991;9:452–462.
120. Patwardhan AG, Li S, Gavin T, et al. Orthotic stabilization of thoracolumbar injuries. Spine 1990;15:654–661.
121. Posner E, White AA, Edwards WT, et al. A biomechanical analysis of the clinical stability of the lumbar and lumbosacral spine. Spine 1982;7(4):374–389.
122. Price C, Makintubee S, Herndon W, et al. Epidemiology of traumatic spinal cord injury and acute hospitalization and rehabilitation charges for spinal cord injuries in Oklahoma, 1988–1990. Am J Epidemiol 1994;139(1):37–47.
123. Reid DC, Hu R, Davis LA, et al. The nonoperative treatment of burst fractures in the thoracolumbar spine. J Trauma 1988;18:1188.
124. Rivlin AS, Tator CH. Effect of duration of acute spinal cord compression in a new acute cord injury model in the rat. Surg Neurol 1978;10:39–43.
125. Roberson JR, Whitesides TE. Surgical reconstruction of late post-traumatic thoracolumbar kyphosis. Spine 1985;10(4):307–312.
126. Roberts J, Curtiss P. Stability of the thoracic and lumbar spine in traumatic paraplegia following fracture

or fracture-dislocation. J Bone Joint Surg Am 1970; 52(6):1115–1130.
127. Rossier AB, Foo D, Shillito J, et al. Posttraumatic cervical syringomyelia. Brain 1985;108:439–461.
128. Saboe LA, Reid DC, Davis LA, et al. Spine trauma and associated injuries. J Trauma 1991;31(1):43–48.
129. Sasso RC, Cotler HB. Posterior instrumentation and fusion for unstable fractures and fracture dislocations of the thoracic and lumbar spine. Spine 1993; 18(4):450–460.
130. Schlegel J, Yuan H, Fredrickson B, et al. Timing of surgical decompression and fixation of acute spinal fractures. Ortho Trans 1992;16:688.
131. Shikata J, Yamamuro T, Iida H, et al. Surgical treatment for paraplegia resulting from vertebral fractures in senile osteoporosis. Spine 1990;15(6):485–489.
132. Shirado S, Kaneda K, Tadano S, et al. Influence of disc degeneration on mechanism of thoracolumbar burst fractures. Spine 1992;17:286–292.
133. Soreff J, Axdorph G, Bylund P, et al. Treatment of patients with unstable fractures of the thoracic and lumbar spine. Acta Orthop Scand 1982;53:369–381.
134. Starr JK, Hanley EN. Junctional burst fractures. Spine 1992;17:551–557.
135. Tencer AF, Allen BL, Ferguson RL. A biomechanical study of thoracolumbar spinal fractures with bone in the canal: Part I. The effect of laminectomy. Spine 1985;10:580–585.
136. Tencer AF, Ferguson RL, Allen BL. A biomechanical study of thoracolumbar spinal fractures with bone in the canal: Part II. The effect of flexion angulation. Spine 1985;10:586–589.
137. Transfeldt EE, White D, Bradford DS. Delayed anterior decompression in patients with spinal cord and cauda equina injuries of the thoracolumbar spine. Spine 1990;15:953–957.
138. Vernon JD, Silver JR, Ohry A. Post-traumatic syringomyelia. Paraplegia 1980;20:339–364.
139. Vernon JD, Silver JR, Symon L. Post-traumatic syringomyelia, the results of surgery. Paraplegia 1983; 21:37–46.
140. Vincent KA, Benson DR, McGahan JP. Intraoperative ultrasonography for reduction of thoracolumbar burst fractures. Spine 1989;14(4):387–390.
141. Watson N. Ascending cystic degeneration of the cord after spinal cord injury. Paraplegia 1981;19:89–95.
142. Weinstein JN, Collalto P, Lehmann TR. Thoracolumbar "burst" fractures treated conservatively: a long-term follow-up. Spine 1988;13:33–37.
143. Weiss M, Bentkowski Z. Biomechanical study in dynamic spondylodesis of the spine. Clin Orthop Rel Res 1974;103:199–203
144. Whitesides TE. Traumatic kyphosis of the thoracolumbar spine. Clin Orthop Rel Res 1977;128:78–92.
145. Willen J, Lindahl S, Nordwall A. Unstable thoracolumbar fractures. Spine 1985;10(2):111–122.
146. Wilmot CB, Hall KM. Evaluation of acute surgical intervention in traumatic paraplegia. Paraplegia 1986; 24:71–76.
147. Wiltse LL. A review of "Stabilization of the lower thoracic and lumbar spine with external skeletal fixation" by Friedrich P. Magerl, MD. Clin Orthop Rel Res 1986; 203:63–66.
148. Yuan HA, Mann KA, Found EM, et al. Early clinical experience with the Syracuse I-plate: an anterior spinal fixation device. Spine 1988;13:278–285.
149. Zdeblick TA, Shirado O, McAfee PC, et al. Anterior spinal fixation after lumbar corpectomy. J Bone Joint Surg Am 1991;73:527–534.
150. Zdeblick TA, Warden KE, Zou D, et al. Anterior spinal fixators. Spine 1993;18(4):513–517.

CHAPTER SEVENTEEN

Rehabilitation of Traumatic Spinal Cord Injury

Christopher Formal

Introduction

Scope of Rehabilitation

Impairment, Disability, and Handicap

Impairment is an abnormality of bodily function, and is determined by the history and physical examination. Physicians are trained to diagnose impairment and the pathology underlying it. An example is paraplegia caused by fracture of T12 (29).

Disability is a restriction of the ability to perform a normal activity. It occurs consequent to an impairment. It is determined less readily by the traditional medical evaluation. A typical disability caused by paraplegia is the inability to walk.

A *handicap* is a disadvantage that limits a person's ability to fulfill a societal role. Thus, the inability to walk is a handicap for a construction worker in that it prevents employment. Inability to walk may not be a handicap (at least as far as employment is concerned) for a secretary.

Rehabilitation medicine is relatively less focused on impairment than are other medical specialties, but it has a stronger attention to disability and handicap. Rehabilitation often involves minimizing disability and handicap in the face of an impairment that may be impossible to modify. With severe impairment (as is common with spinal cord injury), prevention of secondary impairment (such as contracture and pressure ulcer) is also crucial.

The Rehabilitation Team

A clinical "problem list" for a person with spinal cord injury (SCI) may include many items, such as mobility deficit, self-care deficit, neurogenic bladder, neurogenic bowel, spasticity, adjustment, and discharge planning. No single discipline can encompass these, and thus treatment is delivered by a team.

The individual team members may concentrate on different problems. The mobility deficit may be addressed primarily by the physical therapist, and the self-care deficit by the occupational therapist. The physician and nurse manage the neurogenic bowel and bladder. The physician may assume primary responsibility for treating spasticity. The psychologist assists with adjustment problems, and the social worker directs discharge planning.

While certain problems may be addressed primarily by certain team members, any team member may contribute to the resolution of any problem. This distinguishes an interdisciplinary from a multidisciplinary team. Any contribution to the resolution of a problem should be welcomed and not viewed as a battle over "turf."

The team is led by a physician with a special interest in rehabilitation. The team leader has ultimate responsibility for directing medical and rehabilitation management. However, a dictatorial leadership style does not suit an interdisciplinary team.

A team may also include a case manager. This person is responsible for tasks such as scheduling, setting up transportation, and interfacing with insurance companies.

Phases of Care After SCI

Care after SCI can be divided into acute management (pre-hospital and acute hospital care), inpatient rehabilitation, and outpatient follow-up. Each has certain areas of emphasis.

Acute management begins in the field and extends through care in the intensive care unit, including surgery. The goals of this phase include maximizing neurologic recovery (thus minimizing impairment) and achieving medical and spinal stability sufficient to permit mobilization out of bed. Acute management might last several weeks.

Inpatient rehabilitation involves a minimum of several hours out of bed daily, including participation in scheduled therapy sessions. Routine nursing care during nonscheduled hours builds on accomplishments in therapy sessions. For example, a person with paraplegia who has learned to dress in occupational therapy should not depend on the nurses for dressing in the morning. The goals of this phase include maximizing mobility and self-care skills (thus minimizing disability), provision of appropriate equipment, patient and caretaker education, and discharge planning. Inpatient rehabilitation might last 2 months.

Outpatient follow-up includes care by a visiting nursing agency, outpatient physical and occupational therapy, and visits to an interdisciplinary clinic. Goals include assisting with family, educational, and vocational pursuits (thus minimizing handicap), and preventing and managing secondary problems.

The quality of a system of care for SCI can be judged by the degree to which these three phases interact and overlap. For example, long-term issues, such as discharge planning and home modification, should be addressed as early as possible during the acute hospitalization. If the surgeon has confidence in the level of care delivered in the inpatient rehabilitation setting, and is assured of the ability to have involvement during this phase, then transfer can occur earlier. For example, rehabilitation transfer may occur while external stabilization devices are still in place. This can decrease hospital length of stay, which minimizes problems associated with immobilization.

Aspects of the Injury

Epidemiology

Causes of Injury

The most common general cause, accounting for 44.5% of traumatic SCI, is motor vehicle crash (24). More specifically, automobile crashes and motorcycle crashes cause 35.8% and 6.1% of injuries respectively. The second most common general cause is falls, accounting for 18.1% of injuries. The third most common general cause is acts of violence (other than gunshot), which causes 16.6% of injuries. Gunshots are responsible for 14.6%. The fourth most common general cause is sports and recreational injuries, causing 12.7% of injuries; 8.5% are due to diving injuries. Over time, the proportions of SCI caused by motor vehicle crashes and by sports and recreational activities have decreased. The proportions caused by falls and by acts of violence, however, have increased.

Age at Time of Injury

Traumatic SCI is very much a problem in young adults. The mean age at time of injury is 30.7 years, with a median of 24 years and a mode of 19 years. Etiology varies with age. Sports and recreational injuries cause a relatively high percentage—25.8%—of injuries in persons younger than 16. Falls cause a relatively high percentage of injuries in the elderly, accounting for 60.1% of injuries in those 76 and older.

Gender

82.2% of traumatic SCI occurs in males. Sports and recreational injuries cause a greater proportion of the injuries suffered by males compared with females, whereas motor vehicle crashes cause a greater proportion of injuries suffered by females than by males.

Month and Day of Injury

The incidence of traumatic SCI peaks in July and reaches a nadir in February. Much of this pattern appears to result from sports and recreational injuries. Saturday is the most common day of injury.

Ethnic Group

Reporting practices complicate the interpretation of figures regarding ethnic group and traumatic SCI. Whites appear to be relatively under-represented in the SCI population, whereas African-Americans are over-represented. Acts of violence are responsible for a relatively high proportion of SCI in African-Americans.

Incidence and Prevalence

In the United States, the annual incidence of cases that survive until hospitalization is estimated to be 30 to 40 per million. The national prevalence is estimated to be 183,000 to 230,000.

Neurologic Assessment

Overview

The neurologic assessment of SCI begins with determination of motor and sensory function. These data allow determination of the level of the injury, the degree of completeness, and, possibly, a clinical syndrome. Determination of reflex function can provide further information and may be particularly useful in determining a clinical syndrome, such as conus medullaris injury. Imaging and electrophysiologic studies are not routinely required for neurologic assessment. The classification system presented here has been developed by the American Spinal Injury Association (1, 18). It is summarized in Figure 17.1.

Motor Evaluation

Table 17.1 lists key muscle groups for root levels C5 through T1, and L2 through S1. Each of these groups is graded according to the 6 point scale shown in Table 17.2. Each group is tested bilaterally. In addition, the anal sphincter is tested for voluntary contraction.

Sensory Evaluation

Figure 17.2 shows key sensory points for root levels C2 through S4–5. Each dermatome is tested bilaterally for pin and touch sensation. The score is 2 for normal, 1 for impaired, and 0 for absent. If the pin is felt as a touch, without sensation of sharpness, the score for pin sensation is 0. If an area is hypersensitive to pin or touch, the score is 1. In addition to testing of these dermatomes, deep rectal sensation is tested by digital examination. Proprioception should also be tested.

Neurologic Level

The neurologic level specifies the caudal extent of normal function of the spinal cord. A level of C5

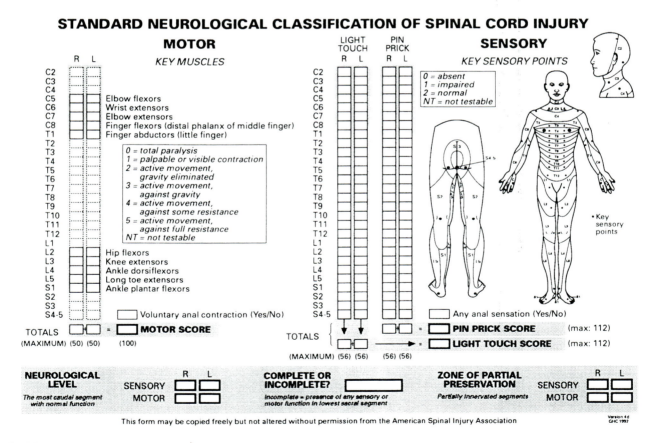

FIGURE 17.1.

Summary of ASIA Standard Neurological Classification of Spinal Cord Injury. Reprinted with permission from American Spinal Injury Association. Standards for neurological and functional classification of spinal cord injury. Rev. ed. Chicago: American Spinal Injury Association, 1992.

TABLE 17.1.
Key Muscle Groups for Root Levels C5–T1 and L2–S1 (1)

Root Level	Key Muscle Group
C5	Elbow flexors (biceps, brachialis)
C6	Wrist extensors (extensor carpi radialis longus and brevis)
C7	Elbow extensors (triceps)
C8	Finger flexors (flexor digitorum profundus) to middle finger
T1	Small finger abductors (abductor digiti minimi)
L2	Hip flexors (iliopsoas)
L3	Knee extensors (quadriceps)
L4	Ankle dorsiflexors (tibialis anterior)
L5	Long toe extensors (extensor hallucis longus)
S1	Ankle plantarflexors (gastrocnemius, soleus)

means that there is normal function through C5, with abnormal function (sensory and/or motor) at the level of C6, and usually below C6. It is also possible to specify a sensory level (which is determined without regard to motor function), and, similarly, a motor level, and a level for each side.

Special consideration is given to the relationship of neurologic level and motor function because of the multiple root innervation of the key muscle groups. For example, the key muscle group for C7 is the elbow extensors (triceps). This group also receives some contribution from C8. Thus, the C7 group could be weak despite entirely normal C7 function. To account for this, by convention, if a key muscle group is tested as at least 3, it is considered to have normal innervation, provided the next most rostral group tests as at least 4.

The term "paraplegia" applies to a level of T1 or below. Thus upper extremity function is spared. "Tetraplegia" (which is preferred over "quadriplegia") applies to a level above T1. The use of "paraparesis" and "quadriparesis" is discouraged; rather, the degree of completeness is conveyed as outlined below.

Degree of Completeness

The degree of completeness is specified by the ASIA Impairment Scale, as described in Table 17.3. A

TABLE 17.2.
Six-point Scale for Grading of Muscle Strength (1)

0 = total paralysis
1 = palpable or visible contraction
2 = active movement, full range of motion (ROM) with gravity eliminated
3 = active movement, full ROM against gravity
4 = active movement, full ROM against moderate resistance
5 = (normal) active movement, full ROM against full resistance
NT = not testable

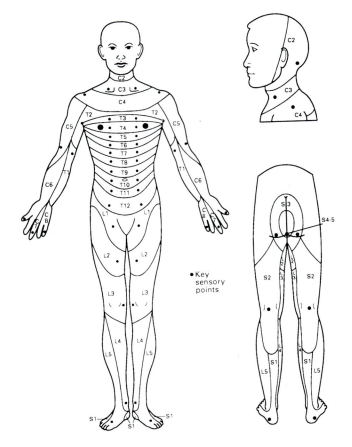

FIGURE 17.2.
Key sensory points. Reprinted with permission from American Spinal Injury Association. Standards for neurological and functional classification of spinal cord injury. Rev. ed. Chicago: American Spinal Injury Association, 1992.

grade of A to E is assigned. The essential determination of whether the lesion is complete or incomplete is based on digital rectal examination and on examination of the S4–5 dermatome. The neurologic status can be summarized by noting the level and ASIA Impairment Scale; e.g., "the injury has caused C5 ASIA Impairment Scale C tetraplegia."

TABLE 17.3.
ASIA Impairment Scale (1)

A = Complete. No sensory or motor function is preserved in the sacral segments S4–5.
B = Incomplete. Sensory but not motor function is preserved below the neurologic level and extends through the sacral segments S4–5.
C = Incomplete. Motor function is preserved below the neurologic level, and the majority of key muscles below the neurologic level have a muscle grade less than 3.
D = Incomplete. Motor function is preserved below the neurologic level, and the majority of key muscles below the neurologic level have a muscle grade greater than or equal to 3.
E = Normal. Sensory and motor function is normal.

Clinical Syndrome

The neurologic examination may suggest a specific site of pathology. The pattern of central spinal cord injury occurs with cervical injury and causes greater loss of function in the upper extremities, especially distally. The Brown-Sequard sydrome is unilateral injury to the cord, causing ipsilateral loss of motor and proprioceptive function and contralateral loss of pain and temperature sense. The anterior cord syndrome causes loss of strength and pin sensation, with sparing of touch and proprioceptive sense. Conus medullaris injury causes flaccid lower extremity paralysis and absent sacral reflexes (such as the anal wink and bulbocavernosus); occasionally, the injury may occur just above the tip of the conus, sparing sacral reflexes. Cauda equina injury causes flaccid lower extremity paralysis and absent sacral reflexes, with a greater propensity for asymmetry than does conus medullaris injury.

Distribution of Impairments

Slightly more than half of injuries result in tetraplegia, and slightly less than half cause paraplegia. The three most common levels are, in order, C5, C4, and C6. For paraplegia, the most common levels, in order, are T12, L1, and T10 (24). Slightly more than half of injuries cause complete lesions.

Neurologic Prognosis

Neurologic prognosis is critical to all involved. This section relates neurologic status upon admission with that occurring later. The separate issue of what a person with a given neurological status can be expected to do is considered later in this chapter.

Changes in ASIA Impairment Scale Grade

The relationship of admission to discharge ASIA Impairment Scale Grade is shown in Table 17.4 (16). A decline occurs in only slightly more than 1% of cases; most remain the same or improve. The major question involves the chances of improvement to a grade of D (which represents recovery of functional strength) in cases admitted with grades of A, B, or C. The percentages are 2.8, 27.6, and 53.3, respectively.

Changes in Level

Changes in level can have great functional implications; the levels C4, C5, C6, and C7 each imply significantly different potential for mobility and activities of daily living. Persons admitted with these levels and motor complete injuries (ASIA grades A and B) are likely to gain a motor level, although not necessarily a sensory level (16).

Other Predictive Factors

Prognostication is difficult for those admitted with ASIA Impairment Scale grades of B. In such cases, preservation of pin sensation suggests a good prognosis (13). It may reflect the proximity of the motor tracts to those carrying pin sense. Prognostication is also difficult for those admitted with grades of C; in these cases, knee extensor strength greater than 3/5 at two months indicates a good prognosis for ambulation, if initial quadriceps strength was 2/5 or less (12). A lower extremity motor score (taken by summing the scores of the 10 lower extremity key muscle groups) of 10 at 1 month predicts ambulation, perhaps with orthoses (46, 47). Incomplete paraplegia with a level of T12 or lower at 1 month suggests a good prognosis for ambulation, as does incomplete paraplegia with hip flexion or knee extension of at least 2/5 at 1 month (46). For patients with tetraplegia and the central cord syndrome, prognosis for ambulation is good if the age is below 50 (41).

Pharmacological Strategies for Preservation of Neurologic Function

In addition to the initial mechanical injury, trauma may have secondary effects on the spinal cord. These effects may be active in the hours or days after injury, and thus may be accessible to intervention.

Methylprednisolone, delivered as an intravenous bolus of 30mg/kg over 15 minutes, followed 45 minutes later by an infusion of 5.4mg/kg/hr for 23 hours, can improve subsequent sensory and motor function (7). This should begin within 8 hours of injury; if the treatment begins later, there could be a deleterious effect (8). The benefit may be caused by inhibition of lipid peroxidation, rather than by its effect at glucocorticoid receptors. Further study, including evaluation of a longer duration of treatment, is in progress (6). GM-1 ganglioside, 100 mg intravenously daily, for 18 to 32 days, beginning within 3 days of injury, may foster improvement in ASIA Impairment Scale grade and in motor strength (23). Gangliosides are present in the membranes of central nervous system cells, and there are several possible mechanisms by which GM-1 ganglioside may help damaged neurons.

TABLE 17.4.
ASIA Impairment Scale Admission Grade related to Discharge Grade. Percentages are given. In the source, the term "Frankel Grade" is used (16). Although there are minor differences, the grading systems are very similar. The ASIA Impairment Scale is currently in broader use.

Admission Grade	Discharge Grade					
	A	B	C	D	E	Unknown
A	88.8	5.0	2.9	2.8	0	0.6
B	4.9	48.9	15.6	27.6	0.7	2.3
C	1.9	0.8	41.4	53.3	1.3	1.3
D	0.5	0.5	0.8	90.3	6.5	1.4

The observation that the beneficial effect occurs in the lower extremities after cervical injuries, as opposed to the upper extremities, suggests that the site of action is in white matter axons rather than in the gray matter.

Other agents may prove beneficial. Tirilazad mesylate is an inhibitor of lipid peroxidation without glucocorticoid activity. It has proven beneficial in experimental SCI (20). Human trials are underway (6).

Strategies for Restoration of Chronically Lost Neurologic Function

Restoration of chronically lost neurologic function can involve improving the activity of damaged neurons that span the lesion, or inducing the regrowth of axons across the lesion. An axon may span the lesion but be nonfunctional because of deficient myelination, which causes conduction block. 4-aminopyridine, which improves the safety factor for conduction by prolonging the duration of the action potiential, has caused temporary improvement in neurologic function in humans with chronic SCI (25).

Transplantation therapy is under investigation in animals (4). Success depends on (in ascending order of difficulty) survival of the graft, formation of new synapses, and integration of the new synapses into the motor and sensory mechanisms of the host. The first problem has been solved in animals, and some preparations form new synapses. In addition, transplantation may have beneficial effects unrelated to the formation of new synapses. Grafts are typically homografts (from the same species) and fetal.

Medical Consequences of the Injury

Deep Venous Thrombosis and Pulmonary Embolus

Incidence

In the absence of prophylactic measures, deep venous thrombosis (DVT) may occur in as many as 81% of victims of SCI (22). Pulmonary embolus (PE) is the third leading cause of death in the first year after SCI (14).

Pathophysiology

Venous stasis after SCI is associated with lower extremity paralysis (38). In addition, a hypercoagulable state has been demonstrated. Whether the third factor of Virchow's triad—intimal injury—is present is not known.

Surveillance

Examination of the lower extremities should be part of the routine daily examination after SCI, and findings should immediately trigger further evaluation, such as duplex scanning. Unfortunately, physical findings are often absent despite extensive thrombosis (22). Duplex scanning (or other noninvasive tests) can be used as a screening tool in those without findings, but it may not be accurate in such asymptomatic cases. Thus, it is difficult to recommend any specific screening regimen (49).

Prophylaxis

Prophylactic regimens can target the etiologic factors of hypercoagulability and stasis. A combination of subcutaneous heparin 5000u every 12 hours (beginning 3 days after injury), and lower extremity compression boots and gradient elastic stockings is reasonable (38). The stockings and compression boots are used 23hrs/day. The heparin should typically be continued for 8 to 12 weeks. The compression boots should be continued for 2 weeks; otherwise their use would interfere with mobilization and rehabilitation.

Autonomic Dysreflexia

Presentation

The combination of paroxysmal hypertension and headache in a person with midthoracic or higher SCI strongly suggests autonomic dysreflexia (AD). There are myriad other manifestations, which may be present, including tingling, feelings of coldness or warmth, a sense of impending catastrophe, diaphoresis, nasal congestion, piloerection, mydriasis, tachycardia and bradycardia, and dysrhythmias. In addition to these manifestations, complications such as atrial fibrillation, seizures, intracerebral hemorrhage, and death can occur. Multiple alternative terms, such as autonomic hyperreflexia, exist for the problem (11, 19, 31, 45). Patient and caretaker education regarding AD is crucial because episodes may occur at home, requiring immediate management without medical personnel.

AD is one of several entities that can present with hypertension and headache. A differential diagnosis includes pheochromocytoma, intracranial pathology, and toxemia of pregnancy.

Pathophysiology

AD occurs when a noxious stimulus below the level of the lesion elicits a sympathetic response. This response is excessive, caused either by loss of supraspinal control or by alterations in neurotransmitter levels or sensitivity to neurotransmitters. When the lesion is mid-thoracic or higher, the splanchnic outflow is involved; apparently, this results in hypertension. Individuals with SCI often have relatively low baseline blood pressures; for example, levels of 140/90 may represent a significant elevation. Regulatory centers in the brain try to compensate for this, resulting in vasodilatation and flushing over the face. Dilatation of the intracranial vessels may cause headache.

Triggering Stimuli

Any noxious stimulus below the level of the lesion can cause the syndrome. Episodes are precipitated most commonly by bladder distention caused by a problem such as a blocked catheter. Rectal distention is another typical cause. Acute medical problems, such as acute abdomen or pulmonary embolus, can present as AD. SCI may mask other manifestations of the problem, such as abdominal pain. Numerous other causes have been reported. Occasionally, the etiology cannot be discerned.

Treatment

When a person with mid-thoracic or higher SCI reports sudden onset of headache, blood pressure should be checked immediately. If possible, the person should assume or be placed in a sitting position, thus raising the head above the heart and using gravity to help control intracranial blood pressure.

A rapid search for the triggering cause is undertaken. The bladder should be considered first. If a catheter is in place, it should be checked for kinking or blockage. If replacement is necessary, the tip of the new catheter can be coated with lidocaine jelly before insertion. If a catheter is not in place, and bladder distention is suspected, a catheter should be passed; as noted, lidocaine jelly may be helpful. If a catheter is in place and is draining properly, but bladder irritation or spasms are suspected as a cause of autonomic dysreflexia, instillation of 30 to 60 cc of 2% lidocaine may be helpful.

If the bladder is not implicated, bowel impaction should be considered. Vigorous disimpaction may exacerbate AD, and application of an anesthetic jelly, such as dibucaine, to the rectum should be performed. The blood pressure should then moderate, and disimpaction can be gently carried out.

If AD is severe, treatment with medication can begin at any time. Sublingual nitroglycerine can be rapidly effective. For severe cases, intravenous nitroglycerine, intravenous nitroprusside, or spinal anesthesia should be considered. Beta blockers are best avoided.

Proper treatment requires accurate diagnosis. For example, if autonomic dysreflexia and toxemia of pregnancy are confused, the outcome will be compromised.

Prophylaxis

Individuals susceptible to recurrent episodes of AD may benefit from prophylactic treatment with a variety of agents, including alpha-adrenergic blockers (such as terazosin), calcium channel blockers, nitrates, guanethidine, and others. Ablative neurosurgical procedures can also prevent episodes in severe cases.

Heterotopic Ossification

Presentation

Heterotopic ossification (HO) involves the formation of periarticular bone. It can occur in parts of the body affected by central nervous system trauma, such as SCI or traumatic brain injury (21, 44). It usually begins in the weeks or months after injury. Presentation can range from subclinical to florid, with swelling and warmth of the extremity, accompanied by loss of joint range of motion, and eventual fusion (Fig. 17.3). HO can mimic and coexist with other problems, such as deep venous thrombosis. When a therapist reports

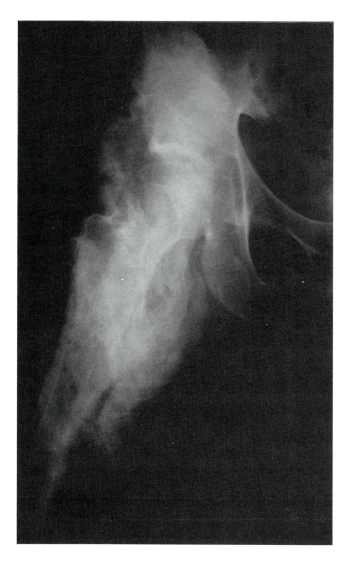

FIGURE 17.3.

Heterotopic ossification about the hip joint after SCI.

loss of joint range at the shoulder, elbow, hip, or knee of a person at risk, HO should always be considered. Detection on bone scan precedes that on plain radiograph. Active HO may also cause an increase in alkaline phosphatase activity. The underlying pathophysiology is not known.

Treatment

Overall goals include minimizing the mass of bone that forms, and maintaining joint range of motion.

While medication may be effective in preventing HO, such prophylactic treatment is not usually recommended after SCI. Drugs are used to limit the progression of HO that has been detected.

Etidronate disodium may prevent the conversion of amorphous calcium phosphate compounds into hydroxyapatite crystals, thus blocking formation of bone. The optimal dose and duration of treatment are not known. Administration of 20 mg/kg po daily for 6 months is reasonable. Occasionally, a rebound follows cessation of therapy. The drug can be given intravenously, but experience with this in the treatment of HO is limited. Indomethacin 25 mg po tid and other nonsteroidal anti-inflammatory agents are also used. Therapeutic irradiation can be considered in severe cases. These interventions are useful only with evolving cases, and will have no effect on mature HO.

Range of motion exercises in cases of HO improve the ultimate joint range of motion. In some cases, the loss of range of motion is not acceptable. Surgical resection of bone may succeed in restoring joint range, or it may create a false but functional "joint". There is a risk of postsurgical recurrence, which can progress to re-ankylosis. Criteria for the timing of surgery are lacking. Surgery carries a high morbidity compared with other orthopedic procedures.

Spasticity

Presentation

Spasticity is a motor disorder with both positive and negative features. Positive manifestations include a velocity-dependent increase in muscle tone during stretch, exaggerated tendon jerks, clonus, positive Babinski sign, and muscle spasms that occur in response to painful or cutaneous stimulation. Negative features include weakness and loss of dexterity (54). Spasticity follows upper motor neuron injury, but the exact pathophysiology is unknown.

Epidemiology

Over half of the persons with chronic SCI experience spasticity (33). Spasticity causes difficulties severe enough to require treatment with medication or surgery in greater than 30% of patients (37). Spasticity appears to be more common in those with ASIA B and C injuries than in those with A or D injuries.

Treatment

Treatment of spasticity is aimed at reducing the positive manifestations, such as increased muscle tone and spasms. Treatment need only be undertaken if these manifestations are disruptive. Occasionally, spasticity can be used to advantage by the individual.

Treatment begins with a regular program of muscle stretching. This temporarily reduces spasticity and also decreases the risk of contractures.

Medications for spasticity either block excitatory neurotransmitters, or facilitate inhibitory transmitters (17, 54). Baclofen is generally the first-line medication. It can be started with a dose of 15 mg po divided into three doses daily, and titrated upward as needed. It is common for an individual to require greater than 100 mg daily in divided doses; a total daily dose of 200 mg can be reasonable in severe cases. This dose must be approached slowly. Sedation is the most common side effect. Abrupt cessation of baclofen can cause a dramatic withdrawal syndrome; this patient should be gradually weaned off the medication.

Clonidine can have a beneficial effect on spasticity. It is started as a dose of 0.05 mg po bid, and can be gradually increased to 0.1 mg po qid. Alternatively, it can be delivered by patch. It can exacerbate orthostatic hypotension.

Diazepam is effective in some cases. It can begin as a dose of 2 mg po tid, and can be titrated as high as 20 mg po tid. Sedation can occur, and tolerance can develop. It should be avoided in patients who have a history of substance abuse.

Dantrolene differs from the preceding agents in that its effect does not involve neurotransmitters. It acts peripherally by uncoupling excitation from muscle contraction. It can be started at 25 mg po bid and can be titrated as high as 100 mg po qid. The risk of hepatitis requires regular monitoring of hepatic enzymes.

There are several invasive modes of spasticity management (54). If a specific group of muscles is causing difficulty (for example, spastic plantar flexors may disrupt a gait pattern, or spastic hip adductors may interfere with perineal hygiene), a nerve block or motor point block may be helpful. Motor point block can be accomplished by injection of phenol or botulinum toxin. The former is less expensive, but injection must be accompanied by electromyographic guidance. In addition, it can occasionally cause persistent sensory symptoms. The latter is more expensive, but the procedure may be easier and potential side effects may be less. The effect of both treatments is on the order of months. Neither method is practical for managing widespread spasticity.

Generalized spasticity that is not amenable to treatment with oral medication can be managed with an implanted baclofen pump. A low dose of baclofen infused into the lumbar subarachnoid space decreases lower extremity spasticity. The medication is diluted by the time it traverses the brain, thus avoiding cognitive side effects.

At all stages in the evaluation and treatment of spasticity, consideration should be given to possible exacerbating factors. Any noxious stimulus, such as urinary tract infection or stone, pressure ulceration, ingrown toenail, or bowel impaction, can worsen spasticity. Indeed, in the presence of sensory impairment, an increase in spasticity can be the presenting sign of an acute illness.

An exacerbation of the underlying neurologic insult can also cause increased spasticity. This could occur with persistently unstable spine, an undiscovered second spinal injury, or post-traumatic cystic myelopathy (5).

Pressure Ulceration

Overview

Persons with spinal cord injury are particularly susceptible to pressure ulceration. In the past, it was a major cause of mortality, and it remains one of the most frequent—perhaps the most frequent—forms of morbidity. It comes to dominate the lives of some patients, and a person who would otherwise be independent at a wheelchair level may be rendered bedfast by persistent ulceration (17).

Pathophysiology

The basic pathophysiology involves the application of a pressure sufficient to block capillary flow over a period sufficient to cause necrosis of tissue (52). SCI predisposes to this because of impaired sensation; the absence of discomfort results in less shifting of weight. Paralysis without associated loss of sensation, as can occur in polio or amyotrophic lateral sclerosis, seems to carry a far smaller risk of pressure ulceration. Whether SCI makes tissue more vulnerable to a given pressure load is uncertain.

In addition to pressure, shear contributes to the development of ulcers. Shear is related to, but distinct from, friction. It results when the skin is displaced in a direction parallel to underlying bone. This can occur when one sits in bed at a 45° angle. Friction holds the skin in place against the mattress, while the underlying sacrum descends because of gravity. The blood vessels between the sacrum and the skin are distorted, and blood flow is interrupted. This may be a mechanism for the development of ulcers in the intergluteal area.

While ulcers are commonly thought to begin at the level of the skin and become deeper as they worsen, not all ulcers behave in this manner. Some may begin with necrosis of deeper tissue, such as muscle, at the interface with bone. Breakdown of the skin would then be a later event. This mechanism may account for ulcers that are small on the surface but undermine beneath.

Location

The most common locations for ulcers after SCI are the sacrum, heels, ischii, and trochanters (53). Early in the course, scapular ulcers are also common, perhaps related to the use of halo or body jacket immobilization.

Evaluation

Accurate description of an ulcer is necessary to follow the progress of treatment. The horizontal dimensions and depth of the ulcer should be recorded. Although depth can also be recorded as a dimension, it may be more meaningful to specify which layers of tissue are involved, such as subcutaneous fat, muscle, or bone. Several systems exist for describing the depth; alternatively, a verbal description may suffice.

Therapeutic decisions are affected by whether underlying osteomyelitis exists. The white count, sedimentation rate, radiograph, and bone scan are of limited use in making this determination. MRI may be more reliable. The definitive study is bone biopsy with pathologic examination and culture.

Prevention

Prevention involves decreasing pressure and the time over which it is applied. Pressure is reduced by the use of specialized surfaces, and time is reduced by frequent changes in position, or by alternating pressure surfaces.

A variety of specialized mattresses and wheelchair cushions are marketed for reducing pressure and decreasing pressure ulcer risk (3, 52). Certain products, such as air-fluidized beds, are effective, but they are practical only in a hospital setting, being too expensive or ungainly for use in the home. Water mattresses, or gel or foam mattress overlays, can be used in the home. Wheelchair cushions can be foam, gel, or air.

A regular turning schedule, which includes repositioning in bed every 2 hours, should be sufficient to avoid pressure ulceration. Position can be alternated between supine, side-lying (though not directly on the trochanter), and, if possible, prone. Certain sophisticated devices, such as rotating beds or alternating pressure mattresses, may be useful in a hospital setting; however, like air-fluidized beds, they generally are not appropriate for home use. Weight shifts should be done every 30 minutes while sitting in the wheelchair. These can be done by push-up, or by leaning forward or to the side. Persons with high tetraplegia can weight shift by a motorized tilt-back or tilt-in-space device.

Prevention depends on proper behavior. Thus, education of the person at risk, as well as caretakers, is crucial.

Local Care

Local care includes debridement of necrotic tissue, maintenance of proper moistness of the wound bed, control of infection, and prevention of outside contamination (3, 52). Debridement can be accomplished with scissors or scalpel. If the necrotic tissue is adherent and difficult to debride mechanically, an enzymatic agent, such as collagenase, can be applied.

A dry wound bed usually is undesirable. A healthy wound heals more rapidly in a moist environment. Thus, dressing, such as dry gauze, which wicks moisture from the bed, may be less effective than calcium alginate preparations, hydrocolloids, and polyurethane films, which retain some of the wound moisture close to the wound bed. The latter two types of dressings are occlusive. Although they have not been found to increase the risk of infection, they should not be used if the wound is grossly infected.

Most ulcers are not infected and need only be cleansed with saline solution. Ulcers that have purulent drainage and a foul odor can be treated with meticulous debridement, more frequent dressing changes, and topical antibiotics, such as silver sulfadiazine, bacitracin, metrinidazole, or combinations of neomycin, bacitracin, and polymixin B. Topical antiseptics should be avoided because of potential for tissue damage.

An infected ulcer associated with fever and spreading infection of soft tissue or bone requires systemic antibiotics. Osteomyelitis may not resolve without operative debridement.

Surgical Treatment

Deep ulcers, or ulcer involving bone, may not heal, may require an unacceptably long period to heal, or may heal in a manner that only predisposes to subsequent breakdown. In such cases, surgery may be preferable.

The goal of surgery is not simply wound coverage. The site must be repaired in a manner that allows it to resist expected pressure and shear. For this reason, coverage by myocutaneous flap is usually the procedure of choice.

Surgery is typically followed by several weeks of relative immobilization. Positioning is selected to avoid pressure or stretch about the surgical site. As healing occurs, massage is used to mobilize the tissue and prevent adhesion to underlying bone. The joints are mobilized to prevent contracture until hip flexion above 90° is achieved.

The flap may be healed sufficiently to allow sitting and weight bearing 2 to 4 weeks after surgery. Initially, sitting is for very short periods and is advanced gradually. Pallor or redness at the operative site that does not resolve with 10 minutes of pressure relief is an indication to decrease the period of sitting (3).

Neurogenic Bladder

Pathophysiology

Severe SCI at any level usually is followed by a period of bladder flaccidity; with injuries of the conus medullaris or cauda equina, flaccidity may be permanent. If the injury is above the conus, bladder reflexes usually return after a period of weeks or months. Filling of the bladder leads to reflex bladder contraction; there is simultaneous reflex contraction of the sphincter mechanism. This lack of coordination between the bladder and the sphincter mechanism is called dyssynergia. It results from the isolation of the pontine micturition center from the spinal reflex arcs. As a result of dyssynergia, high pressures develop within the bladder, and voiding may or may not occur (Fig. 17.4). High pressure voiding can eventually result in lower tract changes, hydronephrosis, reflux, and deterioration of renal function (Figs. 17.5, 17.6) (9, 10, 32).

Management

Bladder drainage by an indwelling catheter is appropriate during the acute phase, when large volumes of fluids are being administered, and urine output is

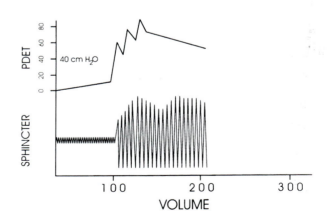

FIGURE 17.4.

Schematic illustration of cystometrogram after SCI occurring above the conus medullaris. Normal bladder capacity is 400 cc. In this case, there is an uninhibited detrusor contraction at a low volume. This is accompanied by increased sphincter activity (dyssynergia). There is voiding, but it occurs at a pressure over 40 cm of water. In an actual study, there would be a tracing of intravesicle pressure, and a tracing of intra-abdominal pressure (taken from a sensor in the rectum) in addition to the tracings above. The machine takes the difference of these two values to calculate detrusor pressure, which is shown here as the top tracing.

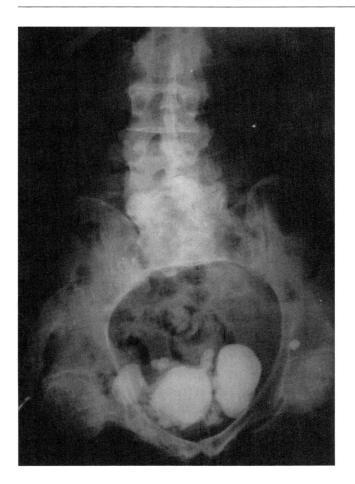

FIGURE 17.5.

Cystogram revealing bladder diverticuli, the result of chronic high pressure bladder voiding, in a man 45 years after SCI.

likely to be high. Intermittent catheterization has been advocated as acute management but runs the risk of bladder overdistention.

Long-term management is influenced by many factors. Concern for the well-being of the kidneys and lower urinary tract must be paramount. Frequently, however, the best method of management is impossible for practical reasons. The optimal drainage method would involve low bladder pressures, low post-void residual urine volume, and minimal instrumentation (9, 10, 32, 39, 51).

Intermittent catheterization can be useful with any type of bladder dysfunction after SCI. The person limits fluids and catheterizes frequently enough to prevent bladder overdistention. Agents such as oxybutinin can prevent reflex voiding and assure low pressure filling. This method is impractical for tetraplegics who lack both adequate hand function and a caregiver to perform the catheterizations.

A bladder with reflex function may be able to empty itself. This is not practical for women because of the lack of an external collecting device. However, men may be able to void by reflex into an external catheter. In most cases, however, reflex voiding involves elevated intravesicle pressures because of the dyssynergic sphincter activity. Occasionally pressures can be decreased by the use of alpha blocking agents, such as terazosin, to decrease internal sphincter activity, and antispasticity agents to moderate external sphincter activity. Pressure can be lowered more definitively by a surgical procedure, such as sphincterotomy or stent placement, to permanently defeat the sphincter mechanism.

Use of a chronic indwelling catheter is a practical method of drainage, but it has been associated with a variety of complications. It is often used by tetraplegic women for whom intermittent catheterization and reflex voiding are not options.

Urinary tract infection is one of the most frequent causes of morbidity after SCI (50). Treatment involves maintenance of a brisk urine output, antibiotics, and assurance of low pressure bladder emptying, which can be achieved by temporary placement of an indwelling catheter. An unsatisfactory response should prompt evaluation for a problem, such as an obstructing urinary tract stone or a renal abscess. A positive urine culture and a urinanalysis showing

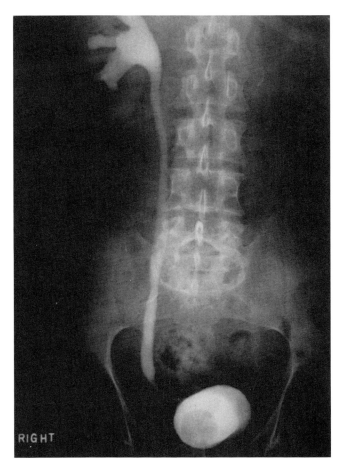

FIGURE 17.6.

Right vesico-ureteral reflux revealed by cystogram of a paraplegic.

bacteria and white cells is common in healthy people with neurogenic bladder; in the absence of symptoms, it does not warrant treatment (39, 43).

Surveillance

Damage to the urinary tract, including loss of renal function, can occur without clinical signs. Annual evaluation of the bladder by cystogram or cystoscopy, and of the kidneys by nuclear scan or ultrasound, can detect subclinical problems, allowing a change in bladder management and prevention of renal failure.

Functional Consequences of the Injury

Areas of Concern

The two general areas of concern regarding function are mobility and activities of daily living. Mobility includes turning in bed, tansferring from surface to surface, and locomotion, whether by ambulation or by wheelchair. Activities of daily living include feeding, dressing, bathing, and bowel and bladder function.

The most widespread tool for measuring function is the Functional Independence Measure (FIM) (16). It is used by ASIA. Abilities are described according to the need for an assistive device or the need for the assistance of another person in doing an activity.

General Approach to Improving Function

Overview

This section summarizes five components of a program for optimizing function after SCI. They are listed in the order of utilization. Reconstructive surgery and functional electrical stimulation are surveyed separately.

Maintenance of Range of Motion

Contractures can compromise function as severely as can loss of strength. Bed positioning and spastic muscular tone favor ankle plantar flexion contractures; other joints develop various other patterns of contracture. In the two most common levels of injury—C5 and C6—sparing of elbow flexors in the absence of extensors can lead to elbow flexion contracture.

The ankle, wrist, and more distal joints can be controlled with splints; more proximal joints are positioned with pillows while in bed and with wheelchair features while sitting. Range of motion exercises should be done at least daily. The hip flexors can be stretched by prone lying. In persons with intact wrist extension but paralysis of finger flexors, modest finger flexion contractures can be allowed to develop; this improves the power of tenodesis grip.

Increasing Strength

At least three mechanisms are available to increase strength after SCI. A partially damaged upper or lower motor neuron can recover; an intact lower motor neuron can adopt, by peripheral sprouting, the muscle fibers of a damaged lower motor neuron; and innervated muscle fibers can hypertrophy through exercise (35). Strengthening exercises are useful in muscles unaffected by SCI (e.g., in upper extremity muscles of paraplegics) that may be required to substitute for paralyzed muscles. Vigorous exercise should be avoided if post-traumatic syringomyelia is suspected; changes in venous pressure associated with straining, especially accompanied by Valsalva, can contribute to syrinx expansion (5). Exhaustive exercise can also be detrimental to partially denervated muscle, and vigorous activity should be avoided unless there is at least three-fifths muscle strength on manual muscle test (26).

Functional Retraining

Functional retraining involves teaching a person to perform an activity in a novel manner as an adaptation to an impairment. For example, a person with paralysis of the legs might learn to roll from supine to sidelying by vigorously rocking the trunk to one side, using momentum to turn the hips and lower extremities. Muscles can be used to move joints that the muscles do not cross. For example, horizontal abduction of the shoulder can extend the elbow by momentum. In certain positions, external rotation of the shoulder can use gravity to extend the elbow and supinate the forearm. In a closed chain system, with the hand fixed, the anterior deltoid and upper pectorals can produce elbow extension (34). With the hands fixed, the triceps, pectoralis major, and latissimus dorsi can elevate the pelvis (42). As noted earlier, if a modest contracture of the finger flexors is allowed to develop, wrist extension can, by tenodesis, cause finger flexion. By a similar mechanism, wrist flexion (which can be powered by gravity) can cause finger extension. Gravity can be used to stabilize the hip in paraplegia standing, in which the hip is locked in extension, anterior to the center of gravity of the body. This posture is fostered by standing with some dorsiflexion of the ankles, which pushes the hips out in front of the body. This is impossible if there are hip flexion or ankle plantar flexion contractures.

Adaptive Equipment

If functional retraining is unable to restore an ability, adaptive equipment may be a substitute. A person with a level of C2 breathes through the use of a ventilator; a person with a level of C4 can shift weight in the wheelchair with a power recliner. With a level of C5, propulsion of a wheelchair is possible if lugs are placed on the handrims. A C6 level allows feeding, writing, or typing by the use of a splint that can hold utensils. A paraplegic is assisted in dressing the lower body by a dressing stick. A level of L3 allows ambulation with the use of ankle-foot orthoses to fix the ankles, and canes to substitute for hip abductors.

Family Training

If adaptive equipment cannot substitute for an activity, a caretaker will be required to help do an activity. Family training is required to learn the skills. Practice can be obtained by having the patient and family spend a night in the hospital's "family room," or by a home pass.

Expected Functional Level for Neurologic Level

Some examples of expected levels of function for given motor levels are listed in Table 17.5. Independence in mobility (at a wheelchair level) and activities of daily living can be achieved with a level of C7.

Reconstructive Upper Extremity Surgery

Reconstructive upper extremity surgery after SCI (tendon transfer surgery) allows a muscle under voluntary control to substitute for a muscle that is paralyzed (28, 30). The main goals are provision of elbow extension and grasp; grasp can be of more than one type. Spasticity and contracture may limit gains, and candidates must be aware of the postoperative period of immobilization, during which hard-won functional abilities may be lost. Analogous procedures are not available for the lower extremity. Transfer of tendons of spastic muscles to correct ankle deformities is not considered here.

The most common level of SCI is C5. The person may have strong elbow flexion, but the extensors are paralyzed. The person is prohibited from raising the hand above the level of the elbow. Benefit is obtained by the use of tendon grafts (which can be harvested from the lower extremity) to attach the posterior third of the deltoid to the triceps. The use of free tendon grafts requires prolonged immobilization while a new blood supply is established.

Grasp can be provided in several ways, and selection may depend on which muscles are available to use as motors. Extensor carp radialis longus is largely spared with C6 injury. It can be transferred to flexor digitorum profundus, assuming that wrist extension will remain strong. Brachioradialis is also spared with C6 injury. It can be transferred to flexor pollicis longus. This provides pinch between the thumb and the radial aspect middle phalanx of the index finger. Pinch can also be provided by tenodesis of the tendon of flexor pollicis longus to the volar surface of the radius, combined with stabilization of the thumb and interphalangeal joint. In this case, pinch occurs when the wrist is extended.

Functional Electrical Stimulation

Electrical current can bring about contraction of muscle that is paralyzed by nerve injury. Muscles can be stimulated in a pattern that results in an activity that is useful for exercise or for improving function: this is called functional electrical stimulation (FES) or functional neuromuscular stimulation (FNS) (27, 36, 48). Muscle that is paralyzed by upper motor neuron injury, with intact lower motor neuron supply, is relatively easy to stimulate. Muscle paralyzed by lower motor neuron injury requires high levels of stimulation and is not used for FES. FES is poorly tolerated in sensate areas. Lower extremity applications are better developed than are systems for the upper extremities.

Sophisticated, practical, commercially available systems have been developed to allow paralyzed lower extremities to pedal a stationary apparatus as a form of exercise. These systems can be used to increase the strength and endurance of muscular response to stimulation and may also have other beneficial effects, such as cardiovascular conditioning, moderation of disuse, osteoporosis, and control of spasticity. However, the programs demand time and effort, and are likely to be indicated in only a minority of persons with SCI.

TABLE 17.5.
Examples of Expected Functional Levels for Motor Levels

Motor Level	Mobility	Self-care
C4	Independent in wheelchair mobility and weight shifts in an accessible environment with a motorized chair	Drinks with long straw after set-up. Can use voice activated environmental control unit to operate appliances
C6	Independent wheelchair propulsion over moderate distances on level surfaces	Independent upper extremity dressing; assistance with lower extremity dressing
C7	Independent transfers and wheelchair propulsion, indoors and outdoors	Independent with equipment
T2–T10	Ambulation, for exercise only, using knee-ankle-foot orthoses and walker	Independent
L3	Independent community ambulation with ankle-foot orthoses and canes or walker	Independent

Several FES systems have been developed that allow ambulation. They vary in their use of orthoses and the types of stimulating electrodes used (these can be surface or intramuscular). Generally, a walker is needed. In an open-loop system, stimuli are delivered according to a pre-set pattern. Alternatively, stimuli can be modified according to feedback (involving, for example, joint position), in which case the system is closed-loop.

Psychosocial Outcome

Adjustment

Depression is not universal after SCI, and health care workers may overestimate its presence (40). It may be less common than after stroke. Attempts to find a pattern of adjustment that people go through after SCI have been unsuccessful.

Long-term survivors of SCI tend to regard their quality of life as good or excellent (50). Even severe disability, with ventilator dependence, is compatible with a positive perceived quality of life (2). Health care professionals who have experience treating severely disabled people underestimate the response of the disabled to measures of quality of life.

Suicide rates are higher for victims of SCI than for the population in general (15). The risk is highest in the first 10 years after injury, after which the suicide rate resembles that of the general population.

Effects Upon Marriage

The majority of people with SCI are single at the time of injury (15). The rate of marriage after SCI is lower than that for an age- and sex-matched group from the general population. Between 10 to 30% of those single at injury will marry in the next 15 years. The rate of divorce for both pre- and post-injury marriages is higher than that of the general population.

Residence

Disposition after SCI has changed remarkably during the past 50 years. Discharge to institutional care is now unusual, and over 90% reside in private residences in the community. The risk of discharge to a facility increases with severity of injury, age, and lack of social supports (15).

Morbidity and Mortality

Long-term Morbidity

The two most frequent causes of morbidity in chronic SCI are pressure ulceration, with an annual incidence of 23%, and urinary tract infection, with an annual incidence of 20% (50). Other morbidity involving the genitourinary system—kidney and bladder stones, autonomic dyreflexia, bladder diverticuli, and hydronephrosis—is common. Musculoskeletal problems, such as contracture, osteoporosis, and fracture, can occur in paralyzed areas of the body. The upper extremities are especially prone to overuse injury, causing shoulder pain and nerve entrapment syndromes.

Mortality

Life expectancy for victims who survive the initial effects of the injury has improved considerably but still remains somewhat below normal (14). The level of injury and completeness of injury both correlate inversely with life expectancy.

The leading cause of death occurring more than 24 hours from injury is pneumonia and influenza. This finding is true for deaths occurring in the first year after injury as well as for deaths occurring later. The risk of dying from pneumonia after SCI is far greater than for the general population. Pneumococcal and influenza vaccination should be considered after SCI.

Non-ischemic heart disease is the second leading cause of death; ischemic heart disease is sixth. The risk is greater than for the general population; therefore, exercise, smoking cessation, and diet modification are even more important than in the general population.

Septicemia is the third leading cause of death. It is the leading cause for persons with paraplegia. The data are not clear on the source of septicemia, but pressure ulceration and urinary tract infection (two of the leading causes of morbidity) are probably common.

The fourth leading cause of death is PE. It is third during the first year after injury, during which time the risk of death from PE is 210 times normal. This finding emphasizes the importance of developing effective prophylactic and surveillance regimens for PE.

Suicide is approximately five times more common than in the general population. Alarmingly, it is the second leading cause of death in those under 30 and the second leading cause in those with paraplegia.

Urinary tract disease was once the most common cause of death after SCI. Modern treatment has greatly diminished this. While we await treatment for the underlying neurologic deficit, further improvements in life expectancy will follow improved prevention and treatment of such complications as pneumonia, heart disease, sepsis, and pulmonary embolus.

References

1. American Spinal Injury Association. Standards for neurologic and functional classification of spinal cord

injury. Rev. ed. Chicago: American Spinal Injury Association, 1992.
2. Bach JR, Tilton MC. Life satisfaction and well-being measures in ventilator assisted individuals with traumatic tetraplegia. Arch Phys Med Rehabil 1994; 74:626–632.
3. Bergstrom N, Bennet MA, Carlson CE, et al. Treatment of pressure ulcers. Clinical practice guideline, No. 15. Rockville, MD: US Department of Health and Human Services, Public Health Service, Agency for Health Care Policy and Research, 1994.
4. Bernstein JJ, Goldberg WJ. Experimental spinal cord transplantation as a mechanism of spinal cord regeneration. Paraplegia 1995;33:250–253.
5. Biyani A, El Masry WS. Post-traumatic syringomyelia: a review of the literature. Paraplegia 1994;32:723–731.
6. Bracken MB. Pharmacological treatment of acute spinal cord injury: current status and future projects. J Emerg Med 1993;11:43–48.
7. Bracken MB, Shepard MJ, Collines WF, et al. A randomized, controlled trial of methylprednisolone or naloxone in the treatment of acute spinal cord injury. N Engl J Med 1990;322:1405–1411.
8. Bracken MB, Shepard MJ, Collins WF Jr, et al. Methylprednisolone or naloxone treatment after acute spinal cord injury: 1-year follow-up data. J Neurosurg 1992;76:23–31.
9. Cardenas DD. Neurogenic bladder. Phys Med Rehabil Clin North Am 1992;3:751–763.
10. Chancellor MB, Kiiholma P. Urodynamic evaluation of patients following spinal cord injury. Semin Urol 1992;10:83–94.
11. Colachis SC III. Autonomic hyperreflexia with spinal cord injury. J Spinal Cord Med 1992;15:171–186.
12. Crozier KS, Cheng LL, Graziani V, et al. Spinal cord injury. Prognosis for ambulation based on quadriceps recovery. Paraplegia 1992;30:762–767.
13. Crozier KS, Graziani V, Ditunno JF Jr, et al. Spinal cord injury: prognosis for ambulation based on sensory examination in those who are initially motor complete. Arch Phys Med Rehabil 1991;72:119–121.
14. DeVivo MJ, Stover SL. Long-term survival and causes of death. In: Stover SL, DeLisa JA, Whiteneck GG, eds. Spinal cord injury. Clinical outcomes from the model systems. Gaithersburg, MD: Aspen, 1995:170–184.
15. Dijkers MP, Abela MB, Gans BM, et al. The aftermath of spinal cord injury. In: Stover SL, DeLisa JA, Whiteneck GG, eds. Spinal cord injury. Clinical outcomes from the model systems. Gaithersburg, MD: Aspen, 1995:185–212.
16. Ditunno JF Jr, Cohen ME, Formal C, et al. Functional outcomes. In: Stover SL, DeLisa JA, Whiteneck GG, eds. Spinal cord injury. Clinical outcomes from the model systems. Gaithersburg, MD: Aspen, 1995:170–184.
17. Ditunno JF Jr, Formal CS. Chronic spinal cord injury. N Engl J Med 1994;330:550–556.
18. Ditunno JF Jr, Young W, Donovan WH, et al. The international standards booklet for neurological and functional classification of spinal cord injury. Paraplegia 1994;32:70–80.
19. Erickson RP. Autonomic hyperreflexia: pathophysiology and medical management. Arch Phys Med Rehabil 1980;61:431–440.
20. Francel PC, Long BA, Malik JM, et al. Limiting ischemic spinal cord injury using a free radical scavenger 21-aminosteroid and/or cerebrospinal fluid drainage. J Neurosurg 1993;79:742–751.
21. Garland DE. A clinical perspective on common forms of acquired heterotopic ossification. Clin Orthop Rel Res 1991;263:13–29.
22. Geerts WH, Code KI, Jay RM, et al. A prospective study of venous thromboembolism after major trauma. N Engl J Med 1994;331:1601–1606.
23. Geisler FH, Dorsey FC, Coleman WP. Recovery of motor function after spinal-cord injury—A randomized, placebo-controlled trial with GM-1 ganglioside. N Engl J Med 1991;324:1829–1838.
24. Go BK, DeVivo MJ, Richards JS. The epidemiology of spinal cord injury. In: Stover SL, DeLisa JA, Whiteneck GG, eds. Spinal cord injury. Clinical outcomes from the model systems. Gaithersburg, MD: Aspen, 1995:21–55.
25. Hayes KC, Blight AR, Potter PJ, et al. Preclinical trial of 4-aminopyridine in patients with chronic spinal cord injury. Paraplegia 1993;31:216–224.
26. Herbison GJ, Jaweed MM, Ditunno JF Jr. Exercise therapies in peripheral neuropathies. Arch Phys Med Rehabil 1983;64:201–205.
27. Jaeger RJ. Lower extremity applications of functional neuromuscular stimulation. Assist Technol 1992;4:19–30.
28. Johnstone BR, Jordan CJ, App B, et al. A review of surgical rehabilitation of the upper limb in quadriplegia. Paraplegia 1988;26:317–339.
29. Kirby RL. Impairment, disability, and handicap. In: DeLisa JA, ed. Rehabilitation medicine: principles and practice. 2nd ed. Philadelphia: JB Lippincott, 1993:40–50.
30. Lamb DW. Reconstructive surgery for the upper limb and hand in traumatic tetraplegia. In: Lee BY, Ostrander LE, Cochran GVB, Shaw WW, eds. The spinal cord injured patient. Comprehensive management. Philadelphia: WB Saunders, 1991:231–243.
31. Lee BY, Karmakar MG, Herz BL, et al. Autonomic dysreflexia revisited. J Spinal Cord Med 1995;18:75–87.
32. Linsenmeyer TA, Stone JM. Neurogenic bladder and bowel dysfunction. In: DeLisa JA, ed. Rehabilitation medicine: principles and practice. 2nd ed. Philadelphia: JB Lippincott, 1993:733–762.
33. Little JW, Micklesen P, Umlauf R, et al. Lower extremity manifestations of spasticity in chronic spinal cord injury. Am J Phys Med Rehabil 1989;68:32–36.
34. Marciello MA, Herbison GH, Cohen ME, et al. Elbow extension using anterior deltoids and upper pectorals in spinal cord-injured subjects. Arch Phys Med Rehabil 1995;76:426–432.
35. Marino RJ, Herbison GJ, Ditunno JF Jr. Peripheral sprouting as a mechanism for recovery in the zone of injury in acute quadriplegia: A single fiber emg study. Muscle Nerve 1994;17:1466–1468.
36. Marsolais EB, Kobetic R, Chizeck HJ, et al. Orthoses and electrical stimulation for walking in complete paraplegia. J Neurol Rehab 1991;5:13–22.
37. Maynard FM, Karunas RS, Adkins RH, et al. Manage-

ment of the neuromusculoskeletal systems. In: Stover SL, DeLisa JA, Whiteneck GG, eds. Spinal cord injury. Clinical outcomes from the model systems. Gaithersburg, MD: Aspen, 1995:145–169.
38. Merli GJ, Crabbe S, Doyle L, et al. Mechanical plus pharmacological prophylaxis for deep vein thrombosis in acute spinal cord injury. Paraplegia 1992;30: 558–562.
39. National Institute on Disability and Rehabilitation Research. The prevention and management of urinary tract infections among people with spinal cord injuries. J Am Paraplegia Soc 1992;15:194–207.
40. Patterson DR, Miller-Perrin C, McCormick TR, et al. When life support is questioned early in the care of patients with cervical-level quadriplegia. N Engl J Med 1993;328:506–509.
41. Penrod LE, Hegde SK, Ditunno JF Jr. Age effect on prognosis for functional recovery in acute, traumatic central cord syndrome. Arch Phys Med Rehabil 1990; 71:963–968.
42. Reyes ML, Gronley JK, Newsam CJ, et al. Electromyographic analysis of shoulder muscles of men with low-level paraplegia during a weight relief raise. Arch Phys Med Rehabil 1995;76:433–439.
43. Stover SL, Lloyd LK, Waites, KB, et al. Neurogenic urinary tract infection. Neurol Clin 1991;9:741–755.
44. Stover SL, Niemann KMW, Tulloss JR. Experience with surgical resection of heterotopic bone in spinal cord injury patients. Clin Orthop Rel Res 1991;263: 71–77.
45. Trop CS, Bennett CJ. Autonomic dysreflexia and its urological implications: a review. J Urol 1991;146: 1461–1469.
46. Waters RL, Adkins RH, Yakura JS, et al. Motor and sensory recovery following incomplete paraplegia. Arch Phys Med Rehabil 1994;75:67–72.
47. Waters RL, Adkins RH, Yakura JS, et al. Motor and sensory recovery following incomplete tetraplegia. Arch Phys Med Rehabil 1994;75:306–311.
48. Weber RJ. Functional neuromuscular stimulation. In: DeLisa JA, ed. Rehabilitation medicine: principles and practice. 2nd ed. Philadelphia: JB Lippincott, 1993: 463–476.
49. Weinmann EE, Salzman EW. Deep-vein thrombosis. N Engl J Med 1994;331:1630–1641.
50. Whiteneck GG, Charlifue, Grankel HL, et al. Mortality, morbidity, and psychosocial outcomes of persons spinal cord injured more than 20 years ago. Paraplegia 1992;30:617–30.
51. Wyndaele JJ. Development and evaluation of the management of the neuropathic bladder. Paraplegia 1995; 33:305–307.
52. Yarkony GM. Pressure ulcers: a review. Arch Phys Med Rehabil 1994;75:908–917.
53. Yarkony GM, Heinemann AW. Pressure ulcers. In: Stover SL, DeLisa JA, Whiteneck GG, eds. Spinal cord injury. Clinical outcomes from the model systems. Gaithersburg, MD: Aspen, 1995:100–119.
54. Young RR. Spasticity: a review. Neurology 1994; 44(suppl 9):S12–S20.

SECTION IV
Degenerative Disorders

CHAPTER EIGHTEEN

Cervical Disc Disease and Cervical Spondylosis

Sanford E. Emery

Introduction

Undoubtedly, cervical disc disease has existed at least as long as man's longevity increased to the point where inevitable degenerative changes in the spine occurred. It is remarkable, however, that much of our understanding of cervical disc disease and development of treatment options has only taken place in the last few decades. This acceleration of knowledge has been driven by technological advancements largely in radiologic and neuroradiologic imaging techniques, allowing us to see the pathologic anatomy and correlate this with patient symptomatology. As in most areas of the spine, many questions have not been answered, and degenerative diseases of the neck and their treatment remain an active area of investigation with continued evolution of diagnostic modalities and treatment options.

Pathophysiology

Paramount to understanding cervical disc disease and its clinical manifestations is to understand the pathophysiology of disc degeneration and disc herniation. The discs function as shock absorbers that undergo biochemical and structural changes with aging. Proteoglycan content shifts to a higher concentration of keratin sulfate versus chondroitin sulfate, and gradual desiccation of the disc occurs. These changes result in loss of height of the disc with alteration of the once perfect biomechanical environment. The end plates adjacent to degenerating discs slowly respond to these changes with formation of chondro-osseous spurs. These spurs occur primarily in the uncovertebral joints but also at the insertion of annular fibers, resulting in transverse osteophytes forming along the rim of the end plate. Facet joint changes with spurring occur as well, which, in conjunction with uncovertebral joint osteophytes, can contribute to foraminal narrowing. Anterior osteophytes along the vertebral bodies commonly occur but are not important with respect to neural compression and rarely are large enough to cause swallowing difficulty. Posterior vertebral osteophytes, however, can lead to canal stenosis with spinal cord compression. These changes of the cervical motion segment resulting in disc narrowing and osteophyte formation can be seen with plain radiographs and is called cervical spondylosis (Fig. 18.1A and B). Cervical spondylosis typically occurs in the older-age groups with an incidence of approximately 50% of people over the age of 50 (12). One need not have spondylotic changes to have cervical disc disease, however, because disc herniations can occur in the absence of radiographically visible disc degeneration or bony changes. Soft disc herniations result when

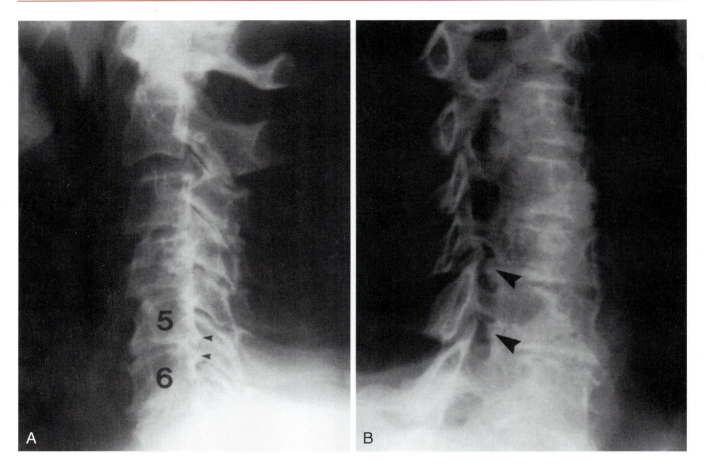

FIGURE 18.1.
A. Lateral radiograph in a 72-year-old woman showing changes of cervical spondylosis. Note the disc narrowing at multiple levels. Posterior osteophytes are well seen at the C5–C6 level (arrows). She has 2-1/2 mm of compensatory subluxation of C2 on C3. **B.** An oblique radiograph in the same patient demonstrates the uncovertebral osteophytes protruding into the neural foramen at C5–C6 and C6–C7 (arrows).

the nucleus pulposus protrudes into the annulus fibrosus region of the disc or extrudes through the outer fibers of the annulus. If large enough, this herniated disc can cause nerve root compression or spinal cord compression depending on the location of the herniation. Typically, soft disc herniations are seen in patients in the third and fourth decades of life, with the older population usually having a combination of disc protrusion plus osteophyte producing neural compression.

With the imperfect biomechanics resulting from cervical spondylosis, some levels may become stiffer than the normal spine. Other motion segments may become hypermobile because of degenerative changes. When hypermobility occurs at levels above stiffer spondylotic segments, it is termed compensatory subluxation (Fig. 18.1A). If the abnormal subluxation is substantial, dynamic compression of nerve roots or the spinal cord can occur, producing clinical symptoms.

Clinical Presentations

In evaluating patients with neck problems relating to cervical disc disease, it is useful to categorize patients into three main diagnostic groups. We will discuss these three groups separately below; however, these are not rigid categories and overlap does occur in any given patient.

Neck Pain Alone

This group of patients report axial neck pain that may be referred to the shoulder or interscapular areas. This referred type of pain should be distinguished from radiating arm pain and neurologic symptoms that suggest radiculopathy. Patients with myelopathy can be distinguished on physical examination. A common cause of neck pain without radiculopathy or myelopathy is from cervical spondylosis changes. As described previously, alterations in the discs with spur formation can result in neck pain. The annulus is believed to be innervated by small nerve fibers that can produce pain (3). Facet joints are synovial joints, and osteoarthritic changes here can produce pain as is true elsewhere in the body. Hypermobility or compensatory subluxation can also cause mechanical neck pain. If the degenerative changes are severe, cervical canal stenosis can result with cord compression. This stenosis does not always manifest as radiculopathy and may not be severe enough to cause myelopathy but can produce neck pain.

In the younger population, mechanical neck pain without radiculopathy or myelopathy is often the result of whiplash-type injuries, such as after motor vehicle accidents. These injuries are to the soft tissues of the neck, and the symptoms typically last for months. Significant trauma such as hyperextension can result in a disrupted disc without frank posterior herniation evident on neuroradiologic studies. Some patients with minor trauma or even no trauma, without any underlying degenerative changes evident, may have discogenic pain. This, however, is a difficult diagnosis to make. Discography has attempted to identify these patients but has very mixed results in the literature (18).

Radiculopathy

This diagnosis connotes nerve root compression. It usually, but not always, occurs in conjunction with neck pain. The location of the radicular pain depends on the level of the root compression in the spine. Neurologic symptoms are common and help confirm the suspected etiology of the symptoms as root compression. These neurologic symptoms include sensory changes symptoms, such as numbness or tingling, and motor symptoms of weakness. Symptoms are typically unilateral but can be bilateral with the appropriate pathologic compression, such as bilateral foraminal stenosis. Patients with radiculopathy often have no traumatic incident to initiate their symptoms. They may wake up one morning with stiffness or pain in their neck and typically develop radicular arm symptoms within a day or two which may be quite severe.

Physical examination of patients with radiculopathy typically shows tenderness to posterior palpation of the spinous processes and paraspinal musculature. Typically, motion is decreased depending on the severity of the pain. Usually these patients cannot extend their neck comfortably because this narrows down the canal and aggravates their symptoms (9). Rotation is usually limited and lateral bending, such as with the Spurling's maneuver, may recreate their arm symptoms. A good neurologic exam is critical in evaluating these patients. Motor testing of the proximal and distal muscle groups bilaterally should always be performed and documented. Sensory changes may be in a dermatomal distribution, although many patients, particularly with cervical spondylosis, may have multiple levels involved, and the sensory abnormalities will not be well defined. Reflex examination of the patient with root compression yields hyporeflexia for that reflex related to the compressed nerve root (i.e., a lower motor neuron problem).

Myelopathy

Cervical myelopathy results from spinal cord compression. The most common cause of this for the North American population is cervical spondylosis with enough osteophytic changes to produce canal stenosis or cord compression. Soft disc herniations without spondylotic changes also occur and, if large enough, can result in clinical manifestations of myelopathy. Other causes include subluxation with dynamic compression of the cord and ossification of the posterior longitudinal ligament. This latter disease is much more common in the Asian race. The posterior longitudinal ligament becomes thickened and ossifies, producing canal narrowing and spinal cord compression either at intermittent levels in the neck or in one continuous strip.

Interestingly, patients with substantial spinal cord compression and severe myelopathy may have no neck pain at all. Many patients do have axial pain, however, and they may have concomitant radicular pain as well. Often, the earliest symptom of myelopathy is a gait disturbance. Patients may note that they are slightly wobbly when turning a corner or getting up and out of a chair. More severe symptoms of gait disturbance include hanging onto walls or furniture for balance or requiring the use of assistive ambulatory devices, such as a cane or walker. Motor weakness is another manifestation of myelopathy. It can occur anywhere in the upper extremities, depending on the level of compression, but often is evident in the distal muscle groups, such as the hand intrinsics. Leg weakness does occur and is typically in the proximal muscle groups. This can manifest as buckling and falling episodes for the patient. The patient may also report sphincter dysfunction usually related to difficulty with urination; this is considered a late sign and corresponds to severe myelopathy.

Spinal cord compression is an upper motor neuron disorder and is characterized by long tract signs. The gait should be evaluated, including toe walking, heel walking, and toe-to-heel tandem gait ("walking the tightrope"). Hyperreflexia should be present, although occasionally, with severe concomitant root compression, one reflex may be decreased. Pathologic reflexes consistent with myelopathy include a positive Hoffman's sign, up-going toes on the Babinski test, and the presence of clonus. As with any of these patients, a specific and thorough motor testing exam should be done, and weakness, often bilateral, in the upper and/or lower extremities may be detected. Decreased sensation may be present in more diffuse nondermatomal patterns than with a one-level root compression problem. Vibratory sense and proprioception should be tested and may be decreased in severe cases.

Differential Diagnosis Considerations

The two most common differential diagnostic entities that produce neck and arm pain involve intrinsic shoulder pathology and peripheral nerve entrapment syndromes. Rotator cuff tendinitis is a common problem that can produce pain in the shoulder, parascapular region, and/or upper arm. Typically, patients with impingement syndrome of the rotator cuff have trouble using their arms overhead and often have trouble sleeping on that particular shoulder. A thorough examination, looking for signs of impingement and tenderness, is helpful in the evaluation. Rotator cuff tears can produce weakness as well as pain and may need to be ruled out with MR imaging or arthrography. A helpful test in the office is subacromial injection with Lidocaine (and often cortisone) to determine if this eliminates their pain, thus pinpointing the etiology of the patient's symptoms.

Peripheral nerve entrapment syndromes include thoracic outlet syndrome, suprascapular nerve palsy, and the more common ulnar cubital tunnel syndrome and carpal tunnel syndrome. All of these can be suspected on the basis of history and physical examination but probably need electrodiagnostic evaluation by an experienced electromyographer to help sort out the various areas of pathology. The double crush syndrome also occurs as a combination of nerve compression anywhere along the nerve from the cervical spine all the way down to the wrist. If two levels of compression can be identified and surgery is indicated, then the most severe area is usually addressed first. If neither area of compression is significantly worse than the other, then the peripheral entrapment syndrome is treated first, given the less complex nature of that procedure compared with cervical spine surgery.

An entity worth mentioning here that is uncommon but can mimic severe radiculopathy is brachial plexopathy (22). Synonyms for this include brachial plexitis or neurologic amyotrophy. Typically, these patients wake up one morning with severe shoulder and arm pain with or without weakness and sensory findings. The etiology of the disorder is unclear. It is generally self-limiting over months, and supportive care during the symptomatic period is indicated.

Other neurologic conditions can mimic cervical disc disease syndromes. Mononeuritis multiplex can be confused with multilevel cervical radiculopathy. Amyotrophic lateral sclerosis and syringomyelia are conditions that at some point in their course may present like cervical myelopathy. The quality and scope of imaging studies generally allow accurate diagnosis, but in many cases, consultation with a neurologist is recommended.

Diagnostic Evaluation

As noted previously, many patients with cervical disc disease can be diagnosed accurately with a thorough physical and history examination. Plain cervical spine films, particularly an anteroposterior and lateral view, should be obtained even on initial evaluation. Oblique views are at times helpful looking for foraminal impingement from uncovertebral hypertrophy but are not routinely necessary. Flexion and extension views should be considered but obtained on a case-by-case basis. With a good history, physical examination, and radiographs, the spine surgeon should have a good working diagnosis for the patient. Whether any further diagnostic measures are needed depends on the suspected diagnosis, the duration and severity of symptoms, and other individual factors.

Our next step for evaluation in patients with radiculopathy or myelopathy is magnetic resonance imaging. This is a noninvasive study that provides good visualization of the soft tissues and the relationship of disc herniations, osteophytes, and even ossification of the posterior longitudinal ligament (OPLL) to the neural elements. Magnetic resonance imaging continues to improve in its resolution; for young patients without spondylotic changes and a simple soft disc herniation, this is the only neuroradiologic study one would generally need (Fig. 18.2A and B). If patients have multiple spondylotic levels with varying degrees of compression, we still often rely on cervical myelography and CT myelography. A subtle root cutoff is best seen on the anteroposterior myelogram, which may not be appreciated with cross-sectional imaging modalities (Fig. 18.3). CT myelography gives the sharpest definition of osteophytic impingement, OPLL, and cord compression compared to magnetic resonance imaging.

Electrodiagnostic tests usually are reserved for patients with differential diagnostic considerations, such as peripheral entrapment syndromes. Cervical discography may be helpful in patients without significant spondylotic changes and suspected discogenic pain. This may occur after a whiplash injury. For discography to be of any benefit, it needs to be

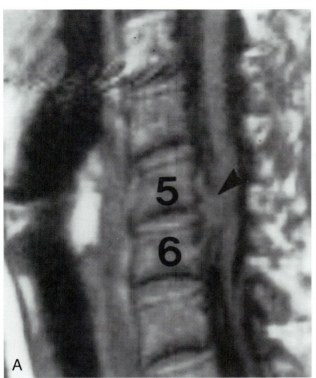 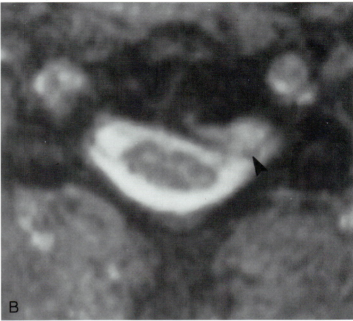

FIGURE 18.2.
A. Sagittal MRI demonstrating a C5–C6 disc herniation in a 44-year-old woman with neck and left arm pain plus significant deltoid and wrist extension weakness. **B.** A large posterolateral soft disc herniation is evident on this T2 weighted transverse image at C5–C6 in the same patient. Note the disc protrusion (arrow), which will severely compress the C6 nerve root in this case.

done by someone experienced with the technique. Reproduction of the patient's pain symptoms from a given level and not from multiple levels may help the surgeon with patient selection. It is a controversial technique, however, and is used sparingly in my practice and at our institution.

Nonoperative Treatment

Most patients with symptoms of neck pain with or without radiculopathy can be managed nonoperatively. For moderate to severe symptoms, initial treatment should consist of the basic triad of a soft collar, anti-inflammatories, and physical therapy modalities including traction. By keeping the neck from extremes of motion, the soft collar helps decrease the dynamic pinching of a compressed root and allows for primary or secondary fatigue or inflammatory changes in the paraspinal muscles and soft tissues to resolve in many cases. Mild narcotic pain medicines may be used in conjunction with anti-inflammatories depending on the severity of the symptoms. Occasionally, a brief cortisone taper may also help alleviate severe root compression symptoms and allow the natural history to take its course if one is early in the clinical presentation. Physical therapy modalities, such as heat and ultrasound, may make the patient more comfortable although it is unclear if it has any significant effect on the natural history. Traction, particularly in younger patients, is often helpful because it allows a pinched nerve root some temporary relief and probably in this way promotes recovery. One should be careful to avoid any traction that might extend the patient's neck. This causes narrowing of the spinal canal as well as the foramen and often will cause an increase in the patient's symptoms (9). For the same reason, we often use the cervical collar in the reverse position such that the narrow strap portion is anterior and the head is in a slightly flexed position. Patients with cervical myelopathy may be immobilized in a soft collar to help prevent dynamic compression of the spinal cord. This, of course, is a temporizing measure as opposed to definitive treatment.

Surgical Indications

For patients with cervical radiculopathy, the two main indications for surgical intervention are pain relief and upper extremity weakness. The vast majority of patients with pain as their predominant problem can undergo a trial of nonoperative measures as outlined previously. The majority of time these measure are successful, and surgery is not nec-

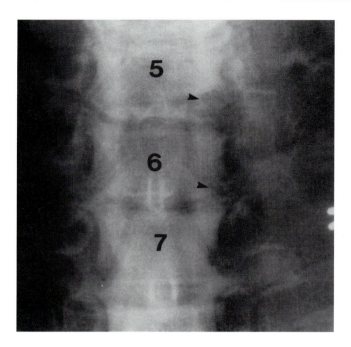

FIGURE 18.3.
Anteroposterior view of a cervical myelogram in a 75-year-old woman with severe radiculopathy showing a significant root cutoff (arrows) at C5–C6 and C6–C7. At times, myelography is superior in demonstrating this pathology compared with magnetic resonance imaging or CT myelography.

essary. When patients have undergone several weeks of nonoperative measures without adequate pain relief or with worsening symptoms, they then become a surgical candidate, provided the appropriate pathology is documented on their neuroradiologic studies. Patients with progressive neurologic deficit need more urgent intervention. Those with profound muscle weakness may need early intervention as well to maximize the chances of root recovery. Mild weakness can be observed after institution of nonoperative measures, but these patients should have frequent reexaminations in the office every 1 to 3 weeks to be sure there is no deterioration and to look for an improving trend. Any patient under consideration for surgical intervention should have appropriate neuroradiologic studies to pinpoint the pathology and allow for appropriate surgical planning.

In patients with cervical myelopathy and demonstrable spinal cord compression on neuroradiologic studies, the recommended treatment is surgical intervention. The natural history of myelopathy is a slow, stepwise deterioration (2). Therefore, once the diagnosis is made, we recommend decompressing the neural elements to halt a decrease in strength and function and allow spinal cord recovery. Although even patients with severe myelopathy can in many instances recover to a significant degree, patients with mild to moderate myelopathy generally have a greater recovery of function.

Surgical indications for patients with neck pain secondary to spondylosis, canal stenosis, or discogenic pain are more limited. If patients have substantial canal stenosis and pain, they may be a candidate for recalcitrant symptoms even if they have no frank radiculopathy or myelopathy. Some patients with severe degenerative changes at one or two levels with neck pain alone can benefit from fusion at those levels, although the best results are obtained if nerve compression symptoms are present as well because the surgical results are more reliable for that patient population (1, 16).

Certain factors come into play regarding a choice of the anterior versus posterior approach for treatment of cervical disc disease disorders. Simple lateral disc herniations may be treated with a posterior laminotomy and discectomy or by anterior discectomy and fusion. For typical posterolateral or central disc herniations, I strongly favor anterior discectomy and fusion (Fig. 18.4A and B). This approach directly addresses the compressive pathology on the cord or root. In patients with spondylotic changes and radiculopathy, again the anterior approach is preferred (1, 6, 19, 21). Disc and osteophytic material can be removed easily and safely, giving a direct decompression of the neural elements. The spondylotic segment can then be stabilized with a bone graft and ultimate fusion. This prevents any recurrent osteophytic changes and minimizes the neck pain that could originate from the degenerative segment. Patients with cervical myelopathy often have cord compression from large osteophytes or ossification of the posterior longitudinal ligament. This often extends down behind the vertebral body. These patients need partial or complete corpectomies followed by strut grafting to adequately decompress the canal from an anterior approach (Fig. 18.5) (4, 7, 14, 17, 23). An alternate approach is multilevel laminectomy. This, however, can result in postlaminectomy instability and kyphosis (13). Laminaplasty has been developed as an alternative to laminectomy. This technique widens the spinal canal to decompress the neural elements yet leaves the lamina as attachments for the posterior paraspinal musculature (8, 10). The author favors this technique in certain cases of congenital canal stenosis at multiple levels where there is no significant anterior indentation of the cord. The patient must have normal lordosis and minimal symptoms of neck pain as well for this procedure to be maximally effective.

Surgical Technique

Anterior Cervical Discectomy and Fusion

This approach was described by Robinson in the mid 1950s (15). It is a slightly anterolateral approach that

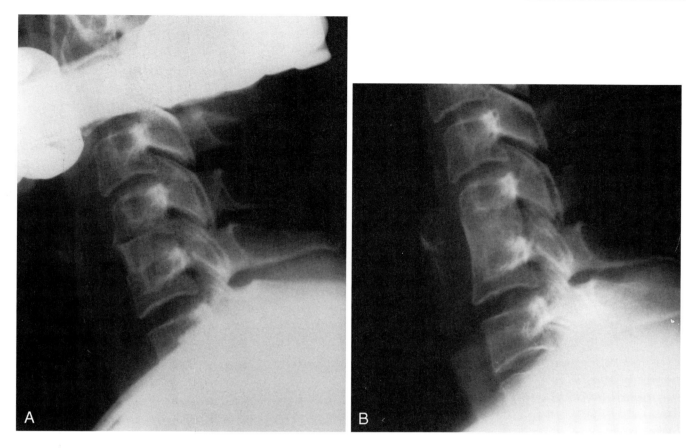

FIGURE 18.4.

A. An early postoperative lateral radiograph of the patient whose MRI is shown in Figure 18.2. Note the Robinson-type bone graft present at the C5–C6 inner space. This graft will maintain the height of the disc space and re-establish the height of the foramen for the nerve roots. **B.** Approximately 2 years postoperatively, this lateral radiograph shows complete consolidation of the iliac graft with remodeling evident.

takes advantage of the fascial planes in the anterior neck. The incision is begun just to the right of the midline and is carried over toward the border of the left sternocleidomastoid. The right side of the incision can be used, but we prefer the left side because the anatomy of the recurrent laryngeal nerve is more consistent here. After making the incision at the appropriate level of the cervical spine, the dissection is carried down through the platysma muscle to expose the superficial layer of the deep cervical fascia. This is incised transversely. The deep layer of the cervical fascia is then incised superiorly and inferiorly, which allows retractors to be slid proximally or distally and essentially enables the surgeon to visualize the entire surgical spine. The interval between the carotid sheath laterally and the trachea and the esophagus medially is identified, and the dissection is carried down to the vertebral column. The pre-vertebral fascia is incised to expose the anterior longitudinal ligament. The longus colli muscles on each side of the spine are coagulated along their edges at the operative levels to prevent bleeding from small veins. At this point, a needle is placed in the disc space, and a radiograph is obtained to ensure the correct surgical level. The anterior annulus of the disc is incised with a knife blade, and the bulk of the disc is removed with tiny curettes and pituitary rongeurs. Headlight illumination is essential as is magnification, either with loupes or the operating microscope. After the bulk of the disk has been removed, the disc space is distracted using a lamina spreader within the disc or using screw post distractors placed into the vertebral body above and below the operative level. By opening the disc space, one can more easily visualize the posterior disc material and posterior longitudinal ligament. The uncovertebral joints should be identified because these are key anatomic landmarks to help limit further lateral dissection and thus avoid possible injury to the vertebral arteries (20). If it is a soft disc herniation without significant osteophytic changes, then after the disc has been removed back to the posterior longitudinal ligament, the decompression is completed. If there are spondylotic changes at this level with root impingement or cord compression from bony pathology, then these ridges or posterior lateral spurs may be removed with

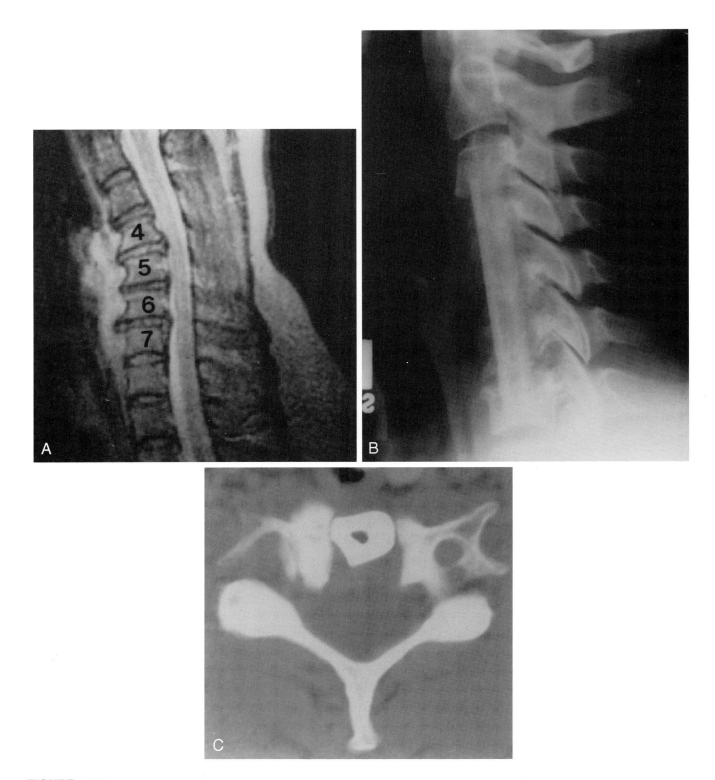

FIGURE 18.5.

A. Sagittal MRI of a 44-year-old woman with cervical kyphosis, spondylosis, and clinical evidence of myelopathy. Her sagittal MRI shows draping of the cord over herniated disc material, particularly at C4–5 with some stenosis present at C5–6 and C6–7 based on transverse sections not shown here. **B.** After a 3-level cervical corpectomy and strut grafting, her lateral cervical spine radiograph shows healing of the fibula graft with correction of her kyphosis. **C.** A postoperative CT scan demonstrates the corpectomy defect, thus enlarging the spinal canal. The fibula strut is seen in cross section within the corpectomy space.

small burrs and curettes. Diamond burrs are used when working near the posterior longitudinal ligament or dura to minimize the risk of a dural tear. After satisfactory decompression, the end plates are abraded with a burr to provide a flattened, bleeding subchondral bone surface. This has been shown to improve the fusion rate and does not result in significant settling of the bone graft (5). The space is measured for height and depth, and a separate incision is made over the anterior iliac crest region. A power saw is used to harvest a full-thickness tricortical horseshoe-shaped bone graft (11). Autogenous bone is preferred because it has superior healing capabilities, particularly in multilevel procedures (24). I use autograft bone exclusively except in very unusual circumstances. The graft is trimmed to the appropriate size and tapped carefully into place with the cortex facing anteriorly. Slight countersinking is important to help prevent dislodgement. Small posterior lips in the back of the vertebral bodies are fashioned with a burr before grafting to prevent posterior migration of the graft. For one-or two-level discectomy and fusion procedures, I do not use any supplemental instrumentation. Because an increasing number of operative levels carries with it an increasing risk of pseudarthrosis, we recommend additional stabilization for three-level discectomy and fusion procedures using an anterior plate and screws to help promote bony union. Patients having discectomy and fusion procedures are generally treated in a rigid two- or four-poster type brace to help limit the range of motion and to promote healing. I recommend 6 weeks of hard collar type of immobilization followed by 1 or 2 weeks of a soft collar as a step-down for comfort. For certain patients who for some reason cannot tolerate a hard collar, anterior plating should provide adequate stability for discectomy and for fusion patients so that a soft collar can be used safely (Fig 18.6A and B).

Some patients with larger osteophytes or segmental OPLL may not adequately be treated by a simple discectomy and fusion, yet may not need a full corpectomy to adequately decompress the operative level. If the osteophytes are large, then a partial or hemicorpectomy may be necessary with removal of the end plate and part of the vertebral body using regular burrs and diamond burrs to remove adequately the posterior osteophytes. Attempting to reach posteriorly behind the vertebral bodies with angled curettes is risky and not recommended. The surgeon can burr down on top of the osteophytes until they are wafer thin and then carefully pick them up with small curettes and pituitary rongeurs. The posterior longitudinal ligament can be left as long as

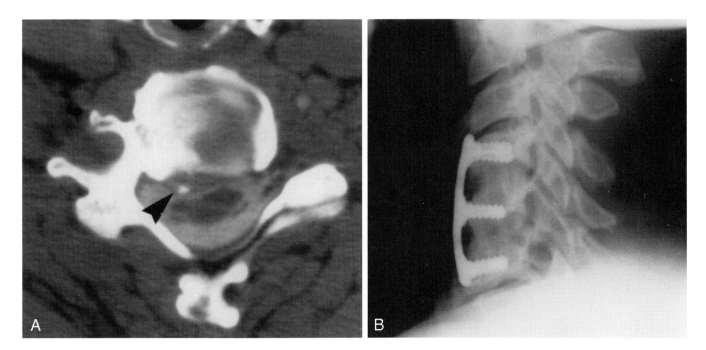

FIGURE 18.6.

A. CT myelogram of this 52-year-old patient shows a right-sided disc herniation at C5–C6 (arrow). Note the spinal cord compression. She had similar pathology at C4–C5 and a 2-level anterior cervical discectomy and fusion was proposed. She had a very short neck with some upper thoracic neuromuscular scoliosis, and fitting with a hard collar would have been extremely difficult. Thus, she was treated with autologous bone grafting plus anterior plate fixation and a soft collar postoperatively (Fig. 18.6B). **B.** Lateral cervical radiograph demonstrating the plate fixation with successful interbody arthrodesis.

it is soft, thus allowing for expansion of the dura. If a partial corpectomy has been done, then an iliac crest graft that is larger in size can be used in the same manner as described previously for a simple discectomy and fusion.

Anterior Corpectomy and Strut Grafting

To reach compressive pathology behind the vertebral body safely, it is necessary to channel out the midportion of the vertebral body, which is called a cervical corpectomy or vertebrectomy. Another indication would be a discectomy and fusion procedure of more than three levels in which the nonunion rate would be unacceptable and a corpectomy with strut grafting would give better results. The surgical approach is the same for a discectomy and fusion. First the discs at the appropriate levels are removed as described previously. It is useful to clean out most of the disc back to the posterior longitudinal ligament to gauge the depth of bone that will need to be taken doing the corpectomy. When the discs above and below the selected vertebrae have been removed, a rongeur can be used to remove some of the anterior part of the vertebrae. Care is taken not to remove bone lateral to the uncovertebral joints. A carbide-tipped burr is used to remove most of the vertebral body at this point back to a thin posterior shell. A diamond burr is then used to further thin the posterior shell. At this point, the thin remnant can be elevated off the posterior longitudinal ligament using small angled curettes and pituitary rongeurs. In this fashion, all compressive discs, bone, and ossified ligament can be removed for the entire width of the spinal canal (Fig. 18.5C). The uncovertebral joint areas can easily be cleaned out of disc materials or osteophytes from this anterior approach as well. When all of the necessary vertebral bodies have been removed in this fashion, the inferior endplate of the proximal vertebra and the superior endplate of the distal vertebra are then prepared for graft seating using a burr. The end plates are flattened to provide a raw bleeding surface. A small posterior lip is left at each end vertebra to prevent any posterior migration of the graft. A small anterior lip is left also to help prevent anterior displacement. At this point, the cervical traction can be increased but generally to not more than 20 pounds. For one-level corpectomies, a full-thickness iliac strut graft is preferred. This is placed into the defect and tapped into a countersunk position. Releasing the traction allows for a snug placement of the graft. For two or more level corpectomy procedures, autogenous fibula is preferred. The fibula can then be seated nicely into the vertebra above and below the decompressed area in a slightly countersunk position (Fig. 18.5B). We do not favor notching the fibula and resting it on the anterior lips of the vertebra because this is prone to fracture the anterior cortex of the vertebra. A small Penrose-type drain is always placed after any anterior procedure in the cervical spine to help prevent hematoma formation. After closure, many of these patients can be maintained in a rigid two-poster type brace. If the vertebral bone is osteopenic or the patient has severe myelopathy, or if posterior instability exists, then a halo vest is recommended.

Posterior Procedures

The surgical approach for posterior cervical spine procedures is straightforward. The incision is placed in the midline and carefully carried down to the tips of the spinous processes. Great care should be taken to stay exactly in the midline to minimize bleeding. Dissecting laterally into the paraspinous muscles results in significantly more bleeding. Periosteal elevators are used to dissect the paraspinal musculature off the appropriate lamina and deep retractors can be placed for exposure. Again, loupe magnification and a headlight are strongly recommended. For a laminotomy, we prefer the keyhole type of technique. At the appropriate interspace, a burr is used to thin the lower edge of the superior lamina and the upper edge of the inferior lamina medial and slightly superior to the facet joint. This hole can be thinned and enlarged with a diamond burr. The thin ligamentum flavum is removed with a small Kerrison rongeur. There often are epidural veins that can be cauterized that cover the lateral edge of the dura and the nerve root in the field. A small Kerrison rongeur can remove any bone laterally for a pure foraminotomy. If the patient has a soft disc herniation, then the nerve root can be elevated gently and the fragment retrieved, using a small incision in the annulus if necessary. This procedure should not result in any late instability because the bulk of the ligamental structures and the facet joints are not violated. After hemostasis is obtained, the wound can be closed and the patient treated in a soft collar for comfort.

For posterior decompression of the spinal canal, a full laminectomy can be performed. This is done carefully with Kerrison rongeurs. The decompression should be wide enough to span the width of the spinal canal. If foraminotomies are performed, then care should be taken not to remove any more of the facet joint than is necessary to minimize the chance of any late postoperative instability (25). Laminaplasty has been developed as an alternative to laminectomy for posterior decompression of the spinal canal (10). There are different techniques for laminaplasty but the basic procedure is to thin the bone with a burr at the junction of the lamina and facet joints to greenstick open the lamina and/or spinous processes. This enlarges the diameter of the spinal canal, thereby relieving the spinal cord compression. I favor the technique from Chiba University in Japan. With this technique, the lateral gutter at the junction of the lamina and facet joints from C3 to C5 is completely burred through. The opposite side at the same levels is then partially burred through. These upper lamina can then be opened with a greenstick hinge on the left side (Fig. 18.7). In a similar fashion, the C6 and C7 lamina are burred through completely, but this time on the opposite side as compared to the top three lamina. It is then hinged on the right side, and then the trapdoor of C6 and C7 is opened to the right, opposite to the top three lamina. To keep these trapdoors open, a hole is placed with a small burr at the inferior right lateral corner of the C5 lamina and another hole at the superior left lateral corner of the C6 lamina. A heavy nylon suture is then placed through these holes and tied such that it tethers the two trap doors in an open position. The C3 lamina is tethered to the C2 spinous process, and the C7 lamina is tethered to the T1 spinous process in a similar fashion. Tiny pieces of cancellous bone obtained from the tips of the spinous processes can be placed in the hinged gutters of each individual lamina to promote healing at this greenstick area. The goal is to avoid an intersegmental fusion, thus preserving neck motion, yet allowing the paraspinal muscles to heal down to the remaining posterior elements to reduce the risk of postlaminectomy instability. These patients can be treated postoperatively in a soft collar for comfort.

Summary

Cervical disc disease is a common problem in primary care, orthopaedic, and neurosurgical practices. A thorough understanding of the anatomy, the common clinical entities and their presentation, and the natural history and treatment options allows the physician and surgeon to successfully treat the majority of these patients. Nonoperative measures for treatment of degenerative disease of the cervical spine are usually successful; however, when surgery is indicated, it can provide excellent functional results and pain relief for the majority of this patient population.

References

1. Bohlman HH, Emery SE, Goodfellow DB, et al. Robinson anterior cervical discectomy and arthrodesis for radiculopathy. J Bone Joint Surg Am 1993;75:1298–1307.
2. Clarke E, Robinson PK. Cervical myelopathy: a complication of cervical spondylosis. Brain 1956;79:483.
3. Cloward RB. The clinical significance of the sinuvertebral nerve of the cervical spine in relation to the cervical spine in relation to the cervical disk syndrome. J Neurol Neurosurg Psychiatry 1960;23:321–326.
4. Emery SE, Bolesta MJ, Bohlman H. Anterior decompression and fusion for cervical spondylotic myelopathy: two to seventeen year follow-up. Orthopaedic Transactions 1994–1995;18(4):1135.
5. Emery SE, Bolesta MJ, Banks MA, et al. Robinson anterior cervical fusion: comparison of the standard and modified techniques. Spine 1994;19:660–663.
6. Gore DR, Sepic SB. Anterior cervical fusion for degenerated or protruded discs. A review of one hundred forty-six patients. Spine 1984;9:667–671.
7. Hanai K, Fujiyoshi F, Kamei K. Subtotal vertebrectomy and spinal fusion for cervical spondylotic myelopathy. Spine 1986;11:310–315.
8. Hase H, Watanabe T, Hirasawa Y, et al. Bilateral open laminaplasty using ceramic laminas for cervical myelopathy. Spine 1991;16:1269–1276.
9. Hayashi H, Okada K, Hashimoto J, et al. Cervical spondylotic myelopathy in the aged patient: a radiographic evaluation of the aging changes in the cervical spine and etiologic factors of myelopathy. Spine 1988;13:618–625.
10. Hirabayashi K, Satomi K. Operative procedure and results of expansive open-door laminaplasty. Spine 1988;13:870–876.
11. Jones AAM, Dougherty PJ, Sharkey NA, et al. Iliac crest bone graft: osteotome versus saw. Spine 1993;18:2048–2052.
12. Kellgren JH, Lawrence JS. Osteoarthritis and disk degeneration in an urban population. Ann Rheum Dis 1958;17:388–397.
13. Mikawa Y, Shikata J, Yamamuro T. Spinal deformity

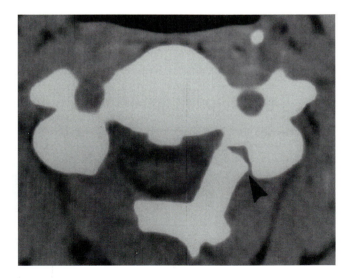

FIGURE 18.7.
CT scan showing a postoperative laminaplasty at the C4 vertebral body level. A greenstick hinge has been created on the left side (arrow), and the lamina has been osteotomized and hinged open from the opposite side. The goal of this is to enlarge the spinal canal and relieve spinal cord compression.

and instability after multilevel cervical laminectomy. Spine 1987;12:6–11.
14. Okada K, Shirasaki N, Hayashi H, et al. Treatment of cervical spondylotic myelopathy by enlargement of the spinal canal anteriorly, followed by arthrodesis. J Bone Joint Surg Am 1991;73:352–364.
15. Robinson RA, Smith GW. Anterolateral cervical disc removal and interbody fusion for cervical disc syndrome. Bulletin Johns Hopkins Hospital 1955;96:223–224.
16. Robinson RA, Walker E, Ferlic DC, et al. The results of anterior interbody fusion of the cervical spine. J Bone Joint Surg Am 1962;44:1569–1587.
17. Saunders R, Bernini P, Shirreffs T, et al. Central corpectomy for cervical spondylotic myelopathy: a consecutive series with long term follow-up evaluation. J Neurosurg 1991;74:163–170.
18. Schellhas K, Smith M, Gundry C, et al. Cervical discogenic pain: prospective correlation of MR imaging and discography in asymptomatic subjects and pain sufferers. Spine 1996;21:300–312.
19. Simmons EH, Bhalla SK, Butt WP. Anterior cervical discectomy and fusion. A clinical and biomechanical study with eight-year follow-up. With a note on discography: technique and interpretation of results. J Bone Joint Surg Br 1969;51:225–237.
20. Smith MD, Emery SE, Dudley A, et al. Vertebral artery injury during anterior decompression of the cervical spine. J Bone Joint Surg Br 1993;75:410.
21. White A, Southwick W, Deponte R, et al. Relief of pain by anterior cervical spine fusion for spondylosis. J Bone Joint Surg Am 1973;55:525–534.
22. Wilbourn AJ. Brachial plexus disorders. In: Dyck PJ, ed. Peripheral neuropathy, 3rd ed. Philadelphia: WB Saunders, 1993:933–934.
23. Yonenobu K, Fugi T, Ono K, et al. Choice of surgical treatment for multisegmental cervical spondylotic myelopathy. Spine 1985;10:710–716.
24. Zdeblick TA, Ducker TB. The use of freeze-dried allograft bone for anterior cervical fusions. Spine 1991;16:726–729.
25. Zdeblick TA, Zou D, Warden KE. Cervical stability after foraminotomy. J Bone Joint Surg Am 1992;74:22–27.

CHAPTER NINETEEN

Thoracic Disc Disease

Michael D. Smith

Introduction and Pathogenesis

Disc degeneration is almost universally present by the sixth decade of life, and thoracic disc degeneration parallels that present in the cervical or thoracic spine. It is a ubiquitous process. It is a natural consequence of the aging process, and it can be observed in the younger age group (4, 19, 21). Such degeneration typically is asymptomatic despite the severity of radiographic findings (10). Similar to degenerative disc disease of the cervical and lumbar spine, the etiology is secondary to the loss of proteoglycan matrix within the substance of the disc itself (3, 6,7). The disc desiccates and loses its biomechanical resilience. The functional spine unit (composed of the disc and the adjacent vertebral bodies) subsequently become stiffer and, as a reparative process, osteophytes and endplate sclerosis form in an effort to stabilize the motion segment. These osteophytes can encroach either the spinal cord or the exiting nerve roots. This degenerative cascade also results in the loss of disc height and shortening of the anterior column. These in turn can result in a progressive thoracic kyphosis if the disc degeneration occurs over multiple segments. The degenerative process is not generally painful, but if there is an irritation or compression of the spinal cord or the nerve roots, consequent symptoms can develop (2, 13, 16, 18).

This chapter provides an overview of this spectrum of degenerative thoracic disease, with an emphasis on those features associated with dysfunction of the spinal cord and the exiting nerve roots.

Definitions

For this chapter, thoracic radiculopathy is defined as a set of symptoms caused by compression of the nerve root. Myelopathy is defined as dysfunction of the spinal cord secondary to extradural compression of the spinal cord caused by herniated disc material or osteophytes, or a combination of both from the degenerative segment.

Diagnosis and Presentation

The clinical diagnosis of thoracic disc disease can be difficult (5, 8, 10, 11, 14, 17). Because the clinical presentation may be caused by either local mechanical effects due to disc degeneration, compression of the spinal cord and subsequent spinal cord syndromes, compression of the thoracic nerve root with radiculopathy, deformity due to incremental loss of disc height, or any of the above in combination, an accurate diagnosis can be an involved undertaking. Clinical presentation of thoracic disc disease can be broadly categorized into four groups: thoracic radiculopathy, local thoracic pain, so-called pseudoradicular pain (defined as radiating low back and leg pain), or thoracic myelopathy. The pain associated with the degenerative thoracic kyphosis is similar to that associated with Scheuermann's kyphosis and Scheuermann's disease and is a subject of different chapters within this text.

Localized Thoracic Pain

Localized thoracic pain caused by thoracic disc degeneration, or so-called mechanical thoracic disc disease, is often difficult to sort out. This difficulty is in part because of nondescript symptoms. Patients typically report vague localized discomfort between the shoulder blades and difficulty sleeping. They have difficulties finding positions of comfort pain with overhead activities, twisting, or playing tennis. Swinging a golf club, cross-country skiing, and swimming tend to aggravate the localized pain because of rotational forces upon the torso. This pain can be confused with cervicogenic or possible lumbar discogenic pain if the disc degeneration is occurring in the geographically approximate regions of the spine. Physical examination is usually unrewarding except for some localizing tenderness of spinous processes, muscle spasms, and pain from trigger points. The diagnosis and localization of thoracic caused by thoracic disc degenerative process is perhaps the most difficult aspects of the management of these patients.

Thoracic Radiculopathy

Thoracic disc radiculopathy has a much more specific presentation. Patients often report burning or lancing or radiating pain, which radiates laterally and anterior. It is strongly dermatome in nature and is rarely bilateral. If it occurs in the mid-portion of the chest on the left, it is often confused with myocardial ischemia. These patients often have extensive cardiac work-up to rule out that entity. Coughing, sneezing, and other Valsalva maneuvers, similar to the cervical and lumbar spine, tend to accentuate the pain. Severely localized tenderness and hyperpathic sensation changes may be found; often the diagnosis of herpes is considered. A discreet sensibility level on pinwheel assessment may be found, but weakness is hard to illicit. Unless a coexistent spinal cord compression exists, the distal neurologic examination is normal.

Lumbar Pseudo-Radicular Syndrome

The so-called lumbar pseudo-radicular pain can be common after a thoracic disc herniation. This in part caused by central compression of the spinal cord. The pain is often bilateral and radiates to the buttocks, low back, and lower limbs. This radiation of pain is caused by nondescript central cord compression, and a component of bilateral referred chest wall pain may exist. The pain may appear to be lumbar in origin on the initial clinical impression, but with specific questioning, often more proximal lumbar dermatomes are involved. Concrete or hard evidence of myelopathy may be absent both on history and physical examinations. The physical examination is variable in that localized tenderness, an ill-defined sensory level, and proximal weakness greater than distal weakness may be present. Occasionally, these patients have a mistaken diagnosis of lumbar spinal disease, and numerous operative procedures may be carried out prior to the diagnosis.

Thoracic Myelopathy

Thoracic myelopathy can be difficult to sort out from cervical spondylitic myelopathy or more global central nervous symptom disorders. There is often a broad-based stumbling buckling gait with bowel and bladder difficulties, bilateral lower extremity weakness, and variable degrees of sensibility loss. There is often a coexistent sensory level to pinwheel, and it is usually bilateral. Thoracic myelopathy may be painless and historically has be confused with other neurologic syndromes, such as multiple sclerosis.

Physical Examination

Physical examination should be done in a systematic and formal fashion. Patients should be undressed, and the spine should be viewed from all aspects to assess for signs of kyphosis or scoliosis. A lateral profile, including forward leaning postures with the arms extended (Adam's test), should be done to assess for Scheuermann's kyphosis and to make an estimate of flexibility in the coronal and sagittal planes. The presence of torso decompensation, thoracic or lumbar prominence, and the overall cervico-sacral compensation should be determined. Presence of deformity changes future treatment recommendations considerably. The posterior midline structures are palpated carefully to see if any geographic pain is present. The paraspinal muscles should be palpated to determine the presence of trigger points, muscle spasms, and local tenderness. A careful pinwheel assessment starting over the lateral aspect of the neck and the trapezial region over the chest to the buttocks should be done to look for sensibility changes. This often is the only presenting objective sign with this disease. A formal graded neurologic examination, including an assessment of proximal muscular weakness (such as hip flexors) and adductors, should be made and documented. The pinwheel assessment of all lumbar dermatomes and abdominal reflexes should be done. The assessment for presence of pathologic cord signs, Babinski signs, and proprioception should be made. Finding any one of the aspects of the neurologic examination to be abnormal, particularly if the upper extremity neurologic assessment is normal, would suggest a localizing thoracic disc lesion, particularly if differential spasticity is prominent.

Radiographic assessment should include anterior/posterior and lateral radiographs to look for the presence of degenerative disc disease or focal osteolytic lesions. The mainstays of imaging for thoracic disc disease include myelography with a follow-up computed tomography scan, or magnetic resonance imaging (MRI). Myelography and computed tomography has the benefit of better visualization of the osseous anatomy. It has the disadvantages of a necessary subarachnoid injection of iodine containing solutions and radiation. MRI in most circumstances has supplanted myelography; it can provide good detail of the spinal canal, nerve roots, and discs, and it allows for a better assessment of intramedullary lesions.

Localization Problems

Difficulties can arise in localizing the disc lesion level (1, 20). For best confidence, the localizing film presented with the MRI scan should include the base of the skull, the entire cervical spine, and the landmark scout views for assigning the gantry positions for the thoracic spine. Errors can occur when this image is then formatted and printed to the film, and then the next set of magnetic images are made. A small time gap exists between these two scans, and patients can move about and invalidate the localized scan. For this reason, it may be necessary to obtain both magnetic resonance imaging and a myelogram with follow-up CT scan to confirm the levels involved. Preoperative chest radiographs should be reviewed to determine the number of ribs and lumbar vertebrae present as well as the presence of associated anomalies, which may make localization difficult.

Thoracic Discography

As an ancillary examination, discography of the thoracic spine is controversial (15). Disc herniations may be central with predominantly spinal cord compression, eccentric with predominantly nerve root decompression, or a combination of both. The diagnostic dilemma is that these findings are not always painful. The presence of the degenerative desiccated nucleus in and of itself is not significant except if it is a focal process and if a patient's pain complaint is suggestive of mechanical pain. Thoracic discography can prove helpful in discriminating patients with amplified chronic pain syndromes and those with clear cut, painful thoracic disc disease. In the former patient, after provocative discography is attempted, numerous levels are severely painful, and no clear cut pattern of pain results. In the latter patient, the discs are typically painless until the involved disc, which correlates with the objective radiographic studies, is severely painful. In that particular individual, simple discectomy and fusion can be very beneficial.

Nonoperative Treatment

The nonoperative treatment of thoracic disc disease has been variably successful. Prolonged attempts are contraindicated in patients with obvious thoracic myelopathy caused by spinal cord compression. Those with thoracic radiculopathy (selective nerve root blocks) with additional instillation of a steroid-containing solution may prove useful. They can occasionally be repeated up to three to four times annually. These blocks can also confirm the diagnosis of radiculopathy and may assure accurate localization of the level. Thoracic epidural steroids have been described, but I have no major experience with them. Various other forms of therapy, such as spinal erector strengthening, physiotherapy, manipulation, chiropractic treatments, transcutaneous nerve stimulation, galvanic stimulation, and acupuncture, have been described with variable success. The reader is asked to review the following reference for further clarification (9).

Indications for Operation

By the time most patients present to the spinal surgeon, they have had a protracted period of symptoms. If these symptoms are relatively acute and short-lived, a trial of cautious nonoperative evaluation may be warranted. Nonsteroidal anti-inflammatory medications, as well as oral or injected steroids, can provide some symptomatic relief. If these methods fail, however, and if further assessment with MRI or CT scanning reveals an obvious disc herniation, the choice is usually distilled down to living with an acceptable amount of disability or having an operation. In patients with thoracic myelopathy, or pseudoradicular symptoms, a spinal cord decompression will be necessary. If a lateral disc herniation presents mainly as radiculopathy, a nerve root decompression can be done. If mechanical disc space disruption and mechanical symptoms are present, a simple anterior discectomy and fusion can be done.

Operative Approach

The operative approach is controversial. Anterior procedures have the benefit of direct exposure, decompression of the spinal canal and nerve roots, and easy application of the fusion. It does have the disadvantage of a thoracotomy. Post-thoracotomy discomfort can be substantial in a small percentage of individuals for an extended period of time. Newer techniques, such as video assisted thoracoscopy, are evolving and may decrease the morbidity and hospitalization (12). Further prospective studies are necessary to determine the true benefits of this approach. The posterior approach has the most efficacy for the treatment of laterally herniated discs. Central disc herniations are best treated anteriorly because posterior spinal canal decompression involves considerable removal of the lamina, facet joint, and pedicles to gain access to the anterior aspect of the spinal canal. This dissection can be destabilizing, particularly if it is done in the apex of a thoracic kyphosis. Modification of the posterior midline procedure, or the so-called lateral extracavitary or costotransversectomy approach, has the benefit of staying out of the chest, and may be best suited in those who have compromised pulmonary function. The overall incidence of neurologic deficits after operation appear to be greater from posterior rather than anterior approaches. Because the anterior approach is best for midline herniations and at least equal in efficacy to the posterior approach for lateral herniation, the anterior approach has gained preference in the recent literature.

Operative Technique

Anterior Transthoracic Decompression and Fusion

Decompression

The patient is intubated with a double lumen endotracheal tube, which allows for selective inflation and deflation of the lungs. If the disc is eccentric, that side is chosen for the approach, however, if the disc is central, the right side is usually preferred because of the location of the aorta and the length of the segmental vessels. The preoperative chest radiograph is reviewed to asses the angle of the insertions of the ribs on the spine. The mid-axial line is determined, and the rib that intersects the line drawn through the disc space to be operated on, as well as the mid-axial line, is selected for thoracotomy. That rib is subperiosteally reflected and removed, and the pleura is opened (Fig. 19.1). The lung is deflated and retracted away from the spine. The presumed disc space is marked with a localizing instrument, and a check radiograph is taken to confirm the operative level. The head of the rib and a one and one-half inch segment of the proximal rib is removed. This exposes the lateral aspect of the pedicle, the costotransverse joint, and the costovertebral joint. This area is debrided carefully of soft tissue. If the preoperative studies suggest that a spinal decompression is necessary, a high speed carbide burr or fine Kerrison punch is used to remove the lateral pedicle cortex. The inner cortex is approached slowly. Once the pedicle is partially excised, the lateral aspect spinal canal is positively identified. The disc space itself need not be developed thoroughly at this time. A high speed carbide burr is used to perform a subtotal corpectomy with a dissection paralleling the disc underneath the spinal canal. The posterior vertebral cortex is identified and thinned cautiously around its perimeter. This cortex is then perforated proximally and distally to the disc space and parallel to the disc space as it crosses underneath the spinal canal. An estimate is made of the mid-portion of the spinal canal, and similar amount of dissection is carried beneath that point to ensure adequate spinal canal decompression. The bridging cortex is perforated on the contralateral side. This creates an island of bone and disc material. This osteocartilaginous herniated disc fragment is pulled away from the spinal canal. At no time are instruments introduced into the spinal canal. This technique obviates the need for spinal canal or cord manipulation and adds safety to the procedure. Once a major disc fragment has been removed, the contralateral base of the pedicle may be palpated with a blunt probe. To increase operative visualization, small dental mirrors may be inserted to inspect the contralateral side, which is hidden from view. Loupes and a surgical head light or operative microscope facilitate dissection.

Division of the posterior longitudinal ligament is controversial, but I typically perform it to assure adequate resection of the endplates and removal of an extruded disc herniation in that region. This is performed by gently developing the plane between the posterior longitudinal ligament and the dura, controlling the epidural veins, and then dividing the thickened and often tenacious ligament under direct visualization using either a fine Kerrison punch, scissors, or knife. Always use carefully placed retractors protecting the dura during the dissection. Once bone and disc material are removed down and over to the contralateral base of the pedicle, an adequate decompression has been assured.

Arthrodesis

The arthrodesis is done by creating mortise type slots in the vertebral bodies above and below and using the previous harvested rib to impact numerous struts. Typically, three to four rib struts can be placed with ease to provide satisfactory anterior column support. The anterior longitudinal ligament and rim of the vertebral bone is not removed, thus preventing kyphosis and collapse in the postoperative period.

Typically, after extensive decompression for herniated discs, there is not enough residual bone for an isolated anterior instrumentation. However, this may be used to obviate the need for postoperative braces. If a suitable low profile rod and screw construct are available, they may be applied at this time. Pledges of gelatin sponges may be placed up between the bone grafts and the dura to aid in postoperative hemostasis. The pleura is then reapproximated, and the chest is closed in a layered anatomical closure. The chest tubes are discontinued when drainage is less than 30 ccs for an 8-hour shift. Most patients benefit from wearing a rigid type of thoracolumbar orthosis for 3 months. The wear usage is typically 6 weeks full-time, followed by 6 weeks only when up and about.

Anterior Transthoracic Discectomy and Fusion

If the preoperative studies suggest that only discectomy is necessary (e.g., patients with isolated mechanical pain, simple discectomy), then, using curettes and other hand instruments, the discectomy should be carried down to but not through the posterior longitudinal ligament. Morsellized bone from the rib is then packed about the decorticated endplates of the intervening vertebral bodies to effect an arthrodesis.

Results

Most patients benefit from thoracic disc operations, and the treatment of thoracic disc disease can be gratifying if the proper patient selection and adherence to precise surgical technique is used. Patients who have objective neurologic compression syndromes, such as myelopathy or radiculopathy, fare better than do those with localized pain. This finding substantiates the impression that operations in general should be done only in patients with neurologic compression, deformities that are likely to be problematic, or instabilities. Pain, despite the attempts of discography to objectify a subjective disorder, is still an elusive feature, and operations in that setting are less precise. If the diagnosis is inaccurate, the treatment is therefore inaccurate and less predictable (2, 8, 10, 12, 13, 14, 17).

Patients with myelopathy generally show substantial degrees of neurologic recovery, but their recovery may be incomplete (Fig. 19.2). Patients with thoracic pain caused by degenerative disc disease fare the least well, in part because the accuracy of the diagnosis is less secure than in those with myelopathy. Thoracic radiculopathy can be treated well by either anterior or posterior approach, and the results are gratifying. Patients with pseudo-radiculopathy tend to have fair to good resolution of their symptoms. This is in part because of the coexistence of other lumbar and adjacent thoracic degenerative disc diseases—these patients therefore tend to have prolonged low-level symptoms (Fig. 19.3).

Complications

Numerous potential complications exist from either nonoperative or operative approaches. Failure to diagnosis or refer a patient with thoracic myelopathy caused by extradural compression, or ascribing a neurologic deficit to that of another cause, such as multiple sclerosis, is common. The results of operation in that scenario are less rewarding than they should be. It is possible to operate on the wrong level if the radiographs are inappropriately interpreted, misread, or obtained, or are unavailable. Post-thoracotomy discomfort is universal for at least several months, but on long-term follow-up, it does not seem to be a major issue with the vast majority of patients. Neurologic deficit related to operative intervention has not occurred in our hands; this may relate to careful spinal canal decompressions and the safety of direct visualization afforded by the operative approach. Non-union occurs in approximately five to seven percent (Fig. 19.4).

The biggest complication from the operative treatment of herniated thoracic discs relates to the results of operation not meeting the patient's preoperative expectation. This complication can be remedied by several means, the first of which is providing a realistic expectation for the patient. Most patients have some persistent and minor problems, such as localized discomforts, occasional twinges of pains, or functional restrictions on long-term follow-up. Although these patients are not perfect, they are perfectly functional, and this difference needs to be understood by the patient. The biggest problems occur

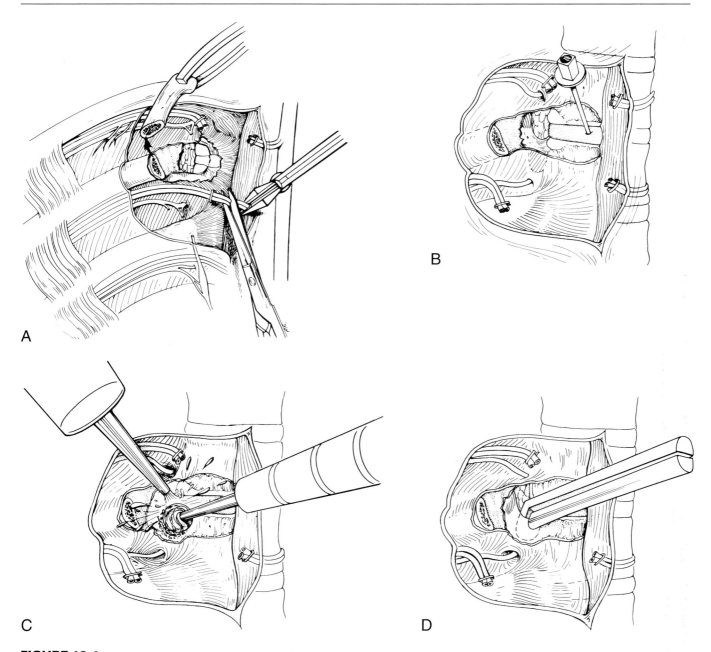

FIGURE 19.1.

A series of line drawings illustrating the transthoracic decompression. **A.** A standard posterolateral thoracotomy with subperiosteal dissection and removal of the rib has been achieved. The rib corresponding to the level of the decompression and fusion has been removed. **B.** Radiographic confirmation using a metallic marker of the proposed level is undertaken if any question of operative level is present. **C.** The soft tissue and the capsule of the costotransverse and costovertebral joint is removed, thus exposing the lateral aspect of the pedicle and its confluence with the transverse process. The pedicle is either partially or completely excised using a small Kerrison rongeur. **D.** Alternatively, a high speed carbide burr or a diamond surfaced burr with continuous water irrigation may be used. The pedicle excision aids to positively identify the lateral aspect of the spinal canal. **E.** The subtotal vertebrectomy is begun by motorized dissection parallel to the end plates and is carried underneath and towards the contralateral side. The dissection is guided by the orientation of the disc, and the visualization of the disc allows the surgeon to maintain a perpendicular orientation to the spinal canal. The posterior vertebral cortex above and below the herniated disc and osteophyte is then perforated carefully along its inferior and superior margins, again parallel to the disc space. The contralateral longitudinal cut is carried out at the base of the contralateral pedicle. **F.** These end plates' perforations create an island of osteophyte and disc herniation. This mobile fragment is then extracted into the previous created corpectomy defect and allows for a satisfactory spinal canal decompression without the introduction of tools or curettes into the spinal canal. Additional reverse angled curettes are used to remove any residual osteophytes on the contralateral portion of the pedicle. The base of the contralateral pedicle is then palpated to assure for adequate side to side spinal canal decompression. **G.** The fusion is begun by creating mortise type cuts in the vertebral bodies above and below. These mortise cuts are suitably wide enough to allow for impaction of multiple rib struts while preserving an anterior column to help avoid postoperative collapse at the segment.

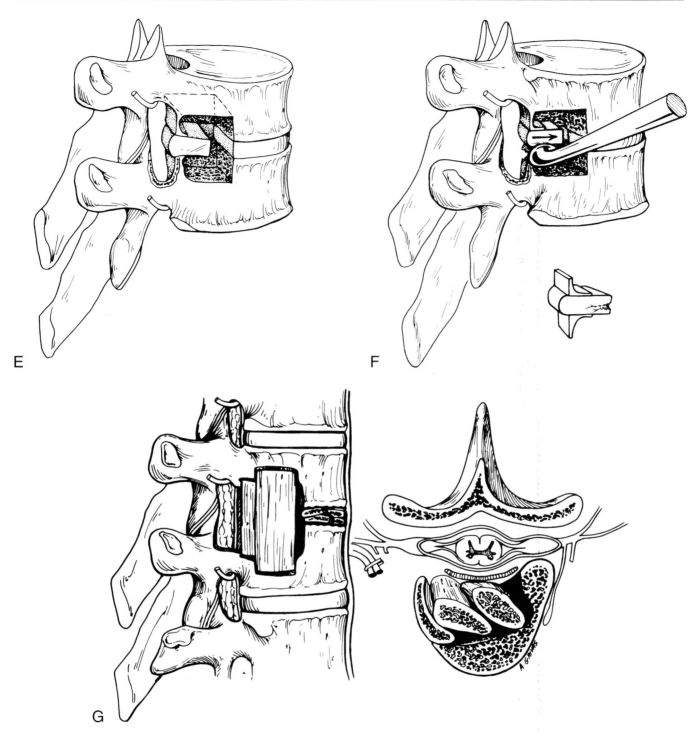

FIGURE 19.1—*continued*

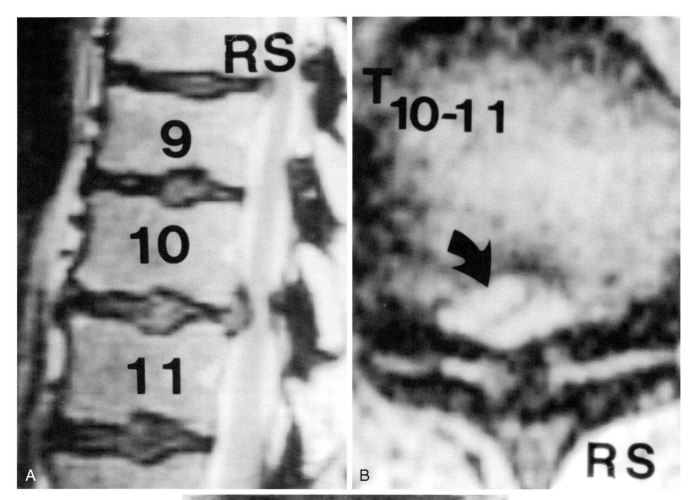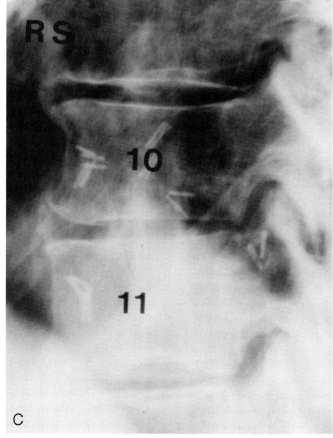

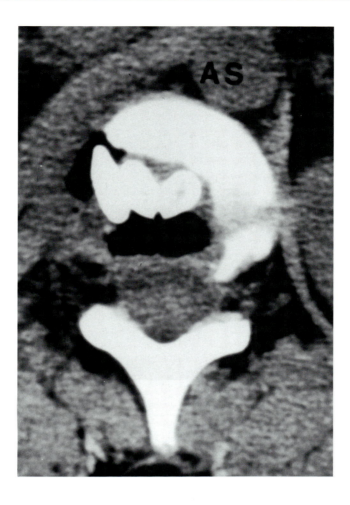

FIGURE 19.3.
A. Another patient who had an anterior decompression and fusion using the technique described in the text. Notice complete anterior decompression of the spinal canal and the numerous tightly fit rib strut grafts.

in the population of patients in which there is reason and benefit for persistent problems, such as impending litigation, worker's compensation, and similar collateral concerns.

Conclusion

Because thoracic disc degeneration is so common and not always painful, in general, operations for the herniated thoracic disc and degenerative disc disease should be considered for those with neurologic compression problems. However, an operation can help patients with focal painful disc segments if proper selection of patients is done. If the preoperative diagnosis accurately suggests a localized painful process, and the operative approach, generally anterior, is carried with careful and complete canal decompression and solid fusion is achieved, the long-term outlook and results can be both gratifying and durable.

FIGURE 19.2.
A 47-year-old male with a history of progressive thoracic pain that radiates in a band-like distribution about the lateral and anterior aspect of his chest with increasing buckling, stumbling and weakness in his legs. **A.** A preoperative sagittal magnetic resonance image demonstrates degenerative disc disease diffusely distributed about the thoracic spine. Additionally, there is an obvious anterior extradural defect at the T10–11 area with severe focal compression of the spinal cord. **B.** An axial image reveals eccentric compression of the spinal cord caused by soft disc material (curved arrowhead). **C.** A postoperative lateral radiograph demonstrating a solid arthrodesis 1 year later. Excellent recovery of the myelopathy ensued.

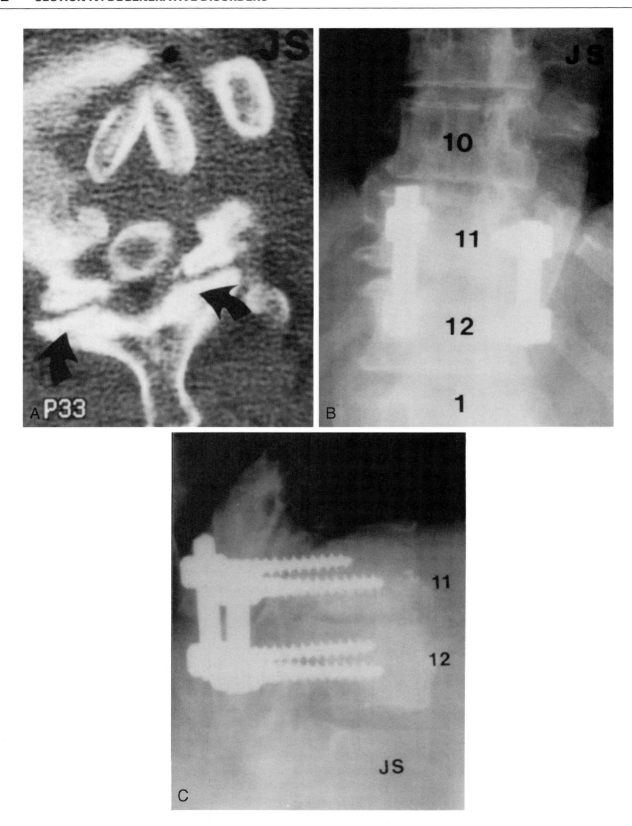

FIGURE 19.4.

A. A fifty-one year old female who had been essentially paraplegic from a large herniation at the T11–12 area. She recovered the ability to ambulate with a cane about the household, but still had significant limitations outside the home. A non-union developed with moderate local pain. An axial computed tomography scan demonstrates the non-union about the rib grafts but an excellent canal decompression. **B** and **C.** A posterior instrumented arthrodesis was done with good relief of the local pain. Pedicle screw instrumentation was used to facilitate vertical ambulation in this morbidly obese woman, and the screws did not require insertion of any fixation devices into the spinal canal.

References

1. Alvarez O, Roque CT, Pampati M. Multilevel thoracic disc herniations. CT and MR studies. J Comput Assist Tomogr 1988;12:649–652.
2. Albrand OW, Corkill G. Thoracic disc herniation. Treatment and prognosis. Spine 1979;4:41–46.
3. Anwad EE, Martin SD, Smith KR Jr, et al. Asymptomatic versus symptomatic herniated thoracic discs: their frequency and characteristics as detected by computed tomography after myelopathy. Neurosurgery 1991;28:180–186.
4. Benjamin V. Diagnosis and management of thoracic disc disease. Clin Neurosurg 1983;30:557–605.
5. Blumenkopf B. Thoracic intervertebral disc herniations: Diagnostic value of magnetic resonance imaging. Neurosurgery 1988;23:36.
6. Boden SD, McCowin PR, Davis DO, et al. Abnormal magnetic-resonance scans of the cervical spine in asymptomatic subjects. A prospective investigation. J Bone Joint Surg Am 1990;72:1178–1184.
7. Boden SD, Davis DO, Dina TS, et al. Abnormal magnetic-resonance scans of the lumbar spine in asymptomatic subjects. A prospective investigation. J Bone Joint Surg Am 1990;72:403–408.
8. Bohlman HH, Zdeblick TA. Anterior excision of herniated thoracic discs. J Bone Joint Surg Am 1988;70:1038–47.
9. Brown CW, Deffer PA Jr, Akmakjian J, et al. The natural history of thoracic disc herniation. Spine 1992;17(6S):S97–S102.
10. Currier BL, Eismont FJ, Green BA. Transthoracic disc excision and fusion for herniated thoracic discs. Spine 1994;3:323–328.
11. Epstein NE, Schwall G. Thoracic spinal stenosis: diagnostic and treatment challenges. J Spinal Disord 1994;3:259–269.
12. Horowitz MB, Moossy JJ, Julian T, et al. Thoracic discectomy using video assisted thoracoscopy. Spine 1994;9:1082–1086.
13. Maiman DJ, Larson SJ, Luck E, et al. A lateral extracavitary approach to the spine for thoracic disc herniation: Report of 23 cases. Neurosurgery 1984;14:178–182.
14. Otani K, Yoshida M, Fujii E, et al. Thoracic disc herniation: surgical treatment in 23 patients. Spine 1988;13:1262–1267.
15. Schellhas KP, Pollei SR, Dorwart RH. Thoracic discography: a safe and reliable technique. Spine 1994;18:2103–2109.
16. Ravichandran G, Frankel HL. Paraplegia due to intervertebral disc lesions: a review of 57 operative cases. Paraplegia 1981;19:133–139.
17. Rogers MA, Crockard HA. Surgical treatment of the symptomatic herniated thoracic disc. Clin Orthop Related Res 1994;300:70–78.
18. Ross JS, Perez-Reyes, Nuria, Masaryk TJ, et al. Thoracic disc herniation: MR imaging. Radiology 1987;165:511–515.
19. Schimel S, Deeb ZL. Herniated thoracic intervertebral discs. J Comput Tomogr 1985;9:141–143.
20. Williams MP, Cherryman GR, Husband JE. Significance of thoracic disc herniation demonstrated by MR imaging. J Comput Assist Tomogr 1989;13:211.
21. Wood KB, Garvey TA, Gundry C, et al. Magnetic resonance imaging of the thoracic spine. J Bone Joint Surg Am 1995;77:1632–1638.

CHAPTER TWENTY

Lumbar Disc Disease

Christopher P. Silveri and Frederick A. Simeone

Introduction

The discussion of lumbar disc disease involves understanding the pathoanatomy and physiology of the intervertebral disc as well as the mechanical and environmental factors that influence its inevitable senescence. Equally important, however, is for surgeons to realize the great socioeconomic impact on the patient if the condition of lumbar disc disease is not fully understood. Pain related to the degeneration of the lumbar disc has caused tremendous economic disability in the Western world, curtailing the productivity of individuals and contributing to the health care crisis. Low back pain accounts for a large proportion of visits to primary care givers, second only to upper respiratory illness, and leads to diminished work time and lost revenues.

The goal of this chapter is to highlight the basic epidemiology, anatomic considerations, diagnostic modalities, and treatment options available for degenerative disc disease. Since Mixter and Barr first noted the pathologic relationship of disc disease with neural compression in the 1930s, great strides have been made in the basic science and clinical understanding of the intervertebral disc (70). What had previously been thought to be compression from chondromas was actually the product of a series of events leading to the overall degeneration of the nucleus pulposus and its supporting structure, the annulus fibrosus. The process of lumbar disc disease leads to varying degrees of symptomatic and clinical manifestations.

Anatomy of the Disc

The intervertebral disc is composed of the nucleus pulposus, a soft hydrated gel-like substance made up of proteoglycan units that electrostatically bond to water molecules, embedded in a superstructure of type II collagen. This central structure of the disc is encapsulated by the annulus fibrosus, which firmly anchors it to the cartilaginous end plates of the vertebrae above and below. The proteoglycan units are large macromolecules made up of numerous glycosaminoglycan constituents, primarily chondroitin sulfate and keratin sulfate, attached to a protein core. Each core is then bound to a hyaluronic acid moiety. The composition of the nucleus pulposus allows for compressibility by virtue of its water content, which is approximately 85% at birth but decreases over the years. The vertebra-disc-vertebra motor unit is efficient in its ability to withstand axial load because of this shock-absorbing characteristic of the disc, allowing it to act as a viscoelastic structure. With age, the disc undergoes a process of collapse, heralded by a subtle change in glycosaminoglycan ratio and an overall decrease in proteoglycan content, leading to less efficient hydrostasis, which negatively affects its function.

The annulus fibrosus is the peripheral supporting structure of the disc and is made up primarily of collagen formed in a latticework of lamellae. These lamellae are arranged at 30° angles to the end plates, which optimizes the ability of the annulus fibrosus to resist torsional stresses and the tensile stress of axial load. Although in the 1970s Kulak elucidated the behavior of the annulus as a uniform concentric structure, more recent investigators have noted the presence of irregularities in the lattice and variations in structure, which is testimony to the complicated nature of this structure (54, 55, 65). With disc dehydration and loss of compressibility, the height of the interspace diminishes, effectively reducing the angle of inclination of the collagen fibers and with it the ability of the annulus to resist tensile forces.

Disc nutrition is contingent on passive diffusion, and its metabolism is facilitated by the osmotic environment created by load transmission across the disc (53). As water moves to and fro, so do nutrients and metabolites. The vertebral end plates also contribute to the nutrition of the disc. It has been suggested that the relatively thin end plates, whose composition of proteoglycans, water, and collagen simulates that of the nucleus pulposus, allow for the transmission of transudates from the osseous vasculature, contributing to disc nutrition (80). Anatomic studies of vertebral end plates show a lack of vascular channels into the disc space after the second decade (16). It is likely that this loss of vasculature marks the beginning of the degenerative process. Disc disease is unusual in adolescents, accounting for less than 3% of surgically proven cases of herniation (13). Diffusion remains as the means of metabolic transport for the disc after childhood, but the reparative processes are severely diminished, and the inevitable degeneration will then progress. Although the pathophysiologic changes that occur in the disc with time contribute to its decline, the mechanical forces imposed on the disc as it is degenerating pose an equally important threat. With disc dehydration comes loss of height and annular laxity, as well as inefficiency in responding to the compressive and tensile loads of daily living. Added stresses of lateral flexion loads, twisting, prolonged sitting, vibrational loads (76), or similar insults can interfere with the diffusion and contribute to disc disease as well. Mechanical effects on the disc are best presented in Nachemson's classic work involving disc pressure measurements (73). Sitting pressures are consistently higher than those in the standing position, and rotation and flexion combined increase the risk of injury (75).

The connection between pain syndromes and this progressive disc disease is difficult to establish, since the degeneration process occurs in many people who remain relatively asymptomatic. Several authors have noted specific anatomic sites in the lumbar spine that they think may be primarily responsible for causing low back pain as well as leg pain. These opinions range from complete exclusion of the disc as a source of pain (100) to causes in facet joints, facet capsules, the annulus fibrosus, the posterior longitudinal ligament, muscle, or muscle fascia, compression of normal roots, presence of tethered inflamed roots, and chemical mediators of radiculitis (39, 41, 68, 82, 94).

Recent studies have helped to clarify the anatomic basis of discogenic pain. Kuslich et al. in 1991 presented the results of performing low back surgery under local anesthesia and directly stimulating each structure under question (56). Their data confirmed that the normal nerve root was insensitive to pain and could be retracted or compressed without any discomfort. Prolonged irritation caused paresthesia but not pain. If the root had been previously inflamed or compressed and exhibited erythema and swelling, manipulation of the nerve reproduced radicular symptoms that had been noted preoperatively. No other stimulation caused radicular-type pain. Two-thirds of patients experienced low back pain on stimulation of the annulus fibrosus or of the posterior longitudinal ligament. This area is richly innervated by the sinuvertebral nerve and is also the area of greatest weakness in the annulus fibrosus and ligamentous support of the disc, which explains why it is both a common location for disc herniation and a painful one (15, 87, 101). Low back pain similar to preoperative symptoms was reproduced by stimulation of the lateral annulus fibrosus in cases in which hypertrophied superior articulating processes of the facet joint were noted to be in contact with the annulus in the lateral recess. Otherwise the facet joint itself and the capsule only occasionally caused low back pain.

As the degenerative process occurs, the annulus fibrosus exhibits the first signs of injury, with circumferential tearing noted on histologic examination (52). In long-standing cases the loss of height leads to increased load on the posterior facet joints, which can potentiate facet arthropathy and osteophyte formation. Horizontal traction spurs also may develop at the level of the disc, indicating segmental instability (63). The initial annular event, along with the areas of weakness in the posterior annulus fibrosus and posterior longitudinal ligament, likely accounts for the propensity for central or posterolateral herniations.

Once the disc is injured to a significant degree, displacement from its central or posterocentral location within the annulus fibrosus can occur. Specific terms are used to describe the different types of herniation. Displacement of a fragment of nucleus pulposus or annulus fibrosus through the tears in the outer one-third of the annulus is called a *disc protrusion*. If the material protrudes beyond the posterior longitudinal ligament, it is said to have *extruded*. Finally, a *sequestered disc fragment* is one that is completely displaced with a free fragment in the canal. Disc bulging, frequently seen on magnetic resonance imaging (MRI) evaluations, is nonspecific, indicating only that disc degeneration has occurred to a degree sufficient to allow a generalized loss of compressive stability in the nucleus/annulus complex.

It is still unclear what makes an individual more susceptible to extrusion, given that more than 30% of asymptomatic individuals will have an abnormal MRI signal indicating degeneration (8). It has also been noted that under extreme compressive loads the vertebral endplates will be injured before the annulus fibrosus, and at extreme torsional positioning the annulus will tear, but nuclear material will not displace (1, 9, 27). When disc herniation does occur, however, the classic locations for it are indicated in Figure 20.1. Posterolateral herniation occurs with the greatest frequency, irritating the exiting nerve below. If the herniation has extruded in the lateral recess of the neural canal or in a far lateral position, the corresponding nerve root above will be compressed either in the axilla against the pedicle or as it exits the foramen. Central herniations can result in localized back pain, single nerve root irritation, or in some cases, if the herniation is large enough, cauda equina syndrome. Although cauda equina syndrome is rare, accounting for only 2.4% of all herniations, the diagnosis must be made immediately. The clinical picture may involve leg and buttock pain, not necessarily radicular in nature, paresthesias, numbness, weakness, and bowel or bladder dysfunction (84).

Epidemiology and Patient Population

If a tree falls in a deserted forest, does it make a sound? It seems relevant to keep this idea in mind when considering the current incidence of disabling back pain in the Western world. Waddell is widely recognized as the first to have noted the epidemic of low back pain ailments in industrial societies. In travels in comparatively underdeveloped areas, he was startled to find an abundance of individuals who actually complained of back pain only after a back pain clinic had been established (88). This is not to say that many did not at one time or another experience such symptoms; it simply suggests that for those distracted by the trials and tribulations of everyday life, the aches and pains of work and play may have seemed quite ordinary.

Low back pain has been estimated to affect 60 to 80% of individuals at one time or another in their lives; figures in this range have been quoted throughout the past four decades (31, 32, 46, 48, 58). The majority will show improvement within 2 to 3 weeks (22). Even though there is little evidence to contradict these numbers, the proportion of the population that is considered permanently disabled continues to rise, and the cost of health care rises with it. Frymoyer emphasizes this point, stating that between 70 and 90% of the total costs related to low back pain are spent on the relatively few individuals who are deemed disabled (31). Although 95% of individuals with low back pain have returned to work after 3 months, the remaining 5% are responsible for over 85% of these costs (28). Most of these patients eventually return to gainful employment, but the statistics show that if they are off work for more than 1 year, the likelihood of returning drops to 20%, and it approaches zero if the disability lasts more than 2 years (3).

Numerous studies have documented several known risk factors or activities associated with low back pain and sciatica. There are both physical or mechanical determinants of low back symptoms as well as psychosocial factors. Commonly noted risk factors for low back pain include repetitive lifting or pulling, exposure to industrial vibrations, prolonged motor vehicle usage, pregnancy, and several ana-

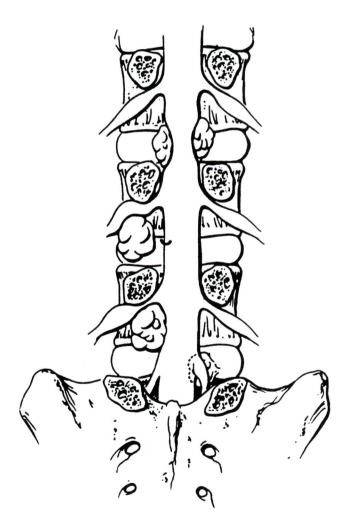

FIGURE 20.1.
A diagram showing a central herniated disc at L3–4 impinging on the cauda equina, a far lateral foraminal herniated disc at L4–5 impinging on the L4 root, an axillary sequestered disc at the L5 root, and a posterolateral herniated disc at L5-S1 impinging on the S1 root.

tomic indices related to obesity, sagittal contour, canal dimensions, and the like (32, 33, 51, 78). Cigarette smoking is also highly associated with these symptoms, as was recently confirmed by the present authors (2). In a comparison between patients with surgically confirmed disc disease and a control population of asymptomatic individuals, 57% of those with disc disease were smokers versus 37% of the control population. It has also been suggested that psychosocial factors may contribute negatively to the symptomatic presentation of low back pain. Most notable are job dissatisfaction, boring work, stress, drug addiction, and compensation cases (31, 86). It is believed that these factors not only may potentiate the symptoms but also may contribute to a patient's being refractory to routine treatment. It is with this in mind that Waddell proposed his description of the nonorganic signs of low back pain (90). These include nonanatomic pain distribution, pain with distraction, stimulation with axial load, and superficial pain or sensory changes. The most important of these signs, however, is overreaction. If signs of this nature make up a large part of the findings in a patient with back or leg pain, further psychosocial testing is indicated.

Natural History

Before considering treatment options for low back pain or leg pain, one must be aware of the natural history of this disorder. In lumbar disc disease the patient usually first notes pain originating in the lower back. It is at a later date that the radiculopathy will appear. This may occur several years later if the process is referable to generalized disc degeneration. During this interval the low back discomfort will wax and wane, often recurring with less intensity. If the symptoms are associated with a more pronounced, yet still mild to moderate disc herniation, the patient classically will describe diminution of the low back symptoms only to be left with leg pain, numbness, or weakness. This is likely explained anatomically in that initial annular fibrosus and local injury elicits pain via the sinuvertebral neural pathways, though the compression on nearby roots is less than that required to produce obstruction of signal transmission, numbness, or weakness. However, once the inflammatory process is in full cascade, the chemical irritants of the nerve manifest themselves. Finally, in cases of severe herniation and extrusion, immediate leg pain, often with minimal back symptoms, will result.

Approximately 5% of the male and 3% of the female population will experience sciatica at some time after they have reach the age of 35 years (98). Hakelius has shown that as many as 75% of these patients will respond to nonsurgical management, improving within 10 to 30 days after the incident. Nineteen percent of the patients in his study required surgical intervention (38). Further confirmation of the natural history of sciatica is revealed in Weber's classic study (92), which is used by most orthopaedic surgeons as the standard reference. Weber randomized a portion of 280 patients with myelographically confirmed herniated discs into a subset of patients treated either conservatively or surgically. All patients with progressive motor paresis or sphincter dysfunction were surgically treated after a period of 14 days of conservative treatment. These patients, as well as those who improved without treatment and who showed no evidence of surgical pathology, were excluded from the primary group. His findings indicate that although the initial results of surgical patients evaluated within the first postoperative year were statistically better than those of the conservative group, further observation revealed no statistical difference in long-term outcome after 4 years. Also noted was that a 3-month trial period of conservative measures despite the presence of motor weakness did not significantly alter the recovery of function postoperatively. Since the study initially excluded those patients with progressive neurological deficit, his conclusion was that muscle weakness alone was a doubtful indication for surgery if its presence had been for an unknown duration. If the onset of weakness is known to be related temporally to the onset of the symptoms, however, and the pressure on the nerve can be relieved immediately after the appearance of the weakness, then surgery is the treatment of choice. This conclusion has also been supported by Hakelius, who found little difference in residual weakness in the final outcome of those treated surgically as compared to those treated nonsurgically (38).

One must always therefore resist the temptation to operate on a patient with an acute herniation who presents with disabling pain if conservative treatment will prove to be equally effective. It is true that their pain relief will be more expedient and quite dramatic if decompression is performed early, but the risk-benefit ratio is clearly in favor of conservative treatment.

Clinical Evaluation

The history and physical examination is, as always, the key to the evaluation, understanding, and treatment of lumbar disc disease. It begins with the initial informal conversation between patient and physician, during which the practitioner can immediately develop a sense of the person's attitudes, fears, and expectations. The patient's socioeconomic background, present work status, sophistication with medical terminology, desire to return to gainful employment, dedication to previous forms of conservative treatment all influence the physician's ability to accurately diagnose and treat the problem. Although not all patients will describe the classic findings, it is important to explore the various avenues known to be characteristic of disc disease and to be able to extrapolate frequently vague complaints to objective pathology.

As previously noted, the initial presenting complaints most often involve symptoms of low back pain. Patients with low back pain will range in age from the very young to the elderly, though those with disc disease are usually between the ages of 30 and 45 years. As with any diagnostic exercise, the differential diagnosis is lengthy, with numerous metabolic, congenital, traumatic, infectious, inflammatory, neoplastic, vascular, and idiopathic disorders that must be ruled out. A careful history and physical examination will exclude most of these disorders; however, one must always remember the adage you cannot see what you do not look for. Fortunately, only a small percentage of patients complaining of back pain have occult forms of cancer or vascular or other medical diseases requiring urgent treatment. Quite often the first clue will come from the age of the patient. It is uncommon for children to complain of low back pain, especially of discogenic origin. When this occurs, one must entertain the diagnosis of spondylolisthesis, discitis, or various neoplastic disorders such as osteoid osteoma, osteoblastoma, and eosinophilic granuloma. Patients over the age of 50 years complaining of pain isolated to the low back are at significant risk for serious medical illnesses, including malignancy and infection (67). This is especially true if the patient complains of persistent, progressive pain unrelieved with recumbency or analgesics. Pain is not always the only complaint. The physician must be able to elicit the appropriate historical facts to confirm or exclude certain diagnoses. Young males with back discomfort without any focal neurologic changes, for example, may complain mostly of morning stiffness that improves with activity. This would suggest ankylosing spondylitis, a seronegative spondyloarthropathy, as opposed to mechanical low back strain. Along the same lines, gait imbalance associated with vague mid and low back discomfort in the elderly may in fact be the expression of cervical myelopathy and not lumbar disease.

The mode of onset and duration of the symptoms is important to establish because it can aid in the assessment of severity, potential for recovery, and success of previous forms of therapy. Quite classically, discogenic back pain with or without radiculopathy will be intermittent in its presentation, usually precipitated by strenuous physical activity and exacerbated by prolonged sitting, moving to a standing position, or bending and twisting, all of which increase disc pressures, as previously noted. Mechanical in nature, it is relieved with rest or limitation of activity. When radiculopathy is present provocative actions such as coughing, sneezing, and other Valsalva maneuvers may acutely exacerbate the leg pain. Middle-aged or elderly patients who describe exacerbation of symptoms with standing or with lying prone and have associated neurogenic claudication from spinal stenosis or lateral recess stenosis will actually improve with flexed postures, which result in widened foramina and diminished neural compression. Postural changes therefore can help the practitioner to formulate an anatomically based understanding of the pain syndrome. Vascular claudication will be excluded from this scenario because standing upright does not relieve the patient's leg pain. In this position, vascular claudication improves with the resting of the gastrocnemius-soleus muscle complex; with stenosis, however, the lumbar lordosis continues to cause compression of neural structures, and it is only with flexion forward or sitting that the canal is sufficiently widened. Bell, who referred to this as the grocery cart sign, summarized the differences between vascular and neurogenic claudication (5).

The relative proportions of back pain versus leg pain are important to establish, because a patient with primarily low back symptoms is less likely to have compressive pathology and therefore less likely to be easily cured with surgery. Many chronically disabled patients will present with numerous complaints, and in distinguishing between back and leg symptoms the practitioner can force the patient to prioritize the complaints and focus on what really hurts. Most patients with long-standing lumbar disc disease will have years of low back complaints, variable and intermittent in nature, before the insidious onset of leg pain. This course has been shown to range from 2 to as many as 10 years of episodic back pain prior to radiculopathy (34, 84, 92).

Understanding the mechanisms of injury and where an injury took place may shed light on other psychosocial causes of prolonged back pain. Secondary gain resulting from litigation or compensation cases will alter the patient's perception of pain and disability and will be a crucial determinant of predicted outcome. If the pain is temporally related to a specific incident at the workplace the clinician must be conservative in the initial treatment plan. This is especially true if the patient is no longer able to perform his or her duties. The success rate of any form of treatment for these patients is diminished by one-third (89). As mentioned earlier, Waddell noted several signs that strongly indicate the need for psychosocial evaluation. Briefly, these include nonanatomic superficial tenderness, axial loading and rotation stimulation tests, distraction tests such as a sitting straight-leg-raising exercise, nonanatomic weakness or sensory deficits, and overreaction in facial expression, verbalization, or muscle tremor. These nonorganic physical signs are harbingers of poor outcomes and, if three or more are present, require further testing to clarify the patient's suitability for surgery. The Minnesota multiphasic personality inventory test (MMPI) is the standard questionnaire used throughout the literature (37). Depression is also a major illness that will negatively affect the treatment of lumbar disc disease. When depression is present some authors believe that it is necessary to treat it as the primary problem and to address the disc disease only after the depression has been controlled (14). Unfortunately, true clinical depression may be subtle and go unnoticed. In order to facilitate the appreciation of this disease, five symptoms have been noted to indicate the potential for depression (5). These are lack or energy (anergy), inability to enjoy oneself (anhedonia), sleep disturbances, spontaneous weeping, and general feelings of depression. Dependency on narcotic medication also will flavor the patients' description of their disability as well as their need for pain relief postoperatively. It is important to clarify exactly how much narcotic use has been necessary to satisfy the patient's needs and from whom he or she has received prescriptions.

Once the frequency, intensity, and location of back pain has been determined, the patient should be challenged to describe specifically and in detail the location and character of any leg pain that may accompany or be distinct from the back symptoms. An effective method is to ask the patient to trace the pain, with one finger, from its most proximal origin to its distal extent. This will provide the examiner the opportunity to determine any dermatomal nature in the pain's distribution. Classically, true radiculopathy has been described as sharp, lancinating pain, and it is usually quite specifically located. The distributions of such lumbar radiculopathy have been well documented and are summarized as follows (45). Involvement of the L1 root primarily results in pain at the inguinal region and inner thigh. As the lower roots are involved, the pain moves anterolaterally about the thigh and eventually into the leg. The L2 root therefore portends a distribution on the anteromedial thigh, and the L3 root covers the anterior thigh to the top of the knee. At this point the more classic L4–S1 patterns predominate, with L4 radiculopathy radiating down the anterolateral thigh across the knee to the medial leg and inner foot. L5 radiculopathy extends down the lateral thigh and lateral calf to the dorsum of the foot and classically involves the great toe. The remaining posterior thigh and posterior calf and lateral foot and sole are served by the S1 nerve root. These parameters are used to identify areas of numbness, dysesthesia, and paresthesia as well.

Finally, it is important to ask in detail whether or not the patient has experienced recent bowel or bladder dysfunction. Cauda equina syndrome, one of the few surgical emergencies in degenerative spinal surgery is potentially disastrous, with a high likelihood of permanent bowel and bladder paralysis. Delay in diagnosis is often the cause of severe disability because it is often accompanied with vague back pain and perianal discomfort, and since multiple roots are involved, specific radicular patterns of leg pain are often absent. Occurring both as an acute massive disc herniation or with a more insidious onset, the classic description of cauda equina syndrome is of low back pain, bilateral sciatica, saddle anesthesia, dysesthesia, lower extremity weakness, and bowel and bladder incontinence (19).

Physical Examination

The physical examination begins the moment the patient walks through the door. Much information can be gleaned from the actions of a patient prior to the formal medical interaction. How a patient conducts himself or herself with office personnel as well as with other patients and the patient's gait and posture moving about the office provide the examiner with invaluable information, especially in cases in which there is evidence of questionable disability, compensation claims, or litigation.

When the patient walks into your office, notice whether the posture is erect, or flexed forward, as is commonly seen with spinal stenosis. Nerve root symptoms will be aggravated with certain positions, especially sitting or leaning forward, and these tend to be avoided with acute symptoms. At times this is so evident that the patient prefers to stand during the interview. The practitioner may also note a subtle list to one side, which may be indicative of axillary or contralateral disc herniation (5, 99). Notice any unusual skin markings or rashes that may signify underlying neurologic abnormalities, such as hairy patches associated with spinal dysraphism, café-au-lait spots associated with neurofibromatosis, or, of course, postoperative surgical scars over the midline or over iliac crest bone graft sites. The overall physical shape and general weight of the patient helps to identify individuals interested in leading active versus more sedentary lifestyles.

Palpation of the spine must specifically incorporate an examination of the midline structures, the supraspinous and interspinous ligaments, the spinous processes, and so on. Inability to palpate all the lumbar spinous processes may indicate occult spondylolisthesis, overlying masses, or swelling from recent trauma. Particular attention should be paid to the paraspinal musculature. In severe cases, a loss of lumbar lordosis may be visually obvious and may manifest itself with unilateral or bilateral muscle spasm. If the patient will allow side-to-side lateral bending, palpation of each paraspinal muscle mass should reveal softening with ipsilateral bending unless involuntary spasm is present. Palpation for sites of tenderness includes the structures above as well as the areas overlying the iliolumbar ligaments, the sciatic nerve between the greater trochanter and ischial tuberosity, the sacroiliac joint areas, and the coccyx. Occult sacroiliitis confirmed by the fabere test (hip *f*lexion, *ab*duction, *e*xternal *r*otation, and *e*xtension) requires immediate attention and can easily be overlooked in favor of the more common diagnosis of sciatica.

The remainder of the examination of the lumbar spine involves range of motion in all planes, flexion, extension, lateral bend, and rotation. These are typically qualitative measurements, since absolute degrees of spinal motion differ with age group. The examiner is usually looking for gross limitations in motion as well as exacerbation of radicular pain with particular motions. To reiterate, spinal stenosis is usually worsened with extension, which effectively closes down the posterior elements, further constricting the neural canal. Disc disease with herniation will be irritated with spinal flexion, and radicular pain should be reproducible with ipsilateral lateral bending or, if an axillary herniation is present, pain will worsen with a contralateral bend. The modified Schober test helps to quantify lumbar spinal range of motion in flexion (64). A point 10 cm above and a point 5 cm below the lumbosacral junction are identified and marked. With flexion the distance between the points should increase by 6 cm or more for the test to be negative.

The neurologic examination of the lumbar spine involves motor evaluation, sensory stimulation, deep tendon reflexes, and various tension signs. As noted earlier, routine posterolateral disc herniations will compress the nerve root below, and far lateral extrusions classically impinge on the exiting root above against its pedicle. To simplify the discussion, the examination will be discussed as one would perform it in the clinical setting, that is, identifying the functions of each root in succession. Severe or prolonged compression of the roots will lead to muscle weakness and eventually atrophy. Examination of the lower extremity muscles can be easily performed with the patient seated on the examination table. The iliopsoas hip flexor muscles are primarily innervated by the L1, L2, and L3 roots and are usually the first major muscle group tested in the lower extremity. Next the quadriceps femoris muscles are tested, noting the function of the L2, L3, and L4 nerves. These two muscle groups are served by multiple roots, and weakness in them can result from any root deficit; however, usually the iliopsoas muscle will gain much of its function from L2, and the quadriceps muscle from L3 and L4. The tibialis anterior muscle is primarily served by the L4 root, although L5 radicular symptoms can sometimes result in foot-drop. Extension of the great toe via the extensor hallucis longus muscle is the most commonly used test for L5 function. Hip abduction function via the gluteus medius muscle is also derived from the innervation of the L5 root. Finally, the examination of the S1 root involves motor testing of the gastrocnemius-soleus muscle complex, the great toe flexors (flexor hallucis longus and brevis muscles), and the foot everters (peroneus longus and brevis muscles). Although rarely tested, the gluteus maximus is also innervated by the S1 root. The most sensitive way to test the plantar flexor muscles is to have the patient perform repetitive heel raises. In this way early fatiguing will be evident as compared to the unaffected side.

The sensory examination is usually a confirmatory test of the patient's historical complaints of numbness or paresthesia. It is less objective than the motor testing but proves to be important when dealing with medical diseases such as diabetes mellitus and its associated polyneuropathies. Preoperative documentation of such diffuse sensory deficits is evidence of profound systemic disease, which will adversely affect the eventual outcome of any decompressive lumbar spine surgery (42, 83). Despite adequate release of the involved roots, it is likely that the preexisting microvascular disease will undermine the nerve roots' ability to respond to the decompression. Poor clinical outcomes may also be attributed to the failure to recognize neuropathic changes that are secondary to the diabetes and hence not affected by the decompressive surgery.

In summary, the L1 dermatome involves the superior aspect of the thigh into the groin. The L2 root supplies innervation down the anteromedial thigh, and compression of the L3 root produces sensory abnormalities along the anterior thigh to the knee. It is only with involvement of the lower roots that the sensory examination is distinct. The L4 root supplies the medial leg and instep, the L5 root the lateral border of the leg to the dorsum of the foot, and the S1 root the posterior calf and lateral aspect of the foot along with the sole. The sacral roots S2–S5, rarely tested in cases of degenerative disc disease, circumferentially surround the anus and can be tested if cauda equina syndrome is suspected or in cases of spinal trauma. The inner portion of the anus is served by S4 and S5 and the middle and outer portions by S3 and S2, respectively.

The deep tendon reflexes, when asymmetric, offer reliable clues to the affected roots. However, one must not be confused by symmetrically diminished reflexes, as they can be normal in certain individuals. This portion of the examination is only reliable if distinct differences are noted from side to side. It is also helpful, as in motor testing, to use repetitive testing of certain reflexes to uncover a dampening or fatiguing character that ordinarily would not be realized with single attempts, especially if the deficit is subtle. Again, medical illnesses or advanced age may result in diminished reflexes, though these should be equal bilaterally. The most commonly tested reflexes are the patellar tendon reflex, primarily innervated by the L4 nerve root, and of the Achilles tendon reflex, subserved by the S1 root. There are possible variations here, for in some cases the L3 root plays a greater role in the knee reflex. It is rare that the practitioner tests for an L5 reflex change, but if desired the tibialis posterior muscle tendon reflex can be elicited by gently tapping the tendon just above the ankle with the foot in eversion and mild dorsiflexion.

By far one of the most convincing confirmatory signs of a compressed nerve root is the successful use of one of the tension signs. Several authors have expounded on the diagnostic certainty obtained when a clinical examination is corroborated by a positive nerve root tension sign. Hirsh and Nachemson classically described their improved diagnostic ability when objective findings are coupled with provocative tests and myelographic data (40). They were able correctly to predict a herniated disc 55% of the time with objective neurologic findings only, as confirmed by surgically documented root compression. With the addition of a positive tension sign, however, their correct diagnoses rose to 86%, and when accompanied by radiographic data as well, it was 95%. In a review of 2504 operations, Spangfort reported that the straight-leg-raising sign was positive in over 90% of cases (84). The classic straight-leg-raising test is performed with the patient supine and the examiner passively elevating the patients leg with the knee locked in extension. Usually the test can be reproduced with the patient sitting, as one would perform the remainder of the examination. With elevation of the limb, the patient is asked whether or not the radicular symptoms or leg pain is exacerbated by this maneuver. Back pain alone in not indicative of a positive test, nor is discomfort from tight hamstring musculature. The examiner must also be cognizant of excessive lumbar lordosis or hip extension, which may be the patient's mechanism to diminish the painful symptoms. A variant of this test includes the addition of foot dorsiflexion to further exacerbate the radiculopathy. There are several other types of tension signs that are reviewed in the literature (81). The standard test is the formal supine straight-leg-raise or its variant, the seated test described above, which have been associated with the name Lasègue. These primarily involve traction of the L5 or S1 roots. The contralateral or well leg straight-leg-raise also stretches these roots, and if positive strongly suggests an axillary herniation involving the opposite root. Those roots more cephalad have been shown to move minimally or not at all with these maneuvers. To test these roots the examiner may use the femoral nerve stretch test to elicit pain involving the L2–L4 roots. This is best performed with the patient on lying on the contralateral side. In this position the examiner stabilizes the pelvis with one hand and then slowly extends the hip using the thigh and flexed knee as a lever. In a positive test, pain is reproduced along the anterior thigh.

Regardless of the position of the patient, provocative tests such as these further support the diagnosis of a herniated nucleus pulposus. This is especially sensitive in the young patient, who lacks significant lateral recess stenosis to confound the diagnosis. In patients over 30 years of age a positive test, although significant, is not as clearly associated with solely a disc herniation. In addition, older patients may not exhibit a positive straight-leg-raise test despite the presence of a disc herniation. Spangfort showed that in patients under 30 years of age, the lack of a straight-leg tension sign in patients with sciatica predictably excluded the presence of the diagnosis of a herniated disc (84).

The remainder of the physical examination should of course include the complete musculoskeletal review, keeping in mind that various hip and knee arthropathies may mimic lumbar radicular pain. The examination of the cervical spine is also important because occasionally symptoms referable to cervical myelopathy may manifest themselves as lower extremity complaints. Performing a peripheral vascular examination is vital in all potential surgical candidates, for not only may the symptoms of peripheral vascular disease or associated medical illnesses mimic those of neurogenic disc disease, but also the examination may reveal occult limb-threatening disease. When indicated by the physician's clinical suspicion, a thorough abdominal and rectal examination may disclose masses or tenderness that later prove to be the cause of the original complaints and allows for prompt referral to a medical or surgical specialist.

Radiologic Evaluation

The role of radiologic testing is to confirm a previously determined provisional diagnosis. All too often patients arrive in the surgeon's office already having obtained an outpatient MRI examination, without having had a complete physical examination or even plain film examination. As noted earlier, the best indication for surgical intervention is when an objective neurologic finding is associated with a positive tension sign and confirmed with a positive radiologic finding. Those radiologic tests include plain films, computerized tomograms (CTs), myelograms, and magnetic resonance imaging.

The role of routine screening x-ray films of the lumbar spine has recently come under question. In this age of cost containment, several authors have noted the inefficiency and low prognostic yield on surveillance films. Given the favorable natural history of low back pain it has been suggested that routine radiographs in atraumatic situations be delayed for an initial treatment period of 8 weeks (60). During this time many patients will show improvement. Certainly in primary care settings it is reasonable to begin treatment with a presumed diagnosis, and if improvement is not seen within a specified period of time then the workup can ensue. In many surgeons' offices, however, a referral pattern is set up so that the initial evaluation by the surgeon is in fact a follow-up visit for the patient, and neglecting to rule out other, more malignant forms of pathology at this time may be questionable. There is usually no urgency, however, and the surgeon can see the patient again in follow-up prior to obtaining his or her own radiologic studies. In order to facilitate this decision process, Deyo and Diehl have formulated guideline criteria for ordering plain radiographs (20). These include patient's age over 50 years, history of trauma, cancer, night pain, rest pain, weight loss, drug and alcohol abuse, steroid usage, elevated temperature, neurologic deficits, or indications of ankylosing spondylitis. Although theoretically accepted, medicolegal ramifications may preclude the strict adherence to these guidelines.

Before considering the use of any of the more advanced modes of radiologic investigation it is important to review the various studies that have revealed the incidence of abnormalities in the asymptomatic population. The report by Hirsh and Nachemson referred to earlier (40) has been the landmark study emphasizing the need to support one's provisional diagnosis with objective findings, tension signs, and, most important, a directed positive finding on myelogram. For some time the contrast myelogram, initially oil based but now with a water-soluble agent, was the "gold-standard" test by which all others were compared (Fig. 20.2). Since then, with the advent of magnetic resonance imaging and improvements in computed tomography, these less invasive and much more sophisticated studies have become more popular and more specific. Their popularity has risen because of their noninvasiveness, outpatient status, the ability through MRI to visualize the soft tissue anatomy with extreme precision, including the spinal cord, disc material, epidural contents, bony or fat infiltration with tumor or osteomyelitis, sagittal multiplane imaging, and the ability through both CT

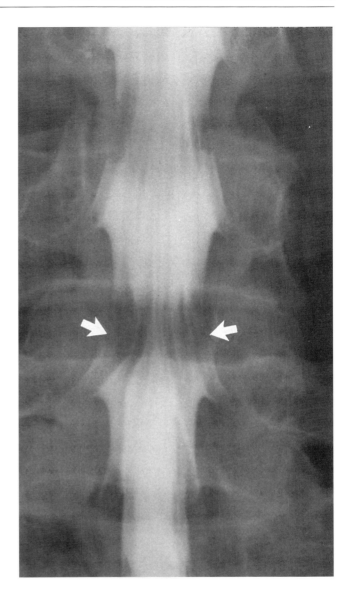

FIGURE 20.2.

Anteroposterior myelography shows decreased filling of L5 roots bilaterally (arrows). This patient had a moderately large central herniated disc.

and MRI to visualize the lateral extent of the roots, their foramina, bony confines, and possible lateral disc herniation otherwise missed on myelograms (Fig. 20.3). Despite these advantages, again, it is necessary to use these studies as confirmation of previously suspected pathology, as in all cases abnormal findings may be identified in clearly asymptomatic individuals. All three studies have significant false positive rates. In reviewing 300 patients undergoing oil-based myelograms for posterior fossa tumors, Hitselberger and Witten found a 37% rate of abnormal findings in the spine, with 24% involving disc abnormalities in the lumbar spine (43). This was later verified with computed tomography by Wiesel et al.,

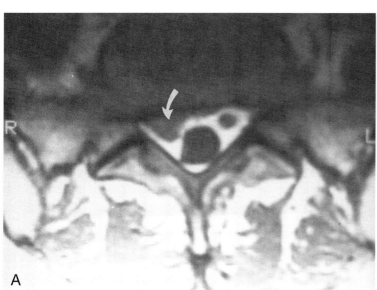
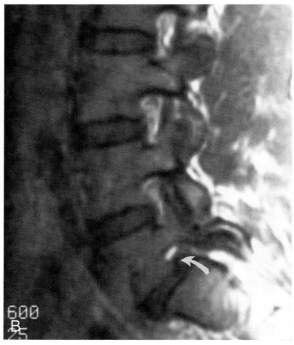

FIGURE 20.3.

A. An axial MRI showing a posterolateral L5-S1 herniated disc impinging on the S1 root (arrow). **B.** A sagittal MRI showing an L5-S1 foraminal herniated disc impinging on the L5 root (arrow).

who found a 37% incidence of disc abnormalities in 50 normal volunteers (95). More recently MRI findings were shown to be equally sensitive in the asymptomatic, with an overall 33% false positive rate, with 20% in patients under 60 years old having a disc herniation (8). Jensen et al. in 1994 also found a significant abnormality rate in asymptomatic subjects, with 38% having an abnormality at more than one level (50).

As the techniques and software continue to improve, so will the accuracy and definition of these studies. From the outset the versatility of the multiplanar CT and MRI evaluations seemed to outpace the less sophisticated myelogram. In many cases this is in fact true. Modic et al. reviewed the overall efficacy of all three studies and concluded that for disc disease and spinal stenosis the MRI was more accurate than myelograms (82.3% versus 71.4%), and virtually equivalent to CT (82.3% versus 83%) (72). Since many practitioners combine myelograms with postmyelographic CT scans to visualize the lateral recesses and bony elements, it would seem logical that the diagnostic accuracy would improve with similar combinations with MRI. In the same study Modic confirmed this theory and noted a combined increase in accuracy with MRI and CT that proved equal to the combination myelogram and CT (92.5% versus 89.4%). Given the invasive nature of myelograms and the labor-intensive multiple imaging required, it appears reasonable to suggest that the CT/MRI combination is more attractive to patients. However, with differences in imaging quality of the various MRI centers in a community, and with the extensive experience with myelograms and postmyelographic CT scans in some centers, there still may be a selective role for the latter combination, especially in the evaluation of central and lateral recess stenosis in the elderly. At present, however, the MRI has come to provide a significant advantage in the evaluation of sequestered disc herniations, soft tissues of the spine, especially at the thoracolumbar junction, tumors, and osteomyelitis (66, 71). Also, in the back-pain patient for whom treatment has failed, gadolinium-enhanced MRI images facilitate the differentiation of epidural fibrosis versus retained or recurrent disc herniation (7, 10, 25, 29). MRI or CT can be the definitive test prior to taking the patient to surgery. These imaging studies are important in defining the type and location of the herniated disc, which is paramount in the surgical patient (Fig. 20.1).

Discography at present is controversial. A discogram is performed on an awake patient by inserting a needle through the midline into the center of the disc. The disc is then injected with a known quantity of water-soluble contrast material while the patient's symptoms are being monitored. Plain radiographs of the lumbar spine are examined for extrusion of the contrast material, degeneration of the disc contents, and other abnormalities.

In centers at which large numbers of patients with back and leg pain are treated, lumbar discography is not frequently performed. The reasons for this include difficulty in performing the test, a high percentage of false positives, uncertainties about the use of the patient's response as a part of the test, and the lack of universal acceptance of the results. To many, the sophistication of modern CT and MRI studies, complemented with water-soluble contrast myelography, render the value of the discogram relatively insignificant. Though not substantiated by statistical data, it is the senior author's impression that in many instances discography is used when the examiner is looking for some type of "abnormal" test results, particularly to fit the accident-related etiology, or to give credence to a chronic pain syndrome. There seem to be few occasions on which the discogram can genuinely add to the discussion of the cause of the patient's symptoms. In a comparison of MRI and discography at 264 disc levels in 90 patients with incapacitating back and leg pain, Birney et al. found an 86% agreement between the two tests. MRI was more sensitive (100%) than discography (86%) in the detection of disc herniation. Although the discogram was more likely to show findings of "disc degeneration," the exact meaning of this abnormality was not discussed (6). The precise value of this test and its ability to elucidate the patient's complaint remain highly speculative.

Conservative Treatment of Disc Disease

Dillin in 1994 passionately outlined the troubles and frustrations of any scientist or thinker who dares to approach the conundrum of back pain and its nonsurgical treatment (24). Although it is one's hope always to rest one's clinical decisions on truths based in science, he states that at this time we can only rely on our common sense. The literature, although replete with papers on the topic, has not yet provided us with any absolute understanding of disc disease process or its treatment. The practitioner is guided only by the desire to alleviate the patient's suffering quickly and efficiently, and certainly to do no harm. However, the role of conservative versus operative treatment for disc disease, unless specifically directed toward the treatment of isolated extruded disc herniations, is fraught with potential failure. In reality, the conservative route may simply be a means of symptomatically allowing the patient to play the odds and win a war of attrition over low back pain. To become victor is to overcome the physical deconditioning, medicinal dependency, and psychological weakness of disabling pain by maximizing those activities that have some basis, at least in common sense, for providing improvement in mental and physical health.

It was the logical approach that gave us the Pennsylvania plan (Fig. 20.4) (98). Formulated through an analysis of numerous cases of back-pain patients for whom treatment had failed, it was an algorithm by which the practitioner could efficiently diagnose and treat ailments of lumbar disc disease and minimize unwarranted surgery and extraneous radiologic tests. It was a means of providing order to the decision-making process and of standardizing such treatment, and it continues to assist the practitioner in this task.

Rest and immobilization are basic tenets in the treatment of many musculoskeletal injuries. The idea of diminished pain and inflammation is always balanced with the potential loss of motion and atrophy of tissues. The very argument for bed rest and immobilization in the treatment of low back ailments and sciatica has been challenged, leaving the patient with seemingly contradictory advice. It is known that intradiscal pressures diminish with recumbency (73). Prolonged recumbency, however, has been believed to potentiate osteoporosis and other diseases of disuse (99). Deyo, Diehl, and Rosenthal have supported the idea that some rest is beneficial but that too much is not necessarily better. Their conclusion was that 2 days of bed rest rather than 7 days allowed for a higher rate of return to activities and less time away from work (21). Wiesel's study of 980 military trainees with low back pain also documented that to some degree bed rest is beneficial (96). Neither study, however, dealt with the addition of radiculopathy to the picture. With an understanding of the natural history of sciatica, the extrapolation—based on common sense—can be made. In the end it is our intuition that tells us that initially bed rest is necessary, in order to moderate the acute inflammation of back pain and sciatica, but a graduated program of increasing activity must be maintained. The use of traction devices, although advocated by some, has had no clear support in the literature and has been shown by others to have no affect on the natural course of sciatica (57, 93). Weber et al. showed no statistically significant difference with or without traction on final outcome, eventual spinal mobility, motor deficits, and the like.

The role of drug therapy in the treatment of lumbar disc disease is a necessary topic of discussion, both for the attributes of analgesic use as well as the dangers of inappropriate administration. The agents available include various nonsteroidal anti-inflammatory drugs (NSAIDs), narcotics, steroids, muscle relaxants, and anxiolytics/antidepressants. The cause of most pain production likely has to do with the irritation or inflammation of local structures damaged during the process of disc degeneration, stimulation of local sensory nerves by pressure or chemical irritants, or direct inflammation of local nerve

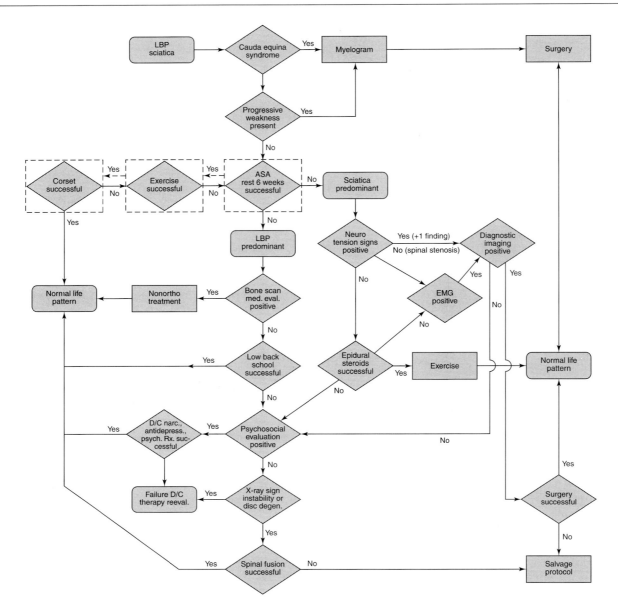

FIGURE 20.4.

Pennsylvania Plan algorithm for low back pain and leg pain. (Reprinted with permission from Rothman RH, Simeone FA. The spine. 3d ed. Vol. 1. Philadelphia: WB Saunders, 1992.)

roots, producing radiculopathy. The mainstay of the pharmacologic outpatient treatment of these factors is the use of aspirin or NSAIDs. With proper medical follow-up to minimize the detrimental side effects, the physician can take advantage of the ability of these agents to decrease prostaglandin synthesis and diminish chemotactic factors of inflammatory cells and their mediators. Contraindications to their extended use may exist, however, because of their potent effects on renal function, coagulation, and exacerbation or initiation of peptic ulcer disease.

In some instances—for example, when acute resolution of pain is needed to maintain the patient's work schedule—the anti-inflammatory effects of enteral steroids may be instituted. In fact, they are so effective that they may produce an artificial perception of improvement, which leads to disappointment when the steroids are discontinued. If steroids are administered, they must be used sparingly and only for short durations in order to prevent local and systemic complications such as Cushinoid syndrome, avascular necrosis, ulcer disease, and so on. The senior author recommends the following schedule as both safe and effective: dexamethasone, 6 mg 4 times a day on day 1, 4 mg 4 times a day on day 2, 2 mg 4 times a day on day 3, 1 mg 3 times a day on day 4, 0.75 mg twice a day on day 5, 0.5 mg twice a day on day 6, and 0.5 mg once a day on day 7. This gradual tapering may reduce the rebound that can occur with abrupt discontinuance of this medication.

The use of muscle relaxants is less than scientific, and its efficacy is speculative. Bed rest and NSAIDs remain the best way to remedy muscle spasm. Certainly in those patients who exhibit the clinical signs of depression it may be useful to attempt a trial of antidepressant medication to break the negative cycle. The clues to evaluating the symptoms in such a patient were reviewed earlier and are usually associated with those experiencing chronic symptoms. If the symptoms are severe, psychiatric evaluation should not be delayed.

Another means of nonoperative therapy is the use of epidural steroid injections. Over the years various studies have addressed the effectiveness of this form of treatment. Since it was first introduced by Evans in 1930, the general consensus in the literature is that results were favorable over the short course; however, studies have also concluded that there is no role for epidural steroid injections in lumbar radicular pain (17, 23, 26). At present, many clinicians still rely on this treatment in cases of refractory radicular pain in patients who are not clear candidates for decompressive surgery and often in patients with spinal stenosis for whom the risks of surgery are too great. The usual treatment plan is to administer a series of three injections at 1-week intervals. Several side effects are possible, including spinal headache, hypotension, and exacerbation of symptoms, so their judicious use is recommended.

Facet joint injections have for years been another commonly discussed mode of treating the low back syndrome. Although there have been studies to implicate the facet capsule as a source of pain and others have noted pain production with percutaneous distension of these joints, there have been no studies to support statistically the predictive value of their use (12, 49, 61).

The general treatment recommendations of chronic low back pain in most cases involves encouraging the patient to participate in exercise therapy. It has long been believed that people who regularly enjoy aerobic exercise develop a stronger sense of wellness and good health and often a better outlook. It also has positive effects on overall body weight and muscle conditioning. Cady et al. have been frequently cited as having shown that firefighters who have been most aerobically fit have had no recurrences in episodes of low back pain, unlike those who were considered least physically fit (11). The exact mechanism by which exercise extends a protective effect over the spine is not known. Whether due to endorphin release, weight loss, erector spinae muscle strength, or overall conditioning, the benefits are real and common sense dictates that the use of exercise in the treatment of chronic back pain is reasonable (4, 59).

Surgical Treatment of Lumbar Disc Disease

The indications for surgical excision of herniated lumbar discs, as mentioned earlier, are maximized when a specific neurologic deficit is combined with a focal radiologic study and a tension sign. The treatment for radiculopathy, with focal or advancing neurologic sequelae, unresponsive to 3 months of conservative treatment is definitive and often rewarding. The problematic patients are those who do not have advanced deficits or who appear partially or totally disabled due to pain; this is especially true if the sole complaint is back pain. There are no definite criteria that can be applied to each patient. The evaluation of these more complex individuals requires an experienced physician to assimilate and prioritize the various physical, psychological, economic, and personality factors evident in each encounter. These includes age, activity level, goals in life, degree of perceived incapacitation, employment profile, presence or absence of depression, expectation from medical or surgical treatment, and willingness to accept less-than-optimal results. Certain factors in the patient profile will not be altered despite the most precise surgical techniques—the patient's mood, conception of illness, disability, and willingness to relinquish his or her symptoms. For this reason the senior author has made an effort not to operate on patients with work-related injuries, nor on those involved in litigation, unless there is advancing neurological deficit. Poor results in this group are common, and the uncertainties involved make it difficult for the surgeon to deal properly with patients who are involved in compensation and litigation.

Surgery is considered in well-motivated patients who have responded incompletely to nonoperative therapy and who remain unable to perform activities important to them. When back pain predominates without obvious signs of instability, or when radiculopathy appears less specific and without precise abnormal radiologic findings, the patient must be willing to accept a less-than-perfect result, especially in the face of the known natural history of repeated waxing and waning of symptoms. He or she must be made aware of the risks of the surgery and weigh these against the possibility of prompt relief. If the patient is unwilling to understand these choices, too anxious to have surgery, exhibits overt signs of secondary gain, has a psychological predisposition to a low threshold for pain, or has an examination without radiologic specificity, then a longer course of conservative, nonsurgical treatment is the only wise option.

There is a more positive side to the story. The most gratifying aspect of patient care in this specialty is likely to come from patients treated surgically for herniated discs and radiculopathy. The various surgical alternatives available include standard discectomy techniques and microdiscectomy, with other treatment options such as percutaneous discectomy and chymopapain chemonucleolysis. The surgical approaches to the patient with lumbar disc disease should all require the same indications for surgery. Micro techniques are no different in their absolute indications than standard laminectomy. The percutaneous or chemonucleolysis approaches, however, have stretched these indications and usually require less severe (nonextruded or contained) disc protrusions to maximize their effectiveness. This, however, challenges the natural history of the disease and its known ability to resolve in these instances. Herein lies the controversy. The general indications for decompression of root compression via formal or microdiscectomy are in those patients with increasing neurological deficits, profound bowel or bladder dysfunction, failure of appropriate, monitored conservative treatment, or recurrent episodes of sciatica, all of which require specific physical examination findings, absolute radiologic confirmation, and preferably the presence of a tension sign, especially in the young. The outcomes of such treatment have been well documented for standard discectomy, with 90 to 95% good-to-excellent results, as well as with microdiscectomy alternatives, with 88 to 96% good-to-excellent results (35, 40, 47, 84, 85, 97). The possible added complications of using a limited exposure such as nerve root or dural injury, or the inability to fully evaluate the pathology, can be minimized through the judicious use of surgical magnification, appropriate intraoperative radiologic confirmation of level, and the maintaining of one's attention to detail and the dogged quest to find clearly observable root compromise at the operative level. If the surgeon is disappointed with the degree of pathology found intraoperatively, it is likely that the level is incorrect.

The alternatives to formal discectomy, namely, chemical ablation of the disc space (chemonucleolysis) or percutaneous disc removal, remain controversial, with several advocates and numerous more conservative skeptics. In chemonucleolysis chymopapain is injected into the disc space to degrade enzymatically the nucleus pulposus. This in turn decompresses the disc volume and secondarily reduces the pressure on the bulging or herniating material. The indications for this technique are limited. These include large herniations filling more than 50% of the sagittal canal, pedunculated disc fragments, or sequestered free fragments (69). Chemonucleolysis would be precluded by additional bony encroachment seen on CT scan or calcification of the disc fragment. Thus it would seem to the skeptic that the procedure is best indicated for small disc protrusions that often respond to conservative treatment. However, there continue to be studies in support of the efficacy of the technique, and these note success rates approaching 75% (30, 62, 91). Given the lower success rate, many contraindications, and the potential complications, including anaphylaxis, nerve injury, and discitis, standard or microdiscectomy techniques remain the treatment of choice for the herniated disc.

Percutaneous or arthroscopic techniques, too, have not approached the established success rates of the open procedures. The documented rates range from 55 to 85% (18, 36, 77). The future may bring improved techniques, with arthroscopic visualization minimizing risk and improving the root decompression. At present, however, the open techniques prevail.

Finally, the indications for fusion in the lumbar spine are limited in disc disease. Radiologic evidence of instability in the patient with back or leg pain often requires surgical fusion. Fusion is also required in cases in which the removal of facets and foraminotomies are required for adequate decompression of neural structures, resulting in an unstable motor segment, and in cases of neural arch defects associated with disc disease. The debate, however, is focused on those problem patients who exhibit disabling pain with no objective findings other than disc degeneration. Although the literature has yielded no clear findings on the validity of discography in the evaluation of possible diseased discs, there are many who rely on it to indicate patients who are candidates for fusion, and at present this usage is not clearly based in science (44, 79). Given the litigious climate of recent years as well as the abundance of disability claims and new scrutiny of lumbar surgery, fusion surgery, and instrumentation, it appears evident that a conservative approach to these individuals will best serve both the patient and the practitioner.

References

1. Adams MA, Hutton WC, Stoff JRR. The resistance to flexion of the lumbar intervertebral joint. Spine 1980;3:245–253.
2. An HS, Silveri CP, Simeone FA, et al. Cigarette smoking as a risk factor for cervical and lumbar disc disease. J Spinal Disord 1994;7:369–373.
3. Anderson G, Svenson H, Oden A. The intensity of work recovery in low back pain. Spine 1983;8:880–884.
4. Astrand, PO. Exercise physiology and its role in disease prevention and in rehabilitation. Arch Phys Med Rehabil 1987;68:305.

5. Bell G. Diagnosis of lumbar disc disease. Semin Spine Surg 1994;6(3):186–195.
6. Birney TJ, White JJ Jr, Berens D, et al. Comparison of MRI and discography in the diagnosis of lumbar degenerative disc disease. J Spinal Disord 1992; 5(4):417–423.
7. Boden SD, O'Malley S, Sunner JL, et al. Contrast enhanced MR imaging performed after successful lumbar disk surgery. Radiology 1992;182(1):59–64.
8. Boden SD, Davis DO, David DD, et al. Abnormal magnetic resonance scans of the lumbar spine in asymptomatic subjects: a prospective investigation. J Bone Joint Surg Am 1990;72:403–408.
9. Brinckmann P. Injury of the annulus fibrosus and disc protrusions. Spine 1986;11:149–153.
10. Bundschuh CV, Modic MT, Ross JS, et al. Epidural fibrosis and recurrent disc herniation in the lumbar spine: MR imaging assessment. Am J Neuroradiol 1988;9:169–178.
11. Cady LD, Bischoff DP, O'Connell ER, et al. Strength and fitness and subsequent back injuries in firefighters. J Occup Med 1979;21:269.
12. Carette S, Marcoux S, Truchon R, et al. A controlled trial of corticosteroid injections into facet joints for chronic low back pain. N Engl J Med 1991;325:1002–1007.
13. Clarke NMP, Cleak DK. Intervertebral lumbar disc prolapse in children and adolescents. J Pediatr Orthop 1983;3:202–206.
14. Coventry EC. Psychiatric aspects of chronic back pain. Semin Spine Surg 1989;1(1):35–42.
15. Coventry MB, Ghormley RK, Kernohan JW. The intervertebral disc: its microscopic anatomy and pathology. Part 1. J Bone Joint Surg Am 1945;27:105–112.
16. Coventry MB, Ghormley RK, Kernohan JW. The intervertebral disc: its microscopic anatomy and pathology. Part 2. J Bone Joint Surg Am 1945;27:233–247.
17. Cuckler JM, Bernini PA, Wiesel SW, et al. The use of epidural steroids in the treatment of lumbar radicular pain. J Bone Joint Surg 1985;67A:63–66.
18. Davis GW, Onik G, Helms C. Automated percutaneous discectomy. Spine 1991;16:359–363.
19. DePalma AF, Rothman RH. The intervertebral disc. Philadelphia: WB Saunders, 1970.
20. Deyo RA, Diehl AK. Lumbar spine films in primary care: current use and effects of selective ordering criteria. J Gen Intern Med 1986;1:20.
21. Deyo RA, Diehl AK, Rosenthal N. How many days of bed rest for acute back pain? A randomized clinical trial. N Engl J Med 1986;315:1064.
22. Deyo RA, Loeser J, Bigos S. Herniated lumbar intervertebral disc. Ann Intern Med 1990;112:598–603.
23. Dilke TWF, Burry HC, Grahame R. Extradural corticosteroid injection in the management of lumbar nerve root compression. BMJ 1973;2:635.
24. Dillin W. Acute back pain and sciatica: conservative treatment. Semin Spine Surg 1994;6(3):196–215.
25. Dina TS, Boden SD, Davis DO. Lumbar spine after surgery for herniated disc: imaging findings in the early post-operative period. Am J Roentgenol 1995; 164(3):665–671.
26. Evans W. Intrasacral epidural injection in the treatment of sciatica. Lancet 1930;2:1225.
27. Farfan H, Cossette J, Robertson G. The effects of torsion on the lumbar intervertebral joint. J Bone Joint Surg 1970;52:468–497.
28. Fishgrund JS, Montgomery DM. Diagnosis and treatment of discogenic low back pain. Orthop Rev 1993 (March):311–318.
29. Fitt GJ, Stevens JM. Postoperative arachnoiditis diagnosed by high resolution fast spin-echo MRI of lumbar spine. Neuroradiology 1995;37(2):139–145.
30. Fraser RD. Chymopapain for the treatment of intervertebral disc herniation: the final report of a double-blind study. Spine 1984;9:815–818.
31. Frymoyer JW, Cats-Baril WL. An overview of the incidence and costs of low back pain. Orthop Clin North Am 1991;22(2):263–271.
32. Frymoyer JW, Pope MH, Clements JH, et al. Risk Factors in low back pain. J Bone Joint Surg 1983;65A:213–218.
33. Frymoyer JW, Pope MH, Costanza MC, et al. Epidemiologic studies of low back pain. Spine 1980; 5:419–423.
34. Garfin SR, Glover M, Booth RE, et al. Laminectomy: review of the Pennsylvania Hospital experience. J Spinal Disord 1988;1:116.
35. Goald HJ. Microlumbar discectomy: follow-up of 477 patients. J Microsurg 1980;2:95–100.
36. Goldstein TB, Mink JH, Dawson EG. Early experience with automated percutaneous lumbar discectomy in the treatment of lumbar disc herniation. Clin Orthop 1989;238:77–82.
37. Graham JR. The MMPI: A practical guide. New York: Oxford University Press, 1977.
38. Hakelius A. Prognosis in sciatica: a clinical follow-up of surgical and non-surgical treatment. Acta Orthop Scand 1970;129(Suppl):1.
39. Hirsh C. An attempt to diagnose the level of disc lesion clinically by disc puncture. Acta Orthop Scand 1948;18:132–140.
40. Hirsh C, Nachemson A. The reliability of lumbar disc surgery. Clin Orthop 1963;29:189–195.
41. Hirsh C, Ingelmark BE, Miller M. The anatomical basis for low back pain. Acta Orthop Scand 1963;33:1–17.
42. Hirsh LF. Diabetic polyradiculopathy simulating lumbar disc disease: report of four cases. J Neurosurg 1984;60:183–186.
43. Hitselberger W, Witten R. Abnormal myelograms in asymptomatic patients. J Neurosurg 1968;28:204.
44. Holt EP. The question of lumbar discography. J Bone Joint Surg 1968;50A:720.
45. Hoppenfeld S. Orthopedic neurology. Philadelphia: Lippincott, 1977.
46. Horal J. The clinical appearance of low back disorders in the city of Gothenburg, Sweden. Acta Orthop Scand Suppl 18, 1969.
47. Hudgins WR. The role of microdiscectomy. Orthop Clin North Am 1983;14:589–603.
48. Hult L. Cervical, dorsal, and lumbar spinal syndromes. Acta Orthop Scand 1954;24:174–175.
49. Jackson R, Montesano P, Jacobs R. Facet joint injections in mechanical low back pain patients. Proceed-

ings of International Society for Study of the Lumbar Spine. Orthop Trans 1986;10:509.
50. Jensen MC, Brant-Zawadzki MN, Obuchowski N, et al. Magnetic resonance imaging of the lumbar spine in people without back pain. New Engl J Med 1994; 331(2):69–73.
51. Kelsey JL, Hardy RJ. Driving of motor vehicles as a risk factor for acute herniated lumbar intervertebral disc. Am J Epidemiol 1975;102:63–73.
52. Kirkaldy-Willis W, Wedge J, Young-Hing K. Pathology and pathogenesis of lumbar spondylosis and stenosis. Spine 1978;3:319–328.
53. Kraemer J, Kolditz D, Gowin R. Water and electrolyte content of human intervertebral discs under variable load. Spine 1985;10:69–71.
54. Kulak RF, Belytschko TB, Schulta AB, et al. Non-linear behavior of the human intervertebral disc under axial load. J Biomech 1976;9:377.
55. Kurz LT. The pathogenesis and natural history of lumbar disc disease: disc degeneration and herniation. Semin Spine Surg 1994;6:170–179.
56. Kuslich, SD, Ulstrom CL, Michael CJ. The tissue origin of low back pain and sciatica: a report of pain response to tissue stimulation during operations on the lumbar spine using local anesthesia. Orthop Clin North Am 1991;22(2):181–187.
57. Larsson V, Choler V, Lidstrom A, et al. Autotraction for treatment of lumbago-sciatica. Acta Orthop Scand 1980;51:791–798.
58. Lawrence JS. Disc degeneration: its frequency and relationship to symptoms. Ann Rheum Dis 1969; 28:121–138.
59. Lewis IW, Cannon JT, Liebeskind JC. Opioid and nonopioid mechanisms of stress analgesia. Science 1980; 208:623.
60. Liang M, Komaroff AL. Roentgenograms in primary care patients with acute low back pain: a cost effective analysis. Arch Intern Med 1982;142:1108.
61. Lora J, Long D. So-called facet denervation in the management of intractable back pain. Spine 1976;1:121.
62. Lorenz M, McCulloch JA. Chemonucleolysis for herniated nucleus pulposus in adolescents. J Bone Joint Surg 1985;67A:1402–1404.
63. MacNab I. The traction spur: an indicator of segmental instability. J Bone Joint Surg Am 1971;57:663.
64. Macrae IF, Wright V. Measurement of back movement. Ann Rheum Dis 1969;28:584.
65. Marchand F, Ahmed A. Investigation of the laminate structure of lumbar disc annulus fibrosus. Spine 1990; 15:402–410.
66. Masaryk TJ, Ross JS, Modic MT, et al. High resolution MR imaging of sequestered lumbar intervertebral disks. Am J Neuroradiol 1988;9:351–358.
67. Mazanec DJ. Differential diagnosis of low back pain and sciatica. Semin Spine Surg 1994;6(3):180–185.
68. McCarron RF, Wimpee MW, Hudkins PG, et al. The inflammatory effect of nucleus pulposus. Spine 1987;12:760–764.
69. McCulloch JA. Microsurgery and chemonucleolysis. Semin Spine Surg 1994;6(4):243–255.
70. Mixter WJ, Barr JS. Rupture of the intervertebral disc with involvement of the spinal canal. N Engl J Med 1934;211:210.
71. Modic MT, Feiglin DH, Piraino DW, et al. Vertebral osteomyelitis: assessment using MRI. Radiology 1985;157:157.
72. Modic MT, Masaryk TJ, Boumphrey F, et al. Lumbar herniated disc and canal stenosis: prospective evaluation by surface coil MR, CT, and myelography. Am J Neuroradiol 1986;7:709.
73. Nachemson AL. The load on lumbar disks in different positions of the body. Clin Orthop 1966;45:107–122.
74. Nachemson AL. The lumbar spine: an orthopaedic challenge. Spine 1976;1:59–67.
75. Nachemson AL, Elfstrom G. Intravital dynamic pressure measurements in lumbar discs: a study of common movements, maneuvers, and exercises. Scand J Rehabil Med 1970;2(Suppl 1):1.
76. Ohshima H, Tsuji H, Hirano N. Water diffusion pathway, swelling pressure, and biomechanical properties of the intervertebral discs during compression load. Spine 1989;14:1234–1244.
77. Onik G, Mooney V, Maroon JC, et al. Automated percutaneous discectomy: a prospective multi-institutional study. Neurosurgery 1990;26:228–233.
78. Ostgaard HC, Andersson GBJ, Karlson K. Prevalence of low back pain during pregnancy. Spine 1991; 16:549–552.
79. Osti OL, Fraser RD. MRI and discography of annular tears and the intervertebral disc degeneration: a prospective clinical comparison. J Bone Joint Surg 1992; 74B:431–435.
80. Roberts S, Menage J, Urban J. Biochemical and structural properties of the cartilage end-plate and its relation to the intervertebral disc. Spine 1989;14:166–173.
81. Scham SM, Taylor TK. Tension signs in lumbar disc prolapse. Clin Orthop 1971;75:195.
82. Shealy, CN. The role of the spinal facets in back and sciatic pain. Headache 1974;14:101.
83. Simpson JM, Silveri CP, Balderston RA, et al. The results of operations on the lumbar spine in patients who have diabetes mellitus. J Bone Joint Surg 1993; 75A:1823–1829.
84. Spangfort EV. The lumbar disc herniation: a computer aided analysis of 2, 504 operations. Acta Orthop Scand 1972;142(Suppl):61.
85. Spengler DM, Freeman CW. Patient selection for lumbar discectomy: an objective approach. Spine 1978; 4:129–134.
86. Svensson HO, Andersson GBJ. Low back pain in 40–47 year old men: frequency of occurrence and impact on medical services. Scand J Rehabil Med 1982;14:47.
87. Tsuji H, Hirano N, Ohshima H, et al. Structural variation of the anterior and posterior annulus fibrosus in the development of human lumbar intervertebral discs: a risk factor for intervertebral disc rupture. Spine 1993;18:204–210.
88. Waddell G. Spine pain and disability determination. In: Frymoyer JW, ed. The adult spine: Principles and practice. New York: Raven, 1991.
89. Waddell G, Kummel EG, McCulloch JA, et al. Failed

lumbar disc surgery and repeat surgery following industrial injuries. J Bone Joint Surg 1979;61A:201–207.
90. Waddell G, McCulloch JA, Kummel E, et al. Nonorganic physical signs in low back pain. Spine 1980; 5:117–125.
91. Watters WS, Mirkovic S, Boss J. Treatment of the isolated lumbar intervertebral disc herniation: microdiscectomy vs. chemonucleolysis. Spine 1988; 13:360–362.
92. Weber H. Lumbar disc herniation: a controlled, prospective study with ten years of observation. Spine 1983;8:131–140.
93. Weber H, Ljungren A, Walker L. Traction therapy in patients with herniated lumbar intervertebral discs. J Oslo City Hosp 1984;34:61–70.
94. Weinstein J. Neurogenic and nonneurogenic pain and inflammatory mediators. Orthop Clin North Am 1991; 22(2):235–246.
95. Wiesel SW, Bell GR, Feffer HL, et al. A study of computer assisted tomography. Part I. The incidence of positive CAT scans in an asymptomatic group of patients. Spine 1984;9:549.
96. Wiesel SW, Cuckler JM, Deluca F. Acute low back pain: objective analysis of conservative therapy. Spine 1980;5:324–330.
97. Williams RW. Microlumbar discectomy. Spine 1978; 3:175–182.
98. Wisneski RJ, Rothman RH. The Pennsylvania Plan II: An algorithm for the management of lumbar degenerative disease. Instr Course Lect (AAOS) 1985:17–36.
99. Wisneski RJ, Garfin SR, Rothman, RH. Lumbar disc disease. In: Rothman RH, Simeone FA, eds. The spine. 3d ed. Philadelphia: WB Saunders, 1992:671–746.
100. Wyke B. The neurology of low back pain. In Jayson MIV, ed. The lumbar spine and back pain. 2d ed. Tunbridge Wells, England: Pitman, 1980:265–339.
101. Yoshizawa H, O'Brien JP, Smith WT, et al. The neuropathology of intervertebral discs removed for low back pain. J Pathol 80;132:95–104.

CHAPTER TWENTY ONE

Spinal Stenosis

Howard S. An and Thomas G. Andreshak

Introduction

The onset of back and radicular pain in the elderly population signals the development of degeneration of the intervertebral disc and the underlying pathophysiology of spinal stenosis. The complex array of symptoms and signs differs between individuals and may vary temporally in an individual patient. The narrowing of the spinal canal that occurs in stenosis may be asymptomatic but generally presents as varying degrees of lower extremity weakness, pain, dysesthesias, and dysreflexias. New research is focusing on compression of the cauda equina and nerve roots. The structural relationship between the neural elements and the discs, facets, hypertrophic ligaments, and bony abnormalities is better understood.

Mixter and Barr confirmed in 1934 that disc degeneration may be the primary factor for sciatica symptoms in patients with spinal stenosis (84). Subsequently, in 1954, Verbiest introduced the concept of lumbar spinal stenosis with a narrowed spinal canal compressing the neural elements (127). Verbiest and, independently, Kirkaldy-Willis, contributed immensely to the understanding of spinal stenosis and the underlying pathophysiologic concepts (63–66, 128, 129).

The spinal canal can become narrowed or undergo stenosis in several locations, including the central spinal canal, the lateral recess, and the intervertebral foramen. The degree and location of the stenosis produce the various clinical presentations, from single root radiculopathy to multilevel symptoms.

Spinal stenosis may be divided into two groups: congenital and acquired stenosis (Table 21.1). Congenital stenosis occurs in achondroplastic dwarfs and in those with an idiopathic narrowed canal (29, 100–102, 138). The congenital stenosis in achondroplasia will not be addressed here; in this chapter the degenerative changes associated with idiopathic or developmental narrowing will be discussed.

Acquired stenosis develops from many conditions and may be secondary to degenerative stenosis, iatrogenic causes, trauma, defects of the pars interarticularis, and various other causes (3, 13, 27, 28, 30, 51, 61, 102, 132).

Pathophysiology

The phenomenon of pain in spinal stenosis is easy to understand as it is related to instability of the spinal motion segments, nerve root compression, and degeneration of the intervertebral discs and facets. Questions are raised, though, as to why not all patients with spinal stenosis are symptomatic, or why individual variation exists in clinical presentation. Spinal stenosis is part of the aging process, and the changes it brings are found in a majority of the asymptomatic population.

The posterior ramus and the sinuvertebral nerves of the spine have been implicated as the source of pain in spinal stenosis (26, 57, 117, 119). Inflammation of these nerves is plausible as a cause of pain, but it has been difficult to study the process, and thus

TABLE 21.1.
Classification of Spinal Stenosis

I. Congenital-developmental stenosis
   a. Idiopathic (hereditary)
   b. Achondroplastic
II. Acquired stenosis
   a. Degenerative
   b. Combined congenital and degenerative stenosis
   c. Spondylolytic/spondylolisthetic
   d. Iatrogenic (e.g., postlaminectomy, postfusion)
   e. Posttraumatic
   f. Metabolic (e.g., Paget's disease, fluorosis)

their involvement may not be significant. Venous stasis has been postulated as a cause of pain in spinal stenosis. Arnoldi et al. demonstrated vertebral venous hypertension in patients with spinal stenosis (3). This theory is questioned for many reasons. The lumbar spine has a large anastomotic plexus, and the veins are valveless, so stasis should not be significant. Pain is relieved by postural changes and can occur rapidly. This should not occur in stasis, where relief would be expected to arrive slowly and not simply through flexion in the erect position. Rapid venous decompression by postural changes should not occur.

Compression of the cauda equina has been demonstrated to be a direct cause of symptomatic spinal stenosis. Schonstrom and associates used cadaveric spines and circumferential bands to narrow the cauda equina (114–116). A minimal cross-sectional area of 77 ± 13 mm^2 at L3 was needed for the neural elements in the dural sac. A further decrease in cross-section would result in an increase in pressure along the nerves. The midlumbar spine required a narrowing to 50% of the normal area to increase pressure significantly and presumably to a point at which symptoms would occur. Rydevik and associates confirmed this 50% value by demonstrating alterations in nerve root and capillary function with pressures above 50 mm Hg (92, 93, 95, 112). Because of the variability in the size of the lumbar spinal canal, in the size of the nerve roots, and in the induced pressures with variations of cross-sectional area, this may explain the diverse presentation of signs and symptoms in individuals and the population. Rydevik and associates demonstrated that mechanical compression of spinal nerve roots leads to neurologic changes in circulation, conduction, and transport (21, 92, 94, 95, 109–112). Delamarter and colleagues confirmed earlier studies by finding that with a 50% or greater constriction of the cross-sectional area, motor and sensory deficits were observed (23).

Studies of the vascular supply of the cauda equina and peripheral nerve roots give a more plausible explanation of symptoms in spinal stenosis. A region of hypovascularity occurs at the area of intersection of the central and radicular blood systems within the cauda equina and spinal nerve roots (98, 99). The dorsal root ganglion has an extensive vascular network and increased vascular permeability, which indicates an increased metabolic function (4, 96, 99). Clinical symptoms may result from the vascular and nutritional deficiencies that occur because of compression, fibrosis, edema, ischemia, inflammation, and reduced metabolism. Although the exact pathoetiology is not fully known, the degenerative processes in the spine result in the mechanical and physiologic changes, compression, ischemia, altered metabolism, and neural inflammation that characterize the pain and neural symptoms of spinal stenosis.

Pathoanatomy

Intervertebral Disc

The main determinant of the onset of spinal stenosis and the cascade of related symptoms is disc degeneration (64, 66, 67, 69). Kirkaldy-Willis and associates promoted the three-joint complex concept (63, 64, 66, 67). The disc acts as one of the joints, and the facets comprise the posterior joints of the tripod configuration. A change in one of the joints leads to abnormal stresses in the other joint complexes, and with the disc as the primary dysfunctional unit the arthritic process of the facets is accelerated and promotes further disc degeneration. Videman et al. have shown that in 20% of degenerative spines, facet degeneration precedes disc degeneration (130).

The intervertebral disc degenerates with increasing age, and disc degeneration can be observed radiologically with increasing frequency as a population ages (62). Many of the changes of the aging and degenerating disc may not be pathologic and remain asymptomatic without any definite signs (18, 49). Disc degeneration is characterized by a bulging annulus fibrosus, which narrows the central anterior spinal canal and may be associated with a frank herniation. Bony osteophytes, ligament buckling, and facet hypertrophy may slowly progress and cause the stenosis. The normal spinal canal has an anteroposterior diameter of 12 mm or more and a cross-sectional area of 77 ± 13 mm^2 (115, 116). The shape of the spinal canal may have a significant role in the etiology of stenosis and in symptomatic patients with relatively early degeneration of the disc. The spinal canal may be round, ovoid, or trefoil-shaped. The round canal is most favorable, whereas the trefoil canal leaves the lumbar roots prone to compression in the lateral recess (31, 32, 104, 105, 136); the development of symptoms is not a certainty with a trefoil canal, however (71).

As the intervertebral disc ages, the annulus fibrosus becomes more distinct and the gelatinous nucleus pulposus is less differentiated from the annulus (18, 41, 49, 126). Circumferential tearing is the first stage in the degenerative cycle, as shown by Kirkaldy-Willis and associates (64). The circumferential tears combine and expand, with subsequent radial tears evident. The disc and hence the intervertebral space collapses because of biochemical and mechanical changes in the disc. Dehydration of the disc occurs with a concomitant breakdown and loss of collagen and proteoglycans. Collapse and fissuring occur and lead to posterior bulging of the disc along the posterior longitudinal ligament. These changes occur in the more mobile spinal segments of L5-S1 and L4–5 initially and then progress cephalad.

Nachemson classified intervertebral disc degeneration into four grades on the basis of the progressive loss of the nucleus, indistinct nucleus-annular border, fissuring of the annulus, and marginal formation of osteophytes (87). Miller et al. found in a collection of autopsy specimens that L5-S1, L4–5, and L3–4 were typically the most degenerative discs and that 97% demonstrated degeneration by 50 years of age. The first appearance of degeneration was in the third decade in females and in the second in males (82). The fibrous border of the nucleus coalesces with the annular fibers, and after the second decade this border becomes indistinct, with subsequent desiccation, cellular degeneration, cavitation, and calcium deposition (19, 25). Fibrocartilage replaces the nuclear material. The mechanical properties of the annulus become altered. The collagen fibrils of the annulus provide tensile strength, whereas those of the nucleus are generally loosely organized and subsequently increase in diameter and density with age (15). The proteoglycans of the nucleus provide the compressive resistance of the disc and allow variation in hydration.

Water comprises about 80% of the intervertebral disc. The annulus fibrosus is made up of about 78% water and the nucleus about 85%. The percentage falls to around 70% with degeneration (37, 45, 54, 89, 90). Urban and McMullin demonstrated that proteoglycan and water content decrease with age, vary with spinal level, and are greater in the nucleus pulposus (125). This hydration is dependent on the ratio of collagen to proteoglycan rather than age.

The proteoglycans of the disc, especially the nucleus, are composed of glycosaminoglycans of keratan sulfate and chondroitin sulfate attached to a protein core. They are able to aggregate with hyaluronic acid and to link proteins. In aging and degeneration, the proteoglycan content decreases, aggregation decreases, and the ratio of keratan sulfate to chondroitin sulfate increases (1, 45, 54, 77, 83, 89, 125). Changes in the proteoglycan components of the disc are a result primarily of proteolysis, and this is believed to play a role in the degeneration of the intervertebral disc. Disc degeneration is a remodeling process in response to mechanical alterations and not a simple deteriorating process.

Facets

Degeneration of the lumbar disc places the facet joints at risk for deterioration as a result of the increased mechanical stresses (5, 73, 76). The joints collapse concomitantly with the disc height, leading to overriding of the articular surfaces (139). The neuroforamen is narrowed in cross-sectional area and impinges on the spinal nerve root as it exits (86). With the collapse of the disc and overriding of the facets, posterior subluxation or retrolisthesis of the superior vertebral body occurs, which may entrap the nerve root in the foramen between the hypertrophic facets, vertebral osteophytes, pedicle, and bulging annulus. The osteophytes may trap and impale the nerve root and increase the stenosis (70). The bony configuration of the pedicles in the lower lumbar spine may explain the frequent symptoms of the lower lumbar nerve roots. The pedicles in the upper lumbar spine are concave on the inferior surface and tend to be smaller in diameter than those of the lower lumbar spine, which are larger and transversely oriented (120). The pedicle thereby takes up more space in the degenerative narrowed neuroforamen. The caudal migration of the pedicle with disc degeneration may trap the nerve root between the pedicle superiorly and the bulging disc and osteophytes inferiorly. The vertebral body and facets limit the neuroforamen anteriorly and posteriorly, respectively, so any change or degeneration in one of the components will compromise the space available for the nerve root. Facet arthritis occurs as in other synovial joints and generally is bilateral.

Facet degeneration may lag behind disc degeneration, and posterior subluxations may occur, or degeneration may be concurrent, and the gradual realignment of the facets occurs with anterior subluxation of the superior vertebral body (34, 35, 38, 58, 106). The iliolumbar ligaments attach to the L5 body and transverse processes and are believed to act as a checkrein, allowing more motion at the L4–5 level and the subsequent increase in subluxation that is observed at that segment (72). The stenosis increases statically and dynamically with the increase in disc degeneration, facet degeneration, subluxations, and generalized disc and ligamentum flavum bulging. Traction osteophytes have been linked to and identified as a sign of this instability of the lumbar spine (79).

Zones of Stenosis

An understanding of the pathologic anatomy of spinal stenosis is important in relating the findings of the history and physical examination to areas of neural impingement, interpreting imaging studies, and planning surgical approaches. Spinal stenosis can be divided into central stenosis and lateral stenosis.

Central stenosis is found at the intervertebral level and is caused by hypertrophic facets, ligamentum flavum buckling or hypertrophy, disc protrusion, and degenerative spondylolisthesis. Forty percent cases of central stenosis are secondary to soft tissue changes (8). The cauda equina is compressed centrally from the anterior-posterior direction at the intervertebral disc level. The discs bulge posteriorly, and the hypertrophied ligamentum flavum and facet joints intrude posteriorly. Multilevel stenosis is common. Imaging studies such as magnetic resonance imaging (MRI) or myelography can vividly demonstrate the pathoanatomy of central stenosis. Intrathecal contrast from the surrounding bone and soft tissue created by T2-weighted images in MRI or with injectable contrast medium in myelography demonstrate where the cerebrospinal fluid (CSF) around the roots of the cauda equina is obliterated. In computed tomography (CT), midsagittal lumbar canal diameters of less than 10 mm are indicative of absolute stenosis, and diameters of less than 13 mm are indicative of relative stenosis (129). Midsagittal lumbar canal diameters are not as reliable as the cross-sectional dimensions at the level of the intervertebral disc, as most cases of degenerative spinal stenosis involve the facet joints and disc space. The lumbar epidural fat is usually obliterated in central spinal stenosis, although a small amount of fat may be preserved in the midline posterior to the dural sac, even in severe stenosis. In lumbar symptomatology, neurogenic claudication is usually the result of central canal stenosis.

Lateral stenosis is a common cause of lumbar radicular symptoms. The lateral lumbar spinal canal includes the nerve root canal (lateral recess) and the intervertebral foramen. Together they form a tubular canal through which the nerve root exits the spinal canal. Lee et al. have divided the lateral lumbar spinal canal into three anatomic zones: entrance zone, midzone and exit zone (Fig. 21.1) (71). The entrance zone is the subarticular area medial to the pedicle and is synonymous with the lateral recess area; the midzone is located under the pars interarticularis and the pedicle; and the exit zone is synonymous with the intervertebral foramen.

The entrance zone is located underneath the superior articular process of the facet joint and medial to the pedicle. The entrance zone is the cephalad aspect of the more commonly known lateral recess, which begins at the lateral aspect of the thecal sac and runs obliquely downward and laterally toward the intervertebral foramen. The lateral recess is bordered laterally by the pedicle, posteriorly by the su-

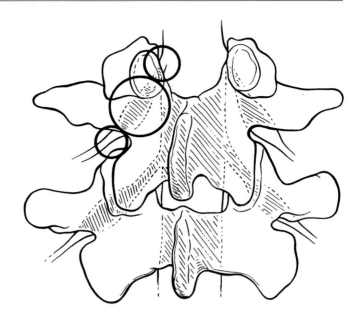

FIGURE 21.1.

A diagram of three zones of the lateral spinal canal: entrance zone proximally, mid-zone under the pars interarticularis, and the exit zone of the intervertebral foramen.

perior articular facet, and anteriorly by the posterolateral surface of the vertebral body and adjacent intervertebral disc. The medial border of the lateral recess is formed by the thecal sac. The narrowest portion of the lateral recess is between the superior border of the pedicle and the broad portion of the superior articular facet. The nerve root in this region is covered by the root sleeve and surrounded by cerebrospinal fluid. The lateral margin of the nerve root sleeve contacts the medial cortical bone of the pedicle, and the medial margin of the nerve root is surrounded by epidural fat tissue. The normal lateral recess measurements have been well delineated by CT. A lateral recess height of 5 mm or more is normal. A height of 2 mm or less is pathologic and a height of 3–4 mm is suggestive of lateral recess stenosis (17). Narrowing of the entrance zone or lateral recess with nerve root compression is most commonly caused by a posterolaterally herniated disc, which compresses the nerve root as it emerges from the dural sac. Another common cause of nerve root compression is a hypertrophic superior articular process, also known as lateral recess syndrome, superior facet syndrome, or nerve root canal stenosis (Fig. 21.2). These two causes account for the majority of cases of lateral spinal stenosis.

The midzone is located under the pars interarticularis and just below the pedicle. It is bounded anteriorly by the posterior aspect of the vertebral body and posteriorly by the pars interarticularis. The medial boundary is open to the central spinal canal. The nerve roots normally run obliquely downward through the lateral recess into the intervertebral foramen. The nerve root travels around the subpedicular notch and comes into contact posteriorly with the ventral wall of the pars interarticularis, where the ligamentum flavum is attached. CT provides accurate information on the pars interarticularis and shows the adjacent nerve root under the pars. In midzone stenosis a defect in the pars interarticularis is most commonly responsible for nerve root compression. For instance, in isthmic spondylolisthesis the L5 nerve root may be entrapped by the fibrocartilaginous tissue at the L5 pars defect. Another common cause of midzone stenosis is pedicular kinking. As the nerve root exits just inferomedial to the pedicle, kinking of the nerve root by the pedicle may be responsible for radiculopathy. This phenomenon is more common in patients with scoliosis or spondylolisthesis, in which one pedicle may be lower than the other because of rotatory deformity of the vertebral body or asymmetric collapse of the disc space.

The exit zone is formed by the intervertebral foramen. The lumbar intervertebral foramen, which is shaped like an inverted teardrop, forms a tunnel that connects with the spinal canal. It is bounded superiorly and inferiorly by the pedicles of the adjacent vertebrae. The posterior boundary is formed by the pars interarticularis and the ligamentum flavum. The anterior boundary is formed by the posteroinferior margin of the superior vertebral body, the posterior margin of the intervertebral disc, and the posterosuperior margin of the inferior vertebral body. The normal foraminal height varies from 20 to 23 mm, and the width at the upper foraminal area varies from 8 to 10 mm (49, 51). The ventral and dorsal nerve roots occupy 23 to 30% of the area of the foramen and lie anterior to the dorsal root ganglion (DRG). The DRG lies within the superior lateral portion of the lumbar

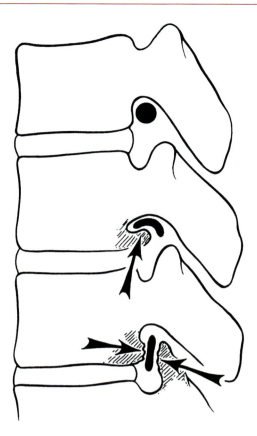

FIGURE 21.3.
A diagram of intervertebral foraminal stenosis by osteophytes (midlevel) and a subluxating facet joint (lowest level) in the exit zone.

intervertebral foramen and directly below the pedicle in 90% of lumbar levels (51). Foraminal height of less than 15 mm and posterior disc height of less than 4 mm are associated with nerve root compression 80% of the time (49).

In exit zone or foraminal stenosis the nerve root can be impinged in an up/down or front/back fashion (Fig. 21.3). This can occur secondary to subluxation of the superior articular facet, a laterally herniated disc or protruding annulus fibrosus, or an uncinate spur from the posterolateral vertebral body. The nerve root may also be compressed at more than one site.

Clinical Presentation

History

Clinical presentation of spinal stenosis may mimic other degenerative processes. Common disorders in the differential diagnosis include peripheral neuropathy, vascular disease, and lumbar disc disease. Peripheral vascular disease is most commonly misdiagnosed because of neurogenic claudication symptoms.

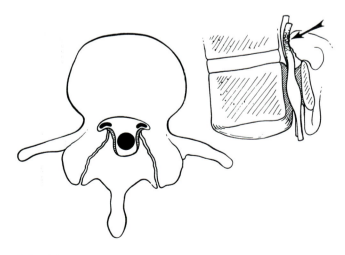

FIGURE 21.2.
A diagram of entrance zone stenosis, showing subarticular entrapment of the nerve root.

Degenerative spinal stenosis, the most common form, usually presents with an onset in patients whose age is in mid-50s to early 60s. Females present with greater frequency than males and include those with degenerative spondylolisthesis as well (16, 40, 46, 47, 122). The usual presenting symptom is not back pain but leg pain. The leg pain may be true sciatica, with complaints in one extremity along a dermatomal distribution. Sensory, motor, and reflex changes may occur with the fifth lumbar root, the most commonly involved. Symptoms of neurogenic claudication are most commonly described at initial presentation. The pain classically radiates to the buttocks and thighs and progressively radiates below the knees to the feet. Symptoms increase with activity. The symptoms are described classically as pain, burning, numbness, tingling, cramping, and weakness in both lower extremities, but it may occur in only one (36, 66). Extension of the spine, such as in walking and standing, exacerbates symptoms, whereas flexion, in leaning forward or lying down, relieves symptoms (74).

Vascular claudication must be distinguished from the neurogenic claudication symptoms of spinal stenosis (Table 21.2). The pain from peripheral vascular disease starts distally with cramping and pain in the calves and progresses proximally; relief is obtained by standing still. The distance walked before onset of pain is fixed, whereas it is variable in spinal stenosis. Pulses may be absent and skin changes may be noted in vascular disease. Peripheral neuropathy is differentiated by a history of diabetes, hypersensitivity in the feet with proximal extension, night pain with no relation to activity, stocking-glove distribution of sensory changes, and weakness with posterior column involvement. Bladder dysfunction occurs in only 3 to 4% of cases.

TABLE 21.2.
Comparison of Vascular with Neurogenic Claudication

	Vascular	**Neurogenic**
Claudication distance	Fixed	Variable
Relief after stop walking	Immediate	Not immediate
Relief of pain	Standing	Flexion or sitting
Walk uphill	Pain	No pain
Bicycle ride	Pain	No pain
Type of pain	Cramp and tightness	Numbness, ache, sharp
Location and radiation	Distal to proximal	Proximal to distal
Pulses	Absent	Present
Bruit	Present	Absent
Skin	Loss of hair, shiny	Normal
Atrophy	Rare	Occasional
Weakness	Rare	Occasional
Back pain	Uncommon	Common
Limitation of extension	Uncommon	Common

Back pain is common in stenosis but is not the underlying cause for seeking medical attention. The back pain of spinal stenosis is insidious in onset, arthritic in quality, and mechanical in nature, occurring with activity. Radiation to the buttock is characteristic and, the pain is "tight" and burning in quality. The pain is aggravated with extension of the spine and relieved by flexion. Patients note relief with pillows under the knees in bed, leaning on a walker, counter, or shopping cart, and propping a leg up while standing. The pain is increased in those with degenerative spondylolisthesis (9).

Physical Examination

Spinal stenosis is not usually confirmed by any definitive signs or findings in the physical examination, which may be confusing when attempting to formulate the actual diagnosis or to understand the basis of presenting complaints.

The gait may show a forward flexed posture with limited pelvis rotation. A shorter stride is sometimes noted. Palpation of the lower back usually does not reveal any tenderness. There is rarely any spasm, as seen in disc herniations. Point tenderness over the sacroiliac joints or the sciatic notch may be noted. Range of motion shows good forward flexion but limited and painful extension. Brieg has shown through studies with cadavers that extension results in a shortened spinal canal, a broadening of nervous tissue, a shortening and broadening of the ligamentum flavum, posterior disc protrusion, and interference of the microcirculation of the cauda equina and nerve roots (12).

The results of the neurologic examination in the patient with spinal stenosis may be normal (78). The L4–5 level is most commonly involved, so any sensorimotor changes are likely to be in this distribution. Motor strength testing is usually unremarkable and may show mild weakness in the extensor hallucis longus muscle or the tibialis anterior muscle. Atrophy and weakness are more common in long-standing disease but may be seen more frequently in lateral recess stenosis. Again, the fifth lumbar root is most often involved. Exercise, walking, or stair climbing may induce the symptoms. The straight-leg-raising test is often negative in cases of stenosis, unlike in patients with disc herniation. Reflex testing is unreliable.

The relative absence of physical findings requires that the diagnosis of spinal stenosis be confirmed by radiologic imaging studies, which help to clarify the confusing picture of the patients symptoms.

Radiologic Findings

Plain x-ray film examination of patients with spinal stenosis will reveal many findings consistent with spinal column degeneration, including disc space narrowing, facet arthrosis, degenerative scoliosis or spondylolisthesis, spondylosis, and spinous process settling. These may occur in many combinations (20, 59, 66, 74, 123). An abnormality is not necessarily the cause of the patient's complaints (42, 137). The examination should include anteroposterior and lateral views, and flexion-extension lateral views may be considered in patients with segmental spinal instability. Verbiest divided the midsagittal canal diameter measurement into three groups: *(a)* 10 mm or less, pure absolute stenosis; *(b)* 10–12 mm, pure relative stenosis; and *(c)* mixed stenosis (127). Degenerative spondylolisthesis occurs more commonly in females than males, at a ratio of 4:1, and is six to nine times more common at the L4–5 interspace. Forward displacement is usually less than 30% and usually occurs in the fifth to sixth decade (106). A loss of lumbar lordosis is noted, with an increase in the lumbosacral angle. The increased stress thus placed at the L4–5 level and the stabilizing effect of the iliolumbar ligaments predispose the L4–5 level to slippage (16). The degree of slippage is not correlated degree of symptoms.

Instability is usually seen radiographically in flexion-extension radiographs (Fig. 21.4). The horizontal displacement or angular motion between two segments or destruction of anterior or posterior structures is believed to represent instability or the loss of the spine's ability to maintain vertebral relationships (103, 133).

Imaging studies that allow the cross-sectional area of the spinal canal to be measured or evaluated represent the current technique in confirming the diagnosis of spinal stenosis. CT and MRI scans are best for identifying the location and degree of canal stenosis. As mentioned earlier, the shape of the canal has been implicated in the pathology of spinal stenosis; the shape may be circular, oval or trefoil in configuration (24). Approximately 15% of lumbar spinal canals are trefoil in shape (108). The lateral recesses are more likely to be narrowed in the trefoil canal, resulting in stenosis of the nerve root (33). CT scanning has been used in identifying central and lateral recess stenosis (Fig. 21.5). Absolute stenosis is defined by a lateral recess diameter of 3 mm or less and relative stenosis of 3–5 mm (17). Bolender and colleagues used CT and myelography to measure the dural sac and concluded that absolute stenosis occurred when cross-sectional area was 100 mm² or less (8).

Myelography is believed to have a high specificity and sensitivity in identifying spinal canal stenosis. Bell and associates found that myelography was superior to CT scanning in confirming spinal stenosis (6). The myelographic appearance of spinal stenosis is an "hourglass" constriction at one or more levels

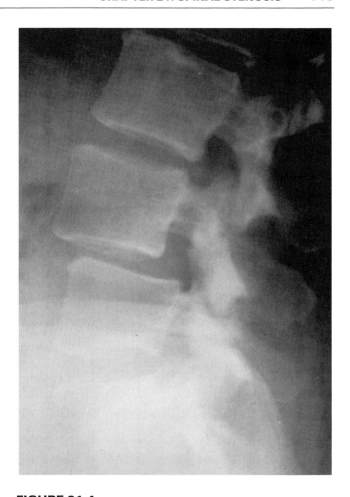

FIGURE 21.4.

Instability is usually seen radiographically in flexion-extension radiographs. A horizontal displacement of more than 4 mm is indicative of instability.

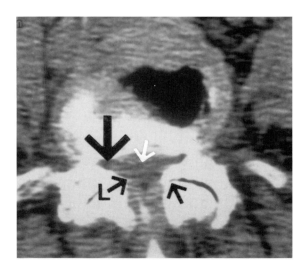

FIGURE 21.5.

Axial CT scan of central lumbar spinal stenosis, showing facet hypertrophy (black arrow), ligamentum flavum (black arrow with L), and bulging disc (white arrow). The lateral recess is narrowed bilaterally (large black arrow).

(81, 91, 121, 124). Myelography allows the patient to be scanned in extension and possibly in hyperextension to reproduce the pathology. False-positive results are common, however, as reported by Hitselberger in 24% of asymptomatic patients (55). False-positive CT results were also fairly significant in an asymptomatic group of patients tested by Wiesel and associates (134). Individuals over the age of 40 years had an incidence of 50% (diagnosis of herniated nucleus pulposus and stenosis), and the overall incidence was 35.4%. Combining CT scanning and myelography has not been shown to be statistically better than either study alone, but they are complementary in the surgical evaluation (Fig. 21.6) (131). The shape of the lumbar intervertebral foramen is not well demonstrated by transaxial CT scans. Sagittal reconstruction images may help to identify the bony abnormalities of the intervertebral foramen (Fig. 21.7).

Magnetic resonance imaging has rapidly become a valuable tool in the study of the spine. MRI does not use radiation, it produces images in sagittal, axial, and coronal planes, and it allows variation in technique to define and differentiate neural tissue and water content. Modic and colleagues evaluated the relative accuracies of imaging techniques in spinal stenosis and found that MRI was comparable to CT and myelography and that the accuracy of MRI and CT combined was 92.5% (85). CT and MR imaging of the lateral recess and spinal canal has been well defined by An and colleagues and helps to differentiate the causes of nondiscogenic lumbar radiculopathy (2, 50). Bowden and colleagues reported false-positive scans in asymptomatic volunteers (11). In those over 60 years of age 21% were found to have stenosis, and in all groups 30% of MRI scans showed signs of abnormalities. As with all of the imaging studies, in the older patient population there is a higher incidence of false-positive results, so correlation of the clinical examination with the diagnostic studies is important.

T1-weighted MRI scanning provides the best images of the spinal anatomy. The cortical bone that outlines the vertebral body has a negligible signal intensity, and the fatty marrow in the cancellous bone produces a higher signal intensity on T1-weighted images. However, cortical margins seen in MRI are less distinct than in CT. In T1-weighted images the intervertebral disc produces a low signal intensity with darker outer annular fibers, which merge with the posterior longitudinal ligaments. Parasagittal images show nerve roots as low-signal-intensity structures within the high-intensity signal of fat in the intervertebral foramen. T2-weighted images demonstrate the fibrocartilage in the nucleus pulposus and inner annulus fibrosus with high signal intensity and the outer, primarily collagenous, annulus with low signal intensity. Changes in the signal intensities of the fibrocartilage reflect changes in the proteoglycans concentrations in the intervertebral disc. With the advent of gradient echo imaging or fast spin-echo techniques, the use of T2-weighted spin-echo studies has decreased.

Central canal stenosis by ligamentum flavum hypertrophy and facet disease is also well demonstrated in MRI (Figs. 21.8 and 21.9). MRI shows disc bulging, which compromises the spinal canal anteriorly, and hypertrophy of the facets and ligamentum flavum,

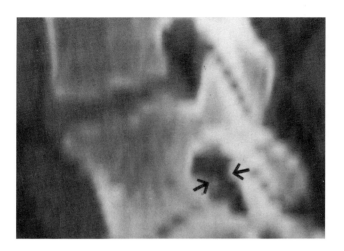

FIGURE 21.7.

A sagittal reconstructed CT scan of the intervertebral foramen, showing osteophytes narrowing the space available for the nerve root.

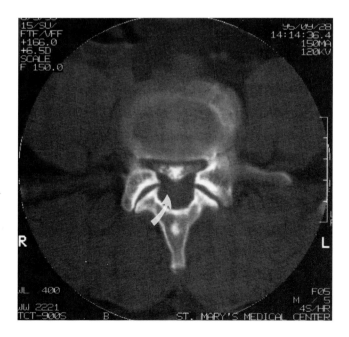

FIGURE 21.6.

Postmyelography CT scan showing central stenosis with significant ligamentum flavum hypertrophy (arrow).

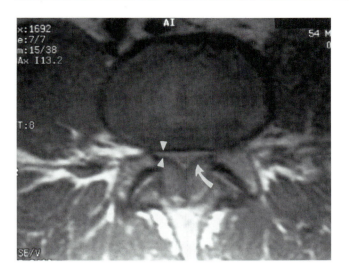

FIGURE 21.8.
Axial T1-weighted MRI showing severe central stenosis with hypertrophic ligamentum flavum (arrow) and narrow lateral recess (arrowheads).

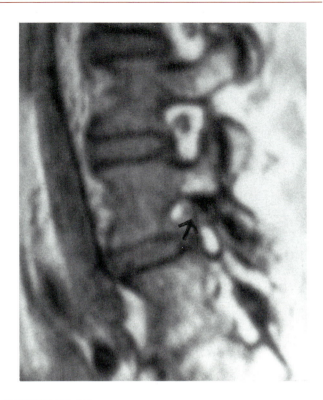

FIGURE 21.10.
Parasagittal T1-weighted MRI showing decreased fat and protruding disc in the intervertebral foramen of L4–5 (arrow).

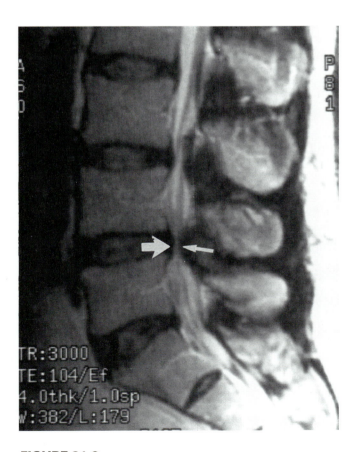

FIGURE 21.9.
Sagittal T2-weighted MRI of central stenosis, showing compression of the thecal sac by bulging disc (large arrow) and hypertrophy of the ligamentum flavum (small arrow).

which indents the spinal subarachnoid space posteriorly. The sagittal T1-weighted images may show the epidural fat in the spinal canal posterior to the dural sac even in severe stenosis. T2-weighted axial images demonstrate narrowing of the cross-sectional area of the spinal canal and a decrease or absence of subarachnoid CSF signal at the stenotic levels. Lateral recess stenosis by the hypertrophy of the superior facets is also demonstrated by MRI, although CT is better for lateral recess measurement. Intervertebral foraminal stenosis is best visualized in parasagittal scans, which show the nerve root compressed or deformed by a laterally herniated disc or facet subluxation with ligamentum flavum impingement on the nerve root (Fig. 21.10). A useful indication of significant foraminal stenosis is the absence of the well-defined perineural fat signal on the parasagittal T1-weighted images. Axial images may also show the narrowing of the intervertebral foramen or foraminal disc herniation (Fig. 21.11).

Treatment

Nonoperative Treatment

Spinal stenosis is a slow, progressive disease, and in the early stages the intermittent symptoms of neural

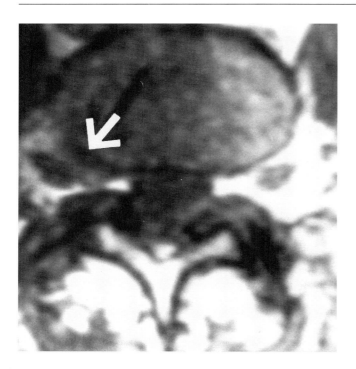

FIGURE 21.11.
Axial T1-weighted MRI showing disc and osteophyte protruding in the foramen, obliterating the fat anterior to the nerve root (arrow).

tissue inflammation can be relieved through nonsurgical treatments (7). The stenosis does not resolve, however, and many who are symptomatic will eventually require surgical intervention. The initial guidance a patient should receive is instruction on modifying activities and staying in shape physically and aerobically. Bed rest should be avoided because of its detrimental effects on the musculoskeletal system and on general health. Modification of activities entails avoiding those that involve bending, twisting, lifting as well as unnecessary walking that induces the symptoms. This limitation usually eases pain and results in some satisfaction. Physical therapy plays a role at this stage as well in stretching and isometrically strengthening muscles that have atrophied from disuse. Modalities such as heat, ultrasound, whirlpool, and massage all may help to alleviate the exacerbations of stenosis and the general degeneration of the spinal column. Aerobic conditioning helps to maintain cardiovascular fitness in this somewhat sedentary population. Endogenous endorphin release from aerobic conditioning exercise also helps to ease pain and to avoid the sedation and depressive effects of narcotics.

Narcotic medication and most muscle relaxants should be avoided in the elderly population, as they promote depression and sedation.

The elderly, with increasing medical problems, pain, decreased function, diminishing support groups, and insomnia, are frequently depressed and exhibit signs of clinical depression. The use of low doses of antidepressant medications can relieve some of the neurogenic pain, allow a more restorative sleep cycle and subsequent daytime activity, and help to reduce some of the depressive symptoms.

Anti-inflammatory medications may be used to reduce the inflammation associated with neural compression and degeneration of the discs and facet joints. This may allow increased activity and more effective rehabilitation. Careful monitoring of the gastrointestinal, hepatic, and renal systems is imperative over the long term, as risks of diminished function and damage may occur insidiously. Epidural steroids or oral steroid "dose paks" may relieve some of the pain and inflammation and allow aerobic conditioning and increased function. Although this is temporary and not a cure for the stenosis, it may provide some indication of the severity of nerve compression and inflammation by its effects on the patient's symptoms.

Operative Treatment

Patients with increasing symptoms should be aware that usually their condition will not progress to paralysis or bowel and bladder dysfunction, and that if activities are curtailed symptoms are generally relieved. The issue becomes one of quality of life and the level of function and activity desired. Many of the symptomatic patients unwilling to limit their activities may become candidates for surgical decompression. Nonsurgical treatment rarely provides long-term relief.

Spinal stenosis surgery can be very demanding and complex for the surgeon because of the various pathoanatomic variations involved. Meticulous technique and a comprehensive understanding of spinal anatomy and the pathophysiology of stenosis are critical to achieving nerve decompression and subsequent good results (16, 43, 44, 66, 97, 118).

The technique of spinal stenosis surgery starts with proper positioning of the patient. The most common position is the kneeling position with the abdomen hanging free. This position reduces intraabdominal pressure and decompresses the epidural venous plexus, which allows better visualization of the neural structures and minimizes postoperative hematoma and perineural scarring. This position allows a variation of the posture of the lumbar spine, and with relative hyperextension the anatomic structures closely mimic the patient's symptomatic posture of ambulation. This allows an adequate decompression to be performed and complete relief of pain should be expected when the patient is ambulatory and erect (10).

A standard posterior midline incision is made

through the skin at the appropriate levels determined by preoperative imaging studies and careful clinical examination (Fig. 21.12). Intraoperative x-ray films may be taken for localization of levels. Attention to careful subperiosteal dissection is required to maintain a relatively blood-free field, and electrocautery is used to release the muscle attachments. Self-retaining retractors provide compression on the muscular vessels to minimize continuous oozing into the operative field. Infiltration of the layers with an epinephrine solution may limit bleeding intraoperatively.

The levels involved, the nerves to be decompressed, and the location of the pedicles—the landmark of the course of the nerve roots—should be well identified. Attention to preoperative x-ray films and imaging studies is crucial if transitional vertebrae are present so that the correct levels are addressed. Dissection centrally may then be performed using curettes, rongeurs, and Kerrison or Lexcel punches. Removal of the lamina and surrounding ligamentum flava allows adequate central stenosis decompression in most instances (Fig. 21.13). The dissection starts centrally from the caudal lamina and proceeds ceph-

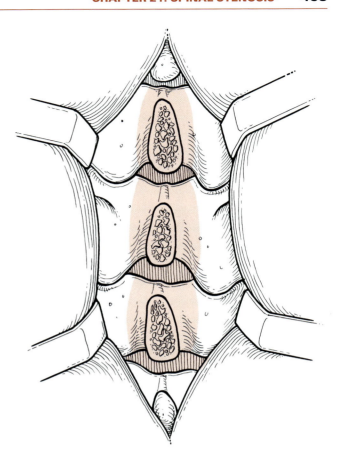

FIGURE 21.13.

Removal of the lamina and surrounding ligamenta flava allows adequate central stenosis decompression.

alad (Fig. 21.14). Cottonoid patties may be placed to displace the dural sac and release adhesions. Angled elevators are used to release adherent ligamentum and dura. The Kerrison rongeur should be seated well under the bone and ligament, and direct dorsal pressure should be directed away from neural elements. This will minimize dural tears or cutting invaginations of the dural sac (Fig. 21.15). Meticulous attention to obtaining hemostasis should be of primary concern to afford adequate constant visualization of neural elements and facilitate surgery. A bipolar cautery device diminishes the heat and current transfer to neural elements and may minimize the occurrence of perineural scarring.

Dissection proceeds caudal to cephalad and then proceeds laterally and caudally, addressing the appropriate nerve roots (Figs. 21.16 and 21.17). The subarticular recess or lateral recess is the area in need of decompression in the majority of patients. Hypertrophy of the superior facet, bulging of the annulus fibrosus, lateral herniations, and slippage of the vertebra all lead to nerve root impingement laterally (80). The anatomic structure to assist in the process is the pedicle. The nerve root exits inferomedial to the pedicle, anterior to the facet complex, and with

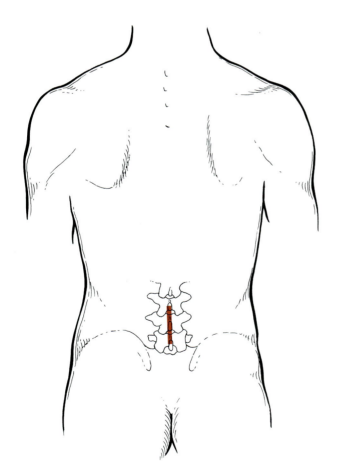

FIGURE 21.12.

A standard posterior midline incision is made through the skin at the appropriate levels.

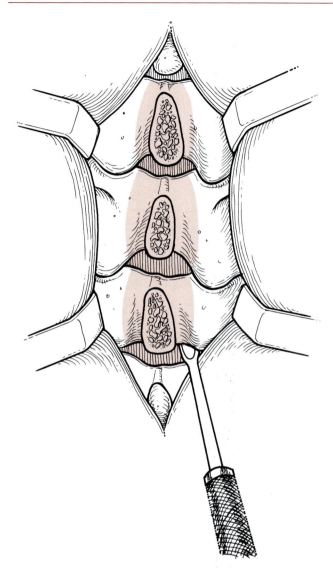

FIGURE 21.14.

The dissection starts centrally from the caudal lamina and proceeds cephalad. An angled curette is used to separate the ligamentum flavum from the inferior aspect of the lamina, and a Kerrison rongeur is used to proceed with laminectomy.

aggressive. Less than 50% of each facet should be violated if needed to preserve stability (Fig. 21.19). The nerve root should be checked for mobility; at the level of the disc space the dural sac should move medially 1 cm. This dissection will eliminate the symptoms in the majority of patients. A concurrent herniated disc and foraminal or extraforaminal compression should also be ruled out if a nerve root is not believed to be completely free. The accuracy of decompression is vital to good results, and experience with good operative judgment must be obtained. The dictum to "think nerve," as coined by Tile and associates, remains the best guideline (44, 122).

In cases of foraminal entrapment the nerve remains tethered and does not mobilize well (Fig. 21.20). An angled elevator or hook may help to differentiate whether the offending tissue is bone, disc, or soft tissue. The facet joint may need to be removed to decompress the nerve from entrapment between the superior facet of the vertebra below and the pos-

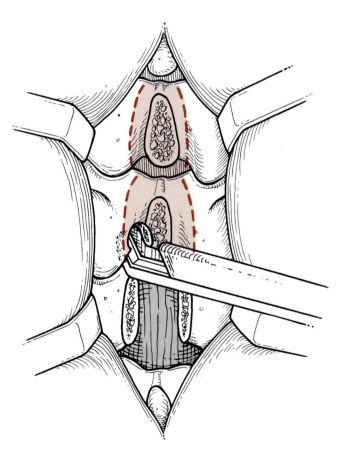

FIGURE 21.15.

The Kerrison rongeur must be used cautiously to avoid dural tears. Cottonoid patties may be placed to displace the dural sac and release adhesions. Angled elevators are used to release adherent ligamenta and dura. The Kerrison rongeur should be seated well under the bone and ligament, and direct dorsal pressure should be directed away from neural elements.

the annulus as the anterior wall. Pedicle "kinking" of the nerve root may occur and be responsible for the compression. Partial or complete excision of the pedicle may be necessary. The medial facets and entrance to the foramen is undercut using a 45° Kerrison punch (Fig. 21.18). The lateral border of the nerve root is identified and protected during all aspects of dissection in the lateral recess. This undercutting is best performed from the opposite side of the operative field. Instruments should be as close to parallel as possible to the nerve root to minimize cutting or grabbing the nerve root. Blind placement into the foramen to undercut is not to be tolerated. Decompression should be piecemeal in its progress and not too necessary in any decompressive laminectomy for degenerative spondylolisthesis (14, 16, 22, 39, 48, 52, 53, 60, 88). Wiltse and associates identified two factors that they believed contributed to a postoperative slip: *(a)* disc height greater than 6 mm preoperatively, and *(b)* the extent of facet excision (75). Further review by Wiltse and White led to criteria for fusion in spinal stenosis surgery: *(a)* age less than 60 years with degenerative spondylolisthesis and aggressive facet excision; *(b)* age less than 55 years with degenerative spondylolisthesis; and *(c)* age less than 50 years with isthmic spondylolisthesis (133a). Herkowitz and Kurz reported a prospective study of 50 patients in which they found that 96% had excellent to good results with fusion, compared to 44% with decompression alone (53).

After reviewing the literature, Garfin and colleagues have identified trends that may be used as predictors of postoperative instability: *(a)* a larger preoperative slip; *(b)* decompression across a normal disc space height; *(c)* greater than 50% excision of each facet at a single level; *(d)* increased number of decompressed levels; *(e)* penetration of a disc space at a decompressed level; and *(f)* female sex (44).

Preoperative indicators of stabilizing factors in-

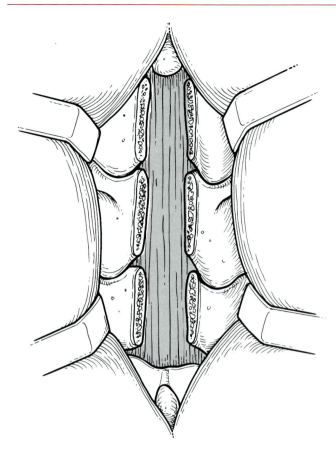

FIGURE 21.16.
Laminectomy decompresses the central canal stenosis.

terolateral aspect of the vertebral body or pedicle above. The nerve root may be impinged by a lateral disc bulge or herniation and the pedicle. This is treated by lateral disc excision and possibly pedicular excision. The nerve is frequently seen exiting the canal in a perpendicular direction rather than the usual oblique course (107).

In degenerative spondylolisthesis and scoliosis other mechanisms of nerve entrapment are recognized. Wiltse described impingement of the L5 root between the ala of the sacrum and the transverse process of L5 (135). This impingement, termed a "far-out syndrome," occurs mainly in degenerative scoliosis and in isthmic spondylolisthesis. Degenerative spondylolisthesis entraps the L5 nerve root between the vertebral body of L5 and the inferior facet of L4 that has eroded through the superior facet of the subjacent vertebra.

Inadequate nerve root decompression is usually the cause of failed spinal surgery for stenosis. A systematic approach to each of the nerve roots and levels of involvement will minimize poor results if adequate decompression is performed. An excessive decompression may lead to instability and iatrogenic or progressive spondylolisthesis and the need for surgical fusion. Many authors believe that a fusion is

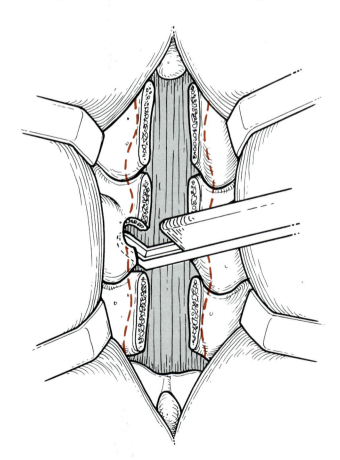

FIGURE 21.17.
The subarticular recess or lateral recess decompression is done using the Kerrison rongeur.

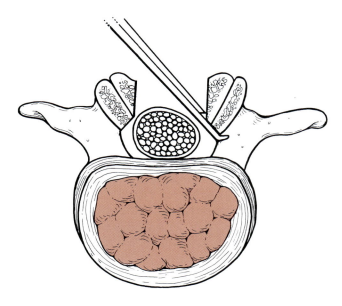

FIGURE 21.18.
The medial facets and entrance to the foramen is undercut using a 45° Kerrison punch. The lateral border of the nerve root is identified and protected during all aspects of dissection in the lateral recess. This undercutting is best performed from the opposite side of the operative field. Instruments should be as close to parallel as possible to the nerve root to minimize cutting or grabbing the nerve root.

clude significant osteophytes, calcified annulus fibrosus, capsule, and ligamentum flavum, and a high intercristal line, whereas instability may be heralded by traction spurs and asymmetrically narrowed discs (56).

In patients with degenerative scoliosis, fusion may be indicated for multilevel decompression or when multiplanar instability is demonstrated with lateral olisthesis. San Martino reported on patients with lumbar scoliosis who did not undergo fusion after surgical decompression and had good to excellent results in 1 to 4 years' follow-up (113). Longer follow-up studies are needed.

The technique of spinal fusion should not be undertaken lightly, as pseudarthrosis may lead to pain and subsequent symptoms of instability if spinal integrity was compromised through decompression. Dissection to the tips of the transverse processes is performed and the appropriate facet joints are meticulously cleaned of cartilage. All soft tissue is cleaned along the transverse process, lateral aspect of the superior facets, pars interarticularis, lamina, and ala, and the bone is decorticated to bleeding bone. Morselized cancellous bone is packed into this lateral gutter, ensuring bone contact on the transverse process and ala (68).

Various spinal implants may be used to augment the fusion and provide initial stability after an exten-

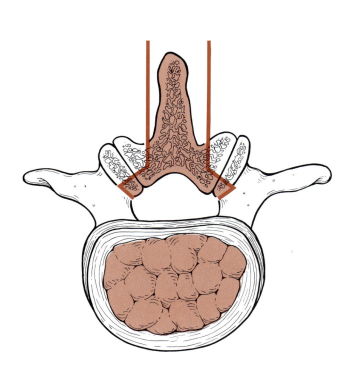

FIGURE 21.19.
Decompression should undercut the superior facet such that less than 50% of each facet is violated to preserve stability.

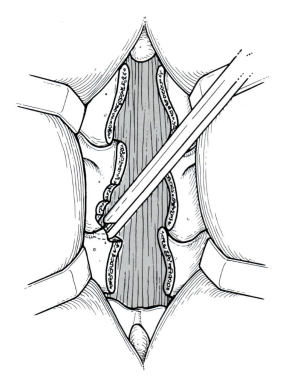

FIGURE 21.20.
Foraminal decompression is performed if the nerve root remains tight or compressed in the foramen.

sive decompression. Operative reduction of olisthesis with newer modular instrumentation is now possible, particularly when pedicular systems are used. These pedicular systems have implant rigidity, allow short segment fusions to preserve motion segments, and allow the maintenance of lumbar lordosis. The importance of the fusion should not be overlooked with the use of instrumentation, and meticulous technique is crucial to obtaining a solid fusion.

References

1. Adams P, Muir H. Qualitative changes with age of proteoglycans of human lumbar disc. Ann Rheum Dis 1976;35:289–295.
2. An HS, Haughton V. Nondiscogenic lumbar radiculopathy: imaging considerations. Semin Ultrasound CT MR 1993;14:414–424.
3. Arnoldi CC, Brodsky A, et al. Lumbar spinal stenosis and nerve root entrapment syndromes: definition and classification. Clin Orthop 1976;115:4–5.
4. Arvidson B. Distribution of intravenously injected protein tracers in peripheral ganglia of adult mice. Exp Neurol 1979;63:388–410.
5. Badgley CE. The articular facets in relationship to low back pain and sciatic radiation. J Bone Joint Surg 1941;23A:481–496.
6. Bell G, et al. A study of computer assisted tomography: comparison of metrizamide myelography and computed tomography in the diagnosis of herniated lumbar disc and spinal stenosis. Spine 1984;9:552–556.
7. Bell G, Rothman R. The conservative treatment of sciatica. Spine 1984;9:54.
8. Bolender N, Schonstrom N, Spengler D. Role of computed tomography and myelography in central spinal stenosis. J Bone Joint Surg 1985;67A:240–246.
9. Bolestra M, Bohlman H. Degenerative spondylolisthesis. Instr Course Lect 1989;10:157–169.
10. Booth RE. Spinal stenosis. Instr Course Lect (AAOS) 1986;35:420–435.
11. Bowden S, Davis D, et al. Abnormal MRI scans of the lumbar spine in asymptomatic subjects. J Bone Joint Surg 1990;72A:403–409.
12. Brieg A. Biomechanics of the central nervous system. Stockholm: Almquist & Wiksell, 1960.
13. Brodsky AE. Post-laminectomy and post-fusion stenosis of the lumbar spine. Clin Orthop 1976;115:130.
14. Brown M, Lockwood S. Degenerative spondylolisthesis. Instr Course Lect 1983;28:162–169.
15. Buckwalter JA. The fine structure of human intervertebral disc. In: White AA III, Gordon SL, eds. Symposium on idiopathic low back pain. St. Louis: Mosby, 1982:108–143.
16. Cauchoix J, Benoist M, Chassaing V. Degenerative spondylolisthesis. Clin Orthop 1976;115:122–129.
17. Ciric I, et al. The lateral recess syndrome. J Neurosurg 1980;53:433–443.
18. Coventry MB, Ghormley R, Kernohan J. The intervertebral disc: its microscopic anatomy and pathology. Part III. Pathologic changes in the intervertebral disc. J Bone Joint Surg 1945;27A:460–474.
19. Coventry MB, Ghormley R, Kernohan J. The intervertebral disc: its microscopic anatomy and pathology. Part II. Changes in the intervertebral disc concomitant with age. J Bone Joint Surg 1945;27A:233–247.
20. Crock HV. Isolated lumbar disc resorption as a cause of nerve root canal stenosis. Clin Orthop 1976;115:109.
21. Dahlin L, Rydevik B, et al. Changes in fast axonal transport during experimental nerve compression at low pressures. Exp Neurol 1984;84:29–36.
22. Dall B, Rowe D. Degenerative spondylolisthesis: its surgical management. Spine 1985;10:668–672.
23. Delamarter R, Bohlman H, et al. Experimental lumbar spinal stenosis: analysis of the cortical evoked potentials, microvasculature, and histopathology. J Bone Joint Surg 1990;72A:110–120.
24. Dommisse G. Morphological aspects of the lumbar spine and lumbosacral region. Orthop Clin North Am 1975;6:163–175.
25. Eckert C, Decker A. Pathologic studies of intervertebral discs. J Bone Joint Surg 1947;29A:447–454.
26. Edgar M, Ghadially J. Innervation of the lumbar spine. Clin Orthop 1976;11:35.
27. Ehni G. Significance of the small lumbar spinal canal: cauda equina compression syndromes due to spondylosis. Part 1. Introduction. J Neurosurg 1969;31:490–494.
28. Ehni G. Significance of the small lumbar spinal canal: cauda equina compression syndromes due to spondylosis. Part 4. Acute compression artificially induced during operation. J Neurosurg 1969;31:507–512.
29. Eisenstein S. Measurements of the lumbar spinal canal in two racial groups. Clin Orthop 1976;115:42.
30. Eisenstein S. The morphometry and pathologic anatomy of the lumbar spine in South African Negroes and Caucasoids with specific reference to spinal stenosis. J Bone Joint Surg 1977;59B:173–180.
31. Eisenstein SM. The trefoil configuration of the lumbar vertebral canal. J Bone Joint Surg 1980;62B:73–77.
32. Eisenstein S. Lumbar vertebral canal morphometry for computerized tomography in spinal stenosis. Spine 1983;8:187–191.
33. Epstein J, et al. Sciatica caused by nerve root entrapment in the lateral recess. J Neurosurg 1972;36:584–589.
34. Epstein J, et al. Degenerative spondylolisthesis. J Neurosurg 1976;44:139.
35. Epstein NE, Epstein J, et al. Degenerative spondylolisthesis with an intact neural arch: a review of 60 cases with an analysis of clinical findings and the development of surgical management. Neurosurgery 1983;13:555–561.
36. Evans J. Neurogenic intermittent claudication. BMJ 1964;2:985–987.
37. Eyring EJ. The biochemistry and physiology of intervertebral disk. Clin Orthop 1969;67:16–28.
38. Farfan HF. The pathological anatomy of degenerative spondylolisthesis in a cadaver study. Spine 1980;5:412.

39. Feffer H, Wiesel S, et al. Degenerative spondylolisthesis: to fuse or not to fuse. Spine 1985;10:287–289.
40. Fitzgerald J, Newman P. Degenerative spondylolisthesis. J Bone Joint Surg 1976;58B:184.
41. Friberg S, Hirsch C. Anatomical and clinical studies on lumbar disc degeneration. Acta Orthop Scand 1949;19:222–242.
42. Frymoyer J, et al. Spine radiography in patients with low back pain. J Bone Joint Surg 1984;66A:1048–1055.
43. Garfin S, Glover M, et al. Laminectomy: a review of the Pennsylvania Hospital experience. J Spinal Disord 1988;1:116–133.
44. Garfin S, Herkowitz H, et al. Nonoperative and operative treatment. In: Rothman RH, Simeone FA, eds. The spine. 3d ed. Vol 1. Philadelphia: WB Saunders, 1992:869.
45. Gower W, Pedrini V. Age-related variations in protein-polysaccharides from human nucleus pulposus, annulus fibrosus, and costal cartilage. J Bone Joint Surg 1969;51A:1154–1162.
46. Grabias S. Current concepts review: the treatment of spinal stenosis. J Bone Joint Surg 1980;62A:308–313.
47. Hall S, Bartleson J, et al. Lumbar spinal stenosis: clinical features, diagnostic procedures, and results of surgical treatment in 68 patients. Ann Intern Med 1985;103:271–275.
48. Hanley EN. Decompression and distraction-derotation arthrodesis for degenerative spondylolisthesis. Spine 1986;11:269.
49. Hasegawa T, An HS, Haughton VM, et al. Lumbar foraminal stenosis: critical heights of the intervertebral discs and foramina. J Bone Joint Surg 1995;77A:32–38.
50. Hasegawa T, An HS, Haughton V. Imaging anatomy of the lateral lumbar spinal canal. Semin Ultrasound CT MR 1993;14:403–413.
51. Hasegawa T, Mikawa Y, Watanabe R, et al. Morphometric analysis of the lumbosacral nerve roots and dorsal root ganglia by magnetic resonance imaging. Spine 1996;21:1005–1009.
52. Herkowitz H, Garfin S. Decompressive surgery for spinal stenosis. Semin Spine Surg 1989;1:163–167.
53. Herkowitz H, Kurz L. Degenerative spondylolisthesis with spinal stenosis: prospective study comparing decompression versus decompression and intertransverse process fusion. J Bone Joint Surg 1991;73A:802–808.
54. Hirsch C, Paulson S, et al. Biophysical and physiological investigations on cartilage and other mesenchymal tissues. Acta Orthop Scand 1952;22:175–181.
55. Hitselberger W, Witten R. Abnormal myelograms in asymptomatic patients. J Neurosurg 1968;28:204–206.
56. Hopp E, Tsou P. Postdecompression lumbar instability. Clin Orthop 1988;227:143–151.
57. Inman VT, Saunders JB. Referred pain from skeletal structures. J Nerv Ment Dis 1944;99:660–667.
58. Johnson KE, Willner S, Johnsson K. Postoperative instability after decompression for lumbar spinal stenosis. Spine 1986;11:107–110.
59. Jones RA, et al. The narrow lumbar canal: a clinical and radiological review. J Bone Joint Surg 1968;50B:595–605.
60. Kaneda K, Kasamma H, et al. Follow-up study of medial facetectomies and posterolateral fusion with instrumentation in unstable degenerative spondylolisthesis. Clin Orthop 1986;203:159–167.
61. Karpman RJ, et al. Lumbar spinal stenosis in a patient with diffuse idiopathic skeletal hypertrophy syndrome. Spine 1982;7:598–603.
62. Kellgren JH, Lawrence JS. Osteoarthrosis and disc degeneration in an urban population. Ann Rheum Dis 1958;17:388–397.
63. Kirkaldy-Willis WH, et al. Lumbar spinal nerve entrapment. Clin Orthop 1982;169:171–178.
64. Kirkaldy-Willis WH, Wedge JH, et al. Pathology and pathogenesis of lumbar spondylosis and stenosis. Spine 1978;3:319.
65. Kirkaldy-Willis WH, Farfan HF. Instability of the lumbar spine. Clin Orthop 1982;165:110.
66. Kirkaldy-Willis WH, Paine KW, et al. Lumbar spinal stenosis. Clin Orthop 1974;99:30–50.
67. Kirkaldy-Willis WH. The relationship of structural pathology to the nerve root. Spine 1984;9:49.
68. Knapp D, Jones E. Use of cortical cancellous allograft and posterior spinal fusion. Clin Orthop 1988;229:99–105.
69. Knuttsen S. The instability associated with disc degeneration in the lumbar spine. Acta Radiol 1944;25:593.
70. Lancourt J, Glenn W, Wiltse L. Multiplanar computerized tomography in the normal spine and in the diagnosis of spinal stenosis. Spine 1979;4:379–390.
71. Lee CK, Rauschning W, Glenn W. Lateral lumbar spinal canal stenosis: classification, pathologic anatomy, and surgical decompression. Spine 1980;13:313–320.
72. Leong JC, Luk K, et al. The biomechanical functions of the iliolumbar ligament in maintaining stability of the lumbosacral junction. Spine 1987;12:669–674.
73. Lewin T. Osteoarthritis in lumbar synovial joints: a morphologic study. Acta Orthop Scand 1964;73 (Suppl):31.
74. Lipson S. Clinical diagnosis of spinal stenosis. Semin Spine Surg 1989;1:143–144.
75. Lombardi J, Wiltse L, et al. Treatment of degenerative spondylolisthesis. Spine 1985;10:821–827.
76. Lorenz M, Patawardhan A, VanDerby R. Load-bearing characteristics of lumbar facets in normal and surgically altered spinal segments. Spine 1983;8:122–130.
77. Lyons H, Jones E, et al. Changes in the protein-polysaccharide fractions of nucleus pulposus from human intervertebral disc with age and disc herniation. J Lab Clin Med 1966;68:930–939.
78. MacNab I. Spondylolisthesis with an intact neural arch: the so-called pseudospondylolisthesis. J Bone Joint Surg 1950;32B:325.
79. MacNab I. The traction spur: an indication of segmental instability. J Bone Joint Surg 1971;53A:663.
80. MacNab I. The pathogenesis of spinal stenosis. Spine: State of the Art Reviews 1987;1:369–382.
81. McIvor GW, Kirkaldy-Willis WH. Pathologic and myelographic changes in major types of spinal stenosis. Clin Orthop 1976;115:72–76.
82. Miller J, Schmatz C, Schultz AB. Lumbar disc degen-

eration: correlation with age, sex, and spine level in 600 autopsy specimens. Spine 1988;13:173–178.
83. Mitchell PE, Hendry N, Billewicz WT. The chemical background of intervertebral disc prolapse. J Bone Joint Surg 1961;43B:141–151.
84. Mixter WJ, Barr JS. Rupture of the intervertebral disc with involvement of the spinal canal. N Engl J Med 1934;211:210.
85. Modic M, Masaryk T, et al. Lumbar herniated disc disease and canal stenosis: prospective evaluation by surface coil MR, CT, and myelography. Am J Roentgenol 1986;147:757–765.
86. Mooney V, Robertson S. The facet syndrome. Clin Orthop 1976;115:149–156.
87. Nachemson A. Lumbar intradiscal pressure. Acta Orthop Scand 1960;(Suppl 43):43–44.
88. Nasca R. Surgical management of lumbar spinal stenosis. Spine 1987;12:809–816.
89. Naylor A. The biophysical and biochemical aspects of intervertebral disc herniations and degeneration. Ann R Coll Surg Engl 1962;31:91–114.
90. Naylor A, Horton W. The hydrophilic properties of the nucleus pulposus of the intervertebral disc. Rheumatism 1955;11:32–35.
91. Nelson MA. Lumbar spinal stenosis. J Bone Joint Surg 1973;55B:506.
92. Olmarker K, Rydevik B, et al. Compression-induced changes of the nutritional supply to the porcine cauda equina. J Spinal Disord 1990;3:25–29.
93. Olmarker K, Rydevik B, et al. Graded compression of the porcine cauda equina modifies nerve root nutrition, blood flow, and impulse conduction. Transactions of the Orthopaedic Research Society, 33d Annual Meeting, San Francisco, January 1987.
94. Olmarker K, Rydevik B, et al. Edema formation in spinal nerve roots induced by experimental, graded compression: an experimental study on the pig cauda equina with special reference to differences in effects between rapid and slow onset of compression. Spine 1989;14:569–573.
95. Olmarker K, Rydevik B, et al. Effects of experimental, graded compression on blood flow in nerve roots: a vital microscopic study on the porcine cauda equina. J Orthop Res 1989;7:817–823.
96. Olsson Y. The involvement of vasa nervorum in the diseases of peripheral nerves. In: Vinken PJ, Bruyn GW, eds. Handbook of clinical neurology. Vol. 12. Vascular diseases of the nervous system. Part II. New York: American Elsevier, 1972:644–664.
97. Paine K. Results of decompression for lumbar spinal stenosis. Clin Orthop 1976;115:96–100.
98. Parke W, Gammell K, Rothman R. Arterial vascularization of the cauda equina. J Bone Joint Surg 1981;63A:53–62.
99. Parke W, Watanabe R. The intrinsic vasculature of the lumbosacral spinal nerve roots. Spine 1985;10:508–515.
100. Porter RW, et al. Measurements of the spinal canal by diagnostic ultrasound. J Bone Joint Surg 1978;60B:481–484.
101. Porter RW, Hibbert C. Relationship between the spinal canal and other skeletal measurements in a Romano-British population. Ann R Coll Surg Engl 1981;63:437.
102. Porter RW, Wicks M, Hibbert C. The size of the lumbar spinal canal in the symptomatology of disc lesion. J Bone Joint Surg 1978;60B:485–487.
103. Posner I, White A, et al. A biomechanical analysis of the clinical stability of the lumbar and lumbosacral spine. Spine 1982;7:374–389.
104. Postacchini F, Ripani M, Carpano S. Morphometry of the lumbar vertebrae: an anatomic study in two Caucasoid ethnic groups. Clin Orthop 1983;172:296–303.
105. Rauschning W. Normal and pathologic anatomy of the lumbar root canals. Spine 1987;12:1008–1019.
106. Rosenberg NJ. Degenerative spondylolisthesis. J Bone Joint Surg 1975;57A:467.
107. Rosenblum BR. The perpendicular nerve root sign. Spine 1989;14:118–119.
108. Rothman RH, Simeone FA. Lumbar disc disease. In: Rothman RH, Simeone FA, eds. The spine. 2d ed. Philadelphia: WB Saunders, 1982:508–585.
109. Rydevik B, Brown M, Lundborg G. Pathoanatomy and pathophysiology of nerve root compression. Spine 1984;9:7–15.
110. Rydevik B, Lundborg G, Bagge U. Effects of graded compression on intraneural blood flow: an in vivo study on rabbit tibial nerve. J Hand Surg 1981;6:3–12.
111. Rydevik B, Nordberg G. Changes in nerve function and nerve fibre structure induced by acute, graded compression. J Neurol Neurosurg Psychiatry 1981;43:1070–1082.
112. Rydevik B, Pedowitz R, et al. Effects of acute, graded compression on spinal nerve root function and structure: an experimental study of the pig cauda equina. Spine 1991;16:487–493.
113. San Martino A, D'Andria F, San Martino C. The surgical treatment of nerve root compression caused by scoliosis of the lumbar spine. Spine 1983;8:261–265.
114. Schonstrom N, Bolender N, et al. Pressure changes within the cauda equina following constriction of the dural sac. Spine 1984;9:604–607.
115. Schonstrom N, Hansson T. Pressure changes following constriction of the cauda equina: an experimental study in situ. Spine 1988;13:385–388.
116. Schonstrom N, Lindahl S, et al. Dynamic changes in the dimensions of the lumbar spinal canal: an experimental study in vitro. J Orthop Res 1988;7:115–121.
117. Sinclair D, Feindel W, et al. The intervertebral ligament as a source of segmental pain. J Bone Joint Surg 1948;30B:515.
118. Spengler DM. Current concepts review: degenerative stenosis of the lumbar spine. J Bone Joint Surg 1987;69A:305.
119. Stillwell DL. Nerve supply of vertebral column. Anat Rec 1956;125:139–142.
120. Sutro CJ. Lumbar facets—spinal stenosis and intermittent claudication: a mini review. Bull Hosp Jt Dis 1979;40:13.
121. Teng P, Papatheodorou C. Myelographic findings in spondylosis of the lumbar spine. Br J Radiol 1963;36:122.
122. Tile M, McNeil S, et al. Spinal stenosis: results of treatment. Clin Orthop 1976;115:104–108.

123. Tsukamoto Y, Onitsuka H, Lee K. Radiologic aspects of diffuse idiopathic skeletal hyperostosis in the spine. Am J Roentgenol 1977;129:913–918.
124. Uden A, et al. Myelography in the elderly and the diagnosis of spinal stenosis. Spine 1985;10:171–174.
125. Urban JP, McMullin JF. Swelling pressure of the lumbar intervertebral discs: influence of age, spinal level, composition, and degeneration. Spine 1988;13:179–187.
126. Van Den Hoof A. Histological age changes in the anulus fibrosus of the human intervertebral disk. Gerontologia 1964;9:136–149.
127. Verbiest H. A radicular syndrome from developmental narrowing of the lumbar vertebral canal. J Bone Joint Surg 1954;38B:230–237.
128. Verbiest H. Further experiences on pathologic influence of a developmental narrowing of the lumbar vertebral canal. J Bone Joint Surg 1956;38B:576–583.
129. Verbiest H. Pathomorphologic aspects of developmental lumbar stenosis. Orthop Clin North Am 1975;6:177–196.
130. Videman T, Malmivaara A, Mooney V. The value of the axial view in assessing discograms: an experimental study with cadavers. Spine 1987;12:299–304.
131. Voelker JL, Mealey J, et al. Metrizamide-enhanced computed tomography as an adjunct to metrizamide myelography in the evaluation of lumbar disc herniation and spondylosis. Neurosurgery 1987;20:379–384.
132. Weisz G. Lumbar spinal canal stenosis in Paget's disease. Spine 1983;8:192–198.
133. White A, Panjabi M. Clinical biomechanics of the spine. Philadelphia: Lippincott, 1978.
133a. White A, Wiltse L. Postoperative spondylolisthesis. In: Weinstein P, Ehni G, Wilson C, eds. Lumbar spondylosis: Diagnosis, management, and surgical treatment. Chicago: Year Book Medical Publishers, 1977:184–194.
134. Wiesel SW, et al. A study of computer assisted tomography: the incidence of positive CAT scans in an asymptomatic group of patients. Spine 1984;9:549–551.
135. Wiltse LL, Guyer RD, et al. Alar transverse process impingement of the L5 spinal nerve: the far-out syndrome. Spine 1984;9:31–41.
136. Winston K, Rumbargh C, et al. The vertebral canal in lumbar disc disease. Spine 1984;9:414.
137. Witt I, Vestegaard A, Rosenklit A. A comparative analysis of x-ray findings of a lumbar spine in patients with and without lumbar pain. Spine 1984;9:398–400.
138. Yamada H, Nakamura S, et al. Neurological manifestations of pediatric achondroplasia. J Neurosurg 1981;54:49–57.
139. Yang K, King A. Mechanism of facet load transmission as a hypothesis for low back pain. Spine 1984;9:557–565.

CHAPTER TWENTY TWO

Functional Restoration of Back and Neck Work-Related Injuries

Tom G. Mayer

Introduction

A critical aspect of planning functional restoration treatment to individuals with cervical and/or lumbar soft tissue work-related injuries is the recognition of similarities and differences in the anatomy and physiology of these two spinal areas. Disability related to cervical injuries occurs less frequently than that due to low back pain. These two conditions together, with their associated extremity neurologic alterations, account for 60 to 65% of all cases of disability, proportions that give rise to the need for a common guide to the evaluation of permanent impairment (4, 11, 21, 22, 60). Anatomic similarities include the three-joint complex controlling joint motion and the bilateral departure of extremity segmental nerve roots. However, the spinal cord is a factor only in the cervical spine region, which engenders the physiologic corollary that significant upper motor neuron injury is only a risk in insults to the cervical spine. Physiologic similarities involve the relative size and stabilization of the anatomic structures to accept the load of the head (cervical) or trunk (lumbar), and the relative freedom of mobility (compared to the thoracic spine) created by a segmented conduit supported by musculotendinous soft tissue structures. It is this latter characteristic that probably accounts for their greater susceptibility to degenerative disc and facet disease and the higher likelihood of the development of disabling symptoms.

Work-related injuries are often related to job demands unique to the symptomatic area. For example, sedentary jobs requiring persistent static positioning (sitting, writing, driving) and upper-extremity activities (reaching, pushing over the shoulder, etc.) are frequently related to cervical spine symptoms. In the lumbar spine, by contrast, heavy activities requiring repetitive transmission of load from the hands through the trunk (lifting, carrying, etc.), particularly in bent or rotated positions, are generally associated with symptom development. A recognition of these similarities and differences is necessary before designing a rehabilitation program for a specific spinal disorder (see Tables 22.1 and 22.2).

Functional restoration of the injured worker with spinal disorders in a workers' compensation setting creates special problems distinct from general health issues. These are related more to the potential for chronic disability than to the injured musculoskeletal region. Emerging concepts in assessment and care require some definition in order to provide a broader context of nonoperative assessment, treatment, and prevention.

The first major point is that the severity of a musculoskeletal injury in the workers' compensation industrial setting is much more dependent on the de-

TABLE 22.1.
Similarities Between Cervical and Lumbar Regions

1. Three-joint complex (disc and posterolaterally oriented diarthrodial joints) positioned to maximize mobility while protecting neurologic structures
2. Laterally placed neuroforamina
3. Posterior ramus innervation of posterolateral musculoskeletal structures
4. Anterior ramus innervation of a single extremity
5. Size and orientation of structures related to biomechanical loads commonly encountered
6. Good resistance to compression, but low resistance to bending/twisting movements
7. Degenerative disease and/or disc injury frequently associated with nerve root compression

TABLE 22.2.
Differences Between Cervical and Lumbar Regions

Condition	Cervical	Lumbar
Motion	3 planes (sagittal/coronal/axial)	Mainly 2 planes (sagittal/coronal)
Upper motor neuron injury	Common (spinal cord vulnerable)	Unlikely (cauda equina)
Muscular support	Paravertebral musculature dominant	Both paravertebral and abdominal support
Biomechanical links	Linked to shoulder girdle function	Linked to hip/pelvis function
Associated peripheral nerve entrapment and/or vascular engorgement	Common (associated "double crush" carpal tunnel, cubital tunnel, thoracic outlet syndromes)	Unusual association

velopment of chronic symptoms and the resultant disability created than on the inciting event. This observation runs counter to experience with severe orthopaedic trauma. The vast majority of worker injuries to the musculoskeletal system involve the "soft tissues" with "sprains and strains" of musculoligamentous tissues, which, in most cases, have a relatively brief healing period. When healing is incomplete or delayed, leading to permanent impairment of important supporting elements, there are greater socioeconomic costs in terms of loss of human productivity, cost of medical care, and disability-related indemnity benefits. Most studies demonstrate that the mean cost of low back pain care is more than 10 times greater than the median cost, implying that the relatively small number of chronic cases comprise the majority share of social and financial cost.

With the notion of chronological severity in mind, the demarcation of treatment into three distinct levels is useful. *Primary treatment* is that generally applied in acute cases, designed for symptom control and usually involving the so-called "passive modalities" (temperature modalities, electrical stimulation, manipulation, etc.) and sometimes accompanied by low-intensity supervised exercises and education. The vast majority of patients entering the health care system require this treatment and no more. *Secondary treatment* is appropriate in the post-acute phase and is the first level of reactivation treatment of medium intensity. It generally involves more restorative exercise and education designed to prevent the onset of deconditioning, and it is usually provided by physical/occupational therapists with available consultative psychological, disability management, and physician services. *Tertiary treatment* is appropriate for the small number of chronically disabled patients requiring physician-directed, intensive, interdisciplinary team treatment with multiple professionals on-site and available for treatment of all participants. Programs are usually organized along the lines of the CARF Pain Management guidelines (Commission on Accreditation of Rehabilitation Facilities) but may follow many diverse patterns. Functional restoration is one of the modes of tertiary treatment with proven outcomes in workers' compensation settings in multiple venues, and as such it is the focus of discussion in this chapter.

Functional restoration involves several concepts not generally considered part of conservative care. The first of these is *deconditioning*. Disuse and immobilization lead to numerous deleterious physical effects on joint mobility, muscle strength, endurance, and soft-tissue homeostasis. A corollary to this problem is the lack of visual feedback to complex spinal structures, necessitating quantification of function technology not specifically required in extremity rehabilitation.

The second major issue involves *psychosocial and socioeconomic factors* in disability that often accompany chronic and postoperative spinal disorders. Disability refers to the inability to perform all of the usual functions of daily living and is frequently linked to prolonged episodes of severe spinal pain. Various treatment interventions are designed to cope with the psychosocial and socioeconomic factors involved in total or partial disability. Psychosocial assessment is often necessary to identify these factors and to guide treatment. In addition to psychosocial problems originating in persistent pain and disability, latent psychopathology may also be activated by these issues. Psychiatric interventions, including use of psychotropic drugs and detoxification from narcotic and tranquilizer habituation, may become necessary.

Finally, primary and secondary treatment alone may be insufficiently effective to deal with chronic dysfunction, and programmatic care delivered by an interdisciplinary team will often prove desirable, if it is available. Such tertiary approaches will be considered separately.

Quantification of Physical and Functional Capacity

The quantitative assessment of function is an essential aspect of developing an effective treatment program for disabling spinal disorders. In the extremities there is relatively good visual feedback of functional capacity. Joints are easily seen, mobility is subject to goniometric measurements, and the muscle bulk is subject to tape measurements. Right/left comparisons between normal and abnormal sides can almost always be made. This concept of visual feedback led to the development of progressive resistance exercises nearly 40 years ago (13), and the patient's participation in rehabilitation dramatically affects physical function after extremity injury. More sophisticated isotonic, isometric, and isokinetic training methods have recently come into play and have greatly enhanced the technology and effectiveness of "sports medicine" extremity rehabilitation. However, in contrast to cardiovascular (a "hidden organ system") reconditioning, where measurement and training are intimately linked, functional quantification has played a relatively small role in extremity musculoskeletal rehabilitation.

In the spine there is inadequate direct visual feedback of physical capacity. Yet this deficiency has not been generally recognized by clinicians who must continue to rely on subjective self-report or physical measurements that are either inaccurate or irrelevant. One example might include goniometric spine mobility, in which the lack of recognition of cumulative effects of spine and hip motion or the absence of observable end points have led to serious problems of accuracy and reproducibility in these compound joint measurements (34, 48). Irrelevant measurements include tests of physical functional capacity that apply primarily to acute injury, such as spasm, or those that apply to questions of surgical intervention, such as leg raising and neurological changes. Recurrent spasm or deformity generally does not imply a new injury in the postoperative or chronic back pain patient. Rather, it results from disuse leading to low functional capacity arising from irritable, atrophic musculature and stiff, hypomobile joints. Positive neurologic findings are sometimes a result of perineural fibrosis in postoperative patients rather than of acute nerve root impingement necessitating surgical intervention or epidural injection. As we shall see, these physical examination findings are poor guides to the physical functional capacity of the low back, though their more accurate descendants are necessary for objective quantification as part of a sports medicine treatment program.

As in the extremities, the critical physical capacity measurements are mobility, strength, endurance, and the ability of the involved "functional unit" to coordinate its activities with adjacent units to perform musculoskeletal and neurological tasks. In the case of the spine, this involves lifting, bending, twisting, walking, and carrying. Though other measurement methods may ultimately be available and useful, those currently available to the clinician will be covered here and may be more extensively reviewed elsewhere (23, 25, 41, 43, 46).

It should not be surprising that physical deficits are found in postsurgical patients and patients with chronic pain. Most parts of the body respond to disuse by developing a "deconditioning syndrome" with components of joint stiffness, muscle atrophy, loss of endurance and connective tissue integrity, and, if inactivity is extreme, a loss of cardiovascular fitness (1, 2). There may be pain associated with restoration of physical functional capacity, with the amount of pain generally in proportion to such factors as the amount of posttraumatic scarring, the degree of loss of functional capacity, and the current psychological makeup of the patient's personality, including attitude to injury.

Physicians have possibly fostered the development of the deconditioning syndrome rather than correcting it, since our customary advice is usually to "do only those things that don't hurt." For example, patients are encouraged to permanently keep the back immobile, using either prolonged bracing, alternative activities (e.g., touching the floor by squatting rather than bending), "stabilization" to hold injured segments rigid, or resting whenever pain occurs. Though these maneuvers may temporarily relieve or prevent painful episodes, they are ultimately counterproductive, for they lead to a progressive decline in physical functional capacity, which predisposes to recurrent injuries.

Range of Motion

The commonly used goniometric techniques for the measurement of extremity motion are invalid and unreliable in the spine. Trunk motion is a compound movement combining intersegmental and hip motion components. Thus, a patient with a completely fused spine can often bend forward to perform toe touches using hip motion alone. Though we are as yet unable to measure intersegmental motion noninvasively, inclinometers may be used to separate the hip from the lumbar spine motion component and derive valuable information (48). As in all functional capacity measurements, range-of-motion techniques must be compared to a normal database, and there must be an "effort factor." For range of motion, this effort factor is the comparison of the hip motion component to the supine straight-leg-raising measurement (23).

In the sagittal plane the inclinometers, which are

available in mechanical or computerized forms from various manufacturers, may be positioned at two points or moved from one point to another (Fig. 22.1) (4, 34, 43). Measurements are taken in both flexion and extension and checked through the effort factor of leg raising.

The effort factor is not the same as a "faking or malingering factor" in that there are many reasons for limitation of effort on any single test. These include pain, fear of reinjury, physiologic perception of excessive load, neuromuscular inhibition, psychological factors of anxiety/depression, or conscious effort to mislead. In addition to sagittal movement of the spine, coronal motion can be assessed just as easily, simply by rotating the inclinometer 90 degrees in the axial plane. Rotation may also be measured, though the very small range of lumbar rotation makes this a far less reliable test (23, 43). If done in a standardized manner, with good effort, the techniques are highly reproducible. However, with suboptimal patient effort, considerable variability is noted on repeated measurements.

The measurement techniques are used for several purposes. For a one-shot assessment of function, the technique can demonstrate the actual range of motion in the T12-S1 segment during sagittal and coronal plane bending. Progress in the functional restoration program can be documented by multiple tests, and the inclinometer techniques are now incorporated into the new American Medical Association (AMA) "Guides for the Evaluation of Permanent Impairment" (3, 4). Suboptimal effort may lead to more careful scrutiny of other components of the functional capacity test battery. However, even in the presence of poor effort, the determination of probable "normal" or "abnormal" motion can be made by comparing the spine and hip motion ratios. In the normally mobile spine, the sequence of forward bending generally involves spine flexion considerably more than hip flexion during the initial phases until the spine is "hanging on its ligaments," at which point hip motion increases (43). If a normal spine/hip ratio exists, even in the presence of suboptimal effort, the clinician can usually conclude that normal spine mobility would have been present if the patient had provided sufficient effort. However, in the presence of an abnormal spine/hip ratio, with or without good effort, some physiologic limitation of spine mobility may be present (postfusion ankylosis or postoperative/disuse stiffness).

Initial objections to the use of this technique is that the dual inclinometers are more cumbersome to use

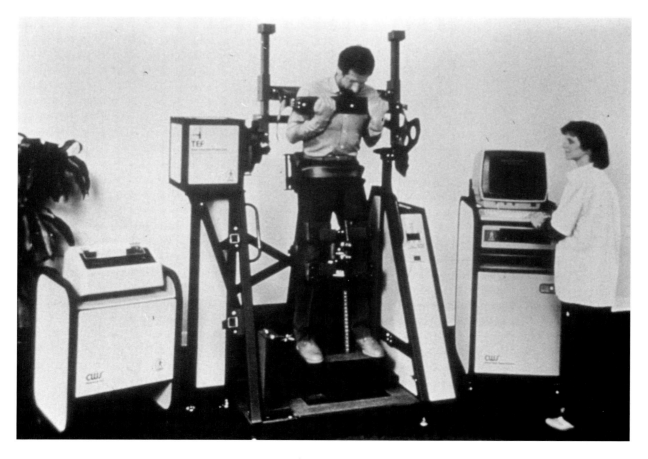

FIGURE 22.1.
The Cybex Trunk Extension/Flexion (TEF) unit is a dedicated sagittal isokinetic (and isometric) trunk strength testing device.

than a typical goniometer. However, there are now multiple equipment manufacturers for both mechanical and electronic inclinometers, some of which use only a single movable measuring head and provide the capacity for internal calculation. Clear instructions are provided in the body of the AMA Guides and forms for repeated measurements (for effort-related consistency documentation) are provided for the use of physicians or allied health personnel performing the test. Once mastered, the technique is less time-consuming than obtaining a blood pressure measurement. Many physicians will prefer to have these measurements made by assisting therapists, nurses, or technicians, particularly since repeated measurements can produce eye-opening results. The simple technique of marking the T12-L1 interspace, placing the hands over the iliac crest with index and thumb producing a plane parallel to the floor (as described elsewhere [48]), and estimating relative inclination can provide the clinician with an expedient approximation of spine/hip differential mobility.

As in all other physiologic measurements, there is some variation in the normal population. Interestingly, our normative data show that the mean true lumbar motion is almost identical between the sexes, even though females tend to have higher hip and straight-leg-raising mobility components. Patient values are expressed as a "percent normal" as related to mean scores of the normal subject population, normalized for such factors as age and sex (or body weight in strength/endurance tests). This system allows the clinician to judge the significance of small variations from the anticipated value, but more important, to track the progress of the functional restoration process from one examination to the next (8, 33, 36, 37, 38, 45).

Cervical and Trunk Strength

Several devices are now commercially available for assessing isometric, isoinertial, or isokinetic trunk strength in the sagittal and axial planes. Two devices, separating the sagittal and torsional motion components, are used in our setting. Sagittal plane (flexion/extension) testing can take place either in a dedicated unit or in a lower-cost and more flexible attachment to a standard Cybex (Lumex, Inc., Ronkonkoma, NY) dynamometer (Fig. 22.1 and 22.2). A rotation testing device is only available in a dedicated unit (Fig. 22.3). Similar isokinetic devices are produced by

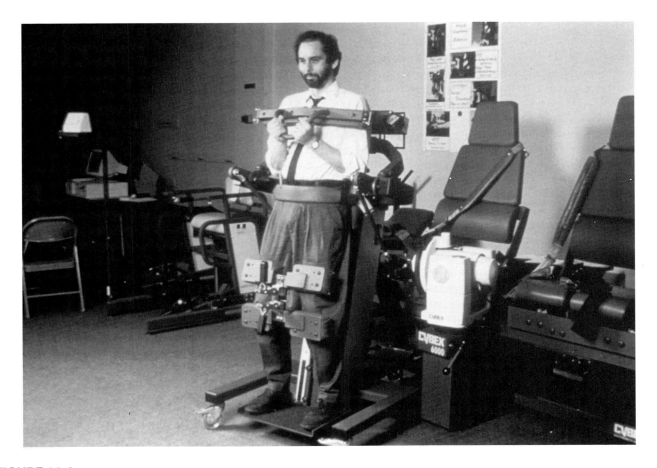

FIGURE 22.2.
The Cybex Trunk Modular Component (TMC) is a separate component that can be fitted onto a standard Cybex 6000 dynamometer to permit measurement of sagittal trunk strength identical to the system provided with the TEF unit.

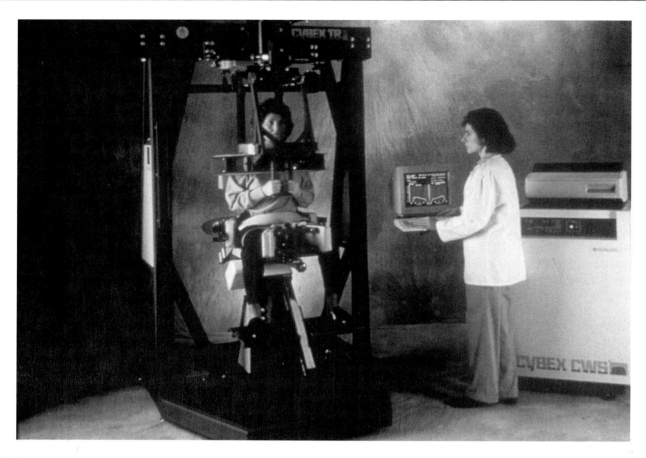

FIGURE 22.3.

The Cybex Trunk Rotation (TR) device measures thoracolumbar isokinetic and isometric axial torques.

several manufacturers, and unique isoinertial and isometric devices are available from other manufacturers. In the cervical spine, in contrast, few measurement tools are available, with only one manufacturer producing a dedicated device. Isometric measurements using hand-held dynamometers must suffice in most instances (8, 26, 34, 35, 38, 44–47).

Strength testing devices isolate the cervical and thoracolumbar portions of the "biomechanical chain" involved in transmitting forces from head and hands to the ground. For trunk strength, using different techniques in each machine, the pelvis and lower extremities are stabilized below, and the upper thorax at the level of the shoulder girdle (midthoracic) is stabilized above. This allows the isolation of the torques produced through that vulnerable portion of the vertebral biomechanical chain spanning the shoulder girdle to the pelvis. It should be clear to the clinician that there is no intent to make either the stabilization or the mode of movement (isometric/isokinetic) truly physiologic. Rather, the devices control as many physiologic variables as possible by isolating the anatomic/functional unit and controlling speed/acceleration/distance, thus leaving only torque and effort as major independent variables. The goal is to improve test discrimination by sacrificing "real-world" simulations. As in strength testing, endurance estimates can be made by repetitive dynamic efforts within established protocols that assess the ability to sustain maximal effort and the degree to which recovery occurs in a fixed time period. Such endurance protocols are built into the testing routines of several of the commercial products.

Though a detailed discussion is beyond the scope of this chapter, it is clear that major differences exist in trunk strength in both sagittal and axial planes, between a normal subject and a patient population. Moreover, through efforts at functional restoration with a sports medicine approach, trunk strength in the patient population can be markedly improved.

Cardiovascular Fitness

The inactivity that leads to deconditioning in patients with low back pain also produces a decline in cardiovascular fitness. Bicycle and upper-body ergometry has long been used to measure the cardiovascular response to a measured work load. Significant deficits in aerobic capacity are frequently present in chronic and postoperative low back pain patients, somewhat proportional to the length of disability and the degree of inactivity. Such inactivity may also produce deconditioning problems of upper and lower extremity fatigue, rather than by problems of cardiovascular fitness. However, this can usually be distinguished by noting the heart rate achieved at the point of voluntary test termination as well as by comparing the upper- and lower-body ergometry results. In most deconditioned patients, however, an exaggerated heart rate response to relatively low work loads is usually the limiting factor and a submaximal stress test results. Such testing leads to an estimate of aerobic capacity and a determination as to which aerobic capacity and/or lower and upper extremity strength training needs to be added to the functional restoration program.

Functional Task Measurements

While the foregoing tests of mobility, strength, and aerobic capacity have focused primarily on the injured functional unit, the measurement of functional tasks have a more practical application. The body is certainly capable of functioning in the presence of rigidity, as in the case of a patient with a completely fused thoracolumbar spine. Using the spine as a rigid vertical column imposes functional demands for substitution for other anatomical structures, such as squatting and whole-body rotation to accommodate limitations in spine bending and twisting. Gait modifications may also be necessary to accommodate losses to the "spinal engine" for locomotion (19). Functional task measurements help the clinician to assess how the body performs as a whole, rather than how the injured region or joint is functioning in isolation. For the thoracolumbar spine, relevant functional tasks involve the transmission of load through the trunk down to the ground, specifically in such activities as floor-to-waist lifting, bending, twisting, and carrying. For the cervicothoracic spine, activities that involve maintenance of head position and use of the shoulder girdle are relevant, including waist-to-overhead lifting, reaching, and static head and shoulder positions (driving, word processing, etc.) (12, 39).

There is, however, a price to be paid for taking "real-world" measurements. The large number of independent variables needed in measuring a "total body activity" decreases reliability and discrimination for test results. For this reason, more than one measurement is necessary to make such functional task measurements truly objective.

Such is the case in the measurement of lifting capacity. Because of its perceived importance as an injury mode in industry, the ability to lift has become the measurement of greatest concern to those involved in ergonomic analysis for functional limitations and job redesign. We use several measurements to give a full picture of lifting capacity, including isokinetic and isometric measuring devices. Isometric measurements are currently employed extensively for industrial use as compiled under National Institute of Occupational Safety and Health (NIOSH) guidelines. These tests are very simple to perform and have a large industrial database to accompany them. Unfortunately, isometric tests are nondynamic and have been proved not to correlate well with dynamic tests (29). In addition, it has been suggested that isometric tests may be likely to produce injury themselves because they involve "pulling against an immovable object."

Isokinetic devices are capable of performing both isometric and isokinetic measurements at multiple speeds over distances from floor to overhead. The isokinetic technique, also intentionally nonphysiologic, stabilizes the speed/acceleration variable that is used in part by most trained lifters to attain higher forces. Though the measuring technique is different, the principle of comparison to a large normal database with an acceptable "effort factor" is now well accepted. Isokinetic strength tests allow effort verification through comparison of curve consistency, termed "average points variance," on the basis of comparisons made as often as every 50 milliseconds. Such comparisons have been shown to have a high sensitivity (20). Some correlation between extensor trunk strength deficits and floor-to-waist lifting capacity deficits exists, but the style of lifting can produce significantly higher lifting capacity measurements than isolated trunk strength measurements in a well-motivated, functionally deconditioned individual. Similarly, an anxious or fearful patient, particularly if the patient has been educated "never to lift anything more than a teacup," may show a paradoxical discrepancy in which lifting capacity measurements are considerably lower than those anticipated on the basis of isolated trunk strength measurements.

Finally, an isoinertial or psychophysical lifting protocol (27, 57) has been modified for use at the Productive Rehabilitation Institute of Dallas for Ergonomics (PRIDE) facility to assess a patient's frequent lifting capacity. The protocol gradually increases weight in a timed test. The cervical test involves waist-to-shoulder lifting, and the lumbar test involves floor-to-waist lifting of "bricks in a box," based on the normal population data for peak weight lifted, force to body weight, work performed, power consumed, endurance time, and final heart rate (30–32).

Positional and activity tolerance is another area of interest in functional task measurement for return to work in its broadest sense. Patients with spine injuries often cannot tolerate prolonged static positioning (sitting/standing) and often report an inability to perform various tasks such as squatting, kneeling, walking, carrying, or climbing. We have devised a timed obstacle course requiring use of multiple positions in an attempt to assess the patient's tolerance of daily living activities individually and in combination. Obstacle course tests include pushing, pulling, crawling, squatting, twisting, climbing, reaching, and bending. Unfortunately, commercial devices are not yet available. Patient observation through a testing or training session can give the therapist an idea of the patient's tolerance of various static positions. Because of lack of corroborative tests, these measurements are somewhat less "objective" than the preceding functional measurements.

Measurement of cervical and lumbar isolated physical capacity as well as whole-body relevant functional performance is the key to guiding any tertiary care treatment program. The measurement of function sets the initial level of training according to a computerized exercise progression program (unique to the PRIDE environment). The progression then follows an expert system process based on patient performance from that starting point, normalized to age, sex, and a height/weight variable. Frequent repeated measurement of function ascertains subjective assessment of both progress and outcomes, which will ultimately be relevant to the limitations for work, the measurement of permanent impairment, and the risk of recurrent injury. The measurement of function is a difficult and time-consuming task and is currently limited by suboptimal standardization. In time, however, the benefits of refining these techniques will undoubtedly raise the level of expertise of physicians and allied health personnel engaged in this type of treatment. Significant improvement in performance can then be anticipated.

Psychosocial Barriers to Recovery

In a work environment, when injury is associated with compensation for disability, physical problems are frequently not the only factor to be considered in organizing a treatment program. Many psychosocial and socioeconomic problems may confront the patient recovering from a spinal disorder, particularly if disability from a productive lifestyle is associated with the industrial back pain. The patient's inability to see a "light at the end of the tunnel" may produce a severe situational depression, often associated with anxiety and agitation. The back injury itself may be a sign of emotional conflicts involving rebellion against authority or job dissatisfaction (6, 7, 58). Personality changes may be manifested in anger, hostility, and noncompliance directed at the therapeutic team. Minor head injuries, organic brain dysfunction from age, alcohol, or drugs, or limited intelligence may produce organic cognitive dysfunctions that may interfere with recovery. A variety of personality disorders, such as sociopathy, may also complicate treatment (15, 16, 17, 24, 41, 61).

Many chronic spinal disorders exist within a "disability system." Workers' compensation laws were initially devised to protect workers' income and provide timely medical benefits following industrial accidents. Employers ultimately agreed to this because of a compensatory benefit; in return for providing these worker rights, they were absolved of certain consequences of negligence, generally including cost-capped liability for any injury, no matter how severe, and set by state statute. As in any compromise situation, certain disincentives to rational behavior may emerge. One outcome of a guaranteed paycheck while Temporary Total Disability persists is that there may be no clear incentive to an early return to work. A casual approach to surgical decision-making and rehabilitation may lead to further deconditioning, both mental and physical, thus making ultimate recovery more problematic. Complicating matters even further is the observation that no group (other than the employer) has any verifiable financial incentive to return patients to productivity as soon as possible. In consequence, an odd assortment of health professionals, attorneys, insurance companies, and vocational rehabilitation specialists may have limited motivation to combat foot-dragging on the disability issue. Altering the contingencies may correct some of the problems. However, this assumes that the present system has not already evolved to a near-perfect balance of interests, or that legislators will respond to changes in outlook regarding optimal patient care.

Early efforts to distinguish between "functional" (nonorganic) and "organic" low back pain did not meet with success. The complex nature of chronic pain makes it difficult to clearly categorize component factors as purely physical or purely psychological. Instead, chronic pain must be understood as an interactive, psychophysiological behavior pattern in which the physical and the psychological constantly overlap and intertwine. The focus of psychological evaluation of the low back pain patient therefore must shift away from "functional" versus "organic" distinctions to the identification of important psychological characteristics with behavioral motivators of each patient. These characteristics will obviously affect a patient's disability and his or her response to treatment efforts. Identification of such characteristics will facilitate treatment planning and assist with the prediction of treatment outcome. Though space does not permit an extensive review of the various instruments used for psychological assessment, a description of some basic instruments commonly used within the PRIDE system may be useful here.

Quantified Pain Drawing: The pain drawing provides a nonverbal assessment tool for pain location, severity, and subjective characteristics (50). Patients are encouraged to freely display all of their pain and rate its intensity along a 10 cm line. Scoring employs an overlay that reliably quantifies pain by dividing the human drawing into a series of boxes, yielding a score for the trunk, extremities, and "outside the body" pain (10, 34). This latter dimension is useful for identifying pain magnifiers as well as suggesting the possibility of somatic delusions in rare cases. Such a pain drawing provides an easy and reliable method for documentation of changing pain perception on repeated measurements in response to treatment.

Million Visual Analog Scale: This analog scale consists of 15 questions relating to perceptions of pain and disability (49). Responses are recorded by placing a mark along a 10 cm line that represents an index of severity. Scores are easily obtained using a ruler or grid. This scale is particularly useful because of its nonverbal form of expression, and its ease of administration and reproducibility make it ideal for monitoring progress through repeated administrations. Extremely exaggerated responses that do not correlate with clinical assessment may also indicate the need for further, in-depth psychological evaluation.

Beck Depression Inventory (BDI): The BDI consists of 21 items pertaining to symptoms of depression, such as sleep disturbance, sexual dysfunction, weight change, and anhedonia. It is very brief and easy to complete, and it has a cumulative scoring system that takes less than 1 minute to complete. The BDI is designed to identify cognitive factors of depression and, along with the Hamilton Depression Rating Scale, can provide the clinician with valuable information about the existence and severity of depression in the low back pain patient (5, 52, 53, 61). The BDI's ease of administration makes it easy to use on repeated visits, offering the clinician a relatively simple means of observing depressive symptoms and treatment progress.

Minnesota Multiphasic Personality Inventory (MMPI): The MMPI is one of the oldest and most frequently used indices of psychological functioning. Its first three clinical scales, Hypochondriasis (Hs), Depression (D), and Hysteria (Hy), provide valuable information in the evaluation of the chronic low back pain (CLBP) patient. Relative elevations of these three clinical scales can alert the clinician to the possibility of important problems such as symptom magnification, poor insight into emotions, and defenses based on denial and somatization tendencies. Many ancillary scales have been developed within the MMPI that also provide specific information pertinent to CLBP treatment. Notable among these are the McAndrews (Mac) and Ego Strength (Es) scales. The Mac scale helps to identify patients with alcoholic or drug-dependent personalities, which may assist the treatment team in preventing drug habituation. The Es scale is designed to identify patients with limited emotional resources who might lack the motivation and personal responsibility to adequately benefit from an intensive treatment regimen. Many articles document correlations between various behaviors and certain scales, of which these are but a few examples.

Other Psychological Assessments: The Structured Clinical Interview for DSM-IV diagnosis (SCID) is an interview test designed to help a trained mental health provider reach a DSM-IV psychiatric diagnosis. The most important are the Axis I and II diagnoses, which occur very commonly in chronic spinal disorders (54). The Hamilton Depression Rating Scale is a clinician-administered test that supplements the self-report of the BDI. A nonstructured clinical interview by clinicians helps to focus on the various critical issues that are the essential barriers to recovery that must be addressed. Many of these may be social (child care or transportation problems), specifically affecting the patient's ability to participate in rehabilitation, or they may involve financial, psychological, legal, and employer-related issues. Similar interviews performed by disability managers are quite useful in evaluating the occupational aspects of ongoing disability, with this role being taken under different training circumstances by occupational therapists, social workers, vocational rehabilitation specialists, or rehabilitation nurses. Tests that evaluate an individual's education and skills, including the Wechsler Adult Intelligence Scale–Revised (WAIS-R) are also commonly used in assessment designed to achieve an outcome of returning the chronically disabled worker back to a productive lifestyle.

The Tertiary Care Treatment Plan for Functional Restoration

Functional restoration is a type of tertiary care that uses the physical/functional capacity and psychosocial assessments described in detail previously to organize a physician-directed interdisciplinary team treatment approach to restoring patients to productivity. Multiple disciplines are required on-site, with all patients having the benefit of access to each specialized group of health providers in an intensive program individualized to the initial assessments (9, 18, 23, 25, 28, 46, 47, 55, 56, 59). An additional feature of functional restoration programs is the attention to outcome monitoring for all patients, with structured clinical interviews at a minimum follow-up interval of 1 year. These interviews focus on specific objective factors of cost and disability (17, 34, 41, 44, 51).

Following the initial assessment, a preprogram phase of treatment is initiated on a once or twice weekly basis. The duration and frequency of this phase are determined by the degree of deconditioning and any psychosocial barriers that would interfere with participation in the 3-week intensive phase. In this phase, the physical and occupational therapists are involved primarily in confidence building to overcome the limitation of physical performance that might derive from inhibition and fear of injury, and mobilization and stretching to prepare the patient for the intensive muscle training portion of the program. Psychologists and disability managers deal with psychological (e.g., depression and/or substance dependence) and social (e.g., financial, transportation, family responsibilities) barriers to program participation, respectively. Utilization ranges from 2 to 6 weeks and is followed by the program's intensive phase. During this portion of the program, the patient participates in a 3-week 10-hour/day program consisting of reconditioning, work simulation, disability management, and a cognitive-behavioral program (17, 34, 40, 41).

The reconditioning and work simulation aspects of the program involve physical and occupational therapists using active (not passive) treatment modalities. Quantification is necessary for these aspects of the program, since they provide the initial levels of exercise from which a progressive resistive program emerges. The indirect assessments confirm functional deficits and psychosocial barriers to effort, leading to a combination of education and exercise training to resolve the deconditioning syndrome. Initial treatment is directed toward mobilizing and strengthening the "weak link" in the biomechanical chain, and whole-body work simulation integrates the performance of this link with other parts of the body that have been deconditioned simply by inactivity.

The cognitive-behavioral multimodal disability management program focuses initially on diagnosis of psychosocioeconomic barriers to functional recovery in the given individual through the assessment mentioned above, and then on specific treatments for problem areas. The initial treatment may be pharmacologic, involving detoxification from habituating opiate and tranquilizer medications, use of antidepressants and anti-inflammatory medications, and occasionally major tranquilizers. Remaining treatments include a cognitive-behaviorally based program of education and counseling, including stress management, that is time limited and aggressively oriented toward sequential goal-setting. Failure to meet mutually prearranged goals may result in dismissal from the program (an event currently occurring in about 5% of comprehensive program admissions). In practice, education and counseling accounts for approximately one-half of total program time, with the remainder spent in physical training.

Outcome Monitoring

Though space does not permit additional details of how each member of the interdisciplinary team treats patients, the reader should now recognize that tertiary care involves medically directed interdisciplinary team treatment based on a therapy plan that is individualized for patient needs by the initial evaluation. Following termination of the intensive phase of treatment, the patient's ultimate socioeconomic outcomes depend on the maintenance of treatment goals. Patients generally achieve a much higher level of physical and functional capacities, which must be continued in a Fitness Maintenance Program, for which the patient is educated, based on the training level he or she has achieved under staff supervision. Repeated objective physical quantification leads to feedback to the patient on maintenance of physical capacity, which can be correlated with job demands to make inferences on the risk of future injury. Relevant pieces of durable medical equipment or memberships in appropriately equipped fitness centers may be suggested for patients. In addition, PRIDE performs routine one-year scheduled follow-up telephone interviews as a regular part of its program. The interview includes information on working status, additional health care utilization, resolution of compensation issues (long-term disability, Social Security Disability, permanent partial/total disability, etc.), and injury recurrence (14, 42). The interviews must be performed in the context of possible remaining barriers to full disclosure by the patient, thus necessitating further investigation through contacts with employers, attorneys, family members, or third party payers in some cases. Combining the follow-up interview information with preprogram demographic data on the same subjects can provide valid statistical comparisons of the ability of a comprehensive functional restoration program to deal with disability and cost. Since the chronic low back and neck pain patient ultimately accounts for 80% of the costs of degenerative spine problems through a combination of medical treatment, lost productivity, indemnity, and government support, program evaluation, including involvement of other members of the disability system, provides a major resource to clinicians, employers, health care planners and legislators alike.

Though functional restoration of the chronic patient is the area of highest anticipated "bang for the buck" in work-incurred spinal disability, employers and government agencies are often slow to effect change in their policies. While the Boeing study clearly demonstrates (6, 7, 58) that job dissatisfaction/personnel relations problems may be the best (or only) predictor of back "injury," the use of the medical system to avoid responsibility for good personnel relations has become endemic in some industries. These employers and government agencies may find it easier to ascribe back injury to the "costs of doing business" and pass these expenses on to the consumer or taxpayer. An adversarial and rancorous relationship more often than not alters the status of the patient from an employee to a claimant. Lest we too quickly fall into the trap of labeling the injured worker who seeks redress from perceived punitive employer actions as a "faker" or "malingerer," we must consider the multitude of factors in the evolution of the workers' compensation and personal injury situations themselves.

It is appropriate here to consider briefly some of the aspects of the employer/employee relationship that are vital to the reader's understanding of the behavior of the injured worker. While manipulativeness, opportunism, and low motivation characterize some patients' behavior, their actions are usually conditioned by perceived grievances in the essentially adversarial workers' compensation system. Employer-employee conflict is often played out through their respective representatives (the insurance carrier and the plaintiff's attorney) in a contest over medical benefits, job retention rights, and disability-related indemnity benefits tied to perceived permanent impairment. The other participants in the disability system may have a variety of personal and business interests that can diverge in certain critical areas from the best interest of the injured worker. As such, the interdisciplinary team's education on the particular rules of the workers' compensation venue can be an important aspect of treatment to assist the patient in escaping the maze of chronic disability. In this regard, the tertiary care provider is the only disinterested party capable of assisting the patient in formulating a problem-solving solution. In this way, tertiary care facilities accomplish specific socioeconomic benefits of interest to the injured worker as well as to the society around him. In so doing, the assessment and tertiary treatment of the chronically disabled worker leads to tertiary prevention, in which the most dismal consequence of permanent disability of the young and potentially productive worker is avoided. Since spinal disorders are the primary cause of disability in people under the age of 45 years in most industrialized countries, an average of 25 to 30 years of taxpayer-supported welfare benefits (Social Security Disability Income (SSDI), long-term disability, unemployment insurance, social welfare, food stamps, etc.) can be prevented by judicious application of tertiary care to the identified chronically disabled worker. Ultimately, application of tertiary care to the large reservoir of "permanently disabled" spinal disorder patients offers a major challenge to society's ability to create jobs and an opportunity to save billions of dollars in unnecessary welfare payments for nonproductivity.

In selected cases, tertiary care may be appropriate even before a maximum normal soft tissue healing period (4 to 6 months postinjury) has been completed. While secondary treatment is usually preferable for patients before they have had 4 months of disability, the availability of effective tertiary care with cost- and duration-limited programs may make them desirable for selected cases even before 4 months have passed. In particular, with more aggressive employer involvement through transitional work return programs, with the recognition of early psychosocial stressors potentially leading to enhancement of disability, and with the advent of treatment guidelines to inform health providers and administrative agencies of demonstrated ways to achieve treatment goals, tertiary treatment (at least in a limited form) may be instituted within 6 to 8 weeks of injury/disability in selected cases. A variety of criteria may be used to distinguish the suitability of secondary or tertiary care in these cases, including the match between physical capacity and job demands, recent prior injury, age, other medical conditions, preexisting psychosocial barriers, and job availability. Progressive education of health providers to the more advanced approaches to rehabilitation of injured workers is the best method to advance program effectiveness and ensure quality of care.

We must conclude that the future of rehabilitation of chronically disabled workers with neck and back pain lies in finding solutions that involve cooperation among stakeholders in the workers' compensation system. The injured worker must be given an opportunity for appropriate medical care, rehire, and compensation for any injury that meets legal compensability criteria. The employer must continue to be protected from excess liability and from the "secondary gain" potential for exploitation of a situation in which relief from the obligation to work (disability) is financially compensable. If objective structural documentation cannot provide adequate means for assessing impairment, scheduled or functional assessment–based awards may be considered. Surgical treatment must be carefully evaluated, not purely on the basis of pain or structural considerations but in terms of the impact it will have in a workers' compensation system. This includes the impact on the socioeconomic outcomes discussed above. Partnerships between surgeons and rehabilitation specialists, based not on higher utilization but rather on proven outcomes, will probably become the rule rather than the exception. Surgeons will have to consider the likelihood that their surgery will be judged by these outcomes in workers' compensation, so that their ultimate objective will become a surgically treated and functionally restored patient who can return to work as a productive taxpaying citizen. If this goal is not achieved, further incursions into surgical practice questioning the indications for surgical treatment in spinal disorders can be anticipated. Surgical treatment of a structural lesion alone can never be expected to produce return to work in complex, chronically disabled patients. A partnership between surgeon and careful providers of secondary and tertiary care, however, coupled with appropriate surgical and nonoperative patient selection, can be anticipated to reduce pain and achieve socially responsible outcomes, even for injured workers with spinal disorders who have limited education and skills. Accomplishing these goals is the challenge for the next decade.

References

1. Abenhaim L, Belanger A, Bloch R, et al. Scientific approach to the assessment and management of activity-related spinal disorders: a monograph for clinicians. Report of the Quebec Task Force on Spinal Disorders. Spine 1987;12(7S):S1–S59.
2. Akeson W, Amiel D, Abel M, et al. Effects of immobilization on joints. Clin Orthop 1987;219:28–57.
3. American Medical Association Guides to the evaluation of permanent impairment. 3d ed. Engleberg A, ed. Chicago: AMA Press, 1988.
4. American Medical Association. Guides to the evaluation of permanent impairment. 4th ed. Doege T, ed. Chicago: AMA Press, 1994.
5. Beck A, Steer R, Garbin W. Psychometric properties of the Beck Depression Inventory: twenty-five years of evaluation. Clin Psychol Rev 1988;8:77–100.
6. Bigos S, Spengler D, Martin N, et al. Back injuries in industry: a retrospective study. II. Injury factors. Spine 1986;11:246–251.
7. Bigos S, Spengler D, Martin N, et al. Back injuries in industry: a retrospective study. III. Employee-related factors. Spine 1986;11:252–256.
8. Brady S, Mayer T, Gatchel R. Physical progress and residual impairment quantification after functional restoration. Part II: Isokinetic trunk strength. Spine 1994;18:395–400.
9. Cady L, Bischoff D, O'Connel E, et al. Strength and fitness and subsequent back injuries in firefighters. J Occup Med 1979;21:269–272.
10. Capra P, Mayer T, Gatchel R. Adding psychological scales to assess back pain. J Musculoskel Med 1985;7:41–52.
11. Carroll R, Hurst L. The relationship of thoracic outlet syndrome and carpal tunnel syndrome. Clin Orthop 1992;164:149–153.
12. Curtis L, Mayer T, Gatchel R. Physical progress and residual impairment after functional restoration. Part III: Isokinetic and isoinertial lifting capacity. Spine 1994;18:401–405.
13. DeLorme T, Watkins A. Progressive resistance exercise: Technic medical application. Appleton Century Crofts, 1951.
14. Garcy P, Mayer T, Gatchel RJ. Recurrent or new injury outcomes after return to work in chronic disabling spinal disorders. Tertiary prevention. Efficacy of functional restoration treatment. Spine 1996;21:952–959.
15. Gatchel R, Mayer T, Capra P, et al. Quantification of lumbar function. Part 6: The use of psychological measures in guiding physical functional restoration. Spine 1986;11:36–42.
16. Gatchel R, Mayer T, Capra P, et al. Million Behavioral Health Inventory: its utility in predicting physical function in patients with low back pain. Arch Phys Med Rehabil 1986;67:878–882.
17. Gatchel R, Mayer T, Hazard R, et al. Editorial: Functional restoration: pitfalls in evaluating efficacy. Spine 1992;17:988–995.
18. Gould J, Davies G, eds. Orthopaedic and sports physical therapy. St. Louis: Mosby, 1985.
19. Gracovetsky S, Farfan H. The optimum spine. Spine 1986;11:543–573.
20. Hazard R, Reid S, Fenwick J, et al. Isokinetic trunk and lifting strength measurements: variability as an indicator of effort. Spine 1988;13:54–57.
21. Hohl M. Soft-tissue injuries of the neck in automobile accidents: factors influencing prognosis. J Bone Joint Surg 1974;56A:1675–1682.
22. Hurst L, Weissberg D, Carroll R. The relationship of the double crush to carpal tunnel syndrome. J Hand Surg 1985;10(2):202–204.
23. Keeley J, Mayer T, Cox R, et al. Quantification of lumbar function. Part 5: Reliability of range-of-motion measures in the sagittal plane and an in vivo torso rotation measurement technique. Spine 1986;11:31–35.
24. Kinney R, Gatchel R, Polatin P, et al. The high prevalence of major psychiatric disorders in chronic low back pain patients: an objective evaluation study. In: Transactions of the International Society for the Study of the Lumbar Spine, annual meeting, Boston, June 15, 1990.
25. Kishino N, Mayer T, Gatchel R, et al. Quantification of lumbar function. Part 4: Isometric and isokinetic lifting simulation in normal subjects and low-back dysfunction patients. Spine 1985;10:921–927.
26. Kohles S, Barnes D, Gatchel R, et al. Improved physical performance outcomes following functional restoration treatment of chronic low back pain patients: early versus recent training results. Spine 1990;15:1321–1324.
27. Kroemer K. An isoinertial technique to assess individual lifting capability. Human Factors 1983;25:493–506.
28. Langrana N, Lee C. Isokinetic evaluation of trunk muscles. Spine 1984;9:171–175.
29. Marras W, King A, Joynt R. Measurements of loads on the lumbar spine under isometric and isokinetic conditions. Spine 1984;9:176–198.
30. Mayer T, Barnes D, Kishino N, et al. Progressive iso-

inertial lifting evaluation: I: An Erratum. Spine 1990; 15:5.
31. Mayer T, Barnes D, Kishino N, et al. Progressive iso-inertial lifting evaluation. Part I: A standardized protocol and normative database. Spine 1988;13:993–997.
32. Mayer T, Barnes D, Nichols G, et al. Progressive iso-inertial lifting evaluation. Part II: A comparison with isokinetic lifting in a disabled chronic low back pain industrial population. Spine 1988;13:998–1002.
33. Mayer T, Brady S, Bovasso E, et al. Noninvasive measurement of cervical tri-planar motion in normal subjects. Spine 1993;18:2191–2195.
34. Mayer T, Gatchel R. Functional restoration for spinal disorders: The sports medicine approach. Philadelphia: Lea & Febiger, 1988.
35. Mayer T, Gatchel R, Betancur J, et al. Trunk muscle endurance measurement: isometric contrasted to isokinetic testing in normal subjects. Spine 1995;20:920–926.
36. Mayer T, Gatchel R, Keeley J, et al. Optimal spinal strength normalization factors among male railroad workers. Spine 1993;18:239–244.
37. Mayer T, Gatchel R, Keeley J, et al. A male incumbent worker industrial database. Part I: Lumbar spinal physical capacity. Spine 1994;19:755–761.
38. Mayer T, Gatchel R, Keeley J, et al. A male incumbent worker industrial database. Part II: Cervical spinal physical capacity. Spine 1994;19:762–764.
39. Mayer T, Gatchel R, Keeley J, et al. A male incumbent worker industrial database. Part III: Lumbar/cervical functional testing. Spine 1994;19:765–770.
40. Mayer T, Gatchel R, Mayer H, et al. Objective assessment of spine function following industrial accident: a prospective study with comparison group and one-year follow-up (Volvo Award in Clinical Sciences, 1985). Spine 1985;10:482–493.
41. Mayer T, Gatchel R, Mayer H, et al. A prospective two-year study of functional restoration in industrial low back injury: an objective assessment procedure. JAMA 1987;258:1763–1767.
42. Mayer T, Gatchel R, Prescott M. Functional restoration socioeconomics outcomes: the PRIDE Outcome Tracking System. In: Bejjani FJ, ed. Occupational musculoskeletal medicine. Philadelphia: JB Lippincott, in press.
43. Mayer T, Kishino N, Keeley J, et al. Using physical measurements to assess low back pain. J Musculoskel Med 1985;6:44–59.
44. Mayer T, Mooney V, Gatchel R. Contemporary care for painful disorders: Concepts, diagnosis, and treatment. Philadelphia: Lea & Febiger, 1991.
45. Mayer T, Pope P, Tabor J, et al. Physical progress and residual impairment quantification after functional restoration. Part I: Lumbar mobility. Spine 1994;18:389–394.
46. Mayer T, Smith S, Keeley J, et al. Quantification of lumbar function. Part 2: Sagittal plane trunk strength in chronic low-back pain patients. Spine 1985;10:765–772.
47. Mayer T, Smith S, Kondraske G, et al. Quantification of lumbar function. Part 3: Preliminary data on isokinetic torso rotation testing with myoelectric spectral analysis in normal and low-back pain subjects. Spine 1985; 10:912–920.
48. Mayer T, Tencer A, Kristoferson S, et al. Use of noninvasive techniques for quantification of spinal range-of-motion in normal subjects and chronic low-back dysfunction patients. Spine 1984;9:588–595.
49. Million R, Nilsen K, Jayson MIV, et al. Evaluation of low back pain and assessment of lumbar corsets with and without back supports. Ann Rheum Dis 1981; 40:449–454.
50. Mooney V, Cairns D, Robertson J. A system for evaluating and treating chronic back disability. West J Med 1976;124:370–376.
51. Nachemson A. Work for all. Clin Orthop 1983; 179:77–82.
52. Polatin P. Functional restoration for the chronically disabled low back pain patient. J Musculoskel Med 1990;7:17–39.
53. Polatin P, Gatchel R, Barnes D, et al. A psychosociomedical prediction model of response to treatment by chronically disabled workers with back pain. Spine 1989;14:956–961.
54. Polatin P, Kinney R, Gatchel R, et al. Psychiatric illness and chronic low-back pain: the mind and the spine—which goes first? Spine 1993;18:66–71.
55. Pope M, Frymoyer J, Andersson G. Occupational low back pain. New York: Praeger, 1984.
56. Smith S, Mayer T, Gatchel R, et al. Quantification of lumbar function. Part 1: Isometric and multi-speed isokinetic trunk strength measures in sagittal and axial planes in normal subject patients. Spine 1985;10:757–764.
57. Snook S, Campanelli R, Hart J. A study of three preventive approaches to low back injury. J Occup Med 1978;20:478–481.
58. Spengler D, Bigos S, Martin N, et al. Back injuries in industry: a retrospective study. I. Overview and cost analysis. Spine 1986;11:241–245.
59. Thompson N, Gould J, Davies G, et al. Descriptive measures of isokinetic trunk testing. J Orthop Sports Phys Ther 1985;7:43–49.
60. Upton A, McComas A. The double crush in nerve entrapment syndrome. Lancet 1973;32:359–361.
61. Ward N. Tricyclic antidepressants for chronic low back pain: mechanisms of action and predictors of response (Volvo Award in Clinical Sciences, 1986). Spine 1986; 11:661–665.

SECTION V

Adult Deformities and Miscellaneous Disorders

CHAPTER TWENTY THREE

Adult Scoliosis

Richard A. Balderston, Todd J. Albert and Alexander R. Vaccaro

Introduction

Adult scoliosis is a spinal deformity with the Cobb angle measuring greater than 10° in the coronal plane in a patient older than 20 years of age. The patients discussed in this chapter had onset of their deformity before skeletal maturity, with persistence and possible worsening of the deformity after the age of 20 years (57). In another group of patients who previously had straight spines, that is, a Cobb angle less than 10° at the age of 20 years, deformity developed as a result of degenerative disease. In patients who have this type of degenerative scoliosis the deformity develops more commonly in the lumbar spine; however, there are surgical considerations that must be taken into account, assuming that all adult patients have some degree of degenerative disease.

Epidemiology and Natural History

In a study group of adult patients with an average age of 61 years, Vanderpool et al. (67) found a prevalence of 6% of deformity as visualized in the coronal plane. However, in this study, curve definition was set at 7° or greater. Patients who had osteoporosis had a 36% incidence of spinal deformity, and more than 30% of these patients had proof of coronal plane worsening secondary to fracture and degenerative disease.

In 1981 Kostuik and Bentivoglio reviewed 5000 intravenous pyelograms and found roughly a 4% incidence of scoliosis of 10° or greater in the lumbar spine (33). In this patient group 86% of the diagnoses were idiopathic scoliosis, with the remainder being degenerative scoliosis.

Curve progression in the adult patient with idiopathic scoliosis has been well defined. Several authors have demonstrated that curves in the adult patient will frequently progress (12, 42, 43, 45, 47, 50, 54). In a landmark study by Weinstein and Ponseti, 40-year follow-up data were gathered for patients who had idiopathic curve patterns (12, 69). Patients who had a curve magnitude between 50° and 75° were found to have the highest risk for progression in both the thoracic and lumbar spine. Thoracic curves with a Cobb angle of this degree at the initiation of the study progressed an average of slightly less than 30° over the 40-year period. Thoracolumbar curves increased an average of 22° over the same period. These figures represent an overall average for participants in the study, and although many patients did not progress, some progressed 1° to 2° per year over the course of the study. In the lumbar spine curves in which the L5 vertebra was seated above the intercristal line and in those curves with lumbar apical rotation greater than 33°, the worst prognosis over a long-term follow-up period could be expected. If the lumbar or thoracolumbar curve was not balanced at the beginning of the follow-up period, a higher incidence of progression was found. Recently Korovessis et al. reviewed 91 patients with lumbar scoliosis and observed them for 2 years (31). They found that the factors that increase the risk of lumbar curve worsening were lateral olisthesis of the apical vertebrae, ratio of the Cobb angle divided by the number of vertebrae within the curve (Harrington factor) (26), and the amount of wedging of the disk spaces within the curve expressed by the total disk height on the convex side divided by the total height on the concave side. The factors that were not prognostic in this study included lumbar scoliotic Cobb angle, lumbar lordosis, rotation of the apical lumbar vertebrae, and sacral inclination.

The cause-and-effect relationship of low back pain and scoliosis in the lumbar spine is not well defined (59, 60, 70). In the Weinstein study, there were no findings of increased incidence of thoracic pain as compared to curve magnitude (69). Kostuik and Bentivoglio noted an increase in incidence of low back pain in 59% of their 189 patients with scoliosis diagnosed on intravenous pyelogram (33). When these patients were matched for age, sex, and occupation with 100 patients without scoliosis, however, the incidence of pain was found to be the same in both populations. Of those patients who had pain, 44% had mild episodes, 49% moderate pain, and 7% had severe pain. The correlation with age was similar, with the maximum severity appearing between the ages of 40 and 60 years. The authors did explain that in patients who had curves greater than 45° in the lumbar spine there was statistically a more significant degree of incapacitating pain than in those who had curves less than 45° or in subjects in the control group.

Cochran et al. have defined the risk of low back pain in patients who have had surgery for idiopathic scoliosis with fusion into their lumbar spine (10). For patients who had a fusion ending at L2 or L3, the incidence of low back pain was no different from that in a control population. For patients who had a fusion ending at L4, the level of low back pain was increased.

Diagnosis

For the adult patient with an adolescent curve pattern that arose before skeletal maturity, the history is the most important aspect of the overall evaluation. The first area of inquiry includes a history of all previous treatment. When was the diagnosis made? What was the Cobb angle, and what were the end vertebrae at the time of initial assessment? Did the curve progress during adolescence, and if so, to what level? Was observation, bracing, or surgery ever recommended to the patient? Most of the patients who are currently in their 40s or 50s would have been told by their physician at the age of 19 years that there was little or no chance of their scoliosis ever progressing because at that time it was thought that progression did not occur in adults.

A history of curve progression can be ascertained from the patient or from those people who have been in contact with the patient frequently over the past several years. Questions for the patient concerning progression should include: Do you feel that you're leaning more to one side? Do you feel you are losing your waistline on one side, or that your hip is becoming more prominent on one side? Do you feel that you have become shorter? How tall were you when you graduated from high school in comparison with your current height? Does it seem that you've become fatter without an increase in weight? Do you have to hem your clothes differently or have you had to have them adjusted because you felt that one leg was becoming longer than the other? Often patients complain of increased fatigue because they must expend more energy in their attempt to stand without decompensation. Serial x-ray films should be obtained and will tell this story with more precision than historical data.

A history of back pain is frequently elicited, and the examiner must be precise in the definition of location and intensity. Does the pain originate at the lumbosacral junction, iliac crests, sacroiliac joints, or distal sacrum? Or is the pain associated with a thoracolumbar prominence, rib hump, thoracic or thoracolumbar spine in the midline? How often does the pain occur and how severe is it? What medication is required to obtain some relief from the pain? Is the patient able to work when the pain occurs? If not, how many days have been missed from work because of the pain?

Pain occurring in the region of the lumbar spine may also be referred to the posterior buttocks or to the proximal half of the posterior or lateral thigh. True radicular pain may be defined as any pain radiating below the knee or pain radiating into the anterior thigh. Adult patients with scoliosis frequently present with an L3, L4, or L5 radiculopathy related to the concavity of a lumbar curve or to the concavity of the compensatory lumbosacral curve. The examiner must be extremely precise in the definition of the feeling of numbness or sharpness of the pain. How far can the patient walk before the symptoms become severe? Is the pain made better with rest and worse with activity? Does extension of the lumbar spine increase the symptoms? A pain questionnaire is a valuable adjunct in evaluating the condition of patients who have either back pain, radicular pain, or both.

Pulmonary function should be evaluated in all patients who have thoracic or thoracolumbar curves. All patients should be asked whether they have had increasing shortness of breath during periods of exertion such as climbing stairs or aerobic exercise. Certainly a history of asthma should be ruled out. In patients who have congenital or neuromuscular curves, this type of problem is much more common, but pulmonary dysfunction has been documented in patients who have thoracic curves greater than 60° (31). Patients who have significant thoracic or thoracolumbar lordosis and an early onset of idiopathic scoliosis are also at high risk for pulmonary compromise. Pulmonary function tests are recommended for any patient with a history of shortness of breath that has been increasing, with thoracic curvatures greater than 60°, with congenital or paralytic scoliosis, or with concomitant pulmonary disease such as asthma or asbestosis.

One final assessment that should be made for every patient is a psychological one. While many patients have learned to live with their deformity, there may be significant life circumstances such as a divorce or a new job that have brought the patient to focus on his or her spine again. Indeed, there may be no change in the patient's spine, but because the patient has had a significant alteration in lifestyle, the issue of the spinal deformity has resurfaced. Also, patients may be afflicted with depression, which may be caused by a multitude of factors. Some assessment must be made of the patient's general feeling of well-being. For many patients, increasing back pain may be a sign of increasing depression, and back pain may be improved simply by treating the depression.

The physical examination of the patient with adult scoliosis focuses on several areas. Careful palpation of the entire spine and pelvis must be performed to determine whether there are any tender areas over the rib hump, thoracolumbar prominence, individual spinous processes of the entire thoracolumbar spine, iliolumbar ligament, sacroiliac joint, sciatic notch, lateral iliac crests, and greater trochanters. Often percussion of the spine is extremely helpful when trying to identify a painful segment.

Spinal alignment and deformity are defined in several ways. A plumb line is used to determine the position of the C7 spinous process with respect to the gluteal cleft. In the standing position, the relative heights of the shoulders and iliac crests are measured. Also in the standing position, the degree of rotatory malalignment is noted by measuring any asymmetry of the shoulders in the sagittal plane. The patient is asked to bend forward, and the examiner must view the spine from four different directions. The location of a thoracic rib prominence and any lumbar asymmetry are noted with respect to level and angulation. In the standing position, lateral bending is performed by the examiner to determine how supple the curvatures are and to determine if pain is elicited or reproduced with forced side bending. Any degree of loss of lumbar lordosis or hip or knee flexion in the standing position should be noted.

A neurologic assessment of the lower extremity should be performed, with an evaluation of each spinal nerve from L3 to S1. In addition, any calf asymmetries, foot deformities, or hyperreflexia should be noted. These findings are more likely to be abnormal in patients who have unusual curve patterns such as left thoracic "idiopathic" curves.

Any areas of abnormal skin pigmentation, dimpling, or hair distribution should be noted. Patients who have ocular abnormalities, high arched palate, and/or hyperlaxity of the joints should be examined further for connective tissue disorder.

The roentgenographic assessment of patients who have any coronal deformity with a Cobb angle greater than 10° should include a 36-inch cassette posteroanterior and lateral view to evaluate the entire thoracolumbar spine in the standing position. Only with these views can one ascertain completely the degree of deformity as measured by Cobb angle in the standing position and the degree of decompensation in both the coronal and sagittal planes. Spot anteroposterior and lateral films of the lumbar spine in the supine position should be taken for any patient who has a lumbar spinal deformity. In adult patients supine films provide more specific assessment of enlarged or subluxated facets, disc narrowing or sclerosis, or subtle congenital anomalies. Spondylolysis or spondylolisthesis should be ruled out in all patients.

Bending films are usually not recommended unless surgery is being considered. At our center bending films are usually taken in the supine position. Traction films may be of value to determine whether distraction produces decompensation. In any patient with a kyphotic deformity, the lateral hyperextension view is mandatory. In patients who have degenerative disease of the lumbar spine, flexion/extension views in the lateral decubitus position are necessary to rule out subtle degrees of instability that may affect the lower limit of fusion.

For the assessment of low back pain or radiculopathy, magnetic resonance imaging has been extremely helpful in ruling out tumor or infection. Great care must be taken in the diagnosis of herniated disc because of the three-dimensional complexity of the scoliotic curvature. Myelography and postmyelogram computed axial tomography may be necessary to define the exact position of spinal nerve compression. A bone scan may be helpful in younger patients who have a mild painful curve to rule out osteoid osteoma or other tumor. Discography may be used to assess pain levels in patients with scoliosis when fusion is being considered (32). Grubb et al.

demonstrated that discs that were painful on discography in patients with adult scoliosis would frequently not be considered for fusion using traditional methods for deciding the lower limits of fusion (23–25). It was Grubb's recommendation that discography be performed for patients who have painful scoliosis so that the scoliosis fusion levels would not be too short.

Indications for Surgery

The indications for surgery in adult patients who have thoracic scoliosis include: curve progression; back pain in the area of the spinal curvature unresponsive to nonoperative care; progressive respiratory decompensation in patients who have no history of concomitant respiratory disorder; and progressive loss of neurologic function and muscle fatigue due to increased decompensation in the coronal or sagittal plane (8, 14, 28, 35, 36, 49, 53, 64, 66). Patients at our center who have had more than 10° of documented progression of a thoracic curve are considered for spinal stabilization. These patients may also have increased fatigue due to muscle imbalance associated with coronal or sagittal plane decompensation. Patients who have significant axial pain in the area of their scoliosis and who have a curvature greater than 60° may be assisted by spinal stabilization. Patients in this category can expect an 80 to 85% chance of improvement of their pain, but they must be cautioned that there is a 15 to 25% chance that their back pain will be no better after thoracic fusion surgery. Patients who have rotatory and lateral olisthesis, localized pain, and decompensation may be assisted by fusion surgery.

The patients with thoracic scoliosis who require surgery have a posterior operation only for scoliosis less than 70° and kyphosis less than 55–60°. If a patient has either kyphosis greater than 55–60° or scoliosis greater than 70–75°, an anterior fusion is added to the surgical regimen of posterior fusion and instrumentation. If patients have a single degenerative disc that is locally tender or a compression fracture from osteopenia producing a local kyphosis that is tender, then anterior surgery may also be performed at the same sitting as the posterior surgery.

Patients who have progression of lumbar curve with associated coronal plane decompensation have a high risk of future disability and increasing back pain. In the thoracolumbar and lumbar spine the indications for surgery are similar, but there is a much higher incidence of axial pain that may or may not be associated with the scoliosis. As has been mentioned, discography may be very helpful in this patient group to determine fusion levels.

If decompression surgery is contemplated for a patient who has idiopathic scoliosis, and decompression is planned for an area near the apex of the patient's lumbar curvature, then consideration must be given to a fusion of the curve that will stabilize the spine and prevent future progression. Lumbar decompressive surgery in the apex of a lumbar curve carries a high risk of producing progression if the curve is not stabilized concomitantly. Low back pain may be caused by degenerative disc disease of the lumbosacral junction in an area where there is no significant curvature. Occasionally the lumbosacral junction may have a compensatory curvature that may be associated with foraminal stenosis and radiculopathy. In these circumstances, foraminotomy and fusion at the lumbosacral junction may be indicated.

Surgical Treatment

How Adult Scoliosis Surgery Differs From Adolescent Scoliosis Surgery

The first major issue that must be addressed in the adult patient is osteopenia. The adult spine, especially in females, is subjected to the continuous loss of bone mineral content in all parts of the thoracic and lumbar vertebrae, including the vertebral body, pedicles, lamina, facet joints, and transverse and spinous processes. Subsequently, when the surgeon applies a force through a hook or wire there is less mass per unit or area to dissipate the force of fixation to the spinal column at the bone-metal interface. Significant problems that may occur because of osteopenia include fracture of the bone at the metal-vertebra interface and compression fractures of the end vertebrae from force concentration at the end vertebrae. The force concentration is enhanced with increasing rigidity in the implant that is used.

To neutralize this effect the surgeon may consider multiple strategies to achieve a well-fixed surgical construct. The first general principle is to increase the surface area of force application at the bone-metal interface. Implants that use wire fixation at the spinous processes have a higher risk of loss of fixation in adults than in adolescents. An implant that employs multiple hooks or screws places less force per unit of area at the bone-metal interface than a construct that uses only a few hooks and interspinous wires. In adults sublaminar wire fixation is usually more effective than interspinous wire fixation. If the spinal implant system uses primarily hooks for fixation, then additional hooks must be added in adults who have a curved pattern similar to one of the more common adolescent forms. Because the forces are greatest at the ends of the surgical construct, it is usually more efficacious to add additional hooks in these areas.

If the deformities are in the lumbar spine, consideration may be given to fixation with pedicle screws. At this point we have not used pedicle screw fixation in this area of the spine for adults with thoracic scoliosis.

The risk of posterior element fracture in the intraoperative, perioperative, and postoperative periods is much higher in adults than in adolescents because of osteopenia. Care must be taken that end vertebrae not rely on transverse process fixation for ultimate maintenance of correction. For adults with idiopathic scoliosis we have used a closed thoracic laminar hook for upper-level fixation on the convex side of the curvature; we have not had problems with laminar fracture of this hook. Also in patients with osteopenia for whom significant correction is achieved, bracing after surgery for a period of 3 to 5 months is strongly recommended.

The second major factor that must be addressed in comparing adult to adolescent curvatures is the stiffness of the adult spine. Loss of disc hydration with concomitant disc degeneration, loss of water content of the ligamentous and tendinous structures about the spine, and weakening of the tendon-bone and ligament-bone attachments all contribute to an increasing mechanical stiffness of the thoracolumbar spine. All of these factors contribute to the fact that the correction that can be achieved in the adult is usually considerably less than in an adolescent. The correction rate for right thoracic curves in adolescents may be between 70 and 90%, but the rate for patients in their fourth, fifth, or sixth decade of life may be 35 to 50%. Patients' expectations may be extremely high in this regard, and care must be taken to educate them on the anticipated correction of their Cobb angle.

Because of differential stiffness of the spine, coronal plane balance is much more of a problem in adults than in adolescents. The first major factor that affects the result of coronal balance is the flexibility of the curvature construct. Bending and traction views are often helpful in determining the extent of correction that may be achieved. Though there still may be significant deviation of the apical vertebrae, ideally the end result will place both ends of the surgical construct within the Harrington stable zone. In most King type I and type II curves (30), right thoracic curve instrumentation will shift the thorax to the left to a variable degree from the preoperative situation. Thus in adult patients who are decompensated to the right, the surgeon has an easier time of producing a more balanced coronal plane than in the patient who is initially decompensated to the left. This situation brings us to the second major factor that hinders achievement of coronal plane balance in adults, which is the ability of the lower lumbar spine to compensate for curve correction above it. In adolescents the fractional lumbosacral curve will usually be corrected to the point at which coronal plane balance is not a problem. However, with the disc degeneration, facet hypertrophy, and arthritis in adults, the lower lumbar spine is not as supple and hence will not be as receptive to thoracic and thoracolumbar curve correction. The surgeon may anticipate this problem with a review of right and left side bending films of the middle and lower lumbar spine. For the same reason, the surgeon must always take into account leg length discrepancy and pelvic obliquity since these factors are more important in adults than in adolescents.

Sagittal plane considerations are equally crucial when comparing the adult to the adolescent patient. Fusion in adolescents may frequently be performed to the L4 level with a primary distractive force. The L4–5 and L5-S1 discs, the hip capsules, and the ligaments of the pelvis are supple and allow for a sagittally balanced spine despite fixation in distraction to L4. It is extremely unusual that the adult patient will tolerate a primary distractive force down to the L4 or L5 level. At this point it is safe to say that distraction as a primary corrective force in the lumbar spine is contraindicated in the adult patient. Thus, with thoracic correction, primary distraction can be used safely to the L1 or L2 level, but at the L3 level a compression force is usually used. The Cotrel-Dubousset or similar device is ideal for this purpose, as distraction and compression can be carried out as primary fixation modes on the same rod.

Another sagittal plane problem that may develop in adults is kyphotic deformity above the level of the fused segment, particularly if the fusion stops at the apex of the curve. This problem frequently occurs in the T8 to T11 region. Such a complication is rare in the adolescent.

Management of Thoracic Curves

Surgery for adult scoliosis requires an instrumentation system that allows for maximum versatility in determining points of fixation and in the application of force to achieve correction. The Cotrel-Dubousset device has revolutionized the ability to achieve both correction and fixation (13). This surgical principle is much more necessary in adult surgery, in which interspinous wiring will not provide reliable fixation.

For King type III right thoracic curves the choice of end vertebrae should result in the ends of the fusion lying in the Harrington stable zone (Figure 23.1). Bending films are helpful in analyzing which vertebrae will lie within this column at the end of the surgical procedure. Lateral films should also be examined to determine the amount of kyphosis; if focal kyphosis is determined at any level, then the instrumentation construct should be lengthened to span the entire kyphotic segment. The right side bending film is used to determine the position of intermediate

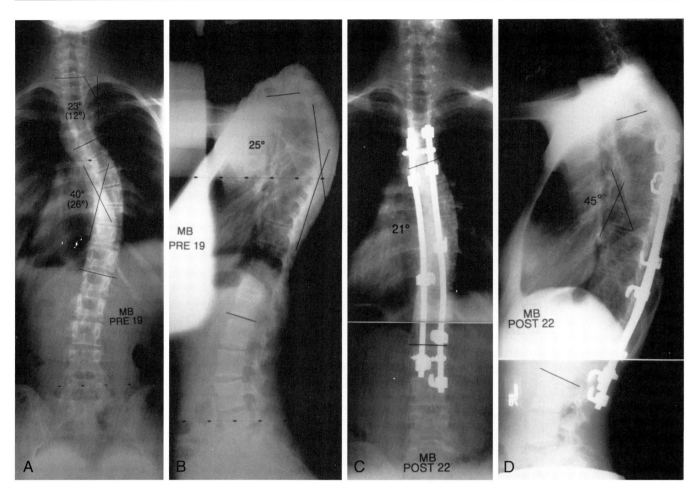

FIGURE 23.1.
This 20-year-old female demonstrated 15° progression of her thoracic curve between ages 17 and 20 years. Her curvature is a type III curve pattern, as her left upper thoracic curve was supple. Postoperative x-ray films at 1-year follow-up demonstrate maintenance of curve reduction and fixation. Shoulder levels are maintained equal by the supple thoracic upper curve.

hooks on the left-sided rod. Those discs that do not open appreciably and are the most rigid will be spanned by an open pedicle and open laminar hook, usually from four to five levels. If significant deviation of the apical vertebrae is seen, consideration may be given to extending the fusion with a small compression construct on the left-sided rod that is placed initially. A left-sided lower compression construct will serve to decrease the risk of junctional kyphosis and translate the thorax to the left side. After insertion of the left-sided rod, rotation of that rod is then considered. As has been mentioned previously, with significant arthritis and disc degeneration the amount of rotation that can be achieved in the adult patient is usually considerably less than in the adolescent; the total amount of rotation possible may be only 20° to 45°. The final hook seating is then achieved on the left-sided rod by distracting the intermediate hooks and then distracting the end vertebrae hooks of the right thoracic curve. The last seated hook on the left-sided rod is in a compression mode if required in the lower thoracic or thoracolumbar segment. The right-sided rod is placed in a classic Cotrel-Dubousset configuration with substitution of a closed thoracic laminar hook down going at the superior aspect of the right-sided rod (58).

For right thoracic left lumbar or right thoracic thoracolumbar curve patterns the Cotrel-Dubousset or similar segmental instrumentation is most efficacious. While distracting in the thoracic spine to achieve correction of the scoliosis and to lengthen the posterior elements of a hypokyphotic segment, the same rod may be used to compress the convexity of a lumbar curve, producing curve correction and simultaneously shortening the posterior elements to increase lumbar lordosis. The end vertebrae for the left-sided rod in the thoracic spine are usually similar to those for a type III curve. Lower hooks are chosen for the lumbar spine to achieve coronal balance and end vertebrae within the Harrington stable zone.

Again, the left-sided rod is always inserted first, with the goal of achieving sagittal plane contour and rotation in order to produce simultaneous posterior column lengthening of the thoracic curve and posterior column shortening of the left lumbar or thoracolumbar curve. After rod rotation, apical compression of the thoracolumbar curve is carried out, followed by distraction of the thoracic curve.

For King type II curves in which there is significant flexibility in the lower lumbar segment, Shufflebarger has recommended partial instrumentation and fusion of the flexible lumbar curve (58). This pattern is a variation in which partial compression is carried out on the lower aspect of the left-sided rod. Often the end vertebrae can be brought into Harrington's stable zone by only partially correcting the lumbar curve.

The surgeon must carefully examine the shoulder levels for each patient with a King type V curve pattern and be very wary when the patient's left shoulder is higher than the right. A distraction force on the left side of the patient's spine with a left shoulder that is already higher will lead to a disastrous result with shoulder imbalance. Careful examination of bending films in the upper thoracic region is necessary to determine how flexible this upper curve is. In most patients with this configuration, surgical reconstruction requires a temporarily placed right-sided concave distraction rod that is initially placed in the upper thoracic spine in an attempt to correct this curvature and elevate the right shoulder. The left-sided rod is then placed, with care being taken to add an upper compression construct on the convexity of the upper left thoracic curve. The patient must be warned that the shoulder asymmetry may not improve even after this procedure. The final surgical construct may include an incorporation of the upper right-sided rod in a three-rod construct or removal of the right upper thoracic rod and insertion of a longer rod to include the entire construct.

Right thoracic curves that are greater than 85° to 100° frequently require special rod constructs. Two separate rods may be utilized to achieve the function of the intermediate and end vertebral hooks on a less severely scoliotic right thoracic curve. Right side bending films in these cases usually demonstrate five or six segments that are rigid. A short concave rod with closed pedicle and laminar hooks at each end is used to achieve correction of the apical vertebrae. A second rod is then placed, with the end vertebrae chosen in routine fashion. Distraction is carried out on both rods in a sequential manner to achieve maximum correction. The rods are then connected with transverse loading devices, and a right-sided neutralization rod may be inserted.

In general, any patient with kyphosis greater than 55° in the thoracic spine requires an anterior release and fusion. For adult patients the principles of kyphosis surgery take precedence over a purely coronal plane operation. That is, the sagittal plane in these patients is much more important than the coronal plane, both in correction and in maintenance of stabilization. For patients who have significant kyphosis, consideration should be given to insertion of the right-sided convex rod first. Multiple fixation points are chosen to achieve posterior column shortening with compression that is done on the convex side of the curvature to simultaneously produce scoliosis reduction. The surgeon must remember that the correction of coronal plane problems with a compression construct will achieve less correction per unit of force in the coronal plane than a corresponding distraction force. The compression force must have at least two to three fixation points on either side of the apex of the kyphosis.

Management of Lumbar Curves

Segmental fixation for adult lumbar scoliosis is used in two groups of patients. The first group comprises patients who have significant thoracolumbar or lumbar curves and have suffered progression of their curvature, increased decompensation, or increased pain. The second group comprises patients with degenerative scoliosis producing primarily sciatica. In the first group instrumentation is used to correct deformity and provide stability in a partially corrected position. The critical issues are lordosis maintenance, coronal plane balance, and consideration of loss of anterior middle column height due to disc degeneration.

In patients with thoracolumbar curvature, hook fixation sites may be used to provide compression on one side of the curve to correct both the sagittal and coronal planes. In general, this compression force allows correction of coronal plane deformity when the force is applied to the convexity of the scoliosis curve pattern. When using hook or vertebral body screw fixation in the lumbar spine, distraction as an initial force is almost never used. Distraction force in the lumbar spine will only produce increased lumbar kyphosis. Rod rotation maneuver from the concave side of the lumbar curvature will also help to correct the scoliotic deformity and enhance lumbar lordosis. If sublaminar wires are used in addition to the hooks, they should be placed in the concave side of the curvature to help in derotating the lumbar vertebrae. In adult patients a minimum of one fixation site for each lumbar vertebra attached to a thoracolumbar fusion is mandatory. For curvatures extending to the L3 or L4 level, the number of fixation sites may include a vertebral body screw and a hook (Fig. 23.2).

In patients who have degenerative lumbar scoliosis and require surgery because of sciatica, the option

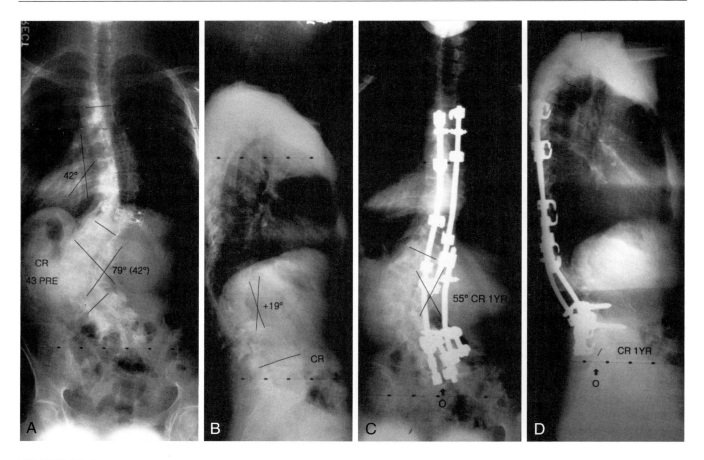

FIGURE 23.2.

A–D. This 43-year-old female has a 5-year history of progressive shortening decompensation to the left and forward flexion deformity. Over a course of 10 years she has noted gradually increasing pain at the thoracolumbar junction. Postoperative x-ray films at 1-year follow-up demonstrate improved balance in both the coronal and sagittal planes. Vertebral body screws were used to stabilize the last segment, where fusion was attempted at L4–5.

of hook utilization is usually not present. In patients who do not have significant problems with coronal or sagittal plane balance, fixation and fusion of the lumbar spine may be confined to only those areas where decompressive surgery has been performed. Vertebral body screw instrumentation may be utilized to achieve partial correction of coronal Cobb angle deformity. In patients who have significant local kyphosis or who have a loss of sagittal balance on standing, lateral 36-inch cassette film analysis should be performed in considering the insertion of structural grafts to increase anterior column height and to improve sagittal balance and decrease stress on the vertebral screw rod construct.

Long Fusions to the Sacrum

The fusion of the pediatric or adult patient spine to the sacrum is fraught with significant technical difficulties and has an increased surgical complication rate (34, 61). However, the advent of new instrumentation systems has made fixation to the sacrum easier with the use of segmental fixation to the iliac wings. This represents significant advances from Luque's original technique for sacropelvic fixation using L-rods, sublaminar wiring to the S1 lamina, and spearing of the cortices of the posterior ileum with a simple 90° lateral bend of the inferior end of the rod (14).

The Galveston technique developed by Allen and Ferguson for neuromuscular spinal deformities represented a significant advance in iliac fixation (2). The tip of the iliac rod ending anterior to the axis of rotation and flexion extension provides a more stable buttress to hold the spine to the pelvis. This system, as with all current fixation systems utilizing iliac fixation, rests in instrumenting but not fusing across the sacroiliac joint. This remains a theoretical disadvantage, as the "windshield-washer" phenomenon has not become clinically significant. Early reports of fusion to the sacrum utilizing Harrington fixation showed very poor clinical results with unacceptably high complication rates and unsatisfactory functional results (15).

It has become well understood that fusion to the sacrum is improved with a combined anterior and posterior approach to lessen the pseudarthrosis rate and with the use of multisegmental fixation, which often includes pedicle screws in addition to Galveston-type fixation across the pelvis into the iliac wings. The standard instrumentation montage to the sacrum now includes anterior structural allograft for at least the lowest two interspaces (L4–5 and L5-S1) to enhance lumbar lordosis and open the disc space, and pedicle screw fixation posteriorly with Galveston outriggers connected with I-bolt connectors for TSRH (Texas Scottish Rite Hospital) instrumentation, domino connectors for Cotrel-Dubousset instrumentation, and I-rod connectors for Isola iliac screws (Fig. 23.3) (48).

The use of pedicle fixation alone to the sacrum with augmentation has led in the past to very high instrumentation and fusion failure, the inability to balance the plane deformity, and a relatively poor functional outcome, according to the report of Devlin et al. (15). Before the advent of segmental pedicle screw fixation with the domino Galveston-type montage, Saer, Winter, and Lonstein reported an improved fusion rate and a lower instrumentation failure rate using the Luque-Galveston fixation method in adults in whom fusion to the sacrum was performed (55). The technique of Luque-Galveston fixation using Luque wires and/or dominoed Cotrel-Dubousset rods is well-described elsewhere (40).

It is important when harvesting a graft during this procedure that care is taken not to harvest from the thickest part of the ileum, where standard grafting procedures are often performed. This is the best part of the bone for insertion of Galveston-type fixation and should be preserved as such. In long fusions to the sacrum it is usually necessary to supplement autograft bone with some allograft.

Postoperative bracing is not necessary when a Galveston technique is used if segmental fixation is obtained and bone purchase is good. When bone stock is poor or inadequate pelvic fixation is obtained, custom-molded thoraco-lumbar-sacral orthoses with leg extension are necessary as an adjunct to the internal fixation. We generally recommend full-time brace wear (23 of 24 hours per day), with careful attention paid to the skin. Bracing is only used in adults who are severely osteopenic or if bilateral Galveston fixation is not possible secondary to prior graft harvesting. In these cases the leg extension brace is placed on the extremity without the iliac rod. The duration of bracing depends on the appearance of the fusion but is usually a minimum of 3 months.

Thoracoplasty

The rib prominence that is usually on the right side in patients with thoracic curves is dependent on many variables. Of course curve magnitude is directly related to chest wall deformity and makes the right side of the chest more prominent. Vertebral body rotation will enhance the posterior projection of the thoracic ribs at the apex of the curve. Many patients with severe curves have a smaller absolute thoracic rib cage volume, and their prominence may be less apparent.

Measurement of the thoracic prominence has been detailed by numerous authors. On forward bending, one can measure the difference between the most prominent or posteriorly projecting aspect of the ribs and its counterpart on the opposite side. Another way to estimate the degree of deformity is to use an inclinometer to measure the angle formed by the chest cage with the patient bending forward 90°. Patients may mention their rib prominence for a number of reasons. For most patients, there is some difficulty with clothing and with the alterations that are necessary to make the clothing appear more normal. Many patients will frankly admit that they consider the posterior prominence of the thoracic rib cage unsightly, and they are very conscious of the presumed negative image they project. For other patients, the prominence may be painful during activities that require an upright position or when the rib prominence is in contact with a hard surface.

The primary considerations for thoracoplasty in patients with significant prominence include cosmetic result, additional fusion mass, and diminished pain at the site of the prominence. Of these factors, the major advantage for the patient is the additional amount of autologous bone that could be added to the thoracic fusion bed. However, most patients are highly satisfied with the diminution of the posteriorly projecting ribs. If there is pain associated with the thoracic prominence, this symptom may be diminished with removal of the ribs. For most rib resection surgeries our technique involves a separate incision at the posterior axillary line. The muscle fibers of the latissimus dorsi muscle are usually sectioned longitudinally with cautery to expose the rib prominences. Subperiosteal dissection is carried out along each rib that is prominent from the transverse process of the thoracic vertebrae to the midaxillary line. The rib is then sectioned and removed. Each rib is then divided into small strips and placed into the fusion bed. Usually four to six ribs are removed in the area of greatest rotation. If an anterior thoracotomy has been performed before the posterior surgery and rib resection, care must be taken that the incision for the thoracotomy does not intersect the incision for the thoracoplasty, as a skin slough may occur in the angle between the two incisions. Once the ribs have been removed, the retractors are then taken out and any areas of prominence are palpated. Frequently there are rib edges that are left or prominent transverse processes that may be removed from either

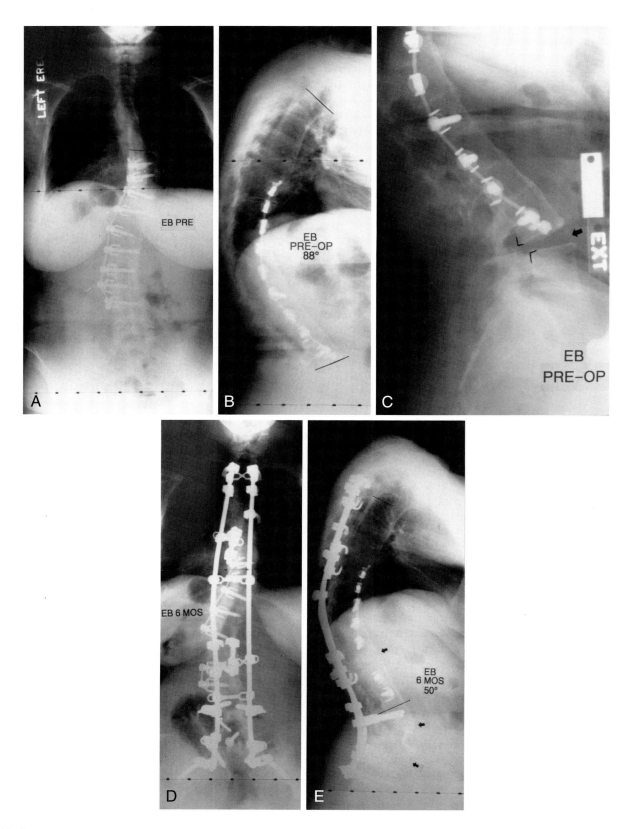

FIGURE 23.3.

A 35-year-old white female 20 years after anterior thoracolumbar fusion with a Dwyer device presents with severe low back and leg pain. A retrolisthesis is seen at L4–5 and significant kyphosis across the fusion area. Discography was positive at L4–5 and L5-S1. Anterior-posterior spinal osteotomy and fusion extension to the sacrum were carried out with structural grafting anteriorly and Galveston augmented fixation posteriorly. Good restoration of sagittal balance and relief of pain were obtained.

the thoracoplasty incision or the midline incision. In this way the surgeon can then sculpt the remaining bony edges to diminish any acute prominences. Other possible techniques include thoracoplasty from a thoracotomy approach and rib resection through a percutaneous trocar.

The complications of thoracoplasty in adult scoliosis are few. The most common problem is a pneumothorax that is produced acutely at the time of subperiosteal dissection of one of the ribs. If a thoracotomy has been performed for anterior discectomy and fusion through the right side of the chest, then a chest tube will already be in place on the right side, and this type of small puncture is not a significant problem. However, if anterior surgery has not been performed, then a chest tube should be inserted at the time that the surgeon notices a discontinuity of the parietal pleura. Lenke et al. have demonstrated that pulmonary function in these patients is significantly diminished both immediately after surgery and at 2-year follow-up (37). Thus in patients with severe deformity who have significantly diminished pulmonary function studies, thoracoplasty must be considered with great caution, as the procedure in itself produces significant loss of lung capacity.

Medical Complications of Scoliosis Surgery

Respiratory complications of scoliosis surgery in the adult can occur from either anterior or posterior surgery (6, 11, 22, 27, 44, 52, 65). These include atelectasis, pneumonia, pleural effusion, pneumothorax, chylothorax, hemothorax, acute respiratory distress syndrome, respiratory failure, pulmonary thromboembolism, and fat embolism.

Pneumothorax can occur during posterior surgery when dissection is carried out too aggressively in the intertransverse process area of the thoracic spine. Additionally, pointed retractors used in the thoracic spine can penetrate too deeply and injure the pleura, causing a pneumothorax. Treatment entails chest tube insertion and negative pressure suction. Knowledge of this complication and surveillance with a chest x-ray film examination is important. After anterior thoracotomy, all patients have a chest tube placed for anterior drainage to treat the pneumothorax that occurs with the incision of the parietal pleura. The chest tube is removed when drainage has decrease significantly and the residual pneumothorax is resolved. A chest film is always obtained after removing the chest tube. Chylothorax and/or chyloperitoneum can occur after an anterior approach to the thoracic or lumbar spine (11, 44, 51). These complications should be recognized at the time of surgery and the stump of the affected lymphatic duct ligated. The development of this kind of complication is difficult to treat postoperatively and often requires insertion of drainage catheters and potentially the use of sclerosing agents.

Pulmonary embolism is less common in spinal surgery than in pelvic and extremity surgery. We use antiembolism stockings and pneumatic compression hose at the time of anesthetic induction for prophylaxis. The diagnosis of pulmonary embolism requires prompt heparinization. In patients in whom anticoagulation therapy is contraindicated, the placement of a caval filter may be necessary.

Other postoperative pulmonary problems such as pneumonia or atelectasis are more frequent in patients who have anterior thoracotomies or thoracolumbotomies. The incidence of these complications can be decreased by ensuring that the lung is fully inflated after intercostal repair sutures have been placed and prior to the final closure of the chest after the anterior procedure. Additionally, aggressive postoperative pulmonary toilet with incentive spirometry and early mobilization when possible also help in preventing these pulmonary complications.

Postoperative ileus is relatively common following scoliosis surgery, particularly those surgeries requiring that the retroperitoneal space be violated. We routinely use nasogastric suction intra- and postoperatively in patients requiring anterior lumbar approaches. We do not discontinue nasogastric suction until the patients have active bowel sounds and/or have passed flatus. The slow readministration of oral feedings is undertaken postoperatively, narcotic use is kept to a minimum, and early mobilization and ambulation is encouraged when possible. All these interventions help to minimize the risk of prolonged ileus.

Ileus, which can be treated expectantly, should not be confused with true mechanical obstruction of the bowel. In the scoliosis patient who has undergone significant correction with instrumentation or casting, superior mesenteric artery syndrome should be thought of when symptoms of nausea and vomiting are present (3, 5, 7, 27, 56). This is caused by an obstruction of the third portion of the duodenum when the angle between the superior mesenteric artery and the aorta narrows and compresses that part of the bowel. Barium swallow radiological examination is diagnostic. Superior mesenteric artery syndrome usually can be successfully treated with nasogastric suction, placement in the left lateral decubitus position, and occasionally modification of a cast if necessary. Surgical intervention is only necessary if prolonged nonoperative treatment fails.

Acute cholecystitis should be entertained as a diagnosis when the postoperative scoliosis patient presents with acute abdominal pain in the right upper quadrant early in the postoperative period (18). Diagnosis is made with a cholecystogram or an abdominal ultrasound examination, and surgical intervention may be necessary.

Urinary retention and urinary tract infection is the most common medical complication for scoliosis patients in the postoperative period. Prolonged use of indwelling catheters or repeated instrumentation of the urinary tract increase the risk of this complication; additional prolonged recumbency and use of narcotics add to the risk. Prompt diagnosis with urinalysis and urine culture are necessary, and appropriate antibiotic treatment should be instituted. Hydronephrosis can be seen remotely after anterior surgery in the lumbar spine for scoliosis due to retroperitoneal fibrosis (9).

The syndrome of inappropriate antidiuretic hormone secretion (SIADH) has been reported following scoliosis fusion (4, 16). The patients present with hyponatremia, oliguria, and a very concentrated urine. Treatment involves fluid restriction.

Scoliosis surgery involves large exposures across the spine with multiple areas of exposed bone. This can lead to excessive blood loss requiring a significant transfusion. The scoliosis surgeon should be aware of the possibility of disseminated intravascular coagulation (DIC) as a causative factor of excessive bleeding (52). DIC is diagnosed on the basis of elevated prothrombin (PT), and partial thromboplastin time (PTT), thrombocytopenia, a low fibrinogen level, and high levels of fibrin split products. Rapid reinfusion of fresh frozen plasma, cryoprecipitate, platelets, and red blood cells is often necessary to treat DIC.

Viral infection with hepatitis B or C, human immunodeficiency virus, and cytomegalovirus are possible with a homologous transfusion of blood or blood products. We routinely have our patients predonate autologous blood for scoliosis surgery and utilize cell saver blood salvage intraoperatively. Meticulous surgical technique also helps in preventing excessive intraoperative blood loss.

The risk of retrograde ejaculation exists in an anterior lumbar procedure for scoliosis. This is a result of injury to the sympathetic plexus, which is usually a plexiform mesh of nerves or a single nerve in the presacral area running anterior to the aorta and coursing down into the pelvis over the bifurcation of the aorta. Injury to this plexus occurs most frequently during fusions of L5-S1. The sympathetic plexus is responsible for bladder neck closure during ejaculation. Failure of closure of the bladder neck causes the ejaculate to travel in a retrograde fashion into the bladder. Fusion at L5-S1 should be done with careful predissection bluntly over the discs utilizing Kittner dissectors and avoidance of electrocautery at this level. Retrograde ejaculation is rare and almost always corrects over time. However, male patients should be warned about this complication preoperatively if they are to undergo anterior lumbar fusions.

Outcome Studies

The field of medical outcomes assessment has gained increasing popularity in recent years (19, 29, 38, 46). These studies concentrate on the centrality of the patients in determining their own outcome from our medical interventions. These studies have been pioneered by the medical community but are now being pursued in other fields such as orthopaedics and spinal surgery. One of the principle tools used in this type of study is the Medical Outcome Study (MOS) Short-Form 36 (SF-36). This outcome instrument has been studied extensively and has been shown to be reliable, valid, and a statistically sound measure of function status, that is, well-being and general health perception (17, 20, 21, 39, 41, 62, 63, 68). This outcome form is generic and therefore allows comparison between different disease states and/or interventions. We have used this form to assess the outcome of adult scoliosis fusion in our patient population.

In 1991 we began a prospective study using the SF-36 (1). Of 68 adult deformity patients, we obtained full follow-up with preoperative and postoperative SF-36 scores for analysis in 55 patients (81% retrieval). The mean age of the patient population was 37.1 years, the group was predominately female (85.3%); and we obtained an average follow-up of 22.5 months. One-quarter of the patients had revision surgery, and 75% were primary adult deformity patients. Nine percent of the patients were kyphotic, and the remainder were purely scoliotic. Fusion was performed in 67.6% of the patients for pain and progression, in 16.2% primarily for pain, and in 16.2% for progression only. Fusion was to L4 or L4 in 29 of the 55 respondents, and to more cranial levels in the remaining 26. Twenty-nine patients were less than 40 years of age, and 26 were greater than 40 years.

The SF-36 has nine separate outcome scores within it, each graded on a 0 to 100 scale in which higher scores represent better functional outcome or less pain (68). Significant improvements were seen in physical functioning, social functioning, pain, and perceived health change.

This study demonstrated that adult scoliosis fusion is useful and beneficial to patients in terms of a generic outcome measure, with four of the nine outcome measures in the SF-36 significantly improving. We also compared outcomes of scoliosis patients with those of patients undergoing primary total hip or knee arthroplasty as well as primary lumbar laminectomy for radiculopathy due to herniated discs. For this comparison, we used only primary adult scoliosis fusion patients. Using a complex statistical analysis and both parametric and nonparametric models, we found total hip arthroplasty and laminectomy to show greater improvements for patients in the pain, energy, and social functioning variables of the SF-36 than scoliosis patients. Total knee arthroplasty patients also had significantly improved pain scores in comparison to the scoliosis patients. These analyses controlled for age, sex, and preoperative SF-36 scores between the groups, which affected the postoperative SF-36 score. This study did point out that the SF-36 may not be the best instrument for measuring the outcome of adult scoliosis fusion; the SF-36 places a high premium on pain relief and restoration of function, which are primary goals of total joint arthroplasty and laminectomy for severe radiculopathy. There is no measure in the SF-36 score that awards points for the prophylactic effect of halting progression with a successful scoliosis fusion or for the added prophylactic pulmonary benefits that scoliosis fusion provides. It is clear that as we continue to improve our assessment techniques for medical interventions and use these techniques to assess the outcomes of adult scoliosis fusion, we must create disease-specific and sensitive instruments that take into account the known benefits of scoliosis surgery.

References

1. Albert TJ, Purtill J, Mesa J, et al. Health outcome assessment before and after adult deformity surgery: a prospective study. Spine 1995;20(18):2002–2004.
2. Allen BL, Ferguson RL. L-rod instrumentation for scoliosis in cerebral palsy. J Pediatr Orthop 1982;2:87–96.
3. Barner HB, Sherman DC. Vascular compression of the duodenum. Surg Gynecol Obstet 1963;117:103.
4. Bell GR, Gurd AR, Orlowski JP, et al. The syndrome of inappropriate anti-diuretic hormone secretion following spinal fusion. J Bone Joint Surg 1986;68A:720–724.
5. Bisla RS, Louis HJ. Acute vascular compression of the duodenum following cast application. Surg Gynecol Obstet 1975;140:563–566.
6. Brown LP, Stelling FH. Fat embolism as a complication of scoliosis fusion. J Bone Joint Surg 1974;56A:1764.
7. Bunch W, Delaney J. Scoliosis and acute vascular compression of the duodenum. Surgery 1970;67:901.
8. Byrd JA III, Scoles PV, Winter RB, et al. Adult idiopathic scoliosis treated by anterior and posterior spinal fusion. J Bone Joint Surg 1987;69A:843–850.
9. Cleveland RH, Gilsanz V, Labowitz RL, et al. Hydronephrosis from retroperitoneal fibrosis and anterior spinal fusion. J Bone Joint Surg 1978;60A:996.
10. Cochran T, Irstram L, Nachemson A. Long-term anatomic and functional changes in patients with adolescent idiopathic scoliosis treated by Harrington rod fusion. Spine 1983;8:576–584.
11. Colletta AJ, Mayer PJ. Chylothorax: an unusual complication of anterior thoracic interbodies spinal fusion. Spine 1982;7:46–49.
12. Collis DK, Ponseti IV. Long-term follow-up of patients with idiopathic scoliosis not treated surgically. J Bone Joint Surg 1969;51A:425–445.
13. Cotrel Y, Dubousset J, Guillaumat M. New universal instrumentation in spinal surgery. Clin Orthop 1988;227:10–23.
14. Dawson EG, Caron A, Moe JH. Surgical management of scoliosis in the adult. J Bone Joint Surg 1973;61A:1151–1161.
15. Devlin VJ, Boachie-Adjei O, Bradford DS, et al. Treatment of adult spinal deformity with fusion to the sacrum using CD instrumentation. J Spinal Disord 1991;4:1–14.
16. Elster AD. Hyponatremia after spinal fusion caused by inappropriate secretion of anti-diuretic hormone (SIADH). Clin Orthop 1985;194:136–141.
17. Feinstein AR, Josephy BR, Wells CK. Scientific and clinical problems in indexes of functional disability. Ann Intern Med 1986;105:159–160.
18. Floman Y, Micheli LJ, Barker WD, et al. Acute cholecystitis following the surgical treatment of spinal deformities in the adult. Clin Orthop 1980;151:205–209.
19. Fossel AH, Roberts WN, Sledge CB. Cost-effectiveness of total joint arthroplasty in osteoarthritis. Arthritis Rheum 1986;29(8):937–943.
20. Fries JF, Spitz P, Kraines RG, et al. Measurement of patient outcome in arthritis. Arthritis Rheum 1980;23(2):137–145.
21. Geigle R, Jones SB. Outcomes management: a report from the front. Inquiry 1990;27:7.
22. Gittman JE, Buchaman TA, Fisher BJ, et al. Fatal fat embolism after spinal fusion for scoliosis. JAMA 1983;249:779–781.
23. Grubb SA, Lipscomb HJ, Suh PB. Results of surgical treatment of painful adult scoliosis. Spine 1994;19:1619–1627.
24. Grubb SA, Lipscomb HJ. Diagnostic findings in painful adult scoliosis. Spine 1992;17:518–527.
25. Grubb SA, Lipscomb HJ, Coonrad RW. Degenerative adult onset scoliosis. Spine 1988;13:241–245.
26. Harrington PR, Dickson JH. An eleven-year clinical investigation of Harrington instrumentation: a preliminary report on 578 cases. Clin Orthop 1973;93:113–130.
27. Hughes JP, McEntire JD, Setze TK. Cast syndrome. Arch Surg 1974;108:230.
28. Johnson JR, Holt RT. Combined use of anterior and posterior surgery for adult scoliosis. Orthop Clin North Am 1988;19:361–370.
29. Katz ME, Harris WJ, Levitsky K, et al. Methods for assessing condition-specific and generic functional status outcomes after total knee replacement. Medical Care 1992;30(5):240–252.
30. King HA, Moe JH, Bradford DS, et al. The selection of fusion levels in thoracic idiopathic scoliosis. J Bone Joint Surg 1983;65A:1302–1313.
31. Korovessis P, Piperos G, Sidiropoulos P, et al. Adult idiopathic lumbar scoliosis. Spine 1994;19:1926–1932.
32. Kostuik JP. Decision-making in adult scoliosis. Spine 1979;4:521–525.
33. Kostuik JP, Bentivoglio J. The incidence of low back pain in adult scoliosis. Spine 1981;6:268–273.
34. Kostuik JP, Hall BB. Spinal fusions to the sacrum in adults with scoliosis. Spine 1983;8:489–500.

35. Kostuik JP, Israel J, Hall JE. Scoliosis surgery in adults. Clin Orthop 1973;93:225–234.
36. Kostuik JP. Recent advances in the treatment of painful adult scoliosis. Clin Orthop 1980;147:238–252.
37. Lenke LG, Bridwell KH, Blanke K, et al. Analysis of pulmonary function and chest cage dimension changes following thoracoplasty in idiopathic scoliosis. Spine 1995;20:1343–1350.
38. Liang MH, Katz JN, Phillips C, et al. The American Academy of Orthopaedic Surgeons Task Force on Outcome Studies. J Bone Joint Surg 1991;73A:639–646.
39. Liang MH, Larson MG, Cullen KE, et al. Comparative measurement efficiency and sensitivity of five health status instruments for arthritis research. Arthritis Rheum 1985;28:542–547.
40. Lonstein JE. The Galveston technique using Luque or Cotrel-Dubousset rods. Orthop Clin North Am 1994;25(2):311–321.
41. Luque ER, Carduso A. Treatment of scoliosis without arthrodesis or external support. Orthop Trans 1977;1:37.
42. Nachemson A. A long-term follow-up study of non-treated scoliosis. Acta Orthop Scand 1983;39:489–500.
43. Nachemson A. Adult scoliosis and back pain. Spine 1979;4:513–517.
44. Nakai S, Zielke K. Chylothorax: a rare complication after anterior and posterior spinal correction (a report of six cases). Spine 1986;11:830–833.
45. Nilsonne U, Lundgren KD. Long-term prognosis in idiopathic scoliosis. Acta Orthop Scand 1968;39:455–465.
46. O'Boyle CA. Assessment of quality of life in surgery. Br J Surg 1992;79:395–398.
47. Perennou D, Marcelli C, Herisson C, et al. Adult lumbar scoliosis. Spine 1994;19:123–128.
48. Perra JH. Techniques of instrumentation in long fusions to the sacrum. Orthop Clin North Am 1994;25(2):287–300.
49. Ponder RC, Dickson JH, Harrington PR, et al. Results of Harrington instrumentation and fusion in the adult idiopathic scoliosis patient. J Bone Joint Surg 1975;57A:797–801.
50. Pritchett JW, Bortel DT. Degenerative symptomatic lumbar scoliosis. Spine 1993;18:700–703.
51. Propst-Proctor SL, Rinsky LA, Bleck EE. The cisterna chyli in orthopaedic surgery. Spine 1983;8:787–792.
52. Raphael BG, Lakner H, Engler GL. Disseminated intravascular coagulation during surgery for scoliosis. Clin Orthop 1982;162:41–46.
53. Robin GC, Span Y, Steinberg R, et al. Scoliosis in the elderly: a follow-up study. Spine 1982;7:355–359.
54. Rogala EJ, Drummond DS, Gurr J. Scoliosis: incidence and natural history: a prospective epidemiological study. J Bone Joint Surg 1978;60:173–176.
55. Saer EH, Winter RB, Lonstein JE. Long scoliosis fusion to the sacrum in adults with non-paralytic scoliosis: an improved method. Spine 1990;15(7):650–653.
56. Scandalakis JE, Akin JT, Milsap JH, et al. Vascular compression of the duodenum. Contemporary Surgery 1977;10:33.
57. Shands AR Jr, Eisberg HB. The incidence of scoliosis in the state of Delaware. J Bone Joint Surg 1955;37:1243–1249.
58. Shufflebarger HL. Fusion levels and hook patterns in thoracic scoliosis with CD instrumentation. SRS Proceedings, Amsterdam, Netherlands, 1989:388.
59. Simmons EH, Jackson RP. The management of nerve root entrapment syndromes associated with the collapsing scoliosis of idiopathic lumbar and thoracolumbar curves. Spine 1979;4:533–541.
60. Simmons EH, Jackson RP, Stripinus D. Incidence and severity of back pain in adult idiopathic scoliosis. Spine 1983;8:749–756.
61. Sponseller PD, Cohen MS, Nachemson AL, et al. Results of surgical treatment of adults with idiopathic scoliosis. J Bone Joint Surg 1987;69A:667–675.
62. Stewart AL, Greenfield S, Hays RD, et al. Functional status and well-being of patients with chronic conditions: results from the Medical Outcomes Study. JAMA 1989;272(7):907–913.
63. Stewart AL, Hays RD, Ware JE. The MOS Short General Health Survey: reliability and validity in patient populations. Medical Care 1988;26(7):724–735.
64. Swank S, Lonstein JE, Moe JH, et al. Surgical treatment of adult scoliosis: a review of two hundred and twenty-two cases. J Bone Joint Surg 1981;63:268–287.
65. Uden A. Thromboembolic complications following scoliosis surgery in Scandinavia. Acta Orthop Scand 1979;50:175–178.
66. Van Dam BE, Bradford DS, Lonstein JE, et al. Adult idiopathic scoliosis treated by posterior spinal fusion and Harrington instrumentation. Spine 1987;12:32–36.
67. Vanderpool DW, James JIP, Wynne-Davies R. Scoliosis in the elderly. J Bone Joint Surg 1969;51A:446–455.
68. Ware JE, Sherbourne CD. The MOS 36-item Short-Form Health Survey (SF-36). Medical Care 1992;30(6):473–483.
69. Weinstein SL, Ponseti IV. Curve progression in idiopathic scoliosis. J Bone Joint Surg 1983;65:447–455.
70. Winter RB, Lonstein JE, Denis F. Pain patterns in adult scoliosis. Orthop Clin North Am 1988;19:339–345.

CHAPTER TWENTY FOUR

Sagittal Plane Abnormalities in Disorders of the Adult Spine

Roger P. Jackson

Introduction

Standing sagittal balance and lumbopelvic alignments are important considerations in spinal arthrodesis, especially with the increasing use of instrumentation and other implants designed for the lumbosacral region. Segmental fixation systems have the capacity to significantly alter alignments and relationships of the spinopelvic axis. This is true whether or not instrumentation is performed to the sacropelvis. Studies of sagittal spinal balance and of lumbopelvic alignments and relationships are therefore potentially helpful. Although values for vertebral angular alignments have been reported, physiologic relationships of the spinopelvic axis have not been well established or defined. It is often advantageous to first measure "normal" asymptomatic subjects for such alignments and relationships. The data from this research can then be used in the analysis of other studies, particularly those involving patients with specific spinal disorders. In doing so, different treatments of these disorders can be more completely compared, especially with respect to patient outcome.

Normative Data Studies for Spinal Alignments

Studies for normal standing kyphosis and lordosis have been published (Table 24.1). Bernhardt and Bridwell reported segmental and total kyphosis and lordosis measurements in a group of 102 asymptomatic patients (55 females and 47 males) with an average age of 12.8 years (range, 4.6 to 29.8 years) who had been screened for possible scoliosis (2). Stagnara et al. had earlier reported similar segmental angular measurements for kyphosis and lordosis in a volunteer group of 100 asymptomatic French subjects (43 females and 57 males) between the ages of 20 and 29 years (38). In addition to kyphosis and lordosis measurements, Stagnara et al. also had published values for standing sacral base slope and had noted a correlation between the sacral slope and lordosis (38). Both of these normative data studies were done on standing lateral radiographs of the entire spine. The mean values, standard deviations, and ranges reported in these studies for standing segmental and total kyphosis and lordosis, as well as sacral slope are shown in Table 24.1.

Jackson and McManus evaluated an older asymptomatic group of 100 normal volunteers (50 females and 50 males) with an average age of 38.9 years (range, 20 to 63 years) for thoracic kyphosis and segmental and total lumbar lordosis on standing radiographs (13). In addition, they evaluated the radiographs for thoracic apex, standing pelvic rotation through the hips as measured by the sacral slope, and sagittal spinal balance. Figure 24.1 is a standing 36-inch lateral radiograph of the spine and pelvis showing the measurements made and the method used by

TABLE 24.1.
Sagittal Plane Normative Data, Mean Measurements (SEM, range)

	Stagnara et al. n = 100; 43F, 57M (ages 20 to 29 yrs)	Bernhardt and Bridwell n = 102; 55F, 47M (ages 4.6 to 29.8 yrs)	Jackson and McManus n = 100; 50F, 50M (ages 20 to 63 yrs)	Peterson et al. n = 50; 25F, 25M (ages 22 to 63 yrs)
(T1–T12)		+41	+42.1 (8.9, +22 to +68)	+47.1 (9.7, +26 to +75)
T1–2		+1		
T2–3		+3		
T3–4		+3.5		
T4–5	+5 (4, −2 to +17)	+5		
T5–6	+5 (4, −2 to +23)	+5		
T6–7	+6 (4, +1 to +22)	+5		
T7–8	+5 (4, 0 to +22)	+5		
T8–9	+4 (5, −5 to 36)	+4		
T9–10	+3 (5, −6 to +24)	+3		
T10–11	+2 (5, −5 to +17)	+3		
T11–12	+2 (5, −7 to +17)	+2.5		
T12–L1	+1 (5, −7 to +17)	+1		
L1–2	−2 (5, −13 to +13)	−4	−1.7 (4.2, −12 to +11)	−1.9 (3.5, −8 to +7)
L2–3	−7 (5, −17 to +7)	−7	−7.0 (4.3, −18 to +5)	−7.2 (4.0, −15 to +1)
L3–4	−11 (5, −26 to 0)	−13	−11.3 (3.8, −19 to 0)	−12.0 (3.4, −20 to −6)
L4–5	−15 (6, −2 to −10)	−20	−16.5 (5.0, −28 to +3)	−17.0 (4.4, −29 to −10)
L5–S1	−21 (6, −35 to −10)	−28	−24.6 (6.2, −39 to −11)	−24.0 (5.4, −37 to −12)
(L1–S1)	−56 (10, −79 to −33)	−72	−60.9 (12.0, −88 to −31)	−62.1 (10.8, −86 to −41)
Sacral Slope	41 (35, 35 to 71)		50.4 (7.7, 28 to 68)	47.9 (6.7, 35 to 61)
Lumbar Apex		L3–4 disc		L3–4 disc
Thoracic Apex		T6–7 disc	T7–8 disc	T7 body
C7 Plumb Line			−0.05 cm (2.5, −6 to +6.5)[a]	+0.38 cm (2.1, −5.7 to +5.2)[a]
Hip Axis to Plumb				−3.9 cm (2.1, −8.8 to +0.5)[a]
Pelvic Angle				17.4 (5.5, 5.0 to 29.0)
Pelvic Radius				13.5 cm (8.6, 11.4 to 15.0)

SEM = Standard error of the mean.
All data in degrees unless otherwise indicated (+ is kyphotic, − is lordotic).
[a] + is anterior to reference point, − is posterior to reference point for plumb line.

Jackson and McManus in their evaluation of the adult volunteers (13). The radiographs were taken such that C7 as well as the pelvis, with both acetabula, were seen on the films. The volunteers were asked to stand up straight, but relaxed, with their knees fully extended. Their arms were horizontal to the floor with the hands holding onto an adjustable-height bar positioned at chest level. This helped to stabilize the spine, improve visualization of the individual vertebrae, and minimize positioning effects on normal standing kyphosis and lordosis. Each radiograph was measured for segmental and total lordosis from L1 to S1 as well as for total thoracic kyphosis from T1 to T12 (Cobb method from the superior endplate of T1 to the inferior endplate of T12). Again the thoracic apex was determined. A sagittal plumb line was suspended from the center of the C7 vertebral body, and its perpendicular distance and direction from the posterior superior corner of the S1 vertebral body were recorded (Fig. 24.2); the distance was measured in centimeters, and a positive or negative sign indicated an anterior or posterior direction, respectively, for the plumb line from the reference point. This positive or negative plumb line measurement was used as a determinant for sagittal spinal balance. In addition, sacral inclination or slope was measured as the angle between the plumb line and a line drawn along the back of the proximal sacrum (Figs. 24.1 and 24.3). This was also considered to be a determinant for standing hip extension with sacropelvic rotation around the acetabula (Fig. 24.3).

Jackson and McManus indicated that the plumb line was dropped from the center of the C7 vertebral body because this point was located with greater confidence on the 36-inch standing lateral radiographs in the sometimes difficult to visualize cervicothoracic junction (13). In addition, they found that the odontoid process and/or auditory canals were frequently not seen on the radiographs and also that these structures could and did vary or translate more with neck posture than did C7 or T1. Also T1 was often more difficult than C7 to visualize with confidence, and so C7 was chosen as the proximal reference point for the sagittal balance measurements. As a reference point from which to measure sagittal spinal balance with respect to the plumb line, the au-

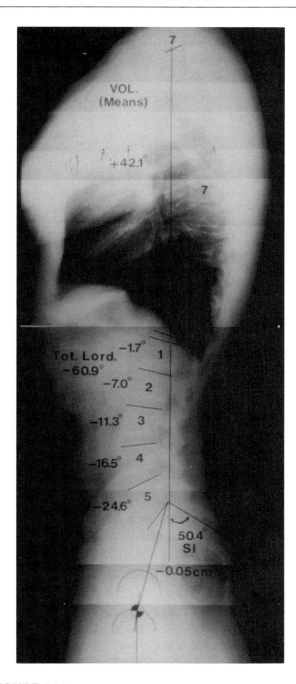

FIGURE 24.1.
Standing 36-inch lateral radiograph of the spine and pelvis showing the method and mean measurements for the 100 adult volunteers. (Reprinted with permission from Jackson RP, McManus AC. Radiographic analysis of sagittal plane alignment and balance in standing volunteers and patients with low back pain matched for age, sex, and size: a prospective controlled clinical study. Spine 1994; 19(14):1611–1618.)

nation or slope (Figs. 24.1 and 24.3). This method of measuring sacral slope had also been reported previously (7). Finally, the middle of the vertebral body or intervertebral disc most closely transected by the sagittal plumb line was recorded when the authors measured and evaluated each radiograph (Fig. 24.1).

The normative data results, displayed in fre-

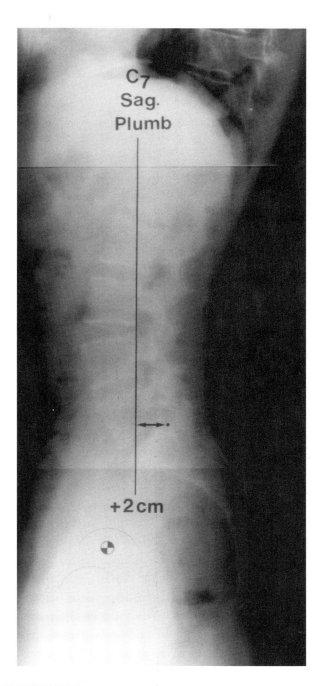

FIGURE 24.2.
Method used to measure sagittal spinal balance. A plumb line is dropped from the center of the C7 vertebral body, and its perpendicular distance and direction from the posterosuperior corner of the S1 vertebral body is recorded. The axis is centered between the acetabula (see Fig. 24.1).

thors chose the posterior superior corner of S1, as it proved to be an easy and consistent point to identify distally. This point was also on the line drawn along the sacral endplate to measure lordosis and along the back of the proximal sacrum to measure sacral incli-

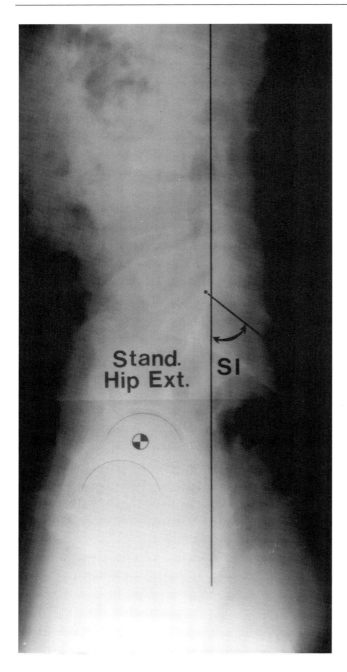

FIGURE 24.3.
Method used to measure sacral inclination (SI) or slope. The SI angle between the vertical line (C7 plumb line) and the line drawn along the back of S1 and S2 is determined. This angle is also considered to be a determinant for standing hip extension with pelvic rotation around the axis centered between the acetabula.

35, 38). As the hips flex with sitting or positioning, studies have shown significant decreases in both total and segmental lordosis, the latter occurring primarily in the lower lumbar spine (1, 33, 34, 39, 40). In addition to total lumbar lordosis, Jackson and McManus also found significant correlations for sacral slope and segmental lordosis in their standing volunteers (13). The significant Pearson correlation coefficients reported by Jackson and McManus for standing sacral slope with segmental and total lordosis were as follows: L1–2, $r = -.30$ ($P = .0020$); L2–3, $r = -.40$ ($P = .0001$); L3–4, $r = -.35$ ($P = .0040$); L4–5, $r = -.49$ ($P = .0001$); L5-S1, $r = -.28$ ($P = .0043$); and L1–S1, $r = -.70$ ($P = .0001$) (13). These standing studies indicated that as both segmental and total lordosis decreased, the sacropelvis rotated posteriorly around the acetabula, resulting in a more vertical sacral slope with an associated increase in standing hip extension, and vice versa. This relationship has been found to be true not only for standing, but again also for sitting and for prone positioning on various surgical frames or tables. As the hips are flexed, the pelvis begins rotating posteriorly with respect to the lumbar spine, and there is a significant decrease in both segmental and total lordosis (1, 33, 34, 39, 40). These findings and relationships are more fully described in this chapter in the section on positioning studies.

In their adult volunteer study Jackson and McManus reported a mean total lordosis from L1 to S1 of $-60.9°$ (standard error of the mean [SEM] 12.0°; range, $-88°$ to $-31°$) (Table 24.1) (13). Total lordosis was not related to sex (specifically, females did not have more lordosis). Total lordosis was also not related to age. In addition, mean segmental lordosis as a percentage of total lordosis was as follows: L1–2, 2.2%; L2–3, 11.1%; L3–4, 18.6%; L4–5, 27.1%; and L5-S1, 41.3%; more than two-thirds of lordosis occurred between L4 and S1. Segmental lordosis at any level was also not related to age. Segmental lordosis was found to be significantly different between each adjacent motion segment at the .01 level. Mean sacral slope was 50.4° (SEM 7.7°; range, 28° to 68°). Older volunteers tended to stand with a more vertical sacrum ($P = .0589$) and, therefore, more hip extension. The mean C7 sagittal plumb line measurement was -0.05 cm (SEM 2.5; range, -6 to $+6.5$ cm). Also, older volunteers stood with their plumb lines more anterior ($P = .0092$). Mean thoracic kyphosis from T1 to T12 was $+42.1°$ (SEM 8.9°; range, $+22°$ to $+68°$). Thoracic vertebral/disc apex was found to occur more commonly at the level of the T7–8 disc space in this study (Fig. 24.9), and at the T6–7 level in the Bernhardt and Bridwell study, which involved younger subjects referred for possible scoliosis (2).

quency distribution graphs for the variables evaluated by Jackson and McManus in their study, are shown in Figures 24.4 to 24.9 (13).

Several studies of normal subjects have shown a close association between standing pelvic rotation, or sacral slope, and total lumbar lordosis (5, 13, 18,

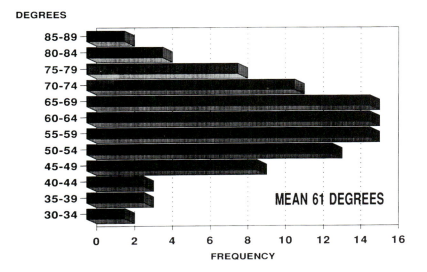

FIGURE 24.4.
Frequency distribution graph for standing total lordosis in degrees (L1–S1, Cobb Method) and mean lordosis of the 100 adult volunteers. (Reprinted with permission from Jackson RP, McManus AC. Radiographic analysis of sagittal plane alignment and balance in standing volunteers and patients with low back pain matched for age, sex, and size: a prospective controlled clinical study. Spine 1994;19(14):1611–1618.)

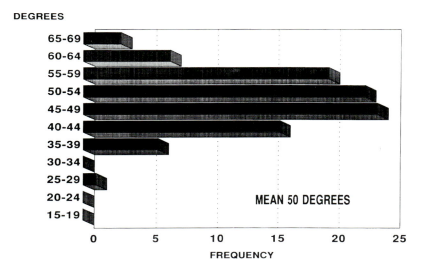

FIGURE 24.5.
Frequency distribution graph for standing sacral inclination or slope in degrees and mean slope of the 100 adult volunteers. (Reprinted with permission from Jackson RP, McManus AC. Radiographic analysis of sagittal plane alignment and balance in standing volunteers and patients with low back pain matched for age, sex, and size: a prospective controlled clinical study. Spine 1994;19(14):1611–1618.)

Definitions and Determinants of Sagittal Spinal Balance

Physiologic relationships of the spinopelvic axis have been studied recently by Peterson et al. (35). These authors evaluated the spines of 50 asymptomatic normal adult volunteers without hip or spinal pathology (25 males, 25 females, mean age 39.4 years, mean height 67 inches, mean weight 168 pounds). For each subject a standing 36-inch lateral radiograph of the pelvis and entire spine was measured by two observers to determine apex and degree of total thoracic kyphosis (Cobb method from T1 to T12, Fig. 24.1), segmental and total lumbar lordosis, and apex of lumbar lordosis. Additional measurements involved sacral inclination or slope (angle $\beta°$ between a line drawn along the back of the proximal sacrum and a plumb line centered at C7), and sagittal balance

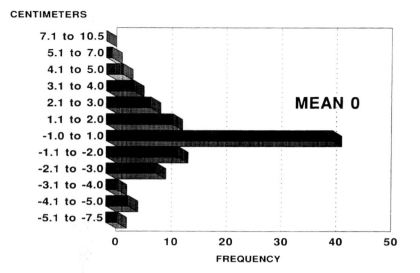

FIGURE 24.6.
Frequency distribution graph for the standing C7 sagittal plumb line measurements in centimeters and mean measurement of the 100 adult volunteers. (Reprinted with permission from Jackson RP, McManus AC. Radiographic analysis of sagittal plane alignment and balance in standing volunteers and patients with low back pain matched for age, sex, and size: a prospective controlled clinical study. Spine 1994;19(14):1611–1618.)

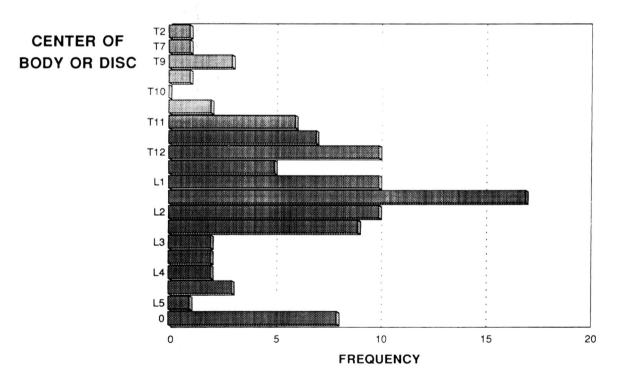

FIGURE 24.7.
Frequency distribution graph for the center of the vertebral body or disc space most closely crossed by the vertical C7 sagittal plumb line of the 100 adult volunteers. Zero means that no vertebral body or disc space was crossed by the plumb line. (Reprinted with permission from Jackson RP, McManus AC. Radiographic analysis of sagittal plane alignment and balance in standing volunteers and patients with low back pain matched for age, sex, and size: a prospective controlled clinical study. Spine 1994;19(14):1611–1618.)

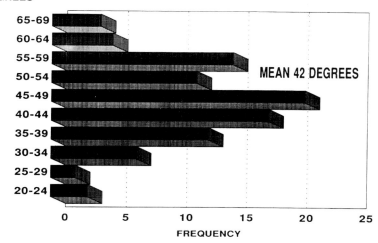

FIGURE 24.8.
Frequency distribution graph for standing total kyphosis in degrees (T1–12, Cobb method) and mean kyphosis of the 100 adult volunteers. (Reprinted with permission from Jackson RP, McManus AC. Radiographic analysis of sagittal plane alignment and balance in standing volunteers and patients with low back pain matched for age, sex, and size: a prospective controlled clinical study. Spine 1994;19(14):1611–1618.)

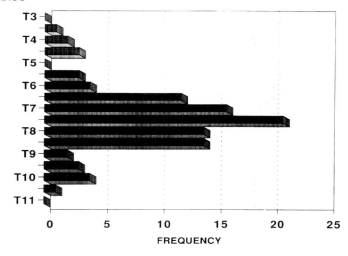

FIGURE 24.9.
Frequency distribution graph for the standing thoracic apex (body or disc) determined in the 100 adult volunteers. (Reprinted with permission from Jackson RP, McManus AC. Radiographic analysis of sagittal plane alignment and balance in standing volunteers and patients with low back pain matched for age, sex, and size: a prospective controlled clinical study. Spine 1994;19(14):1611–1618.)

(perpendicular distance B, measured in centimeters, from the posterosuperior corner of S1 to the C7 plumb line, or A, from the center between the acetabula to the plumb line) (Fig. 24.10). The distance from the center between the acetabula to the S1 reference point was also recorded in centimeters as the pelvic radius r, and the angle formed by the intersection of the radius with the plumb line was recorded in degrees as the pelvic angle $\alpha°$. Twenty percent of the study group was randomly selected and remeasured by each observer. The data were statistically analyzed for intra- and interobserver reliability, normative data, and significant relationships. The intra- and interobserver findings were highly correlated and not significantly different, indicating very good reliability for the data.

Peterson et al. found the following mean values for the sagittal spinal alignments measured: total T1–T12 kyphosis, +47°; segmental lordosis at L1–2, −1.9°; L2–3, −7.2°; L3–4, −12.0°; L4–5, −17.0°;

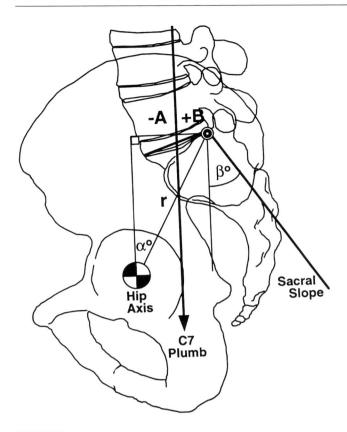

FIGURE 24.10.
Drawing showing method used to measure standing lumbopelvic alignments and balance. The angle $\beta°$ is sacral slope. The hip axis is centered between the acetabula, as shown. The letter "r" is the pelvic radius measured as the distance between the hip axis and the reference point on the posterosuperior corner of S1. The letters "A" and "B" are the perpendicular distances from the hip axis and from the reference point to the C7 plumb line, respectively. The angle $\alpha°$ is the pelvic angle measured between a line parallel with the C7 plumb line and the pelvic radius. (Reprinted with permission from Peterson MD, Jackson RP, McManus AC. Standing sagittal balance, alignments, and lumbopelvic relationships. Part I: A study of adult volunteers [Abstract]; and Peterson MD, Jackson RP, McManus AC. Standing sagittal balance, alignments, and lumbopelvic relationships. Part II: A study of patients with spinal disorders [Abstract].)

L5-S1, −24.0°; and total L1–S1 lordosis, −62.1°; C7 plumb line, +0.38 cm anterior to the S1 reference point or −3.9 cm posterior to the center between the acetabula; sacral slope, 47.9°; pelvic angle, 17.4°; and pelvic radius, 13.5 cm (35). Many of the mean values are similar to those previously reported in other studies (Table 24.1) (2, 13, 38).

Peterson et al. found thoracic kyphosis to have a positive correlation with total lordosis as well as with segmental lordosis at all levels studied, that is, as kyphosis increased or decreased, so did lordosis (35). Stagnara et al. and Jackson et al. found similar correlations (18, 38). In the Peterson et al. study significant correlations ($P < .05$) were also found for sagittal spinal balance (measured as the perpendicular distance from the S1 reference point to the plumb line) with segmental lordosis at L4–5 and L5-S1, total lordosis, pelvic angle, and the perpendicular distance from the center between the acetabula to the plumb line and to S1 (Fig. 24.10) (35). In their study sagittal balance was not found to be correlated with the thoracic or lumbar apex, degree of kyphosis, or segmental lordosis at L1–2, L2–3, L3–4. Other significant lumbopelvic relationships found in this study, again, included correlations for sacral slope with segmental (L1–2, L3–4, and L4–5) and total lordosis. Also, correlations existed for sacral slope ($\beta°$) with pelvic angle ($\alpha°$) and the perpendicular distance from the center between the acetabula to S1 (A + B) (Fig. 24.10). Sacral slope ($\beta°$) was not correlated with thoracic or lumbar apex, degree of kyphosis, perpendicular distance from the center between the acetabula to the plumb line (A), or measurement of sagittal balance (B). The mean pelvic radius (r) was not significantly different between the sexes and showed no correlation with height or weight. Correlation analyses of ratios using measured values as numerators and the pelvic radius as the denominator produced the same relationships previously noted.

The Peterson et al. study showed that as lower segmental lordosis increased, the lumbar spine translated anteriorly with respect to the plumb line, the S1 reference point moved anteriorly along an arc defined by the pelvic radius centered through the acetabula, and the sacropelvis appeared to be better balanced over the hips in the sagittal plane (35). As lordosis decreased, the sacral slope became more vertical as the sacropelvis rotated posteriorly along this same arc around the acetabula, standing hip extension increased, the pelvic angle increased as the S1 reference point moved away from the plumb line, and the perpendicular distance (A + B) from the center between the acetabula to S1 increased (Fig. 24.11). In normal adult volunteers with a full complement of compensatory mechanisms for spinal balance, the authors of this study found that the distance from the center between the acetabula to the plumb line was fairly constant and not correlated with lordosis (segmental or total) or sacral slope, suggesting that the other parameters adjusted around this relationship to keep the center of gravity over the hips in the sagittal plane. These studies supported the theory that the sacrum acts as a sixth lumbar vertebra with an additional restraint of having to translate along an arc defined by the pelvic radius centered through the hips, i.e., sacral translation around the hip axis (Fig. 24.10).

The Peterson et al. study is important because mean values for physiologic standing sagittal balance, alignments, and lumbopelvic relationships are defined and significant correlations identified. The authors noted that some correlations may represent possible compensatory mechanisms for preserving sagittal spinal balance. It was their recommendation

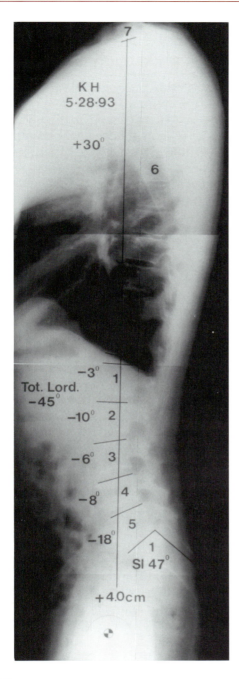

FIGURE 24.11.
Patient with degenerative lumbar disc disease and low back pain. There is a shift of segmental lordosis with an increase at L1–2 and L2–3 and a decrease at L4–5 and L5-S1. Sacral inclination (SI) measures 47° and the C7 plumb line +4.0 cm. The axis is centered through the hips. The thoracic apex is at T6. (Reprinted with permission from Jackson RP, Peterson MD, McManus AC. Standing sagittal balance and lumbopelvic relationships in adult volunteers and patients with degenerative lumbar disc disease, scoliosis, and spondylolisthesis. Presented at the annual meeting of the Scoliosis Research Society, Portland, Oregon, September 1994.)

that the perpendicular distance from some reference point on S1 to a plumb line be measured, as this seems to provide a more clinically useful evaluation of sagittal spinal balance. The authors also suggested that by studying such correlations and relationships it may be possible to further define and understand sagittal balance in patients with different spinal disorders.

In summary, normative data for sagittal spinal balance and segmental alignments should be considered in the evaluation of standing lateral radiographs. The following are believed to be important factors for assessment: thoracic kyphosis (total, segmental, and the distribution); thoracic apex (vertebra or disc); lumbar lordosis (total, segmental, and the distribution); lumbar apex (vertebra or disc); plumb line for sagittal balance (where, if at all, it crosses the spine and its relationship to a reference point on the sacrum as well as the defined axis through the hips); sacral slope for standing hip extension (since the sacropelvis rotates around the axis through the hips); pelvic angle and radius measurements; and a careful consideration for the center of gravity in the sagittal plane, which is generally located globally above the axis through the hips in the subject who is standing upright and balanced. Because the ranges and standard deviations of the normative data vary so much, clinical applications and decisions should be made cautiously and individualized. The present author agrees with Stagnara et al., who noted that in interpreting the results of all these studies, the range of normal values is probably more important than the published mean values (38).

Sagittal Plane Abnormalities in Specific Spinal Disorders

At this point it is important to recognize that sagittal spinal alignments and balance are different. Significantly abnormal segmental alignments or "malalignments" may exist, and yet the spine can still be balanced regionally and globally. This involves the use of compensatory mechanisms that have not been particularly well studied or defined. In the frontal plane the spine appears to be straight and stable; however, in the sagittal plane the spine is not straight and appears to be inherently unstable. Therefore, spinal balance is critically important in this plane, and an understanding of it is perhaps somewhat more complex. It is also important to note that the center of gravity and the plumb line are different. The center of gravity is difficult to determine on routine standing lateral radiographs; the plumb line, however, can be easily measured. In most cases the plumb line is well behind the center of gravity; however, the two do tend to move in the same direction in the balanced and unbalanced states. Generally, the closer the two are together, the better the global balance.

Studies of Patients with Degenerative Lumbar Disc Disease

Jackson and McManus also studied 100 adult patients with low back pain and degenerative lumbar disc disease (13). The group of patients was matched for age, sex, and size with the authors' normative data control group of 100 adult volunteers. In this prospective controlled clinical study, the patients (mean age 39.4 years; range, 22 to 60 years) and the volunteers (mean age 38.9 years; range, 20 to 63 years) had no prior lumbar spine surgery, no isthmic spondylolisthesis, and no clinical deformity. All of the patients had the chief complaint of low back pain of a mechanical nature for at least 6 weeks in duration. As in the control group, there were 50 males and 50 females. The same methodology that was used for measuring the volunteers was used to measure the patients. The authors again chose a sagittal plane plumb line suspended from the center of the C7 vertebral body, and the same reference point at the posterosuperior corner of S1 was used.

In this study Jackson and McManus reported significant differences ($P < .05$) between the asymptomatic volunteers and patients with discogenic low back pain. Total lordosis was less in the patients ($-56°$) than in the volunteers ($-61°$) ($P = .0065$). Again, total lordosis was not related to age or sex in either group. The patients also had significantly less segmental lordosis at L3–4 and L5–S1, and more at L1–2 in comparison with the volunteers. In addition, mean segmental lordosis as a percentage of total lordosis was significantly increased at the L1–2 level for the patients. The patients had a significantly lower or more vertical sacral slope ($47.2°$) than the volunteers ($50.4°$), indicating that they stood with somewhat more standing hip extension. Also, older patients tended to stand with an even greater sacral inclination, that is, further posterior pelvic rotation around the acetabula and more hip extension. As in the volunteers, significant correlations were found in the patients between sacral slope and both segmental and total lordosis. The authors reported that in the patient group the following correlations for sacral slope with segmental and total lordosis were found: L3–4, $r = -.36$ ($P = .0001$); L4–5, $r = -.27$ ($P = .0060$); L5–S1, $r = -.30$ ($P = .0026$); and L1–S1, $r = -.50$ ($P = .0001$). A review of the data from these patients further confirmed that with reductions in both segmental and total lordosis the sacropelvis rotated posteriorly around the hips, apparently as a compensatory mechanism to maintain or adjust balance. These relationships or correlations may have contributed to make balance between the 2 groups not significantly different. While many sagittal alignments for the volunteers and the patients were different, again, spinal balance was not. Thoracic kyphosis was also the same in both groups. However, thoracic apex for the patients occurred more commonly one level higher than that observed in the volunteers (see Fig. 24.9).

In this study the patients demonstrated an actual and a percentage shift of segmental lordosis from the lower to the upper lumbar spine (Fig. 24.11) (13), which was in addition to their standing with a more vertical sacrum or increased posterior sacropelvic rotation. The authors suggested that these subtle but significant changes could represent compensations for the differences in the segmental alignments measured between the patients and the volunteers. Hasday et al. reported a similar finding in their study of gait abnormalities arising from iatrogenic loss of lumbar lordosis secondary to Harrington distraction instrumentation for lumbar fractures (7). In a small group of patients these authors found that posterior pelvic rotation with "hip hyperextension," when available, was the favored compensatory mechanism for loss of lumbar lordosis; otherwise, knee flexion and forward lean of the trunk were seen. With advancing age and hip disease, the possibility for posterior pelvic or sacropelvic rotation diminishes. These factors need to be carefully considered in the overall evaluation and management of the patient, especially if fusion to the sacropelvis is being planned.

Jackson and McManus pointed out in their studies that a considerable amount of segmental lordosis occurred at the L5-S1 level (13). In a review of the literature the authors found that lordosis was measured in different ways and from different levels. Measurement from L1 to L5 was not uncommon. Numerous other studies have also reported a considerable amount of segmental lordosis at the L5-S1 level (1, 2, 5, 38, 40). With this fact apparent, it would seem most appropriate to measure lordosis down to S1, otherwise a significant amount of segmental lordosis will be left unaccounted for or not evaluated.

Additional Comparative Studies in Disorders of the Adult Spine

Sagittal balance, alignments, and lumbopelvic relationships in patients with different spinal disorders have been evaluated by Jackson et al. and Peterson et al. (18, 35, 36). Jackson et al. studied three groups of patients who had diagnoses of degenerative lumbar disc disease with the chief complaint of low back pain; thoracic, thoracolumbar, or lumbar idiopathic and degenerative scoliosis with back pain; or L5-S1 symptomatic isthmic spondylolisthesis (18). The three patient groups were compared to the authors' control group of 100 adult volunteers studied previously (Table 24.2). All patients in each group were randomly selected, with an effort being made to match the three patient groups as closely as possible for age with the volunteer group. In addition, the pa-

TABLE 24.2.
Sagittal Angulations (in Degrees, Cobb Method): Total Thoracic Kyphosis and Segmental and Total Lumbar Lordosis Mean Measurements (SEM, Range)

Level	Volunteers (n = 100)	Degenerative Disc (n = 100)	Scoliosis (n = 30)	Spondylolisthesis (n = 30)	ANOVA (P values)
T1–T12	+42.1 (8.9, +22 to +68)	+42.6 (10.1, +20 to +70)	+35.2 (13.0, +10 to +62)	+42.0 (9.6, +18 to +61)	$P = .0041$
L1–2	−1.7 (4.2, −12 to +11)	−2.9 (4.5, −17 to +12)	−0.4 (4.9, −8 to +12)	−3.4 (4.9, −14 to +9)	$P = .0142$
L2–3	−7.1 (4.3, −18 to +5)	−7.2 (3.8, −17 to +3)	−5.4 (3.4, −13 to +2)	−7.5 (3.4, −14 to −1)	(n.s.)
L3–4	−11.3 (3.8, −19 to 0)	−9.8 (3.7, −17 to +4)	−10.7 (7.2, −29 to +2)	−12.3 (4.2, −22 to −3)	$P = .0158$
L4–5	−16.5 (5.0, −28 to +3)	−15.2 (5.3, −30 to −3)	−16.7 (6.2, −27 to −1)	−20.6 (5.6, −34 to −9)	$P = .0001$
L5–S1	−24.6 (6.2, −39 to −11)	−21.5 (7.5, −37 to −5)	−25.1 (7.4, −37 to −9)	−23.7 (9.6, −43 to +3)	$P = .0128$
L1–S1	−60.9 (12.0, −88 to −31)	−56.3 (11.5, −84 to −24)	−58.6 (12.4, −79 to −24)	−67.6 (11.5, −84 to −40)	$P = .0001$

From Jackson RP, Peterson MD, McManus AC. Standing sagittal balance and lumbopelvic relationships in adult volunteers and patients with degenerative lumbar disc disease, scoliosis, and spondylolisthesis. Presented at the annual meeting of the Scoliosis Research Society, Portland, Oregon, September 1994.
SEM = Standard error of the mean.
+ is kyphotic, − is lordotic.
ANOVA = Analysis of Variants

TABLE 24.3.
Segmental Lordosis as Percentage of Total Lordosis (Cobb method)

Level	Volunteers (n = 100)	Degenerative Disc (n = 100)	Scoliosis (n = 30)	Spondylolisthesis (n = 30)	ANOVA (P values)
L1–2	2.2	4.6	0.7	4.3	$P = .0087$
L2–3	11.1	12.6	9.1	11.0	$P = .0388$
L3–4	18.6	17.6	17.7	18.2	(n.s.)
L4–5	27.1	27.3	28.9	31.5	(n.s.)
L5–S1	41.3	38.5	44.8	34.9	$P = .0069$

From Jackson RP, Peterson MD, McManus AC. Standing sagittal balance and lumbopelvic relationships in adult volunteers and patients with degenerative lumbar disc disease, scoliosis, and spondylolisthesis. Presented at the annual meeting of the Scoliosis Research Society, Portland, Oregon, September 1994.
Statistically significant shifts or changes in the percentages of segmental lordosis between the groups occurred primarily in the proximal lumbar levels and at the L5–S1 level.
ANOVA = Analysis of Variants

tients with degenerative lumbar disc disease were also matched for sex with the volunteers. None of the patients had had prior back surgery, and all were between the age of 20 and 63 years. Among the 30 patients with scoliosis, 28 were female and two were male, and their mean age was 38.0 years. Eighteen had idiopathic curves, and 12 had degenerative curves, with the major curves measuring from 20° to 77°. Among the 30 patients with spondylolisthesis, 14 were female and 16 were male, and their mean age was 36.3 years. Twenty-three had a grade I slip and seven had a grade II slip. All of the patients were studied with the same methodology used for the volunteer control group and had the same measurements made for comparisons. The patients also had additional measurements made, depending on their primary spinal disorder. The data were analyzed statistically and reviewed for significant differences, relationships, and correlations within and among the groups.

Interesting differences ($P < .05$) were found among the four groups in this study. These included differences in total and segmental lordosis (Table 24.2) and segmental lordosis as a percentage of total lordosis (Table 24.3). Scoliosis patients had less segmental lordosis at L1–2 and more at L5–S1 (Fig. 24.12), whereas patients with degenerative lumbar disc disease and with spondylolisthesis had more lordosis at L1–2 and less at L5–S1 (Figs. 24.11 and 24.13). Spondylolisthesis patients had significantly more total lordosis ($P = .0001$). The scoliosis patients had almost three-fourths of their lordosis between L4–S1, whereas the remaining groups had approximately two-thirds of their total lordosis between L4 and S1. In spondylolisthesis patients the L4–S1 lordosis was distributed somewhat equally between the two motion segments, that is, less at L5–S1 and more at L4–5 (Fig. 24.13), which was different from the other three groups. Total lordosis and kyphosis, again, had a positive correlation in all groups except for spondylolisthesis. Stagnara et al. and Peterson et al. also found the same correlation in their adult volunteers (35, 38). In this Jackson et al. study, spondylolisthesis patients had increased lordosis, but not kyphosis, which again was different from the other three groups (18).

Jackson et al. found C7 sagittal plumb line measurements for spinal balance to not be different among their study groups (18). The spondylolisthesis patients, however, did tend to stand with a more positive sagittal balance as defined in this chapter (Fig. 24.13). This finding, coupled with the previous find-

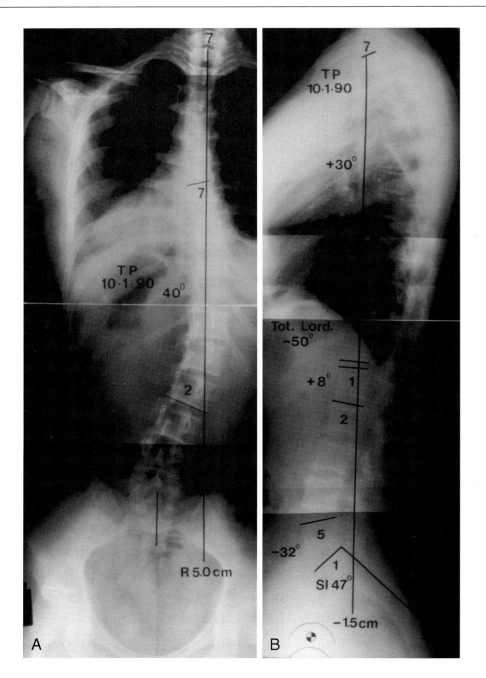

FIGURE 24.12.

A and **B.** Anteroposterior and lateral standing radiographs of patient with right thoracolumbar scoliosis in the frontal plane. In the sagittal plane there is a decrease in segmental lordosis at L1–2 with an actual kyphosis of +8° at this level and an increase in segmental lordosis at L5-S1, which measures −32°. As a group, the scoliosis patients had less proximal segmental lumbar lordosis and more distal lumbar lordosis. (From Jackson RP, Peterson MD, McManus AC. Standing sagittal balance and lumbopelvic relationships in adult volunteers and patients with degenerative lumbar disc disease, scoliosis, and spondylolisthesis. Presented at the annual meeting of the Scoliosis Research Society, Portland, Oregon, September 1994.)

ing that spondylolisthesis patients had increased lordosis but not kyphosis, suggests that with anterior L5 translation on S1, the center of gravity moves forward along with the plumb line, and that spondylolisthesis patients increased their total lordosis, but not their total kyphosis, as compensatory mechanisms for global balance. In this study total and segmental lordosis were found to have some positive correlations with the plumb line in all groups except the patients with degenerative lumbar disc disease. In the scoliosis and spondylolisthesis groups, L5-S1 segmental lordosis was significantly correlated with the plumb line. In these two groups, as L5-S1 lordosis increased, the plumb line was found to fall more posteriorly. The scoliosis and spondylolisthesis groups appeared to adjust lumbosacral segmental lordosis to

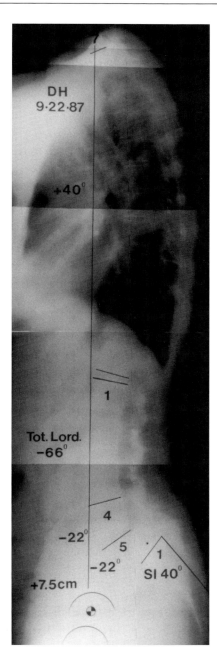

FIGURE 24.13.
Standing lateral radiograph of patient with grade II spondylolisthesis at L5-S1. Total lordosis from L1 to S1 measures −66° with a fairly equal distribution of segmental lordosis at L4–5 and L5-S1. As a group, the spondylolisthesis patients had increased total lumbar lordosis with less segmental lordosis at L5-S1 and more at L4–5 in comparison with adult volunteers. (From Jackson RP, Peterson MD, McManus AC. Standing sagittal balance and lumbopelvic relationships in adult volunteers and patients with degenerative lumbar disc disease, scoliosis, and spondylolisthesis. Presented at the annual meeting of the Scoliosis Research Society, Portland, Oregon, September 1994.)

help balance the spine in the sagittal plane, which was not the case for the degenerative lumbar disc disease group and the volunteer group. There was no correlation between the plumb line and sacral slope or between the plumb line and kyphosis in any group.

Significant standing lumbopelvic relationships were found for both total and segmental lordosis versus sacral inclination (slope) or sacropelvic rotation in the Jackson et al. study. Total lordosis and sacral slope again had strong negative correlations in all four groups. As total lordosis decreased, the sacral inclination became more vertical, that is, the sacropelvis rotated posteriorly around the acetabula, and standing hip extension increased. Segmental lordosis also had significant similar negative correlations with sacral slope in all four groups. As segmental lordosis decreased, the sacral inclination or slope again became more vertical (or decreased, as measured in these studies), and vice versa. In the volunteer groups these correlations existed at all five motion segments studied: in the degenerative lumbar disc disease patients at the L5-S1, L4–5, and L3–4 motion segments; in the spondylolisthesis patients at the L3–4 and L1–2 motion segments; and in the scoliosis patients at the L1–2 motion segment.

Jackson et al. concluded from these studies that significant correlations for sagittal balance and alignments existed and that the correlations appeared to be different for and between the various spinal disorders studied in comparison with the control group. Some of the correlations identified appeared to represent compensatory mechanisms for achieving or maintaining sagittal spinal balance in the different groups studied. Sagittal balance measurements were not different among the groups and were correlated with lordosis measurements in all but the degeneration lumbar disc disease group. Sagittal balance, sacral slope, and kyphosis measurements were not correlated in any group, and sacral slope and lordosis measurements, both segmental and total, were correlated in all four groups. The authors suggested that by comparing such correlations and relationships it may be possible to better understand sagittal balance in normal subjects and in patients with different spinal disorders.

Peterson et al. conducted further analyses of standing sagittal balance, alignments, and lumbopelvic relationships in a subset involving 50 of the 100 degenerative lumbar disc disease patients studied by Jackson et al. as well as the same 30 scoliosis and 30 spondylolisthesis patients, and they compared these studies with the normative data collected from their 50 normal adult volunteers reported previously in this chapter (18, 35, 36). The same methodology, measurements, and statistical analyses were carried out in all groups. In this study 20% of the data collected were analyzed for intra- and interobserver reliability. The reliability studies revealed high correlations within and between the two observers and no significant differences.

The Peterson et al. mean measurements for the degenerative lumbar disc disease patients were as follows: total T1–T12 kyphosis, +43°; segmental lordosis at L1–2, −2°; L2–3, −7°; L3–4, −11°; L4–5, −17°; L5-S1, −20°; and total L1–S1 lordosis, −57°; C7 plumb line, +0.4 cm anterior to S1 or −4.7 cm posterior to the center between the acetabula; sacral slope, 43°; pelvic angle, 19°; and pelvic radius, 13.6 cm (36). Mean measurements for the scoliosis patients were as follows: total T1–T12 kyphosis, +37°; segmental lordosis at L1–2, 0°; L2–3, −6°; L3–4, −10°; L4–5, −17°; L5-S1, −24°; and total L1–S1 lordosis, −57°; C7 plumb line, −0.2 cm posterior to S1 or −4.8 cm posterior to the center between the acetabula; sacral slope, 49°; pelvic angle, 20°; and pelvic radius 13.3 cm. Mean measurements for the spondylolisthesis patients were as follows: total T1–T12 kyphosis, +42°; segmental lordosis at L1–2, −3°; L2–3, −8°; L3–4, −12°; L4–5, −21°; L5-S1, −23°; and total L1–S1 lordosis, −66°; C7 plumb line, +1.4 cm anterior to S1 or −3.8 cm posterior to the center between the acetabula; sacral slope, 43°; pelvic angle, 22°; and pelvic radius, 13.7 cm.

Significant differences ($P < 0.05$) were again seen between the adult patient groups and the adult volunteers in these Peterson et al. studies (35, 36). Patients with degenerative lumbar disc disease stood with less total and less L5-S1 segmental lordosis (similar to the Jackson et al. [18] and Jackson and McManus [13] studies); scoliosis patients stood with less total and less segmental lordosis at L1–2 and L3–4; and spondylolisthesis patients stood with more total and more L4–5 segmental lordosis. Again, as a proportion of total lordosis, degenerative lumbar disc disease patients and spondylolisthesis patients stood with about two-thirds of their total lordosis between L4 and S1; in spondylolisthesis patients lordosis was distributed fairly equally between these two motion segments, that is, less at L5-S1 and more at L4–5; and scoliosis patients had almost three-quarters of their lordosis between L4 and S1. Scoliosis and spondylolisthesis patients had significantly less thoracic kyphosis, which was believed to be structural in scoliosis and perhaps compensatory in spondylolisthesis patients. Spondylolisthesis patients stood with a significant increase in pelvic angle and degenerative lumbar disc disease patients with a more vertical sacral slope. Again, measurements of sagittal spinal balance were not significantly different between groups. Significant relationships were found to exist between segmental lordosis and sagittal balance. The perpendicular distance from the S1 reference point to the plumb line (sagittal spinal balance) was significantly correlated with L4–5 lordosis in degenerative lumbar disc disease patients in this study, but not in the Jackson et al. study (18). Again, L5-S1 lordosis in the scoliosis and spondylolisthesis patients was significantly correlated with balance. This plumb line measurement of spinal balance was also related to the pelvic angle for the spondylolisthesis patients. The perpendicular distance from the center between the acetabula to the plumb line was significantly correlated only with segmental lordosis at L5-S1, and then only in scoliosis patients. Again, sagittal spinal balance, as defined in this study and in this chapter, was not correlated with thoracic kyphosis, nor with total lumbar lordosis in any patient group.

In the Peterson et al. study significant lumbopelvic relationships were found in all patient groups (36). Total lordosis and sacral slope remained highly correlated in each group. This was also true in the volunteers (35). Segmental lordosis and sacral slope also had similar correlations: in spondylolisthesis patients at L1–2; in degenerative lumbar disc disease patients at L2–3 and L3–4; and in scoliosis patients at L1–2, L2–3, and L4–5. Segmental lordosis at L5-S1 was inversely related to the pelvic angle in spondylolisthesis and degenerative lumbar disc disease patients. There were no significant correlations between sacral slope and measurements of spinal balance by the plumb line in any patient group. The mean pelvic radius was again not significantly different between sexes and showed no significant correlation to height, weight, or diagnosis. Correlation analyses of ratios using measured values as numerators and the pelvic radius as the denominator produced the same relationships.

These Jackson et al. and Peterson et al. studies showed that despite definite differences in sagittal segmental and regional alignments, global spinal balance was not significantly different between normal adult volunteers and the adult patients studied (18, 35, 36). Preservation of sagittal spinal balance appeared to be a result of changes primarily in lower lumbar lordosis, sacral slope, and pelvic angle. Correlation analysis indicated that as lower segmental lordosis at L4–5 and L5-S1 increased, the lumbar spine translated anteriorly with respect to the plumb line. To accommodate for sagittal spinal malalignments and adjust for balance, patients with degenerative lumbar disc disease tended to increase L4–5 lordosis, when possible, whereas scoliosis and spondylolisthesis patients increased L5-S1 lordosis on a segmental percentage basis. The authors' analyses showed that lumbopelvic relationships were related to lumbar alignments, that is, as total or segmental lordosis decreased, the sacropelvis rotated posteriorly and the sacrum became more vertical, but not to sagittal spinal balance, which was maintained and largely unaffected in most cases. These authors suggested that changes in sacropelvic rotation probably did not act as the primary compensatory mechanism in preservation of physiologic sagittal balance when other segmental spinal shifts or adjustments were possible and sufficient.

These studies are also important in their providing further mean values for standing sagittal balance, alignments, and lumbopelvic measurements in patients with degenerative lumbar disc disease, scoliosis, and spondylolisthesis. In addition, and equally important, significant correlations for standing sagittal alignments and spinal balance were identified. The authors concluded from their studies that loss of lower lumbar lordosis resulted in other, perhaps less desirable, compensatory mechanisms being used for maintaining balance, when available. They suggested that by studying such correlations and relationships it might be possible to further understand and better treat patients with different spinal disorders, both nonoperatively and operatively, especially with the use of spinal instrumentation systems. They also pointed out that junctional stresses and degenerative changes above and below a fusion, with or without instrumentation, could be related as much to spinal alignment as rigidity. If this were true, it would have significant clinical implications, as well as possible application.

Comparative Studies: Standing Versus Recumbent Extension Lateral Lumbar Radiographs

Very little data have been published on differences in sagittal alignments within and between groups of patients with different spinal disorders. In addition, and just as unfortunately, standing films for evaluation of the sagittal plane are often not taken or are not available in the assessment of such patients. Nelson et al. conducted a study with the objectives of (a) quantitating and comparing total and segmental lordosis for two different spinal diagnoses—isthmic spondylolisthesis and degenerative lumbar disc disease; (b) determining and comparing the lordosis measurements on standing neutral and recumbent extension lateral lumbar radiographs within each patient group; and (c) determining intra- and interobserver reliability of Cobb measurements for segmental and total lordosis on the standing and recumbent films (32). The authors evaluated 30 patients with spondylolisthesis and 30 with degenerative lumbar disc disease. Inclusion criteria for this study were no prior back surgeries in either group and grade I or II slips in the spondylolisthesis group. The spondylolisthesis patients included 18 males and 12 females, with a mean age of 37.5 years. Twenty-one patients had a grade I slip and nine had a grade II slip. The degenerative lumbar disc disease group included 16 males and 14 females, with a mean age of 35.9 years. Total and segmental lordosis measurements (Cobb method from the superior endplates of adjacent vertebrae and from L1 to S1) were made twice by two observers on both the standing neutral and recumbent extension lateral lumbar radiographs for each patient. The results of this study are shown in Table 24.4.

As the data in the table demonstrate, total and segmental lordosis were greater in spondylolisthesis patients than in degenerative lumbar disc disease patients on both the standing neutral and recumbent extension lateral films (32). Measurements on the

TABLE 24.4.
Segmental and Total Lumbar Lordosis Mean Measurements (SEM): Standing Neutral Versus Recumbent Extension Lateral Lumbar Radiographs in Patients with Spondylolisthesis and Degenerative Lumbar Disc Disease

	Spondylolisthesis (n = 30)			Degenerative (n = 30)			Total (n = 60)		
	Standing	P	Extension	Standing	P	Extension	Standing	P	Extension
Observer 1									
L1–2	3.7 (4.5)		4.8 (3.3)	2.6 (3.4)	*	4.2 (3.4)	3.1 (4.0)	*	4.5 (3.3)
L2–3	7.5 (3.2)	*	9.7 (3.4)	7.9 (3.7)		8.8 (3.7)	7.7 (3.4)	*	9.2 (3.6)
L3–4	11.3 (3.5)		11.2 (3.2)	10.3 (3.6)		11.7 (2.7)	10.8 (3.6)		11.5 (2.9)
L4–5	19.5 (5.4)		18.2 (4.0)	15.9 (4.0)		15.8 (5.0)	17.7 (5.1)		17.0 (4.7)
L5–S1	26.7 (10.2)	**	30.7 (9.6)	23.9 (6.9)	**	26.2 (7.0)	25.3 (8.8)	**	28.5 (8.6)
L1–S1	68.5 (11.8)	**	74.7 (13.0)	60.9 (11.8)	**	67.0 (10.1)	64.7 (12.3)	**	70.9 (12.2)
Observer 2									
L1–2	3.3 (4.9)		5.2 (4.3)	3.4 (4.7)	**	5.8 (5.8)	3.3 (4.7)	**	5.5 (5.1)
L2–3	7.5 (3.4)	**	10.3 (3.9)	7.9 (3.5)	**	10.3 (3.7)	7.7 (3.4)	**	10.3 (3.8)
L3–4	12.2 (4.2)		12.5 (4.1)	10.8 (3.8)		12.1 (3.1)	11.5 (4.0)		12.3 (3.6)
L4–5	20.8 (5.8)		19.3 (4.7)	15.2 (4.6)		15.8 (4.9)	18.0 (5.9)		17.6 (5.1)
L5–S1	23.6 (9.7)	**	28.7 (9.3)	21.1 (7.7)	**	24.6 (7.2)	22.4 (8.8)	**	26.7 (8.5)
L1–S1	67.5 (11.4)	**	76.1 (13.8)	58.7 (11.0)	**	68.6 (11.4)	63.1 (12.0)	**	72.4 (13.1)

From Nelson LM, McManus AC, Jackson RP. Standing neutral versus recumbent extension lordosis in patients with spondylolisthesis and degenerative lumbar disc disease (Abstract).
SEM = Standard error of the mean.
All measurements lordotic degrees (Cobb method).
* $P < .05$
** $P < .01$

standing radiographs revealed that the increased lordosis occurred primarily between L3 and S1. Overall, 64% of total lordosis was located at the lowest two levels. In evaluating intra- and interobserver reliability in this study, "agreement" of two measurements at the same level was defined as within plus or minus 5°. Interobserver agreement on the standing films was greater than 85% at each level from L1 to L5, 71.7% at L5-S1, and 68.3% for total (L1–S1) lordosis. Interobserver agreement on the recumbent films was greater than 95% at each level from L1 to L5, 81.7% at L5-S1, and 76.7% for total (L1–S1) lordosis. Intraobserver reliability was 95% overall on standing films and 98% on recumbent extension films.

The Nelson et al. study showed again that spondylolisthesis patients had more total lordosis than did degenerative lumbar disc disease patients (32). While having significantly greater L5-S1 segmental lordosis than degenerative lumbar disc disease patients, spondylolisthesis patients also had a proportionately larger percentage of their total lordosis at the L4–5 level. The authors noted that such a relative increase in L4–5 lordosis could represent an attempt at compensation for the anterior displacement of L5 on S1, as could an increase in total lordosis.

Both the intra- and interobserver reliabilities in the Nelson et al. study were higher on recumbent extension than on standing neutral lateral radiographs (32). Reliabilities on standing films were lower at the lowest two levels. According to the authors, these findings were likely a result of a greater divergence of x-ray beams at the lower levels as well as possible increased motion artifact from patient unsteadiness with standing in this study. Both factors would make the identification of measured landmarks more difficult on the standing films. Despite small differences, the authors believed that recumbent extension films could be used in studying and comparing lordosis when standing lateral films were unavailable. They concluded by recommending that lumbar spine fusion studies include an assessment of lordosis, both total and segmental, preoperatively and postoperatively. They believe that lumbar lordosis is important and that it should be preserved and maintained in all patients undergoing reconstructive lumbar spine surgery.

Positioning Studies in Patients Under Anesthesia and in Awake Volunteers

How patients are positioned at surgery is extremely important as this largely determines the sagittal alignment, especially in the lumbar spine. Studies addressing the effect of operative position on lumbar lordosis are therefore not only interesting but also clinically important and relevant. Peterson et al. evaluated the effect of operative position on lumbar lordosis in a group of patients under general anesthesia (34). To determine how the "90–90" position and the prone position affect sagittal alignment, two patient groups were analyzed by these authors. All patients were selected from the practice of the same surgeon (RPJ). Inclusion criteria for this study required adequate preoperative radiographs (standing 36-inch lateral spine) and intraoperative radiographs (lateral lumbar spine, L1 to the sacrum) in either the "90–90" position on a Hastings frame ($n = 20$), or the prone position on a Jackson table ($n = 20$). Radiographs were measured twice by two observers using the Cobb method for total and segmental lordosis between L1 and S1. The data were analyzed for intra- and interobserver error and for significant changes in total and segmental lordosis between preoperative and intraoperative radiographs. Intraobserver measurements of total and segmental lordosis were highly correlated (mean $r = .87$, $P \leq .01$) and not significantly different. Interobserver measurements were also highly correlated (mean $r = .84$, $P \leq .05$); however, mean standing segmental lordosis at L5-S1 was different ($P < .01$). Standing segmental lordosis at all other levels, standing total lordosis, and intraoperative measurements were not significantly different in this study.

For the "90–90" group the radiographic mean segmental and total lordosis measurements in the standing position were: L1–2, −2.7°; L2–3, −6.4°; L3–4, −9.6°; L4–5, −13.5°; L5-S1, −20.5°; and L1–S1, −52.7°. Mean segmental and total lordosis measurements in the "90–90" position on the Hastings frame were: L1–2, −2.4°; L2–3, −3.2°; L3–4, −4.0°; L4–5, −5.6°; L5-S1, −18.4°; and L1–S1, −33.6°. In comparison with standing, segmental lordosis was significantly reduced ($P < .01$) at all levels except L1–2, which showed no significant change (Fig. 24.14). Total lordosis also was significantly reduced ($P < .01$).

For the prone group the radiographic mean segmental and total lordosis measurements in the standing position were: L1–2, −4.2°; L2–3, −6.5°; L3–4, −10.4°; L4–5, −14.8°; L5-S1, −25.7°; and L1–S1, −61.7°. Mean segmental and total lordosis measurements in the prone position on the Jackson table were: L1–2, −4.4°; L2–3, −5.7°; L3–4, −9.2°; L4–5, −13.9°; L5-S1, −29.2°; and L1–S1, −62.8°. In comparison with standing, segmental lordosis at L5-S1 was significantly increased ($P < .01$). Segmental lordosis at all of the other levels and total lordosis showed no significant change (Fig. 24.15).

Peterson et al. concluded that preservation of normal segmental alignment during reconstructive lumbar spine surgery is important and is largely determined by intraoperative positioning (34). Although the "90–90" position often gave the impression of maintaining lordosis, this was not necessarily so. It

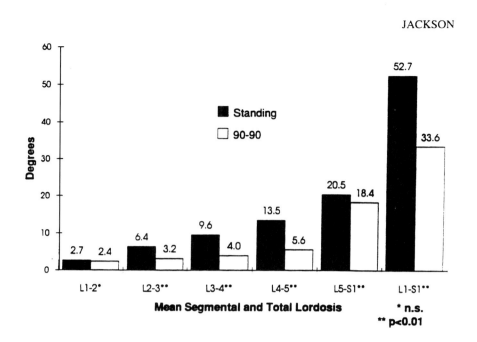

FIGURE 24.14.
Bar graph comparing mean segmental and total lordosis in degrees (Cobb method) measured on lateral radiographs in 20 patients standing preoperatively and at surgery in the 90–90 position on a Hastings frame. Lordosis is significantly decreased at all levels except at L1–2. (Reprinted with permission from Peterson MD, Nelson LM, McManus AC, Jackson RP. The effect of operative position on lumbar lordosis: a radiographic study of patients under anesthesia in the prone and 90–90 positions. Spine 1995;20(12):1419–1424.)

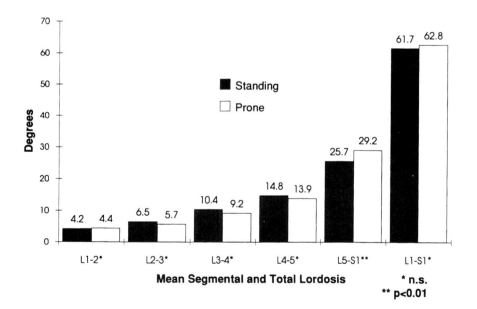

FIGURE 24.15.
Bar graph comparing mean segmental and total lordosis in degrees (Cobb method) measured on lateral radiographs in 20 patients standing preoperatively and positioned prone at surgery on a Jackson table. Segmental lordosis is not different at L1–2, L2–3, L3–4, and L4–5. L5–S1 segmental lordosis was significantly increased on the Jackson table and total lordosis slightly increased. (Reprinted with permission from Peterson MD, Nelson LM, McManus AC, Jackson RP. The effect of operative position on lumbar lordosis: a radiographic study of patients under anesthesia in the prone and 90–90 positions. Spine: 1995;20(12):1419–1424.)

was postulated by the authors that hip flexion produced ligament and muscle tethering across or between the back of the hip joints and ischia, resulting in posterior pelvic rotation that reduced total and segmental lumbar lordosis. These changes were most prominent at the L4–5 level, where lordosis was decreased by nearly 60% in this study and total lordosis was reduced by over one-third. Patients in the prone position, however, showed no change in segmental lordosis above the lumbosacral level. Segmental lordosis at L5-S1 actually increased, and total lordosis was preserved. The authors suggested that this may be a result of anterior pelvic rotation promoted by several factors, including (a) less hip flexion, (b) ligament and muscle tethering on the anterior iliac crests across and in front of the hips, and (c) the location and function of the hip and proximal thigh pads designed for the Jackson table. Here too the authors noted that interobserver differences in segmental lordosis at L5-S1 were likely due to difficulty in identifying the same sacral landmarks. Given that no significant intraobserver differences existed, the authors found that the significant changes in lordosis measured were valid in their study.

This Peterson et al. study concluded that the "90–90" position on the Hastings frame was associated with significant reduction of total and segmental lordosis, most pronounced at the L4–5 level, and that positioning on a Jackson table maintained the standing sagittal alignment of the lumbar spine and increased lumbosacral lordosis. This study supported findings published previously by Tan et al. (40)

Nelson et al. studied the effects of positioning on lumbar lordosis in a group of 17 awake volunteers examined prospectively (33). The authors' objectives were to measure total and segmental lordosis on standing lateral radiographs and on lateral lumbar radiographs taken in four different operative positions. The positions studied were on the Relton-Hall frame, Hastings frame, chest rolls, and the Jackson table. Total and segmental lordosis between L1 and S1 were measured twice by two observers using the Cobb method. Data were analyzed for intra- and interobserver reliability and for changes in total and segmental lordosis among the radiographs in the five different positions. The authors' data here too showed that the intra- and interobserver measurements were reliable and reproducible. Lordosis was decreased in all four operative positions in comparison with standing in these awake volunteers, but it was better maintained on the Jackson table (Table 24.5).

Stephens et al. carried out similar comparative studies for the sagittal lumbar alignment produced by different operative positions, in a study that also involved normal, healthy, awake subjects (39). Ten volunteers under the age of 30 years with no prior history of lumbar disease had lateral lumbar radiographs taken in four different positions: standing; prone on a Jackson table with the hips slightly flexed; prone on an Andrews table with the hips flexed 60°; and prone on the Andrews table with the hips flexed 90°. Lumbar lordosis was measured at all motion segments from L1 to S1 for all subjects in each position.

The authors found an average total lumbar lordosis from L1 to S1 in the standing position of 51.7° (39). Mean contribution from L1 to L4 was 24.2°, and from L4 to S1, 27.5°. Average total lumbar lordosis on the Jackson table was 52.7°, with 26.1° contributed from L1 to L4 and 26.6° from L4 to S1. There was no statistically significant difference between standing and positioning on the Jackson table. In fact, total lordosis was slightly increased on the Jackson table (again, Peterson et al. found the same thing [34]). Average lumbar lordosis on the Andrews table with 90° of hip flexion was only 17°, with L1 to L4 contributing 8.3° and L4 to S1 contributing 8.7°. On the Andrews table with 60° of hip flexion, average total lordosis was 27.3°, with 16.2° measured between L1 and L4 and 11.1° between L4 and S1.

In the Stephens et al. study, the difference be-

TABLE 24.5.
Segmental and Total Lumbar Lordosis Mean Measurements (SEM) in Volunteers ($n = 17$, Cobb method): Lateral Lumbar Radiographs, Standing Neutral Versus Four Prone Positions

	Standing	Jackson	Chest Rolls	Relton-Hall	Hastings
L1–2	3.4 (4.1)	4.6 (3.0)	2.6 (3.9)	2.0 (2.5)	1.2 (3.0)[d]
L2–3	7.0 (3.7)	7.6 (2.0)	5.2 (2.5)	4.2 (2.5)[a,c]	1.9 (2.5)[a,c]
L3–4	10.9 (2.7)	9.9 (2.5)	7.2 (2.0)[a]	6.9 (3.0)[a,d]	3.7 (1.9)[a,c]
L4–5	16.3 (3.7)	13.2 (3.2)[a]	12.1 (3.3)[a]	9.2 (3.3)[a,c]	3.7 (2.0)[a,c]
L5–S1	27.6 (4.7)	25.4 (5.2)[b]	24.6 (4.5)[a]	21.4 (5.5)[a,c]	16.9 (7.7)[a,c]
L1–S1	65.9 (7.9)	60.8 (7.7)[b]	51.7 (10.2)[a,c]	43.7 (10.7)[a,c]	27.5 (10.9)[a,c]

From Nelson LM, Peterson MD, McManus AC, et al. Effect of positioning on lumbar lordosis: a prospective study of awake adult volunteers (Abstract). Hip position: Jackson, 30° flexion; chest rolls, neutral; Relton-Hall, 60° flexion; Hastings, 90° flexion.
SEM = Standard error of the mean.
All measurements lordotic degrees.
[a] Significantly different ($P < .01$) compared to standing.
[b] Significantly different ($P < .05$) compared to standing.
[c] Significantly different ($P < .01$) compared to Jackson table.
[d] Significantly different ($P < .05$) compared to Jackson table.

tween lordosis on the Jackson table and both positions on the Andrews table was statistically significant (39). There was also a significant difference between lordosis measured for both positions on the Andrews table in comparison with standing. Decreasing the amount of hip flexion on the Andrews table produced a significant increase in lumbar lordosis. The authors concluded from their data that for lumbar or lumbosacral fusions using instrumentation, physiologic sagittal spinal alignment can best be maintained by: *(a)* positioning on the Jackson table; and *(b)* avoidance of positions producing hip flexion.

As did Peterson et al., Stephens et al. confirmed and supported the findings previously reported by Tan et al. (40), who had also studied 10 awake volunteers with no prior history of back pain. The volunteers in the Tan et al. study were positioned prone on chest rolls, the Andrews frame, the Hastings frame, and a four-poster spinal frame. Total lordosis from L1 to S1 was measured as well as segmental lordosis at each level. Mean measurements for standing total lordosis and for the various positions evaluated were as follows: standing, $-55.6°$; chest rolls, $-45.8°$; Hastings frame, $-29.6°$; four-poster frame, $-28.3°$; and Andrews frame, $-23.8°$. Positioning on chest rolls lost a mean of around 10° of lordosis, but the difference was not statistically significant in this small study group. All of the other positions showed a statistically significant loss of lordosis, and again, the Andrews frame realized the largest reduction (40).

In summary, preservation of lumbar lordosis is important for some spinal procedures, and positioning of the patient should be carefully assessed, especially when using spinal instrumentation or other implants. From these studies it is shown that sagittal segmental alignment in the lumbar spine is largely dependent on how the patient is positioned, and this would seem to be especially so for patients relaxed or paralyzed under general anesthesia.

Spinal Fixation and Manipulation with Instrumentation

Though positioning of the patient is very important, force application after fixation with spinal instrumentation can also significantly change spinal alignments and balance. Various strategies and techniques can be used to segmentally realign the spine and to improve balance in different spinal disorders. The present author has defined and developed intrasacral fixation and in situ rod contouring principles and techniques for the correction of spinal malalignments and the improvement of segmental, regional, and global balance (9–17, 20–25). Intrasacral fixation and in situ contoured corrections are concepts and techniques largely based on: *(a)* analyses of the sagittal plane studies done by this author, and *(b)* his evolving understanding of the biomechanics governing the instrumental spine (8, 13–26, 32, 35, 36). Posterior spinal instrumentation with rigid implant–implant fixation shifts the segmental axes of angulation in the middle spinal column posteriorly and away from the center of gravity in the sagittal plane (Figs. 24.16 and 24.17). Specifically, the axes are shifted to the necks of the screws, if used, and to the posterior rods or plates. With the use of stiffer and stronger implants, the axes become less active with loading. Also, more unloading of the anterior and middle spinal column occurs. This is true for both static and cyclic loading within the elastic limits of the implants. However, with stiffer and stronger implants the stresses on the implants and bone-implant interfaces are increased.

The center of gravity for sagittal spinal balance is anterior to the sacrum and generally located globally over the axis through the hips when standing upright (Figs. 24.16 and 24.17) (13). The more posteriorly the rods and plates are positioned in the spine, and in the sagittal plane, the longer and stronger are moment arms acting on them, especially at the lumbosacral level (Fig. 24.16). A biomechanical advantage can be created by inserting the rods and plates, and therefore the axes or potential axes, closer to the center of gravity (Fig. 24.17). In addition, the distal ends of these implants are of a much lower profile since they are actually well within the sacrum.

With the intrasacral fixation technique providing increased fixation and long lever arms across the lumbosacral level, and with the use of stiff, strong ductile rods, then application of in situ contouring principles for spinal corrections is possible (12, 14, 15, 20, 21). Contouring creates a "translating axis" in the rod for correction. The axis can be "adjusted" along the rod, and an "adjustable contoured translating axis" (ACTA) can be achieved. Lordotic contouring of the rod in the lower lumbar spine and at the lumbosacral level causes anterior sacropelvic rotation through the hips and ventral translation of the lumbar spine with associated segmental angulation, where desired (13, 18, 36). As a result, the center of gravity in the sagittal plane is shifted posteriorly, further reducing the moment arms acting on the rods (Fig. 24.17). At the same time, better segmental, regional, and global alignments and balance can be realized, especially with respect to the lumbopelvic relationships discussed in this chapter.

Changes in Segmental Alignments Following Spinal Fusion

Hardacker et al. have studied preoperative and postoperative segmental lumbar lordosis in uninstrumented and instrumented solid lumbosacral fusion

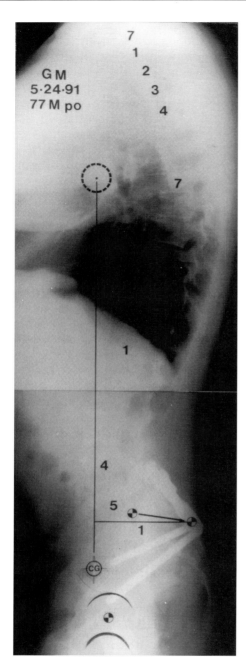

FIGURE 24.16.
Standing lateral radiograph of patient following L4-to-sacrum fusion with a Galveston construct for sacropelvic fixation. Constrained posterior spinal instrumentation shifts the segmental axis or potential axis of angulation at L5-S1 posteriorly to the rod and away from the center of gravity, as shown. With the implants in this position longer moment arms can act on them. (Reprinted with permission from Jackson RP. Intrasacral fixation: principles and techniques [Abstract].)

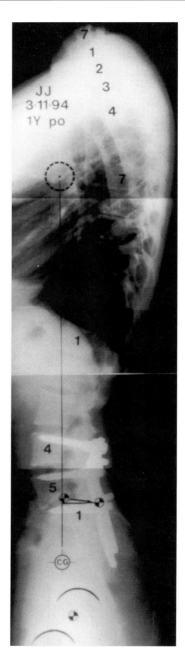

FIGURE 24.17.
Standing lateral radiograph of patient following L4-to-sacrum fusion with intrasacral fixation technique for sacropelvic fixation. With constrained posterior spinal instrumentation the segmental axis or potential axis of angulation at L5-S1 moves posteriorly to the rod and away from the center of gravity, as shown. Positioning the implants deep in the sacrum and closer to the center of gravity results in shorter moment arms acting on them. This can create a biomechanical advantage in comparison with other techniques (Fig. 24.16). With in situ contouring of this construct, segmental lordosis at L4–5 and L5-S1 can be increased and the center of gravity shifted more posteriorly toward the rods. (Reprinted with permission from Jackson RP. Intrasacral fixation: principles and techniques [Abstract].)

patients (6). These authors stated that a primary goal in reconstructive lumbar surgery was to obtain solid fusion, preferably with anatomically correct alignments in all three planes. They noted that much attention had been paid to sagittal spinal malalignment with long fusions into the lumbar spine, and the development of the iatrogenic "flatback syndrome" with its sequelae (7, 27–31, 37, 41). However, they pointed out that little attention had been paid to the sagittal spinal alignment of shorter lumbar and lumbosacral fusions, i.e., segmentally "flat fusions."

The Hardacker et al. study reviewed 119 bilateral posterolateral one-level, two-level, and three-level solid lumbar fusions to the sacrum. Criteria for inclusion in the study were that on recumbent Ferguson and lateral flexion-extension lumbar radiographs, taken a minimum of 2 years postoperatively, two separate observers concluded that solid fusion had been obtained. The authors noted that although sagittal spinal alignment is best assessed on standing lateral radiographs, such a study had not been obtained for many of their patients, but all had recumbent extension lateral lumbar films taken preoperatively and postoperatively. The study of standing versus extension films by Nelson et al. had shown that segmental lordosis was not significantly different at L3–4 and L4–5 and only about 4° different at the L5-S1 level (32). Hardacker et al. thought therefore that a valid comparison could be made using recumbent extension lateral lumbar films.

The 119 patients in the Hardacker et al. study were divided into three fusion groups: group 1, uninstrumented ($n = 37$); group 2, instrumented with standard constructs ($n = 42$; 22 with Cotrel-Dubousset (CD) rods and screws and 20 with bilateral translaminar facet screws); and group 3, instrumented with intrasacral fixation followed by in situ rod contouring using Jackson benders ($n = 40$). Indications for fusion included failure of conservative care and continued disabling low back pain with a diagnosis of lumbar segmental instability, spondylolisthesis, and/or symptomatic degenerative lumbar disc disease with and without disc herniation and/or stenosis. Attention to intraoperative positioning and preservation of lumbar lordosis was carried out in each instrumented case. All of the patients were operated on by the same surgeon (RPJ). All uninstrumented and standard instrumented patients were braced to solid fusion. Group 3 patients, who had intrasacral fixation, required no bracing. The data reviewed included age, sex, levels fused, and the number of prior surgeries. Preoperative and postoperative pain and functional outcome scores on self-assessment analog scores were compared. Segmental lordosis at all levels fused was measured preoperative and postoperatively using the Cobb angle method on the extension lumbar radiographs. Average follow-up for all patients was 54.8 months (range, 24 to 148 months). The preoperative and postoperative mean total segmental lordosis measurements of all levels fused for the three groups are shown in Table 24.6.

The total segmental lordosis change (a minus sign indicates loss of lordosis) and average number of levels fused for each group in the Hardacker et al. study were as follows: group 1, $-385°$, average levels fused 1.7; group 2, $-545°$, average levels fused 2.0; and group 3, $-67°$, average levels fused 2.0. Group 3 was significantly different from group 1 and group 2 ($P = .01$). The three groups differed with regard to age, number of prior surgeries, and levels fused, and hence a comparison of pain and functional capacity assessment analog scores for the different groups is not statistically appropriate. However, group 1 patients had the most favorable factors for outcome and group 3 the least. Despite these differences, group 3 patients did as well or better than the other two groups on all of the self-assessment analog scales and, again, they also had significantly more lordosis over the levels that were operated on.

Hardacker et al. found that group 1 and group 2 patients (uninstrumented and instrumented fusions) lost statistically significant degrees of segmental lordosis at the levels operated on ($P < .01$), and group 3 patients (fusions with intrasacral fixation and in situ rod contouring techniques) maintained the de-

TABLE 24.6.
Preoperative Versus Postoperative Additive Segmental Lordosis Mean Measurements (Cobb method): One-, Two-, and Three-Level Solid Posterior Lumbosacral Fusions

Levels	Pre-op	Post-op		Significance Level
Group 1 (fusion in situ without implants, $n = 37$)				
L5–S1	25.8	14.6	($n = 12$)	$P < .01$
L4–S1	28.0	17.8	($n = 24$)	$P < .01$
L3–S1	48.0	43.0	($n = 1$)	—
Group 2 (standard constructs/sacral fixations, $n = 42$)				
L5–S1	13.4	9.4	($n = 7$)	(n.s.)
L4–S1	35.2	21.1	($n = 29$)	$P < .01$
L3–S1	47.0	30.0	($n = 6$)	$P < .05$
Group 3 (intrasacral fixation/contoured in situ, $n = 40$)				
L5–S1	23.8	25.1	($n = 9$)	(n.s.)
L4–S1	38.1	35.1	($n = 22$)	(n.s.)
L3–S1	43.3	41.9	($n = 9$)	(n.s.)

From Hardacker JW, Jackson RP, Nelson LM, et al. Loss of segmental lordosis in instrumented and uninstrumented solid lumbosacral fusions (Abstract).
All measurements lordotic degrees.
Standard constructs involve one pair of bilateral screws for sacral fixations.
The additive segmental lordosis change (minus = loss) and average number of levels fused for each group was as follows: Group 1, $-385°$, average levels fused 1.7; Group 2, $-545°$, average levels fused 2.0; Group 3, $-67°$, average levels fused 2.0. Group 3 was significantly different from Group 1 and Group 2 ($P < .01$).

grees of preoperative segmental lumbar lordosis at the levels operated on without significant change (6). The authors concluded that in lumbar spine fusions care should be taken to maximize and preserve preoperative levels of segmental lordosis. In their study this was only achieved in the group 3 patients.

Jackson et al. studied a group of patients who between August 1979 and August 1987 underwent bilateral posterolateral one-, two-, and three-level lumbar fusions to the sacrum without instrumentation (19). To be included in this study, a minimum 2-year clinical and radiographic follow-up was required, as well as two observers concluding solid fusion on postoperative recumbent anteroposterior Ferguson and lateral flexion-extension lumbar radiographs. A preoperative recumbent lateral extension lumbar radiograph was also required for comparison, as well as preoperative and postoperative self-assessment analog pain and functional capacity scores and pain drawings for outcomes analysis. In this study patients with anterior interbody fusion and posterior lumbar interbody fusion (PLIF) procedures were not included. During this period a total of 192 patients underwent one-, two-, and three-level uninstrumented fusions and were possible candidates for the study. Of these, 160 were excluded for the following reasons: 76 had no preoperative extension film available or taken; 32 were not solidly fused; 28 had follow-up of less than 2 years, or were lost to contact, or deceased; 15 had chymopapain injection within 1 year before the surgery; seven patients had bone growth stimulators; and two had free-floating lumbar fusion. A total of 32 patients met the criteria. All of the patients had the same surgeon (RPJ). All were ambulated soon after surgery in a brace.

Jackson et al. noted that although sagittal spinal alignment is best assessed on standing lateral radiographs, many patients did not have such a study; however, all had preoperative and postoperative recumbent lateral extension lumbar films for comparison. The authors used the study of Nelson et al. (32) to extrapolate from standing neutral to recumbent extension measurements and to support their methodology and comparisons in this study.

Of the 32 patients in the study 18 were male and 14 were female. At index surgery, the mean age of the patients was 41.5 years (range, 21 to 66 years). Average follow-up time was 83 months (range, 36 to 148 months). The primary preoperative diagnoses were as follows: degenerative lumbar disc disease, with stenosis (7 patients), with herniated nucleus pulposus (11 patients), and without herniated nucleus pulposus or stenosis (2 patients); grade I isthmic spondylolisthesis (4 patients); degenerative spondylolisthesis with stenosis (1 patient); pseudarthrosis with stenosis (4 patients), and without stenosis (3 patients). The diagnosis of stenosis and/or herniated nucleus pulposus involved the performance of laminectomy and/or discectomy surgery at the involved level(s), unilaterally or bilaterally. All of the isthmic spondylolisthesis patients had L5 laminectomy. Nineteen patients (59%) had a total of 31 lumbar spine surgeries (average, 1.6 per patient) prior to their index surgery (resulting in solid fusion). A total of 54 levels were fused. Eleven patients had a one-level fusion, 20 a two-level fusion, and one a three-level fusion. The preoperative versus postoperative total segmental lordosis mean measurements for the one-, two-, and three-level fusions were as follows: L5-S1, 26.4° versus 16.9° ($n = 11$, $P < .01$); L4-S1, 30.7° versus 22.6° ($n = 20$, $P < .01$); L3-S1, 52° versus 58° ($n = 1$). Across all the levels fused, a total of 263° of lordosis was lost, a finding similar to that of the Hardacker et al. study (6).

In this Jackson et al. study a change in segmental lordosis at a given level following fusion was not related to laminectomy with or without discectomy (19). Of the 54 levels fused, 18 levels had fusion only: five levels gained an average of 2.8° of lordosis, one stayed the same, and 12 lost an average of 7.7° of lordosis. Nineteen levels had fusion with laminectomy only: six levels gained an average of 5.3° of lordosis, one stayed the same, and 12 lost an average of 7.9° of lordosis. Seventeen levels had fusion with laminectomy and discectomy: three levels gained an average of 5.0° of lordosis, and 14 levels lost an average of 7.4° of lordosis. Overall the total loss of lordosis was as follows: fusion only (18 levels), 97°; fusion with laminectomy only (19 levels), 72°; fusion with laminectomy and discectomy (17 levels), 94°.

Outcomes analysis in this study found 25 patients to be a little to a lot "better," two to be the same, and five to be worse. Those with one-level fusions did better than those with two-level fusions; however, the outcomes may have been influenced by the fact that only 36% of one-level fusion patients had prior surgeries (one or more), as compared with 70% of the two-level fusion patients. Pain frequency was improved 14%, pain severity 23%, work capacity 35%, and limitations in social and recreational activities 32%, with a mean overall improvement of only 26% on the self-assessment analog scales used.

In these two studies Hardacker et al. and Jackson et al. commented that their work was the first they could find comparing segmental lumbar lordosis before and after short one-, two-, and three-level lumbosacral fusions for degenerative disc disorders and instabilities involving low-grade isthmic and degenerative spondylolisthesis, spinal stenosis, herniated nucleus pulposus, and pseudarthrosis with disabling low back pain (6, 19). Jackson et al. stated in their study that the loss of lordosis was not related to the performance of a laminectomy or discectomy at a given level (19). Possible explanations offered were postoperative bracing, iatrogenic muscle injury, and other causes. The authors of these studies, again, stated that approximately two-thirds of total lordosis is normally distributed between the lower two discs. They found that in situ fusion surgery did not appear to maintain the normal sagittal alignments between L4 and S1 in most of their patients. The long-term clinical consequences for such loss of segmental lordosis at the levels operated on and for the levels above were not part of their present studies. The authors stated that the loss of lordosis was both undesirable and worrisome. Also, the authors of these studies commented that the overall clinical results were not as good as expected in the solidly fused groups of patients with loss of segmental lordosis.

Jackson et al. concluded that one- and two-level uninstrumented solid lumbosacral fusions lost significant segmental lordosis at the levels operated on ($P < .01$) and, again, stated that the changes in lordosis could not be explained by the other procedures performed at a given level, that is, laminectomy and/or discectomy (19). The authors stated that a more careful assessment of preoperative and postoperative segmental lordosis may be indicated, especially when reporting outcome studies. Again, Hardacker et al. found better clinical outcomes in the patients with more segmental lordosis at the lumbar levels fused (6).

Spondylolisthesis

Jackson et al. reported on the clinical results and standing radiographic sagittal spinal alignments in spondylolisthesis before and after surgery (23). Twenty-eight consecutive patients with symptomatic L5-S1 spondylolisthesis had bilateral fusion to the sacrum using lumbosacral rod-screw instrumentation with intrasacral fixation and in situ rod contouring techniques. Five patients also had interbody fusions. The proximal end of the instrumentation was to L5 in 11 patients, to L4 in 15 patients, to L3 in one patient, and to L2 in one patient. There were 16 males and 12 females, and the mean of their ages was 37.8 years (range, 20 to 61 years). The following grades of spondylolisthesis were treated: 17 at grade I, eight at grade II, two at grade III, and one at grade V.

The patients in this study were instrumented with intrasacral fixation techniques distally for increased sacral fixation, and the rods were contoured in situ to create a "translating axis" for lumbosacral manipulation and correction, as described above. The authors stated that such contouring was possible because of the use of stiff, strong ductile rods and the increased fixation and long lever arms provided by the intrasacral fixation technique. Correction by contouring of the rods with screws provided for additional lordosis and further foraminal decompression, according to the authors. This was accomplished with the lever arms acting through both the screws and intrasacral rods, creating sacropelvic rotation through the hips. Selective monosegmental vertebral angulation with intervertebral extension moments across the lumbosacral level in the sagittal plane were developed at the time of manipulation. The authors stated that it was important that complete bilateral L5-S1 facetectomies and foraminotomies be performed prior to contouring for lumbosacral manipulations. When the screws were locked on the rod and contouring carried out, the axis of angulation was shifted to the rod and translated with the ductile rod as it was deformed. Again, this created a "translating axis" for correction. Posterior spinal column shortening resulted without collapse or compression in the middle column or neuroforamina because of where the axis was located with the screws locked on the rods. Bracing was only selectively done.

All of the patients in this study had preoperative and postoperative standing 36-inch lateral radiographs for comparison. The following measurements in the sagittal plane were compared: kyphosis (Cobb method from T1 to T12), lordosis (Cobb method from the superior endplates of L1 to S1), spinal balance (perpendicular distance from the posterosuperior corner of S1 to the C7 sagittal plumb line), and sacral inclination or slope (a line drawn along the back of the proximal sacrum and its angle of intersection with the plumb line) as a measure of pelvic angulation or standing hip extension in the sagittal plane (Figs. 24.1, 24.2, 24.3, and 24.4). Also, L5-S1 slip angle (measured between a line drawn parallel with the L5 superior endplate and a line perpendicular to the one drawn along the back of the proximal sacrum), and percentage of slip were recorded.

The 28 patients in this study had an average clinical and radiographic follow-up of 34 months (range, 24 to 52 months). All 28 were found to have a solid fusion on the basis of recumbent anteroposterior Ferguson and lateral flexion-extension lumbar radiographs postoperatively at last follow-up. Three patients required a second surgery to achieve solid fusion (nonunion in two and delayed healing in one). The authors reported no broken screws. Also no rod or screw pullouts in the sacrum were reported, and this was believed to be due primarily to the use of the intrasacral fixation technique. A broken rod was seen in two patients, both with solid fusions. The use of a "contoured translating axis" with resultant lumbosacral manipulation was also found to be safe, according to the authors. There was one neurologic complication encountered in this series (patient with grade V slip reduced to grade II). All of the patients were better postoperatively, with no clinical failures reported, as determined by self-assessment pain drawings and analog pain and functional capacity comparisons preoperatively and postoperatively. The mean pain and functional capacity assessments were significantly improved ($P < .0001$). Preoperative versus postoperative standing lateral radiographic mean measurements were: kyphosis, $+43°$ versus $+44°$ (P value not significant); lordosis, $-64°$ versus $-70°$ ($P = .0002$); C7 sagittal plumb, $+1.4$ cm versus $+0.1$ cm ($P = .0526$); sacral inclination, $48°$ versus $55°$ ($P = .0012$); slip angle at L5-S1, $-20°$ versus $-30°$ ($P = .0023$); percentage slip, 27% versus 9.4% ($P = .0001$).

Jackson et al. concluded that the intrasacral fixation technique for the implants distally appeared to provide increased fixation clinically (23). They stated that in situ contouring of a stiff, strong ductile rod using Jackson benders provided a "translating axis" for segmental correction and gave selective lumbosacral angulation, where desired. The authors felt that these techniques helped to create the significant postoperative changes measured in their sagittal plane analysis studies.

Scoliosis

Jackson and McManus performed a clinical assessment, including radiographic sagittal plane analysis, in a difficult and challenging group of patients with lumbar and thoracolumbar scoliosis treated with a long fusion from the thoracic spine to the sacrum (17). The authors reviewed 15 consecutive adult patients with painful lumbar and thoracolumbar curves, degenerative and idiopathic, who had posterior spinal instrumentation and fusion to the sacrum using lumbosacral pedicle screws, intrasacral fixation, and in situ rod contouring techniques. Only one patient underwent anterior surgery with interbody fusion, and none had anterior fusion across the lumbosacral level. The proximal end of the instrumentation was to T11 in five patients, to T10 in six patients, to T9 two patients, to T3 in one patient, and to T2 in one patient (revised from T9 to this level). There were 13 females and 2 males, and the mean of their ages was 59 years (range, 35 to 73 years).

In this study, the authors stated that corrections by rod contouring provided for additional lordosis and further foraminal decompression and were believed by the authors to give more intraoperative control of the deformity in three planes (17). The corrections were found to be safe, and no neurologic complications were encountered. Jackson and McManus also stated that posterior column shortening resulted, at least in the lumbar spine, without clinical collapse or compromise of the middle column or neuroforamina occurring (17). When screws were used in the lumbar spine, contouring was carried out because rotation of the rod was difficult and did not control torsion of the spine unless direct derotation forces in the transverse plane were also applied to the screws. This was true whether instrumentation was done down to the sacrum or not. Postoperative bracing was only selectively carried out, usually in the more osteoporotic patients.

In this study average clinical and radiographic follow-up was 24 months (range, 18 to 40 months). The 15 consecutive patients reported a mean 40% improvement in pain on preoperative versus postoperative self-assessment analog pain scores ($P = .0385$). Eight broken rods and two broken screws (both sacral) in six patients were documented. Four patients with one broken rod each had minimal loss of correction and improved clinical results at the time of review. Two patients were reported to have symptomatic pseudarthroses with associated bilateral broken rods, as well as loss of correction and were considered clinical failures. The authors felt that the high rate of implant breakage was a result of not having performed anterior fusions in these patients with long constructs to the sacrum. No rod or screw pullouts in the pelvis were reported, primarily because of intrasacral fixation for the instrumentation distally, the authors stated. Cobb measurements on standing 36-inch anteroposterior radiographs of the 15 major lumbar and thoracolumbar curves averaged $35°$ preoperatively (range, $12°$ to $82°$), and $17°$ postoperatively (range, $0°$ to $62°$) ($P = .0001$). The following preoperative and postoperative sagittal plane measurements were also compared on standing 36-inch lateral radiographs: L1 to S1 lordosis (Cobb method from the superior endplates of L1 and S1), sagittal balance, sacral inclination or slope, and thoracic kyphosis (Cobb method from T1 to T12), as described earlier (Figs. 24.1, 24.2, 24.3, and 24.4). The preoperative versus postoperative mean measurements reported were: thoracic kyphosis, $+26°$ versus $+44°$ ($P = .0001$); total lordosis, $-33°$ versus $-54°$ ($P = .0017$); sagittal balance, $+4.5$ cm versus $+0.1$ cm ($P = .0486$); and sacral inclination, $44°$ versus $46°$ (P value not significant).

Jackson and McManus concluded that the techniques of intrasacral fixation for the instrumentation distally in scoliosis appeared to provide increased fixation clinically (17). Also, in situ contouring of the stiff, strong ductile rod and screw constructs for corrections with "translating axes" was found to be effective and safe. This was similar to what they had reported for spondylolisthesis (23). The authors felt that these techniques resulted in the significant postoperative changes measured in the sagittal plane with increased total lordosis, a posterior shift of the plumb line with improved spinal balance, and an overall increase in total thoracic kyphosis that approached near normal values, as reported above. However, for long-term stability and maintenance of the corrections obtained by these techniques, the authors stated that solid anterior interbody fusions are required.

Kyphosis

Jackson and McManus have also evaluated segmental and total kyphotic and lordotic spinal alignments before and after the surgical correction of developmental thoracic hyperkyphosis using in situ rod contouring techniques (24). Specifically, the authors were interested in looking at preoperative and postoperative total kyphosis and total lordosis as well as the junctional changes in the open motion segments above and below the instrumentation used to correct the deformities, and then comparing the results with normative data. They reviewed 10 consecutive patients who had surgery between July 1986 and June 1990 and were instrumented with CD implants. All the patients were skeletally mature at surgery, except one who had refused bracing and had become progressively worse. Three patients had anterior release and interbody fusions preceding their posterior procedure. Criteria for selection in the study were: (a) chief complaint of kyphotic deformity with or without progression; (b) diagnosis of developmental thoracic hyperkyphosis with lumbar hyperlordosis; and (c) no instrumentation or fusion below L2. Patients with kyphoscoliosis, prior surgery, or congenital, posttraumatic, osteoporotic, pathologic, or iatrogenic hyperkyphosis were excluded. Clinical evaluation included pain and functional capacity assessments on analog scales with outcomes analysis. All of the patients were examined with standing 36-inch lateral radiographs of the entire spine preoperatively and postoperatively. Limits of kyphotic deformity (end vertebra) were determined and measured by the Cobb method. Lumbar lordosis was measured from L1 to S1, also by the Cobb method. The segmental angulation between the last instrumented vertebra and the next uninstrumented vertebra at the proximal and distal ends of the construct was measured between superior adjacent endplates by the Cobb method. Segmental angulation at the distal end of the construct was also evaluated by measuring the intervertebral disc angle; this was done by drawing two lines parallel to the superior and inferior endplates above and below the distal junctional open motion segment disc space and measuring the angle between them. Levels of deformity and levels of instrumentation recorded for this study are shown in Table 24.7.

In this study there were 7 females and 3 males, and the mean of their ages at surgery was 25 years (range, 11 to 44 years). One patient was lost to any further follow-up 17 months after surgery. The remainder of the patients had a minimum 2-year follow-up after surgery. The average follow-up for all patients was 55 months (range, 17 to 92 months). Nine patients were satisfied with the cosmetic result and one was dissatisfied. Seven of the 10 patients had pain preoperatively ranging from only mild to dull on the analog self-assessment pain scale. Using the same self-assessment pain scale postoperatively, backache was reported to be better in three, the same in six, and one grade worse in one patient. Functional capacity in terms of work and social activity limitations was better in five and the same in five postoperatively. Complications involved prominent hardware in four patients (one revised, one removed). There were no hardware failures, neurologic complications, pseudarthroses, or infections found in this study. Preoperative kyphotic deformity averaged +75.5° (range, +66° to +100°) and postoperatively averaged +45.3° (range, +31° to +69°) ($P = .0001$). Preoperative lumbar lordosis (L1 to S1) averaged −80.8° (range, −67° to −95°) and postoperatively averaged −62° (range, −44° to −74°) ($P = .0009$).

TABLE 24.7.
Kyphotic Deformity, Levels Measured (Cobb method) and Levels Instrumented (10 Patients)

	Pre-op (degrees)	Post-op (degrees)	Levels Measured	Levels Instrumented
Group 1 (4 Patients)				
1	70	38	T4–L1	T4–L2
2	66	31	T1–11	T1–12
3	70	43	T3–12	T3–12
4	72	44	T3–L1	T3–L1
Group 2 (6 Patients)				
5	100	69	T2–L1	T2–L1[a]
6	77	46	T2–L2	T2–L2
7	72	51	T2–L1	T3–L2[a]
8	76	52	T3–L1	T1–L2[a]
9	75	45	T3–L1	T3–L2
10	74	43	T3–L2	T3–L2
Mean	75.5	45.3	($P < .0001$)	
Range	66–100	31–69		

From Jackson RP, McManus AC. Evaluation of junctional kyphosis following surgical correction for developmental thoracic hyperkyphosis (Abstract).
[a] Anterior followed by posterior procedure

At the proximal open motion segment adjacent to the most upper instrumented level in this study, there was a mean postoperative kyphosing change of +10.9° (range, +6° to +18°), as measured by the Cobb method at last follow-up (Table 24.8). All of the constructs used bilateral hooks on the most proximal vertebra instrumented consisting of supralaminar hooks or transverse process–pedicle hook "claw" constructs. The most proximal vertebra instrumented was the end vertebra measured for the deformity in eight of the 10 patients (Table 24.7). At the distal end of the construct four patients had bilateral infralaminar hooks only (group 1) and six had bilateral infralaminar hooks plus bilateral screws at the same level (group 2). The mean postoperative kyphosing change

TABLE 24.8.
Postoperative Junctional Segmental Angulation in Instrumented Hyperkyphosis (10 Patients, Cobb Method)

Proximal Open Motion Segment		
Mean Kyphosing Change	+10.9°	(Range +6° to +18°)
Mean Segmental Angulation	+6.7°	(Range +4° to +10°)
Levels: C7–T1 (2), T1–2 (2), T2–3 (5), T3–4 (1)		(Normal range 0° to +3°)
Distal Open Motion Segment		
Hooks Only, 4 Patients (Group 1)		
Mean Kyphosing Change	+14.3°	(Range +10° to +18°)
Mean Segmental Angulation	+7.0°	(Range −5° to +14°)
Levels: T12–L1 (2), L1–2 (1), L2–3 (1)		(Normal range 0° to −7°)
Hooks and Screws, 6 Patients (Group 2)		
Mean Kyphosing Change	+11.8°	(Range +8° to +14°)
Mean Segmental Angulation	+2.3°	(Range −8° to +9°)
Levels: L1–2 (1), L2–3 (5)		(Normal range −3° to −7°)

From Jackson RP, McManus AC. Evaluation of junctional kyphosis following surgical correction for developmental thoracic hyperkyphosis (Abstract).
+ is kyphotic or kyphosing, − is lordotic.
The instrumentation created junctional kyphosis in both the proximal and distal open motion segments.

distally following instrumentation in group 1 was +14.3° (range, +10° to +18°) and in group 2, +11.8° (range, +8° to +14°) by the Cobb method at last follow-up (Table 24.8). However, the mean disc angle measured in group 1 was +9.3° (range, +6° to +11°) and in group 2, only +0.5° (range, −3° to +8°). In group 1, two patients were instrumented distally to the actual end vertebra of the deformity and in two patients one vertebra more distal to the end vertebra measured for the deformity (Table 24.7). In group 2, three patients were instrumented to the end vertebra of the deformity and three patients one vertebra more distal (Table 24.7). (Again, none of the constructs extended below L2 in this study.)

Jackson and McManus pointed out that infralaminar hooks at the distal end of the construct, loaded in compression for correction toward the apex of the deformity, caused junctional kyphosis in the adjacent open disc space. They believed that this was because all of the forces were acting in the posterior column behind the segmental axis of angulation at this junctional uninstrumented and open distal motion segment. They indicated that this tended to angulate the most distally instrumented vertebra too much in flexion, thereby causing compression anteriorly in this adjacent open intervertebral disc and perhaps segmental stretching of the ligaments posteriorly at this level. By adding screws in the distal end vertebra, compressive force application throughout the three columns of the caudal motion segment was possible after completion of in situ rod contouring with Jackson benders. This appeared to reduce the postoperative junctional kyphosing effect of the instrumentation distally in this open disc space as well as to increase the fixation in this vertebra. Their recommended method for choosing the most distal end vertebra to instrument at surgery entails: (a) inclusion of the vertebra transected by the C7 sagittal plumb line on a preoperative standing lateral radiograph of the entire spine; and (b) addition of one vertebra more distal to the end vertebra measured for the kyphotic deformity by the Cobb method on this standing radiograph. Also, instrumentation of the most distal vertebra should include bilateral screws for the biomechanical reasons presented, according to these authors. A method or methods to reduce junctional kyphosing effects of the instrumentation at the proximal end of the construct following surgery needs further evaluation and study, the authors concluded. Whether or not the in situ contouring of the rods contributed to the junctional kyphosis is something that is still being studied by the authors.

In summary, Jackson and McManus stated that in the correction of thoracic kyphotic deformity, (a) the instrumentation is frequently prominent and can apparently be symptomatic; (b) postoperative junctional kyphosis often results and can be problematic; and (c) the use of bilateral screws at the lower end of the construct increases the fixation, but more important, it reduces kyphosis in the open disc space adjacent to the distal end of the instrumentation. The authors found good correction with normalization of kyphosis and lordosis postoperatively when compared with their previously reported mean data of adult volunteers.

Thoracolumbar Burst Fractures

Ebelke et al. and Jackson reviewed a group of 25 consecutive burst fracture patients treated with posterior pedicle instrumentation for reduction and stabilization (3, 15). Ten patients were instrumented with standard hook, screw, and rod constructs without in situ rod contouring, and 15 were instrumented with a six-screw/two-distal hook construct that was contoured in situ for fracture correction (15, 21, 25). The contoured corrections were shown to be safe by these authors. Angular kyphotic change at the fracture site was found to be better in the contoured group, both in terms of initial correction and maintenance of correction. The group of 10 patients treated with standard constructs and techniques had a mean preoperative kyphosis of 17°, and at last follow-up, 16°. The group of 15 patients treated with in situ rod contouring techniques had a mean preoperative kyphosis of

16°, and only 3° at last follow-up. The differences were significant ($P < .05$). The authors pointed out that it was important both to correct and to maintain normal sagittal spinal alignments when possible. They advocated using normative segmental spinal alignment studies for comparison of the preoperative and postoperative angular measurements in patients, as defined and recommended by Farcy et al. (4).

Conclusions

With a better understanding of sagittal spinal alignment, normative data, including standard deviations and ranges, treatment of spinal deformities, instabilities, degenerative conditions, and other disorders can be more carefully evaluated and compared. Typical and somewhat characteristic sagittal plane abnormalities exist for different disorders of the adult spine. It is helpful to recognize the existing abnormalities and compensations prior to any treatment and to not aggravate them with the intervention. By maintaining or correcting for fairly normal segmental alignments, better regional and global balance of the spine can be realized and less desirable or undesirable compensatory mechanisms minimized. This is thought to be especially so for the lumbopelvic alignments and relationships defined and discussed in this chapter.

References

1. Andersson GBJ, Murphy RW, Ortengren R, Nachemson AL. The influence of backrest inclination and lumbar support on lumbar lordosis. Spine 1979;4(1):52–58.
2. Bernhardt M, Bridwell KH. Segmental analysis of the sagittal plane alignment of the normal thoracic and lumbar spines and thoracolumbar junction. Spine 1989;14(7):717–721.
3. Ebelke DK, Jackson RP, Hess WF, et al. CD pedicle instrumentation for improved burst fracture fixation and reduction with in situ extension contouring of the rods. VIII Proceeding of the International Congress on Cotrel-Dubousset Instrumentation, 1991. G.I.C.D. Textbook. Sauramps Medical, 1992:45–54.
4. Farcy JPC, Weidenbaum M, Glassman SD. Sagittal index in management of thoracolumbar burst fractures. Spine 1990;15(9):958–965.
5. Gelb DE, Lenke LG, Bridwell KH, et al. An analysis of sagittal spinal alignment in 100 asymptomatic middle and older aged volunteers. Spine 1995;20(12):1351–1358.
6. Hardacker JW, Jackson RP, Nelson LM, et al. Loss of segmental lordosis in instrumented and uninstrumented solid lumbosacral fusions (Abstract).
7. Hasday CA, Passoff TL, Perry J. Gait abnormalities arising from iatrogenic loss of lumbar lordosis secondary to Harrington instrumentation in lumbar fractures. Spine 1983;8(5):501–511.
8. Jackson RP, Cain JE. Correction and stabilization of kyphotic deformity in spondylolisthesis. V Proceeding of the International Congress on Cotrel-Dubousset Instrumentation, 1988. G.I.C.D. Textbook. Sauramps Medical, 1989:131–134.
9. Jackson RP, Hamilton AC. CD screws with oblique canals for improved sacral fixation: a prospective clinical study of the first fifty patients. VII Proceeding of the International Congress on Cotrel-Dubousset Instrumentation, 1990. G.I.C.D. Textbook. Sauramps Medical, 1991:75–86.
10. Jackson RP, Ebelke DK, McManus AC. The "sacroiliac buttress" and new methods for correction with CD pedicle instrumentation. VIII Proceeding of the International Congress on Cotrel-Dubousset Instrumentation, 1991. G.I.C.D. Textbook. Sauramps Medical, 1992:135–159.
11. Jackson RP, McManus AC. The "iliac buttress": a computed tomographic study of sacral anatomy. Spine 1993;18(10):1318–1328.
12. Jackson RP. Jackson intrasacral fixation and segmental corrections with adjustable contoured translating axes. In: Errico TJ, ed. Spine: State of the art reviews. Philadelphia: Hanley & Belfus, 1994;8(2):307–341.
13. Jackson RP, McManus AC. Radiographic analysis of sagittal plane alignment and balance in standing volunteers and patients with low back pain matched for age, sex, and size: a prospective controlled clinical study. Spine 1994;19(14):1611–1618.
14. Jackson RP. Insertion of intrasacral rods for sacral fixation and spinal correction with in situ rod contouring techniques. In: Bridwell KH, DeWald RL, eds. Textbook of spinal surgery. 2nd ed. Philadelphia: Lippincott-Raven, 1997:2187–2209.
15. Jackson RP. Lumbar burst fractures: fixation with pedicle instrumentation and reduction by adjustable contoured translating axes using in situ Jackson benders. In: Bridwell KH, DeWald RL, eds. Textbook of spinal surgery. 2d ed. Philadelphia: Lippincott-Raven, 1997:1881–1898.
16. Jackson RP. Jackson sacral fixation and contoured spinal correction techniques. In: Margulies JY, Floman Y, Farcy J-PC, and Neuwirth MG, eds. Lumbosacral and Spinopelvic Fixation. Philadelphia: Lippincott-Raven, 1996:357–379.
17. Jackson RP, McManus AC. Radiographic sagittal plane analysis in lumbar and thoracolumbar adult scoliosis instrumented to the sacrum with new techniques. Presented at the annual meeting of the North America Spine Society, San Diego, California, October 1993.
18. Jackson RP, Peterson MD, McManus AC. Standing sagittal balance and lumbopelvic relationships in adult volunteers and patients with degenerative lumbar disc disease, scoliosis, and spondylolisthesis. Presented at the annual meeting of the Scoliosis Research Society, Portland, Oregon, September 1994.
19. Jackson RP, Nelson LM, Hardacker JW, et al. Loss of segmental lordosis in uninstrumented solid lumbosacral fusions (Abstract).
20. Jackson RP. Intrasacral fixation: principles and techniques (Abstract).

21. Jackson RP. In situ contouring for spinal corrections: principles and techniques (Abstract).
22. Jackson RP. Cotrel-Dubousset instrumentation for spondylolisthesis: new techniques (Abstract).
23. Jackson RP, Ebelke DK, McManus AC. Clinical results and standing radiographic sagittal plane analysis in spondylolisthesis instrumented to the sacrum with new techniques (Abstract).
24. Jackson RP, McManus AC. Evaluation of junctional kyphosis following surgical correction for developmental thoracic hyperkyphosis (Abstract).
25. Jackson RP. Biomechanics of lumbar burst fracture reductions with short segment screw fixation systems (Abstract and video).
26. Jackson RP, the Midwest Spine Foundation. Translating axes of segmental spinal motion in three planes (Abstract and video).
27. Kostuik JP, Hall BB. Spinal fusions to the sacrum in adults with scoliosis. Spine 1983;8:489–500.
28. Kostuik JP, Maurais GR, Richardson WJ, et al. Combined single stage anterior and posterior osteotomy for correction of iatrogenic lumbar kyphosis. Spine 1988; 13:257–266.
29. Kostuik JP. Treatment of scoliosis in the adult thoracolumbar spine with special reference to fusion to the sacrum. Orthop Clin North Am 1993;19:371–381.
30. La Grone MO. Loss of lumbar lordosis: a complication of spinal fusion for scoliosis. Orthop Clin North Am 1988;19:383–393.
31. Luk KD, Lee FB, Leong JC, et al. The effect on the lumbosacral spine of long spinal fusion for idiopathic scoliosis: a minimum 10-year follow-up. Spine 1987; 12:996–1000.
32. Nelson LM, McManus AC, Jackson RP. Standing neutral versus recumbent extension lordosis in patients with spondylolisthesis and degenerative lumbar disc disease (Abstract).
33. Nelson LM, Peterson MD, McManus AC, Jackson RP. Effect of positioning on lumbar lordosis: a prospective study of awake adult volunteers (Abstract).
34. Peterson MD, Nelson LM, McManus AC, Jackson RP. The effect of operative position on lumbar lordosis: a radiographic study of patients under anesthesia in the prone and 90–90 positions. Spine 1995;20(12):1419–1424.
35. Peterson MD, Jackson RP, McManus AC. Standing sagittal balance, alignments, and lumbopelvic relationships. Part I: A study of adult volunteers (Abstract).
36. Peterson MD, Jackson RP, McManus AC. Standing sagittal balance, alignments, and lumbopelvic relationships. Part II: A study of patients with spinal disorders (Abstract).
37. Shufflebarger HL, Clark CD. Thoracolumbar osteotomy for postsurgical sagittal imbalance. Spine 1992; 17(Suppl):S287–S290.
38. Stagnara P, De Mauroy JC, Dran G, et al. Reciprocal angulation of vertebral bodies in a sagittal plane: approach to references for the evaluation of kyphosis and lordosis. Spine 1982;7(4):335–342.
39. Stephens GC, Wilber RG, Yoo JU. Comparison of lumbar sagittal alignment produced by different operative positions. Presented at the annual meeting of the Scoliosis Research Society, Portland, Oregon, September 1994.
40. Tan SB, Kozak JA, Dickson JH, et al. Effect of operative position on sagittal alignment of the lumbar spine. Spine 1994;19(3):314–318.
41. Willers U, Hedlund R, Aaro S, et al. Long-term results of Harrington instrumentation in idiopathic scoliosis. Spine 1993;18:713–717.

CHAPTER TWENTY FIVE

Degenerative Lumbar Spondylolisthesis

Harry N. Herkowitz

Introduction

Degenerative lumbar spondylolisthesis is a common condition occurring in the older population (Fig. 25.1). The incidence is higher in females than in males. Although a previous report suggested black females to be the most prone, other studies have disputed this (11, 12, 25). The most common level of involvement in isthmic spondylolisthesis is L5-S1, whereas in degenerative lumbar spondylolisthesis L4–5 is most often involved, followed by L3–4. In addition, the incidence of a double degenerative spondylolisthesis is 5%, with simultaneous involvement of L3–4 and L4–5. The reasons that degenerative spondylolisthesis does not occur at L5-S1 are: *(a)* the iliolumbar ligaments support the L5 vertebra, preventing forward migration; *(b)* the L5 vertebra sits within the pelvic brim below the intercristal line and is protected from stresses affecting the other lumbar vertebrae; *(c)* the coronal orientation of the L5-S1 facet joints acts as a block to forward migration of the L5 vertebra.

The earliest description of this condition dates to the 19th century, and the first description in the modern literature appeared in a report by Junghanns in a German journal (3, 16). The condition was defined in the North American literature by MacNab in 1950, with the modern term "degenerative spondylolisthesis" coined by Newman shortly thereafter (21, 22).

Pathogenesis

The etiology and pathogenesis of degenerative spondylolisthesis involve hormonal factors and structural alterations. The hormonal factors center on estrogen release and its relaxing effect on the ligaments and soft tissues in general, and specifically on the supraspinous and interspinous ligaments and the annulus fibrosus of the spinal motion segment. The structural alterations include factors that increase stress across the motion segment and reduce its structural integrity as well as developmental anatomy that predisposes to vertebral slippage.

While the L5 vertebra remains protected within the pelvic brim, the L4 vertebra is subjected to stresses that can lead to its forward migration, especially when structural alterations such as sacralization are present along with osteoarthritis of the facet joints.

The pathogenesis of degenerative spondylolisthesis begins with degeneration of the intervertebral disc. This in turn increases micromotion of the L4–L5 spinal segment, which leads to degeneration and loss of structural integrity of the L4–L5 facet joints. The developmental anatomical orientation of the facet joints in the sagittal plane associated with the osteoarthritis of the joints, in combination with the loss of ligamentous support, allows the vertebra to slide forward (Fig. 25.2) (9). Because the stresses

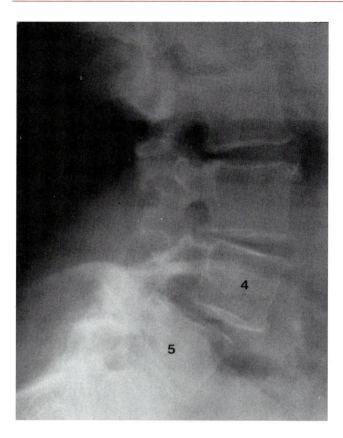

FIGURE 25.1.
Lateral lumbar radiograph demonstrating an L4-L5 degenerative spondylolisthesis.

across the normal facet joint amount to as much as 33% of the applied axial load, it is not surprising that forward slippage occurs when the factors listed above are present (29).

It is important to know the natural history of the condition so that a rational treatment plan can be undertaken. According to Matsunaga et al., in a group of patients who had degenerative lumbar spondylolisthesis and were observed over a 10-year period, an increase in the amount of slippage occurred in 30% of individuals (20). Unlike in isthmic spondylolisthesis, the amount of slip did not exceed 30% of the vertebral body width. No specific factors could be identified that predisposed to progressive slippage, although in females the slip progressed more than in males, and the progression in those who engaged in physical labor tended to be greater than that in sedentary individuals. The clinical symptoms were intermittent, with the severity and duration of symptoms different for each patient.

The symptoms and signs of degenerative lumbar spondylolisthesis are those associated with spinal stenosis (10). These consist of back pain associated with leg pain that may be unilateral or bilateral and is either radicular or the more classic neurogenic claudication associated with spinal stenosis. The symptoms are mechanical, that is, precipitated by activity and improved with rest. Although back pain may be a significant component of the patient's complaints, it is usually the leg symptoms that bring the patient to the doctor. The back pain complaints associated with the instability of spondylolisthesis may be more severe than those associated with degenerative stenosis alone.

The leg symptoms are generally consistent with a radiculopathy. In an L4–5 degenerative spondylolisthesis, leg symptoms usually follow an L5 pattern. However, they may be described as diffuse aching, heaviness, or numbness. This may simulate vascular claudication, but pulses are present and leg symptoms begin proximally and travel distally, whereas in vascular claudication this pattern is reversed. Lower extremity weakness occurs in 15% of cases and usually originates in L5 or L4. Rarely is profound weakness present.

If long tract signs are present, neural compression may be present in the cervical or thoracic spine; it is not uncommon to see compression simultaneously in the cervical and the lumbar spine. Bladder complaints are common in the older age group but are attributable to spinal stenosis only in a small percentage of cases.

Diagnosis

The diagnostic workup consists of plain radiographs, imaging studies, and electrodiagnostic testing. Plain

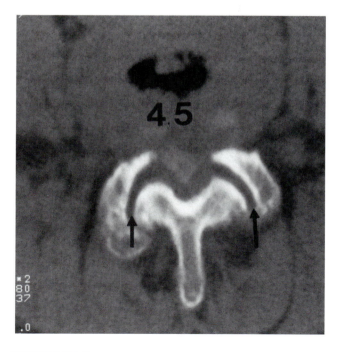

FIGURE 25.2.
Axial image of CT scan at L4-L5 depicting sagittal orientation of left and right facet joints.

radiographs demonstrate lumbar osteoarthritis in addition to the spondylolisthesis and also rule out other pain sources, including tumor, infection, metabolic disorders, Paget's disease, and hip joint arthritis. Degenerative spondylolisthesis is most often seen at L4–5, followed by L3–4. The oblique films do not demonstrate a pars interarticularis defect. A standing lateral film may show the spondylolisthesis not otherwise present on a supine lateral radiograph. The degree of slippage usually does not exceed 30% of the adjacent vertebral body width. Preservation of lordosis is seen in most cases, although some reduction is not uncommon as a result of the diffuse osteoarthritis that tends to flatten the lumbar spine.

Flexion extension lateral films are routinely obtained in cases of spondylolisthesis. These are taken in a standing position with the patient in a maximally flexed and extended position. In cases in which it is difficult for the patient to cooperate, supine bending films are obtained.

The measurements taken on the flexion-extension lateral films follow the technique illustrated by Dupuis (7). Excessive translational movement is defined as more than 4 mm of combined forward and backward motion (Fig. 25.3), and excessive angular motion is defined as endplate angular change greater than 10° compared to the endplate above and below (Fig. 25.4).

Imaging studies consist of computed tomography (CT), myelography with and without CT, and magnetic resonance imaging (MRI). CT provides a detailed view of the bony pathology better than it does

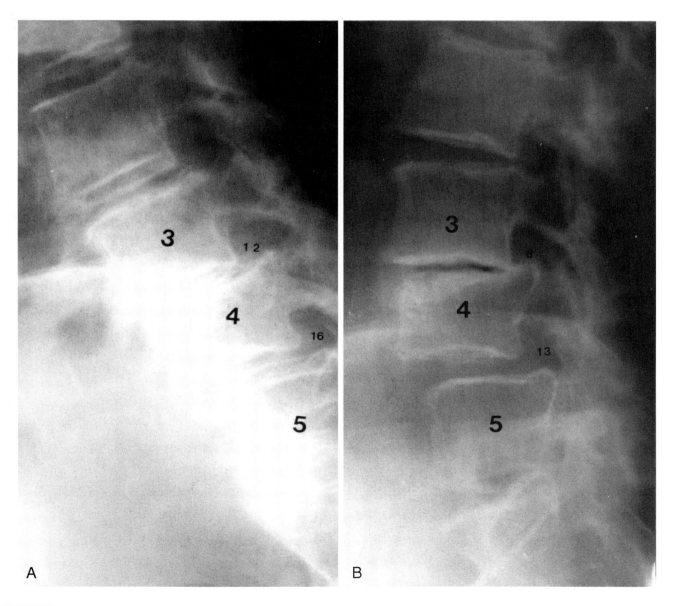

FIGURE 25.3.

A. Lateral flexion radiograph depicting spondylolisthesis measuring 12 mm at L3–4 and 16 mm at L4–5. **B.** Lateral extension radiograph depicting spondylolisthesis reducing to 8 mm at L3–4 and 13 mm at L4–5.

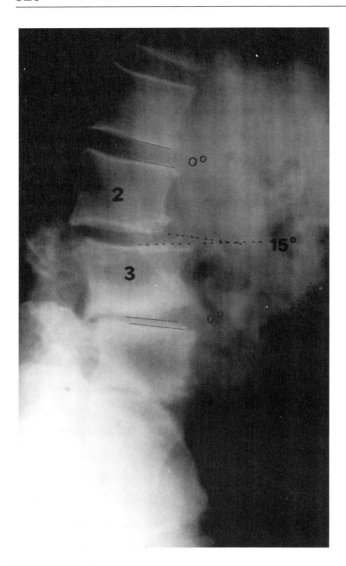

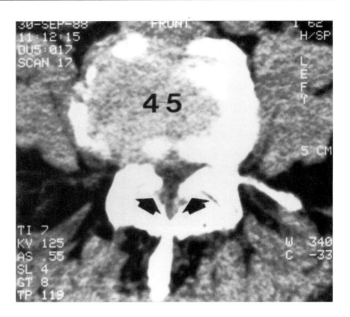

FIGURE 25.5.
Axial CT scan at L4-L5 demonstrating spinal stenosis by encroachment of the facet joints on the dural sac at L4-L5 (arrows).

FIGURE 25.4.
Lateral flexion radiograph status after decompressive laminectomy demonstrating 15° of endplate angulation at L2–3 compared to 0° at L1–2 and L3–4.

of soft tissue abnormalities (Fig. 25.5). Volume averaging of the various tissue densities may lead to a false interpretation, and therefore pathology should be confirmed on both soft tissue and bone windows, or additional studies may be warranted. The routine CT scans are obtained from L3 to S1. For evaluation of spinal stenosis they should be obtained from L1 to S1 since stenotic compression occurs at L1–2 and L2–3 in 10% of cases.

Although myelography has traditionally been the gold-standard contrast study for the lumbar spine, its use has decreased significantly with the development of MRI. It remains a useful test in spinal stenosis in the following situations: *(a)* when scoliosis is associated with stenosis, myelography combined with CT provides optimal images for central and recess stenosis (Fig. 25.6); *(b)* since some of the myelo-

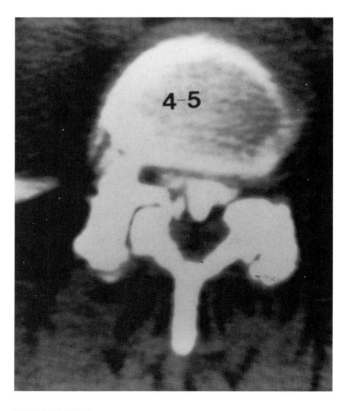

FIGURE 25.6.
Axial myelo-CT scan at L4-L5 demonstrating severe constriction of the dural sac by the facet joints.

graphic images are obtained in the standing extended position, stenosis may be demonstrated on that view when it was not evident on a supine imaging study; and *(c)* flexion-extension myelography may reveal stenosis not evident on static images. Flexion-extension MRI has limited availability at present.

The disadvantages of myelography are the potential side effects of nausea, seizure, and allergy to contrast medium. Nausea is quite common (30%) and responds to hydration and an antiemetic agent. In addition, myelography is an invasive procedure with the inherent risks associated with needle insertion.

Magnetic resonance imaging is the study of choice for most spine imaging. It provides a comprehensive assessment of the nerves and discs, from the conus medullaris to the sacrum (Fig. 25.7). It is noninvasive and does not involve radiation exposure. The disadvantages, however, are: *(a)* claustrophobia, which prevents 15% of patients from taking the test; *(b)* the quality of MRI scans varies considerably among imaging centers; and *(c)* it does not provide optimal imaging when significant deformity is present, such as in scoliosis. Regardless of which imaging modality is chosen, there is a significant percentage of false-positive results (2, 15, 28). The clinical picture must correlate with the imaging studies.

Electromyography (EMG) is used when a question of neuropathy arises, such as in a patient who has diabetes mellitus and spinal stenosis. The EMG is helpful in defining the extent of the neuropathic condition.

Nonoperative Treatment

The nonoperative treatment of degenerative spondylolisthesis is similar to that of spinal stenosis. This consists of restricted activity with only a short course of bed rest (1 to 3 days). Nonsteroidal anti-inflammatory drugs or aspirin are also recommended for a short period of time. Bracing the patient with a lumbosacral corset for 3 to 6 weeks may provide a splinting effect, aiding recovery. Physical therapy in the form of pelvic traction, heat, ultrasound, and massage may provide some relief of back and leg symptoms. This may be instituted for a period of 3 to 6 weeks at three times per week.

Epidural steroid injections may be used for patients who have radiculopathy and who have not responded to other modalities. Usually a series of up to three injections is given. A home exercise program is an essential component of conservative treatment. Appropriate exercises include stretching, active flexion, and aerobic exercise such as walking, swim exercise, or bicycling. It is recommended that one of these be performed for 30 minutes every other day.

Most patients who have degenerative spondylolisthesis with or without spinal stenosis respond to nonoperative treatment. Approximately 20% of patients, however, are afflicted to such a degree that their quality of life declines as they can no longer do the things they enjoy. It is this group of patients for whom surgery may be considered.

Surgical Treatment

The indications for surgical intervention are: *(a)* persistent or recurrent back and leg pain that is unresponsive to nonoperative treatment; *(b)* progressive neurologic deficit (rare), including bladder dysfunction; *(c)* significant reduction in quality of life over an extended period (1 year or more). In addition to

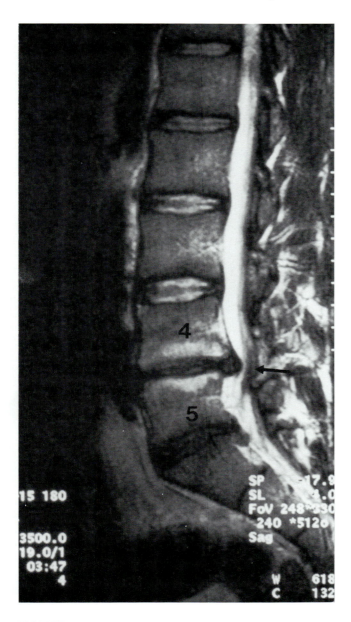

FIGURE 25.7.
Sagittal T2-weighted MRI scan of the lumbar spine demonstrating stenosis at L4–5 due to disc herniation and thickening of the ligamentum flavum (arrow).

the clinical indications, a confirmatory imaging study consistent with the clinical examination is necessary before proceeding with surgery (11, 12).

The surgical procedures available for patients who have degenerative spondylolisthesis with associated spinal stenosis are a decompressive laminectomy alone or a decompressive laminectomy associated with an arthrodesis (11, 13, 14).

Unlike a disc herniation, in which the pathology is isolated to a small portion of the motion segment, spinal stenosis affects the entire central canal, with facet hypertrophy and thickened ligamentum flavum along with nerve root compression in the lateral recess in most cases (Fig. 25.8). With the addition of spondylolisthesis, further entrapment may occur between subluxated vertebral body, annulus fibrosus, pedicle, or superior facet. Some authors advocate a limited decompression in which only a small portion of the lamina and ligamentum flavum is removed (23). The decompressive procedure must address all of the pathology to ensure adequate decompression of the central canal and lateral recesses.

For an L4–5 spondylolisthesis with spinal stenosis, a minimum of one-half of the lamina of L4 and one-half of the lamina of L5 should be removed. This allows adequate decompression of the central canal since the maximal central compression is between the L4–L5 facet joint. If imaging studies reveal further compression proximally or distally, then the laminectomy should be extended appropriately. For decompression of the L5 nerve root, a partial L4–L5 facetectomy should be performed. This involves removing the medial one-half of the facet and accompanying lateral portion of the ligamentum flavum (Fig. 25.9). If the nerve root remains immobile, then further bony removal is required until the nerve root is mobile and a probe easily passes through the root foramen. In rare situations, this may involve removing the pars interarticularis. If compression of the L4 nerve is present, then a complete laminectomy of L4 is necessary. In addition, a small portion of the L3–L4 facet joint may have to be removed to completely free the L4 nerve root. Since nerve entrapment may be related to a combination of sources—for example, L4–5 annulus fibrosus, vertebral body, superior facet, or pedicle—a careful analysis must be made preoperatively so that these sources of nerve impingement can be identified.

In 5% of cases an associated disc herniation is present. Usually a hard, bulging annulus fibrosus is noted but does not require removal. Satisfactory results after a decompressive laminectomy alone have been reported in 60 to 90% of patients (3, 6). However, residual or recurrent pain in the back or legs or both has been noted in as many as 73% of patients. Residual low back pain is reported more frequently than leg pain (14). This may be a result of residual instability or the development of increased olisthesis postoperatively (6, 8). Postoperative progressive olisthesis leads to mechanical instability or recurrent stenosis or both. This may result in a return of low back pain or radicular or neuroclaudicatory symptoms. By definition, degenerative spondylolisthesis implies that the facet joints of a motion segment and the supporting capsular ligaments are compromised. A decompressive laminectomy with partial facet excision

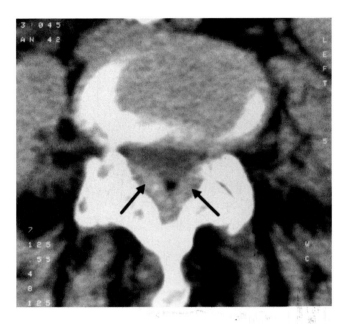

FIGURE 25.8.

Axial CT scan at L3-L4 showing thickened ligamentum flavum encroaching on the central canal.

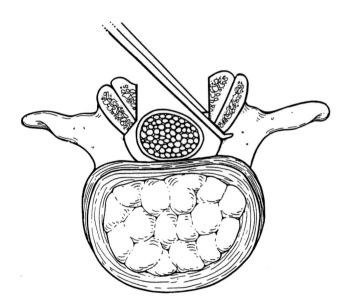

FIGURE 25.9.

A. Cross-section schematic of spinal stenosis demonstrating hypertrophic facet joints. **B.** Removal of the medial one-half of the facet joints (dotted line) decompresses the central canal and lateral recess while maintaining stability.

further destabilizes the weakened segment, leading to progressive olisthesis. The addition of an arthrodesis at the time of decompressive laminectomy addresses the instability.

Although some authors advocate the use of an interbody fusion, the overwhelming majority recommend an intertransverse process arthrodesis (27). The technique of harvesting the bone from the iliac crest and placing it on the transverse processes has been previously described (17) (Fig. 25.10–25.13). Autogenous bone graft has been shown to provide a significantly better fusion rate than allograft bone (1).

Support for the addition of an arthrodesis following a decompressive laminectomy when degenerative spondylolisthesis is present was first reported by Lombardi et al. in 1985 (18). They divided their patients into three groups: those treated with a radical decompressive laminectomy, those treated with a decompressive laminectomy with preservation of the facet joints, and those treated with a decompressive laminectomy with intertransverse process fusion. The best outcomes were in those patients with an arthrodesis. In 1991 Herkowitz and Kurz published a prospective study comparing decompressive lami-

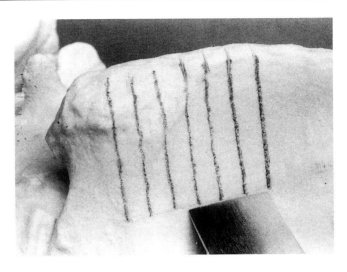

FIGURE 25.11.

Lateral view of pelvis showing curved osteotome connecting vertical cuts at the ventral aspect. This horizontal cut yields uniform strips of corticocancellous bone graft material.

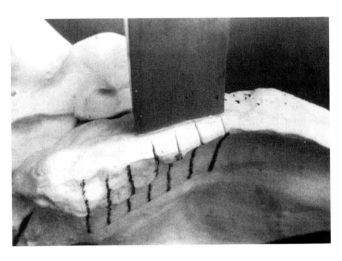

FIGURE 25.12.

Crestal view of pelvis depicting curved osteotome beginning at the medial margin of the vertical cuts.

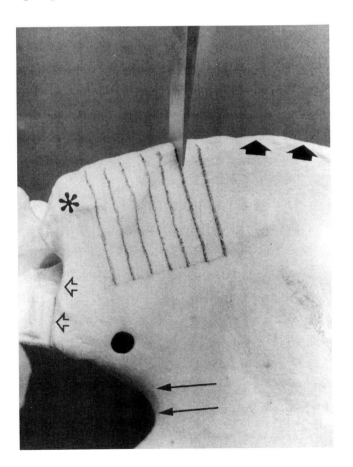

FIGURE 25.10.

Lateral view of pelvis indicating the posterior iliac spine (asterisk), the iliac crest (short solid arrows), and the sciatic notch (long solid arrows). The straight osteotome is used to make successive vertical cuts approximately 7 mm apart.

nectomy to laminectomy with fusion (11). The results were superior for the group with the fusion. Since then other authors have substantiated the value of adding an arthrodesis at the time of laminectomy (1, 5, 24).

Although the overall outcome is significantly better when concomitant fusion is performed, there does remain a role for decompression alone. In those patients with an osteoarthritic stiff spine, it would be unlikely that progressive instability would occur. Sanderson and Wood reviewed 31 elderly patients who had undergone decompressive laminectomy alone for spinal stenosis. Nineteen of these patients had degenerative spondylolisthesis. A satisfactory

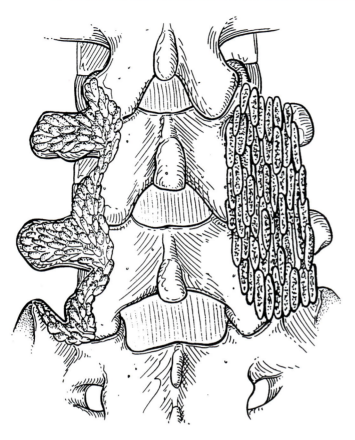

FIGURE 25.13.
Schematic representation of bridging of the L4 to sacrum by strips of corticocancellous bone graft.

outcome was noted in 84% of the patients with no further olisthesis (26).

Spinal Instrumentation

What is the role of spinal instrumentation in the older patient population? The goals of internal fixation are to improve the fusion rate, to reduce the number of levels requiring fusion, to reduce rehabilitation time, and to improve functional outcome. Historically, fixation systems have consisted of hooks and rods anchored to the vertebrae. This has often resulted in longer fusions than necessary and led to a loss of lumbar lordosis because of the distraction placed on the spine by the rods. The use of lumbar pedicles as an anchor for rods or plates provides biomechanically superior fixation points, often allowing a shorter arthrodesis than traditional fixation devices. In addition, the lack of lamina from the decompressive procedure and the presence of osteopenia in the older population makes pedicle fixation the optimal system for stabilization following decompressive laminectomy when spinal instrumentation is believed to be necessary (Fig. 25.14).

The critical issue in adding instrumentation following the intertransverse arthrodesis is whether the fusion success will increase and the clinical outcome will be improved. This must be balanced against the added costs of the instrumentation and the potential complications that may occur.

Few studies have appeared in the literature addressing instrumentation for spinal stenosis associated with degenerative spondylolisthesis. Zdeblick compared noninstrumented fusions to semirigid and rigid instrumented fusions in 124 patients, of whom 56 had a diagnosis of degenerative or isthmic spondylolisthesis. This series demonstrated better fusion rates in the rigidly instrumented group (31). Unfortunately, no breakdown of the number of degenerative spondylolisthesis patients was made. Complications in that series consisted of two screws and one rod linkage loosening and three screws poorly inserted without sequelae.

Bridwell et al. compared three treatment groups with degenerative spondylolisthesis (4). One group had a decompressive laminectomy alone; the second and third groups had an arthrodesis, and the third group also had instrumentation. This series demonstrated better results with instrumentation, although the series was not large enough to be statistically significant. In 1993 a scientific committee composed of representatives of various specialty societies was formed to develop and oversee the "Historical Cohort Study of Pedicle Screw Fixation in Thoracic, Lumbar, and Sacral Spinal Fusions" (30). Data were collected from 314 spine surgeons across the United States. A total of 3498 cases were collected for degenerative spondylolisthesis and thoracic and lumbar fractures. As part of the committee's work, a meta-analysis of degenerative spondylolisthesis was performed by Mardjetko et al. (19). They reviewed over 20 years' worth of articles on the subject. Although not a true scientific study, certain trends were noted. Rates of satisfactory outcomes for decompression alone, decompression with fusion, and decompression with instrumented fusion were 69%, 90%, and 86%, respectively. The fusion rates for the series without instrumentation and the series with instrumentation were 86% and 93%, respectively. No surgical complications were reported from the decompression/fusion group without instrumentation. A complications rate of 10% was reported for the series with an instrumented fusion.

From the meta-analysis, it appears that the clinical outcome is improved with fusion, and the addition of instrumentation does not improve clinical outcome but does improve the fusion rate. However, surgically related complications were noted only in the series with instrumentation.

The cohort study itself (30) collected data from more than 300 surgeons on 2684 patients who had

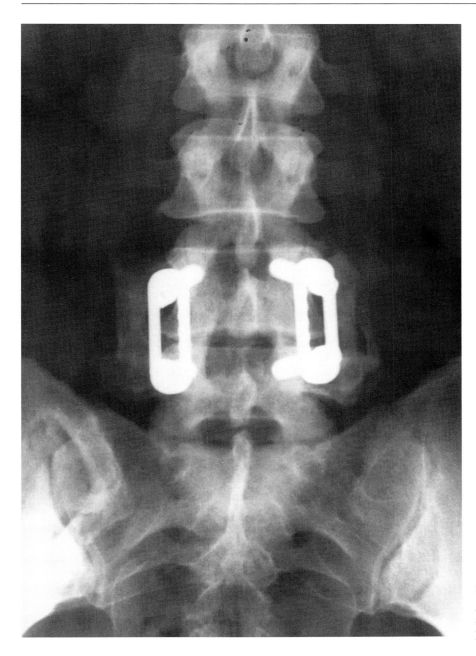

FIGURE 25.14.
Anteroposterior radiograph demonstrating spine plates at L4-L5 with solid posterolateral fusion.

lumbar spondylolisthesis and spinal stenosis. Eighty-one percent (2177 patients) were in the pedicle screw treatment group. Satisfactory outcome was judged by restoration of function and relief of pain. The results for function for the group with pedicle instrumentation was 87%, as compared with 90% for the noninstrumented group. The results for pain relief were 84% versus 92%, respectively. Neither function nor pain relief results were statistically significant when comparing the instrumented group and the noninstrumented groups.

The fusion rates for the noninstrumented group and for the pedicle screw group were 70% and 89%, respectively, and were statistically significant. The rate of postoperative complications from infection was 3% in both groups, and screw-related complications included instrument failure in 7%. Vascular injury and neural injury occurred in less than 0.5% of the cases.

The reoperation rate in the noninstrumented group was 15%, as compared to 18% in the pedicle screw group. Reoperations in the pedicle screw group were primarily for hardware removal. The pedicle screw group also had a higher reoperation rate for adjacent level degeneration than the noninstrumented group. Attempts to obtain a solid fusion accounted for 6% of the reoperations in the pedicle screw group and 5% in the noninstrumented group.

In summary, the data collected by the cohort study indicate that clinical outcomes are similar for the pedicle screw group and the noninstrumented group except that back pain recurrence is higher in the noninstrumented group. Fusion rates were higher in the pedicle screw group than in the noninstrumented fusions. Complication rates were similar in both groups. One aspect that was not evaluated was the costs involved for each group. This includes hardware costs, costs of reoperation, and complications. In this age of cost-conscious medicine, cost-benefit ratio is a significant factor to consider in determining optimal treatment. Randomized prospective analysis of pedicle screws versus noninstrumented fusion for degenerative spondylolisthesis with spinal stenosis currently under way will determine the most effective surgical treatment for this condition.

Conclusions

1. Symptomatic degenerative spondylolisthesis with spinal stenosis in most cases does not require surgery.
2. MRI is the optimal imaging study for this disorder.
3. In most cases, surgical management should consist of a decompressive laminectomy with intertransverse process arthrodesis.
4. The addition of pedicle screws improves the fusion rate but may not improve the clinical outcome.

References

1. An H, Lynch K, Toth J. Prospective comparison of autograft vs. allograft for adult posterolateral lumbar spine fusion: differences among freeze-dried, frozen, and mixed grafts. J Spin Disord 1995;8:131–135.
2. Boden S, Davis D, Dina T, et al. Abnormal magnetic resonance scans of the lumbar spine in asymptomatic subjects. J Bone Joint Surg 1990;72A:403–408.
3. Bolestra M, Bohlman H. Degenerative spondylolisthesis. Instr Course Lect (AAOS) 1989;38:1–20.
4. Bridwell K, Sedgewick T, O'Brien M, et al. The role of fusion and instrumentation in the treatment of degenerative spondylolisthesis with spinal stenosis. J Spin Disord 1993;6:467–472.
5. Caputy A, Lessenhop A. Long-term evaluation of decompressive surgery for degenerative lumbar stenosis. J Neurosurg 1992;77:669–676.
6. Dall BE, Rowe DE. Degenerative spondylolisthesis: its surgical management. Spine 1985;10:668–672.
7. DuPuis PR, Yong-Hing K, Cassidy JD, et al. Radiologic diagnosis of degenerative lumbar instability. Spine 1985;10:262–276.
8. Feffer H, Wiesel S, Cuckler J, et al. Degenerative spondylolisthesis: to fuse or not to fuse. Spine 1985;10:286–289.
9. Grobler L, Robertson P, Novotny J, et al. Etiology of spondylolisthesis: assessment of the role played by lumbar facet joint morphology. Spine 1993;18:80–92.
10. Herkowitz HN. Spinal stenosis: clinical evaluation. Instr Course Lect (AAOS) 1992:183–185.
11. Herkowitz HN, Kurz LT. Degenerative spondylolisthesis with spinal stenosis: a prospective study comparing decompression with decompression and intertransverse arthrodesis. J Bone Joint Surg 1991;73A:802–808.
12. Herkowitz HN. Spine update: degenerative lumbar spondylolisthesis. Spine 1995;20:1084–1090.
13. Herkowitz HN. Lumbar spinal stenosis: indications for arthrodesis and spinal instrumentation. Instr Course Lect (AAOS) 1994:425–435.
14. Herron LD, Trippi AC. L4-L5 degenerative spondylolisthesis: the results of treatment by decompressive laminectomy without fusion. Spine 1989;14:534–538.
15. Hitzelberger W, Witten R. Abnormal myelograms in asymptomatic patients. J Neurosurg 1968;28:204–206.
16. Junghanns H. Spondylolisthesis ohne spaalt in zwischengelenstuck. Archiv fur Orthopaedische und Unfall-Chirurgie 1930;29:118–127.
17. Kurz LT. Lumbar intertransverse process spinal fusion. Operative Techniques in Orthopaedics 1991;1:69–76.
18. Lombardi J, Wiltse L, Reynolds J, et al. Treatment of degenerative spondylolisthesis. Spine 1985;10:821–827.
19. Mardjetko SM, Collolly DJ, Shott S. Degenerative lumbar spondylolisthesis: a meta-analysis of literature, 1970–93. Spine 1994;19:2256S–2265S.
20. Matsunaga S, Sakou T, Morizono Y, et al. Natural history of degenerative spondylolisthesis. Spine 1990;15:1204–1210.
21. MacNab I. Spondylolisthesis with an intact neural arch: the so-called pseudo-spondylolisthesis. J Bone Joint Surg 1950;32B:325–333.
22. Newman PH. Spondylolisthesis: its causes and effects. Ann R Coll Surg 1955;16:305–323.
23. Postacchini F, Cinott G, Perugia D, et al. The surgical treatment of central lumbar stenosis. J Bone Joint Surg Br 1993;75:386–392.
24. Postacchini F, Cinott G. Bone regrowth after surgical decompression for lumbar spinal stenosis. J Bone Joint Surg Br 1992;74B:862–869.
25. Rosenberg NJ. Degenerative spondylolisthesis. J Bone Joint Surg 1975;57A:467–474.
26. Sanderson PL, Wood D. Surgery for lumbar stenosis in old people. J Bone Joint Surg Br 1993;75B:393–397.
27. Takahashi K, Kitahara H, Yamagata M, et al. Long-term results of anterior interbody fusion for treatment of degenerative spondylolisthesis. Spine 1990;15:1211–1215.
28. Wiesel S, Tsourmas T, Feffer H, et al. A study of computer assisted tomography: the incidence of positive CAT scans in an asymptomatic group of patients. Spine 1984;9:549–551.
29. Yang K, King A. Mechanism of facet load transmission as a hypothesis for low back pain. Spine 1994;9:557–565.
30. Yuan H, Garfin S, Dickman O, et al. A historical cohort study of pedicle screw fixation in thoracic, lumbar, and sacral spinal fusions. Spine 1994;19:2279S–2296S.
31. Zdeblick T. A prospective randomized study of lumbar fusion. Spine 1993;18:983–991.

CHAPTER TWENTY SIX

Spinal Neoplasms

Robert F. McLain

Introduction

Although many spinal column tumors still cannot be cured by surgical therapy, appropriate surgical treatment can provide most patients with increased survival and significantly improved quality of life. Failure to appropriately diagnose, stage, or take a biopsy specimen in a spinal lesion may, on the other hand, lead to premature deterioration and death. When combined with improved systemic therapies, aggressive surgical approaches have led to improved short-term and long-term outcomes in appropriately selected patients and now offer a reasonable likelihood of functional improvement, pain relief, local tumor control, and in many cases, cure of the disease.

Pathogenesis

Spinal neoplasms may arise from any of the soft or hard tissues that make up the spinal column, or they may arise at distant sites and metastasize to the spinal column by hematogenous or lymphatic routes, or through direct extension. Primary spine tumors include primary tumors of bone, marrow elements, connective tissues, muscle, and cartilage, primary lesions arising in the spinal cord or its coverings, or contiguous spread of tumors of the paraspinal soft tissues and lymphatics. Regional or distant spread of metastatic disease may occur with almost any malignancy but is most common with adenocarcinomas of the lungs, breasts, prostate, kidneys, thyroid, and gastrointestinal tract (41).

Incidence

Both metastatic and primary tumors occur in all age groups and at all levels of the spinal column. However, metastatic tumors are far more common than primary lesions, accounting for skeletal disease in 40 times as many patients as all forms of primary cancer combined. Between 50 and 70% of patients with carcinoma will develop skeletal metastases prior to death; as many as 85% of all women with breast carcinoma will develop skeletal metastases during the course of their disease (46). On the other hand, primary tumors of the spine are rare. Certain tumors, such as chordoma, plasmacytoma, or osteoblastoma, do show a predilection for the spinal column, but these comprise a small proportion of all spinal tumors.

Presentation

Tumors of the spinal column may remain asymptomatic or mildly symptomatic for long periods. Symptoms that do develop are usually a consequence of one or more of the following: *(a)* expansion of the cortex of the vertebral body by tumor mass, with fracture and invasion of paravertebral soft tissues; *(b)* compression or invasion of adjacent nerve roots; *(c)* pathologic fracture as a result of vertebral destruction; *(d)* development of spinal instability; and/or *(e)* compression of the spinal cord (40). Rapidly progressive symptoms of pain or neurologic compromise are associated with the more malignant, rapidly destructive tumors, whereas patients who present with symptoms that have progressed slowly over the years will typically have slowly growing tumors with a better long-term prognosis.

Age

The increasing incidence of metastatic disease with increasing age is well known, and it clearly holds true for spinal tumors as well. Systemic neoplasms such as myeloma and lymphoma also usually occur after the fifth decade of life. Similarly, primary spinal neoplasms show a strong relationship between age and malignancy; in patients older than 21 years of age, more than 70% of primary tumors are malignant, whereas in those under 21 years of age, the majority of lesions are benign (115).

Location

Location of the lesion within the vertebra also differs between benign and malignant disease. The majority of malignant tumors, both primary and metastatic, originate anteriorly, involving the vertebral body and possibly one or both pedicles. The predilection of metastatic tumors for the vertebral body is related to the vascular supply of the spine; backflow through the vertebral venous system (Batson's plexus) allows tumor cells from the abdominal cavity (prostate, colon, kidneys) to seed directly to the vertebral body (37). Strictly posterior localization, even when more than one level is involved, is more typical of benign lesions.

Diagnosis

Although back pain is a common, nonspecific symptom in patients of all ages, certain risk factors may alert the clinician to the presence of a spinal neoplasm as the underlying cause of a patient's pain.

Pain is by far the most common presenting complaint of patients with spinal column tumors, whether primary or metastatic (Table 26.1). More than 80% of patients will complain of either back pain or radicular pain, or a combination of the two. Night pain is a common finding, and particularly ominous. Pain associated with neoplasm tends to be progressive and unrelenting in character and does not have a close association with activity, as does mechanical back pain. Pain tends to be well localized to the spinal segment involved and may be reproduced by pressure or percussion over that area. Radicular symptoms are seen alone in approximately 10% of patients but are more frequently seen in combination with weakness, autonomic dysfunction, or in combination with back pain itself. Radicular symptoms may simulate those seen in cases of herniated nucleus pulposus, leading to confusion in di-

TABLE 26.1.
Common Presenting Symptoms in Patients with Spinal Neoplasia

Presenting Symptoms	Overall Incidence	Subgroups
Pain (back or leg pain)	85%	
Back Pain Only		30%
Radicular Pain Only		10%
Pain and Weakness		28%
Pain with Mass		11%
Pain, Bowel and Bladder		5%
Motor Weakness	42%	
Weakness Only		8%
Pain and Weakness		29%
Mass	16%	
Mass Only		5%
Painful Mass		11%
Incidental Findings	2%	

agnosis and treatment. In such cases, symptoms associated with lumbar and sacral neoplasms are usually unrelenting and progressive and are not relieved by rest or recumbency, as in cases of true disc herniation (100).

Although structural deformities are rarely associated with spinal tumors, scoliosis may arise from paraspinal muscular spasm. Scoliosis is sometimes associated with osteoid osteoma or osteoblastoma, and typically these patients present with localized paravertebral pain, paravertebral muscle spasm, and limitation of motion. The onset and progression of this type of scoliotic deformity may be rapid (50). Scoliotic curves associated with neoplasm are usually correctable early on, but may become structural if neglected for prolonged periods of time (79). Neurologic deficits are common in patients with spinal tumors. Weakness may be present at the time of presentation in nearly one-half of all patients, but it is rarely the first symptom observed, and it rarely presents alone. Depending on the tumor type, significant back pain may persist for months or years before lower extremity weakness becomes apparent. Nonetheless, as many as 70% of all patients will manifest clinical weakness by the time the correct diagnosis is established. In order to make the correct diagnosis before myelopathy is present, physicians must have a high index of suspicion in patients with persistent back pain, with nonmechanical characteristics or radicular pain, and particularly in any patient with a history of a known previous malignancy (2, 30, 95).

Imaging Techniques

High-quality roentgenograms are still the initial test of choice when a neoplasm of the spine is suspected. Good-quality anteroposterior and lateral views of the symptomatic segment of the spine may be sufficient to identify many characteristics of tumor growth or bone destruction and may even be enough to establish a diagnosis in some tumor types. When the specific tumor cannot be identified in plain roentgenograms, the benign or malignant nature of the lesion may often be implied from the pattern of bone destruction. Even when a specific diagnosis cannot be suggested, plain roentgenograms will demonstrate some abnormality suggestive of neoplasm over 90% of the time (115).

In patients with persistent or suspicious symptoms but normal or equivocal roentgenographic findings, a bone scan may be helpful. Because roentgenographic evidence of bony destruction is not apparent until after 30% to 50% of trabecular bone has been destroyed, the technetium-99m bone scan is far more sensitive in detecting small spinal lesions, provided that there is some osteoblastic response in the surrounding bone (21). The bone scan cannot differentiate among fracture, infection, and neoplasm, however, and it frequently provides false-positive results in the presence of osteoarthritis. False-positive scans are therefore most prevalent in the older population most at risk for metastatic disease (8, 13, 114). Information obtained from a bone scan must be carefully correlated with the clinical findings, roentgenographic findings, and the clinician's suspicions before a diagnosis can be confirmed. Although bone scans lack specificity, patterns of uptake showing multiple areas of skeletal involvement are virtually diagnostic for metastatic disease in a patient with a known primary malignancy. In any case, the bone scan is helpful in localizing areas of interest so that more sophisticated techniques such as computed tomography can be used efficiently to diagnose spinal pathology.

Computed tomography (CT) may provide visualization of spinal lesions at an earlier point in their development, before extensive bony destruction or intramedullary extension has occurred and before cortical erosion has progressed to the point of impending fracture. Because it demonstrates bony involvement far more reliably than plain radiographs or magnetic resonance imaging (MRI), CT is vital in planning surgical approaches and tumor resection. It will also demonstrate characteristic features of soft-tissue calcification, which may be pathognomonic for some tumor types.

Myelography, which in the past was the "gold standard" for the evaluation of epidural metastases and cord compression, has been largely replaced by magnetic resonance imaging. MRI is noninvasive, readily available at almost all centers, and safe. It has been proved highly useful in evaluating a variety of spinal diseases, and it demonstrates soft tissue contrasts better than does CT. The ability to obtain multiplanar images enhances the diagnostic and treatment planning capabilities of the surgeon considerably. MRI provides a better delineation of soft-tissue tumor extension and demonstrates adherence or invasion of paravertebral structures better than does CT or myelography. Although CT reconstructions are constantly improving, direct sagittal and coronal images obtained through MRI are superior to reconstructions available though CT, and they directly depict the spinal cord without the aid of intrathecal contrast material (31). By varying the MRI technique, the radiologist may provide considerable information regarding the vascularity or tissue density of the tumor and the presence of edema or hemorrhage surrounding the tumor, and may distinguish between infection and tumor. Finally, because MRI provides an imaging analysis of the entire spinal column and is highly sensitive for spine tumors, it is superior at identifying multilevel disease.

Biopsy Techniques

Three forms of biopsy procedure are available to the surgeon: excisional, incisional, and needle biopsy or aspiration. Occasionally a posterior lesion may prove suitable for an excisional biopsy, but most lesions of the spinal column will require either an incisional or needle biopsy.

Needle biopsy procedures are subject to sampling errors and provide a small specimen for evaluation. The primary role of needle biopsy is confirmation—confirmation of metastatic disease, of recurrence of a known lesion, or of sarcomatous histology in an otherwise classic clinicoradiologic presentation of osteosarcoma (71). When the differential diagnosis is limited to lesions that are easily distinguished histologically, a needle biopsy may be ideal. In more complex lesions and in those with a more subtle differential diagnosis, the specimen obtained will often prove inadequate (103).

The incisional biopsy procedure should be the last step in staging the pathology, performed just before or at the time of definitive surgical resection. As with extremity tumors, the biopsy incision should be placed so that it may be excised with the tumor during the definitive procedure. A small longitudinal incision in the midline or paravertebral line should be used; transverse incisions over spine tumors should be avoided (Fig. 26.1). During dissection the overlying tissue should be handled very carefully, and hemostasis must be meticulous. All tissues contaminated during the biopsy or by subsequent hematoma must be excised if surgical control is to be expected (103). Bone should not be removed or windowed during a biopsy procedure unless absolutely necessary. Once the tumor is exposed, an adequate sample of tissue must be obtained. The specimen should be large enough to allow histological and ultrastructural analysis as well as immunological staining. The mar-

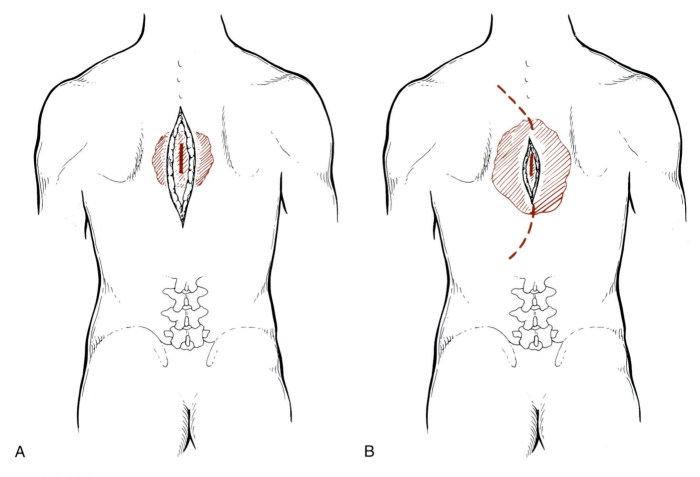

FIGURE 26.1.
Posterior incisions for tumor biopsy and excision. **A.** For bony lesions or tumors with minimal to moderate soft tissue mass, a midline biopsy incision serves well. Dissection is restricted to one hemilamina or the other to minimize tissue exposure. The subsequent incision for definitive resection will include the entire biopsy tract with a margin of normal tissue. **B.** For tumors with a large soft-tissue mass, a curvilinear incision may be required for the definitive resection. In these cases the longitudinal biopsy incision may be placed off the midline, over the bulk of the paraspinal mass. Broad flaps can then be developed, allowing the surgeon to maintain a margin around masses that extend on both sides of the midline.

gin of the soft-tissue mass is often most helpful because central portions of the tumor may be necrotic. The specimen should be obtained with a sharp scalpel; the surgeon must take care not to crush or distort the tissue, and electrocautery must not be used on tissues to be examined. It is crucial to maintain the architecture of the tissue during the biopsy procedure.

Tumors

Primary Tumors of Bone

Primary bone and soft-tissue tumors rarely arise in the spine. Of 82 primary neoplasms seen over a 50-year period at the University of Iowa, 31 benign and 51 malignant spinal lesions were identified, representing eight different benign and nine malignant tumor types (115). Survival rates vary most dramatically with the benign or malignant nature of the tumor, but not all benign tumors are survivable. The five-year survival rate in the Iowa series was 86% in patients with benign tumors and 24% in patients with malignancies (115). Patients with high-grade malignancies usually do not achieve a prolonged survival, even with aggressive systemic therapy. Patients with slower-growing, more locally aggressive tumors may experience a much greater overall survival but will still succumb to disease if local control is not achieved (3).

Benign Primary Tumors

Osteochondroma

This lesion is more a defect in bone formation than a true neoplasm. Vertebral involvement occurs in approximately 7% of patients with osteochondromatosis, but neurologic compromise is rare (56). Over 60% of symptomatic osteochondromas arise in the cervical spine, with another 19% in the thoracic spine at or above the T6 level (49, 57, 102). When cord compression does occur, routine roentgenograms may not be adequate because the cartilage cap producing the compression is radiolucent and may not be visualized without myelography or MRI. Because of the very slow progression of the compressive lesion, excision of the tumor, en bloc or piecemeal, provides excellent recovery of neurologic function with little likelihood of recurrence. Persistent neglect of these tumors can result in paralysis over time and occasionally in the death of a patient with a high cervical lesion. Enchondromas rarely produce any symptoms but may occasionally present a diagnostic puzzle requiring further workup or biopsy analysis (84).

Osteoblastoma and Osteoid Osteoma

Osteoblastoma and osteoid osteoma are benign neoplastic lesions that are frequently found in the spine, usually involving the posterior vertebral elements (50, 60). Patients usually present in their second or third decade, most commonly complaining of back pain that is unrelenting and unrelated to activity and often most noticeable at night. Although aspirin may provide dramatic relief of symptoms, the lack of any response to aspirin does not rule out the diagnosis.

Osteoid osteoma, by definition less than 2 cm in diameter, is easily obscured among the overlapping shadows of the vertebral column, and radiographic demonstration is difficult. Computed tomography demonstrates the lesion very well once the vicinity is known, but the most sensitive method of locating an osteoid osteoma is by a bone scan. The technetium-99m bone scan provides accurate localization of the lesion, permitting an early diagnosis and prompt treatment (79). Osteoblastomas are characterized by expansion of the overlying cortical bone, maintaining a thin rim of reactive bone between the lesion and the surrounding soft tissue. These lesions become considerably larger than osteoid osteomas and may be quite apparent on plain radiographs. Either lesion may be associated with a painful scoliosis.

Excision of either of these lesions provides reliable pain relief and resolution of spinal deformity in most patients (50, 82). When complete excision is not feasible, curettage and bone grafting of vertebral osteoblastomas has provided satisfactory long-term results (34, 60). Some investigators have recommended instrumentation and fusion for large, long-standing scoliotic curves, but this need not be done at the time of tumor excision.

Hemangiomas

Vertebral hemangiomas occur in approximately 10% of patients with spinal neoplasm, but they are rarely symptomatic or of clinical importance. The surgeon should not rush to attribute symptoms of mechanical or chronic back pain to these lesions. Reports of deformity or pain associated with vertebral hemangiomas are uncommon, but cases of nerve root and cord compression have been documented with large lesions. Plain films typically show prominent vertical striations produced by the abnormally thickened trabeculae of the involved vertebral body. These lesions are radiosensitive and frequently respond to radiotherapy alone. When vertebral fracture or cord compression develops and surgical treatment is considered, angiography is indicated to establish the vascular source for the tumor, to identify the primary vascular supply to the cord (the artery of Adamkiewicz), and for consideration of preoperative embolization or operative ligation (7).

Giant Cell Tumors

These slow-growing, locally aggressive tumors are usually seen in patients in their third and fourth decades. Plain radiographs often demonstrate an area of focal rarefaction, though some show a more geographic, lytic appearance with marginal sclerosis (Fig. 26.2). The tumor matrix generally has a "ground glass" appearance, which may be difficult to distinguish from a low-grade malignance such as chordoma. Giant cell tumors are most commonly found in the vertebral body, and they tend to expand the surrounding cortical bone as they enlarge. Computed tomography is especially important in the preoperative staging of these tumors. Because they have a strong tendency to recur locally, complete excision is key to eradicating these lesions. CT and MRI are also crucial in identifying recurrences and should be used routinely in postoperative follow-up.

Because of their locally invasive nature, giant cell tumors of the spine have a high rate of recurrence; in the Iowa series, two-fifths of patients died as a result of aggressive recurrence (115). Other investigators have reported better results in treating these tumors, however, and have even suggested that lesions of the spine are less aggressive than tumors of the extremities (16, 89). Prolonged disease-free survival has been reported following tumor resection, with radiation therapy recommended for patients with incomplete excision or documented recurrence (88). Good disease-free survival rates have been obtained with more aggressive surgical resection, without the risks of irradiation (89). Marcove et al. have recommended adjuvant cryotherapy to improve results in sacral giant cell tumors without the risks of radiation therapy or destructive radical excisions (59).

Eosinophilic Granuloma

Eosinophilic granuloma is a benign, self-limiting condition most commonly seen in children before the age of 10 years. Its cause is unknown. Vertebral involvement occurs in approximately 10 to 15% of

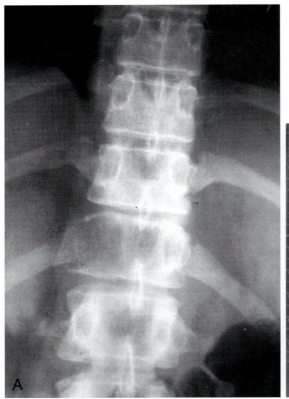 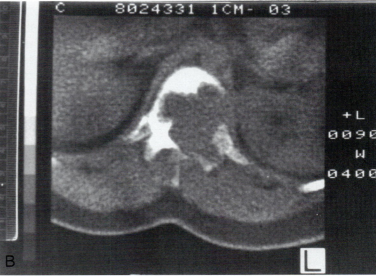

FIGURE 26.2.
Giant cell tumor. **A.** Plain roentgenogram of T12 giant cell tumor. Classic findings include the destruction of the left pedicle, expansion and lysis of the left hemivertebra, and the ground-glass appearance of the tumor itself. **B.** Computed tomography clearly demonstrates the destruction of the left hemivertebra and pedicle and reveals a geographic pattern to the bony destruction. Although the left-side vertebral cortex is breached, there is no associated soft-tissue mass.

cases and can be seen in any of the triad of syndromes of isolated eosinophilic granuloma, Hand-Schüller-Christian disease, and Letterer-Siwe's disease (24, 74). The vertebral body is typically involved, and bony destruction may produce a classic vertebra planum or "coin lesion" following complete collapse of the vertebra (Fig. 26.3) (11, 93). This appearance is not pathognomonic; a similar picture can be produced by either infection or Ewing's sarcoma. With such a broad differential, the importance of obtaining an adequate biopsy specimen before beginning treatment cannot be overstated. To assure an adequate specimen and to allow definitive treatment at the same procedure, open biopsy is recommended (24, 33, 93). Low-dose radiotherapy (5 to 10 Gy) has been advocated in the past, but this may be avoided in most patients. Many lesions will heal completely without any treatment other than a biopsy procedure.

Neurologic symptoms may develop with or without associated vertebral collapse, and may be severe. In these patients, the established course of biopsy followed by irradiation and immobilization remains the most widely accepted (33). As long as treatment is instituted without delay, recovery of neurologic function is usually excellent.

Aneurysmal Bone Cysts

Aneurysmal bone cysts rarely involve the vertebrae, but when they do, they are found most commonly in the lumbar spine, involving the posterior vertebral elements in approximately 60% of cases. Aneurysmal bone cysts have a tendency to involve adjacent vertebrae and may invest parts of three or more vertebrae in sequence. Radiographs typically demonstrate an expansile, osteolytic cavity with strands of bone forming a bubbly internal appearance. The cortex is often eggshell thin and blown out. When total excision is not feasible, curettage provides a high rate of cure. Although recurrence develops in as many as 13% of cases, these may be successfully treated by a second curettage or excision (43).

Malignant Primary Tumors

Osteosarcoma

Approximately 2% of all primary osteogenic sarcomas arise in the spine. Treatment of these lesions is challenging, and outcomes have traditionally been poor regardless of surgical approach or adjuvant ther-

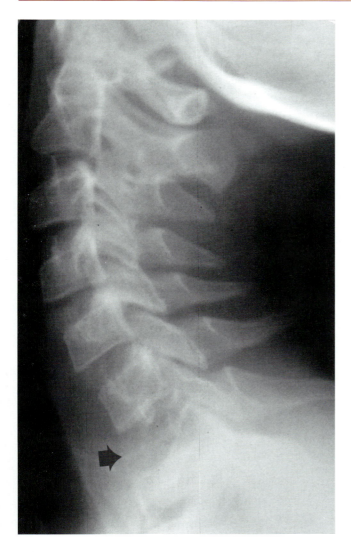

FIGURE 26.3.
Eosinophilic granuloma in a 12-year-old girl. In this patient the C7 vertebral body has been reduced to a thin wafer of calcified tissue (arrow). Needle biopsy examination confirmed the diagnosis, and the patient was treated in a brace until healing was complete.

apy. Median survival following diagnosis of an osteogenic sarcoma of the spine has ranged from 6 to 10 months in previous series (1, 89).

Primary osteosarcoma arises within the vertebral body in over 95% of cases. Radiographs demonstrate cortical destruction, soft tissue calcification, and periosteal reaction, with vertebral collapse in some cases. Tumor extension may produce a soft-tissue mass in the paraspinal region and may also result in spinal cord or cauda equina compression due to an intraspinal soft-tissue mass. Computed tomography and MRI studies are often necessary to demonstrate soft-tissue extension and to clearly outline vascular or cord involvement for preoperative planning.

Traditionally therapy has consisted of limited tumor excision, spinal cord decompression, and radiotherapy. More recently investigators have advocated a more aggressive surgical approach in hopes of improving survival and local control (100, 115). The results of small series suggest that this approach may provide a significant benefit for selected patients (109). Of seven patients undergoing wide resection or vertebrectomy followed by radiotherapy, four remained alive at a mean follow-up time of 52 months, three of whom had no evidence of recurrent disease. Although such results indicate that a more aggressive surgical approach may result in longer survivals, no conclusions may be drawn at present regarding our ability ultimately to cure these malignancies.

Ewing's Sarcoma

Approximately 3.5% of Ewing's sarcomas arise in the spinal column (119). Although the prognosis is generally worse for spinal lesions than for extremity lesions, long-term survival has been reported in cases of spinal Ewing's sarcomas (86).

The radiographic diagnosis of Ewing's sarcoma in the spine may be difficult, as the permeative appearance of the tumor is difficult to distinguish in x-ray films of the spine. In more advanced disease, with vertebral collapse and vertebra planum, the tumor may be indistinguishable from eosinophilic granuloma (Fig. 26.4) (80, 81). Neurologic deficits are common patients with Ewing's sarcoma; in one series 64% presented with neurologic compromise (80). MRI and CT are valuable in identifying the level of cord compression and distinguishing between bony involvement and metastasis to the epidural space, a rare but documented phenomenon (90, 92).

Surgical treatment is indicated for decompression of neural elements and stabilization of the vertebral column, but effective therapy must also include multiagent chemotherapy and high-dose radiotherapy to obtain both local and systemic control. With current regimens of multimodal therapy, excellent local control and encouraging disease-free survival rates are obtainable (51).

Chordoma

Chordoma is a relatively rare malignancy arising out of notochordal remnants within the spinal column. Chordomas occur predominantly in patients in the fifth or sixth decade of life. They are most commonly seen in the sacrococcygeal and suboccipital regions of the spine but occasionally arise from notochordal rests within the vertebral body in the thoracic or lumbar region (48, 70). The tumor is characterized by a slow but relentless local progression and tends to metastasize late in its course. Chordomas may reach a considerable size before they are recognized, and patients may present with symptoms of constipation, urinary frequency, or nerve root compression related to extensive tumor spread. In sacrococcygeal tumors,

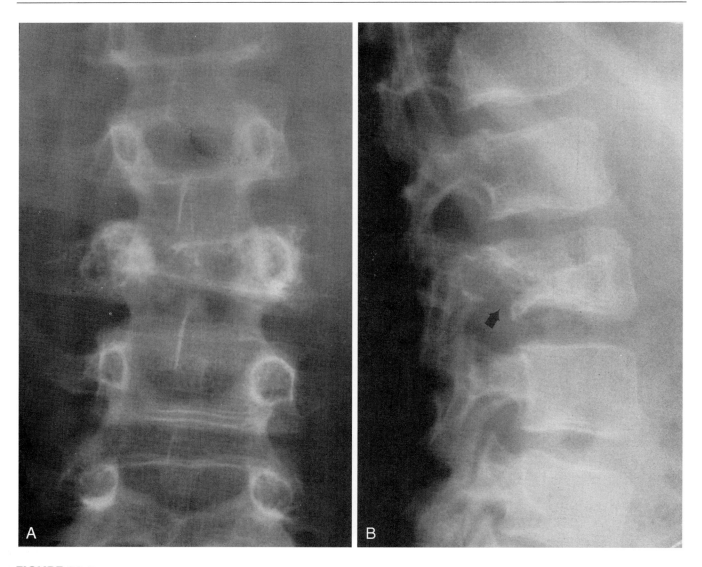

FIGURE 26.4.
Ewing's sarcoma in a 13-year-old boy. **A.** Anteroposterior roentgenogram demonstrates collapse of L2 vertebral body with loss of left pedicle definition. This presentation is indistinguishable from eosinophilic granuloma, and the patient age is ideal for either diagnosis. **B.** Lateral view of same lesion. Posterior half of vertebral body suggests a permeative destructive process (arrow).

a firm, fixed mass can usually be palpated on rectal examination (Fig. 26.5).

Because of the locally aggressive nature of these tumors and their propensity for local recurrence, surgical extirpation is the only curative procedure, and a wide margin must be obtained at the time of the initial resection. A biopsy procedure should not be performed until all other appropriate staging studies have been completed, and then the procedure must be directed through a posterior approach. The biopsy procedure should never be carried out through the rectal wall.

At the time of definitive treatment, the biopsy incision tract must be excised en bloc with the tumor. Kaiser et al. demonstrated that simply exposing the tumor during resection dramatically increased the recurrence rate of this tenacious lesion from 28% to 64% (48). Local recurrence of chordoma is a grim prognostic sign, dramatically reducing the likelihood of cure. To limit the risk of local recurrence, the indicated procedure for sacrococcygeal chordoma is a high sacral amputation, maintaining a cuff of normal bone above the tumor (106). Carried out though a posterior approach, this aggressive surgical technique has provided a significant improvement in overall survival rates, with acceptable morbidity and surprisingly little functional loss for the patient. The approach requires the sacrifice of the sacral roots above the lesion, but bowel and bladder function can be maintained as long as the S2 roots are spared bilaterally or the S2 and S3 roots are spared unilaterally (28, 84).

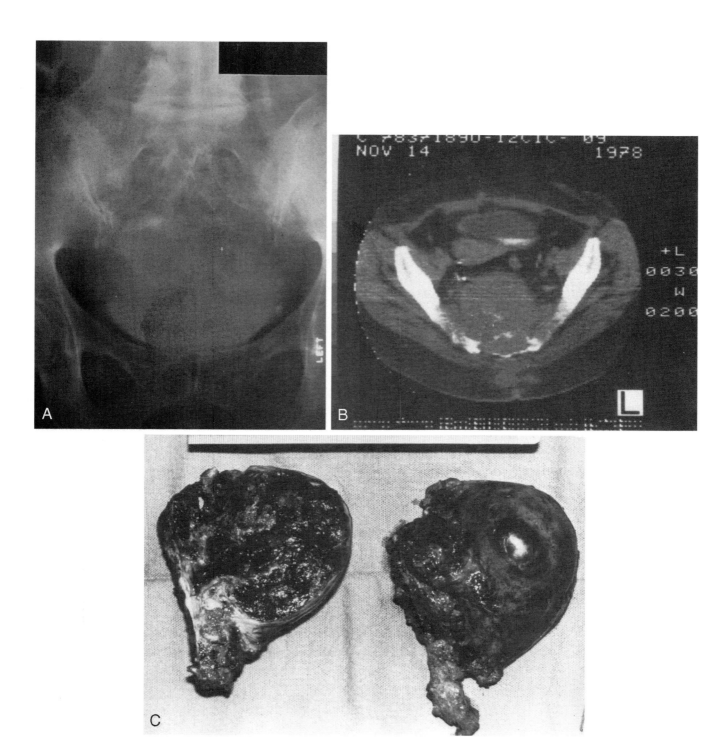

FIGURE 26.5.

Chordoma. **A.** Anteroposterior roentgenogram of a 68-year-old man with a long history of sacral pain and progressive constipation. Destruction of the sacrum is revealed by loss of cortical outline caudal to the sacroiliac joints and rarefaction of the S2–S4 bodies. Bowel gas, overlying soft tissues or abdominal contents, and obesity can make it difficult to see these changes clearly. **B.** Computed tomography clearly demonstrates the large soft-tissue mass typically associated with sacral chordoma. This mass is easily palpated on rectal examination but should never be approached in a transrectal biopsy examination. **C.** Transsacral amputation at the S2 level provided a narrow margin proximal to the tumor. A combined anterior/posterior approach allows the general surgeon to develop a plane between the tumor and the rectum while the orthopaedist performs the tumor resection.

Chondrosarcoma

Approximately 10% of chondrosarcomas arise in the spinal column or the sacrum (17). Chondrosarcomas are slow-growing and locally invasive, and they are relatively resistant to both radiotherapy and chemotherapy. Because of their high incidence of local recurrence, lesions of the vertebral column have a poor prognosis overall (45).

Chondrosarcoma is characterized radiographically by extensive bony destruction, a soft-tissue mass, and flocculent calcifications within that soft tissue (44). Because local extension is so important to local control and prognosis, CT and MRI information is crucial to establishing a surgical plan, demonstrating any invasion of great vessels and encroachment on the spinal cord.

Although long-term survivals have been described after intralesional excisions, with the use of high-dose radiotherapy to improve survival, a wide surgical margin is usually required to provide local cure for the patient with chondrosarcoma (96, 105). Although this is usually difficult to achieve, an attempt at wide excision is warranted, and it gives the patient the best chance of local control. Curettage and intralesional excisions provide little hope of either local control or long-term survival.

Solitary Plasmacytoma

Whether solitary plasmacytoma is an entity in and of itself or simply a less aggressive form of multiple myeloma is unclear—both are manifestations of a continuum of B-cell lymphoproliferative diseases. However, the natural history of solitary plasmacytoma is clinically distinct from that of multiple myeloma, particularly when the spine is involved, and the two entities may be considered separately when discussing prognosis and treatment (Fig. 26.6).

True solitary plasmacytomas are rare, comprising only 3% of all plasma cell neoplasms (14). Patients with multiple myeloma and spinal column involvement rarely survive a year and never achieve four-year survival; patients with solitary plasmacytoma, however, have a significantly better short-term and long-term outcome (113). The five-year survival rate in spinal solitary plasmacytomas may be as high as 60% (63). Though the majority of these lesions will eventually disseminate into multiple myeloma with a subsequently lethal course, survivals of 20 years or more have been reported in the literature (63, 91, 115).

The most appropriate treatment for solitary plasmacytoma of the spine remains radiotherapy. Because the lesion is highly radiosensitive, surgical treatment has less influence on overall outcome than it does in other tumor types and is necessary more for stabilizing the spine and reducing the pain. Although some authors have recommended prophylac-

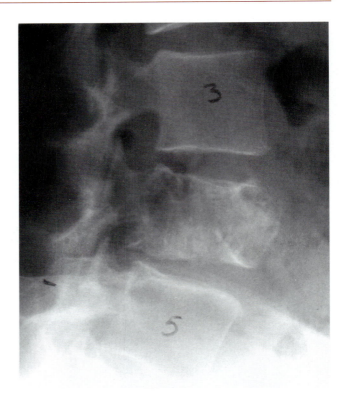

FIGURE 26.6.
Solitary plasmacytoma. Extensive vertebral lysis with expansion of the cortex circumferentially is typical of this lesion.

tic spinal stabilization prior to radiotherapy, vertebral collapse and neurologic compromise are rarely seen during therapy. Because the dissemination of myeloma may occur after many years of disease-free survival, routine follow-up with MRI and immunoglobulin studies is indicated for an indefinite period.

Lymphoma

Lymphoma of the spine may occur as a skeletal manifestation of systemic disease or an isolated primary bony tumor. Lymphomas account for a large number of spinal neoplasms requiring treatment. As with plasmacytoma, surgical treatment may be required to decompress the spinal cord or nerve roots or to provide skeletal stabilization and pain relief. Systemic therapy and radiotherapy remain the keystones of overall disease control, however.

Metastatic Tumors

Of all lesions of the spinal column, particularly in adults, the vast majority are from metastatic disease (17). Skeletal metastases and spinal metastases are most commonly the result of carcinoma of the breast, lung, prostate, kidney, thyroid, or gastrointestinal tract. Multiple myeloma is considered a metastatic lesion in many series. Breast, lung, myeloma, and prostate tumors comprise approximately 60% of all spinal column metastases requiring treatment. Tumors of the gastrointestinal tract actually result in more spinal metastases than do thyroid tumors.

The clinical behavior of the specific primary tumor dictates the prevalence of its metastases and ultimately determines the clinical significance for each patient. Patients with breast and prostate carcinomas typically have a prolonged survival and hence often require treatment of their subsequent spinal metastases. Patients with pulmonary malignancies frequently have a very short survival and may succumb so rapidly that little more than supportive care is indicated in treating their spinal disease. Patients with gastrointestinal carcinoma, which tends to metastasize to the liver and lungs long before it involves the spine, often die from their disease before their spinal lesions become clinically apparent or symptomatic. Patients with renal neoplasms, on the other hand, may develop spinal metastases early, and frequently they require treatment of these lesions.

Although spinal disease may be the initial presentation for a few patients with adenocarcinoma, most patients have been diagnosed months or years before symptoms of spinal involvement become apparent (30, 98). Whenever a patient with a history of previous malignancy develops symptoms of persistent back pain or neurologic compression, metastatic disease must be suspected. Patients with a previously diagnosed carcinoma should be observed closely, and if symptoms suggesting spinal disease arise, a bone scan and MRI are indicated.

Children's Tumors

Children suffer from a significantly different distribution of tumor types. Primary malignant lesions are uncommon in the pediatric spine. Nearly 70% of primary bone tumors in the pediatric spine are benign. Ewing's sarcoma of the spine is the most common primary malignancy, but is more often a metastatic lesion than a primary lesion (115). Metastatic disease is still the most common malignancy of the spine, and neuroblastoma alone accounts for 20 to 30% of all pediatric spine tumors seen (26, 54, 110). Neuroblastoma, embryonal cell carcinoma, and sarcoma may spread to the spine either through distant metastasis or contiguous spread from the primary lesion. These are highly aggressive neoplasms, and the patient's prognosis is poor overall regardless of treatment.

Leukemia may also present as a focal lesion of the vertebral column. Persistent back pain and vertebral collapse may be seen secondary to leukemic infiltrates (85). Children with leukemia manifest a variety of nonspecific constitutional symptoms in addition to musculoskeletal pain, including lethargy, anemia, and fever, and the correct diagnosis is difficult to make. Radiographic findings are not characteristic: studies may be interpreted as normal, or they may demonstrate focal lytic lesions, sclerotic geographic lesions, or isolated periosteal reactions without obvious bony destruction. Similarly, results of radionuclide scans can be unreliable in patients with leukemia (10).

In addition to treating the neoplasm itself, the spine surgeon must be aware of the potential for spinal deformity following treatment of pediatric spine tumors. Vertebral destruction and collapse may result in focal kyphosis in pediatric patients as well as in adults. Postlaminectomy kyphosis may likewise result in severe and progressive kyphosis. Kyphotic deformities developed in 46% of children treated at the Mayo Clinic, with the highest incidence in the cervical and cervicothoracic spine (121). The younger the child is at the time of laminectomy, or the more segments involved, the more severe the eventual deformity is likely to be (65). Rib resection or hemibody irradiation at an early age may cause iatrogenic scoliosis in 25 to 50% of children with spinal metastases (61, 83). Freiberg et al. noted that when laminectomy, radiation therapy, and chemotherapy were combined, the incidence of spinal deformity was 100% (27). Scoliotic deformities may also develop as a result of painful benign lesions such as osteoid osteoma and osteoblastoma, and some of these curves can become structural over time. Scoliotic deformities secondary to acquired paraplegia are also common and tend to be more severe in children with earlier onset of paralysis and higher levels of cord injury. The surgical management of children with spinal column tumors must anticipate the later development of deformity and seek to minimize it through early bracing or surgical stabilization.

Spinal Cord Compression

Spinal cord compression is a relatively common occurrence in either primary or metastatic disease, and it may result from direct compression by the enlarging soft-tissue mass, fracture and retropulsion of bony fragments into the canal, severe kyphosis following vertebral collapse, or intradural metastases (4). Of these, the most common cause of cord compression is mechanical pressure by tumor tissue or bone extruded from the collapsing vertebral body (40). Symptomatic cord compression occurs in 5 to 20% of patients with widespread carcinoma (12, 99).

Early recognition of spinal cord compression is critical to effective intervention and prevention of permanent injury (36). Patients usually complain of persistent and progressive back pain, radicular symptoms or "girdle" pain, weakness in the lower limbs, sensory loss, and, late in the course, loss of sphincter control. The prognosis for neurologic recovery is determined by (a) tumor biology, (b) pretreatment neurologic status, and (c) location of the lesion within the spinal canal (99). Although metastatic lesions typically demonstrate behavior similar to their parent lesions, this is not always true; some metastases may be far more invasive or rapid growing than the primary lesions from which they come. It is the biological behavior of the metastases that determines the likelihood of spinal cord compression. Acute spinal cord compression typically occurs as the result of rapid soft tissue expansion or vertebral erosion and pathological fracture, and has a poorer prognosis for recovery after treatment. Patients who have cord compression that has come on slowly and progressed over weeks or months have a much better prognosis for recovery (40).

The goal with treatment of any patient is to maintain ambulatory function and sphincter control. Because posttreatment outcome is so clearly related to the pretreatment neurologic status, it is of primary importance to identify impending spinal cord compression early and institute treatment immediately. Between 60 and 95% of patients who are ambulatory at the time of diagnosis will retain that function following treatment; only 35% to 65% of paraparetic patients and less than 30% of paraplegic patients will regain ambulatory function after treatment, whether surgical or not (2, 22, 36, 42, 53, 58, 73). Rapid progression of neurologic compromise is also an ominous sign. When symptoms of neurologic compromise progress from earliest onset to a major deficit in less than 24 hours, the prognosis for recovery is poor, irrespective of treatment. On the other hand, a slowly evolving neurologic deficit, one that progresses over a course of months, has a far more favorable prognosis for recovery following treatment, either with radiation or surgery (40).

The location of the neoplasm within the vertebral body or spinal canal determines the symptoms and signs of neurologic compression, and it dictates which surgical approach is most appropriate for treatment. Cord compression is most common in cases of thoracic lesions, where the spinal cord is relatively large in relation to the vertebral canal. Also, anterior vertebral lesions are more likely to result in vertebral collapse and extrusion of fracture fragments into the canal, and hence tumors of the anterior and middle columns of the spine are associated with more frequent and more profound neurologic injuries than tumors of the posterior column.

Spinal cord decompression can provide dramatic improvement in neurologic function, even in patients who have advanced deficits, depending on how rapidly deterioration has progressed. In these patients, the surgical approach used has a significant impact on outcome. In the past, radiation therapy has been the standard treatment for cord impingement by metastatic disease, and surgical decompression was used as an adjuvant therapy, usually consisting of a laminectomy and removal of whatever tumor could be reached laterally or through the pedicle. Even when combined with radiotherapy, the results of laminectomy have been found in some series to be little better than those of radiotherapy alone and often result in iatrogenic spinal instability or acute cord injury (30, 40, 94). Overall, satisfactory outcomes can be expected in 29% to 48% of patients treated with posterior decompression (Table 26.2). In one study, satisfactory results (maintenance of am-

TABLE 26.2.
Outcome Following Spinal Cord Decompression in Tumor Patients: Comparison of Anterior and Posterior Surgical Approaches

Study	Patients	% Improved	% Satisfactory
Posterior Decompressions			
Gilbert et al., 1978 (30)	65	45%	46%
Hall and MacKay, 1973 (36)	123	30%	29%
Kostuik et al., 1988 (53)	30	36%	37%
Nather and Bose, 1982 (73)	42	13%	29%
Sherman and Waddell, 1986 (94)	149	27%	48%
Siegal and Siegal, 1985 (97)	25	39%	39%
White and Panjabi, 1971 (118)	226	38%	37%
Wright, 1963 (122)	86	35%	33%
Total	746	Mean = 33%	Mean = 37%
Anterior Decompressions			
Fidler, 1986 (22)	17	73%	78%
Harrington, 1988 (42)	77	84%	73%
Kostuik et al., 1988 (53)	70	73%	84%
Manabe et al., 1989 (58)	28	82%	89%
Siegal and Siegal, 1985 (97)	75	80%	80%
Sundaresan et al., 1985 (107)	160	80%	78%
Total	427	Mean = 79%	Mean = 80%

The number in parentheses following each study is its reference number, as listed at the end of the chapter.

bulatory function and sphincter control) were obtained in 46% of patients treated with laminectomy and radiotherapy, in comparison with 49% for patients treated with radiotherapy alone (30). The fact that less than one-half of the patients treated with posterior decompression, with or without radiotherapy, achieve a satisfactory outcome is discouraging. Furthermore, the complications of multilevel laminectomy are considerable in their own right.

The results of surgical decompression through the anterior approach have been far more favorable and now offer a genuine improvement over radiotherapy alone (97). Satisfactory outcomes range from 73% to 89% using a primarily anterior approach. The reason for this improvement over the standard laminectomy approach is that spinal cord compression most commonly occurs from anteriorly based lesions; the posterior approach simply cannot adequately address anterior compression of the spinal cord.

Indications

With the improvement of adjuvant therapies and the widespread acceptance of more aggressive surgical techniques, the indications for surgical intervention have expanded. Currently it is recommended that operative treatment be considered in any patient who has *(a)* an isolated primary or metastatic spinal lesion or a solitary focus of recurrence; *(b)* a pathologic fracture or deformity producing neurologic symptoms or intractable pain; *(c)* radioresistant tumors—metastatic or primary; and/or *(d)* segmental instability of the spinal column following radiotherapy (23, 40, 53, 58, 99, 107, 115). Surgery is also indicated when the nature of the primary tumor has not been discovered or the diagnosis is in doubt, or when a tumor relapses following maximal radiotherapy or progresses during radiotherapeutic treatments. Recommendations for surgical intervention presume that the patient is healthy enough to survive surgery but are not dependent on an expected long-term survival. Any patient with expectations of surviving 6 weeks or longer and who is not hopelessly bedridden should be given consideration.

Nonoperative Treatment

Patients with metastatic disease are, by definition, systemically ill. Chemotherapy and radiotherapy may result in immunosuppression, thrombocytopenia, radiation enteritis, or neurologic disorders. The preoperative evaluation of these patients should always include consideration of the ramifications of previous treatment and the neoplasm that the patient is suffering. Serum calcium and phosphorus levels must be evaluated serially to detect any development of malignant hypercalcemia (41). Hematologic abnormalities must be identified and corrected and the patient's overall fitness maximized prior to any surgical intervention. Patients with long-standing carcinoma are often cachectic, and despite nutritional support, the risk of surgical mortality must be weighed against the likelihood of incapacitating pain, paralysis, and subsequent mortality if surgical treatment is withheld.

Radiotherapy remains the most appropriate treatment for the majority of patients presenting with spinal column metastases. Different tumor types exhibit very different radiosensitivity, however, and different clones of the same tumor type may exhibit very different responses to radiotherapy as well. Prostatic and lymphoreticular neoplasms are typically quite radiosensitive, and excellent clinical results may be obtained in most patients (6, 67, 111). The majority of metastases from breast carcinoma are also responsive to radiation alone (34, 111). Patients with pulmonary metastases may obtain significant relief of pain and neurologic compromise from radiation therapy, and typically succumb before instability and collapse become a factor. Gastrointestinal and renal neoplasms are often not radiosensitive.

The patient's neurologic status at the time of presentation is an important factor in predicting the relative benefits of radiotherapy versus surgical treatment. Seventy percent of patients who are ambulatory and neurologically intact will remain so following radiotherapy for spinal metastases, but rarely will patients who have lost neurologic function or ambulatory capacity regain it with irradiation alone (111). On the other hand, surgical treatment of metastatic disease provides excellent pain relief in over 80% of patients (42, 53, 76) and a significantly improved chance of restoring neurologic function. Recovery depends to some extent on the surgical approach. When patients undergoing laminectomy and posterior decompression are compared with those undergoing anterior decompression for metastatic spinal cord compression, neurologic improvement and satisfactory outcome is nearly twice as likely with the anterior approach (22, 23, 36, 58, 73, 94, 97, 107). In summary, the decision to intervene surgically in a patient with metastatic disease of the spine must take into account the patient's age, sex, physical condition, underlying tumor, and neurologic status. When selected appropriately, surgery can provide a significant benefit to these patients.

Surgical Treatment

There are a number of surgical approaches available to the spine surgeon in treating tumors of the spinal column. Choosing the correct approach for the given tumor is perhaps the most important step in preoperative planning.

Resection

Although some investigators have advised that extensive surgical procedures are fruitless and should not be attempted, it is clear from others that the ability to resect completely the primary tumor plays a major role in overall patient survival (3, 95, 104, 105, 115). Similarly, the ability to widely resect the tumor may determine the recovery and maintenance of neurologic function. In treating primary spinal neoplasms, the vertebral body, the anterior and posterior longitudinal ligaments, the intervertebral discs, and the dura may all be resected to avoid leaving residual tumor behind. In some cases specific nerve roots may be sacrificed to provide a wide margin of excision. In locally aggressive lesions such a surgical approach is well justified; as in extremity surgery, extirpation provides the best prognosis for local control and cure of the disease.

The vertebral body may be divided into four zones, I–IV (Fig. 26.7). Tumor extension is designated as A–C for intraosseous, extraosseous, and distant tumor spread (116). Zone IA includes the spinous process to the pars interarticularis and the inferior facets. Zone IIA includes the superior and inferior articular facets, the transverse process, and the pedicle from the level of the pars to its junction with the vertebral body. Zone IIIA includes the anterior three-fourths of the vertebral body, and zone IVA designates that portion of the vertebral body between the pedicles and adjacent to the posterior vertebral cortex. Zone IV is that portion of the vertebral body immediately anterior to the spinal cord. Zones IB to IVB are the extraosseous extensions of tumor beyond the boundaries of the cortical bone, and zones IC to IVC designate an associated regional or distant metastases. Surgical outcome and the technical demands of surgical treatment correlate with the zones involved and the extent of the local and distant tumor spread as well as by the type of the tumor and its grade.

Complete radiologic examination, including CT and MRI studies, allows accurate determination of the tumor location and extension and a more informed prediction of the tumor's grade if not its actual tissue type. Surgical planning also depends on early recognition of tumor extension into vital structures. Involvement of the aorta, vena cava, or spinal cord itself may indicate that a tumor is already unresectable prior to surgical exploration. In such cases an alternative plan may be most appropriate for the patient. Evaluation and planning of treatment should follow an algorithm similar to that outlined in Figure 26.8.

Obtaining the widest possible margin is essential in many locally aggressive or malignant tumors, but this can be extremely difficult in type B lesions. IB–IVB lesions of the lumbosacral regions may not be resectable without producing serious neurological deficits. In these cases surgery is marginal at best, and usually intralesional. The decision to attempt a wide or radical resection in these cases must be weighed against the risks, and in some circumstances adjuvant radiotherapy or cryotherapy may represent a more reasonable approach to treatment.

Zone I lesions are best approached posteriorly, and the extent of excision must be based on any soft-tissue extension seen on preoperative studies. Zone II lesions are also more easily excised through a pos-

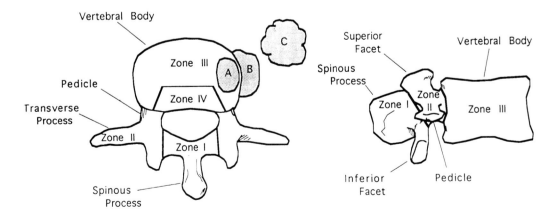

FIGURE 26.7.
Anatomic staging system for vertebral neoplasms. Tumor location within the body is described relative to zones I–IV. Extension of tumor is described as **A.** intraosseous, **B.** extraosseous, or **C.** distant metastasis. Tumors in zone IV must be approached through one or more of the other zones, making their management particularly challenging.

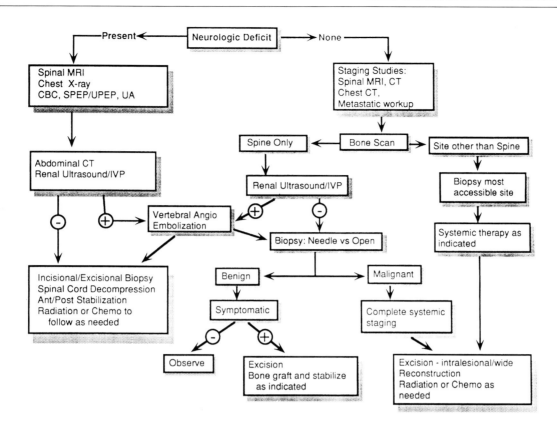

FIGURE 26.8.
Algorithm for assessing and treating spinal column neoplasms.

terolateral approach (55) and should be similarly stabilized. Once laminectomy and excision have been performed, the resulting instability is best minimized though posterior instrumentation of the surgeon's choice with autologous bone graft.

Lesions in zone III should be approached anteriorly. Adequate resection of a type A lesion can be obtained throughout the spinal column, but type B lesions should be carefully analyzed preoperatively to anticipate invasion or adherence to critical adjacent structures. In these cases spinal reconstruction may be performed with or without internal fixation, depending on the extent of the resection and the inherent stability of the residual elements.

Zone IV lesions often require a combined anterior and posterior surgical approach. These lesions typically involve the most inaccessible region of the vertebral body, and they are the most difficult cases to reconstruct. Likewise, these tumors are most likely to result in spinal cord or nerve root compression. Zones I, II, and/or III must be crossed at some point to provide access to zone IV lesions, and more than one zone is usually involved with tumor. Complete excision can be obtained through vertebrectomy, essentially separating zones II from III through combined approaches. In such cases both anterior and posterior stabilization is typically necessary. Even in these cases the tumor resection must be considered marginal at best and frequently may actually be intralesional. Nonetheless, experience has shown that an aggressive approach to tumor control does provide the patient with a more prolonged life span, even if cure cannot be obtained.

Metastatic Disease

When conservative therapy of metastatic disease fails, the physician must determine whether surgery is likely to improve the patient's function, quality of life, or longevity. In cases of severe, intractable pain or neurologic compromise, surgical intervention is often clearly indicated.

In lesions of the cervical spine above the level of C3, the posterior surgical approach is usually most appropriate. In all other regions laminectomy should be restricted to those cases in which the focus of neurologic compression is shown to be primarily posterior (22). When anterior disease occurs, the anterior approach is usually recommended below C3 (Fig. 26.9). As an alternative, some authors recommend a

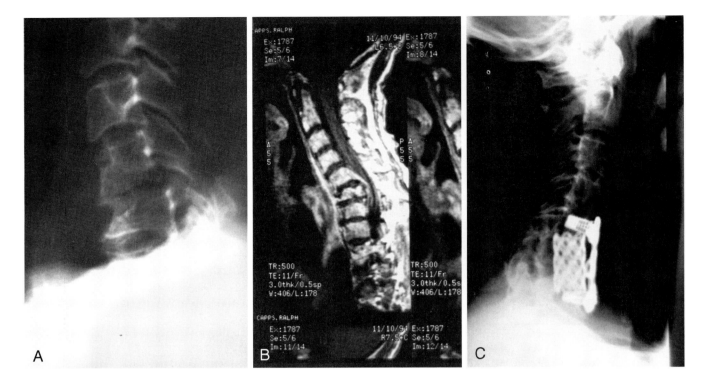

FIGURE 26.9.
Cervical spine metastasis. **A.** Patient with small cell lung carcinoma and metastasis to spine and shoulder. Pain and paresthesias progressed despite radiotherapy, and kyphosis and imminent vertebral collapse is demonstrated on lateral roentgenogram. **B.** Magnetic resonance image shows extent of tumor mass and demonstrates spinal cord compression due to a combination of tumor extension and focal kyphosis. **C.** Surgical treatments include vertebrectomy, spinal cord decompression, and reconstruction with a Moss titanium cage and polymethylmethacrylate. A Morscher anterior plate was applied in this patient to allow early mobilization in the face of an abbreviated life expectancy. Pain and paresthesias resolved and the patient returned to activity within 3 weeks of surgery.

posterolateral approach to lesions involving the thoracic spine, including lesions involving multiple adjacent segments. Costotransversectomy allows an intralesional tumor resection, providing posterolateral decompression, and may be followed by posterior segmental fixation and sublaminar wiring, and sometimes methylmethacrylate augmentation of the vertebral bodies from the posterolateral approach (52, 53). Exposure is somewhat limited from this angle, however, and full decompression of the spinal cord is not usually feasible. In contrast, Harrington has reported excellent results with anterior decompression, followed by stabilization using longitudinal rods and methylmethacrylate in lesions involving up to seven vertebral levels (4). This approach allows a wide vertebrectomy, full decompression of the spinal cord, including resection of involved pedicles if necessary, and allows the widest exposure of the vertebral bodies for stable fixation.

Specific tumors may present a special challenge to the spine surgeon. Renal cell tumors frequently metastasize and demonstrate a highly variable course in terms of both survival and local progression (87, 101). These tumors can be highly vascular, and life-threatening hemorrhage may occur when resection is attempted. Nonetheless, Sundaresan et al. found that patients undergoing complete resection of renal cell tumors had a significantly better survival than those treated with radiotherapy alone. Neurologic improvement was seen in 70% of surgical patients, as compared with 45% of patients treated with radiotherapy alone (108). Preoperative vascular studies and embolization reduce blood loss significantly in these cases and may prove lifesaving in some cases. Two courses of embolization are sometimes necessary to identify all major vessels supplying the tumor and provide the most reliable embolization.

Posterior Approach

As noted above, the benefit provided by laminectomy to patients with spinal cord compression is debatable (30, 75, 95). Although Constans et al. demonstrated some improvement in results with the use of laminectomy with radiotherapy, Gilbert et al. found very little difference between patients treated with radiotherapy alone and those treated with both laminectomy and radiation (12, 30). Nonetheless, the proportion of satisfactory outcomes was less than 50% in each of these studies. It is difficult to directly compare results for anterior and posterior approaches because of the lack of continuity of reported outcome measures, the lack of paired prospective studies, and differences in adjuvant therapy over time. For primarily posterior or posterior-lateral lesions, laminectomy or costotransversectomy is the most direct approach to the tumor, and decompression by this route is logical and effective (Fig. 26.10). Still, there is a clear trend favoring anterior decompression over posterior decompression in terms of neurologic recovery. Of 746 patients treated with posterior decompression, only 38% had a satisfactory neurologic outcome, with even poorer results in those who had a severe preoperative deficit. Although stabilization significantly improved the pain relief and maintenance of neurologic function relative to laminectomy alone, the overall results were still somewhat disappointing (65, 94).

Anterior Approach

Anterior decompression has been used successfully in treating cord compression caused by a variety of different lesions, including fractures, neoplasms, infection, and congenital or acquired deformity. Significant neurologic improvement has been documented in 75 to 93% of patients who underwent anterior decompression for metastatic disease (22, 39, 47).

Siegal and Siegal demonstrated a significant difference in neurologic recovery comparing anterior decompression to posterior decompression in patients with primary and metastatic tumors of the spine. They selected patients for the anterior or the posterior approach on the basis of the location of the tumor in the vertebra. Still, only 40% of patients treated with laminectomy retained or regained the ability to walk, as opposed to 80% of vertebrectomy patients (97). Of 13 paraplegic patients treated by anterior decompression, all but one improved at least one grade in neurologic function, whereas five of 25 patients treated with laminectomy actually deteriorated as a result of treatment. Even though the operative mortality was similar for both approaches, postoperative complications were far more frequent in the laminectomy group, often because of poor healing of surgical incisions made though previously irradiated tissue (97). Of 427 cases of anterior decompression in the literature in which the objective grading of neurologic recovery was reported, 79% had a significant improvement in functional grade, and 77% obtained a satisfactory outcome (65). These results are significant, and they are consistently superior to those seen with posterior decompression, even in carefully selected patients.

The intraoperative stress and intraoperative complications related to anterior surgery are not significantly greater than those for posterior procedures. When the anterior approach is carried out by skilled hands, both blood loss and perioperative complications can be minimized.

Reconstruction

Regardless of the method of decompression, posterior stabilization and fusion are frequently required to prevent early, progressive deformity and to allow incorporation of the bone graft. A wide variety of instrumentation systems have been used in spinal reconstruction, and the surgeon must consider a number of factors when choosing a system for a patient. The selected construct must meet the mechanical demands that it will face after tumor resection. It must compensate for the resection of bony elements or extended decompressions resulting from surgery and permit postoperative imaging in patients in whom this is essential for follow-up (Fig. 26.11).

Distraction instrumentation systems were among the first used to stabilize the spine following tumor resection. First-generation systems such as the Harrington rod provided distraction from the construct ends without segmental fixation and generally had to span several segments to provide adequate spinal stability. These systems still provide suitable fixation for thoracic compression fractures or following laminectomy, and combined with Drummond or sublaminar wires, they provide segmental stability sufficient to treat more significant disruptions or tumor resections. The system is at risk, however, in extensive fractures or tumor cases in which both the anterior and middle columns have been disrupted; in these cases the three-point fixation of the Harrington system cannot counter the excessive bending loads produced by the spine, and hook dislodgment or rod fracture is a significant risk (29, 117). Although studies have shown that longitudinal distraction can reduce some retropulsed bony fragments in trauma cases, distraction rod systems have a limited capacity for decompressing the spinal canal in tumor cases (120). Restoration of sagittal alignment, with reduction of kyphosis, may significantly decompress neural elements, but any retropulsed vertebral fragments that may be compressing the cord are not reduced.

The Luque system using steel rods and sublaminar wires has been shown to provide better fixation in soft bone than the Harrington system (15, 19). This system has been used successfully in cervical, thoracic, and lumbar segments both for degenerative disease and for tumors, and a number of strategies have been developed to use sublaminar wires and the Luque system even following laminectomy and decompression. In these cases laminar wires may be

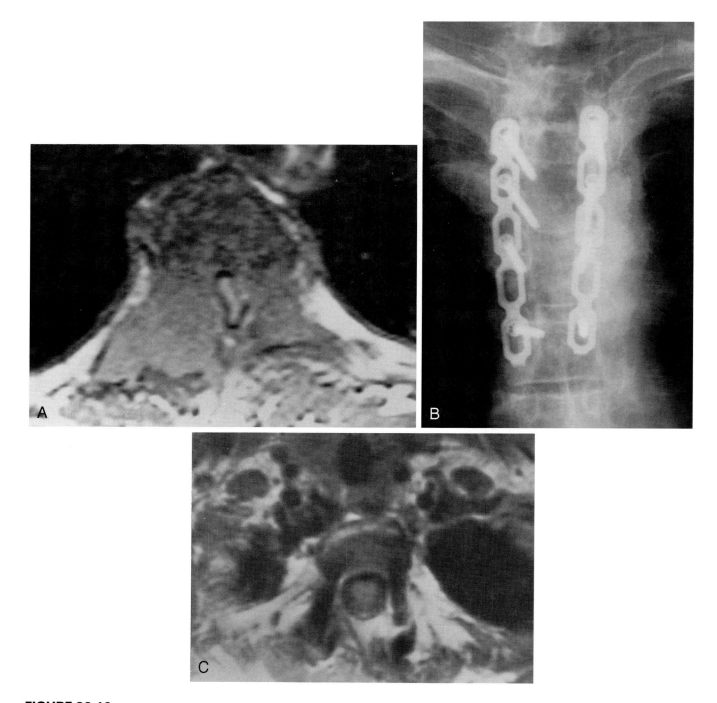

FIGURE 26.10.

Posterolateral thoracic metastasis. **A.** Patient with solitary metastasis from colon carcinoma. Patient presented with back pain, lower extremity weakness, and mild ataxia. Computed tomography shows a large expanding mass in the right pedicle, with diffuse marrow replacement in the body and lamina. Severe spinal cord compression is seen here, illustrating the fact that compression that increases slowly over time may be remarkably well tolerated. **B.** Following posterolateral decompression, necessitating multilevel laminectomies, the spine was stabilized with posterior plates and transpedicular screws. The variable slots in these plates allow placement of 3.7 mm screws exactly down the center of the narrow thoracic pedicles. **C.** The titanium plate and screw construct permits postoperative MR and CT imaging. The patient had excellent recovery from symptoms.

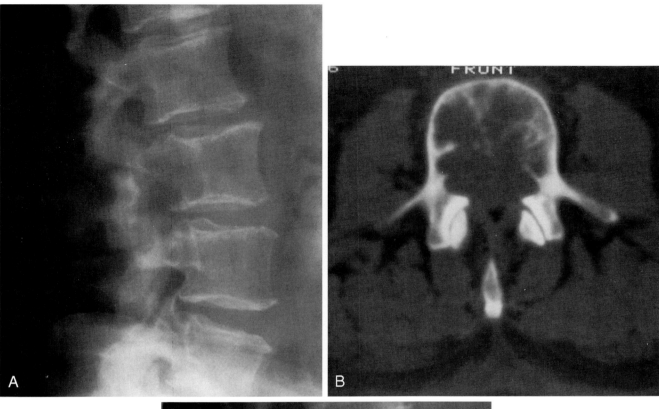
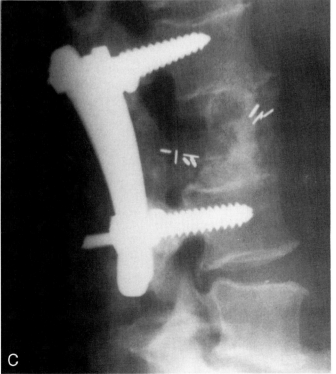

FIGURE 26.11.
Chordoma of L2. **A.** Patient with L2 vertebral lesion involving posterior vertebral body, with destruction of cortex and cancellous bone. **B.** Computed tomography shows that the tumor has replaced most of the vertebral body and disrupted the posterior vertebral cortex but has not entered either pedicle. Although the cauda equina is not compressed, the tumor has entered the canal. This stage B tumor involved both zones III and IV, necessitating an anterior en bloc resection. **C.** After removal of the posterior elements and stabilization with plates and pedicle screws, an anterior vertebrectomy was performed en bloc. A tricortical graft from the iliac crest was used to reconstruct the anterior column defect.

passed under the transverse processes or through the neural foramina at the segments operated on (23). The primary difficulty with the Luque system in tumor care is that the sublaminar wires will slide along the longitudinal rod. The system is therefore unable to deal with axial instability in the way that the distraction systems can. This severely limits the efficacy of Luque rod systems in spine tumor reconstruction.

Currently there are a variety of rod-hook systems available that allow segmental fixation of the spine as well as good axial and torsional support. These instrumentation systems allow the surgeon to combine a variety of sublaminar, pedicle, and transverse hooks with the use of pedicle screws, and they provide the sort of versatility necessary for reconstruction following extensive tumor resections. Many of these systems are now available in titanium, allowing more sensitive postoperative imaging in tumors that have a high risk for local recurrence. The versatility of the systems also allows the surgeon to address multiple levels of vertebral involvement in the same construct, a situation that arises from time to time when dealing with metastatic disease (Fig. 26.12). These constructs can be combined with anterior reconstructions to provide a very satisfying and stable result even in patients with extensive vertebral involvement (72).

Pedicle screw instrumentation has also provided significant benefit in spinal reconstruction. Particularly helpful in patients who have undergone previous laminectomy, pedicle screws allow the surgeon to obtain three-column purchase of the vertebral body through the posterior approach. This allows the surgeon to instrument levels that would otherwise be unobtainable, and also to minimize the number of vertebral segments fused. The use of the variable screw placement (VSP) plate with pedicle screws has allowed surgeons to fuse significantly fewer segments of the thoracolumbar spine than with systems using sublaminar hooks or wires, frequently allowing the surgeon to immobilize only two motion segments when treating primary or metastatic tumors (66). Pedicle screw fixation may also allow the surgeon to limit lumbar fusions even though more extended thoracolumbar and thoracic instrumentation is still required above the tumor. These strategies reduce the disruptive effect of fusion on the lower lumbar spine and may limit the magnitude or risk of subsequent low back pain and disability. When combined with rod systems, pedicle screws significantly extend the versatility of these fixation systems.

Regardless of the fixation system or technique used, posterior instrumentation alone cannot provide a stable construct in all cases. In particular, when laminectomy is superimposed on preexisting anterior and middle column vertebral collapse, the resulting spinal instability can be severe (19). When

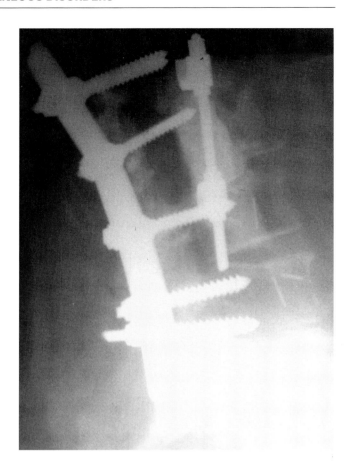

FIGURE 26.12.
Multilevel metastasis in the lumbar spine. Patient with metastatic melanoma to L2 and L4, with cauda equina compression at L2. Anterior decompression at L2 was reconstructed with Harrington rod and polymethylmethacrylate. Posterior instrumentation from L1 to L5 stabilized both pathologic levels, relieving pain and helping the patient to stay mobile and independent for as long as possible.

the anterior weightbearing column is compromised, there can still be substantial vertebral motion in response to physiological compressive and bending loads despite rigid posterior fixation or solid fusion (29). Despite the three-column fixation provided by pedicle screw systems, it is clear that untreated anterior column instability leads to a higher incidence of failure and screw breakage (66). Although supplementing posterior instrumentation with methylmethacrylate has been advocated in the past to provide more rigid fixation, the complications associated with this technique are unacceptably high (18).

Because spine tumor patients have often already undergone regional radiation therapy and are often ill or infirm, there is an increased incidence of wound complications and breakdown associated with posterior implementation. Some authors have suggested that anterior instrumentation should be preferred for spinal reconstructions in these cases. Harrington recommended that posterior instrumentation be restricted to *(a)* cases in which combined anterior and posterior decompression is necessary; *(b)* cases in which lengthy anterior fixation would be inadequate to restore stability; *(c)* individuals with posterior instability produced by tumor lysis or laminectomy; and/or *(d)* cases in which the vertebral lesion is located distal to the L3 level (42). Considering the frequent need for neural decompression in these patients, anterior reconstruction techniques now comprise a major portion of the spine surgeon's repertoire when dealing with vertebral tumors.

The complexity of the anterior resection depends on the tumor type and the surgeon's primary treatment goals. Curettage and intralesional surgery may be adequate in some patients with metastatic disease when the goal is decompression and stabilization but not cure or local control. On the other hand, wide resection of those tumors that have a strong potential for local recurrence requires an aggressive approach to the anterior vertebral structures. Regardless of the technique of vertebrectomy, anterior stabilization must then be carried out, using one of a number of methods for reconstructing the anterior load-bearing spinal column: patients with an expected life span of 6 months or less may be appropriately treated with methacrylate or other synthetic spacer; patients for whom a long-term survival of more than 6 months is expected should undergo reconstruction with bone graft material in anticipation of a solid arthrodesis. Tricortical strut grafting or the use of a titanium cage with morselized autograft material is favored in the treatment of benign or slowly growing tumors when the patient's survival is expected to be measured in years. In advanced metastatic disease, the primary internal strut may be methylmethacrylate or a titanium or metal implant construct. Methacrylate or titanium cages function as an adjunct to stabilization, providing a temporary internal splint in anticipation of eventual bony arthrodesis. If arthrodesis is not obtained, it is only a matter of time before the construct fails; only patients with a very limited life expectancy should be indicated for methylmethacrylate fixation without bone grafting (62). Even in these patients methylmethacrylate should be used in anterior reconstructions rather than posterior reconstructions (77). Here it proves quite resilient and dependable as long as it is reliably anchored into the bone (29). Steinmann pins may be used longitudinally within the anterior construct, both to enhance the bending resistance of the methacrylate strut and to improve fixation to the adjacent vertebral bodies (107). Harrington distraction rods as well as Moe sacral hooks and threaded rods have been used to obtain purchase, and Harrington has used Knodt rods for several years for the same purpose (39, 40, 98).

When methylmethacrylate is used anteriorly to reconstruct the vertebral body, care must be taken to avoid contact between the cement and the dural sack. Using cement in the dough phase allows better control of its placement, and a sheet of absorbable gelatin sponge (Gelfoam) interposed anterior to the dural elements will further shield them (20). A Silastic dam may be used for the same purpose. During the polymerization a steady flow of saline irrigation should be employed to minimize the heat transmitted to the surrounding tissues.

Titanium cages may be used to supplement both methylmethacrylate and autograft reconstructions. The cage is set between the vertebral bodies in the same way that a tricortical graft would be placed. The cage is packed full of bone graft material prior to placement if fusion is intended, and after impaction into the vertebrectomy space an anterior fixation device, such as a Z-plate, a University plate, a Kaneda Rod, and the like, may be applied to stabilize the spinal construct. An additional benefit of the titanium cage construct is that it will not interfere with postoperative imaging in patients in whom local recurrences are a concern.

Conclusions

Improvements in medical and adjuvant therapy for cancer patients has dramatically improved survival rates over the past three decades. Prolonged survivals and improved cure rates ensure that patients with spinal column tumors will continue to require highly sophisticated and aggressive therapies to maintain neurologic function and spinal stability. It is no longer appropriate to assume pessimistically that these patients are near death simply because they have a tumor of the spine, nor to offer them only palliative care. Improved medical management, antibiotics, preoperative planning, along with techniques of preoperative embolization and early postoperative mobilization have made surgical management of these patients much less risky. Vertebrectomy, considered a last alternative in the past, is now coming to be seen as the conservative approach to tumor management in many situations.

Appropriate surgical treatment can have a dramatic impact on function and outcome in patients with tumors of the spinal column and should never be dismissed as an option without serious consideration. Advances in fixation systems, local and systemic therapy, and our understanding of the biology of cancer promise even greater improvements in the future.

References

1. Barwick KW, Huvos AG, Smith J. Primary osteogenic sarcoma of the vertebral column. Cancer 1980;46:595–604.

2. Black P. Spinal metastasis: current status and recommended guidelines for management. Neurosurgery 1979;5:726–746.
3. Bohlman HH, Sachs BL, Carter JR, et al. Primary neoplasms of the cervical spine. J Bone Joint Surg 1986;68A:483–494.
4. Boland PJ, Lane JM, Sundaresan N. Metastatic disease of the spine. Clin Orthop 1982;169:95–102.
5. Brice J, McKissock W. Surgical treatment of malignant extradural spinal tumors. Br Med J 1965;1:1341–1344.
6. Bruckman JE, Bloomer WD. Management of spinal cord compression. Semin Oncol 1978;5:135–140.
7. Bucknill T, Jackson JW, Kendall BE. Hemangioma of a vertebral body treated by ligation of the segmental arteries. J Bone Joint Surg 1973;55B:534–539.
8. Citrin DL, Bessent RG, Greig WR. A comparison of sensitivity and accuracy of the ^{99m}Tc phosphate bone scan and skeletal radiograph in the diagnosis of bone metastases. Clin Radiol 1977;28:107–111.
9. Clain A. Secondary malignant disease of bone. Br J Cancer 1965;19:15–29.
10. Clausen N, Gotze H, Pedersen A, et al. Skeletal scintigraphy and radiography at onset of acute lymphocytic leukemia in children. Med Pediatr Oncol 1983;11:291–296.
11. Compere EL, Johnson WE, Coventry MB. Vertebra plana (Calve's disease) due to eosinophilic granuloma. J Bone Joint Surg 1954;36A:969–980.
12. Constans JP, de Divitiis E, Donzelli R, et al. Spinal metastases with neurological manifestations: review of 600 cases. J Neurosurg 1983;59:111–118.
13. Corcoran RJ, Thrall JH, Kyle RW, et al. Solitary abnormalities in bone scans of patients with extraosseous malignancies. Radiology 1976;121:663–667.
14. Corwin J, Lindberg RD. Solitary plasmacytoma of bone vs. extramedullary plasmacytoma and their relationship to multiple myeloma. Cancer 1979;43:1007–1013.
15. Cybulski GR, Von Roenn KA, D'Angelo CM, et al. Luque rod stabilization for metastatic disease of the spine. Surg Neurol 1987;28:277–283.
16. Dahlin DC. Giant-cell tumor of vertebrae above the sacrum. Cancer 1977;39:1350–1356.
17. Dahlin DC. Bone tumors: general aspects and data on 6,221 cases. 3d ed. Springfield, IL: Thomas, 1978.
18. Denis F. The three column spine and its significance in the classification of acute thoracolumbar spine injuries. Spine 1983;8:817–831.
19. DeWald RL, Bridwell KH, Prodromas C, et al. Reconstructive spinal surgery as palliation for metastatic malignancies of the spine. Spine 1985;10:21–26.
20. Dolin MG. Acute massive dural compression secondary to methylmethacrylate replacement of a tumorous lumbar vertebral body. Spine 1989;14:108–110.
21. Edelstyn GA, Gillespie PJ, Grebell ES. The radiologic demonstration of osseous metastases: experimental observations. Clin Radiol 1967;18:158–164.
22. Fidler MW. Anterior decompression and stabilization of metastatic spinal fractures. J Bone Joint Surg 1986;68B:83–90.
23. Flatley TJ, Anderson MH, Anast GH. Spinal instability due to malignant disease. J Bone Joint Surg 1984;66A:47–52.
24. Fowles JV, Bobechko WP. Solitary eosinophilic granuloma of bone. J Bone Joint Surg 1970;52B:238–243.
25. Francis KC, Hutter RVP. Neoplasms of the spine in the aged. Clin Orthop 1963;26:54–66.
26. Fraser RD, Paterson DC, Simpson DA. Orthopaedic aspects of spinal tumours in children. J Bone Joint Surg 1977;59B:143–151.
27. Freiberg AA, Graziano GP, Loder RT, et al. Metastatic vertebral disease in children. J Pediatr Orthop 1993;13:148–153.
28. Gennari L, Azzarelli A, Quagliuolo V. A posterior approach for the excision of sacral chordoma. J Bone Joint Surg 1987;69B:565–568.
29. Gertzbein SD, MacMichael D, Tile M. Harrington instrumentation as a method of fixation in fractures of the spine. J Bone Joint Surg 1982;64B:526–529.
30. Gilbert RW, Kim JH, Posner JB. Epidural spinal cord compression from metastatic tumor: diagnosis and treatment. Ann Neurol 1978;3:40–51.
31. Godersky JC, Smoker WRK, Knutzon R. Use of magnetic resonance imaging in the evaluation of metastatic spinal disease. Neurosurgery 1987;21:676–680.
32. Graham WD. Metastatic cancer to bone. In: Bone tumours. London: Butterworths, 1966:94–100.
33. Green NE, Robertson WW, Kilroy AW. Eosinophilic granuloma of the spine with associated neural deficit. J Bone Joint Surg 1980;62A:1198–1202.
34. Griffin JB. Benign osteoblastoma of the thoracic spine. J Bone Joint Surg 1978;60A:833–835.
35. Habermann ET, Sachs R, Stern RE, et al. The pathology and treatment of metastatic disease of the femur. Clin Orthop 1982;169:70–82.
36. Hall AJ, MacKay NNS. The results of laminectomy for compression of the cord or cauda equina by extradural malignant tumor. J Bone Joint Surg 1973;55B:497–505.
37. Harada M, Shimizu A, Nakamura Y, et al. Role of the vertebral venous system in metastatic spread of cancer cells to the bone. Adv Exp Med Biol 1992;324:83–92.
38. Harrington KD, Sim Fh, Enis JE, et al. Methylmethacrylate as an adjunct in internal fixation of pathological fractures. J Bone Joint Surg 1976;58A:1047–1055.
39. Harrington KD. The use of methylmethacrylate for vertebral-body replacement and anterior stabilization of pathologic fracture-dislocations of the spine due to metastatic malignant disease. J Bone Joint Surg 1981;63A:36–46.
40. Harrington KD. Current concepts review: metastatic disease of the spine. J Bone Joint Surg 1986;68A:1110–1115.
41. Harrington KD. Metastatic disease of the spine. In: Harrington KD, ed. Orthopaedic management of metastatic bone disease. St. Louis: Mosby, 1988:309–383.
42. Harrington KD. Anterior decompression and stabilization of the spine as a treatment for vertebral collapse and spinal cord compression from metastatic malignancy. Clin Orthop 1988;233:177–197.
43. Hay MC, Paterson D, Taylor TKF. Aneurysmal bone cysts of the spine. J Bone Joint Surg 1978;60B:406–411.

44. Hermann G, Sacher M, Lanzieri CF, et al. Chondrosarcoma of the spine: an unusual radiographic presentation. Skeletal Radiol 1985;14:178–183.
45. Hirsh LF, Thanki A, Spector HB. Primary spinal chondrosarcoma with eighteen-year follow-up. Neurosurgery 1984;14:747–749.
46. Jaffe HL. Tumors and tumorous conditions of the bones and joints. Philadelphia: Lea & Febiger, 1948.
47. Johnson JR, Leatherman KD, Holt RT. Anterior decompression of the spinal cord for neurologic deficit. Spine 1983;8:396–405.
48. Kaiser TE, Prichard DJ, Unni KK. Clinicopathologic study of sacrococcygeal chordoma. Cancer 1984;54:2574–2578.
49. Kak VJ, Prabhaker S, Khosla VK, et al. Solitary osteochondroma of spine causing spinal cord compression. Clin Neurol Neurosurg 1985;87:135–138.
50. Keim HA, Reina EG. Osteoid-osteoma as a cause of scoliosis. J Bone Joint Surg 1986;57A:159–163.
51. Kornberg M. Primary Ewing's sarcoma of the spine. Spine 1986;11:54–57.
52. Kostuik JP. Anterior spinal cord decompression for lesions of the thoracic and lumbar spine: techniques, new methods of internal fixation, results. Spine 1983;8:512–531.
53. Kostuik JP, Errico TJ, Gleason TF, et al. Spinal stabilization of vertebral column tumors. Spine 1988;13:250–256.
54. Leeson MC, Makley JT, Carter JR. Metastatic skeletal disease in the pediatric population. J Pediatr Orthop 1985;5:261–267.
55. Lesoin F, Rousseaux M, Lozes G, et al. Posterolateral approach to tumours of the dorsolumbar spine. Acta Neurochir 1986;81:40–44.
56. Loftus CM, Rozario RA, Prager R, et al. Solitary osteochondroma of T4 with thoracic cord compression. Surg Neurol 1980;13:355–357.
57. Malat J, Virapongse C, Levine A. Solitary osteochondroma of the spine. Spine 1986;11:625–628.
58. Manabe S, Tateishi A, Abe M, et al. Surgical treatment of metastatic tumors of the spine. Spine 1989;14:41–47.
59. Marcove RC, Sheth DS, Brien EW, et al. Conservative surgery for giant cell tumors of the sacrum: the role of cryosurgery as a supplement to curettage and partial excision. Cancer 1994;74:1253–1260.
60. Marsh BW, Bonfiglio M, Brady LP, et al. Benign osteoblastoma: range of manifestations. J Bone Joint Surg 1975;57A:1–9.
61. Martin NS, Williams JW. The role of surgery in the treatment of malignant tumors of the spine. J Bone Joint Surg 1970;52B:227–237.
62. McAfee PC, Bohlman HH, Ducker T, et al. Failure of stabilization of the spine with methylmethacrylate. J Bone Joint Surg 1984;68A:40–46.
63. McLain RF, Weinstein JN. Solitary plasmacytomas of the spine: a review of 84 cases. J Spinal Disord 1989;2:69–74.
64. McLain RF, Weinstein JN. An unusual presentation of Schmorl's node. Spine 1990;15:247–250.
65. McLain RF, Weinstein JN. Tumors of the spine. Semin Spine Surg 1990;2:157–180.
66. McLain RF, Kabins M, Weinstein MN. VSP stabilization of lumbar neoplasms: technical considerations and complications. J Spinal Disord 1991;4(3):359–365.
67. Meissner WA, Warren S. Neoplasms. In: Andeson WAD, ed. Pathology. Vol 1. St. Louis: Mosby, 1966:534–540.
68. Milch A, Changus GW. Response of bone to tumor invasion. Cancer 1956;9:340–351.
69. Millburn L, Hibbs GC, Hendrickson FR. Treatment of spinal cord compression from metastatic carcinoma. Cancer 1968;21:447–452.
70. Mindell ER. Current concepts review: chordoma. J Bone Joint Surg 1981;63A:501–505.
71. Mirra JM, Gold RH, Picci P. Osseous tumors of intramedullary origin. In: Mirra JM, ed. Bone tumors. Philadelphia: Lea & Febiger, 1989:31–33.
72. Montesano PX, McLain RF, Benson DR. Spinal instrumentation in the management of vertebral column tumors. Semin Orthop 1991;6:237–246.
73. Nather A, Bose K. The results of decompression of cord or cauda equina compression from metastatic extradural tumors. Clin Orthop 1982;169:103–108.
74. Nesbit ME, Kieffer S, D'Angio GJ. Reconstitution of vertebral height in histiocytosis X: a long-term follow-up. J Bone Joint Surg 1969;51A:1360–1368.
75. Nicholls PJ, Jarecky TW. The value of posterior decompression by laminectomy for malignant tumors of the spine. Clin Orthop 1985;201:210–213.
76. O'Neil J, Gardner V, Armstrong G. Treatment of tumors of the thoracic and lumbar spinal column. Clin Orthop 1988;227:103–112.
77. Panjabi MM, Goel VK, Clark CR, et al. Biomechanical study of cervical spine stabilization with methylmethacrylate. Spine 1985;10:198–203.
78. Perrin RG, McBroom RJ. Anterior versus posterior decompression for symptomatic spinal metastasis. Can J Neurol Sci 1987;14:75–80.
79. Pettine KA, Klassen RA. Osteoid-osteoma and osteoblastoma of the spine. J Bone Joint Surg 1986;68A:354–361.
80. Pilepich MV, Vietti TJ, Nesbit ME, et al. Ewing's sarcoma of the vertebral column. Int J Radiat Oncol Biol Phys 1981;7:27–31.
81. Poulsen JO, Jensen JT, Tommesen P. Ewing's sarcoma simulating vertebra plana. Acta Orthop Scand 1975;46:211–215.
82. Ransford AO, Pozo JL, Hutton PAN, et al. The behavior pattern of the scoliosis associated with osteoid osteoma or osteoblastoma of the spine. J Bone Joint Surg 1984;66B:16–20.
83. Rate WR, Butler MS, Robertson WW, et al. Late orthopaedic effects in children with Wilm's tumor treated with abdominal irradiation. Med Pediatr Oncol 1991;19:265–268.
84. Rich TA, Schiller A, Suite HD, et al. Clinical and pathologic review of 48 cases of chordoma. Cancer 1985;56:182–187.
85. Rogalsky RJ, Black GB, Reed MH. Orthopaedic manifestations of leukemia in children. J Bone Joint Surg 1986;68A:494–501.
86. Russin LA, Robinson MJ, Engle HA, et al. Ewing's sar-

86. coma of the lumbar spine. Clin Orthop 1982;164:126–129.
87. Saitoh H, Hida M. Metastatic process and a potential indication of treatment for metastatic lesions of renal adenocarcinoma. J Urol 1982;128:916–918.
88. Sanjay BK, Sim FH, Unn KK, et al. Giant cell tumor of the spine. J Bone Joint Surg 1993;75B:148–154.
89. Savini R, Gherlinzoni F, Morandi M, et al. Surgical treatment of giant-cell tumor of the spine. J Bone Joint Surg 1983;65A:1283–1289.
90. Savitz MH, Goldstein HB, Jaffrey IS, et al. Ewing's sarcoma arising in the sacral epidural space. Mt Sinai J Med 1988;55:339–342.
91. Schajowicz F. Tumors and tumorlike lesions of bones and joints. New York: Springer-Verlag, 1981:281–302.
92. Sharma BS, Khosla VK, Banerjee AK. Primary spinal epidural Ewing's sarcoma. Clin Neurol Neurosurg 1986;88:299–302.
93. Sherk HH, Nicholson JT, Nixon JE. Vertebra plana and eosinophilic granuloma of the cervical spine in children. Spine 1978;3:116–121.
94. Sherman RMP, Waddell JP. Laminectomy for metastatic epidural spinal cord tumors. Clin Orthop 1986;207:55–63.
95. Shives TC, Dahlin DC, Sim FH, et al. Osteosarcoma of the spine. J Bone Joint Surg 1986;68A:660–668.
96. Shives TC, McLeod RA, Unni KK, et al. Chondrosarcoma of the spine. J Bone Joint Surg 1989;71A:1158–1165.
97. Siegal T, Siegal T. Surgical Decompression of anterior and posterior malignant epidural tumors compressing the spinal cord: a prospective study. Neurosurgery 1985;17:424–432.
98. Siegal T, Tiqva P, Siegal T. Vertebral body resection for epidural compression by malignant tumors. J Bone Joint Surg 1985;67A:375–382.
99. Siegal T, Siegal T. Current considerations in the management of neoplastic spinal cord compression. Spine 1988;14:223–228.
100. Sim FH, Dahlin DC, Stauffer RN, et al. Primary bone tumors simulating lumbar disc syndrome. Spine 1977;2:65–74.
101. Skinner DG, Colvin RB. Diagnosis and management of renal cell carcinoma. Cancer 1971;28:1165–1177.
102. Slepian A, Hamby WB. Neurologic complications associated with hereditary deforming chondrodysplasia. J Neurosurg 1951;8:529–535.
103. Springfield DS, Enneking WF, Neff JR, et al. Principles of tumor management. Instr Course Lect 1984;33:1–25.
104. Stener B, Johnsen OE. Complete removal of three vertebrae for giant cell tumour. J Bone Joint Surg 1971;53B:278–287.
105. Stener B. Total spondylectomy in chondrosarcoma arising from the seventh thoracic vertebra. J Bone Joint Surg 1971;53B:288–295.
106. Stener B, Gunterberg B. High amputation of the sacrum for extirpation of tumors. Spine 1978;3:351–366.
107. Sundaresan N, Galicich JH, Lane JM, et al. Treatment of neoplastic epidural cord compression by vertebral body resection and stabilization. J Neurosurg 1985;63:676–684.
108. Sundaresan N, Scher H, DiGiacinto GV, et al. Surgical treatment of spinal cord compression in kidney cancer. J Clin Oncol 1986;4:1851–1856.
109. Sundaresan N, Rosen G, Huvos AG, et al. Combined treatment of osteosarcoma of the spine. Neurosurgery 1988;23(6):714–719.
110. Tachdjian MO, Matson DD. Orthopaedic aspects of intraspinal tumors in infants and children. J Bone Joint Surg 1965;47A:223–248.
111. Tomita T, Galicich JH, Sundaresan N. Radiation therapy for spinal epidural metastases with complete block. Acta Radiol Oncol 1983;22:135–143.
112. Torma T. Malignant tumors of the spine and the spinal epidural space: a study based on 250 histologically verified cases. Acta Chir Scand 1957;225(Suppl):1–138.
113. Valderrama JAF, Bullough PG. Solitary myeloma of the spine. J Bone Joint Surg 1988;50B:82–90.
114. Waxman AD. Bone scans are of sufficient accuracy and sensitivity to be part of the routine workup prior to definitive surgical treatment of cancer. In: Van Scoy-Mosher MB, ed. Medical oncology: Current controversies in cancer treatment. Boston: Hall, 1981:69–76.
115. Weinstein JN, McLain RF. Primary tumors of the spine. Spine 1987;12:843–851.
116. Weinstein JN. Surgical approach to spine tumors. Orthopaedics 1989;12:897–905.
117. White AA III, Panjabi MM. Surgical constructs employing methylmethacrylate. In: Clinical biomechanics of the spine. Philadelphia: Lippincott, 1978:423–431.
118. White WA, Patterson RH, Bergland RM. Role of surgery in the treatment of spinal cord compression by metastatic neoplasm. Cancer 1971;27:558–561.
119. Whitehouse GH, Griffiths GJ. Roentgenologic aspects of spinal involvement by primary and metastatic Ewing's tumor. J Can Assoc Radiol 1976;27:290–297.
120. Willen J, Lindahl S, Irstam L, et al. Unstable thoracolumbar fractures: a study by CT and conventional roentgenology of the reduction effect of Harrington instrumentation. Spine 1984;9:214–219.
121. Wong DA, Fornasier VL, MacNab I. Spinal metastases: the obvious, the occult, and the imposters. Spine 1990;15:104.
122. Wright RL. Malignant tumors in the spinal extradural space: results of surgical treatment. Ann Surg 1963;157:227–231.
123. Young RF, Post EM, King GA. Treatment of spinal epidural metastases. J Neurosurg 1980;53:741–748.

CHAPTER TWENTY SEVEN

Intradural Lesions of the Spine

Don M. Long

Introduction

The majority of intradural procedures in the spine are required for treatment of tumors. Correction of congenital abnormalities also often requires an intradural component to the operation. Arachnoiditis is a rare reason for intradural surgery, and an occasional intervertebral disc requires an intradural approach. Every spinal surgeon should understand the indications for a transdural operation. However, the tissue manipulation required once inside the dura is strikingly different from the techniques that are used in extradural procedures. Only those trained and experienced in manipulation of nervous tissue should attempt intradural surgery.

Diagnosis of Intradural Abnormalities

When an intradural lesion is suspected, magnetic resonance imaging (MRI) is the diagnostic tool of choice. Studies should be conducted with and without intravenous gadolinium. Nearly all intradural lesions will be defined accurately.

Meningiomas and schwannomas enhance brightly on MRI and are usually easily identified. They are differentiated by the evidence of dural involvement, which is present only in the meningioma. Epidermoid cysts, dermoid cysts, and lipomas have the characteristics of fat on MRI. The arachnoid cyst can be very difficult to identify. Since its characteristics on MRI are those of cerebrospinal fluid (CSF), an arachnoid cyst will be missed unless cord distortion is seen.

Intramedullary tumors are also best seen on MRI. The ependymomas virtually always enhance with contrast, whereas lower-grade astrocytomas may not. The high-grade astrocytomas usually have patchy areas of enhancement. The rarer hemangioma or hemangioblastoma is normally seen easily.

Congenital anomalies are defined on MRI as well. The characteristics of the Arnold-Chiari malformation are easily appreciated, as are syringomyelia and other forms of congenital anomalies. Arteriovenous malformations may be very difficult to demonstrate on MRI. A finding of large veins in the epidural space may be a clue, but when a diagnosis of arteriovenous malformation is suspected, angiography is likely to be necessary. An intermediate step is to study the cord with computed tomography (CT) myelography. The rare intradural disc herniation is difficult to define in MRI. CT myelography is usually required to make the diagnosis.

Plain x-ray films and plain CT scans are rarely useful with intradural lesions. CT myelography is still required occasionally, however. It is most useful for the diagnosis of arachnoiditis, arteriovenous malformations, and arachnoid cysts.

Tumors of the Spinal Cord and Spinal Nerves

It is traditional to divide tumors of the spinal column into three categories on the basis of their anatomical location: extradural, intradural-extramedullary, and intramedullary (6, 30, 33).

Extradural Tumors

Extradural tumors are virtually always metastatic in origin, though a few primary tumors of the spinal column are known. Since these tumors become intradural rarely, they will not be discussed in detail here. Occasionally a primary or metastatic bone tumor will invade the dura. In this situation it is necessary to excise all involved dura and remove the intradural portion of the tumor by techniques to be described below for intradural-extramedullary lesions, which are more common. The dura is then repaired with a patch, and the remainder of the extradural procedure can proceed as is usual.

Intradural-Extramedullary Tumors

Intradural-extramedullary tumors are typically schwannomas, meningiomas, or myxopapillary ependymomas of the filum terminale. Rarely, a dermoid cyst or hemangioblastoma may be encountered, particularly in the region of the cauda equina. All others are oddities and do not require different surgical maneuvers (6).

Schwannomas

Schwannomas characteristically occur on the posterior roots and thus are located in the posterolateral quadrant (Fig. 27.1). They are best diagnosed by MRI and are rarely mistaken for any other tumor. Schwannomas are most common in the thoracic region, but also occur in the cervical area, with a nearly equal proportion in the lumbar region. They usually occur singly, except in neurofibromatosis (42, 44). Tumors may grow to very large size before significant symptoms develop (10, 11, 19, 32, 46, 48).

It is important to recognize the signs and symptoms of myelopathy. These will be similar for all the tumors to be described and result from nonspecific compression of the spinal cord. Typically patients describe first a gait disturbance. Physical findings may be unremarkable at this stage. Next, subtle changes in posterior column function appear. Patients often say they can no longer walk in the dark, when their feet are not visible. Difficulty ascending stairs or curbs is common. Then hyperreflexia occurs and pathological signs such as the Babinski or Hoffmann signs appear. Later, weakness becomes obvious, a sensory level appears, and finally bowel, bladder, and sex function are likely to be affected. Investigation of the gait disturbance is critical to early diagnosis. Radicular pain sometimes occurs with the early warning signs of the extramedullary tumor and diffuse dermatomal pain can accompany the intramedullary lesion.

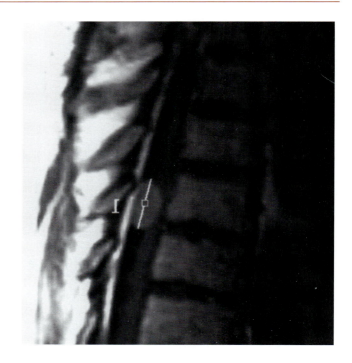

FIGURE 27.1.
Sagittal MRI demonstrates a well-circumscribed rounded mass posteriorly placed with marked spinal cord compression. This was an intradural schwannoma.

Operative Procedures

No matter what the spinal location, surgery is carried out with the patient under general anesthesia and in the prone position. The techniques for cervical and thoracic tumor removal are virtually identical, though the technique required for involvement of a lumbar route is somewhat different and will be described separately. A major extraspinal component may require more lateral exposure.

Localization of the lesion is paramount. In the cervical region this is generally not difficult to do. In the thoracic region x-ray films may be necessary for accurate localization. A midline incision should be planned to allow exposure of at least one segment above and one segment below the superior and inferior margins of the tumor. Muscles are dissected in a subperiosteal fashion bilaterally. I prefer to carry out these operations through a full laminectomy because I think it is safer when spinal cord retraction is required. Certainly some tumors can be removed by hemilaminectomy. Bone should be removed until the upper and lower margins of the tumor are clearly visible. When there is no contraindication, I prefer an operative field one full level above and below. The laminectomy should be wide so that the lateral margin of the tumor in the spinal canal is reached. The extraforaminal portion of the tumor must be judged. When it is substantial, sometimes a second-stage operation is required. However, it is usually possible to follow the tumor out through the neural foramen and remove the extraforaminal expansion by simply expanding the muscular retraction laterally. This is another reason for being certain that the incision is well above and well below the tumor, so that the lateral retraction is possible. I always carry out the intradural removal first so that the cord is no longer compressed during removal of the remainder of the extraspinal tumor.

Immaculate extradural hemostasis is required. The gutters should be packed with hemostatic agents until there is no blood at all. At this point the operating microscope is brought into the field and the remainder of the operation is carried out under appropriate magnification.

The dura should be opened in the midline from above downward, remembering the displacement of the spinal cord. It is extremely important in opening the dura to leave the arachnoid intact so that CSF is not lost and so that no cord herniation or injury with the knife blade occurs. The dural margins should be tied back to bone or retracted by sutures weighted with clamps. This will provide good hemostasis and expose the tumor widely. Then the arachnoid is opened on the lateral side of the tumor from the top to the bottom of the incision. This will usually allow good visualization of the spinal cord and the superior and inferior margins of the tumor. The adhesions of the lateral margin of the spinal cord to tumor should be freed by sharp dissection. If coagulation is used, it should always be on the tumor side, and not near the cord. Then the relationships of nerve roots to the tumor must be identified. All nerve roots not entering the tumor mass should be dissected free. Those that obviously enter the tumor may be cut at this point. Here it is easy to be fooled into thinking that something that is actually dissectable is entering the tumor, so care must be taken to separate all nerve roots possible. Of course in the thoracic region or the upper cervical region, where loss of a single posterior root is unimportant, it may be reasonable simply to cut them all at this point. In the brachial plexus or at the thoracolumbar junction all possible roots must be preserved.

Most of these tumors should undergo intracapsular removal before they are manipulated in order to minimize cord trauma. Enter the tumor near its lateral dural attachment and remove it by ultrasonic dissection, suction, laser, or forceps. When the majority of the tumor has been removed, the capsule can be slowly mobilized and dissected free from spinal cord. Crossed blood vessels should be coagulated near the tumor and cut. I prefer to do most of this with coagulation and sharp dissection rather than blunt dissection, which may injure the cord. These maneuvers will allow the tumor gradually to be extracted from the spinal cord and mobilized from medial to lateral, thus decompressing the cord.

Most of the capsule may now be removed. A cuff will remain exiting from the dura. When in an area in which the anterior roots are important, they should be examined and freed from tumor as well. Then the tumor can be mobilized from the margins of the dura and followed out into the extraforaminal space. Protect the spinal cord with cottonoid so that it is not injured by any movement of the instruments directed toward the extraforaminal component of the tumor. The tumor is followed out into the space through the foramen, and the capsule is gradually mobilized. It must be kept in mind that in the cervical area the vertebral artery is likely to be adherent anteriorly to a sizable tumor mass. The nerve roots should not be injured during the dissection. It is usually possible to free the capsule completely, coagulate it distally, and cut the residual capsule with total removal of the tumor. If the vertebral artery does bleed, it is best controlled by packing. Venous bleeding around the tumor may be substantial as the tumor is debulked and should be packed off as the dissection continues.

If it is impossible to remove all the extraforaminal tumor distally, it is better to stop the procedure at this point and carry out a second-stage removal. This is rarely necessary.

When tumor removal is complete, it is important to reconstitute the dura. The midline incision is easily closed. It is always the large dural defect left by removal of the tumor that is a problem. I prefer to harvest a fascial graft and suture it circumferentially in a watertight fashion, using fine sutures of at least No. 4–0. Pseudomeningocele is an irritating complication that may prolong hospitalization.

If it was necessary to divide an important motor or sensory root, every effort should be made to reapproximate them. If it is not possible to reapproximate the ends, I harvest the greater occipital nerve, or better, the sural nerve, previously prepared for this purpose, to graft an important anterior cervical root. In the lumbar region there is nearly always enough redundant root to gain first-intention approximation. The recovery of function for this rare eventuality has been uniformly good.

The wound is then closed in anatomical layers, as after any spinal operation. If a watertight closure has been obtained, there is no reason to restrict postoperative mobility.

Schwannomas of the Cauda Equina

Treatment of tumors of the cauda equina is somewhat different (Fig. 27.2) (32). They are also approached by the midline and through laminectomy. However, after the dura has been opened the technique changes. The roots of the cauda must be separated

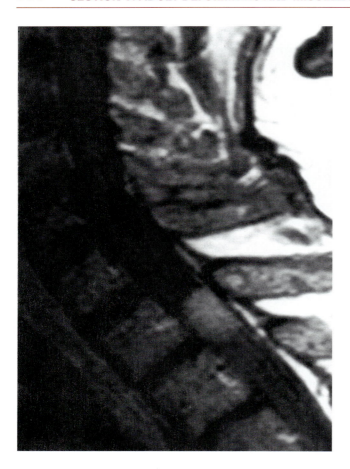

FIGURE 27.2.

Two enhancing lesions are seen within the dura in the cauda equina. Diagnosis: multiple neurofibromas complicating von Recklinghausen disease.

from the tumor, to which they are frequently adherent. This should be done without entering the capsule of the tumor. I prefer to do this sharply with a small cataract knife unless the roots come off easily with blunt dissection. When all of the uninvolved roots are clearly free from the tumor, it should be possible to identify those roots that actually enter and exit the tumor. Some of these tumors will be true neurofibromas. The technique with a neurofibroma does not differ, but it is frequently more difficult in neurofibromas than in schwannomas to isolate the roots that are actually involved in the tumor down to one or a few filaments.

Once the dissection of roots is done, I stimulate the distal root(s) to determine what muscles are involved. The patients have been previously prepared with electromyographic electrodes so that we can determine the involved roots and their importance. Important motor roots will be resutured if their division has been necessary.

Now it is possible to remove the tumor. If the tumor is relatively small and can be easily brought out of the intraspinal space, it can be removed in its entirety. The root above is cut without coagulation or clamping if it is to be reapproximated. If it is not to be reapproximated, it can be clamped and then cut with impunity. The same is true distally. Do not lose the ends of the roots if you plan to try to put them back together. Fine suture tags will help to prevent this embarrassing delay.

When the tumor is large, intracapsular removal may be necessary. The tumor is debulked with ultrasonic suction or bipolar forceps until the residual tumor capsule can be mobilized out of the field and treated as described earlier.

When reconstitution of an important root is necessary, it is usually possible to put it together with one or two fine sutures. There is frequently enough redundant root to bring the two ends together without difficulty. However, grafting may occasionally be required. The dura should be closed in a watertight fashion and the wound repaired as would any other spinal wound.

Intradural Meningiomas

Meningiomas are commonly found in the anterolateral quadrant of the canal (Figs. 27.3 and 27.4). They typically displace the cord posteriorly and laterally.

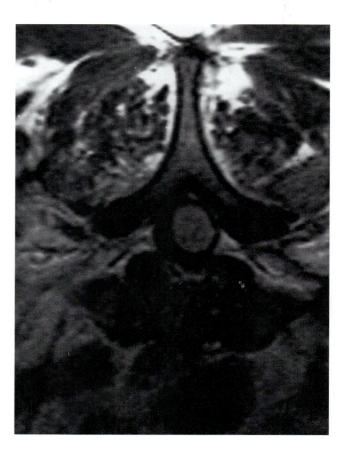

FIGURE 27.3.

Sagittal MRI demonstrates an anterior mass markedly compressing the thoracic cord. There is a broad dural base, but the tumor is rounded and well circumscribed. Diagnosis: meningioma.

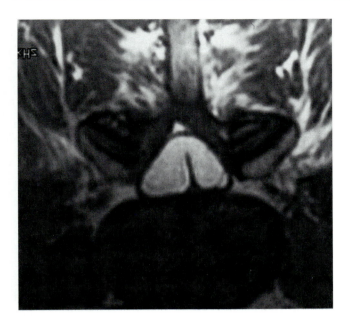

FIGURE 27.4.
There is a posteriorly placed, well-circumscribed mass with a broad dural base and enhancement of dura surrounding the tumor. Diagnosis: meningioma.

Occasionally one may be found directly in front of the cord. It is important to recognize this situation on the preoperative MRI so that an intramedullary tumor is not mistakenly diagnosed (32, 35).

The operation for meningioma is identical to that for schwannoma or neurofibroma until the tumor is actually exposed. The meningioma will not have the same smooth capsule and cannot be dissected free from surrounding structures as easily. Once the meningioma is exposed above and below, the spinal cord should be dissected free from the meningioma throughout the length of the tumor. Nerve roots should be separated as well. Then removal of the meningioma may begin laterally. An intracapsular removal allows the tumor gradually to be dissected free and brought from medial to lateral. The nerve roots will all be salvageable, and so great care should be taken in dissecting them free from the tumor mass. The ultrasonic dissector is the most effective way to remove the tumor, and if there is adequate exposure it will allow the meningioma to be removed with great precision without risk of injury to the spinal cord. Occasionally a meningioma is calcified and virtually rock hard. Such tumors usually have to be cut and removed piecemeal.

When the tumor is all removed, there will be residual involvement of the dura. There are two ways to manage this problem. One is simply to excise the dura and replace the removed dura with a patch. The other is to use a laser to vaporize all residual tumor until only normal dura remains. Total excision carries less risk of recurrence, but it exposes the spinal cord to increased risk. The laser has an excellent capacity for vaporization of tumor, but there remains a higher risk of recurrence. Nevertheless, for most of these tumors I prefer to vaporize all involved dura and coagulate the extradural veins in the area at the same time. To date I have not had a recurrence with this technique.

The closure is identical to that employed for other spinal operations.

Myxopapillary Ependymoma of the Filum Terminale

Myxopapillary ependymomas are exposed in exactly the same way as described for schwannoma. The dura is opened in the midline, and at least one segment above and below the tumor should be exposed. Then the nerves must be dissected from the tumor. With a myxopapillary ependymoma it is extremely important not to spill cells into the subarachnoid space, for implantation may occur and multiple intraspinal metastases may result. Hence I pack off the subarachnoid space with soft cotton before beginning tumor removal. Then, with the use of high magnification, all nerve roots and vessels are dissected from the capsule. This will allow identification of the filum terminale, which can be coagulated and cut above and below the tumor. Small tumors are then lifted out of their bed, making certain that all nerve roots are dissected free. Larger tumors may have to be entered and debulked. These tumors are very soft and the Cavitron will remove them quickly. Be sure not to go through the capsule and injure a nerve root or have the nerve roots caught in the suction of the ultrasonic dissector. Here too, great care must be taken not to spill cells.

Once the tumor removal is complete, copious irrigation should be used to make certain that any cells that have seeded the area are washed out. Only then should the cottonoid dams that have protected the rest of the subarachnoid space be removed and the whole field irrigated again. The dura is then closed in a watertight fashion and the wound closed in the usual way, in anatomical layers (24).

Unusual Intradural-Extramedullary Tumors

Occasionally unusual tumors such as dermoid cysts, epidermoid cysts, or lipomas are encountered (Fig. 27.5) (7, 32). These tumors are removed exactly as described in the preceding section. Dermoids and epidermoids contain noxious materials that must be kept from the subarachnoid space. Other than that, they require no special techniques. The key is to dissect all nerve roots free from the tumor. When the tumor is small, it does not represent a serious problem. Unfortunately, some of these tumors are enormous and may fill the entire spinal canal from the conus medullaris well down into the sacrum. Removal of the cholesterol material that constitutes the bulk of the tumor is not difficult. These large tumors

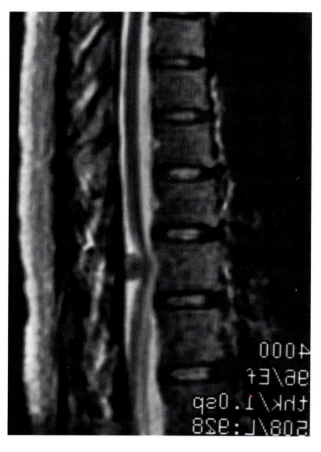

FIGURE 27.5.
A large lumbar lipoma compressing the cauda equina and tethering the spinal cord is seen on sagittal MRI.

should be removed piecemeal after opening the dura to be certain that all of the noxious material is out. Copious irrigation is required after they are removed. The problem with these tumors is the adherence of the capsule to dura and the nerves in a manner that may be undefinable and inextricable. High magnification and a great deal of patience must be used to try carefully to separate the capsular material with adherent arachnoid from nerve roots. This may be an impossible job. It is particularly difficult in patients for whom previous attempts at surgery have failed. These are unusual tumors and should not be approached by anyone who is not thoroughly skilled in their removal and willing to spend the long periods of time required in the tedious dissections. Even so, it may not be possible to cure these tumors.

With large epidermoid tumors I usually leave the dura open so that the tumor can grow into an expanded extradural space without recompressing nerve roots. This technique has resulted in long-term palliation and makes reoperation for evacuation of accumulated cholesterol crystals substantially easier. The remainder of the wound is closed in anatomical layers.

Arachnoid Cysts

Arachnoid cysts are functionally intradural-extramedullary tumors (43). They can be identified on MRI with accuracy now and should be operated on when loculated. Exposure is achieved as for any other tumor, and the dura is opened above and below the mass. Care should be taken not to open the cyst while opening the dura, or it may be very difficult to determine its margins and therefore to remove it totally. These cysts are usually elliptical masses clearly separable from the remainder of the subarachnoid space. Some can be dissected free virtually in their entirety as a tumor and removed. Most will be opened before this, and then the cyst disappears. For this reason it is very important to recognize its extent beforehand, mark it above and below, and then excise all the cyst wall and associated arachnoid until the mass is gone. If any part of the cyst must be left behind, it seems to increase the risk of recurrent loculation. In spite of the most extensive removals of this abnormal arachnoid, there is a tendency for reloculation of CSF in the area. Therefore, it is important to be certain that CSF flow is reconstituted in an unimpeded fashion above and below, posteriorly and anteriorly around the denticulate ligament. Most of these arachnoid cysts occur in the posterior region and are easily accessible. Cutting the denticulate ligament and opening the arachnoid anteriorly decreases the risk that loculation can reoccur. The dura is then closed in a watertight fashion posteriorly and the wound closed in anatomical layers.

Intramedullary Tumors

Typical intramedullary tumors are astrocytomas and ependymomas, which each make up nearly 50% of intramedullary neoplasms. These tumors can be identified with great accuracy with MRI. Cystic components are seen. The extent and nature of the tumor can usually be determined with great accuracy.

There are some other intramedullary oddities that may occasionally be encountered. Granulomatous disease such as sarcoid, intramedullary schwannoma, and inflammatory diseases may mimic these more common intramedullary tumors. Even acute multiple sclerosis may occasionally look like a tumor (32).

The surgery should be planned to be well above and below these tumors. I like to have an operative field two full segments above and two below whenever possible and consider one segment above and below a necessity. The operations are carried out with the patient under general anesthesia and in the prone position. The skin incisions are marked appropriately, and the midline incision is used universally. A typical subperiosteal dissection of muscles from spinous processes and laminae is carried out and a laminectomy is performed. In children, laminoplasty is preferable to laminectomy. If laminectomy is used, posterior fusion should follow in the cervical region in children. Fusion is not usually required in adults. Remember that both children and adults must be observed postoperatively for the development of the hyperextended swan neck syndrome.

Ultrasonography may be used to locate the tumor with accuracy once the laminectomy is complete. The dura is then opened from above down in the midline, and dural retention sutures are used, either in suturing the dura back to the muscle or using clamp-weighted retention sutures. Immaculate hemostasis is required so that there is no bleeding to distract the surgeon and obscure the field during the operation.

From this point forward the operating microscope is used at high magnification. Identify the tumor, if possible, and verify its nature with a frozen section. Sometimes the tumor is wholly intramedullary and cannot be seen. In this case the expanded area of the cord is identified. Ultrasonography is useful to verify the area of the cord that is increased in size, particularly if there is an associated cyst.

Usually the cord is opened in the midline. I prefer very fine (No. 6–0 or 7–0) retention pial sutures to keep the cord open so that it is not traumatized by retraction. Begin in a convenient place where the cord is most abnormal and where it appears that the tumor is closest to the surface. Carry out a midline myelotomy using a fine arachnoid knife and careful midline dissection. Micro-knives (Rosen) are good tools in the avascular plane. Then a biopsy specimen of the tumor can be taken. The astrocytomas are rarely encapsulated, usually infiltrative, and usually difficult to differentiate from spinal cord. They may have a pseudoencapsulated appearance and then can be removed. Ependymomas, by contrast, are well encapsulated and usually separate relatively easily from surrounding cord. Since ependymomas can be cured by surgery and astrocytomas probably cannot, it is extremely important to determine which one is present. The other masses such as sarcoid or acute inflammatory processes generally do not need to be removed, but the biopsy analysis will verify their nature. Oddities such as schwannoma can be removed, as can hemangioblastoma.

Management of High-Grade Astrocytoma

If the tumor is a high-grade astrocytoma, then the prognosis is virtually hopeless at present. No cure has yet been reported (32). However, to preserve function as long as possible, it is usually feasible to remove the bulk of the tumor. They tend to be soft, separable from the remainder of the cord, and removable by suction or ultrasonic dissection.

Another technique used is to carry out this removal in two stages. The first stage is simply midline myelotomy to the extremities of the tumor. The wound is then closed, leaving the dura open. The surgeon returns 7 to 10 days later, when it is usually possible to remove a great deal of tumor that has become exophytic through the long myelotomy. This will often palliate the neurological deficit. However, these tumors tend to spread rapidly, and death from intracranial extension is the rule. Radiation therapy is employed postoperatively, but its effect is uncertain.

Radical cordectomy going well above the tumor has been described. My limited experience with this technique in four patients has been disappointing. Three of the four died of intracranial tumor in less than 1 year. I no longer consider this a standard option.

Management of the Low-Grade Astrocytoma

Most low-grade tumors are not separable from the cord. The myelotomy should be large enough to explore the tumor and determine whether it has a pseudoencapsulated appearance. If it does, it may be possible to separate tumor from cord using precise microsurgical techniques and to remove a substantial part of the mass. Cure is not probable. However, palliation may be obtained for the patient by the removal of a portion of a compressive mass. The attempt to remove tumor is terminated when separation from surrounding tissue becomes too difficult.

All of this removal is carried out using spinal evoked sensory potentials and motor stimulation. Substantial degradation of the responses may lead to cessation of the surgery as well.

When all that is possible has been accomplished, the operation must be terminated. If an excellent decompression has been obtained, it may be possible to close the dura primarily. However, it is more likely that a dural patch will be required. Dorsal fascia, fascia lata, or a dural substitute may be employed and should be circumferentially sutured to the defect precisely. In order to provide maximum decompression I often leave the dural retention sutures in place and suture the patch into the expanded dural pouch. Once this is accomplished, the wound is closed in anatomical layers (13, 27, 29, 50, 51, 55).

Intramedullary Ependymoma

Treatment of ependymomas is quite different from that of the tumors just described. They can be cured surgically, and therefore radical surgery is warranted (Fig. 27.6) (15, 16, 24, 40, 54).

Exposure is performed as described for all other intramedullary tumors. Once the dura is opened and the nature of the tumor identified, its extent should be determined with accuracy using direct observa-

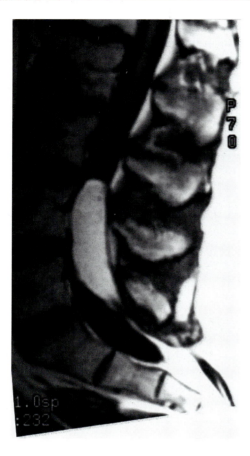

FIGURE 27.6.
Axial MRI demonstrating a well-circumscribed demarcated mass within the substance of the cord. Diagnosis: ependymoma.

tion and ultrasonography. The myelotomy should extend from top to bottom and a little beyond obvious tumor because there tend to be small tails of tumor going up and down the central canal. Again, pial retention sutures are used. The dissection of the overlying cord from capsule can usually be done bluntly or with micro-knives. Blood vessels are coagulated on the tumor side as they are encountered and cut. I prefer to do most of this sharply to reduce the risk of trauma to the cord. Evoked potential and motor stimulation monitoring are used throughout and the technique modified if changes in wave forms or responsivity occur. The tumor mass is gradually isolated from top to bottom and then laterally. It may be necessary to open into the tumor and reduce its bulk if the mass is a particularly large one. The cystic cavities that commonly are associated with these tumors usually occur at the extremities, and we need not be concerned with them during the dissection of the main tumor mass. Remember that these tumors can spread in the subarachnoid space, so if the capsule is entered it is important to create dams above and below to prevent tumor spread. The tumors are dissected free circumferentially. Blood vessels typically enter in the midline anteriorly and should be coagulated as the tumor is removed. Be sure to follow the small extensions that go superiorly and inferiorly so that no tumor is left. If there is a substantial syrinx cavity, the wall should be analyzed by biopsy to be certain that it is not tumor. Usually there is no tumor in the wall of the cavity, but occasionally the cavity will have actually occurred within the capsule of the tumor, and it is important to recognize this so that no tumor is left behind.

When the tumor is completely removed, hemostasis should be obtained without coagulating in the tumor bed. I do not resuture the cord because that may lead to postoperative syrinx formation. The dura is reconstituted in the midline; grafting is virtually never required. The wound then closed in anatomical layers.

It should be kept in mind that these extensive laminectomies in children may lead to a serious postoperative deformity. The surgeon has the option of carrying out the exposure and closure by means of laminoplasty or postoperative fusion using a lateral technique. Either one is satisfactory (4). Details are provided elsewhere in this book.

Radiotherapy is commonly used for tumors in which removal is incomplete. The use of radiotherapy probably compounds the issue of bone deformity because it interferes with appropriate bone growth and maturation. It may also interfere with fusion healing. When the need for radiation is obvious, it is probably better to defer the fusion until after the course of radiation therapy (8, 21, 37, 56).

Hemangioma, Lipoma, and Other Unusual Intramedullary Tumors

Hemangiomas are handled almost exactly like ependymomas. The only difference is in their vascularity. An occasional ependymoma may be so vascular that it appears to be a hemangioblastoma or hemangioma. The tumor should be dissected circumferentially without entering the capsule, coagulating and cutting the feeding blood vessels as encountered. Cure is probable.

Lipomas are quite different. They tend to be intramedullary with exophytic masses outside the cord. Once their nature is identified and they are decompressed, they do not need to be removed. Elimination of the compression, tethering of the spinal cord by removal of the exophytic mass, and a dural graft are all that is required.

Occasionally other rare tumors may be encountered. The intramedullary schwannoma has been mentioned. It is removed in exactly the same way that an ependymoma is approached. Intramedullary meningioma now has been reported. Because of the rarity of this tumor, no surgical rules have been established, but it is probable that such a tumor would be treated in the same way as described for ependymoma (32).

Congenital Anomalies of the Spine

There are four congenital anomalies that routinely require intradural exploration. The Arnold-Chiari malformation and attendant syringomyelia; diastematomyelia; the tethered cord syndrome; and the various forms of arteriovenous malformations (20, 53).

Arnold-Chiari Malformation With and Without Syringomyelia

The Arnold-Chiari malformation includes a congenital deformity of the hindbrain, herniation of the tonsils below the level of the foramen magnum with cervicomedullary compression, and commonly a cystic formation within the spinal cord called syringomyelia. When symptomatic, the treatment includes decompression and dural grafting (12, 17, 23, 25, 26, 38, 41).

Surgery for the Arnold-Chiari Malformation

These operations are carried out with the patient under general anesthesia and in the prone position with the head in skeletal fixation. A skin incision is made from the inion to the spine of C3 or C4, depending on the extent of the tonsillar herniation through the foramen magnum. Bones are exposed by typical subperiosteal dissection until the occipital bones are exposed from mastoid process to mastoid process. The arch of C1 is exposed to a point just medial to the vertebral arteries, and the spine and laminae of C2 are completely exposed to the zygapophyseal joints. In the rare case in which the tonsils are herniated far into the cervical cord, the exposure to one level below the lowest tonsil is required.

A laminectomy is then performed, removing the occipital bone first, then C1, and finally C2. This sequence is usually required because the arch of C1 may be under the rim of the foramen magnum and very difficult to reach. I prefer to remove the posterior rim of the foramen magnum by high-speed drills and rongeurs. The arch of C1 and C2 can usually be removed by rongeurs alone.

Once hemostasis is adequate, the dura is opened in a Y-shaped incision beginning in the midline just above C3, with the arms of the Y emanating from the foramen magnum upward. Remember that dural venous anomalies are extremely common and venous bleeding may be brisk here. It may be necessary to coagulate the edges thoroughly or even apply clips to obtain adequate hemostasis.

This will usually provide adequate decompression. There is considerable disagreement among surgeons about the extent of the decompression necessary. Some believe that all of the potential dural adhesions in the area should be sectioned surgically, whereas others do nothing with them. Some advocate exploration of the posterior fossa and even placement of a small pledget of muscle in the obex to try to prevent CSF from entering the central canal; others omit this step. Some believe that a compressive tonsil should be removed. Others indicate that this is never necessary. The only rule to follow is that the cervicomedullary junction must be decompressed, and it is important to do whatever is required for this.

Once this decompression is satisfactory and it is clear that there is free communication from posterior fossa subarachnoid space into the same space in the cervical spine, closure can follow. A graft of fascia lata, cervical fascia, or dural substitute is formed as a triangle to fit the Y-shaped opening. It is then sutured circumferentially in a watertight fashion. Obtaining a watertight closure is extremely important here. Otherwise a pseudomeningocele is likely to develop. Bony stabilization is usually not necessary, so the remainder of the closure is performed as in any typical cervical spine operation.

Syringomyelia

Management of the syrinx is a matter of considerable debate now (22, 34). The majority opinion seems to be to do nothing directly when an associated symptomatic Chiari malformation has been appropriately decompressed. The supposition is that restoration of normal CSF dynamics around the foramen magnum will cause collapse of the syrinx. The weight of opinion favors this approach at present, but definitive data to support this opinion are still lacking. Other options are to open the syrinx and create a cyst subarachnoid shunt or to open the syrinx and create a shunt into another body cavity, usually the pleura.

Other syringomyelic cysts do not communicate with the fourth ventricle or are not associated with a Chiari malformation and may require direct treatment. Furthermore, small tumors are sometimes associated with large cysts, and it is very important to be certain of the nature of the cyst before deciding that a shunt alone is adequate.

When opening the cyst in a case in which shunting is required, the operation is performed as if for tumor removal, but in a much more limited way. Fortunately, MRI with gadolinium enhancement will identify most tumors, so extensive decompressive laminectomy for exploration is not required. I prefer to operate in the least critical area where the cyst is easily accessible. A one-level laminectomy or even hemilaminectomy is all that is required. The dura is then opened, preferably in the midline, and the presence of the cyst is verified. I then make a very small incision into the cord through the midline raphe and enter the cyst. Do not allow the cyst to empty, or it may be difficult to get the shunts in place. Myelotomy above the denticulate ligament through the thinning that routinely occurs there is an option.

There are a variety of shunts that may be used. I currently use the commercially available lumbar shunt or T-tubes cut to size, without a valve and with multiple holes both inside the cyst and in the subarachnoid space. I place one inferiorly in the cyst and one superiorly, bringing them out through the same midline incision. They should be sutured in position with a fine suture attached to the pia or the arachnoid. The ends must extend well into the subarachnoid space if they are to function. It does no good to place them in the extra-arachnoid subdural space, where they will not flow for long. The dura is then closed in the midline and the wound closed in the usual fashion. If shunting to the pleura or the peritoneum is required, the technique requires only slight modification. The same cystostomy is performed, but a single shunt tube is used, and it is placed such that the majority of the tube is in the dependent portion of the cyst. The catheter is then brought out and tunneled to the appropriate pleural or peritoneal space, and the remainder of the shunt completed.

Since most cases of syringomyelia occur in the higher thoracic or the cervical areas, the pleura is an easily accessible location for the shunt. A convenient space, usually in the posterior axillary line, is identified well below the scapula. The pleura is exposed, and once the catheter has been tunneled from the midline to this incision, a small nick is made in the pleura and the catheter put into the space. It is usually not possible to suture the pleura, so the muscle should be gathered tightly around it, with the sutures being placed after the anesthesiologist has inflated the lung. Both wounds are then closed in anatomical layers. A chest film should be taken immediately after surgery to be certain that no pneumothorax has occurred.

When the peritoneum is the choice for locating the shunt, it is usually necessary to turn the patient over. It is possible to do the posterior operation in the lateral position and then to tunnel around to the side, but I find it easier to do the first operation in the prone position, placing the catheter as described, and then closing the wound with the catheter buried in the subcutaneous space. The patient is then turned to the supine position, and the catheter can then be tunneled the remainder of the necessary distance and placed in the peritoneum through a typical subcostal incision.

Diastematomyelia

This unusual abnormality consists of a spike of bone or a band of heavy, fibrous tissue that divides the dura, usually connecting vertebral body with laminae in the midline (Fig. 27.7). A number of anomalies can occur in diastematomyelia. There may be a temporary split in an otherwise normal cord, or there may be true diplomyelia, with separate divided cords and dural tubes below. MRI and CT scanning are capable of identifying the nature of the anomaly with great accuracy (28).

The operation is carried out with the patient under general anesthesia and in the prone position. These anomalies occur almost exclusively in the thoracic region. A subperiosteal dissection of muscles from spine and laminae is carried out, and the location of the anomaly is identified by x-ray film. A laminectomy to expose the dural tube one segment above and below the anomaly is required. From this point the course of the procedure depends on the nature of the anomaly. The typical abnormality is completely extradural, with an intact dural tube surrounding it on both sides. The first step is to bring in the operating microscope and complete the remainder of the operation under high magnification. A high-speed drill is used to remove the bony spicule by drilling it

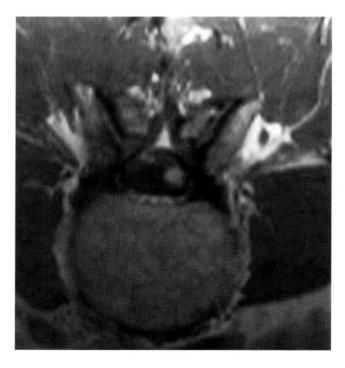

FIGURE 27.7.

The typical sagittal spur of diastematomyelia is seen.

down to the base. Once it is gone nothing further is required if that is the only abnormality. Occasionally the abnormality is truly intradural, in which case the dura must be opened above, on both sides, and below the anomaly so that it is completely exposed. It is then removed with high-speed drill, laser, or small fine rongeurs, depending on its nature. Occasionally a fibrous band can simply be cut anteriorly and posteriorly and removed.

Once the offending mass is removed, nothing else is required. If the dura is opened, it should be reconstituted in a watertight fashion. When the mass has been purely extradural, nothing is required except anatomical closure of the wound.

Tethered Cord Syndrome

There are a number of anomalies in the lumbar region that produce traction on the spinal cord and neurological symptoms. Patients typically present with back pain, leg pain, weakness and/or sensory loss in the legs, and dysfunction of bowel and bladder. Sexual function is often affected before either bowel or bladder abnormalities appear. The anomalies that produce this syndrome lie in a spectrum, beginning with simple enlargement and shortening of the filum terminale so that the spinal cord is in an abnormally low position and stretched by the tight filum to full lipomyelomeningocele. Most of the other intradural anomalies are related, and a single generic operation will suffice for all, with modifications according to what is found.

A clue to the nature of the abnormality is often seen from examination of the back. Birthmarks, hair patches, dimples, and small sinus tracks, frequently associated with subcutaneous lipomas, are seen. Three-dimensional CT scanning and MRI define these abnormalities exactly. The thickened, shortened filum can often be seen, lipomas are identified, the rare associated dermoid is found, and the bony anomalies can be described exactly. The surgeon no longer has to explore, but usually knows exactly what to expect and can plan surgery definitively.

These operations are carried out with the patient under general anesthesia and in the prone position on an appropriate spinal frame or support. A midline incision is made that will expose the area to be repaired. A subperiosteal dissection of muscles from spinous processes and laminae is then carried out, taking care not to enter the dura or injure a nerve root through a bony anomaly. Posterior decompression is required. Occasionally a patient's spine will be unstable enough to require fusion, but this is usually determined from the analysis of the bony anomaly prior to surgery.

If there is a subcutaneous lipoma, it should be removed. These anomalies often have tracks that go down to the dura; these extensions should be followed and all extradural abnormal tissue removed. Do not compromise later skin closure by excessive tissue removal.

Then the dura is opened above the area of abnormality and followed down until the tract can be circumscribed. Sometimes the roots are quite adherent posteriorly, and this must be taken into consideration in opening the dura.

Once the dura is opened a number of associated anomalies may be found. When the abnormality is a thickened, shortened filum terminale, all that is required is to accurately identify the filum, stimulate it to be sure that it is not a nerve root, and then divide it. I prefer to coagulate the filum and take out a centimeter or so to prevent any possibility of readherence. When there is an associated intradural lipoma, the mass must be removed if it is compressive or tethering. Then, using exact microtechniques, the nerve roots must be dissected, at least partially, until the mass of tissue is adequately removed to untether the cord. The mass must be detached circumferentially so that no further tethering can occur. I usually identify the filum and cut it. Sometimes the lipoma and the filum are all the same mass, in which case cutting the filum above and removing all possible lipoma is all that is required. There is no reason to try to remove the lipoma totally because it will not grow, and the goal of the operation is untethering. Sometimes the lipoma and the cord are fused; radical removal is not necessary since untethering is accomplished.

The dura must be closed in a watertight fashion; if a patch is required it should be harvested or a dural substitute used. A generous patch reduces the risk of scarring retethering the cord. Watertight closure is important. Finally, the wound is reconstituted in anatomical layers (28).

Dural Arteriovenous Fistulae and True Arteriovenous Malformations

The arteriovenous malformations involving the spinal cord are of three basic kinds. There is an intramedullary type with multiple feeding arteries and veins, which is generally inextricable from the spinal cord and can only rarely be treated successfully. There is a related form of arteriovenous malformation that is largely extramedullary, though often compressing and invading the spinal cord; total removal of this type is possible. There is the dural fistula, which occurs at the root entry zone and is associated with symptoms secondary to increased venous pressure in the spinal cord. These can almost always be obliterated by simple blockade of the fistula (1).

MRI frequently provides a hint that the diagnosis is one of the forms of arteriovenous malformation.

Myelography may be required to verify the diagnosis. In some patients it is impossible to be certain without spinal angiography, which is also needed to identify feeding vessels. A combination of the three techniques usually defines the malformation completely (2, 3, 5, 18, 31, 36, 57).

Dural Arteriovenous Fistula

The abnormalities usually occur at a single level identified by myelography. Most commonly they are treated by endovascular techniques, which are curative in the majority.

When embolization is not curative, it is possible to obliterate the fistula directly. Careful localization is required to be certain that the exposure is at the proper level. The incision need not be very large. Usually exposing only the segment to be removed is all that is required. A subperiosteal dissection of muscles from spinous processes and laminae is carried out with the patient in the prone position and under general anesthesia. A laminectomy is performed at the level to be exposed, with enough bony removal above and below to be certain that the whole fistula is reached. It is usually possible to find the feeding vessels intradurally and to ligate them, thus eliminating the increased venous pressure in the cord. The fistula itself should be coagulated. If there is any question as to whether the whole fistula has been removed, the whole dura of the root exit area can be excised, and then it is certain that the fistula is gone. Thoracic roots can be sacrificed with impunity when the vascular anatomy is known so that it is certain that in so doing you are not devascularizing the cord. Such radical removal is not possible in lumbar or cervical areas. The wound is then closed in anatomical layers after posterior dural closure.

The Extramedullary Arteriovenous Malformation

Occasionally these large arteriovenous malformations are virtually outside the cord and markedly compressing it. They are then treated as any extramedullary intradural tumor except that their extreme vascularity and high flow means that control of the feeding vessels is mandatory. Usually most, some, or all of these feeders will have been embolized previously and the mass generally devascularized. Then it is straightforward to dissect it from the cord. To do so, it is necessary to carry out the typical laminectomy exposure at least one segment above and below the mass. The dura is opened in the midline and the mass exposed. Using high magnification and careful microdissection, all residual feeding vessels are identified, ligated, and cut. Then the mass is dissected free from underlying cord using fine micro bipolar coagulation and sharp dissection. The separation must be precise, but it is usually not difficult, and the mass can be removed in its entirety. This is curative. The dura is then closed, and anatomical reconstruction of the wound is required.

The Intramedullary Arteriovenous Malformation

Operations on intramedullary arteriovenous malformations are rare. They frequently can be at least partially devascularized by occlusion of feeding vessels, and operation is unlikely except when it appears to be an extramedullary mass. Occasionally a patient with progressive neurological deficit cannot be treated in any way other than excision, and then a rare favorable mass may be excised directly. However, for the most part it is not possible to cure these lesions surgically except at great risk. Occasionally treatment may require exposing one and actually ligating feeding vessels that cannot be embolized appropriately. The operation is no different from that described for the dural fistula.

Transdural Removal of Herniated Disc

There are two indications for the transdural removal of a herniated disc. One is the extradural herniation that simply cannot be reached by an extradural approach. These typically occur in the cervical and thoracic regions. The other indication is the true transdural migration, which occurs characteristically in the lumbar region (39).

Usually MRI will define the pathologic process well enough that a dural exploration is anticipated prior to surgery. Occasionally in the lumbar region the intradural nature of the mass will not be recognized on MRI and discovered only at surgery. All of these operations are carried out with the patient under general anesthesia and in the prone position.

Transdural Removal of Cervical Disc

Transdural removal of a cervical disc is required typically when the disc is to be removed posteriorly because of its largely unilateral nature and because it cannot be extracted from the epidural space. Obviously, if this situation is recognized in advance an operation via the anterior approach is preferable, but frequently in cases of unilateral disc herniation it is anticipated that the disc can be removed from the posterior approach and then it is found that the root cannot be mobilized enough to allow removal of the disc. Then a generous foraminotomy should be carried out in the typical fashion.

Enough of a laminectomy is done above and below to allow a short dural incision; 5 or 6 mm may suffice, and 1 cm is usually more than enough. The dural incision is made vertically just medial to the exit of the root. The intradural exposure then continues.

The root is usually moved upward but sometimes might be depressed interiorly. It may be necessary to cut a denticulate ligament. I prefer to do all of this with the microscope at high magnification. This allows an excellent view of the anterior surface of the dura, and the disc fragment can be identified by direct vision and palpation. With the use of a fine knife, the anterior dura is incised directly over the fragment so that no bleeding will occur. It is usually possible to reach in with a fine forceps and extract the disc fragment as a single piece or in a few large pieces. Sometimes when the disc fragment comes out some epidural bleeding occurs. This should be tamponaded immediately with a hemostatic agent. The anterior dura does not need to be repaired; the posterior dura is sutured in a watertight fashion, and the wound closed in anatomical layers.

Transdural Removal of the Thoracic Disc

Occasional a thoracic disc will present in the same way. Again, if it appears that the disc is too medially placed to be removed by the lateral approach or is intradural, then a transthoracic or costovertebral approach is preferable. However, for many laterally placed discs a transpedicular approach is ideal, and in doing so occasionally a transdural herniation will be encountered or the disc will not be removable without opening the dura.

The spinous processes and laminae are exposed in the usual way. A high-speed drill is used to remove the joint, pedicle, and lateral portion of the laminae. This brings you down to the interspace. Be sure that you are at the right level with radiographic verification before removing the joint and pedicle. Usually at this point all that is required is to retract the dura slightly medially, incise the posterior ligament, and remove the disc, but occasionally the disc is so medially placed that it is not possible to carry out this maneuver. If so, then the dura should be opened exactly as described for the cervical disc; it is opened from root exit to root exit. The subarachnoid space is opened, and the microscope is used to identify the mass anteriorly. The dura is opened anteriorly using a small pointed knife so that the tip is visualized easily, and then the herniated fragments are removed piecemeal with small disc rongeurs. Occasionally one of these masses is actually herniated intradurally, in which case it will be encountered as soon as the dura is opened. It should be extracted with great care to be certain that the large mass does not compromise the spinal cord by compression during the extraction. The anterior dura does not need to be repaired. The posterior dura should be closed and then the wound closed in anatomical layers.

Intradural Lumbar Disc Herniation

Rarely, a lumbar disc herniates intradurally, usually in patients who have undergone one previous operation. MRI will generally reveal that the mass is intradural, so the operation can be planned beforehand as one different from the typical discectomy. When the intradural nature of the mass is not apparent, the traditional discectomy approach must be modified to allow transdural removal.

The operation is carried out by subperiosteal dissection of muscles from spinous processes and laminae. A complete laminectomy is performed to allow exposure of the mass. The dura is opened either in the midline or to one side or the other, depending on the location of the mass. It is best not to attempt this operation through a small incision. In my experience the roots are intimately adherent to the disc mass and you need room to manipulate the nerve roots and free them using microtechniques.

Once the dura is opened, the disc is usually seen immediately. Using a microscope, each individual nerve root is freed from the disc and then gradually teased out of the subarachnoid space. If the mass has been within the dura for a while, its adherence is likely to be substantial.

Once the disc fragment is out, the hole in the ligament in the adherent dura is usually easily seen. An experienced intradural surgeon can remove the remainder of the degenerated disc through this approach. However, for most others it is better to go back to the extradural space and remove any residual degenerated disc in the usual way. There is a great propensity for more disc herniation to occur through this hole, so it is important to remove all degenerated disc material possible, even if it requires a bilateral incision in the ligament and disc removal.

There is no reason to try to repair the dura anteriorly, but if the hole is large, I harvest a small piece of fat and slide it into the interspace to occlude the hole. Then the dura is closed posteriorly and the wound reconstituted in anatomical layers.

Intraneural Disc Herniation

A real oddity that I have encountered on a few occasions is that of a transdural herniation actually occurring within the nerve root. Typically the situation is recognized after the interspace is carefully identified and no mass can be found. Usually the disc mass is hard and can be easily felt, but no amount of root manipulation demonstrates a disc fragment to be removed. Usually the surgeon then thinks that a nerve tumor has been encountered. In order to verify this, it is necessary to incise the dura over the palpable mass. This is done longitudinally so that rootlets are not injured. Then, under high magnification, the rootlets are dissected free and the mass within the nerve is examined. Its nature as disc or tumor usually becomes apparent, and a decision can then be made about how to treat it. If it proves to be a tumor, it should be managed in the same way as described for schwannoma or neurofibroma. However, occasionally these intraneural masses will be discs. In that case, the incision is extended until it goes beyond the disc, and the disc fragment is teased out carefully, with the dissection of nerve rootlets maintained so that none are injured. Then the dura can be closed in the root sheath in a watertight fashion and the remainder of the operation continued as with any disc removal.

Unusual Approaches to Intradural Tumors

Most intradural tumors are approached by the direct posterior route, though occasionally an unusual approach is required, most commonly at the cervicomedullary junction. Intramedullary meningiomas and schwannomas located directly in front of the cervicomedullary junction, for example, may be difficult to expose by a direct posterior approach. In this case a far lateral approach with unilateral removal of the C1-C2 and C1-occipital articulations may be required.

Even more unusual is the direct anterior transoral approach to such a lesion. The descriptions of these unusual operations are included elsewhere in the literature. The transoral operation provides excellent access to the cervicomedullary junction and requires removal of only the anterior arch of C1, the odontoid process, and occasionally the lower third of the clivus. The issue is obtaining a watertight closure, for it may be very difficult or impossible to close the dura. Packing with fat and meticulous closure of the oropharynx coupled with spinal drainage will usually prevent CSF leak, but infection remains a serious issue (9, 45, 52).

What to Do When the Dura Is Inadvertently Opened

An unexpected laceration of the dura during extradural surgery is not uncommon. The loss of spinal fluid may reduce tamponade and lead to excessive extradural bleeding, but usually the dural tear does not reduce the quality of the outcome of surgery. To be certain that this is the case, it is necessary to understand how these openings can be treated. The typical abnormality is just a small pinhole with a patch of arachnoid through it. A single fine suture (No. 4–0 or smaller) suffices to close the defect. If the laceration is larger, it may require several stitches. The important thing is to remove bone until the entire laceration can be visualized, and then to close the margins of the dural tear carefully with fine sutures. Be certain that no nerve roots are adherent around the laceration so that the nerve roots are not incorporated into the closure. Nerve roots tend to pouch through the defect and may have to be held in place with small cottonoid pledgets. A watertight closure should be obtained. Sometimes the laceration is in a place that simply cannot be sutured well. This is particularly true with reoperations or when the laceration is around the nerve root. Posteriorly placed lacerations or defects can be closed by sewing a small graft of fascia or a small pledget of muscle or fat over the hole. Sometimes when the laceration is on the root sheath, attempting to close the dural defect may compromise the root. In this case, packing with fat or muscle is an acceptable alternative. Closing or packing should be adequate to allow the anesthesiologist to increase intrathoracic pressure dramatically without evidence of CSF leak.

When the CSF space has been entered, it is important to reconstitute CSF volume by the injection of saline to recreate the tamponade in the epidural space. Special care must be taken to close the wound solidly so that a pseudomeningocele or cutaneous leak cannot occur.

Conclusions

Most spinal surgery is extradural only, and only few procedures require intradural exploration. It is important to understand that the techniques required for intradural surgery are very different from those used when the operation is extradural only. Extradural operations require that the surgical techniques be directed toward bone removal or reconstruction, whereas intradural techniques focus on the exposed nervous system. The difference between nerve roots covered by CSF and dura and those that are exposed is very important. Intradural procedures should be carried out by surgeons who have been trained to handle nervous tissue and are familiar with both the anatomy and the function of intradural surgery. Most intradural surgery is straightforward and can be planned well in advance; with modern imaging techniques, the diagnosis is nearly always known beforehand. However, there is still an occasional need for an unplanned intradural exploration in the course of an operation that was envisioned as extradural only. The spine surgery team needs a member skilled in intradural surgery as an integral part of its function.

References

1. Anson JA, Spetzler RF. Interventional neuroradiology for spinal pathology. Clin Neurosurg 1992;39:388–417.

2. Anson JA, Spetzler RF. Surgical resection of intramedullary spinal cord cavernous malformations. J Neurosurg 1993;78(3):446–451.
3. Barrow DL, Colohan AR, Dawson R. Intradural perimedullary arteriovenous fistulas (type IV spinal cord arteriovenous malformations). J Neurosurg 1994; 81(2):221–229.
4. Bell DF, Walker JL, O'Connor G, et al. Spinal deformity after multiple-level cervical laminectomy in children. Spine 1994;19(4):406–411.
5. Biondi A, Merland JJ, Hodes JE, et al. Aneurysms of spinal arteries associated with intramedullary arteriovenous malformations. I. Angiographic and clinical aspects. Am J Neuroradiol 1992;13(3):913–922.
6. Brotchi J, Noterman J, Baleriaux D. Surgery of intramedullary spinal cord tumours. Acta Neurochir 1992; 116(2–4):176–178.
7. Chapman PH, Davis KR. Surgical treatment of spinal lipomas in childhood. Pediatr Neurosurg 1993; 19(5):267–275 (discussion 274).
8. Chun HC, Schmidt-Ullrich RK, Wolfson A, et al. External beam radiotherapy for primary spinal cord tumors. J Neurooncol 1990;9(3):211–217.
9. Crockard HA, Sen CN. The transoral approach for the management of intradural lesions at the craniovertebral junction: review of 7 cases. Neurosurgery 28(1):88–97 (discussion 97–98).
10. Dernevik L, Larsson S. Management of dumbbell tumours: reports of seven cases. Scand J Thorac Cardiovasc Surg 1990;24(1):47–51.
11. Dorizzi A, Crivelli G, Marra A, et al. Associated cervical schwannoma and dorsal meningioma: case report and review of the literature. J Neurosurg Sci 1992; 36(3):173–176.
12. Elster AD, Chen MY. Chiari I malformations: clinical and radiologic reappraisal. Radiology 1992; 183(2):347–353.
13. Epstein FJ, Farmer JP. Pediatric spinal cord tumor surgery. Neurosurg Clin N Am 1990;1(3):569–590.
14. Epstein FJ, Farmer JP, Freed D. Adult intramedullary spinal cord ependymomas: the result of surgery in 38 patients. J Neurosurg 1993;79(2):204–209.
15. Ernestus RI, Wilcke O. Spinal metastases of intracranial ependymomas: four case reports. Neurosurg Rev 1990;13(2):147–154.
16. Ferrante L, Mastronardi L, Celli P, et al. Intramedullary spinal cord ependymomas: study of 45 cases with long-term follow-up. Acta Neurochir 1992;119(1–4):74–79.
17. Fiaschi A, Orrico D, Polo A, et al. Cervical arachnoidal cyst with basilar impression and Arnold-Chiari malformation: a case report. Eur Neurol 1992;32(2):91–94.
18. Friedman DP, Flanders AE, Tartaglino LM. Vascular neoplasms and malformations, ischemia, and hemorrhage affecting the spinal cord: MR imaging findings. Am J Roentgenol 1994;162(3):685–692.
19. Friedman DP, Tartaglino LM, Flanders AE. Intradural schwannomas of the spine: MR findings with emphasis on contrast-enhancement characteristics. Am J Roentgenol 1992;158(6):1347–1350.
20. Gundry CR, Heithoff KB. Imaging evaluation of patients with spinal deformity. Orthop Clin North Am 1994; 25(2):247–264.
21. Hulshof MC, Menten J, Dito JJ, et al. Treatment results in primary intraspinal gliomas. Radiother Oncol 1993; 29(3):294–300.
22. Isu T, Chono Y, Iwasaki Y, et al. Scoliosis associated with syringomyelia presenting in children. Childs Nerv Syst 1992;8(2):97–100.
23. Isu T, Sasaki H, Takamura H, et al. Foramen magnum decompression with removal of the outer layer of the dura as treatment for syringomyelia occurring with Chiari I malformation. Neurosurgery 1993;33(5):844–849 (discussion 849–850).
24. Kanzer MD, Parisi JE. Case for diagnosis: myxopapillary ependymoma. Mil Med 1990;155(2):87, 90.
25. Koehler PJ. Chiari's description of cerebellar ectopy (1891), with a summary of Cleland's and Arnold's contributions and some early observations on neural-tube defects. J Neurosurg 1991;75(5):823–826.
26. Lagerkvist B, Olsen L, Carlsson H, et al. The Chiari II malformation in neonates: a prospective study. Eur J Pediatr Surg 1991;1(Suppl 1):48.
27. Li MH, Holtas S. MR imaging of spinal intramedullary tumors. Acta Radiol 1991;32(6):505–513.
28. Linn RM, Ford LT. Adult diastematomyelia. Spine 1994;19(7):852–854.
29. Lunardi P, Licastro G, Missori P, et al. Management of intramedullary tumours in children. Acta Neurochir 1993;120(1–2):59–65.
30. Masaryk TJ. Neoplastic disease of the spine. Radiol Clin North Am 1991;29(4):829–845.
31. McCormick PC. Spinal vascular malformations. Semin Neurol 1993;13(4):349–358.
32. McCormick PC, Post KD, Stein BM. Intradural extramedullary tumors in adults. Neurosurg Clin N Am 1990;1(3):591–608.
33. McCormick PC, Stein BM. Miscellaneous intradural pathology. Neurosurg Clin N Am 1990;1(3):687–699.
34. Milhorat TH, Johnson WD, Miller JI, et al. Surgical treatment of syringomyelia based on magnetic resonance imaging criteria. Neurosurgery 1992;31(2):231–244 (discussion 244–245).
35. Mimatsu K, Kawakami N, Kato F, et al. Intraoperative ultrasonography of extramedullary spinal tumours. Neuroradiology 1992;34(5):440–443.
36. Mullan S. Reflections upon the nature and management of intracranial and intraspinal vascular malformations and fistulae. J Neurosurg 1994;80(4):606–616.
37. Nadeem SQ, Feun LG, Bruce-Gregorios JH, et al. Post radiation sarcoma (malignant fibrous histiocytoma) of the cervical spine following ependymoma (a case report). J Neurooncol 1991;11(3):263–268.
38. Nohria V, Oakes WJ. Chiari headaches [letter; comment]. Neurology 1993;43(6):1272.
39. Ozer AF, Ozek MM, Pamir MN, et al. Intradural rupture of cervical vertebral disc. Spine 1994;19(7):843–845.
40. Pagni CA, Canavero S, Giordana MT, et al. Spinal intramedullary subependymomas: case report and review of the literature. Neurosurgery 1992;30(1):115–117.
41. Payner TD, Prenger E, Berger TS, et al. Acquired Chiari malformations: incidence, diagnosis, and management. Neurosurgery 1994;34(3):429–434 (discussion 434).
42. Pulst SM, Riccardi VM, Fain P, et al. Familial spinal

neurofibromatosis: clinical and DNA linkage analysis. Neurology 1991;41(12):1923–1927.
43. Rabb CH, McComb JG, Raffel C, et al. Spinal arachnoid cysts in the pediatric age group: an association with neural tube defects. J Neurosurg 1992;77(3):369–372.
44. Sanguinetti C, Specchia N, Gigante A, et al. Clinical and pathological aspects of solitary spinal neurofibroma. J Bone Joint Surg Br 1993;75(1):141–147.
45. Sen CN, Sekhar LN. An extreme lateral approach to intradural lesions of the cervical spine and foramen magnum. Neurosurgery 1990;27(2):197–204.
46. Seppala MT, Haltia MJ. Spinal malignant nerve-sheath tumor or cellular schwannoma? A striking difference in prognosis. J Neurosurg 1993;79(4):528–532.
47. Sharma V, Newton G. Cervical intramedullary neurofibroma. J Korean Med Sci 1990;5(3):165–167.
48. Steck JC, Dietze DD, Fessler RG. Posterolateral approach to intradural extramedullary thoracic tumors. J Neurosurg 1994;81(2):202–205.
49. Stein BM, McCormick PC. Intramedullary neoplasms and vascular malformations. Clin Neurosurg 1992;39:361–387.
50. Stiller CA, Bunch KJ. Brain and spinal tumours in children aged under two years: incidence and survival in Britain, 1971–1985. Br J Cancer Suppl 1992;18:S50–S53.
51. Tatter SB, Borges LF, Louis DN. Central neurocytomas of the cervical spinal cord: report of two cases. J Neurosurg 1994;81(2):288–293.
52. Tominaga T, Koshu K, Ogawa A, et al. Transoral decompression evaluated by cine-mode magnetic resonance imaging: a case of basilar impression accompanied by Chiari malformation. Neurosurgery 1991;28(6):883–885.
53. Ulmer JL, Elster AD, Ginsberg LE, et al. Klippel-Feil syndrome: CT and MR of acquired and congenital abnormalities of cervical spine and cord. J Comput Assist Tomogr 1993;17(2):215–224.
54. van Velthoven V, Jost M, Siekmann R, et al. Surgical strategies and results in syringomyelia. Acta Neurochir 1993;123(3–4):199–201.
55. Venkataramana NK, Kolluri VR, Narayana Swamy KS, et al. Exophytic gliomas of the spinal cord. Acta Neurochir 1990;107(1–2):44–46.
56. Whitaker SJ, Bessell EM, Ashley SE, et al. Postoperative radiotherapy in the management of spinal cord ependymoma. J Neurosurg 1991;74(5):720–728.
57. Willinsky R, terBrugge K, Montanera W, et al. Spinal epidural arteriovenous fistulas: arterial and venous approaches to embolization. Am J Neuroradiol 1993;14(4):812–817.

CHAPTER TWENTY EIGHT

Spinal Infections

Bradford L. Currier

Introduction

Advances in radiology, infectious disease, and surgery during the past few decades have dramatically improved the prognosis of patients afflicted with spinal infections. Before the advent of antibiotics, the mortality rate of patients with a neurologic deficit from tuberculous spondylitis was close to 60% (20). With current treatment regimens the rate should be less than 5% (3, 157). Despite this encouraging statistic, spinal infections can still have devastating consequences, and they deserve great respect.

Spinal infections may be classified by the histologic response of the host, the cause or anatomic site of the infection, and the age of the patient. This chapter covers each of these variations and highlights the differences in evaluation, management, and prognosis. Most bacteria induce a pyogenic histologic reaction in the host, and this accounts for the majority of infections encountered in the developed countries. *Mycobacterium, Brucella,* fungi, and syphilis cause a granulomatous response and are more commonly responsible for disease in the lesser-developed countries and in immunocompromised hosts.

Pyogenic Infections

Iatrogenic Infections

Epidemiology and Etiology

The incidence of postoperative infection varies with the procedure. The rate for a simple lumbar discectomy performed with prophylactic antibiotics is approximately 0.7% (60, 123, 160, 220). In one series, microdiscectomy was found to be complicated by infection in 1.4% of cases, in comparison with 0.5% for a standard discectomy (257). In a prospective study of 412 cases of lumbar microdiscectomy, cultures from the cover of the microscope were positive in 12, suggesting that contamination from the microscope may be to blame (268).

Horwitz found that when the discectomy was accompanied by a fusion procedure the infection rate rose from 0.6% to 6.2% (123). Scoliosis fusions performed without hardware had a rate of 2% (161). Instrumentation increased the rate to around 6% (161). The rate varied from zero to 12.9% in different series (1, 6, 17, 63, 98, 161, 260, 286).

Esophageal perforation can occur during exposure of the spine by a retractor or other instrument. If the complication is recognized and treated appropriately, infection may be avoided. Unrecognized cases of esophageal perforation, on the other hand, may cause life-threatening mediastinitis (274). Rupture of the esophagus with subsequent infection can also be caused by a cervical spine fracture or from the sharp edge of a bone graft (145, 214, 287). Not only can instrumentation act as a foreign body, but also hardware fixed to the cervical spine anteriorly can erode the wall of the esophagus and cause an infection (148, 199, 250).

Certain subgroups of patients are prone to developing infections. In Lonstein's series, the infection rate in spinal dysraphics was 57% (161). In another series, the infection rate in myelodysplasia was 7.9%, 2.5% in cerebral palsy, and 1.4% in idiopathic scoliosis (267).

The rate of infection complicating percutaneous procedures is low but not insignificant. In 24 of 135,000 patients undergoing chemonucleolysis, infection was reported to have developed (200). Infection occurred in two of 31 patients who underwent cervical discography. In one of the patients, an epidural abscess developed that led to quadriplegia (38). Transfeldt and others reviewed 7769 spinal procedures performed during a 32-year period (267). The overall infection rate was 2.5%. They found that the rate was higher in posterior procedures (2.6%) than in operations performed anteriorly (0.9%). The rate was 1.5% for patients younger than 20 years of age and 2.7% for patients older than 20 years. The rate was higher in revision surgery (6.8%) and in cases requiring preoperative traction. Faciszewski and others confirmed the low rate of infection (0.6%) complicating anterior spinal fusions (64).

Methyl methacrylate, used to enhance spinal stability, may increase the infection rate (56, 172). Methyl methacrylate decreases chemotaxis of polymorphonuclear leukocytes and impairs the ability of leukocytes to phagocytose and kill bacteria (208, 209).

Late infection of spinal instrumentation can occur by hematogenous seeding. Heggeness and others described six cases in which an infection occurred at least 10 months postoperatively (110). In five of the six cases, a distant focus of infection was identified. Ten additional cases of delayed infection after posterior spinal instrumentation have been reported (226). The authors believed that some delayed infections occur from intraoperative seeding and remain indolent for months to years. Several host risk factors for postoperative infection have been identified. Some factors, such as increasing age, steroid therapy, and immunosuppression, cannot be controlled (197, 211). Factors that can be controlled include malnutrition, morbid obesity, concurrent remote infection, cigarette smoking, and poorly controlled diabetes (44, 189, 198, 211, 212, 255, 265). Whenever possible, preoperative hospitalization should be kept to a minimum. Cruse and Foord found that the infection rate doubled for each additional week that patients were hospitalized before surgery (44).

The surgical team can decrease contamination of the wound by following the guidelines presented by Polk and colleagues (212). Traffic and conversation in the operating room should be kept to a minimum. The operating room doors should be kept closed at all times. Room air should be filtered and exchanged 25 times per hour. Two pairs of gloves, shoe covers, and properly fitted head covers and masks should be worn. The patient's skin should be prepared with a technique proved to decrease bacterial counts. During the procedure, the surgeon can control other local factors that influence the rate of infection by following basic surgical principles. Tissues should be handled gently and the wound edges débrided at the conclusion of the case. Unnecessary delays should not be allowed to lengthen the case. Self-retaining retractors should be periodically released to allow adequate perfusion of the muscles (286). Hematoma formation should be avoided by careful hemostasis, layered wound closure, and, if drains are used, the use of a closed-suction system.

Microbiology and Prophylactic Antibiotics

Staphylococcus aureus is the most frequently isolated organism in postoperative infections. In one series of 22 spinal infections, more than 50% of the cases were caused by *S. aureus* (170). Gram-negative organisms were cultured from 40% of the wounds and multiple organisms were cultured in 59% of the cases. In some cases of presumed postoperative discitis, cultures of specimens from the disc space have negative results despite increased erythrocyte sedimentation rate (ESR) and C-reactive protein (CRP) values and histologic findings consistent with infection. These cases may be caused by slow-growing or low-virulence organisms (76). "Aseptic" or "chemical" discitis may also occur after spine surgery. In these cases the clinical and radiographic findings are similar, but the histology is characterized by dense fibrotic changes rather than inflammation. The ESR and CRP values are generally lower than expected for a "septic" discitis (76). Prophylactic use of antibiotics substantially decreases the rate of infection. Horwitz reported that the rate of infection after discectomy decreased from 9.3% to 1% when antibiotics were given prophylactically (123). In another series the rate was found to decrease from 6% to none with antibiotics (132). The timing of administration of the drugs is important. In Horwitz's series, when the antibiotics were given preoperatively, the infection rate was 0.6%, in comparison with 2.7% when they were administered after the procedure (123). Animal studies confirm that antibiotics are most effective when given before inoculation of the wound (27).

Some surgeons use antibiotics prophylactically for all spine cases; others reserve the use of antibiotics for cases involving instrumentation, immunocompromised hosts, and other high-risk situations (164, 213). Additional doses of drug should be given during long cases, though the appropriate duration of prophylaxis is controversial. The drugs could probably be stopped after the first dose or two, but many surgeons prefer to continue antibiotic therapy until the drains have been removed. Clearly antibiotics should not be continued for more than 48 hours postoperatively (71, 164, 198). The choice of antibiotic is based on many factors, including spectrum of activity, side effects, cost, and pharmacokinetics. Host factors must also be considered, such as preoperative hospitalization, exposure to antibiotics, remote infections, and compromise of the immune system.

Clinical Presentation

WOUND INFECTIONS

Wound infections may be classified as superficial or deep. A superficial infection is characterized by pain and tenderness and the typical signs of infection: erythema, fluctuance, swelling, drainage, and fever. By definition, the infection is located superficial to the deep fascia. The infection may track below the fascia as well, and such extension of the process should be sought at the time of wound exploration (89).

Deep wound infections are more insidious than superficial infections. Progressive back pain out of proportion to the expected postoperative course may be the only symptom. The average time between operation and diagnosis of the infection is 11 days (range, 7 to 16 days) (132). The wound frequently appears completely normal (89). Patients with deep infections are generally febrile, and the temperature is typically higher than that seen with superficial infections (89).

DISCITIS

Patients with postoperative discitis generally follow a benign course in the first week or so after surgery. They typically note initial improvement in leg pain and complain of a normal degree of incisional back pain. In the ensuing weeks or months they complain of increasing back pain and may have a recurrence of leg pain. Occasionally they may complain of fevers, chills, and night sweats, and rarely, if the infection progresses to an epidural abscess, they may note weakness and bowel and bladder dysfunction. The most constant and striking complaint is back pain that is out of proportion to the expected postoperative time course or the findings on examination.

Paralumbar spasm is the most common finding on physical examination. The spine wound generally appears benign. Scoliosis secondary to spasm may be present, and patients may complain of increased back pain with a straight-leg-raising test. If a new neurologic deficit is present, an epidural abscess (discussed later) should be considered and eliminated with a magnetic resonance imaging (MRI) study performed emergently.

Diagnostic Evaluation

LABORATORY TESTS

The ESR and CRP value are normally increased in the early postoperative period after uncomplicated procedures. In one prospective study (Fig. 28.1), the CRP level was normal preoperatively (less than 10 mg/L) and reached a peak on the second day after microdiscectomy (46 ± 21 mg/L) and anterior fusion (70 ± 23 mg/L) and the third day after conventional discectomy (92 ± 47 mg/L) and posterolateral fusion (173 ± 39 mg/L) (266). The CRP levels returned to normal 5 to 14 days after surgery. The ESR reached a peak level 5 days postoperatively and declined slowly and irregularly. The ESR was still increased in some patients 21 to 42 days after surgery. In another study the mean ESR reached peak levels 4 days after surgery and was higher for after fusions (102 mm/h) than after disc surgery (75 mm/h) (128). The values normalized in the majority of patients 2 weeks postoperatively. The peak levels were lower in a separate study (mean ESR 25 mm/h and mean CRP 2.4 mg/L) of patients undergoing discectomy, but the time course for the peak values was similar (243). Patients with postoperative discitis or deep infection typically have elevations of ESR and CRP values that are greater than expected (16, 128, 220, 243). An increasing value for CRP or ESR after 3 or 5 days, respectively, is highly suggestive of infection. The white blood cell count is generally unremarkable but may be increased, especially in deep wound infections (89).

A positive result of Gram stain or culture is diagnostic of infection. Patients with presumed disc-space infections should undergo a biopsy examination (discussed later) before treatment. If a deep wound infection is suspected, aspiration of the wound under strictly sterile conditions is recommended. After a surgical preparation of the wound, a spinal needle can be advanced down to bone (or hardware) and aspirated. If the tap was dry, a new needle can be inserted in another quadrant of the wound and the procedure repeated until fluid is obtained for analysis. If all four quadrants of the wound produce dry aspirates, the examination is considered to have a negative result. If signs of superficial infection are present, the deep aspiration is not performed until the superficial space is clean, because the needle may contaminate the deep space.

It is not necessary to obtain specimens for cultures of a draining wound before taking the patient to the operating room if antibiotics can be withheld until after surgery. Exploration and débridement of the wound should be performed urgently, and tissue samples for cultures can be obtained at surgery.

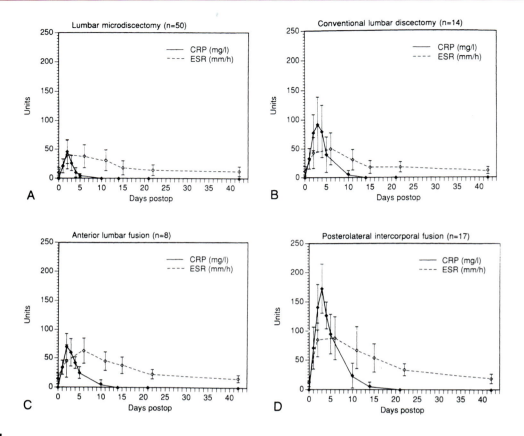

FIGURE 28.1.
Graphs showing the serial mean values of CRP and ESR before and after four types of uncomplicated spinal operations. (From Thelander U, Larsson S. Quantitation of C-reactive protein and erythrocyte sedimentation rate after spinal surgery. Spine 1992;17:400–404.)

IMAGING STUDIES

Plain roentgenograms, computed tomography (CT), and MRI and radionuclide scans all have a role in the diagnosis of discitis and are discussed in the following section on hematogenous osteomyelitis and disc-space infections, because the findings are similar. MRI scans may be misleading in the early postoperative period. Gadolinium enhancement of the endplates, a finding consistent with infection in unoperated cases, is present in nearly 20% of cases at the level operated on following lumbar discectomy (95). Imaging studies are not generally helpful in the diagnosis of wound infections, and treatment should not be delayed while waiting for these studies to be performed.

Management

WOUND INFECTION

Treatment of a wound infection must be aggressive. The patient should be taken to surgery without undue delay and the wound should be opened and explored. If the infection is superficial, the deep fascia should be left intact; samples of the subcutaneous tissues should be cultured and the tissues should be copiously irrigated and débrided. The fascia is then inspected for any signs of communication between the layers. If the fascia is intact and the patient does not have signs of septicemia, some authors recommend leaving the fascia closed and draining the superficial space only. The subfascial plane can be aspirated and left undisturbed if the tap is negative (89). Other authors claim that it is necessary to open and débride (one layer at a time) the wound down to the bone in all cases (170). All devitalized tissue should be removed from the wound. Bone graft that is loosened by the irrigation or grossly infected and cortical pieces of bone that have not become incorporated yet should be removed. It is not necessary or desirable to remove all of the bone graft, because achieving a solid fusion helps to resolve the infection (82, 89, 132, 161). Likewise, the hardware should be left in place unless it has failed (82, 89, 132, 161, 187, 265). Multiple débridements may be required to control the infection.

The technique and timing of wound closure are based on the nature of the infection, host risk factors, clinical response, and appearance of the wound. The options include: *(a)* wound closure over large drains in each layer, *(b)* closure over suction-irrigation tubes, *(c)* open packing with delayed closure, and *(d)* open packing with healing by secondary intention. Thalgott and colleagues developed a classification scheme and protocol for managing postoperative infections in patients with spinal implants (265). The system is based on the adult osteomyelitis classification of Cierny and Mader (33). They stage each case on the basis of two variables: severity of the infection and host response or physiologic class (Table 28.1). They found that 12 of 13 patients with a group 1 infection were successfully managed with a single irrigation and débridement with closure over suction drains. The 16 patients with group 2 infections required an average of three irrigation-débridement procedures. All eight of the patients managed with closed suction-irrigation healed, whereas in six of eight patients whose wounds were closed over drains the initial closure attempt failed. Only two patients were in group 3, and both had a poor result. Flap coverage of the wound was required in both cases. To aid in the management of these severe infections as well as in selected group 2 cases, hyperalimentation is recommended (265).

The suction-irrigation system recommended by Thalgott and colleagues includes a single Jackson-Pratt drain for inflow and a single Hemovac drain for outflow. The irrigation solution is 500 mg vancomycin and 1000 U of heparin in 1 L of isotonic saline, running continuously at 125 mL/h. The system is continued for 3 to 4 days and then converted to suction; the drains are removed on the sixth day (265). My colleagues and I do not use suction-irrigation as frequently now as we did in the past and have found that the majority of postoperative infections can be managed with one or more débridements and closure over suction drains. When suction-irrigation is used, we use normal saline without antibiotics. We do not have any experience with vancomycin and heparin irrigation but caution against using neomycin and other antibiotic solutions that are readily absorbed, because systemic toxicity may occur (Hanssen A, personal communication, 1994).

Glassman and colleagues recommend the use of antibiotic impregnated beads in combination with serial débridement and systemic antibiotics (92). Heller noted that the spine is a highly vascular region and that antibiotic concentrations in seroma fluid are similar to serum levels when the drugs are administered intravenously (Heller JG, personal communication, 1995). He contended that antibiotic beads are unnecessary and that their use requires the additional procedure of removing them.

The keys to successful treatment are early aggressive irrigation-débridement in association with appropriate antibiotic therapy (directed by an infectious disease specialist) and close attention to nutrition and medical management. The principles of wound closure that we follow are to obliterate dead space, to use interrupted nonabsorbable sutures in the fascia, and to use large retention sutures in the skin and paraspinous muscle. Sutures should be left in the skin for a minimum of 3 weeks.

Several authors have been successful in managing refractory wound infections associated with soft-tissue defects by using muscle flaps for coverage (77, 141, 265).

DISCITIS

The management of postoperative discitis is the same as for hematogenous osteomyelitis (discussed in the next section).

Prognosis

The prognosis of a patient treated for postoperative infection is based on the nature of the infection, the health of the host, and the adequacy of treatment. In one series of 22 infections, five cases required reoperation and ten cases were allowed to heal by secondary intention, but all wounds eventually healed (170). There were no deaths, chronic drainage, or osteomyelitis. In the series of Thalgott and colleagues (Table 28.1), all patients in group 1 achieved fusion and had a good result (265). The average hospital stay was 14 days, and the average hospital cost was $42,000. Patients in group 2 averaged 51.6 days in the hospital, and the average cost was $128,000. One patient succumbed to the infection, and three died of underlying conditions. Seventy-five percent of the surviving patients had a good clinical result, and 25% had a pseudarthrosis. The two patients in group 3 had poor results. One achieved a solid fusion but had persistent drainage for 1 year, requiring hardware removal. The other required an anterior graft for

TABLE 28.1.
Clinical Staging System for Spinal Wound Infections

Group	Anatomic Type
1	Single organism (superficial or deep)
2	Multiple organism (deep)
3	Multiple organism with myonecrosis
Class	**Host Response**
A	Normal
B	Local or multiple systemic disease (cigarette smoking)
C	Immunocompromised (ISS 18)

ISS = injury severity score.
From Thalgott JS, Cotler HB, Sasso RC, et al. Postoperative infections in spinal implants: classification and analysis. Spine 1991;16:981–984.

total resorption of the posterior bone graft. In Stambough and Beringer's series, three of 11 patients with deep spinal infections required hardware removal, whereas the hardware was retained in all four superficial spinal infections and all four iliac crest infections (255). Seventeen of 18 arthrodeses fused, and all but one infection eventually resolved.

Hematogenous Vertebral Osteomyelitis and Disc-Space Infection

Epidemiology and Etiology

The incidence of pyogenic vertebral osteomyelitis is increasing (36, 258). This observation may be the result of the increasing prevalence of elderly and immunocompromised individuals in the population. In one series nearly 40% of the cases involved immunosuppressed patients. Vertebral osteomyelitis represents 2 to 7% of all cases of osteomyelitis (31, 146, 221, 230, 280, 289). The disease affects people of all ages and both sexes, but it has a predilection for elderly men (18, 238). Immunocompromised hosts, especially diabetics, are particularly susceptible to the development of vertebral osteomyelitis (18, 84, 238, 258). Young patients who are intravenous drug abusers or seropositive for human immunodeficiency virus (HIV) are more susceptible to infection and represent a growing subgroup of patients with vertebral osteomyelitis (108, 194). Any condition that causes a bacteremia can lead to hematogenous vertebral osteomyelitis. Urinary tract infections and bacteremia secondary to genitourinary procedures are the most frequent causes. Soft-tissue and respiratory tract infections and intravenous drug abuse represent other common sources of spine infections (238, 239).

Microbiology

In the preantibiotic era, *S. aureus* was the causative organism in almost every case of vertebral osteomyelitis (107). Since the introduction of antibiotics, there has been an increase in infections caused by Gram-negative bacilli and low-virulence organisms such as diphtheroids and coagulase-negative staphylococci (242). *S. aureus* now accounts for about 50% of all spine infections (238). The most frequently isolated Gram-negative organisms are *Pseudomonas, Escherichia coli,* and *Proteus* species, which are common sources of urinary tract infections (79, 84, 88, 225). *Pseudomonas aeruginosa* is frequently identified as the pathogen in heroin abusers (154, 239, 288). Anaerobic infection is uncommon and is generally associated with open fractures, infected wounds, foreign bodies, human bites, or diabetes (126, 238). *Salmonella* osteomyelitis is rarely encountered and has a tendency to infect sites of preexisting disease (32, 237).

Pathogenesis

The pathogenesis of adult vertebral osteomyelitis and disc-space infection is the same as that described in a later section on pediatric discitis. The different clinical manifestations result from the anatomic changes associated with aging. The cartilaginous canals in the vertebral endplates of children allow microorganisms nearly direct access to the disc (Fig. 28.2) (284). In adults an infection of the disc space may result from inoculation of the nucleus pulposus by surgery, chemonucleolysis, or discography, but spontaneous infection of the disc is unlikely to occur (91, 134, 256). Segmentation of sclerotomes during development leads to the vascular arrangement of a single artery supplying two adjacent vertebral bodies. Wiley and Trueta demonstrated that bacteria could gain access to the metaphyseal region of adjacent vertebrae through these arteries and cause infection (290). Because the clinical manifestations and treatment of septic discitis and vertebral osteomyelitis are similar, it is best to consider these conditions as part of a spectrum of disease rather than as distinct clinical entities.

Parke and associates demonstrated the peculiar

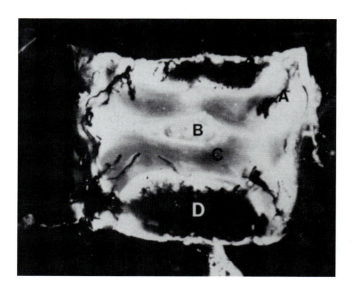

FIGURE 28.2.
Sagittally sectioned human fetal specimen (26 weeks gestation), injected, cleared, and transilluminated, shows cartilage canals and absence of vessels in nucleus pulposus. **A.** cartilage canal, **B.** nucleus pulposus, **C.** hyaline cartilage end plate, **D.** ossified vertebral body ×10. (From Whalen JL, Parke WW, Mazur JM, Stauffer ES: The intrinsic vasculature of developing vertebral end plates and its nutritive significance to the intervertebral discs. J Pediatr Orthop 1985;5:403–410.)

blood supply of the upper cervical spine (207). The odontoid process is surrounded by a rich venous plexus that has lymphovenous anastomoses with the posterior superior nasopharynx. It is postulated that the plexus is responsible for hematogenous infections of the upper cervical spine, including Grisel's syndrome. Grisel's syndrome refers to nontraumatic atlantoaxial subluxation secondary to ligamentous laxity induced by peripharyngeal inflammatory conditions.

The pathogenesis of neurologic compromise associated with vertebral osteomyelitis may be related to direct compression by bone or disc, from spinal instability and deformity or by epidural pus and granulation tissue. The neural tissue may also sustain ischemic damage from septic thrombosis or be impaired by inflammatory infiltration of the dura (134, 146, 238).

Clinical Presentation

The presentation may be acute, subacute, or chronic, depending on the host's resistance and the organism's virulence (134, 146). Before antibiotics were available, two-thirds of patients presented with acute osteomyelitis with signs of severe toxemia (107). A literature review in 1979 indicated that 50% of the patients had symptoms for more than 3 months before presentation, and only 20% had symptoms for less than 3 weeks before seeking help (238).

The most common complaint of patients with pyogenic spine infection is back or neck pain; only about 50% overall have a fever (238). Subacute or chronic infections often have an insidious onset. Vague back pain may be the only symptom, especially when the infection is caused by a low-virulence organism (242). Patients with acute infection have a more striking presentation, with fever, local spine pain, severe spasm, and limited spinal motion. Patients with cervical disease may have torticollis, and those with lumbar involvement may have a hip flexion contracture from psoas muscle irritation, loss of lumbar lordosis, and hamstring tightness (279, 294). The patient may be reluctant to bear weight and the straight-leg-raising test may be positive. Atypical symptoms such as meningeal irritation and pain in the chest, abdomen, hip, or leg occur in approximately 15% of cases (219, 238, 258).

Vertebral osteomyelitis occurs most commonly in the lumbar spine. In a review of the literature, 48% of the cases were found to have been located in the lumbar area, 35% in the thoracic spine, and only 6.5% in the cervical spine (238).

Many patients have some soft-tissue mass or swelling adjacent to the infected vertebrae, but a clinically significant abscess has been uncommon since the advent of antibiotic therapy. The cervical and thoracic regions are more prone to developing an abscess than the lumbar spine (84). Antibiotic therapy has also decreased the incidence of kyphotic deformity of the spine (79, 146).

Infants and intravenous drug abusers generally have a more acute presentation than other subgroups (58, 218, 238, 239). Infants with vertebral osteomyelitis often appear to have toxic responses, high temperature, and systemic signs of illness (58, 218).

Neurologic deficits occur in approximately 17% of patients (238). Predisposing factors for paralysis include diabetes, rheumatoid arthritis, increased age, systemic steroid therapy, and a more cephalad level of infection (57, 146, 238).

Diagnostic Evaluation

The differential diagnosis of pyogenic disc-space infection and vertebral osteomyelitis includes granulomatous infections, metastatic carcinoma, multiple myeloma, trauma, degenerative disease, localized Scheuermann's disease, fractures associated with osteoporosis, and destructive spondyloarthropathy (35, 36, 169, 174, 238). Less common disorders in the differential diagnosis are leukemia, perinephric abscess, neuropathic spinal arthropathy and sarcoidosis (129, 210, 218, 233).

The ESR is increased in more than 90% of patients with pyogenic spine infection (238). An increased ESR is not sensitive or specific for infection but it is a good screening test, and it is also useful for following the response to treatment (36, 79, 134, 238, 242). The CRP value is also a good screening test for infection and may prove to be helpful in the evaluation and follow-up of patients with vertebral osteomyelitis.

The white blood cell count is increased in only 42% of cases overall and is usually normal in patients with chronic infections (84, 238).

Blood cultures have positive results in only 24% of patients with pyogenic infections (238). Urine cultures are not reliable indicators of the pathogen causing a spine infection, because the patient may have a coexistent urinary tract infection with a different organism (79).

Plain roentgenographic findings are characteristic but are not evident until 2 to 4 weeks after the onset of the disease (37, 84, 233). The earliest change seen on plain films is disc-space narrowing. Destructive changes in the end plates and the anterior aspect of the vertebral body are present after 3 to 6 weeks. Tomograms often show abnormalities earlier than plain roentgenograms. If the disease is not treated or the infection is particularly fulminant, progressive collapse of the vertebral body may occur and lead to a kyphotic deformity (Fig. 28.3), especially in infants (58, 218). As the infection is brought under control,

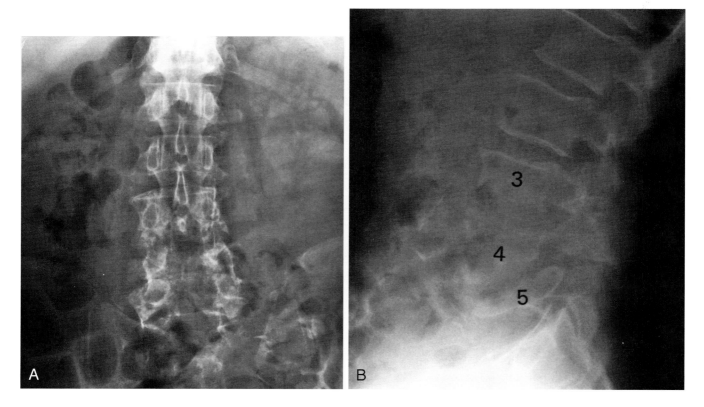

FIGURE 28.3.

A. Anteroposterior and **B.** lateral radiographs show severe destruction (L3, L4, and L5) with L4–5 spondylolisthesis secondary to *S. aureus* disc space infection of L3–4 and L4–5 and L3, L4, and L5 vertebral osteomyelitis.

hypertrophic changes occur at the vertebral margins with sclerosis of the endplates (238). The radiographic findings lag behind the clinical response by 1 or 2 months.

Radionuclide studies allow early detection of spinal infections before plain films become positive (26, 134, 186, 254). Gallium scans show evidence of infection earlier in the course of disease than technetium scans (26, 201). In a study of experimentally induced disc-space infection, bone scans were positive in 23% at 3 to 5 days and in 71% at 13 to 15 days (263). Gallium scans are more useful for following the response to treatment, because they become normal during resolution of the infection; technetium scans remain positive for many months after the disease has resolved (204). Gallium scans have slightly higher specificity than technetium scans (85% versus 78%). Both studies have about 90% sensitivity and 85% accuracy (26, 186). Single-photon emission computed tomography is more sensitive and has better contrast resolution than planar scintigraphy; it also allows three-dimensional localization (261). Gallium scans show increased uptake in a butterfly-shaped area around the spine, whereas technetium scans show uptake diffusely in the area of the infection (100). Indium scans are not particularly helpful in the evaluation of spinal infections, because of their low sensitivity. The specificity is 100%, but the sensitivity is only 17% and the accuracy is 31% (283).

Computed tomography is helpful to differentiate infection from malignancy and to clearly demonstrate the extent of bony destruction and the formation of soft-tissue abscesses (93, 130, 275). The soft-tissue mass frequently seen in the prevertebral area in infections usually surrounds the spine anteriorly, in contrast to neoplasms, which are more likely to have a partial paravertebral soft tissue mass or no extension beyond the vertebra. Neoplasms are more likely than infections to involve the posterior elements and may be osteoblastic, whereas infections are likely to have an osteolytic appearance (275).

Postmyelography CT or MRI is indicated in the presence of neurologic signs or symptoms to eliminate the possibility of epidural and subdural abscesses (these conditions are discussed in a later section). Myelography is invasive, and if it is performed, spinal fluid should be examined to eliminate the possibility of meningitis. MRI allows early diagnosis of infection and recognition of abscess formation without the risk of intrathecal injection (25, 216). This study provides much more anatomic information than radionuclide studies and becomes positive at about the same time as a gallium scan (186). MRI has

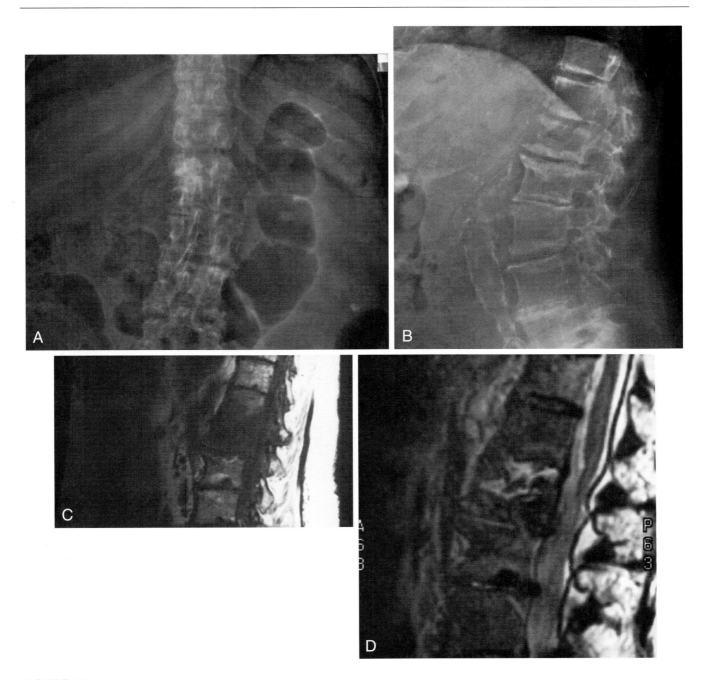

FIGURE 28.4.
Seventy-six-year-old female with rheumatoid arthritis with T12-L1 disk space infection and L1 osteomyelitis. Results of three needle biopsy analyses were negative. Patient underwent anterior vertebrectomy and discectomy and tricortical iliac crest allograft and rib autograft struts from T12-L2. Cultures grew *S. aureus*. Patient was also given the option of 6 weeks of bed rest or posterior fusion, and she elected to undergo surgery. After intravenous antibiotics had been administered for 6 days, a posterior fusion from T10 to L3 with instrumentation was performed. She was treated with 6 weeks of intravenous antibiotics followed by oral antibiotics. She remained neurologically intact, the infection and back pain resolved, and the fusion healed uneventfully. **A.** Anteroposterior and **B.** lateral lumbar spine radiographs show discitis at T12 and L1 and destruction of L1 vertebral body. **C.** T1-weighted sagittal MRI sequence shows decreased signal throughout L1 and across the T12-L1 disc space. The endplates are blurred and indistinct. **D.** T2-weighted sagittal MRI sequence shows high signal within T12-L1 disc and the L1 vertebral body.

96% sensitivity, 93% specificity, and 94% accuracy in detecting vertebral osteomyelitis and is considered to be the diagnostic modality of choice (186).

Modic and colleagues have described the characteristic MRI findings of disc-space infection and vertebral osteomyelitis (Fig. 28.4C–F) (186). In T1-weighted sequences the signal intensity in the peridiscal area is decreased and the margin between

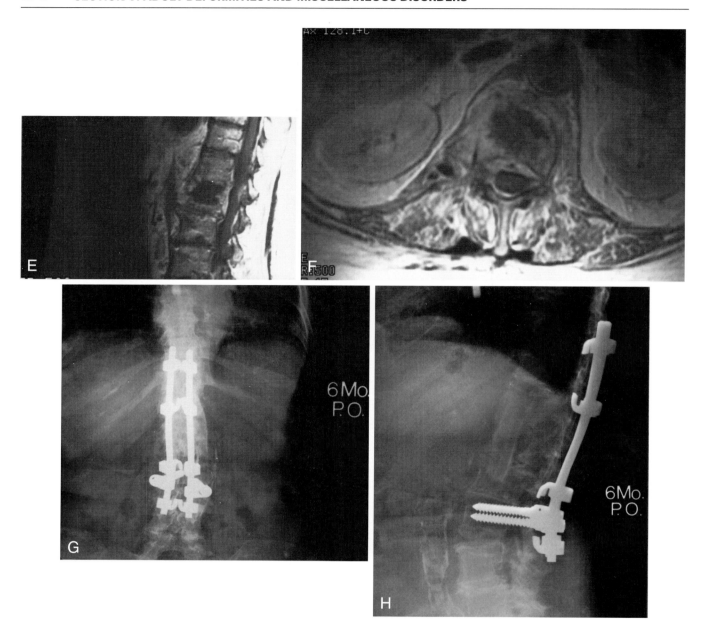

FIGURE 28.4—*continued*

E. T1-weighted sagittal MRI sequence with gadolinium shows enhancement of the T12-L1 disc space and L1 vertebral body. There is a slight amount of enhancing tissue in the anterior epidural space but no compression of the conus medullaris or cauda equina. F. T1-weighted axial MRI sequence with gadolinium shows enhancement of the T12-L1 disc space and the enhancing tissue in the anterior epidural space. There is a small enhancing soft-tissue mass surrounding the anterior aspect of the T12-L1 disc space. G. Anteroposterior and H. lateral radiographs taken 6 months after surgery show solid fusion with incorporation of bone anteriorly and posteriorly.

the disc and the vertebral body is indistinct. In T2-weighted sequences, the signal intensity is higher than normal in the disc and adjacent vertebral bodies, and the intranuclear cleft, the low-intensity central line normally seen in the disc, is generally absent. Gadolinium, a paramagnetic contrast material, causes enhancement of the disc space and allows better delineation of epidural abscesses (217).

The MRI signal abnormalities change with resolution of the infection but the response of unenhanced MRI is too slow to be used to assess the efficacy of treatment (186). Over time the T1-weighted sequences revert from a hypointense signal in the vertebral body to a hyperintense fat signal, and the hyperintense signal on the T2-weighted sequence gradually diminishes. In the healed stage, the disc space is narrowed or obliterated (246, 276). Gadolinium-enhanced MRI is helpful in demonstrating the activity of a spinal infection. Post and colleagues found that dense enhancement indicated active infection, whereas minimal enhancement was seen in cases that were responding to treatment (217).

MRI is able to distinguish tumor from infection in almost all cases. Tumors rarely involve the disc spaces and do not have the typical T1- and T2-weighted changes described above for infection. Contiguous vertebral involvement is seen more frequently in infections than in tumors. Fat planes are often obscured diffusely as a result of edema with infection, whereas they are often intact or only focally altered with tumors (7).

Despite the accuracy of MRI, an absolute diagnosis must be based on bacteriologic or histologic examination of the pathologic tissue (59, 146, 195). The only circumstances in which the diagnosis may be made without a tissue biopsy are in pediatric discitis and when a positive blood culture is found in a patient with signs and symptoms of spinal infection.

Needle biopsy examinations of the spine can be performed safely throughout all regions of the spine (205, 206). A definite diagnosis is possible by a closed needle biopsy examination in 68 to 86% of cases (9, 24, 84, 90, 206, 238). Small-needle aspiration has a considerably lower yield than the larger tissue specimens obtained with a Craig needle (42).

A false-negative closed-needle biopsy result often occurs in patients being treated with antibiotics at the time of the biopsy procedure. If a biopsy analysis is nondiagnostic and the clinical situation allows a delay in treatment, it is reasonable to observe the patient off antibiotics and to repeat the biopsy procedure. Open biopsy procedures have lower false-negative rates, because the surgeon is able to select grossly abnormal tissue and to provide the pathologist with a larger tissue sample (238).

Management

The goals of treatment are to establish the diagnosis, to prevent or reverse neurologic deficits, to relieve pain, to establish spinal stability, to eradicate the infection, and to prevent relapses. Antibiotic therapy and surgery play a major role in the treatment of spinal infections, but attention to good general medical care is still a vital part of the treatment. Associated conditions that compromise wound healing or immune response should be managed aggressively. Proper nutrition and the reversal of metabolic deficits and hypoxia are essential. Diabetes and other systemic illnesses, including coexistent infections, should be brought under control (57).

When possible, the choice of antibiotics should be determined by the culture and sensitivity test results so that the most specific and least toxic agent can be used. Treatment should be withheld until an organism is identified by a biopsy analysis, in case a second biopsy specimen is required. Patients who have systemic toxicity, however, should be treated with maximal doses of broad-spectrum antibiotics as soon as the biopsy procedure has been completed. Antibiotics should be administered parenterally for 6 weeks and followed with an oral course of antibiotics until the disease is resolved. It may be reasonable to switch from parenteral to oral therapy at 4 weeks, but parenteral therapy for less than 4 weeks results in a higher rate of failure (79, 238). It is possible that potent, new oral antibiotics may supplant parenteral treatment of vertebral osteomyelitis in the future, but general use of these agents should await evidence of their effectiveness.

The ESR is a reasonable guide in assessing the therapeutic response and can be expected to decrease to one-half to two-thirds of pretreatment levels by the time of completion of successful treatment (36, 51, 79, 134, 238). Repeat biopsy is indicated if the ESR does not decrease with treatment or if the patient does not respond clinically as expected.

Patients should be immobilized to control pain and to prevent deformity or neurologic deterioration. The length of time for bed rest, the type of orthosis, and the duration of its use all depend on the location of the infection, the degree of bone destruction and deformity, and the response to treatment. Thoracic and thoracolumbar lesions are best managed initially with bed rest until a good response to treatment is noted. Thoracic and thoracolumbar lesions are more likely to cause deformity, and the prognosis for neurologic deficits is worse than in lumbar spine involvement (57, 79). Cervical and cervicothoracic lesions are best immobilized with a halo device. These lesions have a tendency to progress rapidly and to lead to instability. A thoracolumbosacral orthosis with a chin extension may be used for upper thoracic lesions; lower thoracic and lumbar lesions may be immobilized in a device without a chin piece. Most authors recommend bracing for at least 3 to 4 months, but the regimen may be individualized and based on the response to treatment (84).

Surgical treatment is indicated in the following circumstances: *(a)* to obtain a bacteriologic diagnosis; *(b)* to drain a clinically significant abscess (spiking fevers and septic course); *(c)* to treat cases refractory to nonoperative treatment (persistently increased ESR or persistent pain); *(d)* to decompress neural elements in the presence of a neurologic deficit; and *(e)* to prevent or correct spinal deformity or instability (57, 61, 73, 166).

The timing of operation must be individualized. A progressive neurologic deficit or a clinically significant abscess is a surgical emergency, but most spinal infections can be managed in a less urgent time frame.

In nearly all cases, the spine should be approached anteriorly to provide direct access to the infected tissues and to allow adequate débridement. Anterior exposure allows stabilization of the spine by bone grafting, which promotes rapid healing without collapse and facilitates rehabilitation (57, 65, 133, 140, 252). Laminectomy is contraindicated in most cases because it may lead to neurologic deterioration and increased instability (57, 135). Laminectomy may be reasonable in the lumbar spine below the level of the conus medullaris, provided that there is no psoas muscle abscess or extensive anterior destruction of the bodies that requires radical débridement. If a laminectomy is performed, the facets should be preserved and a discectomy should be done.

For lesions in the thoracic or thoracolumbar spine, the transthoracic approach has the advantage of better exposure, allowing more extensive débridement and better decompression of the cord and more effective bone grafting (133, 140). Costotransversectomy or a slightly more extensive posterolateral decompression is recommended when a spine biopsy specimen or minimal decompression with limited grafting is necessary or when gross purulence is expected (29).

After débridement of the infected focus, autogenous iliac crest grafting can be performed during the same procedure. The graft should extend from healthy bone above to healthy bone below (133, 140). Autogenous bone grafting after vertebral body resection in the presence of active infection is safe and effective (291). The iliac crest generally provides a better graft than a rib (118, 133, 223). If a rib is excised in the process of a transthoracic approach, it is often an adequate graft as long as there is not a significant kyphotic deformity or a large segment to span (223).

Fibular grafts have also been used successfully when it is necessary to span large segments (96).

In cases in which there is significant kyphotic deformity, anterior reconstruction with autogenous bone grafts after débridement should be done as a first stage (65, 96, 133, 140, 223). Posterior stabilization and fusion are indicated in cases of more severe kyphosis, spinal instability, or when postoperative bracing is not possible (Fig. 28.4) (96, 133, 135). Posterior instrumentation after anterior débridement and fusion has been shown to be effective (96, 278).

Several cases have been described that have been successfully managed by percutaneous discectomy. Additional studies are required in order to determine the role of percutaneous discectomy for the treatment of spinal infections (87, 264, 293).

Prognosis

Relapse of infection occurs in up to 25% of cases but is much less common if antibiotics are administered for more than 28 days (57, 238). The mortality rate is less than 5% and death is much more likely in the elderly and in those with an underlying disease (57, 238).

Factors that predispose a patient to paralysis include increased age, a more cephalad level of infection, and a history of diabetes mellitus or rheumatoid arthritis (57). Fewer than 7% of patients overall have residual neurologic deficits (238).

Diabetic patients are more likely to have permanent neurologic deficits, and patients with thoracic involvement are the least likely to recover (57, 238). Eismont and associates described the results of surgery on 14 patients with spinal cord paralysis (57). Three of the seven patients who underwent a laminectomy deteriorated, and four remained unchanged. In contrast, half of the patients treated by an anterior procedure recovered normal or nearly normal function, and no patient was made worse by the procedure. The patients with root lesions alone had an excellent outcome with or without surgery.

In selected patients who require surgical treatment for pyogenic osteomyelitis, the prognosis is good after anterior débridement and primary bone grafting in conjunction with a full course of antibiotics (65, 156). In the series reported by Emery and colleagues, six of 21 patients treated surgically had neurologic deficits preoperatively (61). There were no deaths and no relapses, and all of the patients with neurologic deficit recovered. All but one of the patients who underwent fusion had a solid fusion, and one of the two patients who did not have a graft had spontaneous fusion. The mean increase in kyphosis was 3°.

Spontaneous fusion occurs in approximately 50% of patients treated nonoperatively (79, 139, 238). The more cephalad the level of infection, the higher the rate of spontaneous fusion. Almost all cases of cervical infection fuse spontaneously (36, 183).

Deformities of the spine appear to be most common in the thoracic and thoracolumbar area and in cases with involvement of more than 50% of one or more vertebral bodies (Fig. 28.3) (79).

Infants with vertebral osteomyelitis have a poor prognosis and a high recurrence rate (58, 218). Intravenous drug abusers, on the other hand, have a surprisingly good prognosis; in 67 cases reported in the literature, there were no deaths or permanent neurologic sequelae (239). HIV seropositive status does not appear to affect the neurologic outcome of patients with spinal infections (108).

Pediatric Discitis

Epidemiology and Etiology

The peak incidence of pediatric discitis is at age 1 to 5 years, with cases occurring infrequently in juveniles and teenagers (244, 281). The disease has no sex or race predilection. The lumbar spine is involved much more frequently than other regions. Unlike in adult disc-space infection, there are no apparent predisposing factors in the children who develop discitis.

There are many theories concerning the etiology of discitis. Most authors now favor bacterial infection, but viral infection, trauma, and low-grade inflammation have also been proposed as causative factors (4, 54, 182, 251, 253). Pediatric discitis and vertebral osteomyelitis were once thought to be distinct clinical entities. They are now generally regarded as related conditions in the spectrum of disease caused by bacterial infection of the spine (281). The incidence of the two conditions is changing with time. In the 25 years spanned by Wenger's series (281), reported in 1978, discitis and vertebral osteomyelitis were seen with equal frequency. Since that time, the incidence of vertebral osteomyelitis has markedly declined, but discitis is still seen quite frequently (227, 282). The change in rate is thought to be due to several factors. The common practice of liberally prescribing antibiotics for suspected infections has probably diminished episodes of bacteremia that would have led to spine infections. In addition, greater awareness of the conditions and improved diagnostic techniques may have allowed successful treatment of infections classified as discitis that might otherwise have gone on to become vertebral osteomyelitis.

Microbiology and Pathogenesis

Because discitis is usually a benign, self-limited condition, disc-space aspiration is rarely performed, and therefore microbiology data are lacking. In the study by Wenger and colleagues nine patients underwent a biopsy examination (281). Six of the nine cultures grew *S. aureus,* and one of the positive cultures also grew α-hemolytic Streptococcus. The remainder of the specimens were negative, but all of them had histologic evidence of acute, subacute, or chronic inflammation. In other studies approximately 50% of blood cultures or spine biopsies have positive results, and *S. aureus* is the organism identified most frequently (19, 150, 184, 244, 253).

The pathophysiology of pediatric discitis is the same as that of adult disc-space infection. The conditions have different clinical manifestations as a result of the anatomic changes that take place with aging. The nucleus pulposus is an avascular tissue that is metabolically active (23). The disc receives nutrition from diffusion across the endplates and from blood vessels in the annulus fibrosus (23, 106). One early study suggested that blood vessels enter the nucleus pulposus in human fetuses and neonates (106). More recent studies, however, have shown that the nucleus pulposus is always avascular. In the developing spine, the endplate has an orderly arrangement of cartilage canals that contain vascular organs resembling glomeruli (Fig. 28.2) (284). After birth, the cartilage endplates become progressively thinner, and by adulthood most of the vessels of the cartilage canals are obliterated (41, 234).

Wiley and Trueta's injection studies demonstrated that bacteria can spread easily to the metaphyseal region of adjacent vertebrae through the rich arterial anastomosis within and between the vertebral bodies (290). The infection could also begin in the metaphyseal region of one vertebra and spread across the disc by lysosomal destruction of the nucleus pulposus or through the annular vessels. In children, microorganisms have nearly direct access to the nucleus pulposus through the cartilage canals, allowing the infection to begin spontaneously in the disc with little involvement of the adjacent bone.

Clinical Presentation

Most children with discitis present with pain and no history of a prodromal illness. Only about one-half of the patients have a fever. Puig Guri described three different modes of presentation, based on the age of the patient. Children younger than 3 years of age may suddenly refuse to walk. Children of ages 3 to 8 years frequently complain of pain radiating to the abdomen, whereas adolescents are more likely to complain of back or leg pain (219). Infants with vertebral osteomyelitis generally have fulminant infection and present with high fever and systemic signs of illness (58, 218).

Diagnostic Evaluation

On physical examination, a child with discitis often exhibits a rigid posture. The hamstring muscles are usually tight, and the straight-leg-raising test may be positive. When the child extends from a forward flexed position, the normal spinal rhythm is lost.

Useful laboratory studies include complete blood cell count with differential, ESR, and CRP measurement. Plain roentgenograms are frequently normal for the first several weeks after the onset of the illness, but they are helpful to eliminate the possibility of other conditions and to assess spinal alignment. The radiographic findings of discitis include narrowing of the disc space and erosion of the adjacent endplates.

The most sensitive imaging studies are bone scan and MRI. A bone scan is inexpensive and highly sensitive, but it lacks specificity. An MRI is expensive but provides a great deal of useful information. The typical changes of discitis are the same as the findings in adults with disc-space infection (55, 229, 262). The MRI eliminates other disorders in the differential diagnosis, including Scheuermann's kyphosis, epidural abscess, neoplasm, and tumorlike conditions of the spine. Progression of discitis to vertebral osteomyelitis and the presence or absence of an abscess are evident on MRI. The MRI findings in tuberculosis or other granulomatous spinal infections are distinctive, and although not pathognomonic, the changes allow a presumptive diagnosis to be made. (The MRI findings were discussed earlier in the section on adult disc-space infection.) A skin test for tuberculosis, a chest roentgenogram, and a spine biopsy are indicated if a granulomatous infection is considered.

If the bone scan or MRI suggests discitis, blood cultures are recommended. A biopsy analysis is not required unless a granulomatous infection or neoplasm is suspected or the child does not respond to antibiotic therapy as expected.

Management

Pediatric discitis is managed with an empiric course of antibiotics given intravenously and immobilization. The antibiotic chosen must cover *S. aureus;* a first-generation cephalosporin is commonly prescribed for its spectrum of activity, safety, and low cost. The patient may switch to antibiotics given orally when a good clinical response is noted and the ESR or CRP value declines. Orally administered antibiotics are frequently prescribed for 3 to 4 weeks. Some investigators have, on occasion, used orally administered antibiotics exclusively, and the older literature recommended immobilization alone without any antibiotic treatment (19, 227, 253). Most authors now accept the bacteriologic etiology of pediatric discitis and recommend antibiotic therapy in an effort to stop the disease and prevent progression of the infection to vertebral osteomyelitis. Some investigators use antibiotics selectively in children with systemic signs such as fever, increased ESR, or leukocytosis (43, 244).

Immobilization is often recommended for comfort, to decrease the duration of the illness, and to prevent recurrence of the infection. Ring and colleagues reported their experience with 47 children treated for infectious spondylitis (227). The ages of the patients ranged from 7 months to 15 years 8 months (average 4 years 8 months). The patients treated with antibiotics given intravenously and immobilization had a better outcome than those treated without antibiotics or bracing. Of the children who were not braced, prolonged or recurrent symptoms occurred in 18% (4 of 22) receiving antibiotics intravenously, 50% (5 of 10) receiving antibiotics orally, and 67% (4 of 6) receiving no antibiotics. Only one of five children treated with antibiotics given intravenously and bracing had recurrent symptoms after discontinuation of immobilization. Two children were immobilized as the sole form of treatment, and both had recurrence of symptoms when bracing was discontinued.

Most patients with discitis respond rapidly to treatment with antibiotics given empirically and bracing. Children who continue to have clinical signs and symptoms of infection after 3 or 4 days and those who appear septic should undergo computed tomography–directed biopsy to confirm the diagnosis and to determine the sensitivity pattern of the pathogen.

Débridement and fusion are occasionally required to manage patients who fail to respond to antibiotics and bracing. Surgery may also be required to drain a psoas muscle abscess or epidural abscess in association with discitis or vertebral osteomyelitis (122, 182, 227).

Children with significant bony collapse from vertebral osteomyelitis may require a fusion for kyphotic deformity. Hyperextension bracing for 6 months or more may allow restoration of the vertebral body height in younger children, but older children may have persistent or progressive kyphosis requiring anterior and posterior fusion (282).

Infections of the Spinal Canal

Epidural Abscess

Epidemiology and Etiology

The incidence of pyogenic infections in the epidural space appears to be increasing (47, 113, 202). Nussbaum and colleagues reported on 40 patients seen at one institution between 1979 and 1991 (202). A significant increase in the incidence was noted after 1988. They attributed the change to several factors, including an increase in illicit drug use, increasing rates of spine surgery and spinal anesthesia, and a heightened awareness of the disorder. Hlavin and colleagues also documented an increasing incidence of epidural abscess, up to 1.96 patients per 10,000 admissions per year. Most cases occur in adults; the mean age in most series is in the sixth decade of life (47, 48, 113, 202). In a referral setting, an epidural abscess can be expected to occur in about 7% of the spine infections encountered (85). The male-to-female ratio is approximately 1:1, although one study reported a striking male predominance (47, 48, 202).

The primary source of infection can be identified in approximately 60% of cases (47). Infection may occur by hematogenous spread from a remote focus of infection (12, 47, 48, 103, 112, 131, 202), by spread from a contiguous focus of vertebral osteomyelitis, a disc-space infection, or by direct inoculation at the time of operation, epidural steroid injection, lumbar puncture, or epidural catheterization (12, 14, 47, 48, 69, 103, 112, 131, 202). Factors that may be associated with a higher incidence of infection include diabetes mellitus, intravenous drug abuse, prior back trauma, and pregnancy (12, 21, 47, 85).

Microbiology

In the preantibiotic era, *S. aureus* was the pathogen in almost all cases in which the causative organism was known (112). In later series, *S. aureus* accounted for approximately 60% of cases (12, 47, 48, 131, 202). In 166 patients from five series, *S. aureus* accounted for 62%, aerobic streptococci for 8%, *S. epidermidis* for 2%, aerobic Gram-negative rods for 18%, anaerobes for 2%, and other bacteria for 1%; 6% of the organisms were unidentified (12, 47, 103, 112, 131). Intravenous drug abusers are frequently infected with Gram-negative organisms, especially *Pseudomonas,* although one series documented a high percentage of drug abusers infected with *S. aureus* (131, 142, 202).

Pathogenesis and Pathology

Most epidural abscesses occur in the regions of the spinal canal where the epidural space is largest. Dandy's cadaver dissections demonstrated that the epidural space is filled with fat and loose areolar tissue containing numerous veins (46). The size and shape of this space is determined by the variations in size of the spinal cord. In the cervical spine there is almost no fat between bone and dura. Except for a space dorsal to the origin of the spinal nerves, the epidural region is mostly a potential space. Ventrally, the dura is closely applied to the spinal canal from C1 to S2. Posteriorly, the space begins to appear at C7 and gradually deepens along the thoracic vertebrae to a depth of 0.5 to 0.75 cm between T4 and T8. The space tapers between T11 and L2, and its greatest depth is found below L2. The epidural space communicates with the retroperitoneal and posterior mediastinal spaces through the intervertebral foramina (49). The abscess was located posteriorly in 73% of cases and anteriorly in 27% of cases in six series in which the location was recorded (12, 47, 48, 103, 112, 224). A review of the literature in 1987 revealed that the thoracic spine was involved in 51% of cases, the lumbar spine in 35%, and the cervical spine in 14% (47). This distribution has been challenged. One study revealed that the lumbar region was involved either alone or together with other areas in 60% of cases, whereas two other series showed a higher percentage of cases occurring in the cervical spine (48, 202, 224). Because there is no anatomic boundary within the space, the infection can extend the entire length of the spinal canal, but generally it covers only three or four segments (12, 47, 85, 112, 131).

The pathogenesis of the neurologic manifestations is related to direct compression from epidural pus or granulation tissue or to embarrassment of the intrinsic circulation of the cord (12, 21, 22, 112). A microangiographic study in a rabbit model demonstrated that the initial neurologic deficit is related to compression rather than to ischemia (66).

Several authors have identified a correlation between the duration of infection and the gross appearance at operation or postmortem examination. Corradini and colleagues described an early presuppurative phase in which the inflammatory lesion was characterized by an epidural mass of swollen, red, friable fat without any gross pus (40). In patients who have had symptoms for less than 2 weeks, gross pus with varying amounts of red granulation tissue has been identified (12, 21, 40, 47, 235). In patients with symptoms of longer duration, granulation tissue is often identified on the dura (12, 40, 47, 235). In delayed cases with symptoms for 150 days or longer, grayish-white granulation tissue or fibrous tissue has been found (235). Some authors argue that it is not always possible to predict whether pus or granulation tissue is likely to be found at surgery (103, 112, 131).

Clinical Presentation

Patients with an epidural abscess have a highly variable presentation, which causes initial misdiagnosis in approximately 50% of cases (47). Long delays between presentation and definitive treatment are common.

Most authors attempt to distinguish between acute and chronic disease, but this distinction is somewhat arbitrary and probably relates to the virulence of the organism, the resistance of the host, and the type of treatment received before definitive diagnosis. Most patients with an acute epidural abscess present with fever, back pain, and spine tenderness. These signs and symptoms may be lacking in patients with chronic disease (12, 21, 85, 103, 112, 235). Several authors have claimed that the distinction between acute and chronic disease is not clinically relevant (45, 113, 202, 224).

Without treatment, the disease frequently progresses through four stages. The initial symptom is local spine pain, followed by radicular pain, weakness, and, finally, paralysis (21, 40, 112). The transition from one stage to another is highly variable; weakness or paralysis may not develop for many months, or they may occur suddenly and unpredictably in a matter of hours (47, 85).

Nuchal rigidity may occur in patients with an epidural abscess, and therefore this sign is not helpful in distinguishing an epidural abscess from meningitis or spinal cord abscess (12).

Diagnostic Evaluation

Patients with an acute epidural abscess generally appear more systemically ill than those with vertebral osteomyelitis. The white blood cell count and the

ESR generally are increased (85). Patients with chronic disease often appear to have fewer toxic responses, and the white blood cell count is normal (12).

The definitive diagnosis is based on identification of the organism. Culture specimens taken directly from the abscess are positive in approximately 90% of cases. Blood cultures have positive results in 60% of cases, and cultures of spinal fluid yield the organism in approximately 11% of cases (12, 47, 103, 112, 131). Plain roentgenographs frequently are normal unless an established disc-space infection or focus of vertebral osteomyelitis is present (142, 235). Radionuclide studies may be helpful, but they are nonspecific and results may be falsely negative (142). A gallium scan may be slightly more sensitive than a technetium scan (142).

Myelography was the standard imaging modality in the past. It was often necessary to perform injections at sites above and below the abscess to demonstrate the extent of the epidural compression. A high-grade block is commonly seen. The lateral myelogram demonstrates whether the abscess is located anteriorly or posteriorly and is helpful for surgical planning (12, 131, 235). If pus is encountered during needle insertion, a specimen should be taken for a culture, but the thecal sac should not be entered. A second puncture for myelography should be performed at a different level. Cerebrospinal fluid should be sampled at the time of myelography for cell count, glucose measurement, protein measurement, and culture. Bacteria are generally not present in the cerebrospinal fluid unless the epidural abscess is complicated by a subdural abscess or meningitis (12, 131, 235). The spinal fluid generally reflects a parameningeal infection with increased protein content.

Plain computed tomography has a high false-negative rate, and in one study it was diagnostic in only four of nine cases (47). Contrast-enhanced CT has been advocated by some authors (Fig. 28.5C) (8, 155). Unfortunately, it may miss the area of interest unless a myelogram is performed in conjunction with the study.

MRI is now considered the imaging modality of choice (8, 15, 62, 85, 202). It is noninvasive and safe and allows the visualization of the degree of cord compression and extent of abscess in all directions (Fig. 28.5D). The MRI can also provide the diagnosis of disc-space infection or vertebral osteomyelitis. Areas of infection appear as high-signal intensity on T2-weighted images. False-negative results may occur with nonenhanced MRI, especially with extensive abscesses that do not have discrete cephalad and caudad borders (85). The MRI may also be falsely negative in patients with concomitant meningitis, because the signal changes in the abscess may be similar to those in the infected cerebrospinal fluid (216). If the MRI scan is negative, a myelogram and postmyelographic CT study should be performed if an epidural abscess is suspected. Some authors claim that pus has a much higher signal intensity on T2-weighted sequences than granulation tissue and surrounding inflammatory edema (8). Other investigators believe that it is not possible to make such a distinction even with gadolinium-enhanced images (217).

Contrast enhancement is valuable for the detection of an epidural abscess as well as other spine infections, especially if the infection spans multiple segments (216, 217, 236). Follow-up studies on treated infection demonstrated a decrease in abscess size, but enhancement may persist in the disc or epidural space despite clinical improvement (236). This persistent enhancement may represent chronic granulation tissue or scar formation (Fig. 28.5) (236).

Management

An epidural abscess is a medical and surgical emergency. The goals of treatment are to eradicate the infection, preserve or improve the patient's neurologic status, relieve pain, and preserve spinal stability.

A review of the literature from 1970 to 1990 revealed 37 reported cases of epidural abscess that had been treated conservatively (285). These patients represented 6.6% of the cases published during that time frame. Sixty-three percent of the cases were managed successfully; however, some of the patients had disastrous outcomes. Baker and colleagues noted that all five patients in their series who were managed without surgery died (12). Danner and Hartmann described six patients and Hlavin reported on eight patients who required emergent laminectomy for neurologic deterioration while being treated with appropriate antibiotics for epidural abscesses (47, 113). Wheeler and colleagues noted the difficulty in drawing conclusions on the basis of small series and case reports but indicated that the literature does not support medical management for patients presenting with paralysis or septic shock (285). They called for a prospective study to address the indications for nonsurgical management for patients presenting with less severe signs and symptoms. Even the most ardent proponents of nonoperative management of epidural abscesses recommend this approach only in selected cases, namely, patients who *(a)* are poor surgical candidates, *(b)* have an abscess that involves a considerable length of the vertebral canal, *(c)* have no significant neurologic deficit, and *(d)* who have had complete paralysis for more than 3 days (155, 167). These authors think that patients who are deteriorating neurologically should undergo surgery.

Most authors consider surgical decompression in combination with antibiotic therapy to be the treatment of choice in all patients except those who could

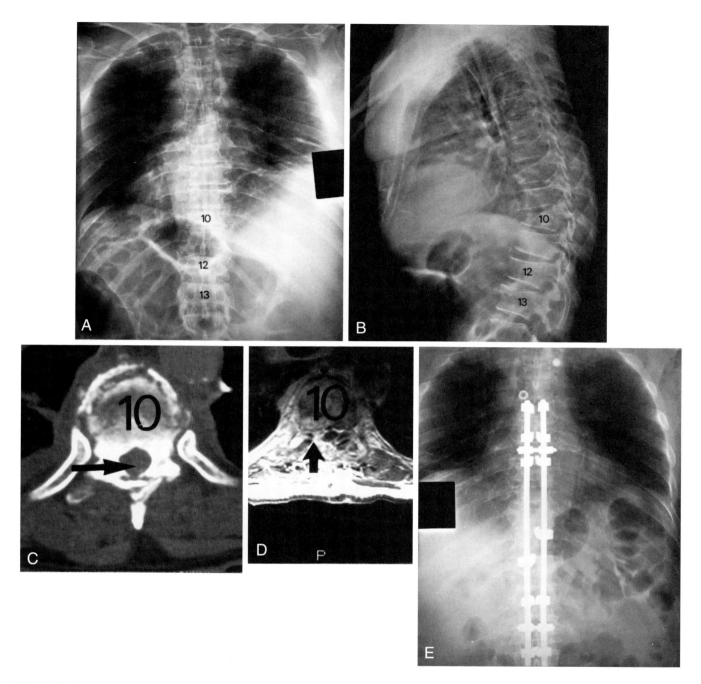

FIGURE 28.5.

Sixty-two-year-old male who fell 15 feet from a tree and suffered compression fractures of T10, T12, and T13 (13 rib-bearing vertebrae). He was neurologically intact and was treated with a thoracolumbosacral orthosis. Four days later he developed an ileus and required colonoscopic decompression. Six days later he developed a fever; blood cultures were positive for *S. aureus,* and he was given intravenous antibiotics. Seven days later he developed dysesthetic pain in the lower extremities, and he was placed on bed rest and observed. Six days later (three and a half weeks following injury) he developed bilateral lower extremity weakness (3–4/5) with long tract signs. A CT myelogram showed a block at T10, and he underwent emergency laminectomy of T8, T9, and T10 and a total facetectomy on the right at T9-T10. Chronic granulation tissue with small amounts of gross pus were found compressing the spinal cord. The wound was closed over drains. Intraoperative cultures grew *S. aureus,* and the patient was treated with intravenous antibiotics for 3 weeks. He then underwent T5-L1 fusion with instrumentation. No gross infection was identified at the time of the fusion. Eleven days later he developed a wound infection of the left iliac crest donor site, which was treated with debridement, open packing, and intravenous antibiotics. Cultures were positive for *Proteus, Enterobacter,* and *Pseudomonas.* His wounds healed and his neurologic deficit improved, but he continued to have back pain and an elevated ESR. One year after the fusion procedure he had spontaneous drainage from his spine wound. Gross pus was found throughout the length of the fusion mass. Hardware was removed and the wound was débrided. Cultures were positive for *Pseudomonas aeruginosa.* A stable pseudarthrosis was found above and below the previous decompression site, but the patient's fusion was solid over the previously unstable segments. His wound was managed with two débridements and closure over suction-irrigation tubes, which were removed 7 days later. He received another course of intravenous antibiotics. At final follow-up 14 months after hardware removal his spine was stable, pain and infection were resolved, and his only neurologic deficit was 4+ out of 5 strength of the left tibialis anterior muscle.

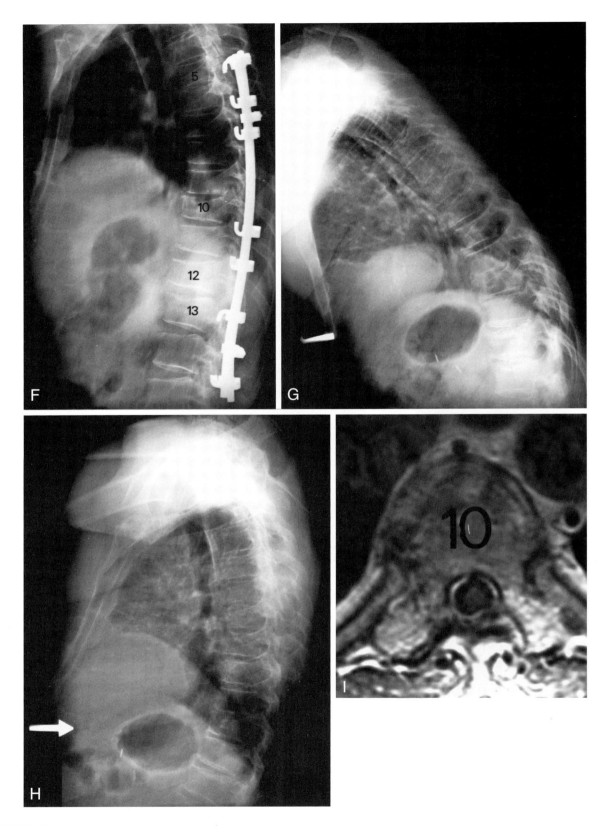

FIGURE 28.5—continued

A. Anteroposterior and **B.** lateral thoracic spine radiographs show compression fractures of T10, T12, and T13. **C.** Post-myelographic CT image shows compression fracture of T10 with near complete block of contrast (arrow) and displacement of the spinal cord to the left by epidural mass. **D.** MRI with gadolinium enhancement performed after thoracic decompression and prior to stabilization. The complete right T9-T10 facetectomy and persistent cord deformation from granulation tissue is seen (arrow). **E.** Anteroposterior and **F.** lateral thoracic spine radiographs show T5-L1 posterior fusion with instrumentation. **G.** Flexion and **H.** extension thoracic spine radiographs taken 10 months following hardware removal show that spine is stable. **I.** Gadolinium-enhanced MRI taken 22 months after surgery shows minimal enhancing epidural fibrosis on the right side of the spinal canal at T10 without any cord compression.

not tolerate operation or those who have had complete paralysis for more than several days. The surgical approach depends on the location of the abscess. Laminectomy is generally the treatment of choice, because the abscess is located posteriorly in most cases (12, 112). The facet joints should be left intact to preserve spinal stability. Intraoperative ultrasonography after laminectomy allows the epidural mass to be localized (216). When the abscess is secondary to a focus of vertebral osteomyelitis, it may be necessary to perform the decompression anteriorly and posteriorly. If the entire epidural mass is located anteriorly, then an isolated anterior approach is appropriate. Instrumentation and fusion may be necessary in cases in which spinal stability has been compromised by the decompression. In these cases, long-term follow-up is essential because of the risk of pseudarthrosis and persistent low-grade infection (Fig. 28.5).

After a laminectomy, the wound may be closed over drains or packed open (12, 47, 112). Some authors recommend closure of the wound and continuous suction-irrigation after laminectomy (86).

In children, extensive laminectomy is undesirable because of the risk of postoperative spinal deformity (70, 125). Irrigation and drainage performed openly through laminotomies or percutaneously have been successful in eradicating epidural abscesses in several case reports. The authors believe that the procedure is reasonable when the abscess is located in the posterior epidural space, when the extent of the abscess is well defined by MRI, and when the abscess consists of pus rather than granulation tissue (30, 49, 125). The technique carries a risk of dural perforation and spread of the infection in the epidural space by the irrigation. If a patient's condition deteriorates during irrigation and drainage, the surgeon should be prepared to perform an emergency open procedure (264).

As soon as the diagnosis is made, specimens should be obtained and antibiotic therapy started immediately on the basis of the Gram stain results and the known bacteriologic cause of the disease. Initial therapy should include a first-line antistaphylococcic agent. Gram-negative organisms should be suspected if there is a history of a spinal procedure or intravenous drug abuse. *S. epidermidis* should also be considered after spinal procedures (47). The definitive antibiotic therapy should be based on the culture and sensitivity results. Antibiotics should be given in maximum dosages for at least 2 weeks, and most authors recommend 3 to 4 weeks of parenteral therapy (12, 47). Antibiotics must be administered parenterally for at least 6 to 8 weeks for coexistent vertebral osteomyelitis or disc-space infection (12, 47).

Prognosis

The natural history of an untreated epidural abscess is relentless progression of symptoms and eventual paralysis and possible death. In the preantibiotic era, the overall mortality rate was between 55 and 70% (21, 22, 185). The outcome of patients with epidural abscess treated with surgical decompression and antibiotics appears to have improved in recent years as a result of improved diagnostic imaging, antibiotic therapy, and surgical techniques. A review of early studies indicated that 39% of patients recovered fully, 26% had residual weakness but were able to ambulate, 22% were paralyzed, and 13% died (47). A combination of five series indicated that 78% of patients undergoing surgery recover fully or with minimal weakness (39, 45, 113, 173, 202, 224).

The prognosis for neurologic recovery depends on the duration and severity of the neurologic deficit (47, 85, 112, 125, 131). Heusner found that most patients with paresis for less than 36 hours had a complete recovery (112). No patient with complete paralysis for more than 36 to 48 hours recovered significant neurologic function (101, 112). Complete sensory loss is also considered to be a poor prognostic factor (101). Patients who have an acute progressive syndrome with complete paraplegia occurring within the first 12 hours have a poor prognosis, presumably on the basis of spinal cord infarction rather than mechanical compression (142). Other associated conditions thought to be poor prognostic factors are diabetes, advanced age, female sex, HIV infection, and associated vertebral osteomyelitis (85, 112, 142).

Several authors have claimed that the distinction between acute and chronic disease has no prognostic significance (45, 113, 202, 224). These groups found no difference in terms of clinical grade on presentation or functional recovery when patients were classified by duration of illness.

Subdural Abscess

Epidemiology and Etiology

Since Sittig first described spinal subdural empyema in 1927, only 44 cases have been described in the literature (153, 248). The condition involves intrathecal infection of the spinal meninges. Similar to other infections of the spinal canal, a subdural abscess may occur by hematogenous spread from a distant focus of infection, spread from a contiguous infection, or by direct inoculation (153, 163).

There is no apparent predilection for any age group, and the female-to-male ratio is approximately 2:1. Pregnant women and diabetic individuals appear to be two groups at risk for infection.

Pathogenesis, Pathology, and Microbiology

The paucity of reported cases prohibits definitive statements about the pathogenesis of this disorder. Autopsy results have been reported in only six cases: five authors specifically stated that spinal cord inflammation was not present (153). The majority of reported cases describe local liquefaction necrosis with wallerian degeneration without evidence of microemboli or inflammation. Levy favored ischemia secondary to spinal cord compression as the pathogenesis of the neurologic sequelae that result from subdural abscesses (153). Most infections are caused by *S. aureus,* although other organisms, including streptococcus, *E. coli,* and *Pseudomonas* have been reported (153).

Clinical Presentation

Fraser and colleagues suggested that a patient with a subdural abscess presents exactly like one with an epidural abscess, except that often there is no spinal percussion tenderness (78). Nearly one-third of patients in the review of the literature by Levy and colleagues complained of spinal tenderness, however (153). In addition, not all patients with an epidural abscess have spinal tenderness, making that feature unreliable for differentiating the two disorders (101, 103). The clinical triad of fever, spinal pain, and spinal cord compression was present in approximately 40% of all cases in the literature (153).

Diagnostic Evaluation

Laboratory analysis results are similar to those in cases of an epidural abscess. The white blood cell count and ESR are generally increased. The cerebrospinal fluid analysis generally is consistent with a parameningeal process with increased protein level and a moderate pleocytosis and low to normal glucose levels (78, 153).

Myelography reveals an intradural extramedullary filling defect, usually with a complete spinal block, and may demonstrate defects at several levels (28, 78, 153, 163). Fraser and colleagues noted that there is no major anatomic barrier in the subdural space, and therefore an abscess in this location could extend more easily than an epidural abscess (78). They believed that the myelographic finding of multiple defects would favor a diagnosis of a subdural abscess over an epidural abscess. Fraser and colleagues also suggested that the radiographic finding of osteomyelitis in association with a myelographic block would favor a diagnosis of an epidural abscess, because an infection in the subdural space is unlikely in association with vertebral osteomyelitis (78).

MRI has been reported to be effective in the diagnosis of subdural abscess. The findings are quite similar to those in an epidural abscess (153). Similarly to the arguments that Fraser and colleagues made for myelography, the findings of adjacent osteomyelitis suggest an epidural abscess, and multilevel or multiply loculated collections favor a diagnosis of subdural abscess (78, 153).

Management

The appropriate treatment for subdural abscess is urgent decompressive laminectomy with irrigation and drainage in conjunction with appropriate antibiotic therapy. Because the vast majority of subdural abscesses are caused by *S. aureus,* the initial antibiotic regimen must cover Gram-positive cocci until culture and sensitivity results are available (153).

Only one documented case has been reported of a patient's improving following antibiotic therapy alone (149). The prognosis of patients treated with surgery and antibiotics is reasonably good. Levy and colleagues collected all cases reported in the literature through 1993 (153). Thirty-two cases were treated with surgery and antibiotics after 1948 and had adequate documentation to assess the response to treatment. Of these patients, 12 made a full recovery, 11 had a marked recovery, four showed moderate recovery, one had mild recovery, and four died.

Intramedullary Spinal Abscess

Epidemiology and Etiology

Intramedullary spinal abscesses are rare infections. Fewer than 100 cases have been reported since Hart first described the condition in 1830 (13, 105).

The male-to-female ratio is approximately 3:1. The average age of affected females is younger than that of male patients (16.9 ± 16.3 years for females, 33.8 ± 19.8 years for males); overall there is a wide age range (7 months to 72 years; mean, 28.9 ± 20.9 years) (13).

Spinal cord abscesses generally occur by hematogenous spread from a distant focus of infection, but, like abscesses in the epidural space, they may be caused by a contiguous infection or by direct inoculation. In contrast to cases of epidural abscesses, most patients are healthy before the onset of infection. A review of the literature revealed that only three of 93 infections occurred in diabetic patients, and only two cases have been reported in patients who were intravenous drug abusers (13).

Microbiology

The agents responsible for abscesses in the spinal cord are similar to the pathogens that cause epidural abscesses. In 56 reported cases in which the organism was identified, staphylococcus was the causative agent in 22 cases and streptococcus was found in 15 cases. The remaining cases were caused by various organisms, including Gram-negative bacteria; in 10 patients, multiple organisms were cultured (13).

Clinical Presentation

Initial symptoms of an intramedullary spinal abscess include weakness (38.6% of patients), spinal pain (36.1%), fever (27.7%), and radicular pain (26.5%). At presentation the majority of patients have weakness (88.9%), and many have sensory loss (47.7%), sphincter disturbance (40%), and fever (25.6%) (13). The rareness of the condition and the unusual constellation of symptoms may lead to a considerable delay in diagnosis. The progressive clinical stages described for epidural abscess are usually not encountered in cases of spinal cord abscess, and the rate of progression of the disease is unpredictable.

The thoracic cord has been involved in 30 of the reported cases, the cervical spine in 16, and the lumbar cord in 12. Nineteen cases have occurred in the thoracolumbar region, 6 have occurred in the cervicothoracic area, and 10 have involved the entire spine (13).

Diagnostic Evaluation

Surprisingly, spinal fluid is often normal or shows nonspecific increases in protein. Occasionally, clear evidence of inflammation or pus is encountered.

Plain computed tomography may show a widened cord and may demonstrate the intramedullary abscess. Myelography and postmyelographic CT usually show a block and a widening of the cord. MRI has been described in only eight patients but is now considered to be the diagnostic method of choice. In addition to a widened cord, the lesion may have signal characteristics typical for infection. The lesion has usually been isointense or hypointense on T1-weighted sequences, and in three of five cases there was increased signal intensity on T2-weighted sequences. The lesions enhanced with gadolinium administration in two of three cases (13).

Definitive diagnosis is made from culture results of a biopsy specimen taken at surgery.

Management and Prognosis

The treatment for a spinal cord abscess is urgent surgical drainage and antibiotic therapy. The disease was universally fatal in the preantibiotic era, and several patients treated later with antibiotics but without surgery also died. Only eight of the 59 patients reported in the literature that have been treated surgically have died. Six of these eight patients did not receive antibiotics postoperatively. With appropriate treatment, the prognosis is favorable: 22% of patients have made a complete recovery, 55.9% have improved, 6.8% were unchanged, one patient deteriorated, and only two patients died (13).

Spinal Infection from Traumatic Injuries

Penetrating Trauma

High-velocity combat injuries require aggressive débridement of the missile tract to prevent infection. Low-velocity gunshot wounds and stab wounds, on the other hand, generally can be treated nonsurgically. Low-velocity gunshot wounds to the spine do not require débridement as long as the bullet does not traverse the colon, esophagus, or pharynx (109, 136, 147, 159, 165, 231, 232, 277, 292). Treatment of gunshot wounds that traverse a contaminated viscus is considerably more controversial. Poret and colleagues described 151 patients with a gunshot wound to the colon and found an increased infection rate in patients who had retained bullet fragments (215). Romanick and colleagues reported that infections developed in seven of eight patients with gunshot wounds traversing the colon (232). Kihtir and colleagues recommended that all patients with low-velocity wounds to the spine with an associated colonic injury undergo routine operative débridement of the spine and missile tract (136). Antibiotic therapy averaged 2 to 5 days in six of the eight patients in that series. Subsequent reports demonstrated a relatively low infection rate when broad-spectrum antibiotics were administered for at least 5 to 7 days (159, 231).

Roffi and colleagues described 42 patients with low-velocity gunshot wounds associated with a perforated viscus (231). In only three of their patients a spinal or paraspinal infection developed. They found that early removal of bullet fragments was unnecessary. Fourteen of their patients had colon perforation; a psoas muscle abscess developed in only two, and no spinal infections developed. They believed that an extended course of antibiotics given intravenously for at least 7 days, providing coverage for Gram-negative and anaerobic organisms, should be adequate.

Kihtir and colleagues had good results with transperitoneal gunshot wounds of the spine, with or without colon injury (136). They recommend irrigation of the missile tract and a 48-hour course of antibiotics without removal of bone fragments. They performed primary repair or resection and entero-enterostomy in all but one of their five patients with colonic injury. Seven of the eight patients in the series by Romanick and associates underwent a colostomy or ileostomy (232). The poor outcome in the Romanick series may be related to the type of surgical treatment as well as inadequate antibiotic therapy (159).

The group at Thomas Jefferson University does not routinely débride spinal wounds after visceral injury. They reported on 295 patients with gunshot wounds to the spine resulting in a neurologic deficit. They found that patients who underwent spine surgery were more likely to develop spinal infections than those who were treated nonoperatively. Patients receiving steroids and those who had sustained multiple gunshot wounds were also more likely to suffer an infection (109). The current recommendations from that group for patients with low-velocity, transperitoneal gunshot wounds to the spine include broad-spectrum antibiotics for at least 5 days and no routine bullet removal or missile tract débridement (159).

Transpharyngeal gunshot wounds are also controversial. Schaeffer and colleagues recommend aggressive management (127, 241). If a pharyngeal wound is identified by endoscopy, they recommend intravenous administration of broad-spectrum antibiotics, neck wound exploration to repair soft tissues and débride the cervical spine, and external immobilization for approximately 6 weeks.

Kupcha and colleagues described 28 patients with low-velocity gunshot wounds to the cervical spine (147). They found that routine exploration without specific indications was not beneficial. They recommend panendoscopy and arteriography for all patients and a short course (less than 7 days) of antibiotics given intravenously. If the bullet traverses the pharynx, they recommend following the guidelines of Schaeffer and colleagues (241). The Thomas Jefferson University group subsequently has found that débridement of the spine wound is not necessary. They recommend endoscopy with individualized management of the esophageal wound, 48 hours of antibiotics given intravenously, and no débridement of the spine (109; Vaccaro A, personal communication, 1995).

Blunt Trauma

Spinal infections are rarely caused by blunt trauma. Kulowski thought that trauma was a predisposing factor in pyogenic vertebral osteomyelitis (146); later studies have not supported that association (84, 194, 233). A history of trauma was present in only 5% of the 207 cases included in Sapico and Montgomery's literature review (238).

Two groups have reported a total of eight cases of vertebral osteomyelitis at the site of a spine fracture (162, 174). Osteomyelitis may develop as a complication of the fracture because the fracture creates a favorable environment for the hematogenous infection. Alternatively, the osteomyelitis may develop within the central portion of an osteoporotic vertebral body, perhaps because the bone is more hyperemic or because of vascular stasis. Infection may then lead to a pathologic fracture of the vertebra without the usual involvement of the disc space (174). This is an infrequent occurrence but should be considered in certain clinical settings. One case report described a patient who became paraplegic from an epidural abscess 48 hours after a burst fracture of T12 (143). The case was presumed to have occurred by hematogenous seeding of *S. aureus* from a focus of cellulitis to the fracture hematoma.

Vertebral osteomyelitis has been reported to occur in the cervical and upper thoracic spine after blunt traumatic esophageal rupture (214, 228). The esophageal injury may be due to direct trauma from bone fragments or vertebral osteophytes, from breakdown of contused esophageal tissue anterior to a fracture site, or from a rapid increase in intraluminal pressure (214, 228).

Granulomatous Infections

Granulomatous infections may be caused by fungi, certain bacteria, and spirochetes (102, 152). These disorders have similarities in clinical presentation and in histologic features. Most bacteria cause pyogenic infections, but bacteria in the order Actinomycetales cause chronic granulomatous infections. This order includes the following families of pathogens: Mycobacteriaceae (genus *Mycobacterium*), Actinomycetaceae (genera *Actinomyces, Arachnia*), and Nocardiaceae (genus *Nocardia*) (152). Tuberculosis is the most common granulomatous spine infection in the world and is described in the following section. The clinical features of the other granulomatous infections are similar to tuberculous spondylitis, and the surgical principles are the same. The chemotherapeutic management of these infections is highly variable and is beyond the scope of this chapter. I strongly recommend enlisting the help of an infectious disease specialist when treating these conditions.

Tuberculosis

Epidemiology and Etiology

The incidence of tuberculous spondylitis varies considerably throughout the world and is generally proportional to the quality of public health services available. In affluent countries the incidence has decreased dramatically in the past 30 years, and until recently the disease was quite uncommon. In 1986 the number of new cases of tuberculosis increased 2.6% for the first time in several decades (68). The growing number of patients immunocompromised by acquired immunodeficiency syndrome (AIDS) or other conditions are thought to be responsible for the resurgence of tuberculosis.

Spinal involvement develops in approximately 50% of patients with tuberculosis (34, 270). A neurologic deficit develops in 10 to 47% of those with tuberculous spondylitis (11, 20, 67, 81, 121, 168). The disease rarely affects children in North America, Europe, and Saudi Arabia, but it is relatively common in African and Asian children. The incidence of infection in infants and young children has been decreasing in Hong Kong (190).

Spinal tuberculosis generally occurs by hematogenous spread from a distant focus of infection. The pulmonary and genitourinary systems are the most frequent sources, but tuberculosis may also spread from other skeletal lesions (37, 81). The spine may also become infected by direct extension from visceral lesions (37).

Pathogenesis and Pathology

There are three major types of spinal involvement: peridiscal, central, and anterior, listed in decreasing order of incidence (52, 53). Atypical forms of spinal tuberculosis include those with neural arch involvement only and rare cases of epidural or intradural tuberculomas without bony involvement (52, 196).

In peridiscal disease, the infection begins in the metaphyseal area and spreads under the anterior longitudinal ligament to involve the adjacent bodies. In contrast to pyogenic infections, the disc is relatively resistant to infection and may be preserved, even with extensive bone loss. In cases with primarily anterior involvement, the infection spreads beneath the anterior longitudinal ligament and may extend over several segments. The scalloping erosion of the anterior aspect of the vertebral body may be from changes in local vertebral body blood supply (11). With central involvement, the disease begins within the middle of the vertebral body and remains isolated to one vertebra. Central lesions tend to lead to vertebral collapse and are therefore the most likely type to produce significant spinal deformity (53).

There are several pathologic findings that distinguish tuberculous spondylitis from pyogenic infections. Large paraspinal abscesses are more common and the disc is more resistant in tuberculous infections. The pathologic changes generally take longer to develop and frequently are associated with greater deformity in tuberculosis (37, 51, 121, 233).

There are several pathogenic mechanisms responsible for the neurologic deficits that may occur with infection. Seddon recognized that the neurologic compromise could occur acutely or chronically (245). "Paraplegia of active disease" results from external pressure on the neural elements or invasion of the dura. Pressure on the spinal cord may arise from an epidural granuloma or abscess, from sequestered bone and disc, or from pathologic subluxation or dislocation of the vertebrae. The paraplegia in chronic cases is caused by pressure on the cord from epidural granulomas or fibrosis or from a ridge of bone anteriorly created by a progressive kyphotic deformity. These mechanisms have been confirmed at surgery or postmortem examination (11, 116, 124).

An epidural granuloma is analogous to a pyogenic epidural abscess. Usually the granuloma arises by spread from the adjacent bone but rarely may occur by hematogenous seeding without any bony involvement (10, 80, 157, 196). Other lesions that may cause a neurologic deficit without bony involvement are tuberculous arachnoiditis, meningitis, and intradural extramedullary and intramedullary tuberculomas (80, 157, 158, 171). Paraplegia from extraosseous disease occurs in approximately 5% of cases (157).

The pathologic features of tuberculous spondylitis may be altered by secondary pyogenic infection that may occur through sinus tracts or after débridement procedures (37).

Clinical Presentation

The classic presentation of a patient with tuberculous spondylitis includes a patient with spinal pain and manifestations of chronic illness such as weight loss, malaise, and intermittent fever. The physical findings include local tenderness, muscle spasm, and restricted motion. The patient may also have a spinal deformity and neurologic deficit. In the lesser-developed countries the complications of neglected disease, such as paraplegia, kyphosis, and draining sinuses, may be the presenting complaints (121, 175–177).

The location of pain corresponds to the site of the disease, which is most frequent in the thoracic region, less common in the lumbar area, and rare in the cervical spine and sacrum (11, 52, 121). Patients may present with an abscess in any one of many locations, including the groin and buttock (53). In 10 to 47% of patients, neurologic deficits develop during the course of their disease (11, 20, 67, 81, 121, 168, 259). The incidence of paraplegia is highest with spondylitis in the thoracic and the cervical spine (52, 259).

A distinct syndrome has been reported in heroin addicts with tuberculous spondylitis. All five patients in one series had an acute toxic reaction with fever, back pain, weight loss, night sweats, and rapidly evolving neurologic deficits (72). All patients had disseminated tuberculosis with involvement of extravertebral sites.

Diagnostic Evaluation

The ESR generally is increased with tuberculous spondylitis. The tuberculin purified protein derivative skin test usually is positive and indicates past or present exposure to *Mycobacterium* (157). Cultures of early morning urine samples may be helpful in cases of renal involvement, and sputum specimens and gastric washings may be positive with active pulmonary disease. These laboratory findings are helpful, but an absolute diagnosis can be made only by biopsy analysis of the spinal lesion or associated soft-tissue mass (140). Because the vertebral lesions frequently are lytic and may be associated with a paraspinal abscess, CT-directed biopsies using a fine needle have proved effective in confirming the diagnosis (188). Aspiration of a subcutaneous abscess may reveal the organism and obviate the need for spinal biopsy.

The earliest finding on plain roentgenographs is bone rarefaction. With peridiscal involvement, disc-space narrowing is followed by bone destruction similar to pyogenic infections. (Fig. 28.6A). With anterior multilevel spine involvement, the anterior aspect of several adjacent vertebrae may be eroded in a scalloped fashion (Fig. 28.6B). Central body involvement generally resembles a tumor with central rarefaction and bone destruction followed by collapse (Figs. 28.6C and 28.7A,B) (53). Occasionally, lumbar spine radiographs demonstrate calcification in the psoas muscle in cases with a long-standing abscess (11).

Radionuclide scanning with technetium or gallium may help to define the extent of disease (240). Unfortunately, radionuclide scans are not sensitive for tuberculous infection. Technetium bone scans are negative in 35% of cases and gallium scans are negative in 70% (157).

Computed tomography is useful to delineate soft tissue changes around the spine and in the canal and clearly demonstrates the extent of bony involvement. MRI is the imaging modality of choice, because it demonstrates the bony and soft tissue involvement and is capable of direct imaging in multiple planes. The intervertebral disc may have a normal signal on MRI, reflecting the resistance of the disc to tuberculous infection. The MRI findings are different from those in pyogenic infections and reflect the pathologic types described earlier (247, 249). The signal changes on T1- and T2-weighted sequences are similar to those described for pyogenic infection (Fig. 28.7C–E) (276). Gadolinium-enhanced scans are helpful in demonstrating abscesses as well as the extent of osseous involvement (138, 217, 276). Enhanced MRI can distinguish abscesses from granulation tissue. A mass with enhancement at the periphery but not the center is generally an abscess, whereas a mass with near-total enhancement is generally granulation tissue (Fig. 28.7F,G) (138).

Management

The goals of management are to eradicate the infection and to prevent or treat neurologic deficits and spinal deformities. Chemotherapy is an integral part of the management of spinal tuberculosis. The only cases in which chemotherapy is not indicated are those in which late-onset paraplegia from progressive deformity has occurred in a patient with healed inactive disease. Drug therapy is usually started preoperatively but may be started after surgery if a biopsy is necessary. The first line of drugs currently in use includes isoniazid, rifampin, pyrazinamide, streptomycin, and ethambutol. The second-line agents that occasionally are used in special circumstances include ethionamide, cycloserine, kanamycin, capreomycin, p-aminosalicylic acid. The choice of agents, dosages, and duration of therapy should be directed by an infectious disease expert. Multiple drugs are used because of the potential for resistance to a single agent. Selection of rational combinations of drugs is based on the mechanism of action and toxicity of the agents (50).

In 1963 the Medical Research Council Committee for research on tuberculosis of the tropics began to investigate the widely divergent forms of treatment available at that time. A subcommittee was established that later became known as the working party on tuberculosis of the spine. This group initiated several large-scale, controlled prospective trials of treatment methods. The design of each study was based on the available resources in areas where tuberculosis was endemic. The conclusion of the Research Council was that the treatment of choice for spinal tuberculosis in developing countries is ambulatory chemotherapy with 6- or 9-month regimens of isoniazid and rifampin. Surgery was recommended only for biopsy or the management of myelopathy, abscesses, or sinuses (178, 180).

Some surgeons recommend surgery for almost all patients, whereas most surgeons recommend surgery in selected cases only (99, 180, 269, 270). In general, I think that the indications for surgery are the same as in pyogenic infection. Neurologic compromise is the primary indication for surgery since anterior decompression and fusion have been shown to lead to higher recovery rates in patients with neurologic deficit than nonoperative treatment alone (11, 67, 157, 168). Surgery should also be performed for biopsy, management of clinically significant abscesses, failed medical therapy, and deformity.

When surgery is necessary, radical débridement and anterior strut graft fusion in association with chemotherapy (Hong Kong operation) is recommended (117, 119, 175). The Medical Research Council compared the Hong Kong operation to débridement alone. At long-term follow-up there was no difference between the groups in terms of neurologic recovery or pain. None of the patients had recurrence or reactivation of tuberculosis. The primary difference was that patients who underwent radical surgery with fusion had slight correction in deformity

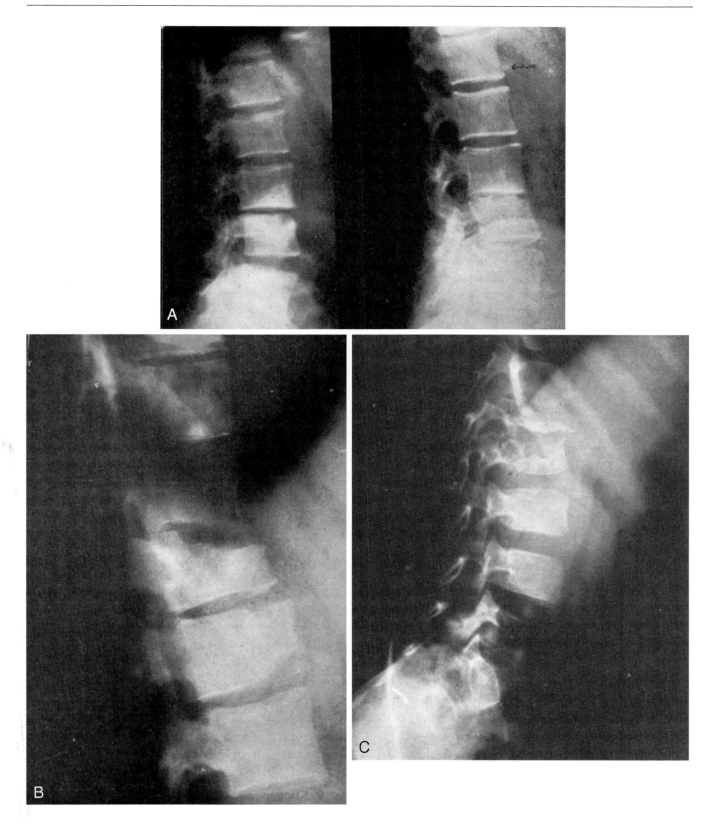

FIGURE 28.6.

Radiographic features of the three types of tuberculous spondylitis. **A.** Peridiscal involvement is characterized by disc-space narrowing followed by variable bone destruction. The radiograph on the left is early in the disease. The radiograph on the right is after resolution of the disease and shows minor deformity. **B.** Anterior multilevel disease is distinguished by scalloped erosions of the anterior aspect of several adjacent vertebrae. In this case, T11, L2, and L1 are involved. **C.** Central involvement resembles a tumor with central body rarefaction and bone destruction followed by collapse. In this radiograph, L1 and L2 are involved. (From Doub HP, Badgley CE. The roentgen signs of tuberculosis of the vertebral body. AJR 1932; 27:827–837).

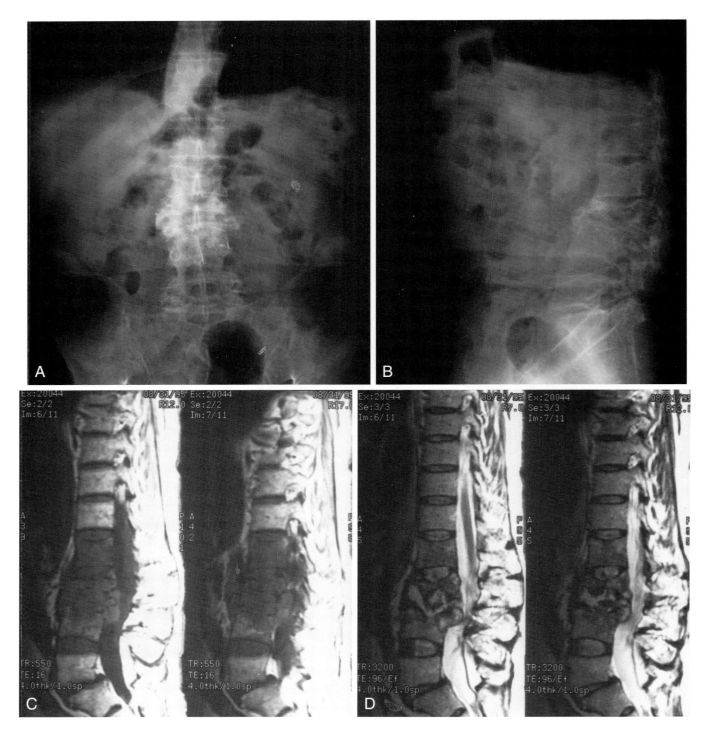

FIGURE 28.7.
Tuberculosis of the lumbar spine. Fifty-two-year-old Mexican man with disseminated tuberculosis was treated with 1 year of therapy with three antituberculous drugs. He presented with progressive low back pain and pseudoclaudication. He was found to have spinal stenosis from collapse of L2 and L3 vertebrae and a sterile psoas muscle abscess. The MRI suggested that the disease was still present, but all cultures and stains taken at operation were negative. **A.** Anteroposterior and **B.** lateral lumbar spine radiographs show collapse of L2 and L3 with kyphotic deformity. **C.** T1-weighted sagittal MRI sequence demonstrates decreased signal in the bodies of L1 to L4, kyphotic deformity, and epidural mass composed of necrotic bone, disc, and purulent debris. **D.** T2-weighted sagittal MRI sequence demonstrates areas of high signal intensity within the L2 and L3 vertebral bodies and in the anterior paraspinal region.

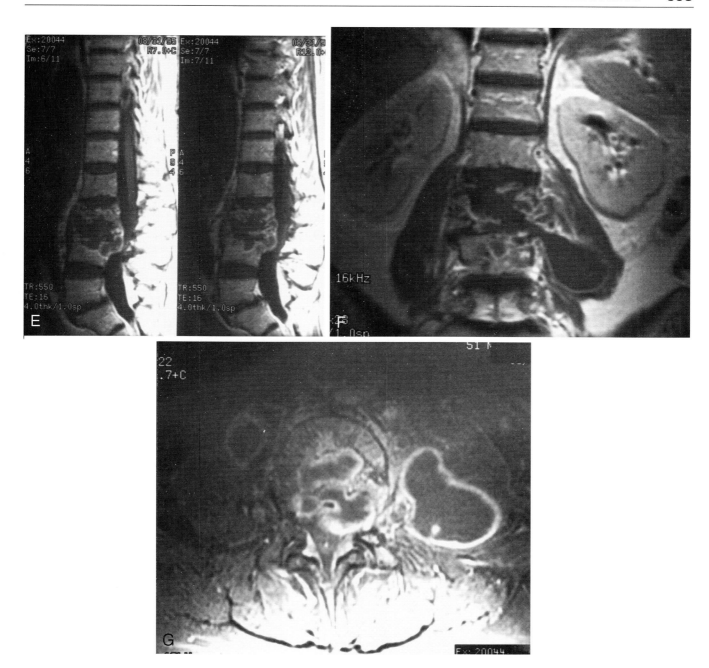

FIGURE 28.7—continued

E. Gadolinium-enhanced T1-weighted sagittal sequence shows enhancement at the periphery of the collapsed and necrotic vertebrae. F. Gadolinium-enhanced coronal MRI sequence shows peripheral enhancement of a low-signal mass within the left psoas muscle. The psoas abscess was found to be a sterile loculation of pus that communicated with the L2-L3 region. G. Gadolinium-enhanced axial MRI sequence shows the same findings noted in E and F.

that was maintained over time, whereas those treated with débridement alone had progressive kyphosis. Significant change was not found when the 6-month evaluations were compared with the 10-year or 15-year follow-up data (181, 273).

Children treated with radical surgery and grafting had less kyphosis at 6-month follow-up than they had preoperatively; the group treated with débridement alone had an increased deformity at 6-month follow-up. There was a tendency for some spontaneous correction during growth in children treated with débridement alone, making the two groups similar when evaluated 15 years postoperatively (271, 272). Other independent studies have demonstrated the effectiveness of débridement and fusion and recommend that procedure over simple débridement alone (11, 75, 115, 121, 133, 140).

When an operation is indicated, it is easier to do

it early, because abscesses tend to dissect along tissue planes. If surgery is delayed, fibrosis makes the procedure technically much more difficult. There is a direct correlation between the duration of neurologic symptoms before operation and the time for recovery from paraplegia (67, 118). Surgery may also be performed for late-onset paralysis associated with cord compression by a hard bony ridge in association with kyphosis.

In the Hong Kong procedure, the spine is approached anteriorly so that the affected area may be dealt with most directly. Débridement, decompression, and fusion in the thoracic spine may be performed through a transthoracic approach, through a costotransversectomy, or through an extrapleural anterolateral approach. The latter has the theoretic benefit of avoiding a tuberculous empyema (97). However, no studies have demonstrated any actual advantage in an extrapleural approach over a standard thoracotomy. In tuberculosis, the periosteum generally is thicker and frequently adherent to the pleura; therefore, it often is necessary to dissect in a subperiosteal plane for exposure. The transthoracic approach is more successful than a modified costotransversectomy. Kirkaldy-Willis and Thomas found that the fusion rate was 95% after a transthoracic approach, and only 78% after a costotransversectomy (140). The mortality was 3% and 8%, respectively. The lumbar spine may be exposed through a retroperitoneal approach. Lesions between C3 and C7 may be approached through the anterior triangle or the posterior triangle. The latter may be preferable in some cases, because abscess cavities often extend into the posterior triangle, making dissection easier (114).

The sequestered bone and caseous material must be débrided back to bleeding bone above and below and back to the posterior longitudinal ligament. The decompression should go back to the dura in cases of neurologic deficit when spinal cord decompression is necessary (179). The angular deformity is corrected by insertion of a strut graft. Autogenous bone grafting at the time of the primary débridement is reliable in adults and children (5, 11, 67, 115, 121, 133, 140, 181, 291). The choice of graft material is based on considerations of graft incorporation and structural support. The grafts used most frequently are iliac crest and rib. Iliac crest is preferable to rib, especially in patients with a large defect (118, 133, 223). Vascularized rib strut grafts have reportedly been effective in children (193). Fibular grafts provide good structural support, but the large amount of cortical bone may be undesirable in cases of infection. In general, autograft is preferred to allograft bone, although there have been no series comparing the two types of graft.

Because of the potential for wound dehiscence in these patients, who are frequently immunocompromised and have poor wound healing potential, the wounds should be closed in layers with interrupted nonabsorbable sutures. In patients with lesions involving more than two vertebral bodies, a period of bed rest followed by external support in a thoracolumbosacral orthosis is recommended until the fusion becomes consolidated (223).

The only indication for a laminectomy in the treatment of spinal tuberculosis is atypical disease involving the neural arch and causing posterior spinal cord compression (83, 135, 196, 245). It is also reasonable in rare circumstances with posterior epidural or intradural tuberculomas without bony involvement (10, 158). In all other cases, laminectomy is contraindicated because the procedure destabilizes the spine and may lead to further deformity and neurologic damage (245).

If a laminectomy is indicated, a fusion should also be performed if any of the facets are removed or if a kyphotic deformity is already present (135). Some authors recommend a posterior fusion in addition to an anterior fusion to eliminate the risk of increasing deformity in children (140, 191). In a long-term follow-up study Upadhyay and colleagues found that a prophylactic posterior spinal arthrodesis is not indicated (273). They followed 33 children, who were aged 10 years or younger at the time of anterior radical resection and fusion, for 15 years. They found that the growth of the posterior portion of the spine does not contribute to the progression of deformity after that procedure. Fountain and associates found that progressive kyphosis developed in only three of 31 children with solid anterior fusions (74). They recommend performing a supplementary posterior fusion only if progressive deformity is noted.

Some authors recommend a two-stage procedure with an instrumented posterior fusion followed by anterior débridement and fusion. The rationale for a two-stage procedure is that after anterior débridement and fusion, a significant portion of the correction is lost in the first 6 to 24 months postoperatively (138, 151). Anterior grafts do not always provide stable fixation, especially in cases in which the graft spans more than two disc spaces (223).

Moon and colleagues reported on 39 adults undergoing a two-stage procedure with the instrumented posterior fusion followed by anterior débridement and fusion either in the same operative setting or in sequential operations (192). They were able to achieve excellent deformity correction without prior anterior release, and the loss of correction did not exceed 3°. The tuberculosis was completely cured in all patients.

Güven and colleagues recommend a single-stage

posterior approach with rigid internal fixation without any anterior procedure (99). They described 10 patients who underwent that procedure. All patients achieved a stable fusion with resolution of the tuberculosis, and the mean loss of correction was only 3.4°. They used pedicle-screw instrumentation in most cases, whereas Moon and associates generally used Harrington distraction rodding or Luque segmental spinal wiring (192). Güven and colleagues do not recommend the single-stage posterior approach when the patient has paraplegia, when a huge abscess requiring drainage is present, or when there is multisegmental involvement (more than two vertebral bodies) (99).

The risk of using spinal instrumentation despite active tuberculous infection was studied by Oga and colleagues (203). They evaluated 11 patients undergoing combined posterior instrumented fusion and anterior débridement and fusion. None of the patients had persistence or recurrence of infection; no kyphotic deformities occurred after operation. The authors also evaluated the adherence properties of *Mycobacterium tuberculosis* and *S. epidermidis* to stainless steel. Scanning electron microscopy showed that the surface of the stainless steel was heavily colonized by staphylococcus and covered with a thick adherent biofilm. In contrast, only a few biofilm-covered microcolonies of *Mycobacterium tuberculosis* were observed. They concluded that posterior instrumentation is not associated with persistence or recurrence of spinal tuberculosis infection.

Rare case reports have documented successful results in treating spinal infections with anterior decompression and fusion with anterior instrumentation (144). Although anterior instrumentation may be effective in selected cases, the author is aware of one unreported case in which anterior instrumentation failed because of the poor bone quality of the vertebral bodies adjacent to the infection. I do not recommend anterior instrumentation in the presence of spinal infection.

Complications of surgical treatment are frequent. The operative risk is greatest in elderly patients with extensive disease. In one series the operative mortality was 2.9%, and an additional 1% of the patients died of the disease later (119). Early complications include wound sepsis, pleural effusion, pulmonary embolism, cerebrospinal fluid fistula into the pleural cavity, ileus, progressive neurologic deficit, damage to the ureter, loss of graft fixation or graft fracture, atelectasis, pneumonia, air leak, Horner's syndrome, and injury to one of the great vessels (120). Late complications include graft resorption, graft fracture, nonunion, and progressive kyphosis (133, 222, 223).

The prognosis of patients treated for tuberculous spondylitis depends on the age and general health of the patient, the severity and duration of the neurologic deficit, and the treatment selected.

Before the advent of chemotherapy, the mortality rate for patients treated nonoperatively was 12 to 43% (2, 52). The rate for patients with a neurologic deficit was close to 60% (20). With the chemotherapeutic regimens now available, the mortality rate should be less than 5% if the disease is diagnosed early, the patient complies with the regimen, and follow-up is frequent (3, 157). The relapse rate should approach zero (157).

Progressive kyphosis is a significant cosmetic deformity and may cause a neurologic deficit, respiratory failure, or cardiac failure. Nonoperative treatment is associated with a significantly higher rate of kyphotic deformity than is surgical management (222). Posterior spinal instrumentation with or without anterior débridement and fusion provides the best results for maintenance of spinal alignment (99, 192, 203). Radical débridement and fusion allow slight improvement in the kyphotic deformity (137, 151, 273). Anterior débridement alone does not prevent kyphotic deformity (273).

The risk factors for a neural deficit include older age, more cephalad level of infection, increased loss of vertebral body height, and absence of paraspinal abscesses (259). These risk factors seem self-evident except for the absence of extensive paravertebral abscess. The authors postulated that the drainage of pus and debris from the spinal canal releases pressure on the cord (259). Patients with neurologic deficit may improve spontaneously without operation or chemotherapy or with chemotherapy alone, but, in general, the prognosis is improved with early operation (11, 81, 83, 157, 168, 269).

In one study, 94% of neurologically impaired patients recovered normal function after anterior decompression; only 79% totally recovered after nonoperative management (157). In a separate study, when patients with a neurologic deficit were operated on only if they failed to respond to an initial course of antibiotics, the overall success rate was 78.5% (269). Patients who have an atrophic cord, as seen on CT myelography preoperatively, usually do poorly after decompression (94).

Patients with cervical spine involvement are at high risk for neurologic deficit but do well after anterior débridement and fusion.

The rate of bony fusion varies with the treatment regimen. Spontaneous fusion occurred in 27% of patients treated with bed rest in a plaster shell without chemotherapy or surgery (52). The fusion rates in patients treated by ambulatory chemotherapy alone were 9% at 6 months, 26% at 12 months, 50% at 18 months, and 85% at 5 years. After débridement without surgical fusion, the rate was almost identical to nonoperative treatment with fusion in 3% by 6 months, 23% by 12 months, 52% by 18 months, and 84% at 5 years. After the Hong Kong procedure, fusion occurred in 28% by 6 months, 70% by 12 months, 85% by 18 months, and 92% at 5 years (179).

References

1. Abbey DM, Turner DM, Warson JS, et al. Treatment of postoperative wound infections following spinal fusion with instrumentation. J Spinal Disord 1995; 8:278–283.
2. Adams ZB. Tuberculosis of the spine in children: a review of 63 cases from the Lakeville State Sanatorium. J Bone Joint Surg 1940;22:860–861.
3. Adendorff JJ, Boeke EJ, Lazarus C. Tuberculosis of the spine: results of management of 300 patients. J R Coll Surg Edinb 1987;32:152–155.
4. Alexander CJ. The aetiology of juvenile spondylarthritis (discitis). Clin Radiol 1970;21:178–187.
5. Allen AR, Stevenson AW. Follow-up notes on articles previously published in the journal: a 10-year follow-up of combined drug therapy and early fusion in bone tuberculosis. J Bone Joint Surg 1967;49A:1001–1003.
6. Allen BL, Ferguson RL. The Galveston experience with L-rod instrumentation for adolescent idiopathic scoliosis. Clin Orthop 1988;229:59–69.
7. An HS, Vaccaro AR, Dolinskas CA, et al. Differentiation between spinal tumors and infections with magnetic resonance imaging. Spine 1991;16(Suppl):S334–S338.
8. Angtuaco EJ, McConnell JR, Chadduck WM, et al. MR imaging of spinal epidural sepsis. AJR 1987;149:1249–1253.
9. Armstrong P, Green G, Irving JD. Needle aspiration/biopsy of the spine in suspected disc space infection. Br J Radiol 1978;51:333–337.
10. Babhulkar SS, Tayade WB, Babhulkar SK. Atypical spinal tuberculosis. J Bone Joint Surg 1984;66B:239–242.
11. Bailey HL, Gabriel SM, Hodgson AR, et al. Tuberculosis of the spine in children: operative findings and results in 100 consecutive patients treated by removal of the lesion and anterior grafting. J Bone Joint Surg 1972;54A:1633–1657.
12. Baker AS, Ojemann RG, Swartz MN, et al. Spinal epidural abscess. N Engl J Med 1975;293:463–468.
13. Bartels RHMA, Gonera EG, van der Spek JAN, et al. Intramedullary spinal cord abscess. Spine 1995; 20:1199–1204.
14. Bergman I, Wald ER, Meyer JD, et al. Epidural abscess and vertebral osteomyelitis following serial lumbar punctures. Pediatrics 1983;72:476–480.
15. Bertino RE, Porter BA, Stimac GK, et al. Imaging spinal osteomyelitis and epidural abscess with short T1 inversion recovery (STIR). Am J Neuroradiol 1988; 9:563–564.
16. Bircher MD, Tasker T, Crawshaw C, et al. Discitis following lumbar surgery. Spine 1988;13:98–102.
17. Blumenthal S, Gill K. Complications of the Wiltse pedicle screw fixation system. Spine 1993;18:1867–1871.
18. Bonfiglio M, Lange TA, Kim YM. Pyogenic vertebral osteomyelitis: disc space infections. Clin Orthop 1973;96:234–247.
19. Boston HC Jr, Bianco AJ Jr, Rhodes KH. Disk space infections in children. Orthop Clin North Am 1975; 6:953–964.
20. Bosworth DM, Pietra AD, Rahilly G. Paraplegia resulting from tuberculosis of the spine. J Bone Joint Surg 1953;35A:735–740.
21. Browder J, Meyers R. Infection of the spinal epidural space: an aspect of vertebral osteomyelitis. Am J Surg 1937;37:4–26.
22. Browder J, Meyers R. Pyogenic infections of the spinal epidural space: a consideration of the anatomic and physiologic pathology. Surgery 1941;10:296–308.
23. Brown MD, Tsaltas TT. Studies on the permeability of the intervertebral disc during skeletal maturation. Spine 1976;1:240–244.
24. Brugieres P, Revel MP, Dumas JL, et al. CT guided vertebral biopsy: a report of 89 cases. J Neuroradiol 1991; 18:351–359.
25. Bruns J, Maas R. Advantages of diagnosing bacterial spondylitis with magnetic resonance imaging. Arch Orthop Trauma Surg 1989;108:30–35.
26. Bruschwein DA, Brown ML, McLeod RA. Gallium scintigraphy in the evaluation of the disk space infections: concise communication. J Nucl Med 1980; 21:925–927.
27. Burke JF. The effective period of preventive antibiotic action in experimental incisions and dermal lesions. Surgery 1961;50:161–168.
28. Butler EG, Dohrmann PJ, Stark RJ. Spinal subdural abscess. Clin Exp Neurol 1988;25:67–70.
29. Capener N. The evolution of lateral rhachiotomy. J Bone Joint Surg 1954;36B:173–179.
30. Cardan E, Nanulescu M. Epidural lavage for extensive epidural suppuration. Anaesthesia 1987;42:1023.
31. Carragee EJ, van der Vlugt T, Billys J. The changing face of pyogenic vertebral osteomyelitis. Presented at North American Spine Society, October 21, 1995, Washington, DC.
32. Carvell JE, Maclarnon JC. Chronic osteomyelitis of the thoracic spine due to *Salmonella typhi:* a case report. Spine 1981;6:527–530.
33. Cierny G, Mader JT. Approach to adult osteomyelitis. Orthop Rev 1987;16:259–270.
34. Cleveland M. Tuberculosis of the spine: a clinical study of 203 patients from Sea View and St. Luke's Hospital. American Review of Tuberculosis 1940; 41:215–231.
35. Cohn SL, Akbarnia BA, Luisiri A, et al. Disk space infection versus lumbar Scheuermann's disease. Orthopedics 1988;11:330–335.
36. Collert S. Osteomyelitis of the spine. Acta Orthop Scand 1977;48:283–290.
37. Compere EL, Garrison M. Correlation of pathologic and roentgenologic findings in tuberculosis and pyogenic infections of the vertebra: the fate of the intervertebral disk. Ann Surg 1936;104:1038–1067.
38. Connor PM, Darden BV. Cervical discography complications and clinical efficacy. Spine 1993;18:2035–2038.

39. Corboy JR, Price RW. Myelitis and toxic, inflammatory, and infectious disorders. Curr Opin Neurol Neurosurg 1993;6:564–570.
40. Corradini EW, Turney MF, Browder EJ. Spinal epidural infection. NY State J Med 1948;48:2367–2370.
41. Coventry MB, Ghormley RK, Kernohan JW. The intervertebral disc: its microscopic anatomy and pathology. Part I: Anatomy, development, and physiology. J Bone Joint Surg 1945;27:105–112.
42. Craig F. Vertebral body biopsy. J Bone Joint Surg 1956; 38A:93–102.
43. Crawford AH, Kucharzyk DW, Ruida R, et al. Diskitis in children. Clin Orthop 1991;266:70–79.
44. Cruse PJE, Foord R. A five-year prospective study of 23, 649 surgical wounds. Arch Surg 1973;107:206–209.
45. Curling OD, Gower DJ, McWhorter JM. Changing concepts in spinal epidural abscess: a report of 29 cases. Neurosurgery 1990;27:185–192.
46. Dandy WE. Abscesses and inflammatory tumors in the spinal epidural space (so-called pachymeningitis externa). Arch Surg 1926;13:477–494.
47. Danner RL, Hartman BJ. Update of spinal epidural abscess: 35 cases and review of the literature. Rev Infect Dis 1987;9:265–274.
48. Darouiche RO, Hamill RJ, Greenberg SB, et al. Bacterial spinal epidural abscess: review of 43 cases and literature survey. Medicine 1992;71:369–385.
49. De Villiers JC, de Clüver PF. Spinal epidural abscess in children. S Afr J Surg 1978;16:149–155.
50. Des Prez RM, Heim CR. Mycobacterium tuberculosis. In: Mandell GL, Douglas RG Jr, Bennett JE, eds. Principles and practice of infectious diseases. 3d ed. New York: Churchill Livingstone, 1990:1877–1906.
51. Digby JM, Kersley JB. Pyogenic nontuberculous spinal infection: an analysis of 30 cases. J Bone Joint Surg 1979;61B:47–55.
52. Dobson J. Tuberculosis of the spine: an analysis of the results of conservative treatment and of the factors influencing the prognosis. J Bone Joint Surg 1951; 33B:517–531.
53. Doub HP, Badgley CE. The roentgen signs of tuberculosis of the vertebral body. AJR 1932;27:827–837.
54. Doyle JR. Narrowing of the intervertebral-disc space in children: presumably an infectious lesion of the disc. J Bone Joint Surg 1960;42A:1191–1200.
55. Du Lac P, Panuel M, Devred P, et al. MRI of disc space infection in infants and children. Pediatr Radiol 1990; 20:175–178.
56. Eismont FJ, Bohlman HH. Posterior methylmethacrylate fixation for cervical trauma. Spine 1981;6:347–353.
57. Eismont FJ, Bohlman HH, Soni PL, et al. Pyogenic and fungal vertebral osteomyelitis with paralysis. J Bone Joint Surg 1983;65A:19–29.
58. Eismont FJ, Bohlman HH, Soni PL, et al. Vertebral osteomyelitis in infants. J Bone Joint Surg 1982;64B:32–35.
59. Eismont FJ, Green BA, Brown MD, et al. Coexistent infection and tumor of the spine: a report of three cases. J Bone Joint Surg 1987;69A:452–458.
60. El-Gindi S, Aref S, Salama M. Infection of intervertebral discs after operation. J Bone Joint Surg 1976; 58B:114–116.
61. Emery SE, Chan DPK, Woodward HR. Treatment of hematogenous pyogenic vertebral osteomyelitis with anterior debridement and primary bone grafting. Spine 1989;14:284–291.
62. Erntell M, Holtas S, Norlin K. Magnetic resonance imaging in the diagnosis of spinal epidural abscess. Scand J Infect Dis 1988;20:323–327.
63. Esses SI, Sachs BL, Dreyzin V. Complications associated with the technique of pedicle screw fixation: a selected survey of ABS members. Spine 1993;18: 2231–2238.
64. Faciszewski T, Winter RB, Lonstein JE, et al. The surgical and medical perioperative complications of anterior spinal fusion surgery in the thoracic and lumbar spine in adults: a review of 1223 procedures. Spine 1995;20:1592–1599.
65. Fang D, Cheung KMC, Dos Remedios IDM, et al. Pyogenic vertebral osteomyelitis: treatment by anterior spinal debridement and fusion. J Spinal Disord 1994; 7:173–180.
66. Feldenzer JA, McKeever PE, Schaberg DR. The pathogenesis of spinal epidural abscess: microangiographic studies in an experimental model. J Neurosurg 1988; 69:110–114.
67. Felländer M. Paraplegia in spondylitis: results of operative treatment. Paraplegia 1975;13:75–88.
68. Fertel D, Pitchenik AE. Tuberculosis in acquired immune deficiency syndrome. Semin Respir Infect 1989; 4:198–205.
69. Fine PG, Hare BD, Zahniser JC. Epidural abscess following epidural catheterization in a chronic pain patient: a diagnostic dilemma. Anesthesiology 1988; 69:422–424.
70. Fischer EG, Greene CS Jr, Winston KR. Spinal epidural abscess in children. Neurosurgery 1981;9:257–260.
71. Fitzgerald RH, Thompson RL. Current concepts review: cephalosporin antibiotics in the prevention and treatment of musculoskeletal sepsis. J Bone Joint Surg 1983;65A:1201–1205.
72. Forlenza SW, Axelrod JL, Grieco MH. Pott's disease in heroin addicts. JAMA 1979;241:379–380.
73. Forsythe M, Rothman RH. New concepts in the diagnosis and treatment of infections of the cervical spine. Orthop Clin North Am 1978;9:1039–1051.
74. Fountain SS, Hsu LCS, Yau ACMC, et al. Progressive kyphosis following solid anterior spine fusion in children with tuberculosis of the spine: a long term study. J Bone Joint Surg 1975;57A:1104–1107.
75. Fountain SS. A single stage combined surgical approach for vertebral resections. J Bone Joint Surg 1979; 61A:1011–1017.
76. Fouquet B, Goupille P, Jattiot F, et al. Discitis after lumbar disc surgery: features of "aseptic" and "septic" forms. Spine 1992;17:356–358.
77. Frank CJ, Brantigan JW, Cronan J. Early primary closure of postoperative spinal infections using a local myocutaneous flap. Presented at the 10th Annual Meeting of the North American Spine Society, October 19, 1995, Washington, DC.

78. Fraser RAR, Ratzan K, Wolpert SM, et al. Spinal subdural empyema. Arch Neurol 1973;28:235–238.
79. Frederickson B, Yuan H, Orlans R. Management and outcome of pyogenic vertebral osteomyelitis. Clin Orthop 1978;131:160–167.
80. Freilich D, Swash, M. Diagnosis and management of tuberculous paraplegia with special reference to tuberculous radiculomyelitis. J Neurol Neurosurg Psychiatry 1979;42:12–18.
81. Friedman B. Chemotherapy of tuberculosis of the spine. J Bone Joint Surg 1966;48A:451–474.
82. Gaines DL, Moe JH, Bocklage J. Management of wound infections following Harrington instrumentation and spine fusion. J Bone Joint Surg 1970;52A:404–405.
83. Garceau GJ, Brady TA. Pott's paraplegia. J Bone Joint Surg 1950;32A:87–95.
84. Garcia A Jr, Grantham SA. Hematogenous pyogenic vertebral osteomyelitis. J Bone Joint Surg 1960;42A:429–436.
85. Gardner RD, Cammisa FP, Eismont FJ, et al. Nongranulomatous spinal epidural abscesses. Orthop Trans 1989;13:562–563.
86. Garrido E, Rosenwasser RH. Experience with the suction-irrigation technique in the management of spinal epidural infection. Neurosurgery 1983;12:678–679.
87. Gebhard JS, Brugman JL. Percutaneous diskectomy for the treatment of bacterial diskitis. Spine 1994;19:855–857.
88. Genster HG, Andersen MJF. Spinal osteomyelitis complicating urinary tract infection. J Urol 1972;107:109–111.
89. Gepstein R, Eismont FJ. Postoperative spine infections. In: Garfin SR, ed. Complications of spine surgery. Baltimore: Williams & Wilkins, 1989:302–322.
90. Ghelman B, Lospinuso MF, Levine DB, et al. Percutaneous CT guided biopsy of the thoracic and lumbar spine. Orthop Trans 1990;14:635.
91. Ghormley RK, Bickel WH, Dickson DD. A study of acute infectious lesions of the intervertebral discs. South Med J 1940;33:347–352.
92. Glassman SD, Dimar JR, Puno RM, et al. Treatment of spinal wound infections using antibiotic impregnated PMMA beads. Presented at the 10th Annual Meeting of the North American Spine Society, October 20, 1995, Washington, DC.
93. Golimbu C, Firooznia H, Rafii M. CT of osteomyelitis of the spine. AJR 1984;142:159–163.
94. Govender S, Charles RW, Naidoo KS, et al. Results of surgical decompression in chronic tuberculous paraplegia. S Afr Med J 1988;74:58–59.
95. Grand CM, Bank WO, Baleriaux D, et al. Gadolinium enhancement of vertebral endplates following lumbar disc surgery. Neuroradiology 1993;35:503–505.
96. Graziano GP, Sidhu KS. Salvage reconstruction in acute and late sequelae from pyogenic thoracolumbar infection. J Spinal Disord 1993;6:199–207.
97. Guirguis AR. Pott's paraplegia. J Bone Joint Surg 1967;49B:658–667.
98. Gurr KR, McAfee PC. Cotrel-Dubousset instrumentation in adults: a preliminary report. Spine 1988;13:510–520.
99. Güven O, Kumano K, Yalçin S, Karahan M, Tsuji S. A single stage posterior approach and rigid fixation for preventing kyphosis in the treatment of spinal tuberculosis. Spine 1994;19:1039–1043.
100. Haase D, Martin R, Marrie T. Radionuclide imaging in pyogenic vertebral osteomyelitis. Clin Nucl Med 1980;5:533–537.
101. Hakin RN, Burt AA, Cook JB. Acute spinal epidural abscess. Paraplegia 1979;17:330–336.
102. Halpern AA, Rinsky LA, Fountain S, et al. Coccidiomycosis of the spine: unusual roentgenographic presentations. Clin Orthop 1979;140:78–79.
103. Hancock DO. A study of 49 patients with acute spinal extradural abscess. Paraplegia 1973;10:285–288.
104. [Reference deleted.]
105. Hart J. Case of encysted abscess in the centre of spinal cord. Dublin Hospital Report 1830;5:522–524.
106. Hassler O. The human intervertebral disc: a microangiographical study on its vascular supply at various ages. Acta Orthop Scand 1970;40:765–772.
107. Hatch ES. Acute osteomyelitis of the spine: report of case with recovery and review of the literature. New Orleans Med Surg J 1931;83:861–873.
108. Heary RF, Hunt CD, Krieger AJ, et al. HIV status does not affect microbiologic spectrum or neurologic outcome in spinal infections. Surg Neurol 1994;42:417–423.
109. Heary R, Vaccaro A, Masa J, et al. Infections following gunshot wounds to the spine resulting in a neurologic deficit. Presented at the 10th Annual Meeting of the North American Spine Society, October 18–21, 1995, Washington, DC.
110. Heggeness MH, Esses SI, Errico T, et al. Late infection of spinal instrumentation by hematogenous seeding. Spine 1993;18:492–496.
111. [Reference deleted.]
112. Heusner AP. Nontuberculosis spinal epidural infections. N Engl J Med 1948;239:845–854.
113. Hlavin ML, Kaminski HJ, Ross JS, et al. Spinal epidural abscess: a 10-year prospective. Neurosurgery 1990;27:177–184.
114. Hodgson AR. An approach to the cervical spine (C3–C7). Clin Orthop 1965;39:129–134.
115. Hodgson AR. Report on the findings and results in 300 cases of Pott's disease treated by anterior fusion of the spine. J West Pacific Orthop Assoc 1964;1:3.
116. Hodgson AR, Skinsnes OK, Leong CY. The pathogenesis of Pott's paraplegia. J Bone Joint Surg 1967;49A:1147–1156.
117. Hodgson AR, Stock FE. Anterior spinal fusion: a preliminary communication on the radical treatment of Pott's disease and Pott's paraplegia. Br J Surg 1956;44:266–275.
118. Hodgson AR, Stock FE. Anterior spine fusion for the treatment of tuberculosis of the spine: the operative findings and results of treatment in the first 100 cases. J Bone Joint Surg 1960;42A:295–310.
119. Hodgson AR, Stock FE, Fang HSY, et al. Anterior spinal fusion: the operative approach and pathological findings in 412 patients with Pott's disease of the spine. Br J Surg 1960;48:172–178.
120. Hodgson AR, Yau ACMC. Anterior surgical ap-

proaches to the spinal column. Recent Adv Orthop 1969;1:289–323.
121. Hodgson AR, Yau A, Kwon JS, et al. A clinical study of 100 consecutive cases of Pott's paraplegia. Clin Orthop 1964;36:128–150.
122. Holliday PO, Davis CH, Shaffner L de S. Intervertebral disc space infection in a child presenting as a psoas abscess: case report. Neurosurgery 1980;7:395–397.
123. Horwitz NH, Curtin JA. Prophylactic antibiotics and wound infections following laminectomy for lumbar disc herniation: a retrospective study. J Neurosurg 1975;43:727–731.
124. Hsu LCS, Cheng CL, Leong JCY. Pott's paraplegia of late onset: the cause of compression and results after anterior decompression. J Bone Joint Surg 1988; 70B:534–538.
125. Hulme A, Dott NM. Spinal epidural abscess. Br Med J 1954;1:164–168.
126. Incavo SJ, Muller DL, Krag MH, et al. Vertebral osteomyelitis caused by *Clostridium difficile:* a case report and review of the literature. Spine 1988;13:111–113.
127. Jones RE, Bucholz RW, Schaefer SD. Cervical osteomyelitis complicating transpharyngeal gunshot wounds to the neck. J Trauma 1979;19:630–634.
128. Jonsson B, Soderholm R, Stromqvist B. Erythrocyte sedimentation rate after lumbar spine surgery. Spine 1991;16:1049–1050.
129. Kalen V, Isono SS, Cho CS, et al. Charcot arthropathy of the spine in long-standing paraplegia. Spine 1987; 12:42–47.
130. Kattapuram SV, Phillips WC, Boyd R. CT in pyogenic osteomyelitis of the spine. AJR 1983;140:1199–1201.
131. Kaufman DM, Kaplan JG, Litman N. Infectious agents in spinal epidural abscesses. Neurology 1980;30:844–850.
132. Keller RB, Pappas AM. Infections after spinal fusion using internal fixation instrumentation. Orthop Clin North Am 1972;3:99–111.
133. Kemp HBS, Jackson JW, Jeremiah JD, et al. Anterior fusion of the spine for infective lesions in adults. J Bone Joint Surg 1973;55B:715–734.
134. Kemp HBS, Jackson JW, Jeremiah JD, et al. Pyogenic infections occurring primarily in intervertebral discs. J Bone Joint Surg 1973;55B:698–714.
135. Kemp HBS, Jackson JW, Shaw NC. Laminectomy in paraplegia due to infective spondylosis. Br J Surg 1974;61:66–72.
136. Kihtir T, Ivatury RR, Simon R, et al. Management of transperitoneal gunshot wounds of the spine. J Trauma 1991;31:1579–1583.
137. Kim BJ, Koh S, Lim Y, et al. The clinical study of the tuberculous spondylitis. J Korean Orthop Assoc 1993; 28:2221–2232.
138. Kim NH, Lee HM, Suh JS. Magnetic resonance imaging for the diagnosis of tuberculous spondylitis. Spine 1994;19:2451–2455.
139. King DM, Mayo KM. Infective lesions of the vertebral column. Clin Orthop 1973;96:248–253.
140. Kirkaldy-Willis WH, Thomas TG. Anterior approaches in the diagnosis and treatment of infections of the vertebral bodies. J Bone Joint Surg 1965; 47A:87–110.
141. Klink BK, Thurman RT, Wittpenn GP, et al. Muscle flap closure for salvage of complex back wounds. Spine 1994;19:1467–1470.
142. Koppel BS, Tuchman AJ, Mangiardi JR. Epidural spinal infection in intravenous drug abusers. Arch Neurol 1988;45:1331–1337.
143. Korovessis P, Sidiropoulos P, Piperos G, et al. Spinal epidural abscess complicated closed vertebral fracture. Spine 1993;18:671–674.
144. Kostuik JP. Anterior spinal cord decompression for lesions of the thoracic and lumbar spine. Techniques, new methods of internal fixation, results. Spine 1983; 8:512–531.
145. Krespi YP, Grossman BG, Berktold RE, et al. Mediastinitis and neck abscess following cervical spine fracture. Am J Otolaryngol 1985;6:29–31.
146. Kulowski J. Pyogenic osteomyelitis of the spine: an analysis and discussion of 102 cases. J Bone Joint Surg 1936;18:343–364.
147. Kupcha PC, An HS, Cotler JM. Gunshot wounds to the cervical spine. Spine 1990;15:1058–1063.
148. Kuriloff DB, Blaugrund S, Ryan J, et al. Delayed neck infection following anterior spine surgery. Laryngoscopy 1987;97:1094–1098.
149. Kurokowa Y, Hashi K, Fujishige M, et al. Spinal subdural empyema diagnosed by MRI and recovered by conservative treatment. NoToShinkei 1989;41:513–517.
150. Lascari AD, Graham MH, MacQueen JC. Intervertebral disk infection in children. J Pediatr 1967;70:751–757.
151. Lee EY, Hahn MS. A study of influences of the anterior intervertebral fusion upon the correct ability of kyphosis in tuberculous spondylitis. J Korean Orthop Assoc 1968;3:31–40.
152. Lerner PI. *Nocardia* species. In: Mandell GL, Douglas RG Jr, Bennett JE, eds. Principles and practice of infectious diseases. 3d ed. New York: Churchill Livingstone, 1990:1926–1932.
153. Levy ML, Wieder BH, Schneider J, et al. Subdural empyema of the cervical spine: clinical pathologic correlates and magnetic resonance imaging. J Neurosurg 1993;79:929–935.
154. Lewis R, Gorbach S, Altner P. Spinal pseudomonas chondro-osteomyelitis in heroin users. N Engl J Med 1972;286:1303.
155. Leys D, Lesoin F, Viaud C. Decreased morbidity from acute bacterial spinal epidural abscesses using computed tomography and nonsurgical treatment in selected patients. Ann Neurol 1985;17:350–355.
156. Lifeso RM. Pyogenic spinal sepsis in adults. Spine 1990;15:1265–1271.
157. Lifeso RM, Weaver P, Harder EH. Tuberculous spondylitis in adults. J Bone Joint Surg 1985;67A:1405–1413.
158. Lin SK, Wu T, Wai YY. Intramedullary spinal tuberculomas during treatment of tuberculous meningitis. Clin Neurol Neurosurg 1994;96:71–78.
159. Lin SS, Vaccaro AR, Reisch S, et al. Low velocity gunshot wounds to the spine with an associated transperitoneal injury. J Spinal Disord 1995;8:136–144.
160. Lindholm TS, Pylkkanen P. Discitis following removal of intervertebral disc. Spine 1982;7:618–622.

161. Lonstein J, Winter R, Moe J. Wound infection with Harrington instrumentation and spine fusion for scoliosis. Clin Orthop 1973;96:222–223.
162. Lowe J, Kaplan L, Liebergall M, et al. Serratia osteomyelitis causing neurological deterioration after spine fracture: a report of two cases. J Bone Joint Surg 1989; 71B:256–258.
163. Lownie SP, Ferguson GG. Spinal subdural empyema complicating cervical discography. Spine 1989; 14:1415–1417.
164. Mader JT, Cierny G. The principles of the use of preventive antibiotics. Clin Orthop 1984;190:72–75.
165. Maier RV, Carrico CJ, Heinbach DM. Pyogenic osteomyelitis of axial bones following civilian gunshot wounds. Am J Surg 1979;137:378–380.
166. Malawski SK, Lukawski S. Pyogenic infection of the spine. Clin Orthop 1991;272:58–66.
167. Mampalam TJ, Rosegay H, Andrews BT. Nonoperative treatment of spinal epidural infections. J Neurosurg 1989;71:208–210.
168. Martin NS. Pott's paraplegia: a report of 120 cases. J Bone Joint Surg 1971;53B:596–608.
169. Maruyama H, Gejyo F, Arkawa M. Clinical studies of destructive spondyloarthropathy in long-term hemodialysis patients. Nephron 1992;61:37–44.
170. Massie JB, Heller JG, Abitbol JJ, et al. Postoperative posterior spinal wound infections. Clin Orthop 1992; 284:99–108.
171. Mathuriya SN, Khosla VK, Banerjee AK. Intradural extramedullary tuberculous spinal granulomas. Clin Neurol Neurosurg 1988;90:155–158.
172. McAfee PC, Bohlman HH, Ducker T, et al. Failure of stabilization of the spine with methylmethacrylate. J Bone Joint Surg 1986;68A:1157.
173. McGee-Collett M, Johnston IH. Spinal epidural abscess: presentation and treatment. Med J Aust 1991; 155:14–17.
174. McHenry MC, Duchesneau PM, Keys TF. Vertebral osteomyelitis presenting as spinal compression fracture: six patients with underlying osteoporosis. Arch Intern Med 1988;148:417–423.
175. Medical Research Council Working Party on Tuberculosis of the Spine. A controlled trial of six-month and nine-month regimens of chemotherapy in patients undergoing radical surgery for tuberculosis of the spine in Hong Kong. Tubercle 1986;67:243–259.
176. Medical Research Council Working Party on Tuberculosis of the Spine. A controlled trial of debridement and ambulatory treatment in the management of tuberculosis of the spine in patients on standard chemotherapy: a study in Bulawayo, Rhodesia. J Trop Med Hyg 1974;77:72–92.
177. Medical Research Council Working Party on Tuberculosis of the Spine. A controlled trial of anterior spinal fusion and debridement in the surgical management of tuberculosis of the spine in patients on standard chemotherapy: a study in two centers in South Africa. Tubercle 1978;59:79–105.
178. Medical Research Council Working Party on Tuberculosis of the Spine. A controlled trial of ambulant out-patient treatment and in-patient rest in bed in the management of tuberculosis of the spine in young Korean patients on standard chemotherapy: a study in Masan, Korea. J Bone Joint Surg 1973;55B:678–697.
179. Medical Research Council Working Party on Tuberculosis of the Spine. Five-year assessments of controlled trials of ambulatory treatment, debridement, and anterior spinal fusion in the management of tuberculosis of the spine: studies in Vulawayo (Rhodesia) and in Hong Kong. J Bone Joint Surg 1978; 60B:163–177.
180. Medical Research Council Working Party on Tuberculosis of the Spine. A comparison of 6 or 9 month course regime of chemotherapy in patients receiving ambulatory treatment or undergoing radical surgery for tuberculosis of the spine. Indian J Tuberculosis 1989;36(Suppl):1–21.
181. Medical Research Council Working Party on Tuberculosis of the Spine. A 10-year assessment of a controlled trial comparing debridement and anterior spinal fusion in the management of tuberculosis of the spine in patients on standard chemotherapy in Hong Kong. J Bone Joint Surg 1982;64B:393–398.
182. Menelaus MB. Discitis: an inflammation affecting the intervertebral discs in children. J Bone Joint Surg 1964;46B:16–23.
183. Messer HD, Litvinoff J. Pyogenic cervical osteomyelitis: chondro-osteomyelitis of the cervical spine frequently associated with parenteral drug use. Arch Neurol 1976;33:571–576.
184. Milone FP, Bianco AJ Jr, Ivins JC. Infections of the intervertebral disk in children. JAMA 1962;181:1029–1033.
185. Mixter WJ, Smithwick RH. Acute intraspinal epidural abscess. N Engl J Med 1932;207:126–131.
186. Modic MT, Feiglin DH, Piraino DW. Vertebral osteomyelitis: assessment using MR. Radiology 1985;157: 157–166.
187. Moe JH. Complications of scoliosis treatment. Clin Orthop 1967;53:21–30.
188. Mondal A. Cytological diagnosis of vertebral tuberculosis with fine-needle aspiration biopsy. J Bone Joint Surg 1994;76A:181–184.
189. Monson TP, Nelson CL. Microbiology for orthopaedic surgeons: selected aspects. Clin Orthop 1984;190:14–22.
190. Moodie AS. Tuberculosis in Hong Kong. Tubercle 1963;44:334–345.
191. Moon MS, Kim I, Woo YK, et al. Conservative treatment of tuberculosis of the thoracic and lumbar spine in adults and children. Int Orthop 1987;11:315–322.
192. Moon MS, Woo YK, Lee KS, et al. Posterior instrumentation and anterior interbody fusion for tuberculous kyphosis of dorsal and lumbar spines. Spine 1995;20:1910–1916.
193. Mosheiff R, Meyer S, Floman Y, et al. Anterior vascularized rib strut graft in the treatment of Pott's disease in the young child. Bull Hosp Jt Dis 1993; 53:61–65.
194. Musher DM, Thorsteinsson SB, Minuth JN, et al. Vertebral osteomyelitis still a diagnostic pitfall. Arch Intern Med 1976;136:105–110.

195. Nagel DA, Albright JA, Keggi KJ, et al. Closer look at spinal lesions: open biopsy of vertebral lesions. JAMA 1965;191:103–106.
196. Naim Ur Rahman, Al Arabi KM, Khan FA. A typical form of spinal tuberculosis. Acta Neurochir 1987;88:26–33.
197. National Academy of Sciences, National Research Council. Postoperative wound infections and the influence of ultraviolet irradiation of the operating room of various other factors. Ann Surg 1964;160(Suppl):1–125.
198. Nelson CL, Green TG, Porter RA. One day versus seven days of preventive antibiotic therapy in orthopaedic surgery. Clin Orthop 1983;176:258–263.
199. Newhouse KE, Lindsey RW, Clark CR, et al. Esophageal perforation following anterior cervical spine surgery. Spine 1989;14:1051–1053.
200. Nordby EJ, Wright PH, Schofield SR. Safety of chemonucleolysis: adverse effects reported in the United States, 1982–1991. Clin Orthop 1993;293:122–134.
201. Norris S, Ehrlich MG, McKusick K. Early diagnosis of disk space infection with 67 Ga in an experimental model. Clin Orthop 1979;144:293–298.
202. Nussbaum ES, Rigamonti D, Standiford H, et al. Spinal epidural abscess: a report of 40 cases and review. Surg Neurol 1992;38:225–231.
203. Oga M, Arizono T, Takasita M, et al. Evaluation of the risk of instrumentation as a foreign body in spinal tuberculosis. Spine 1993;18:1890–1894.
204. Onofrio BM. Intervertebral discitis: incidence, diagnosis, and management. Clin Neurosurg 1980;27:481–516.
205. Ottolenghi CE. Aspiration biopsy of the spine: technique for the thoracic spine and results of twenty-eight biopsies in this region and overall results of 1050 biopsies of other spinal segments. J Bone Joint Surg Am 1969;51:1531–1544.
206. Ottolenghi CE, Schajowicz F, De Schant FA. Aspiration biopsy of the cervical spine: technique and results in thirty-four cases. J Bone Joint Surg Am 1964;46:715–733.
207. Parke WW, Rothman RH, Brown MD. The pharyngovertebral veins: an anatomical rationale for Grisel's syndrome. J Bone Joint Surg 1984;66A:568–574.
208. Petty W. The effect of methylmethacrylate on bacterial phagocytosis and killing by human polymorphonuclear leukocytes. J Bone Joint Surg 1978;60A:752–757.
209. Petty W. The effect of methylmethacrylate on chemotaxis of polymorphonuclear leukocytes. J Bone Joint Surg 1978;60A:492–498.
210. Piazza MR, Bassett GS, and Bunnell WP. Neuropathic spinal arthropathy in congenital insensitivity to pain. Clin Orthop 1988;236:175–179.
211. Polk HC Jr. Principles of preoperative preparation of the surgical patient. In: Sabiston DC, ed. Textbook of surgery: The biological basis of modern surgical practice. 13th ed. Philadelphia: WB Saunders, 1986:87–98.
212. Polk HC Jr, Simpson CJ, Simmons BP, et al. Guidelines for prevention of surgical wound infection. Arch Surg 1983;118:1213–1217.
213. Polk HC, Trachtenberg L, Finn MP. Antibiotic activity in surgical incisions: the basis for prophylaxis in selected operations. JAMA 1980;244:1353–1354.
214. Pollock RA, Purvis JM, Apple DF, et al. Esophageal and hypopharyngeal perforation injuries in patients with cervical spine trauma. Ann Otol Rhinol Laryngol 1981;90:323–327.
215. Poret HA, Fabian TC, Croce MA, et al. Analysis of septic morbidity following gunshot wound to the colon: the missile is an adjuvant for abscess. J Trauma 1991;31(8):1088–1095.
216. Post MJD, Quencer RM, Montalvo BM, et al. Spinal infection: evaluation with MR imaging and intraoperative US. Radiology 1988;169:765–771.
217. Post MJD, Sze G, Quencer RM, et al. Gadolinium enhancing MR in spinal infection. J Comput Assist Tomogr 1990;14:721–729.
218. Pritchard AE, Thompson WAL. Acute pyogenic infections of the spine in children. J Bone Joint Surg 1960;42B:86–89.
219. Puig Guri J. Pyogenic osteomyelitis of the spine: differential diagnosis through clinical and roentgenographic observations. J Bone Joint Surg 1946;28:29–39.
220. Puranen J, Makela J, Lahde S. Postoperative intervertebral discitis. Acta Orthop Scand 1984;55:461–465.
221. Rafto SE, Dalinka MK, Schiebler ML, et al. Spondyloarthropathy of the cervical spine in long-term hemodialysis. Radiology 1988;166:201–204.
222. Rajasekaran S, Shanmugasundaram TK. Prediction of the angle of gibbus deformity in tuberculosis of the spine. J Bone Joint Surg 1987;69A:503–509.
223. Rajasekaran S, Soundarapandian S. Progression of kyphosis in tuberculosis of the spine treated by anterior arthrodesis. J Bone Joint Surg 1989;71A:1314–1323.
224. Redekop GJ, Del Maestro RF. Diagnosis and management of spinal epidural abscess. Can J Neurol Sci 1992;19:180–187.
225. Redfern RM, Cottam SN, Phillipson AP. *Proteus* infection of the spine. Spine 1988;13:439–441.
226. Richards BS. Delayed infections following posterior spinal instrumentation for the treatment of idiopathic scoliosis. J Bone Joint Surg 1995;77A:524–529.
227. Ring D, Johnston CE, Wenger DR. Pyogenic infectious spondylitis in children: the convergence of discitis and vertebral osteomyelitis. J Pediatr Orthop 1995;15:652–660.
228. Ring D, Vaccaro AR, Scuderi G, et al. Vertebral osteomyelitis after blunt traumatic esophageal rupture. Spine 1995;20:98–101.
229. Ring D, Wenger DR. Magnetic resonance imaging scans in discitis: sequential studies in a child who needed operative drainage: a case report. J Bone Joint Surg 1994;76A:596–601.
230. Robinson BHB, Lessof MH. Osteomyelitis of the spine. Guy Hosp Rep 1961;110:303–318.
231. Roffi RP, Waters RL, Adkins RH. Gunshot wounds to the spine associated with a perforated viscus. Spine 1989;14:808–811.
232. Romanick PC, Smith TK, Kopaniky DR, et al. Infection about the spine associated with low-velocity-missile

injury to the abdomen. J Bone Joint Surg 1985;67A: 1195–1201.
233. Ross PM, Fleming JL. Vertebral body osteomyelitis: spectrum and natural history: a retrospective analysis of 37 cases. Clin Orthop 1976;118:190–198.
234. Rudert M, Tillman B. Lymph and blood supply of the human intervertebral disc. Acta Orthop Scand 1993; 64:37–40.
235. Russell NA, Vaughan R, Morley TP. Spinal epidural infection. Can J Neurol Sci 1979;6:325–328.
236. Sadato N, Numaguchi Y, Rigamonti D, et al. Spinal epidural abscess with gadolinium-enhanced MRI: serial follow-up studies with clinical correlations. Neuroradiology 1994;36:44–48.
237. Sandiford JA, Higgins GA, Blair W. Remote salmonellosis: surgical masquerader. Am Surg 1982;48:54–58.
238. Sapico FL, Montgomerie JZ. Pyogenic vertebral osteomyelitis: report of nine cases and review of the literature. Rev Infect Dis 1979;1:754–776.
239. Sapico FL, Montgomerie JZ. Vertebral osteomyelitis in intravenous drug abusers: report of three cases and review of the literature. Rev Infect Dis 1980;2:196–206.
240. Sarkar SD, Ravikrishnan KP, Woodbury DH, et al. Gallium 67-citrate scanning: a new adjunct in the detection and follow-up of extrapulmonary tuberculosis: concise communication. J Nucl Med 1979;20:833–836.
241. Schaefer SD, Bucholz RW, Jones RE, et al. The management of transpharyngeal gunshot wounds to the cervical spine. Surg Gynec Obstet 1981;152:27–29.
242. Schofferman L, Schofferman J, Zucherman J, et al. Occult infections causing persistent low-back pain. Spine 1989;14:417–419.
243. Schulitz KP, Assheuer J. Discitis after procedures on the intervertebral disc. Spine 1994;19:1172–1177.
244. Scoles PV, Quinn TP. Intervertebral discitis in children and adolescents. Clin Orthop 1982;162:31–36.
245. Seddon HJ. Pott's paraplegia: prognosis and treatment. Br J Surg 1935;22:769–799.
246. Sharif HS. Role of MR imaging in the management of spinal infections. AJR 1992;158:1333–1345.
247. Sharif HS, Aideyan OA, Clark DC, et al. Brucellar and tuberculous spondylitis: comparative imaging features. Radiology 1989;171:419–425.
248. Sittig O. Metastatischer Ruckenmarksabscess bei Sepischem Abortus. Z Gesamte Neurol Psychiatr 1927;107:146–151.
249. Smith AS, Weinstein MA, Mizushima A, et al. MR imaging characteristics of tuberculous spondylitis vs. vertebral osteomyelitis. AJR 1989;153:399–405.
250. Smith MD, Bolesta MI. Esophageal perforation after anterior cervical plate fixation: a report of two cases. J Spinal Disord 1992;5:357–362.
251. Smith RF, Taylor TKF. Inflammatory lesions of intervertebral discs in children. J Bone Joint Surg 1967; 49A:1508–1520.
252. Southwick WO, Robinson RA. Surgical approaches to the vertebral bodies in the cervical and lumbar regions. J Bone Joint Surg 1957;39A:631–644.
253. Speigel PG, Kengla KW, Isaacsson AS, et al. Intervertebral disc-space inflammation in children. J Bone Joint Surg 1972;54A:284–296.
254. Staab EV, McCartney WH. Role of gallium 67 in inflammatory disease. Semin Nucl Med 1978;8:219–234.
255. Stambough JL, Beringer D. Postoperative wound infections complicating adult spine surgery. J Spinal Disord 1992;5:277–285.
256. Stauffer RN. Pyogenic vertebral osteomyelitis. Orthop Clin North Am 1975;6:1015–1027.
257. Stolke D, Sollmann WP, Seifert V. Intra and postoperative complications in lumbar disc surgery. Spine 1989;14:56–59.
258. Stone DB, Bonfiglio M. Pyogenic vertebral osteomyelitis: a diagnostic pitfall for the internist. Arch Intern Med 1963;112:491–500.
259. Subhadrabandhu T, Laohacharoensombat W, Keorochana S. Risk factors for neural deficit in spinal tuberculosis. J Med Assoc Thai 1992;75:453–461.
260. Swank SM, Cohen DS, Brown JC. Spine fusion in cerebral palsy with L-rod segmental spinal instrumentation: a comparison of single and two-stage combined approach with Zielke instrumentation. Spine 1979; 14:750–759.
261. Swayne LC, Dorsky S, Caruana V, et al. Septic arthritis of a lumbar facet joint: detection with bone SPECT imaging. J Nucl Med 1989;30:1408–1411.
262. Szalay EA, Green NE, Heller RM, et al. Magnetic resonance imaging in the diagnosis of childhood discitis. J Pediatr Orthop 1987;7:164–167.
263. Szypryt EP, Hardy JG, Hinton CE, et al. A comparison between magnetic resonance imaging and scintigraphic bone imaging in the diagnosis of disc space infection in an animal model. Spine 1988;13:1042–1048.
264. Tabo E, Ohkuma Y, Kimura S, et al. Successful percutaneous drainage of epidural abscess with epidural needle and catheter. Anesthesiology 1994;80:1393–1395.
265. Thalgott JS, Cotler HB, Sasso RC, et al. Postoperative infections in spinal implants: classification and analysis: a multicenter study. Spine 1991;16:981–984.
266. Thelander U, Larsson S. Quantitation of C-reactive protein levels and erythrocyte sedimentation rate after spinal surgery. Spine 1992;17:400–404.
267. Transfeldt EE, Lonstein JE, Winter RB. Wound infections in reconstructive spinal surgery. Orthop Trans 1985;9:128.
268. Tronnier V, Schneider R, Kunz U, et al. Postoperative spondylodiscitis: results of a prospective study about the aetiology of spondylodiscitis after operation for lumbar disc herniation. Acta Neurochir 1992;117: 149–152.
269. Tuli SM. Results of treatment of spinal tuberculosis by "middle-path" regime. J Bone Joint Surg 1975;57B:13–23.
270. Tuli SM, Srivastava TP, Varma BP, et al. Tuberculosis of spine. Acta Orthop Scand 1967;38:445–458.
271. Upadhyay SS, Saji MJ, Sell P, et al. Spinal deformity after childhood surgery for tuberculosis of the spine. J Bone Joint Surg 1994;76B:91–98.
272. Upadhyay SS, Saji MJ, Sell P, et al. The effect of age on the change in deformity after radical resection and

anterior arthrodesis for tuberculosis of the spine. J Bone Joint Surg 1994;76A:701–708.
273. Upadhyay SS, Sell P, Saji MJ, et al. Surgical management of spinal tuberculosis in adults. Clin Orthop 1994;302:173–182.
274. van Berge Henegouwen DP, Roukema JA, de Nile JC, et al. Esophageal perforation during surgery on the cervical spine. Neurosurgery 1991;29:766–768.
275. Van Lom KJ, Kellerhouse LE, Pathria MN, et al. Infection versus tumor in the spine: criteria for distinction with CT. Radiology 1988;166:851–855.
276. Van Tassel P. Magnetic resonance imaging of spinal infections: topics in magnetic resonance imaging 1994;6:69–81.
277. Velmahos G, Demetriads D. Gunshot wounds of the spine: should retained bullets be removed to prevent infection? Ann R Coll Surg Engl 1994;76:85–87.
278. Verska JM, Leung KY, Wagner TA, et al. Primary infections of the spine treated surgically: instrumented vs. non-instrumented. Presented at the 10th Annual Meeting of the North American Spine Society, October 18–21, 1995, Washington, DC.
279. Visudhiphan P, Chiemchanya S, Somburanasin R, et al. Torticollis as the presenting sign in cervical spine infection and tumor. Clin Ped 1982;21:71–76.
280. Waldvogel FA, Medoff G, and Swartz MN. Osteomyelitis: a review of clinical features, therapeutic considerations, and unusual aspects. New Engl J Med 1970;282:198–206, 260–266, 316–322.
281. Wenger DR, Bobechko WP, Gilday DL. The spectrum of intervertebral disc-space infection in children. J Bone Joint Surg 1978;60A:100–108.
282. Wenger DR, Davids JR, Ring D. Discitis and osteomyelitis. In: Weinstein SL. The pediatric spine: Principles and practice. New York: Raven, 1994:813–835.
283. Whalen JL, Brown ML, McLeod R, et al. Limitations of indium leukocyte imaging for diagnosis of spine infections. Spine 1991;16:193–197.
284. Whalen JL, Parke WW, Mazur JM, et al. The intrinsic vasculature of developing vertebral end plates and its nutritive significance to the intervertebral discs. J Pediatr Orthop 1985;5:403–410.
285. Wheeler D, Keiser P, Rigamonti D. Medical management of spinal epidural abscesses: case report and review. Clin Infect Dis 1992;15:22–27.
286. Whitecloud TS, Butler JC, Cohen JL. Complications with the variable spinal plating system. Spine 1989;14:472–476.
287. Whitehill R, Sirna EC, Young DC, et al. Late esophageal perforation from an autogenous bone graft. J Bone Joint Surg 1985;67A:644–645.
288. Wiesseman GJ, Wood VE, Kroll LL. *Pseudomonas* vertebral osteomyelitis in heroin addicts: report of five cases. J Bone Joint Surg 1973;55A:1416–1424.
289. Wilensky AO. Osteomyelitis of the vertebrae. Ann Surg 1929;89:561–570, 731–747.
290. Wiley AM, Trueta J. The vascular anatomy of the spine and its relationship to pyogenic vertebral osteomyelitis. J Bone Joint Surg 1959;41B:796–809.
291. Wiltberger BR. Resection of vertebral bodies and bone grafting for chronic osteomyelitis of the spine. J Bone Joint Surg 1952;34A:215–218.
292. Yoshida GM, Garland D, Waters RL. Gunshot wounds to the spine. Orthop Clin North Am 1995;26:109–116.
293. Yu WY, Siu C, Wing PC, et al. Percutaneous suction aspiration for osteomyelitis: report of two cases. Spine 1991;16:198–202.
294. Zigler JE, Bohlman HH, Robinson RA, et al. Pyogenic osteomyelitis of the occiput, the atlas, and the axis: a report of five cases. J Bone Joint Surg 1987;69A:1069–1073.

CHAPTER TWENTY NINE

Rheumatoid Arthritis and Ankylosing Spondylitis

J. Michael Simpson and Howard S. An

Rheumatoid Arthritis

Rheumatoid arthritis is a chronic systemic inflammatory disorder with a predilection for affecting the smaller joints of the appendicular skeleton in a symmetrical pattern. The disease affects approximately 1% of the population worldwide, with a peak incidence in the fourth through the sixth decades. The ratio of females to males with rheumatoid arthritis is 2:1 (96, 97). The most common area of the spine affected by rheumatoid arthritis is the cervical region, and in particular the occiput-C1-C2 complex.

Pathophysiology

The etiology of rheumatoid arthritis remains uncertain. It is postulated that rheumatoid arthritis develops after some environmental exposure, such as infection, in a genetically predisposed host (78). There appears to be an association between rheumatoid arthritis and class II histocompatibility antigen HLA-DR4 (27). This antigen has been found in 70% of patients with rheumatoid arthritis, but in only 28% of the general population (87). Primary relatives of severely affected individuals have four times the risk of disease. There is a concordance of 30% in monozygotic twins and 5% in dizygotic twins. While an exact cause-and-effect relationship in rheumatoid arthritis remains unknown, the inflammatory process itself has been well described. The current assumption is that synovial cells of patients with rheumatoid arthritis express a new antigen. This chronic antigenic stimulus then triggers the body to produce rheumatoid factor, an immunoglobulin M (IgM) molecule directed against autologous immunoglobulin G (IgG). Approximately 70% of active rheumatoid arthritis patients test positive for IgM anti-IgG. The presence of rheumatoid factor alone in synovial fluid does not produce rheumatoid arthritis, however. There is increasing evidence showing that immunologic mechanisms, including a new complex formation of antigen and antibodies followed by complement binding and polymorphonuclear cell infiltration, are important in the pathogenesis of rheumatoid arthritis (41, 57, 87, 91). Phagocytosis of the immune complexes by polymorphonuclear cells results in release of lysosomal enzymes, oxygen radicals, and arachidonic acid metabolites that produce inflammation and tissue destruction. The influx of fluid in actions of these inflammatory mediators produce the erythema, warmth, and pain that is characteristic of rheumatoid synovitis. This same sequence of events may explain the pathogenesis of rheumatoid nodules and other systemic immune sequelae such as vasculitis.

Rheumatoid pannus represents granulation tissue formed within the synovium from proliferating fibroblasts and inflammatory cells. Pannus is productive of collagenase and other proteolytic enzymes capable of destroying adjacent cartilage, ligaments, tendons, and bone. It is this destructive property that leads to ligamentous laxity, cartilage loss, tendon ruptures, and bone erosion.

Clinical Manifestations

In the majority of patients prodromal symptoms of fatigue, joint stiffness, arthralgia, and myalgia precede actual joint effusions. The small appendicular joints of the hands and feet are typically involved in a symmetric fashion. Large weightbearing joints may also be affected. Multiple joint involvement is typical, though one-third of patients may have monarticular symptoms.

Rheumatoid spondylitis is usually manifested in the cervical spine, but may, though uncommonly, involve the sacroiliac joints. Involvement of the thoracolumbar spine is rare. Cervical spine involvement in the rheumatoid patient has been reported at 25 to 90%, depending on the study and diagnostic criteria (5, 20, 57, 58, 67, 87, 92). The pathologic sequence in the joints of the cervical spine is identical to those that occur peripherally, as proven by biopsy examination (2, 33, 57, 87). The four abnormalities most commonly seen in rheumatoid cervical spine disease are:

1. C1-C2 instability
2. Basilar invagination
3. C1-C2 rotatory subluxation (lateral subluxation)
4. Subaxial subluxation

Atlantoaxial subluxation is the result of severe erosive synovitis of the atlantoaxial and atlantodental joints. Involvement of these articulations occurs more commonly in patients with severe rheumatoid arthritis. Conlon and associates reported a 25% incidence of atlantoaxial subluxation in a hospital population of rheumatoid arthritis patients (20). Radiologic progression has been reported at 40% for atlantoaxial subluxation, but development of neurologic symptoms is significantly less, ranging from 2 to 14% (86, 95). The odontoid process and transverse ligaments are separated by a synovial lined space, which leads to laxity of the transverse ligament. This allows anterior displacement of the atlas, particularly in neck flexion. Clinical manifestations of atlantoaxial subluxation include occipital, retro-orbital, and temporal pain. Headaches and burning sensations along the basiocciput are also common. A "clunking" sensation may also be noticed on neck flexion (Sharp and Purser's sign) (77).

Vertebrobasilar insufficiency may also accompany rheumatoid involvement of the upper cervical spine. The vertebral arteries can be kinked around the anteriorly displaced atlas, producing dizziness, headache, dysphagia, vertigo, visual disturbances, and nystagmus. Sudden temporary episodes of unconsciousness (drop attacks) may also occur in rare cases. Concomitant atherosclerosis may contribute to the development of vertebrobasilar insufficiency.

Although neurologic compromise is thought to be relatively uncommon in cases of atlantoaxial subluxation, myelopathy can occur. Neurologic manifestations may be due to direct soft-tissue or bony impingement of the spinal cord. Other potential sources of neurologic compromise include ischemia from compression of vertebral arteries, anterior spinal arteries, or small arteries that perforate the brainstem and spinal cord (97). Mathews found that long tract signs develop in nearly one-third of patients with atlantoaxial subluxation (59). Myelopathic findings are generally limited to hyperactive deep tendon reflexes but may include incontinence, weakness, sensory loss, and paresis when involvement is severe. Flexion and rotation of the head may produce an electric shock sensation (Lhermitte's sign) into all four extremities.

Lateral (rotatory) subluxation results from asymmetric erosion and collapse of C1 and C2 and occurs from the same destructive rheumatoid involvement of the occiput-C1 and atlantoaxial joints. The principal clinical finding in this group is pain, although neurologic compromise may be seen in more severe forms. This type of subluxation is progressive and may result in a fixed torticollis. Many believe the incidence of C1-C2 rotatory subluxation to be underestimated (20). In one series it accounted for 21% of all atlantoaxial subluxations (14).

Posterior atlantoaxial subluxation is a rare complication of rheumatoid cervical spine involvement, noted in 6.7% of all C1-C2 subluxations in one study (95). Extensive bony erosion or fracture of the odontoid process allows the anterior arch of the atlas to displace posteriorly (42). This displacement may result in myelopathy with compression at the cervicomedullary junction (55).

Basilar invagination, also known as cranial settling, upward migration of the odontoid, vertical subluxation, and atlantoaxial impaction, occurs as a result of bone, ligament, and cartilage destruction at the atlanto-occipital and atlantoaxial joints. Basilar invagination has been shown to progress in 35 to 50% of patients, allowing the cranium to settle on the cervical spine and the odontoid process to project cephalad into the foramen magnum (84, 90, 95). Cranial settling occurs as the result more of bone and cartilage destruction than of ligamentous laxity. Cranial settling can produce severe and chronic occipitocervical pain, which is caused by first and second cervical nerve root compression. The vertically displaced odontoid process can ventrally compress the cranial nerve nuclei in the medulla oblongata and cause dysfunction (28). Compression of branches of the spinal arteries or vertebral arteries may also produce severe neurologic dysfunction and can even be life threatening (93). Only in rare advanced cases of cranial settling can one see facial diplegia, internuclear ophthalmoplegia, spastic quadriparesis, sleep apnea, loss of light touch sensation in the trigeminal nerve distribution, and dysfunction of cranial nerves IX, X, and XII. The odontoid process may also compress the pyramidal tracts in the midline, which are anterior and decussating. Compression of the upper corticospinal tract decussation without compromise of the uncrossed lower-extremity fibers produces a brachial cruciate paralysis, as described by Bell (3). This syndrome produces significant upper-extremity paralysis with normal strength in the lower extremities.

In a review of patients with cranial settling, Menezes and associates found that posterior occipital pain was the primary complaint of all 45 patients studied (62). Myelopathy was noted in 36 patients, blackout spells in 24 patients, brainstem symptoms in 17, and lower cranial nerve palsies in 10 patients. The clinical evaluation of rheumatoid patients in whom cranial settling is severe can be difficult because of multifocal sources of pain and other symptoms. A very careful examination must be carried out in an attempt to elicit silent neurologic involvement. Pyramidal tract signs, including hyperactive reflexes, a positive Babinski sign, and loss of proprioception, are early signs of myelopathy. Rana and associates pointed out subtle involvement of the fifth cranial nerve with rheumatoid involvement of the craniovertebral junction (70). Loss of the corneal reflex, diminished light touch and pain sensation, especially in the first division of the trigeminal nerve, are common subtle findings. These signs probably indicate an involvement of the descending tract of the nucleus of the fifth nerve, which can reach as low as C2.

Death due to spinal cord compression in patients with rheumatoid arthritis is probably underestimated (63). Meijers and colleagues reported on an autopsy study of 104 rheumatoid patients, of whom 11 were found to have C1-C2 subluxation with cord compression. Seven of these 11 patients died suddenly, which represents an estimated 10% rate of fatal medullary compression (61). In a more recent postmortem analysis, Delamarter et al. found spinal cord compression to be the main cause of death in 10 of 11 rheumatoid arthritis patients with paralysis (30). This strongly suggests that once cervical myelopathy is established in patients with rheumatoid cervical disease, who are not surgically decompressed and stabilized, the natural history is one of progression, and the resultant mortality is likely more common than currently reported. Marks and Sharp have reported on 31 patients with rheumatoid arthritis and cervical myelopathy (56). Fifteen of these patients died within 6 months of clinical presentation, and 50% of those treated with a cervical collar died. Surgical stabilization provided a reasonable chance for survival.

For patients presenting with neurologic involvement it is useful to classify the extent of deficit. The classification system described by Ranawat is commonly employed (71). Patients without neurologic deficit are class I; those with subjective weakness, hyperreflexia, and dysesthesias are class II; those with objective weakness and long tract signs are class III. Class III is subdivided into IIIa (ambulatory) and IIIb (quadriparetic and unable to walk). This is important prognostically, as patients with more severe paralysis have poorer outcomes following surgery. Duration of paralysis is not a good predictor of outcome (6).

Radiologic Evaluation

While magnetic resonance imaging (MRI) has dramatically improved our ability to visualize pannus formation and spinal cord impingement, plain roentgenograms remain the primary means of radiologically evaluating the cervical spine of patients with rheumatoid arthritis. Initial radiographic views should include anteroposterior, open-mouth odontoid, and lateral flexion-extension dynamic roentgenograms. Evaluation may sometimes be difficult because of diffuse osteopenia, destructive bony changes, and overlap of bony structures at the craniovertebral junction. In such cases further studies, including conventional tomography, computed tomography (CT), and MRI, are helpful in delineating pathologic anatomy.

In the evaluation of atlantoaxial integrity, lateral flexion-extension views are most helpful. An anterior atlantodental interval of more than 3.5 mm is abnormal and indicative of atlantoaxial subluxation (Fig. 29.1). This distance is measured between the posterior edge of the anterior ring of C1 and the anterior surface of the odontoid process, measured along the transverse axis of the C1 ring (17). Subluxation of more than 10 to 12 mm indicates complete destruction of the atlantoaxial ligamentous complex (36). Anterior atlantoaxial subluxation may result in compression of the cervical spinal cord. Pannus formation around the odontoid process, with or without abnormal sagittal plane motion of the atlantoaxial articulation, may be sufficient to produce spinal cord compression.

It is apparent from multiple reports that the anterior atlantodental interval does not reliably correspond to the development of neurologic deficits (6, 18, 20, 29, 46, 59, 85, 94). Boden has shown that the posterior atlantodental interval (PADI) is the most reliable predictor of both the development and the severity of paralysis (6). This measurement, which is the distance from the posterior aspect of the odontoid

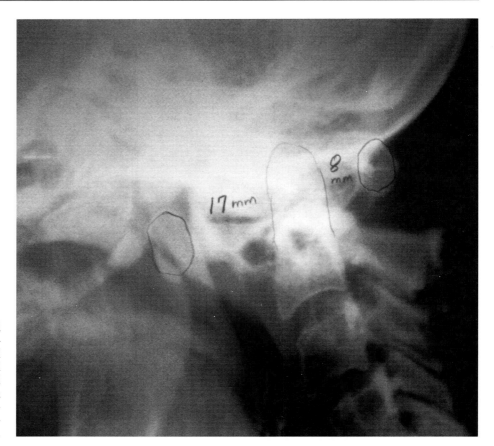

FIGURE 29.1.
Lateral radiograph of a rheumatoid arthritis patient with C1-C2 instability. The atlantodental interval (ADI) is measured to be 17 mm, and posterior atlantodental interval (PADI) is only 8 mm on flexion view. A PADI of 14 mm or less represents a significant risk for development of neurologic compromise.

process to the anterior edge of the posterior ring of the atlas (as measured along the transverse axis of the ring of the atlas), more accurately reflects the space available for the spinal cord (Fig. 29.1). Boden concluded that a PADI of 14 mm or less on plain radiographs represents a significant risk factor for the development and progression of neurologic compromise. If the PADI is 14 mm or less, MRI taken in flexion is advised to evaluate the true space for the spinal cord. However, if there is significant narrowing of the space available for the spinal canal, the flexion MRI procedure may carry the danger of producing neurologic deficits. An MRI taken in extension may allow the visualization of the spinal cord without further spinal cord compression during scanning (Fig. 29.2). If the MRI demonstrates a cervicomedullary angle of 135°, a spinal cord diameter in flexion of less than 6 mm, or a space available for the spinal cord of less than 13 mm, a posterior atlantoaxial fusion should be considered (7).

Lateral subluxation of the atlantoaxial complex is demonstrated on anteroposterior open-mouth views. Lateral mass displacement of C1 more than 2 mm lateral to the mass of C2 is considered abnormal (95). This apparent lateral subluxation usually represents a true rotatory subluxation, which is reflected in the asymmetry of the lateral mass sizes of C1 and C2.

A multitude of measurement techniques have been described to evaluate basilar invagination. This area is often difficult to evaluate on plain radiographs. In such cases additional studies may be required. The traditional measurement of basilar invagination has been McGregor's line, which connects the posterior margin of the hard palate to the most caudal point of the occiput (Fig. 29.3). The tip of the odontoid process should not project more than 4.5 mm beyond this line. McRae's line defines the opening of the foramen magnum (Fig. 29.3). Protrusion of the odontoid process to any degree beyond this transverse diameter is considered abnormal in defining basilar invagination.

Chamberlain's line is drawn from the hard palate to the inner aspects of the posterior rim of the foramen magnum. The odontoid process should not project more than 3 mm above this line, and more than 6 mm is considered definitely pathologic. Symptomatic basilar invagination usually requires significant protrusion. With any of these measurements, polytomography is often required to detail the bony landmarks.

The method described by Fischgold and Metzger evaluates cephalad migration of the odontoid process on the basis of an anteroposterior open-mouth view of the spine (Fig. 29.4) (37). The digastric line connects the right and left digastric grooves (where the mastoid process is connected to the base of the skull).

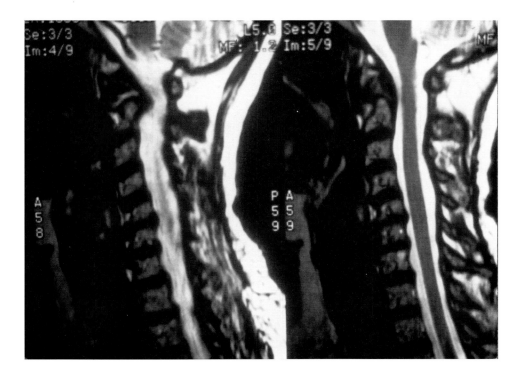

FIGURE 29.2.
Sagittal T2-weighted MRI taken of the same patient as in Figure 29.1 shows that the spinal cord is decompressed in extension.

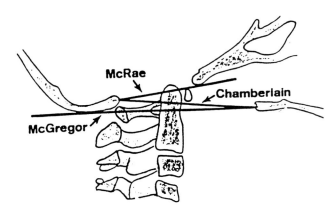

FIGURE 29.3.
Illustration of the lateral upper cervical spine demonstrating McGregor's, Chamberlain's, and McRae's criteria for basilar invagination. McGregor's line is drawn from the posterior margin of the hard palate to the most caudal point of the occiput. The tip of the odontoid process should not project more than 4.5 mm beyond this point. Chamberlain's line is drawn from the posterior lip of the foramen magnum to the dorsal margin of the hard palate. The odontoid process should not project more than 3 mm beyond this point. McRae's line is drawn from the basion to the posterior lip of the foramen magnum. Protrusion of the odontoid process above this line to any degree is considered abnormal.

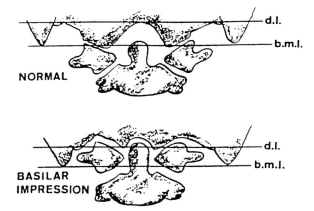

FIGURE 29.4.
Illustrations of normal and basilar invagination on anterior upper cervical anteroposterior tomogram using Fischgold and Metzger lines. The upper line connects the digastric grooves, and the lower line connects the lower poles of the mastoid process. The digastric line should normally be 1 cm or more above the tip of the odontoid process.

This line should be 1 cm or more above the tip of the odontoid process.

Wackenheim's line is drawn along the cranial surface of the clivus. It should normally be tangent to or intersect the tip of the odontoid process. Posterior protrusion of the odontoid beyond this line is indicative of cranial settling (Fig. 29.5).

Clark and associates described "stations" of the atlas, noting the relationship of the anterior arch of C1 to the axis (Fig. 29.6) (17). The station of C1 is determined by dividing the axis into thirds in the sagittal plane and then noting the relationship of the anterior ring of C1 to C2. In a normal individual, the anterior ring of C1 is adjacent to the upper third of C2 (station 1). When the ring of C1 is adjacent to the middle third of C2, it is considered station 2 and indicative of mild cranial settling. Station 3 is considered evidence of severe cranial settling.

Ranawat's criteria for basilar invagination are based on a horizontal line connecting the center of the anterior and posterior arches of C1 (Fig. 29.7) (30). A vertical line is drawn from the center of the C2 pedicle extending along the midaxis of the odontoid process, perpendicular to the horizontal line. Normal values are 17 mm ± 2 in males and 15 mm ± 2 in females. As this interval becomes smaller, the severity of basilar invagination increases (30). The Ranawat and Clark methods are particularly useful because they can routinely be determined on plain roentgenographs.

Finally, Redlund-Johnell described a technique

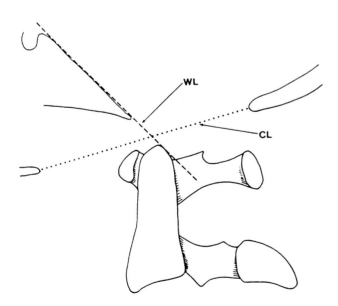

FIGURE 29.5.
Wackenheim's line (WL) is drawn along the cranial surface of the clivus. It should normally be tangent to or intersect the tip of the odontoid process. Protrusion of the odontoid posterior to this line is indicative of cranial settling. Chamberlain's line (CL) is also illustrated.

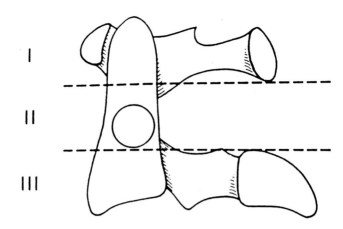

FIGURE 29.6.
The station of the atlas is determined by noting the relationship of the anterior arch of the atlas to the axis by dividing the axis into thirds in the sagittal plane. (Reprinted with permission from Clark CR, Goetz DD, Menezes AH. Arthrodesis of the cervical spine in rheumatoid arthritis. J Bone Joint Surg 1989;71A:381–392.)

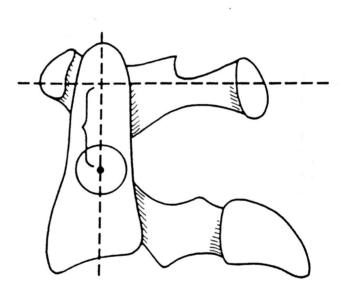

FIGURE 29.7.
The distance described by Ranawat and associates is between the sclerotic ring, which represents the pedicle of the axis, and the transverse axis of the atlas, as measured along the longitudinal axis of the odontoid process. As this distance becomes shorter, the severity of cranial settling increases. (Reprinted with permission from Clark CR, Goetz DD, Menezes AH: Arthrodesis of the cervical spine in rheumatoid arthritis. J Bone Joint Surg 1989;71A:381–392.)

measuring the distance between the sagittal midpoint of the base of C2 and McGregor's line (Fig. 29.8) (72). Normal values for Redlund-Johnell are 34 mm or more for males and 29 mm or more for females. As opposed to the methods of Clark and Ranawat, which describe only the relationship of C1 and C2,

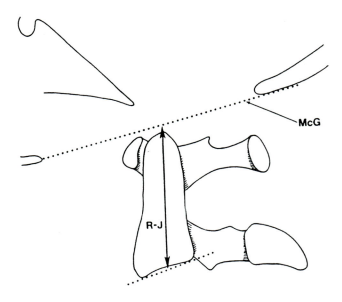

FIGURE 29.8.
The distance described by Redlund-Johnell (R-J) is the minimal distance between the sagittal midpoint of the base of the axis and the McGregor line.

Redlund-Johnell values reflect problems associated with the entire occipitoatlantoaxial complex.

To determine the presence of spinal cord compression radiographically, the physician may resort to cervical myelography followed by computed tomography. However, to study the craniovertebral junction properly the dye must pass through the foramen magnum into the cranium, which may lead to complications secondary to meningeal irritation such as headaches and seizure. This study has been largely replaced by magnetic resonance imaging. MRI provides explicitly detailed information about pannus formation and spinal cord compression and is considered the test of choice for evaluating the craniovertebral junction. Pannus is visualized as having an increased signal intensity on T2-weighted imaging consistent with the edematous process.

Electrophysiologic Testing

Electromyography may be useful in some patients with subaxial disease and a radicular component. In most rheumatoid arthritis patients, however, the upper cervical spine and spinal cord compression is a much more common concern.

Somatosensory evoked potentials (SSEP) are gaining in popularity not only for intraoperative evaluation but also for preoperative clinical assessment of myelopathy. Neurologic evaluation can be difficult in patients who have severe rheumatoid arthritis with polyarticular involvement. Objective testing such as SSEPs can be useful in detecting an overt myelopathy. Lachiewicz has shown that 58% of patients with an irreducible atlantoaxial subluxation or cranial settling demonstrated abnormal cervical cord conduction latencies (51). Not all rheumatoid patients require SSEPs in their evaluation, but testing can be useful in the examination and follow-up of many patients in whom myelopathy is a concern.

Indications for Surgery

Atlantoaxial Subluxation

The treatment of atlantoaxial subluxation is based on several factors, including the patient's general health, severity of symptoms, neurologic dysfunction, and radiologic parameters. First, unremitting pain that fails to improve despite conservative measures is a reason to consider surgical stabilization. Usually intractable pain accompanies significant atlantoaxial subluxation. Secondly, any patient with rheumatoid disease and evidence of myelopathy must be considered for surgery. If the patient is medically stable and fit for such a major procedure, surgical stabilization and possibly transoral decompression should be offered.

For the asymptomatic patient with atlantoaxial subluxation, radiographic parameters are used in determining need for surgical stabilization. While the anterior atlantodental interval is a reasonable measurement for evaluating atlantoaxial subluxation, it has no strong correlation to the development of neurologic deficit. The posterior atlantodental interval has been shown to be the critical diameter in the evaluation of atlantoaxial subluxation. Using plain radiographs as a screening tool, a PADI of 14 mm or less requires further evaluation with MRI in flexion. If the space available for the spinal cord is less than 13 mm, posterior stabilization should be recommended (7). This is particularly true when the atlantoaxial articulation remains hypermobile on flexion-extension views. This diameter, which is a measure of the available space for the cervical spinal cord, has demonstrated statistically significant correlations with the presence and severity of paralysis. In a study by Boden and associates, all patients with a class III neurological deficit had a posterior atlantodental interval of less than 14 mm (6). In contrast, the anterior atlantodental interval was not correlated with the presence or severity of paralysis. Furthermore, the prognosis for neurologic recovery following surgery was not affected by the duration of paralysis but was influenced by the severity of paralysis at the time of the operation. The most important predictor of potential neurologic recovery after surgery was the preoperative posterior atlantodental interval. In patients who had paralysis due to atlantoaxial subluxation, no recovery occurred if the posterior atlantodental interval was less than 10 mm, whereas recovery of at least one neurologic class occurred when the posterior atlantodental interval was at least 10 mm (6). Boden further recommends atlantoaxial stabilization when the cervicomedullary angle is more than 135° or the spinal cord diameter is less than 6 mm in flexion (7).

Basilar Invagination

Like atlantoaxial subluxation, basilar invagination may produce isolated symptoms of neck pain with radiation of symptoms along the basiocciput and headaches. Mild forms of basilar invagination producing such symptoms warrants conservative management. Surgical stabilization may be indicated for those who have severe unremitting pain that fails to improve with conservative measures.

More severe basilar invagination can be associated with any of the severe neurologic sequelae described for C1-C2 subluxation, including sudden death. For patients who develop neurologic compromise secondary to basilar invagination and, in particular, patients demonstrating a progressive quadriparesis, hospital admission is required for purposes of halo traction and serial neurologic evaluation, followed by surgical stabilization and possibly decompression. Conservative treatment of patients with basilar invagination accompanied by signs and symptoms of neural compression carries a significant risk of progressive neurologic impairment and sudden death. For patients who have basilar invagination who do not have neurologic compromise, radiographic criteria must be used in determining the need for surgical stabilization. Multiple reports have confirmed that basilar invagination is associated with a higher frequency of severe neurologic deficit that may not be reversible and could be fatal (15, 16, 31, 44). In the study by Boden and colleagues, it was apparent that patients who had combined atlantoaxial subluxation and basilar invagination were at high risk for the development of neurologic deficit (6). Using McGregor's criteria, these authors found that the severity of basilar invagination alone beyond 5 mm did not appear to affect the prognosis as much as the degree of atlantoaxial subluxation as reflected by the posterior atlantodental interval. No patient in their study who remained intact neurologically had basilar invagination and marked atlantoaxial subluxation. Accordingly, they recommend that when any evidence of basilar invagination is detected in patients who have marked atlantoaxial subluxation, an MRI in flexion should be obtained to quantitate spinal cord compression. If there is any evidence of spinal cord compression, cervical traction is indicated, and if reduction is achieved, a posterior occipitocervical fusion should be performed (7). If cord compression is not relieved with traction, either a C1 laminectomy or a transoral resection of the odontoid process should be considered (25). For asymptomatic patients who have an isolated and fixed basilar invagination without evidence of significant spinal cord compression, observation with close follow-up reevaluations is a reasonable course of action.

Subaxial Disease

In considering the need for surgical stabilization for subaxial involvement in the rheumatoid arthritis patient, the most critical measurement is the available space for the spinal cord. Patients with rheumatoid disease are not immune to the processes of disc degeneration, disc herniation, or spinal stenosis. These conditions can be exacerbated by the development of spinal instability. Again, the critical measurement is the space available for the spinal cord. According to the study by Boden and associates, a sagittal spinal canal diameter of 14 mm or less is considered critical and grounds for further evaluation with flexion-extension MRI (6). If the space available for the spinal cord is less than 13 mm or a significant amount of mobility is present, surgical arthrodesis should be considered. If significant neurologic deficit is present, an anterior decompression and stabilization will likely be required. If the patient has no significant neurologic compromise, an isolated posterior arthrodesis is the procedure of choice (7).

General Surgical Considerations

First and foremost, the overall medical status of the patient must be considered. Many patients are older and have other medical problems in addition to the consequences of their rheumatoid disease. All of these factors must be taken into account when considering patients as candidates for major cervical procedures.

Preoperative traction is occasionally used in patients with cervical instability, usually those who have severe irreducible subluxations with or without neurologic compromise. Skeletal traction with the use of a halo ring provides the best control. Traction may be required for several days, and hence can be associated with the potential medical complications of immobilization. In such cases halo wheelchair traction to avoid prolonged immobilization and bed rest is a good option. Traction should be applied gently; 5 to 10 pounds of weight is generally adequate. The patient is monitored neurologically and radiographically during the process to avoid neurologic sequelae and to assess reduction. For patients with a reducible subluxation and neurologic compromise, neurologic improvement can be seen in the course of just a few days. For patients who improve through skeletal traction, stabilization alone may be all that is required. However, if the subluxation remains unreduced and the patient is neurologically unchanged, a decompressive procedure may be indicated in addition to the stabilization procedure.

The perioperative management of the airway including intubation in patients with rheumatoid arthritis is difficult, for several reasons. The frequent finding of head tilt, instability, and stiffness of the rheumatoid cervical spine combine to compromise the optimum position of the head and neck for intubation purposes. Many of these patients have severe canal compromise, which may further limit the ability of the anesthesiologist to extend the neck and perform routine intubation. Furthermore, common arthritic involvement of the temporomandibular joints and micrognathia result in limited mouth opening. Acquired laryngeal deviation, laryngeal mucosal abnormalities, and the frequent presence of cricoarytenoid and cricothyroid arthritis also distort the anatomy of the airway (47, 48, 54).

Wattenmaker and associates studied the effects of perioperative complications related to the airway in patients with rheumatoid arthritis undergoing cervical spine procedures (92). Fourteen percent of 58 patients who had been intubated without fiberoptic assistance developed an upper-airway obstruction after extubation. In the group of patients intubated with fiberoptic assistance, only one of 70 patients had such complications. The data from their study suggest that edema caused by the trauma of nonfiberoptic intubation was the primary cause of postoperative airway obstruction. It should also be noted that trauma to the airway is not often recognized by the anesthesiologist at the time of intubation. Of the nine patients who had postoperative airway obstruction, only two of the intubations had been noted to be traumatic.

Spinal cord monitoring is routinely applied, and a baseline SSEP tracing is obtained with the patient in a supine position. Patients are then long-rolled into position and secured to the operating table with either halo traction, halo vest, or Mayfield pin-holding headrest. Once the patient's position is secured, a lateral cervical spine radiograph is obtained to verify satisfactory reduction and position of the spine. SSEP tracings are repeated to ensure no positional neurologic compromise.

The surgeon has the intraoperative option of using one of three methods just mentioned to secure the patient's head and neck. Skeletal traction through the halo ring or tongs may be required to maintain reduction, particularly in cases of basilar invagination. If skeletal traction is not required, the patient can be fitted with a posteriorly opened halo ring and vest preoperatively. The patient then can be placed prone on the operating table and the posterior aspect of the vest can then be removed, allowing access to the surgical site. This is a particularly useful technique in patients with poor bone stock, in whom the quality of internal fixation may be compromised. For patients who have good-quality bone, postoperative immobilization in a rigid orthosis may be adequate. For these patients, we prefer to stabilize the patient to the operating table with a Mayfield pin-holding headrest.

Through halo traction or head positioning in extension, the surgeon actively attempts to reduce either the C1-C2 articulation or the basilar invagination. Care must be taken to avoid overextension of the cervical spine, which may make the surgery itself more difficult.

Atlantoaxial Arthrodesis

The patient is placed in the prone position described above. Chest rolls are used to support the torso. The posterior aspect of the head and neck are shaved from the inion and distally. The neck and posterior iliac crest regions are then sterilely prepared and draped.

A midline incision is made from the occiput to the fourth cervical vertebra. The tips of the spinous processes are exposed, and a subperiosteal dissection is carried out along the spinous process and lamina of the C1-C2 articulation. The dissection of C2 is carried out to the junction point of the lamina and facet joint. The arch of C1 should not be exposed more than 1.5 cm from the midline in the adult to avoid injury to the vertebral arteries. Care is taken not to disturb the interspinous ligament of C2-C3. Additionally, great care must be taken not to fracture the often weak posterior ring of C1 while dissecting the posterior atlantoaxial membrane. Some soft-tissue dissection of the basiocciput is required to allow adequate exposure to the superior aspect of the posterior ring of C1. Once this dissection has been completed, a small angled curette followed by a dental elevator is used to dissect subperiosteally under the posterior arch of C1 and/or C2. Spending adequate time with the subperiosteal dissection will greatly facilitate the overall procedure.

Fielding et al. and Simmons advocate the use of a modified Gallie H-graft from the iliac crest, contouring it to fit over the posterior arches of C1 and C2 (Fig. 29.9) (35, 80). A doubled U-shaped 18- or 20-gauge wire is passed under the arch of C1 from inferior to superior. To facilitate passage of the wire, a curved Mayo needle is passed in a reverse fashion under the arch of C1. The blunt eye portion of the needle is passed in a caudal to cephalad direction. A No. 2 silk suture is then placed through the eye of the needle and passed under the arch of C1. The suture is then tied to the loop of 18- or 20-gauge wire, which is then passed. A bone block is taken from the posterior iliac crest and shaped to fit between C1 and C2. The loop of the wire goes over the bone block and the spinous process of C2. The ends of the wire are tightened around the graft between C1 and C2, thus stabilizing the segment. It is important in this technique that the deep cancellous surface of the graft is

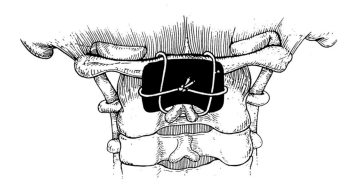

FIGURE 29.9.
Gallie technique modified by Fielding and Simmons. A doubled U-shaped 18- or 20-gauge wire is passed under C1 in a caudal to cranial direction. A bone block is taken from the posterior iliac crest and shaped to fit between C1 and C2. The loop of wire goes over the bone block and the spinous process of C2, and the end of the wire is tightened around the graft between C1 and C2.

contoured to fit over the curved posterior surfaces of C1 and C2 so that the graft is in firm contact with the underlying vertebrae, maximizing surface area contact for graft incorporation. Additional cancellous bone chips are placed lateral to the main graft as far as possible over the lamina.

We generally prefer the Brooks-type fusion (Fig. 29.10) (11). In this technique the posterior atlantoaxial membrane is carefully resected between the arches of C1 and C2 to allow for adequate visualization of the dura. A curved Mayo needle is used to pass a sublaminar No. 2 silk suture at C1 and C2 bilaterally. For the purposes of fixation, a looped 18-gauge stainless steel wire is passed on each side. The suture is tied securely to the loop in the wire and passed in a sequential fashion. To ensure that the wire does not dip anteriorly during the wire passing process, we prefer to visualize the wires in the C1-C2 interlaminar space. A Woodson elevator or a sturdy nerve hook placed under the wire at the interlaminar space with gentle upward traction applied will greatly facilitate the passage of the wires. Once the wires or cables have been passed, the suture is removed and the tips of the wires cut, providing two wires on each side of the C1-C2 segment.

From the posterior iliac crest, a tricortical iliac crest bone graft 3.5 cm long and 2.5 cm wide is obtained using an oscillating saw. This bone graft is then cut in half along its longitudinal axis, creating two wedges of bone measuring approximately 1.25 cm by 3.5 cm. These grafts are then shaped and beveled to fit the interval between the arch of C1 and the laminae of C2. Prior to securing these grafts, a burr is used to lightly decorticate the undersurface of the posterior arch of C1 and the superior surface of the C2 laminae. The two wires on each side are then secured in sequential fashion, providing excellent stability. These bone grafts, wedged between the C1-C2 laminar surfaces, create a "brake shoe" effect, which has been shown to be biomechanically superior in preventing motion in all planes. As an alternative to the use of stainless steel wires, titanium cables are available and can be used in exactly the same fashion and allow for future magnetic resonance imaging.

In some cases the surgeon may not be completely satisfied with the quality of the patient's own iliac crest bone. Several alternatives have been suggested in attempts to augment the stability of the construct. Lipson has suggested reinforcing constructs with metal mesh, wire, and polymethylmethacrylate (55). Recent reports of such augmentations, however, have indicated an association with higher incidences of

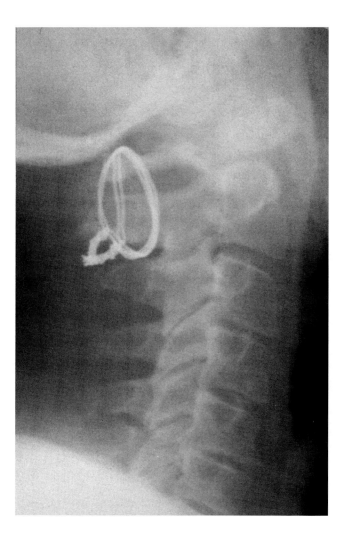

FIGURE 29.10.
Lateral radiograph of a patient who underwent the Brooks-type C1-C2 fusion. A looped 18-gauge wire is passed under the arch of C1 and then under the lamina of C2 on both the right and left sides. Wedges of bone are harvested from the iliac crest and beveled to fit the interval between the arch of C1 and the lamina of the axis. The wires are tightened to secure the graft.

wound dehiscence and infection. In general we have found such constructs to be neither necessary nor advisable in posterior cervical fusions in the rheumatoid arthritis patient. It would be our preference in such patients to augment internal fixation with a halo device. Adequate external immobilization should be carried out for approximately 12 weeks postoperatively.

At the completion of the surgical procedure, the wound should be thoroughly irrigated. Drains are placed, and the patient is given prophylactic antibiotics until they are removed.

Occipitocervical Arthrodesis

Patient positioning and surgical exposure for an occipitocervical arthrodesis are similar to those in an atlantoaxial arthrodesis. The skin incision, however, is extended proximally to allow adequate exposure of the external occipital protuberance. Many surgical techniques have been described. Newman and Sweetnam as well as Perry and Nickel have described an onlay graft technique and reported a high fusion rate (65, 69). Other techniques have included various forms of internal fixation, including Luque rectangles and plate-screw constructs (15, 16, 21, 40, 75). Additionally, anterior approaches have been described, but these may be associated with serious complications and may require long periods of skeletal traction and immobilization (55).

We prefer the rigid-wiring technique described by Wertheim and Bohlman (Fig. 29.11) (95). A midline posterior approach is made, exposing the area from the external occipital protuberance to the fourth cervical vertebra. Sharp subperiosteal dissection is completed, exposing the occiput and the cervical laminae. The external occipital protuberance is thick and represents the ideal location for passage of wires without having to go through both cortical tables of the occiput. A high-speed burr is used to create a trough on both sides of the protuberance at a level 2 cm above the foramen magnum. The transverse and superior sagittal sinuses are cephalad to the protuberance and thus are out of danger. A towel clip is then used to create a hole through the base of this ridge, through only the outer table of the bone. A 20-gauge wire is then looped through the hole and around the ridge. A second wire loop is passed around the arch of C1, and a third is passed through and around the base of the spinous process of C2. Therefore, on each side of the spine there are three separate wires, which are used to secure the bone grafts.

The posterior iliac crest is exposed, and a large, thick, slightly curved tricortical graft of corticocancellous bone of appropriate length and width is obtained. The graft is then carefully divided in half longitudinally and three holes are drilled through each graft. The occiput is decorticated, and the grafts are anchored in place by tightening of the wires. Additional cancellous bone is packed between the two grafts. The wound is closed in layers over suction drains. This technique allows immediate rigid internal fixation and has been associated with minimal operative morbidity while allowing early mobilization of the patient. In Wertheim and Bohlman's study the technique resulted in successful fusion in all 13 patients over long-term follow-up (95). Current mortality rates approximate 10%, which represents significant improvement over earlier studies. This is most likely a result of improved and earlier surgical intervention and improved anesthetic and perioperative management (10, 21, 22, 34, 43, 50, 52, 71, 96).

Successful surgical fusion predictably relieves pain and halts progression of neurologic dysfunction in the vast majority of patients (23, 34, 68, 71, 76, 96). Reports of neurologic improvement have been variable, although Wertheim and Bohlman reported neurologic improvement in all 10 of the patients in their study who had preoperative myelopathy.

Transoral Decompression

Transoral decompression of the anterior spinal cord can be used for patients who show clinical evidence of spinal cord compression and irreducible basilar invagination and/or C1-C2 subluxation. The role of transoral decompression, however, remains unclear in the current literature, as the technique has been associated with high rates of morbidity and mortality (10, 23, 24, 62, 66). We currently reserve the option of transoral decompression for the myelopathic patient who does not respond adequately to skeletal traction or stabilization.

For the transoral approach, the patient is placed in the supine position and the head held in a hyperextended position. While routine tracheostomy is advocated by many, endotracheal anesthesia may be used as well. The soft palate is turned back on itself and held in position with a stay suture. A 5 cm midline incision is then made in the posterior pharyngeal wall, with its center 1 cm inferior to the palpable anterior tubercle of the atlas. The incision is carried down to bone. The posterior wall is then dissected subperiosteally as far lateral as the lateral mass of the atlas and axis, exposing the anterior arch of C1 and the body of C2. The anterior arch of C1 is then removed with a rongeur, exposing the odontoid process. The odontoid is then removed, preferably with a high-speed drill. Excision of a superiorly migrated and posteriorly angulated odontoid process may be difficult. Careful dissection, freeing the odontoid of all soft tissue, is required. If lateral C1-C2 fusion is performed, articular cartilage from the C1-C2 articu-

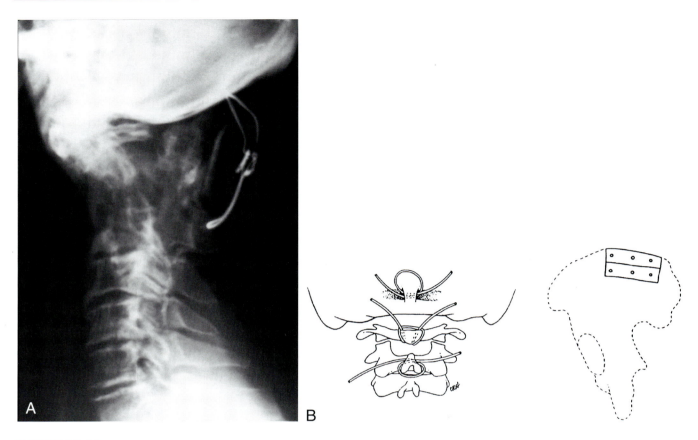

FIGURE 29.11.
A. Lateral radiograph of a patient who underwent posterior occiput–C2 fusion. This 80-year-old male had a previous odontoid fracture with malunion and progressive C1-C2 instability and basilar invagination with myelopathy. Posterior decompression of the C1 ring and occiput–C2 fusion was performed. Myelopathic symptoms resolved and solid fusion was noted at 1-year follow-up. **B.** Illustration of the Wertheim and Bohlman method of wiring for the occipitocervical fusion. A wire is looped around the external occipital protuberance at a level 2 cm above the foramen magnum. A second wire loop is passed around the arch of C1, and a third is passed through and around the spinous process of C2. A large, thick graft from the posterior iliac crest is harvested and holes are drilled. The wires are fed through the holes in the bone grafts and then tightened to provide good fixation.

lation is removed and the defect packed with a wedge iliac crest bone graft. A single-layer closure is recommended by most to allow for drainage. Oral intake is deferred for 6 to 7 days.

Alternatively, a retropharyngeal approach to the base of the skull, as reported by McAfee and colleagues, can be used (60). This avoids the potential contamination of the transoral approach and allows for excision of C2 and fusion of C1 to C3. Bilateral exposure, however, is required for arthrodesis. Resection of the odontoid process should be accompanied by posterior fusion.

Subaxial Subluxation

Subaxial subluxations tend to be more subtle and located at multiple levels, producing a staircase or stepladder type of deformity. The indication for surgery in this particular group of patients is the development of neurologic impairment and, to a lesser extent, pain. It is recommended that the diameter of the spinal canal be evaluated. If the sagittal diameter of the spinal canal is 14 mm or less, surgical stabilization should be considered (6). For the patient who has no neurologic compromise, posterior stabilization alone is sufficient. We prefer the triple-wire technique described by Bohlman with a corticocancellous strip of iliac crest bone. This procedure is well described in Chapter 32 of this volume. For the occasional rheumatoid patient who may have significant anterior neurologic impingement with associated instability, an anterior or combined anterior-posterior approach is indicated.

Complications

Mortality

Perioperative mortality in fusion procedures for atlantoaxial subluxation has been reported as high as 42% in an early series. More recent reports have been encouraging, however, with perioperative mortality rates averaging 10% (19, 22, 34, 48, 50, 52, 71, 91). In most cases, deaths were not directly attributed to the surgical procedure itself but reflect the systemic severity of the underlying disease process. This is especially true for patients who had cardiopulmonary compromise.

Neurologic Deficit

Neurologic compromise resulting from cervical spine surgery in a rheumatoid arthritis patient is uncommon. Preoperative traction to reduce subluxation, careful surgical technique, adequate stabilization, and postoperative immobilization are necessary to avoid this complication. The passing of sublaminar wires is certainly the most critical element in most of these surgical procedures. It can be particularly difficult in patients who have an irreducible C1-C2 subluxation and a preexisting neurologic deficit. Clark and associates reported one case of transient hemiparesis secondary to the passing of the sublaminar wire (17); it resolved spontaneously except for residual hyperreflexia. The use of intraoperative somatosensory evoked potential monitoring is advocated to minimize the potential for neurologic injury.

Pseudarthrosis

Pseudarthrosis remains a problem in attempted C1-C2 fusions in the rheumatoid arthritis patient and may be attributed to several factors. First, the posterior arch of C1 is often eroded in the rheumatoid patient. This leaves a significantly decreased surface area for bony contact with the bone graft and may result in nonunion. Secondly, obtaining rigid fixation may be difficult. The use of a halo device, especially in patients whose internal fixation is compromised by poor bone quality and erosion, is essential. It is crucial that the surgeon devote adequate time and attention to detail in contouring these grafts to the posterior laminar surfaces of C1 and C2. While many surgeons continue to use the Gallie technique in posterior cervical fusion in the rheumatoid arthritis patient, we believe that the Brooks technique provides a biomechanically superior construct and may yield a lower rate of nonunion.

The difficulty in obtaining fusion of the C1-C2 articulation is clearly illustrated in the literature. Success rates have ranged from 50% to 85%. In 1975 Ferlich and associates reported a 50% success rate in fusing C1 to C2 using a Gallie-type wiring technique (34). Bohlman achieved 10 solid fusions in 17 patients (59%) operated on for atlantoaxial subluxation (8). Conaty and Morgan reported 67% satisfactory results in 27 patients who had surgery (19). More recently, Santavirta and associates recognized only two nonunions in 13 patients treated with a Gallie-type fusion (76). Clark and associates reported a 15% rate of nonunion using a Brooks-type fusion augmented posteriorly with polymethylmethacrylate (17).

Occipitocervical fusion has generally met with higher success rates. Clark and associates reported union in all 16 patients treated with an occipitocervical fusion, either for isolated cranial settling or for those with associated atlantoaxial or subaxial subluxation (17). Conaty and Morgan reported only one nonunion in 14 patients (19). Improved fusion rates may reflect prolonged halo immobilization time or larger surface area for graft healing. Other reports have not been as encouraging. Brattstrom and colleagues achieved successful fusion in 58% of their patients but noted a stable fibrous union in another 28% (10). Meticulous decortication, stable wire fixation, large iliac crest bone graft, and postoperative halo immobilization are all important in achieving successful fusion.

Progression of Instability

Late subaxial subluxation below a higher cervical fusion has been reported by several authors (12, 22, 62). Careful preoperative radiographic evaluation is necessary to identify other areas of instability or potential instability. Flexion-extension views of the cervical spine are helpful in delineating areas of potential instability, which, when identified, should be included in an extended fusion mass.

Previously asymptomatic levels may develop subluxation below already fused segments. In one series of 41 patients treated with a cervical arthrodesis, Clark and associates noted subsequent subluxation and displacement in 13 patients (17). Long-term follow-up monitoring for the development of instability is therefore necessary.

Ankylosing Spondylitis

Ankylosing spondylitis is a seronegative spondyloarthropathy affecting both skeletal and extraskeletal tissues. It affects primarily the axial skeleton, including ligaments and articulations of the pelvis and vertebral bodies. It was once believed to affect men predominantly; however, recent evidence suggests that women are affected equally but with less severe involvement. Eighty to ninety percent of patients with ankylosing spondylitis are HLA-B27 positive but only 8% of the general population of American Caucasians is found to have the HLA-B27 antigen (45, 49). This strongly suggests that HLA-B27 antigen is important in the pathogenesis of ankylosing spondylitis. However, its precise role remains unknown. It may resemble or serve as some receptor for an inciting antigen such as a virus. Although incompletely understood, ankylosing spondylitis is generally viewed as an inflammatory disorder incited by environmental or infectious agents and hosts rendered susceptible by HLA-B27 or related antigens (53, 91).

Pathophysiology

The pathophysiology of ankylosing spondylitis, like that of rheumatoid arthritis, remains unclear. The characteristic pathologic picture of ankylosing spondylitis includes inflammation, bony erosion, and ankylosis. The inflammatory infiltrate is generally lymphocytic, and target tissues include both joints and areas of ligament, tendon, and joint capsule attachments (entheses). The sacroiliac, apophyseal, and costovertebral joints are generally involved in the axial skeleton and may eventually become ankylosed. Inflammation of the entheses, termed enthesopathy, manifests itself in the anterior spine through a spectrum of well-defined changes that have been documented both clinically and radiographically (32, 38, 64). These anterior lesions may be classified as either localized or extensive forms of the disease process.

The "Romanus lesion" is an erosion of the anterior and anterior-lateral surface of the vertebral rim at the vascular attachment site of the annulus fibrosus. This lesion represents an anterior spondylitis, which results in a focal osteitis as part of the inflammatory process of ankylosing spondylitis. Damage to these tissues subsequently results in a bony repair process, syndesmophyte formation, and ossification of the annulus fibrosus, which is the hallmark of ankylosing spondylitis (26). Osseous changes of this type in the thoracolumbar spine yield the classic "bamboo spine" appearance in radiologic imaging.

Extensive destructive skeletal lesions can also be seen in ankylosing spondylitis, as first described by Anderson (1). This massive destruction is seen at the discovertebral junction and histologically shows evidence of fibrinoid necrosis. These findings have supported the clinical suspicions of many suggesting that trauma and pseudarthrosis are the cause of the extensive discovertebral lesions in ankylosing spondylitis. Any inflammation represents a reaction to the trauma and tissue damage in that area.

Clinical Manifestations

Ankylosing spondylitis typically occurs in the young healthy adult between the ages of 17 and 35 years. Sacroiliitis is usually the first manifestation of the disease. Symptoms include low back pain and unilateral or bilateral buttock, hip, and thigh pain. Onset is generally insidious. Buttock pain with radiation to the legs is common and may be confused with sciatica, but the pain from ankylosing spondylitis seldom radiates below the knee. Symptoms are generally worse in the morning and improve with exercise. This clinical feature helps in distinguishing ankylosing spondylitis from mechanical low back pain, which generally is worse with activity and improves with rest (73). Patients with ankylosing spondylitis often complain of nocturnal pain that interrupts sleep (45). These patients generally awaken from sleep and feel the need to move around before returning to bed.

Patients with uncontrolled inflammation develop ankylosis of the lumbar, thoracic, and cervical spine. The disease generally progresses in a caudal to cranial direction. Patients may assume a posture of fixed lumbar flexion in an attempt to transfer weight away from the inflamed facet joints (79). In time, fixed lumbar, thoracic, and cervical kyphosis may develop, resulting in severe spinal deformity and functional disability. Compensatory flexion contractures of the hips and knees may develop as the patient attempts to maintain an erect posture. As with the rheumatoid arthritis patient, atlantoaxial instability may also develop and require periodic radiologic evaluation.

There are several extraskeletal manifestations of ankylosing spondylitis that must be considered. Among the most prominent and severe are recurrent iritis, aortitis, and carditis (4, 13, 88). Pulmonary function is not significantly compromised by the limited motion of the costovertebral articulation; however, pulmonary fibrosis is occasionally seen in this patient population. The cause of fibrosis remains uncertain, but some have suspected that colonization of the lung with certain fungi—namely, *Aspergillus*—may be a causative agent (9, 74).

Of particular concern to the spine surgeon in patients with ankylosing spondylitis is spinal deformity. As a result of these severe kyphotic deformities, patients may become functionally disabled, and peripheral vision can be extremely limited. Lumbar kyphosis is most common, followed by thoracic and cervical deformities.

Spinal fracture in the patient with ankylosing spondylitis also presents special problems to the orthopaedic surgeon and can be extremely challenging and fraught with complications and high rates of mortality. Another complication of advanced ankylosing spondylitis is spondylodiscitis, which consists of focal pain accompanying erosive sclerotic changes in adjacent vertebral bodies. As mentioned earlier, it is uncertain whether this is primarily an inflammatory process or the result of trauma. The radiographic appearance of spondylodiscitis, pseudarthrosis, and infectious discitis are very similar.

Neurologic compromise in the patient with ankylosing spondylitis is uncommon. Only in the rare case will ossification of the posterior longitudinal ligament lead to symptomatic lumbar spinal stenosis. Neurologic compromise can, however, be a significant complication of fracture in the patient with ankylosing spondylitis. Finally, instability of the atlantoaxial complex may lead to spinal cord impingement in the most severe cases.

Diagnostic Evaluation of Spinal Deformity in Ankylosing Spondylitis

In assessing any patient who has ankylosing spondylitis with significant spinal deformity, the primary site of deformity must be recognized. Careful clinical and radiologic evaluation of the cervical, thoracic, and lumbar spine and the hips is essential to addressing the patient's deformity correctly.

Ankylosing spondylitis may lead to severe flexion deformities of the spine. The goal in treatment of these patients is early recognition and adequate medical therapy in the attempt to control the disease's progress as well as the associated deformities. However, many of these patients develop significant loss of lumbar lordosis with marked kyphosis in both the thoracic and cervical regions. Patients can become grossly deformed and functionally disabled. Spinal osteotomy may be indicated to correct the deformity and attain an upright posture. It is important to reemphasize that the entire spine as well as the hips must be evaluated to delineate the primary site of deformity. Accurate measurement of the deformity is required in surgical planning. Simmons believes that the most effective and reproducible measurement of deformity is the chin-brow to vertical angle (Fig. 29.12) (80). This angle is measured with the patient attempting to stand in an upright position. Knee and hip joints must be held in a maximally extended position. The first line is drawn from the prominent aspect of the patient's brow to the chin and is compared to a vertical line. The larger the angle, the more severe the deformity.

The major deformity in patients presenting with apparent spinal kyphosis may originate in the hip joint, the lumbar spine, the thoracic spine, or the cervical spine. In some patients more than one of these sites may contribute to the deformity. Once the surgeon rules out hip flexion contracture as a major contributor, attention can be directed toward the spine. The lumbar spine is the most common cause of deformity, followed by the cervical and thoracic regions. Deformities isolated to the lumbar spine are corrected by lumbar osteotomy, usually at the L3-L4 level (81). Most combined lumbar-thoracic kyphotic deformities can also be addressed through a single lumbar osteotomy. However, severe isolated thoracic-level deformity must be addressed at the thoracic level, usually requiring a combined anterior-posterior procedure. Some patients have a deformity occurring primarily in the cervical region. Significant deformity in this region can result in a "chin-on-chest" deformity, severely restricting field of vision and the ability to open the mouth.

General Surgical Considerations in Deformity Surgery for Ankylosing Spondylitis

The indications for correction of spinal deformity in patients with ankylosing spondylitis are somewhat variable and must be individualized to meet the patient's needs and expectations. The degree and primary site of deformity, the patient's age and general medical condition, and the patient's desire to undergo such an extensive procedure with the accompanying risk must be considered. Primary surgical objectives may include a more erect posture, improved field of vision, improved diaphragmatic excursion, decompression of abdominal viscera by elevation of the rib margin, and improved access to the abdomen for surgical procedures.

As mentioned earlier, patients who have ankylosing spondylitis have an increased incidence of aortic stenosis. Preoperative assessment should include pulmonary function studies and evaluation for cardiac murmurs in addition to the standard preoperative workup. Preoperative radiologic studies should include chest, hip, and spine radiographs. When a hip flexion deformity is associated with ankylosis or significant arthrosis, total hip arthroplasty should be performed prior to surgical correction of any spinal deformity. If hip pathology is bilateral, both hips should be replaced concurrently or within a week or so to prevent recurring flexion contracture. Flexion-extension views of the cervical spine are recommended to rule out instability, particularly of the C1-C2 complex.

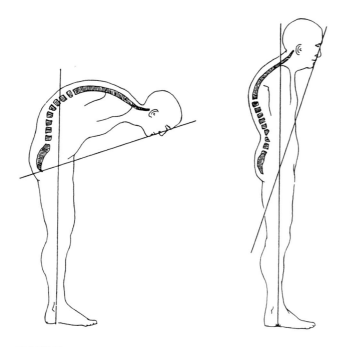

FIGURE 29.12.
Measurement of the chin-brow to vertical angle. This angle is measured from the brow to the chin and compared to the vertical with the patient standing with the hips and knees extended and the neck in its fixed or neutral position.

Many patients who have ankylosing spondylitis have associated long-standing ileitis or colitis. Such a history is important in evaluating the nutritional status of the patient, which may also reflect qualitative changes in bone density. In the event of significant osteopenia, internal spine fixation may be compromised.

Respiratory function must be fully evaluated. Ankylosis of the costovertebral articulation can seriously limit chest expansion. Significant thoracic kyphosis can compromise pulmonary function. A history of smoking increases the difficulties of intraoperative and postoperative pulmonary management.

Intubation of patients with ankylosing spondylitis may be difficult because of limited airway access. Ankylosis of the temporomandibular joints and arytenoid cartilages may occur. Simmons has advocated the use of local anesthesia in attempts to better monitor patients neurologically during the operative procedure (80). Most surgeons, however, prefer general anesthesia except in cervical osteotomies. In difficult cases, awake oral or nasal intubation may be necessary. Only in extreme cases would tracheostomy be needed. Postoperative ventilation may be required, particularly in patients who have preexisting pulmonary compromise.

Lumbar Spine Osteotomy

Patients selected for a lumbar spine extension osteotomy have their primary deformity in the lumbar spine with loss or reversal of lordosis. This deformity may be associated with an accentuated thoracic kyphosis but still be balanced through overcorrection of the lumbar deformity, returning the chin-brow to vertical angle as close to normal as possible. Full correction is required to shift the weightbearing access posteriorly to the osteotomy site. Gravity not only helps to maintain correction, but it also places the osteotomy site under compression, which should stimulate the healing process. The amount of correction to be obtained surgically is determined by the preoperative chin-brow to vertical angle. This angle is transferred to the standing lateral radiograph of the lumbar spine. The apex of the angle is placed at the posterior longitudinal ligament at the L3–4 disc space (which is the center of the normal lumbar lordosis) and projected posteriorly across the lamina to the spinous processes (Fig. 29.13). Measurements are taken at the intersection points at the tips of the spinous processes and the facet joint level. These distances are then used in determining the size of the V-wedge to be resected intraoperatively. A template of this angle can be made and used intraoperatively for evaluation of the osteotomy.

We prefer general anesthesia with the patient in a prone position. The operating table must be modified according to the patient's preoperative deformity. Usually a "jackknifed" position with the apex of the table under the primary spinal deformity is useful, with appropriate bolsters to free the abdomen while protecting bony prominences and neurologic structures of the extremities.

Posterior surgical exposure extends from T12 to the sacrum. Dissection is carried laterally to the transverse processes at the site of the L3-L4 osteotomy. A V-shaped wedge resection osteotomy is completed as recommended by Smith-Peterson and associates (86). Bone cutters are used to remove the spinous processes at the appropriate angle. The ossified ligamentum flavum and appropriate amount of lamina are resected at the L3 and L4 levels. The osteotomy is carried laterally and includes resection of the L3-L4 facet joint bilaterally. The laminae and pedicles are undercut to prevent impingement of the dura or nerve root upon closure of the osteotomy site. It is essential that adequate bone resection be completed in order to obtain full correction of the deformity. In the presence of a small spinal canal (an anteroposterior diameter less than 20 mm as measured in preoperative radiologic studies), it is particularly important to perform a generous posterior decompression. Simmons suggests leaving the central laminectomy area open to avoid compression from impingement or spine in these cases (80).

Once the osteotomy is complete, osteoclasis is achieved by extension of the hips and pelvis while applying anterior pressure to the osteotomy site. An audible crack usually occurs, allowing closure at the osteotomy. Extension of the table from the "jackknifed" position may help to maintain reduction. A lateral radiograph is then taken to verify adequate correction. Occasionally osteoclasis may be difficult to achieve manually. In such instances the dura may be gently retracted and an osteotome passed anteriorly at the level of the disc. Once the osteotome has been passed across the disc space bilaterally, osteoclasis is reattempted. In recalcitrant cases, the pedicle may be resected unilaterally in attempts to weaken the anterior elements to allow manual osteoclasis.

Some surgeons prefer to perform these procedures with the patient in the lateral decubitus position. Such positioning can allow concomitant retroperitoneal exposure of the L3-L4 segment to facilitate osteoclasis in difficult cases. It should not be done routinely, though, since completion of the osteotomy and spinal instrumentation can be difficult in this position.

Instrumentation is used by the majority of spine surgeons in such osteotomy cases. Segmental fixation with multiple pedicle screws and/or hook constructs are typically used and allow for immediate patient

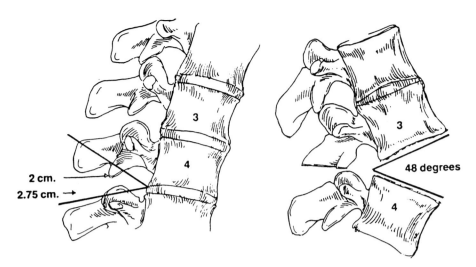

FIGURE 29.13. Illustration of the Smith-Peterson lumbar osteotomy. The angle of correction is obtained through closure of osteotomy and anterior osteoclasis at the L3-L4 level. A V-shaped wedge resection osteotomy is completed. The spinous processes, the ossified ligamentum flavum, and an appropriate amount of lamina are resected at the L3 and L4 levels. The osteotomy is carried laterally and includes resection of the L3-L4 facet joint bilaterally. The laminae and pedicles are undercut to prevent impingement of the dura or nerve root after closure of the osteotomy site. It is essential that adequate bone resection is completed to obtain full correction of the deformity.

mobilization. Because of the high stresses applied to the osteotomy site, it is recommended that brace immobilization with a custom-molded thoracolumbosacral orthosis with a thigh extension be used for 4 to 6 months postoperatively.

Through a single osteotomy site, Simmons has reported a 40 to 104° range of correction with an average of 56° in 90 patients (81). The chin-brow to vertical angle improved from an average of 60° preoperatively to 5° postoperatively.

The most common complication associated with this procedure is neurologic compression. In Simmons's series of 90 patients, seven (8%) developed L3 nerve root or cauda equina compression within 2 to 14 days postoperatively (81). Most of these occurred before the use of internal fixation and preoperative assessment of spinal canal diameter. In patients with these problems, reexploration, decompression, and stabilization should be performed promptly. Such complications can be minimized by thorough preoperative assessment of the spinal canal diameter, generous decompression (especially superiorly), and rigid stabilization. It was reported in Simmons's series that these patients generally do well after secondary decompression (81).

Three of the 90 patients in Simmons's series had nonunion. In one noninstrumented patient, posterior regrafting and instrumentation led to a successful outcome. In two previously instrumented patients, successful fusion was obtained through an anterior spinal fusion.

The osteotomy advocated by Smith-Peterson and Simmons is an open wedge osteotomy, and therefore there may be an inherent risk of stretching neural structures as well as a potential for damage to vital structures from sharp vertebral edges. Thomasen reported a spinal column shortening procedure with the use of a decancellization procedure from the posterior approach (89). The decancellization procedure is performed by removing the posterior elements of L2 or L3 with the pedicle, followed by resection of the posterior vertebral cortex (Fig. 29.14). Thomasen reported 12° to 50° of correction in 11 patients, with five of the 11 having a correction of less than 35° (89). Thomasen's technique is our procedure of choice at this time.

Thoracic Spine Osteotomy

Thoracic-level osteotomies are rarely required in ankylosing spondylitis. As mentioned earlier, almost all patients have some accentuation of their normal kyphosis. If the thoracic-level kyphosis is mild to moderate and associated with a flattened or kyphotic lumbar spine, the overall deformity can be adequately addressed with a lumbar spine osteotomy. For the rare patient who has severe thoracic kyphosis and normal or nearly normal cervical and lumbar lordosis, the primary thoracic deformity must be addressed.

For patients who have severe rigid thoracic kyphosis and complete anterior ossification, an anterior transthoracic approach is first completed. The ossified discs are removed back to the posterior part of the annulus fibrosus, and the space is filled with autogenous cancellous graft. Multiple V-shaped wedge osteotomies are then performed posteriorly as part of a single- or two-stage procedure (Fig. 29.15). The ossified ligamentum flavum and adjacent laminae are resected through the neuroforamina. Compression instrumentation using segmental hook fixation is then performed, and the osteotomy site is closed. Cortical cancellous grafting is completed over the osteotomy sites.

For patients who have incomplete anterior ossification of the thoracic spine or destructive spondylodiscitis, Simmons recommends multiple posterior wedge osteotomies following halo-dependent trac-

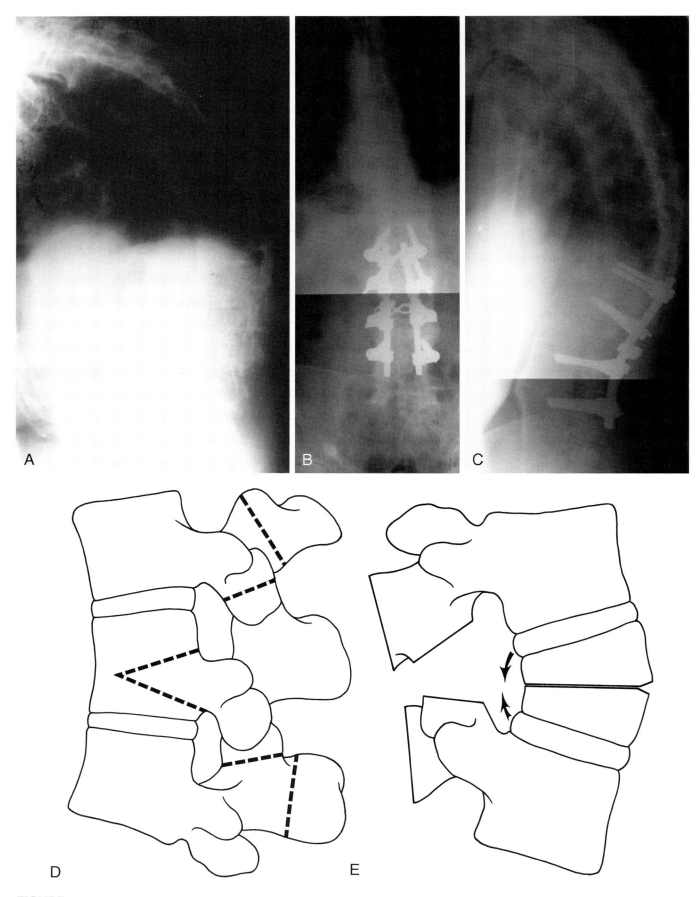

FIGURE 20.14.

A. Lateral radiograph of an ankylosing spondylitis patient with severe sagittal plane imbalance. **B.** Anteroposterior radiograph following an osteotomy at L2 by the Thomasen technique shows the pedicle screw ISOLA instrumentation, which provided a stable fixation. No brace was used postoperatively. **C.** Lateral radiograph shows the osteotomy site at L2 and good correction of the sagittal imbalance. The patient is quite satisfied postoperatively. **D.** and **E.** Illustration of the Thomasen osteotomy with resection of the posterior element and close extension osteotomy of the vertebral body.

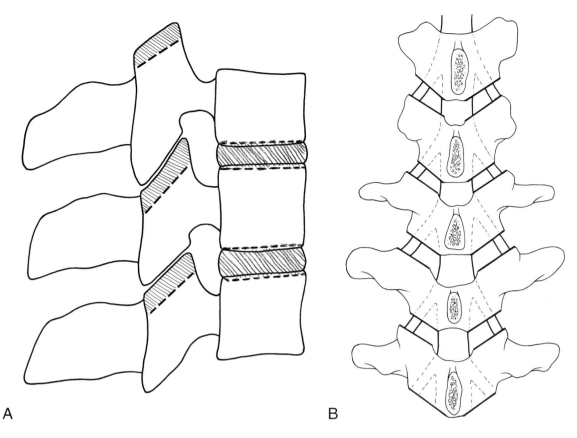

FIGURE 29.15.

Illustration of multiple thoracic osteotomies. **A.** Anterior transthoracic resection of ossified discs is completed at multiple levels. Rib grafts are placed after thorough resections are completed. **B.** Posteriorly, multiple V-shaped osteotomies are completed, depending on the degree of desired correction.

tion in the subgroup of patients with a primary thoracic deformity. This is followed by a second-stage anterior resection of discitis and strut grafting with iliac crest bone graft. Spinal cord monitoring and Stagnara wake-up testing are advocated for thoracic-level osteotomy cases (80).

Cervical Osteotomy

Severe cervical kyphosis in ankylosing spondylitis can be extremely disabling, with marked visual field restriction and interference with mouth opening. Local anesthesia is used in the performance of cervical osteotomies because of the inherent difficulties of intubation with this deformity (Fig. 29.16) (15). The patient is held in a seated position and halo traction applied in line with the deformity. Sedation is given preoperatively and supplemented during the procedure as needed using drugs such as fentanyl or diazepam. After infiltration of the skin with a local anesthetic, an incision is made covering the spinous processes of C5 to T3. The spinous process of C7 and part of those of C6 and T1 are resected (Fig. 29.16A–C). The entire posterior arch of C7, the superior half of T1, and the inferior half of C6 are then removed in a piecemeal fashion. The laminae are undercut above and below to prevent C8 nerve root impingement upon closure. A complete foraminotomy is required over the C8 roots bilaterally with resection of the C7-T1 facet joints. The amount of bone to be resected is based on the preoperative chin-brow to vertical angle. This angle is transferred to the lateral radiograph, with the apex of the angle at the posterior edge of the C7-T1 disc space. Lateral tomography is usually required to identify the landmarks properly. The pedicles of C7 and T1 are exposed, and partial resection may be necessary to protect the C8 nerve root. The bony resections must be made evenly and parallel throughout their length. Overcorrection must be avoided. Once the bony resection is complete, the neck is extended by grasping the halo ring and tilting the head backward. An audible crack usually occurs. Upon closure of the osteotomy the patient is asked to confirm neurologic function with movement of the upper and lower extremities. The patient is also asked about sensory changes along the C8 nerve root distribution. Assessment of both spinal cord and C8 nerve root function is imperative. Just before per-

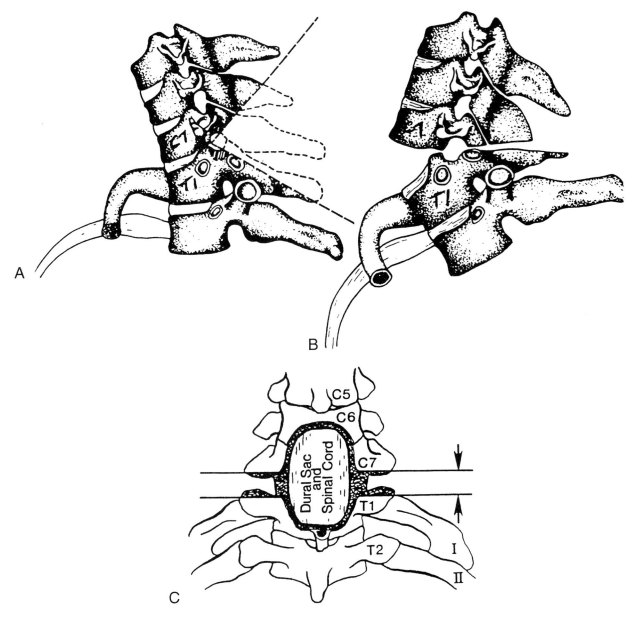

FIGURE 29.16.
Cervicothoracic osteotomy. **A.** Lateral diagram of cervicothoracic spine showing area to be resected. The inferior aspect of the C7 pedicles and the superior aspect of the T1 pedicles are removed to create adequate room for the C8 nerve roots. **B.** Once the osteotomy is completed, osteoclasis is performed through the opening in the ossified disc at C7-T1. **C.** Posterior illustration of laminectomy at C7-T1. The entire posterior arch of C7, the inferior half of C6, and the superior half of T1 are removed. After the laminectomy is completed, the dura, spinal cord, and C8 nerve roots are widely visible. The superior and inferior laminar margins are undercut.

forming osteoclasis, Simmons generally provides additional sedation. Following closure of the osteotomy, Simmons grafts the lateral masses with local bone graft taken from the decompressed site. He then fixes the halo to a body cast, which is worn for approximately 4 months (82). Others prefer internal fixation using various techniques without halo immobilization.

Full correction is usually obtained at the time of the surgical procedure. However, in cases of severe deformity, full correction may be limited by the tightness of the anterior cervical musculature. In such circumstances, halo immobilization will allow further correction approximately 7 to 10 days postoperatively, once the soft tissues have stretched and the overall correction and position of the head has been evaluated by the patient.

Simmons has the most extensive experience with this operation, reporting on 95 patients (82). Thirteen patients developed transient C8 weakness, and five had persistent C8 deficits, one of whom required further decompression, which brought clinical improvement. Other neurologic complications include a transient Horner's syndrome and a mild transient central cord syndrome, which occurred at 2 weeks postoperatively. Four cases of nonunion were noted in this series. Three responded with an anterior cervical fusion, and the fourth required both an anterior cervical fusion and posterior cervical fusion with instrumentation and bone grafting.

Spondylodiscitis

The etiology of spondylodiscitis remains in doubt. Some believe that is a result of the inflammatory processes of ankylosing spondylitis, and others believe there to be a traumatic component resulting in pseudarthrosis. Many of these lesions are found coincidentally on radiographs, and others are seen in follow-up evaluation of known acute fractures. These lesions are often painful and may result in significant spinal deformity. For symptomatic lesions presenting with several months of pain without significant deformity, anterior resection and grafting may be all that is required. For lesions of the thoracolumbar spine accompanied by severe deformity, Simmons advocates an extension osteotomy to diminish stress across the site of spondylodiscitis and induce spontaneous healing (80).

Fractures

Treatment of fractures in patients with ankylosing spondylitis remains a topic of debate and is fraught with a high rate of complications and a high mortality. For any acutely presenting fracture in a patient with ankylosing spondylitis the potential of an epidural hematoma must be considered. Hematoma formation in such a closed space may lead to neurologic compromise necessitating emergent laminectomy for decompression, followed by stabilization.

The majority of fractures in ankylosing spondylitis occur in the cervical spine, but they may occur in the thoracolumbar region, even with minimal trauma. Graham and Van Peteghem reported on 15 patients with ankylosing spondylitis who presented with acute fractures (39). Twelve of these injuries occurred in the cervical spine, two in the thoracic spine, and one in the lumbar region. The mechanism of injury involved only mild forces in six cases, including simple falls from a standing position in four. Of the 12 cervical injuries, 11 had minor neurologic involvement.

Not all fractures are immediately recognized by the patient. Incidental trauma is often ignored, resulting in relatively minor complaints of discomfort (83). Without recognition of the fracture, deformity may follow. In any patient with ankylosing spondylitis who presents with a new deformity or persistent pain, occult fracture must be suspected. Tomography is often required to fully evaluate the suspected areas of trauma, particularly at the cervicothoracic junction. Given the transverse nature of most fractures, translocation may occur, resulting in neurologic compromise.

Optimal treatment is controversial. Many reports emphasize conservative management. Surgical treatment of cervical fractures in some series have noted mortality rates of 50%, in comparison with 25% in nonoperative series. Clearly surgery is indicated in cases of progressive neurologic deficit secondary to epidural hematoma. For patients who have incomplete neurologic deficit, decompression and stabilization may be contemplated. With today's advancements in spinal fixation and improved perioperative management, many believe that aggressive surgical management may lead to early mobilization and avoid the secondary complications of prolonged bed rest, including pneumonia, deep venous thrombosis, pulmonary emboli, and decubitus ulcers. Such aggressive treatment is particularly indicated for the patient who has a complete spinal cord injury.

References

1. Anderson O. Rontgenbilder Vid Spondylarthritis Ankylopoetica. Nord Med 1937;14:2000.
2. Ball J, Sharp J. Rheumatoid arthritis of the cervical spine. In: Hill AGS, ed. Modern trends in rheumatology, vol. 2. New York: Appleton-Century-Crofts, 1971.
3. Bell HS. Paralysis of both arms from injury of the upper portion of pyramidal decussation: "cruciate paralysis." J Neurosurg 1970;33:378–380.
4. Bergfeldt L, Edhag O, Vedin L, et al. Ankylosing spondylitis: an important cause of severe disturbances of the cardiac conduction system. Am J Med 1982;73:187–191.
5. Bland JH. Rheumatoid arthritis of the cervical spine. J Rheumatol 1974;3:319.
6. Boden SD, Dodge LD, Bohlman HH, et al. Rheumatoid arthritis of the cervical spine: a long-term analysis with predictors of paralysis and recovery. J Bone Joint Surg 1993;75A:1282–1297.
7. Boden SD. Rheumatoid arthritis of the cervical spine: surgical decision making based on predictors of paralysis and recovery. Spine 1994;19:2275–2280.
8. Bohlman HH. Atlantoaxial dislocations in the arthritic patient: a report of 45 patients. Orthop Trans 1978; 2:197.
9. Boushea DK, Sundstrom WR. The pleuropulmonary manifestations of ankylosing spondylitis. Semin Arthritis Rheum 1989;18:277–281.
10. Brattstrom H, Elner A, Granholm L. Case report: transoral surgery for myelopathy caused by rheumatoid arthritis of the cervical spine. Ann Rheum Dis 1973; 32:578–581.
11. Brooks AL, Jenkins EB. Atlanto-axial arthrodesis by the

wedge compression method. J Bone Joint Surg 1978; 60A:279–284.
12. Bryant WJ, Inglis AE, Sculco TP, et al. Methylmethacrylate stabilization for enhancement of posterior cervical arthrodesis in rheumatoid arthritis. J Bone Joint Surg 1982;64A:1045.
13. Bulkley BH, Roberts WC. Ankylosing spondylitis and aortic regurgitation: description of the characteristic cardiovascular lesion from study of eight necropsy patients. Circulation 1973;48:1014–1027.
14. Burry HC, Tweed JM, Robinson RG, et al. Lateral subluxation of the atlanto-axial joint in rheumatoid arthritis. Ann Rheum Dis 1978;37:525–528.
15. Cantore G, Ciappetta P, Delfini R. New steel device for occipito-cervical fixation: technical note. J Neurosurg 1984;60:1104–1106.
16. Castaing J, Gouaze A, Plisson JL. Technique of cervico-occipital arthrodesis by iliac graft screwed into occipital bone. Rev Chir Orthop 1963;49:123–127.
17. Clark CR, Goetz DD, Menezes AH. Arthrodesis of the cervical spine in rheumatoid arthritis. J Bone Joint Surg 1989;71A:381–392.
18. Cohen C. Fatal dislocation of the cervical spine in rheumatoid disease. Gerontol Clin 1969;11:239–243.
19. Conaty JP, Morgan ES. Cervical fusion in rheumatoid arthritis. J Bone Joint Surg 1981;63A:1218–1227.
20. Conlon PW, Isdale IC, Rose BS. Rheumatoid arthritis of 333 cases. Ann Rheum Dis 1966;25:120–126.
21. Cregin, JCF. Internal fixation of the unstable rheumatoid cervical spine. Ann Rheum Dis 1966;25:242–252.
22. Crellin RQ, MacCable JJ, Hamilton EBD. Severe subluxation of the cervical spine in rheumatoid arthritis. J Bone Joint Surg 1970;52B:244–251.
23. Crockard HA, Essigman WK, Stevens JM, et al. Surgical treatment of cervical cord compression in rheumatoid arthritis. Ann Rheum Dis 1985;44:809–816.
24. Crockard HA, Pozo JL, Ransford AO, et al. Transoral decompression and posterior fusion for rheumatoid atlanto-axial subluxation. J Bone Joint Surg 1986;68B: 350–356.
25. Crockard HA, Calder I, Ransford AO. One stage transoral decompression and posterior fixation in rheumatoid atlantoaxial subluxation. J Bone Joint Surg 1990; 72B:682–685.
26. Cruickshank B. Pathology of ankylosing spondylitis. Clin Orthop 1971;74:43.
27. Cush JJ, Lipsky PE. The immunopathogenesis of rheumatoid arthritis: the role of cytokines in chronic inflammation. Clinical Aspects. Autoimmune 1987;1:2–13.
28. Davidson RC, Horn JR, Herndon JH, et al. Brain-stem compression in rheumatoid arthritis. JAMA 1977; 238:2633–2634.
29. DeAndrade JR, MacNab I. Anterior occipito-cervical fusion using an extra-pharyngeal exposure. J Bone Joint Surg 1969;69A:1621–1626.
30. Delamarter RB, Dodge L, Bohlman HH, et al. Post mortem neuropathologic analysis of eleven patients with paralysis secondary to rheumatoid arthritis of the spine. Orthop Trans 1988;12:54.
31. El-Khoury GY, Wener MH, Menezes AH, et al. Cranial settling in rheumatoid arthritis. Radiology 1980;137: 637–642.
32. Dihlmann W. Current radiodiagnostic concepts in ankylosing spondylitis. Skeletal Radiology 1979:179–188.
33. Eulderink F, Meijers KAE. Pathology of the cervical spine in rheumatoid arthritis: controlled study of 44 spines. J Pathol 1976;120:91–108.
34. Ferlich DC, Clayton ML, Leibholt JD, et al. Surgical treatment of the symptomatic unstable cervical spine in rheumatoid arthritis. J Bone Joint Surg 1975;57A: 349–354.
35. Fielding JW, Hawkins, RJ, Ratzan SA. Spine fusion for atlantoaxial instability. J Bone Joint Surg 1976;58A: 400–407.
36. Fielding JW, Cochran G, Van B, et al. Tears of the transverse ligament of the atlas: a clinical and biomechanical study. J Bone Joint Surg 1974;56A:1983–1991.
37. Fischgold H, Metzger J. Etude radiographique de l'impression basilaire. Rev Rheum 1952;19:261–264.
38. Frank P, Gleeson JA. Destructive vertebral lesions in ankylosing spondylitis. Br J Radiol 1975;48:755–758.
39. Graham B, Van Peteghem PK. Fractures of the spine in ankylosing spondylitis: diagnosis, treatment, and complications. Spine 1989;14(8):803–807.
40. Grob D, Dvorak J, Manohar M, et al. The role of plate and screw fixation in occipitocervical fusion in rheumatoid arthritis. Spine 1994;19:2545–2551.
41. Gruhn WB, McDuffie FC. Studies of serum immunoglobulin binding to synovial fibroblast cultures from patients with rheumatoid arthritis. Arthritis Rheum 1980;23:10–16.
42. Halla JT, Harden JG, Vitek J, et al. Involvement of the cervical spine in rheumatoid arthritis. Arthritis Rheum 1989;32:652–659.
43. Hamblen DL. Occipito-cervical fusion: indications, techniques, and results. J Bone Joint Surg 1967;49B:33–45.
44. Henderson DR. Vertical atlanto-axial subluxation in rheumatoid arthritis. Rheumatol Rehabil 1975;14:31–38.
45. Hochberg M. Epidemiology. In: Calin A, ed. Spondyloarthropathies. Orlando: Grune and Stratton, 1984:21–42.
46. Hopkins JS. Lower cervical rheumatoid subluxation with tetraplegia. J Bone Joint Surg 1967;49B(1):46–51.
47. Jurik AG, Pendersen V. Rheumatoid arthritis of the crico-arytenoid and crico-thyroid joints: a radiological and clinical study. Clin Radiol 1984;35:233–236.
48. Keenan MA, Stiles CM, Kaufman RL. Acquired laryngeal deviations associated with cervical spine disease in erosive polyarticular arthritis: use of the fiberoptive bronchoscope in rheumatoid disease. Anesthesiology 1983;58:441–449.
49. Khan, MA. Genetics of HLA-B27. Br J Rheumatol 1988; 27(Suppl 2):6–11.
50. Lachiewicz PF, Inglis AE, Ranawat CS. Methylmethacrylate augmentation for cervical spine arthrodesis in rheumatoid arthritis. Orthop Trans 1967;11:7.
51. Lachiewicz PF, Schoenfeldt R, Inglis A. Somatosensory evoked potentials in the evaluation of the unstable rheumatoid cervical spine: a preliminary report. Spine 1986;11:813–817.
52. Larsson SE, Toolanen G. Posterior fusion for atlanto-

52. axial subluxation in rheumatoid arthritis. Spine 1986; 11:525–530.
53. Lawrence JS. The prevalence of arthritis. Br J Clin Pract 1963;17:699–705.
54. Lawry, GV, Finerman ML, Hanafee WN, et al. Laryngeal involvement in rheumatoid arthritis: a clinical, laryngoscopic, and computerized tomographic study. Arthritis Rheum 1984;27:873–882.
55. Lipson SJ. Cervical myelopathy and posterior atlantoaxial subluxation in patients with rheumatoid arthritis. J Bone Joint Surg 1985;67A:593–597.
56. Marks JS, Sharp J. Rheumatoid cervical myelopathy. QJM 1981;50:307–319.
57. Marmion BP. Infection, autoimmunity, and rheumatoid arthritis. Clin Rheum Dis 1978;4:565–578.
58. Martel W, Duff IF, Preston RE, et al. The cervical spine in rheumatoid arthritis: correlation of radiographic and clinical manifestations (Abstract). Arthritis Rheum 1964;7:326.
59. Mathews JA. Atlantoaxial subluxation in rheumatoid arthritis. Ann Rheum Dis 1974;33:526–531.
60. McAfee PC, Bohlman HH, Riley LH Jr, et al. The anterior retropharyngeal approach to the upper part of the cervical spine. J Bone Joint Surg 1987;69A:1371–1383.
61. Meijers KAE, Cats A, Kremer HPH, et al. Cervical myelopathy in rheumatoid arthritis. Clin Exp Rheumatol 1984;2:239–245.
62. Menezes AH, Van Gilder JC, Clark CR, et al. Odontoid upward migration in rheumatoid arthritis. J Neurosurg 1985;63:500–509.
63. Mikulowski P, Wollheim FA, Rotmil AP, et al. Sudden death in rheumatoid arthritis with atlantoaxial dislocation. Acta Med Scand 1975;198:445–451.
64. Murray RO, Jacobsin HG. The radiology of skeletal disorders. London: Churchill Livingstone, 1981.
65. Newman P, Sweetnam R. Occipito-cervical fusion: an operative technique and its indications. J Bone Joint Surg 1969;51B:423–431.
66. Olerud S, Sjostrom L. Dens resection in a case of vertical impression of the dens in the foramen magnum. Acta Orthop Scand 1986;57:262.
67. Pellici POM, Ranawat SC, Tsarairis P, et al. A prospective study of the progression of rheumatoid arthritis of the cervical spine. J Bone Joint Surg 1981;63A:342–350.
68. Peppelman DO, Kraus DR, Donaldson WF, et al. Cervical spine surgery in rheumatoid arthritis: improvement of neurologic deficit after cervical spine fusion. Spine 1993;18:2375–2379.
69. Perry J, Nickel VL. Total cervical spine fusion for neck paralysis. J Bone Joint Surg 1959;41A:37–60.
70. Rana NA, Hancock DO, Taylor AR, et al. Upward translocation of the dens in rheumatoid arthritis. J Bone Joint Surg 1973;55B:471–477.
71. Ranawat CS, O'Leary P, Pellici PM, et al. Cervical spine fusion in rheumatoid arthritis. J Bone Joint Surg 1979; 61A:1003–1010.
72. Redlund-Johnell I, Pettersson H. Radiographic measurements of the cranio-vertebral region. Acta Radiol 1984;25:23–28.
73. Resnick D, Niwayama G. Diagnosis of bone and joint disorders. Philadelphia: WB Saunders, 1981;2:982–985.
74. Rosenow E, Strimlan CV, Muhm JR, et al. Pleuropulmonary manifestations of ankylosing spondylitis. Mayo Clin Proc 1977;52:641–649.
75. Sakov T, Kawaida H, Morizono Y, et al. Occipitoatlantoaxial fusion using a rectangular rod. Clin Orthop 1989;239:136–144.
76. Santavirta S, Slatis P, Kankaanpaa U, et al. Treatment of the cervical spine in rheumatoid arthritis. J Bone Joint Surg 1988;70A:658–667.
77. Sharp J, Purser DW. Spontaneous atlanto-axial dislocation in ankylosing spondylitis and rheumatoid arthritis. Ann Rheum Dis 1961;20:47–77.
78. Silman AJ. Rheumatoid arthritis and infection: a population approach. Ann Rheum Dis 48:707–710.
79. Simkin PA, Downey DJ, Kilcoyne RF. Apophyseal arthritis limits lumbar motion in patients with ankylosing spondylitis. Arthritis Rheum 1989;31:798–802.
80. Simmons EH. Surgery of the spine in rheumatoid arthritis and ankylosing spondylitis. In: Evarts CM, ed. Surgery of the musculoskeletal system. New York: Churchill Livingstone, 1983;2:85.
81. Simmons EH. Kyphotic deformity of the spine in ankylosing spondylitis. Clin Orthop 1977;128:65–77.
82. Simmons EH. The surgical correction of flexion deformity of the cervical spine in ankylosing spondylitis. Clin Orthop 1972;86:132–143.
83. Simmons EH, Duncan CP. Fracture of the cervical spine in ankylosing spondylitis: an analysis of its influence on severe deformity for spinal osteotomy. Clin Orthop 1978;133:227–239.
84. Slatis P, Santavirta S, Sandelin J, et al. Cranial subluxation of the odontoid process in rheumatoid arthritis. J Bone Joint Surg 1989;71A:189–195.
85. Smith PH, Benn RT, Sharp J. Natural history of rheumatoid cervical luxations. Ann Rheum Dis 1972;31: 431–439.
86. Smith-Peterson MN, Larson CB, Aufranc OE. Osteotomy of the spine for correction of flexion deformity in rheumatoid arthritis. J Bone Joint Surg 1945;27:1–11.
87. Stastny P. Association of the B-cell alloantigen DRw4 with rheumatoid arthritis. N Engl J Med 1978;298:869–871.
88. Stewart SR, Robbins DL, Castles JJ. Acute fulminant aortic and mitral insufficiency in ankylosing spondylitis. N Engl J Med 1978;299:1448–1449.
89. Thomasen E. Vertebral osteotomy for correction of kyphosis in ankylosing spondylitis. Clin Orthop 1985; 194:142–152.
90. Thompson RC, Meyer TJ. Posterior surgical stabilization for atlantoaxial subluxation in rheumatoid arthritis. Spine 1985;10:597–602.
91. Utsinger PD, Zvaifler NJ, Weiner SB. Etiology of rheumatoid arthritis. In: Utsinger PD, Zvaifler NJ, Ehrlich GE, eds. Rheumatoid arthritis: Etiology, diagnosis, and management. Philadelphia: Lippincott, 1985:21.
92. Wattenmaker I, Conception M, Hibberd P, et al. Upperairway obstruction and perioperative management of the airway in patients managed with posterior operations on the cervical spine for rheumatoid arthritis. J Bone Joint Surg 1994;76A:360–365.
93. Webb F, Hickman J, Brew D. Death from vertebral artery

thrombosis in rheumatoid arthritis. Br J Med 1968;2:537–538.
94. Weissman BNW, Aliabadi P, Weinfeld MS, et al. Prognostic features of atlantoaxial subluxation in rheumatoid arthritis patients. Radiology 1982;144:745–751.
95. Wertheim SB, Bohlman HH. Occipitocervical fusion: indications, technique, and long-term results in thirteen patients. J Bone Joint Surg 1987;69A:833–836.
96. Zeidman SM, Duckner TB. Rheumatoid arthritis: neuroanatomy, compression, and grading of deficits. Spine 1994;19:2259–2266.
97. Zvaifler NJ. Rheumatoid arthritis: epidemiology, etiology, rheumatoid factor, pathology, pathogenesis. In: Schumacher HR, ed. Primer on the rheumatic diseases. 9th ed. Atlanta: Arthritis Foundation. 1989.

CHAPTER THIRTY

Sacral Disorders

Todd E. Siff and Stephen Esses

Sacral Anatomy

The sacrum is composed of five vertebrae that become fused during development. The anterior surface is concave in both the sagittal and frontal planes. The lateral aspect of the upper sacrum is concave and articulates with the ilium. Anteriorly are four pairs of foramina, called the anterior or pelvic sacral foramina. Running transversely between each pair of foramina is a ridge that represents the site where the vertebrae became fused. The upper part of the first sacral vertebra is called the sacral promontory. The area lateral to the pelvic foramina is called the pars lateralis. Superiorly, at the level of the first sacral vertebra, the pars lateralis is large and is called the ala.

On the posterior aspect of the sacrum the foramina (posterior sacral foramina) are smaller. A ridge of bone runs longitudinally in the midline, representing the fusion of the sacral spinous processes, and is called the sacral median crest. Inferiorly, some bone is absent on the posterior aspect in the midline, which is referred to as the sacral hiatus.

The sacrum is stabilized by the sacroiliac joints and by the lumbosacral ligament. This ligament is a thick band that extends from the anterior-inferior aspect of the transverse process of the last lumbar vertebra to the lateral surface of the sacrum. It is sometimes referred to as the sickle ligament.

Sacral Tumors

Introduction

Tumors of the sacrum and presacral space are rare. The incidence of sacral tumors among all bone tumors varies from 1% to 3.5%. In three large hospital series, sacral and presacral tumors accounted for a combined incidence of 1 per 46, 000 admissions (5, 17).

The history plays an important role in diagnosing sacral tumors. The most common complaint is diffuse low back pain; pain is typically worse at night and is not alleviated with recumbency. The pain is described as pain at rest that is unaffected by the patient's physical movements. Late in the course of the disease urinary and bowel incontinence is a complaint. The complaint of diffuse pain in the absence of neurologic signs can be confused with coccydynia. The history of this disease can be misleading, and the nonspecific nature of the patient's complaints can result in a delay in proper diagnosis and allow for progression of tumor growth.

In many cases the physical examination is not especially helpful. There are no pathognomonic signs. Local tenderness over the sacral region is common. One of the most important elements of the physical examination is the rectal examination. Upon careful rectal examination, a swelling or a mass can occasionally be detected. The gait is usually normal, though if there is nerve root involvement or vertebral destruction, the gait will be affected. The history and physical examination of a patient with a sacral tumor most likely will not lead to the diagnosis of a sacral tumor, but it should alert the examiner to the need for further investigation.

Radiographic findings of these tumors are often missed because of the overlying gas pattern and bowel contents obscuring the lesion. To optimize a search for a sacral lesion, the bowel must be thoroughly prepared. Other diagnostic tests of value are the high-resolution computed tomography (CT) scan for delineating bony destruction, magnetic resonance imaging (MRI) for identifying soft-tissue involvement and neural compression, and a bone scan. A myelogram is useful to delineate extradural extension. Angiography is an important test prior to surgery to assess the vascularity of the tumor.

After a complete history and physical examination and radiologic studies have been completed, a biopsy should be performed for definitive diagnosis. Generally a frozen-section biopsy is preferable. It is important not to contaminate the tissue planes during the biopsy. Before performing the biopsy, consideration should be given to performing the definitive surgical procedure at the same sitting in the event of a positive frozen section. The definitive surgical procedure will minimize the risk of tumor implantation and spread of the tumor by excising the biopsy tract.

Most lesions can be accessed through a midline vertical posterior approach via the posterior elements of the lower sacral vertebrae. Sometimes the coccyx must be resected to achieve better exposure. The anterior approach is rarely used, because of the increased risk of tumor cell implantation and difficulty in excising the biopsy tract. An open biopsy of an anterior lesion may be done through a lower midline abdominal incision or an oblique incision from near the left costal margin to near the pubic symphysis.

Sacral tumors are divided into two groups: benign and malignant. The benign tumors include aneurysmal bone cysts, osteoblastomas, giant cell tumors, osteochondromas, and sacral cysts. The malignant tumors include chordomas, chondrosarcomas, metastatic carcinomas, marrow tumors (myeloma and Ewing's sarcoma), and other primary malignant tumors.

Benign Sacral Tumors

Benign sacral tumors are generally asymptomatic. These tumors are often first realized on examination following trauma or on routine rectal or pelvic examination. The benign sacral tumors are categorized into three stages: stage 1 (latent), stage 2 (active), and stage 3 (aggressive). The majority of osteoblastomas and aneurysmal bone cysts are stage 1 or 2. In large, narrowly marginated stage 2 or stage 3 benign sacral tumors such as aneurysmal bone cysts or giant cell tumors, there is a significant risk of hemorrhage or neurologic deficit. Staging is important when considering treatment options.

Aneurysmal Bone Cyst

An aneurysmal bone cyst is a cystic, vascular process that expands and destroys bone. The incidence of aneurysmal bone cysts in the sacrum is 3.7% from a total of 134 found in one study (5). These cysts are more common in females; they predominate in the second to third decades of life and are uncommon after the age of 30 years. Some remain latent, and others are aggressive and mimic sarcoma. In some cases an aneurysmal bone cyst can be a disabling condition. The clinical presentation is variable, depending on the size of the cyst and on the presence of pathological fractures.

The diagnosis is aided through imaging studies. A pathognomonic radiographic finding is a localized expansion of bone with development of a thin peripheral rim of bone, which is seen well on a CT scan. This narrow rim of bone distinguishes the edge of the lesion and separates it from adjacent normal soft-tissue structures. The aneurysmal bone cyst can expand into adjacent vertebrae. They can be seen in any part of the skeleton, but predominate in the metaphysis of long tubular bones and in the vertebral column. Bone scans show increased uptake around the periphery and decreased uptake at the center of the vertebrae. An angiogram will show vascular activity around the periphery of the lesion and relative avascularity at the center of the vertebrae.

Biopsy confirms the diagnosis. Open biopsy is preferable, although fine-needle biopsies can be valuable if adequate tissue is obtained. On gross examination of the lesion, the surrounding thin rim of bone can be easily broken through with an osteotome. The inner region contains unclotted blood and various amounts of soft tissue.

On a pathological examination of the vertebrae, blood-filled cavernous sinuses, benign spindle cells, and new bony trabeculae can be seen at the center. Multinucleated giant cells can be found in these lesions, but they are smaller than those found in giant cells tumors. Histiocyte and foam cells are also found. The peripheral rim of new bone is quite cellular, with bone formation and resorption often adjacent to large vascular lakes.

The differential diagnosis for aneurysmal bone cysts includes giant cell tumor and telangiectatic osteosarcoma. The pathogenesis of this lesion is unknown, although some speculate it to be a result of local change in vascular hemodynamics (10).

Giant Cell Tumor

Giant cell tumors in the sacrum are a rare clinical entity. The incidence in the spine and sacrum has been estimated to be between 4% and 12% of all giant cell tumors (4). The sacrum is the fourth most common location for this tumor. The clinical impact of giant cell tumors occurs with neurologic impairment. Giant cell tumors occur predominantly in the upper sacral segments and often extend to the sacroiliac joint. These tumors have an eccentric location, which helps in differentiating them from sacral chordomas. The radiographic characteristics of the sacral giant cell tumor are similar to those it has when located elsewhere in the body. Radiographically, giant cell tumors appear as homogeneous, oval or round, lytic lesions with occasional trabeculations. The margins are hazy without a sclerotic border or periosteal reaction. The upper sacrum lesions can present with soft-tissue extensions. The delay in radiographic suspicion of these tumors results from the difficulty in seeing the lytic lesions in the thickness of the sacral bone.

On gross examination, it is difficult to differentiate the giant cell tumor from other vertebral body tumors. This tumor is typically soft and homogeneous, with a central cystic, necrotic, or rubbery area. The color ranges from light to dark brown to bloody.

The histological hallmarks of the giant cell tumor, which are not unique to the sacral tumor, are the sheets of mononuclear cells situated among numerous multinucleated osteoclast-like giant cells. The nuclei of the giant cells are round or oval and are not spindly. Necrosis is often found in giant cell tumors. These tumors are difficult to treat, but local resection with or without postoperative radiation is mainstay of treatment (Fig. 30.1).

Other Benign Tumors

Other benign tumors include osteochondromas, osteoblastomas, sacral meningiomas, neurofibromas, and intraspinal lipomas. Osteochondromas and sacral meningiomas are very rare. Osteoblastomas and neurofibromas have been occasionally noted in the sacrum. Intraspinal lipomas are believed to be congenital; they are seen with defects in the laminae and may be extensions of subcutaneous lipomas. They pose significant danger when surgical removal is delayed until adulthood, when there is a significant risk for neurologic compromise.

Malignant Sacral Tumors

Unlike benign sacral tumors, malignant sacral tumors typically present with pain. This pain is distributed along the sacrococcygeal region, the lower back, and the rectal area, with radiations down to the legs. This characteristic pain has been estimated to occur in 65% to 90% of malignant tumors, with a mean duration of preexisting pain of 6 to 12 months. Bowel and bladder dysfunctions are seen in approximately 15 to 20% of patients who have these lesions (8). The majority of malignant sacral tumors can be detected on rectal examination.

Chordoma

The sacrococcygeal chordoma is a rare, fatal malignant tumor. Chordomas have been shown to arise from infancy through old age, though approximately one-half of the cases are found in the fifth through the seventh decades of life. It is typically slow-growing and destructive locally. The embryonic notochord is thought to be the progenitor of the chordoma. The chordomas arise either in the sacrococcygeal area or in the basiocciput as a result of the persistence of notochord in the fused bones of the sacrum and basiocciput. The discovery of this tumor is often delayed, because the early symptoms are often insidious and vague.

The most common complaint is pain, centered either in the lower back or in the sacrum. The nature of the sacral pain varies and may be dull, sharp, continuous, or intermittent. Patients may also complain of back pain or perineal pain and numbness. Other symptoms that may be present are fecal and urinary difficulties, including constipation, tenesmus, rectal bleeding, urinary frequency, urgency, difficulty starting the stream, and both urinary and fecal incontinence. If the lesion impinges on the pelvic nerves, paresthesias and anesthesia can result. When the symptoms progress, they can become intractable and at times disabling. On physical examination, a presacral tumor mass can usually be detected through a rectal examination. The mass is usually firm, fixed to the sacrum, and does not involve the rectal mucosa. Diminished perianal sensation can also occur, though motor loss is unusual. The radiographic features include bone destruction and the appearance of a soft-tissue mass, which is usually directed anteriorly. Typically the bony involvement entails destruction of several segments of the sacrum. In the literature, reports on the amount of calcification has ranged from 40 to 80% (15). The calcification is usually amorphous and located peripherally. The size of the soft-tissue mass is usually much larger than the amount of bony destruction. Remodeling can occur around a slowly growing lesion, which results in expansion of the sacrum. Irregular areas of osteolysis can be seen around the sacrum. These chordomas commonly spread to the adjacent vertebrae without involving the intervertebral disc. CT and MRI are helpful in defining both the bony component and the soft-tissue involvement, respectively (Fig. 30.2).

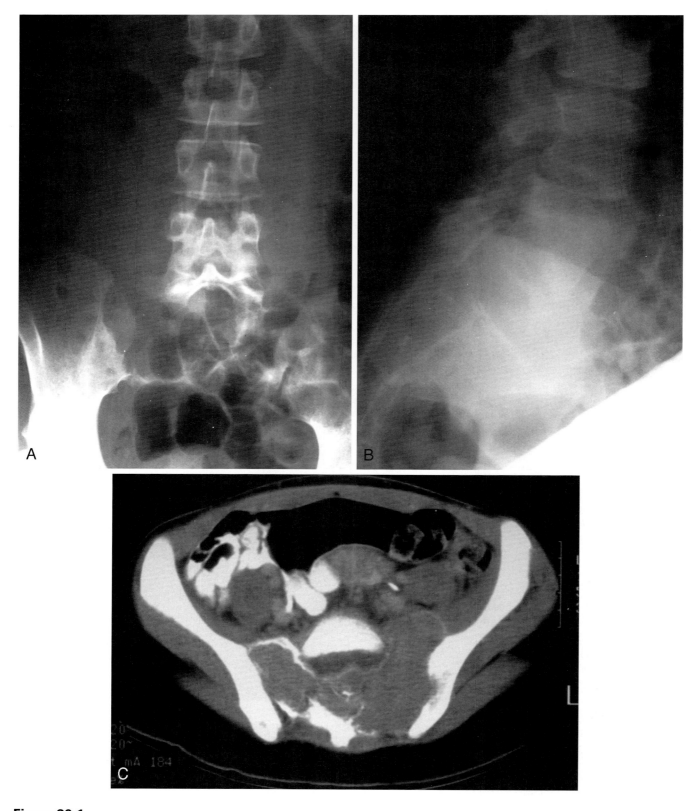

Figure 30.1.
Giant cell tumor of the sacrum in a 20-year-old female with severe back pain and weakness of left L5 and S1 roots. **A.** Anteroposterior radiograph shows destructive process of the sacrum, including the left sacroiliac joint. **B.** Lateral radiograph shows destructive lesion of the entire sacrum. **C.** CT scan clearly demonstrates the extent of the lesion, which involves the left sacroiliac joint, the spinal canal, and the neural foramina. The lesion extends into the retroperitoneal space anteriorly on the left side.

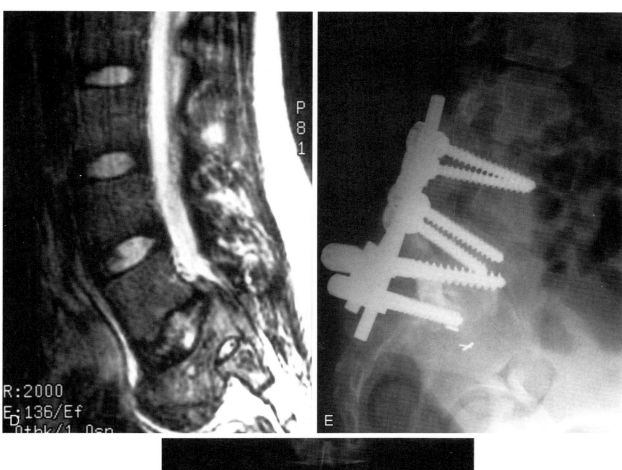
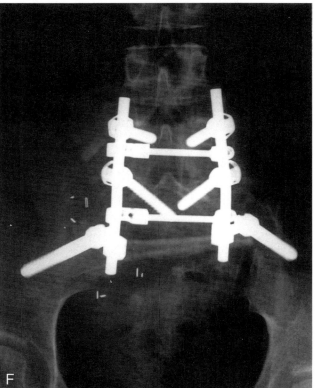

Figure 30.1—*continued*

D. Sagittal T2-weighted MRI shows the large lesion extending into the spinal canal. **E.** and **F.** The patient underwent posterior excision of the entire sacrum, sparing all the nerve roots. A fibula strut graft was placed anterior to the thecal sac, extending from one ilium to the other. Pedicle screws at L4 and L5 and iliac screws are used to stabilize the lower lumbar spine to the ilium. The patient was allowed to ambulate immediately, and good healing and the maintenance of stabilization were noted. Postoperative radiation therapy was given 3 months after the surgery. No recurrence of disease is noted at 1 year after surgery. (Courtesy of Howard S. An.)

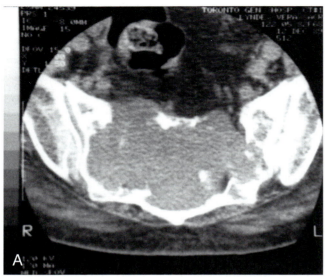

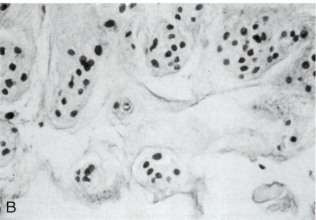

Figure 30.2.

A. CT scan showing sacral chordoma with invasion of the left sacroiliac joint and extension through the anterior cortex. **B.** Histologic preparation of sacral chordoma demonstrating physaliferous ("soap bubble") cells.

Bone scans are not of much use, since they rarely show positive uptake in the tumor. Before surgery, angiography is helpful in determining the vascular status of the tumor.

The presence of a midline sacral tumor demonstrating radiographic evidence of bone destruction accompanied by a soft-tissue mass suggests a chordoma. A biopsy then should then be performed to confirm this diagnosis. The preferred approach for open biopsy is via the posterior route. In planning, the surgeon must prepare to carry out a radical resection immediately following the biopsy should the biopsy results be positive for chordoma. On gross examination a chordoma is typically lobulated and soft but can vary from semiliquid to firm. Usually it is gray and semitransparent. Hemorrhage, whether recent or old, can discolor the tumor. The soft-tissue component of the chordoma can be substantial because of its slow growth. A pseudocapsule forms within the soft tissues and completely surrounds the tumor. This pseudocapsule is derived from the anterior aspect of the periosteum, which is intact and elevated.

The microscopic hallmark of this tumor is the vacuolated physaliferous cells; these "soap bubble" cells form a unique lobular arrangement with prolific vacuolated cytoplasm. They have intracytoplasmic mucus droplets in different sizes that stain for glycogen and mucin. The mucin is expelled from the vacuoles and spreads between the cells. The presence of both intra- and extracellular mucin production is important in differentiating the chordoma from a cartilaginous tumor. A narrow extension of the clear cytoplasm surrounds the nucleus. The nucleus can also be vacuolated. Binucleate forms and multinucleated giant cells are present in most of these tumors (Fig. 30.2). Mitotic figures are rare. It has been postulated that the stellate cell is the primary neoplastic cell, which metamorphoses into the physaliferous cell through a process of cisternal dilatation and internal secretion (11). Another characteristic feature of the chordoma is the syncytial strands of cells with unclear cell boundaries within an expanse of mucin.

The differential diagnosis of a chordoma includes giant cell tumor, metastatic carcinoma, ependymoma, and chondrosarcoma. As with all malignant tumors, defining the extent of spread of the chordoma is vital. Technetium bone scans are helpful in delineating the local involvement of the tumor. Other useful imaging tests include MRI, barium enema radiography, angiogram, intravenous pyelogram, and chest roentgenograms. Before treatment intervention, the extent of the chordoma must be completely defined. After treatment, the patient must be regularly followed up to monitor for any recurrence or metastases. Chordomas have a strong predilection for local recurrence. The rate of distant metastases has been reported to be between 10% and 27% (9). Chordomas metastasize to soft tissues, lymph node, lung, bone, liver, and other abdominal organs. There has been no established relationship between mode of treatment and the propensity of the tumor to metastasize. However, because of the devastatingly aggressive course of the sacral chordoma, metastases generally have little impact on long-term survival. The discovery of a sacrococcygeal chordoma early on is vital to the survival of the patient. Chordomas metastasize late in their course, so early intervention offers the best chance for long-term survival.

Chondrosarcoma

Chondrosarcomas are found in adults between the ages of 30 and 60 years. The sacrum represents an area of a potential primary focus or a location for metastatic spread. The behavior of chondrosarcomas is not well understood. They can appear as a primary tumor, or they can form as a result of malignant degeneration of a benign bone neoplasm. Pain is the chief complaint and lasts for several months to years. Because of the nonspecific nature of the symptoms, these tumors often stay localized for several years and grow dramatically or metastasize before they are diagnosed. It is not uncommon for the presentation to be heralded by neurologic deficits. Gradual loss of bowel, bladder, and sexual function are often seen.

Radiographic studies typically reveal a mass with differing degrees of calcification. Chondrosarcomas first cause local destruction centered in the vertebral body with later spread to the posterior elements. In the plain radiograph shown in Figure 30.3, the local bony destruction is seen with calcification. The CT scan is better able to delineate the bony destruction.

Unfortunately, the pathological examination of chondrosarcomas does not offer much benefit. Predicting the behavior of these tumors solely on the basis of the histology or staging system has not been reliable because of the variability in biological behavior from benign local growth to aggressive metastatic disease. It is dangerous to differentiate benign cartilage neoplasms from low-grade malignancies, which may continue to a fulminating systemic disease, solely on the basis of histology or staging criteria. Using biochemical features of neoplastic cartilage in combination with histological criteria is a more useful predictor of biologic progression (13). The differential diagnosis for chondrosarcomas should always include osteosarcoma.

Metastasis

The sacrum serves as an important site for metastasis. The majority of intraspinal extradural tumors are metastatic. The lung, breast, prostate, kidney, and lymphoma are sources of metastatic spread to the sacrum. The source of metastasis is either hematogenous or by local spread. The rectum and genitourinary organs can metastasize to the sacrum via the venous system, the lymph vessels, or direct spread. A distinguishing feature between hematogenous and local metastasis to the sacrum is vertebral involvement. In hematogenous spread of the disease the center of the vertebra is affected, whereas in local spread the vertebral cortex is involved. The prognosis for metastatic involvement to the sacrum is grim. The treatment is palliation, but pain control is extremely difficult. In some cases, local radiation treatment is attempted for palliation. The life expectancy after discovery of a metastasis to the sacrum is 2 years.

Treatment

Stage 1 and 2 sacral tumors, such as osteoblastomas and aneurysmal bone cysts, can be treated with intralesional curettage or marginal excision through a posterior approach. In large, narrowly marginated

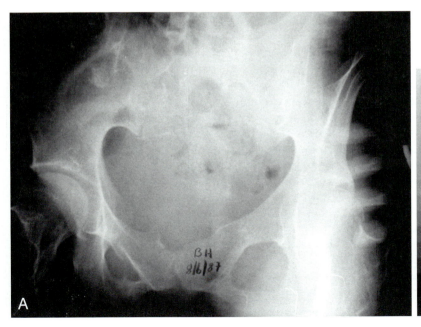
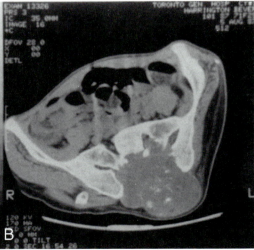

Figure 30.3.
Comparison of chondrosarcoma in **A.** plain radiograph and **B.** CT scan. The local destruction of sacral bone is seen with some suggestions of calcification in the plain radiograph. In the CT scan, better definition of the sacral and adjacent pelvic destruction and calcification within the tumor mass is seen.

stage 2 or stage 3 benign sacral tumors, such as aneurysmal bone cysts or giant cell tumors, intralesional curettage and occasionally adjunctive radiotherapy are valid options.

The treatment of choice for newly discovered and recurrent aneurysmal bone cysts is marginal excision involving curettage and bone grafting. Treatment considerations include the location, size, signs and symptoms, and spread of the disease. The course of aneurysmal bone cysts is unpredictable. The recurrence rate after marginal excision is 20%. However, the recurrence is often not significant, mainly noted in imaging studies and having no clinical impact. Some aneurysmal bone cysts subside spontaneously despite the persistence of radiologic abnormalities. However, some recurrences are noted to destroy the bone graft and progress to marked disability. Radiation therapy is employed in these refractory cases.

The treatment choices for giant cell tumors are numerous and controversial, though complete surgical resection remains the treatment of choice. Wide resection of the tumor has consistently produced better results than marginal curettage. However, when anatomic considerations do not allow the complete resection of the tumor a more limited approach is advisable. In this instance, gross resection of the tumor followed by careful curettage of the remaining tumor, decompression of the neural elements, and radiation therapy to eradicate any remaining tumor is recommended. Most advocate excising the biopsy tract to avoid any spreading of the tumor. The critical decision of whether the tumor should be approached by an abdominal or a perineal approach should be made on the basis of whether the examining finger can reach the superior limit of the tumor from the perineal approach.

In extensive sacral resections, nerve considerations are important. The unilateral sacrifice of the sacral nerves with the preservation of the contralateral sacral nerves has not been shown to cause functional impairments (10). The interruption of the pudendal nerve supplying the sphincters similarly does not cause any difficulties with urinary and fecal incontinence. However, the bilateral interruption of all the sacral nerves except for S1 impairs the urinary bladder and urethral sphincter control. Additionally, most genital functions except for ejaculation will be affected. The urinary and fecal difficulties can be managed by regular self-catheterizations and fecal disimpactions. Preservation of bilateral S1 nerve roots does not greatly affect motor function. In addition, transection of the sacrum above the level of the first sacral foramina does not significantly alter pelvic stability and strength. Ambulating is unaffected on level ground, though climbing is affected as a result of the partial impairment of the gluteus maximus muscle.

The primary modality of treatment for the sacrococcygeal chordoma is resection. Wide resection of the tumor with adequate margins can lead to eradication of the tumor. The approach to the resection of the chordoma, as in any other malignant tumor, depends on its size and location. The different approaches are the anterior, the posterior, and the combined approach. Common to all of these is the potential for significant blood loss.

The main indication for the anterior approach is the presence of adhesions in the presacral space formed from previous surgery or radiation treatment. For the anterior approach, the patient is placed in the supine position. After the sterile preparation and draping of the patient, a standard retroperitoneal dissection is carried out through a standard left paramedian incision. This may be modified to a midline or right paramedian incision, depending on the location of the tumor. On the basis of preoperative imaging, a decision is made as to whether to ligate one or both internal iliac arteries. This is done to facilitate the exposure and to control bleeding.

More often, the tumor is approached from a posterior incision. A commonly used posterior approach is that advocated by the Mayo Clinic (7). The patient is placed in the prone position. Through a perianal skin incision and a perineal dissection, the approach is begun above the tumor so as not to contaminate the wound with tumor cells. If the tumor is present posteriorly, both the midline skin and a part of the subcutaneous tissue along with the sacrum may have to be sacrificed. The pelvic organs are mobilized to protect them from later sacral resection. Unless the tumor extends more proximally, the ilium and sacrum are osteotomized at the S2-S3 level. The pudendal nerve, sacral nerves, and proximal nerve roots are identified and spared. The sacrum and the coccyx are then removed. Drains are placed in the large space created by the resection of the sacrum. The gluteal muscles may be used to fill in this defect. With this technique, the Mayo clinic reports a 28% recurrence rate with an en bloc resection and a 64% recurrence when violating the tumor. Complications include bladder dysfunction and fecal incontinence, with a gradual disappearance of these complications over time. It is important not to allow the contamination of normal tissue with spillage of the tumor. Most advocate excising the biopsy tract to avoid any spreading of the tumor.

A variation of the Mayo posterior approach involves placing the patient in the lithotomy position. The rectum and the anal canal are then mobilized. After a thorough bowel preparation in the operating room, a purse-string suture is placed around the anus. The anal canal and rectum are dissected away from the presacral space through a posterior perineal incision. Placing a lap pad behind the rectum after mobilization protects the rectum. The biopsy tract is excised. The surgery is completed with the patient in the prone position (16).

The third option is the combined anterior and posterior approach (6). The patient is placed in the lateral position. An oblique incision is made extending between the left iliac crest and costal margin. The left colon is freed and moved anteriorly and to the right along with the rectum. The iliac vessels and left ureter are identified. The middle sacral vessels and lateral sacral veins are sacrificed with suture ligation. Then a posterior incision is made over the sacrum, and skin flaps are fashioned. The gluteal muscles are separated from their iliac attachments. The presacral space is accessed by cutting the anococcygeal ligaments. The next step involves incising the sacroiliac, sacrotuberous, and sacrospinous ligaments and the piriformis muscles. The sacrum is osteotomized. The nerve roots below the resected sacrum are sacrificed. The tumor is resected. The wound is then closed.

Another option in the combined anterior and posterior approach involves placing the patient in a supine position. Using an incision that extends between the left iliac crest and the left costal margin, a careful dissection down to the tumor is performed. Ligation of one or both of the internal iliac arteries is then carried out. Using an osteotomy, resection of the sacral tumor is done. After this is accomplished and prior to turning the patient, a marker is placed on the sacrum where the osteotomy was performed. This helps with orientation after placing the patient in a prone position. Dissection down to the tumor is then done from the posterior side. The osteotomy and resection of the tumor are then completed.

Other modes of treatment do not meet with much success. Although radiation therapy is very useful for palliative considerations, it is believed that it does not alter the long-term prognosis of the patient with this disease. Currently, preoperative treatment with radiation is being investigated. Postoperative radiation treatment significantly reduces the risk of tumor contamination during resection. Chemotherapy is not thought to play a role in the treatment of chordomas.

Chondrosarcomas are generally radioresistant, and they do not respond well to chemotherapy. The primary treatment for chondrosarcomas is surgical ablation. However, due to the size of these tumors and the areas of involvement in the spine, wide resection is not always possible. In these cases, repeated local debulking procedures should be performed.

Results

The outlook for malignant sacral tumors is poor. The median survival is 5 years for sacral lesions, and it varies from 20 to 40% at 10 years (16). The only mode of treatment is surgical resection. Hence diagnosing the tumor early on by paying close attention to the history of the patient is vital. This should be followed up with biopsy and surgery if necessary.

Fractures

Sacral fractures are rare, comprising only 1% of all fractures affecting the spinal column. In most instances they are associated with other injuries. Therefore, in a multiply traumatized patient it is of the utmost importance to adequately examine both the patient and the roentgenographs to determine whether a sacral fracture is present. Bruising over the buttock or pain on rectal examination may be indicative of a sacral injury.

Many classifications have been proposed for sacral injuries. The most commonly used is the Denis classification, which arranges the fractures according to location (Fig. 30.4). Zone 1 fractures involve the ala without injury to the foramina or the central canal. Zone 2 fractures involve one or more of the sacral foramina but do not involve the sacral canal. Zone 3 fractures involve the sacral canal and are almost always transverse.

In general, neurologic injury is rare in zone 1 injuries. Zone 2 injuries can be associated with nerve root injury, particularly when there is displacement

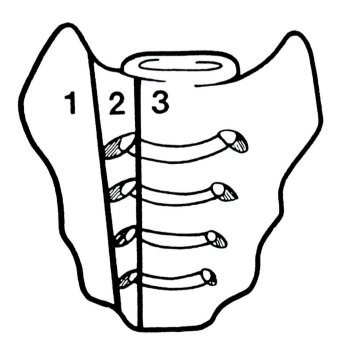

Figure 30.4.

Denis classification of sacral fractures: zone 1—the region of ala; zone II—the region of the foramina; and zone III—the region of the central canal.

at the fracture site. Most zone 3 fractures are associated with significant neurologic deficits.

Treatment

The treatment of sacral injuries is guided by two major goals. The first is to provide stability in those instances in which trauma has created instability. The second is to optimize neurologic recovery when there has been significant neurologic injury. Many sacral fractures are associated with injury to the sacroiliac joints or to the pelvis. Often this creates an unstable fracture pattern and mandates internal fixation.

Neurologic impairment can be associated with ongoing compression of neural elements. In this case surgical management is usually indicated. Surgical technique involves a posterior midline incision with exposure of the dorsal aspect of the sacrum. Unroofing of the sacrum then allows hematoma evacuation and neural decompression. In some cases in which bone has been retropulsed into the canal, it is possible to use a bone punch or tamp to push the bony fragments anteriorly.

Sacroiliac Joint Problems

Fracture-Dislocation

Sacral fracture-dislocations represent a rare but dangerous phenomenon. This type of injury is the result of a very high-energy insult. Most sacral fracture-dislocations result from vertical shear injuries. Consequently these injuries have a high morbidity and mortality. Other injuries accompanying sacral fracture-dislocations often include damage to the urinary tract, disruption of the rectum, vagina, and bowel, and injury to the diaphragm. Neurologic involved is always an important consideration. Patterson and Mortar studied a series of 633 patients who sustained pelvic injuries, some of whom had sacral fractures. Overall they found 3.5% to have some neurologic impairment (12), though they did not report any consistent neurological injury. The neurological injuries included damage to the lumbosacral plexus, the sciatic nerve, the femoral nerve, the gluteal nerve, the obturator nerve, and the cutaneous nerves of the thigh. The mortality has been estimated to be approximately 20% (2). Posterior instability of the sacroiliac complex can be seen radiographically by a gap posteriorly in the sacroiliac complex, an avulsion of the transverse process of L5, and/or an avulsion of the ischial spine.

The treatment of sacral fracture-dislocations is the subject of some controversy. Several reports of bilateral sacral fracture-dislocations describe successful nonoperative treatment. These case reports typically involve a patient who has been in an accident and has sustained multiple and severe injuries. Because of the critical condition of the patient, however, no sacral surgery is performed, and good results have been described. Carl and Thomas reported on such a case, noting only four other cases of bilateral sacroiliac joint fracture-dislocation in the literature. Three of the four patients were treated nonoperatively, and one had an open reduction and internal fixation. Three of the patients retained functional capacity and one patient (in a nonoperative case) died as a result of the traumatic injuries initially sustained. Carl and Thomas's patient had good results. Carl and Thomas thus concluded that nonoperative treatment can lead to a functional result (1).

Usually surgical correction is advocated for fracture-dislocations of the sacrum. The most basic surgical treatment involves closed reduction followed by the application of a triangular frame. If an acceptable closed reduction is not achieved, then an open reduction and internal fixation of one or both of the sacroiliac joints is done. The open reduction and internal fixation can be accomplished with lag screws or cobra plates along with a simple external frame or plate fixation of the pubic symphysis.

For complex, unstable sacroiliac joint fracture-dislocations, open reduction and internal fixation is indicated. Such injuries include multiple rami fractures and diastasis accompanied by an iliac fracture. Generally, two approaches are used for these types of fracture-dislocations. One option is to perform an open reduction and internal fixation of the iliac fracture and sacroiliac disruption followed by the placement of a simple external frame. The other option involves using the triangular frame in conjunction with internal fixation of the iliac fracture. A contraindication to anterior internal fixation is the presence of multiple rami fractures. An exception to this is in young women with multiple fractured rami. In these cases, plate fixation is preferred, using a bilateral ilioinguinal approach (3).

To provide anterior exposure of the hemipelvis, the ilioinguinal incision is preferred. Anterior stabilization is accomplished by placing a two-hole plate or four-hole plate between the sacral ala and the adjacent lateral ilium. Another option entails placing lag screws through the lateral aspect of the ilium into the sacral ala and the first sacral body. Using an ilioinguinal incision, a careful dissection is performed subperiosteally along the inner table of the ilium. It is important to be careful in preserving the L5 nerve root. Injuries involving single interruptions of the pelvic ring are easily reached through the posterior approach. Using the triradiate or iliofemoral approach and continuing the lateral incision, lag screws can be placed through the sacroiliac joint. The surgical approach is as follows. The patient should be positioned so that the wide part of the superior aspect of the ilium is parallel with the floor. The incision is begun next to the posterosuperior spine of the ilium. To expose the ilium or sacrum, the incision must be carried either more medial or lateral, respectively, to the spine of the ilium. The gluteus maximus is reflected superiorly. Then the periosteum is elevated to provide exposure for the surface of the ilium. For unstable sacroiliac disruptions, the sacroiliac crest is approached medial to the iliac crest. To expose the sacrum, the erector spinae and the multifidus muscles must be removed. Being able to palpate the inferior aspect of the sacroiliac joint allows in obtaining adequate reduction of the joint.

Stabilization of the sacroiliac joint is accomplished by placing two 6.5 mm cancellous lag screws with washers through the lateral ilium into the sacral ala and the first sacral body. To prevent rotational movement, a two- or three-hole plate can be used. The cancellous screws can be inserted with the use of a C-arm. Predrilling facilitates cancellous screw placement. Careful attention must be directed to the sacral nerve roots, the cauda equina, neurovascular structures, and the rectum, all of which lie anterior to the sacrum. With a 3.2 mm drill bit, a hole is begun perpendicularly to the ilium, superior and posterior to the roof of the greater sciatic notch, and directed through the superficial and deep iliac cortices. The drill is advanced approximately to 45 to 60 mm; if the drill bit penetrates the deep sacral cortex, there is risk to the soft tissues. To achieve optimal stability, a 50 mm or longer lag screw with a 32 mm thread length is used. The second screw is predrilled at a point 2.5 cm superior and posterior to the first screw and directed toward the first sacral body. To avoid the first sacral nerve root, direct the drill bit superior to the first anterior sacral foramen (3). CT scanning can be used to check the position of the sacral screws.

Sacral Arthritis

Ankylosing Spondylitis

One of the essential features of ankylosing spondylitis is involvement of the sacroiliac joint. Typically ankylosing spondylitis is bilateral and symmetric. Sacroiliitis represents an early phase in the development of this disease. The early radiographic appearance will demonstrate a widened joint articulation. As the disease develops, a broad area of sclerosis appears on the iliac side of the joint with larger subchondral erosions. Bony bridges span the joint space, forming isolated areas of intact cartilage. During the advanced stages of the disease, the sacral bones will fuse and the periarticular sclerosis disappears. Another feature of ankylosing spondylitis is involvement of the ligamentous part of the sacroiliac joint. This involvement can progress to bony erosions and proliferation.

Psoriatic Arthritis

Involvement of the sacroiliac joint is also prominent feature of psoriatic arthritis. Psoriatic arthritis usually is bilateral and symmetric. It typically affects synovial cartilaginous joints and entheses. The presence of joint-space narrowing or widening is characteristic. Areas of erosion develop in marginal areas in a central direction, often resulting in a whittled deformity of the involved articulation (14). Early pathologic changes, which are similar to those seen in ankylosing spondylitis, involve subchondral bony erosions and ill-defined sclerosis. Psoriatic arthritis differs from ankylosing spondylitis in that (a) intraarticular bony ankyloses are less common in psoriatic arthritis, and (b) blurring and eburnation of opposing sacral and iliac surfaces within the ligamentous portion of the sacroiliac joint are more common in psoriatic arthritis. The sacroiliac joint abnormalities are frequent. These findings may be bilateral and asymmetric or unilateral in distribution. In general, the characteristic findings of Reiter's syndrome are identical to those found in psoriatic arthritis.

The treatment for sacral arthritis is conservative. If conservative therapy fails to control the severe symptoms, then a surgical alternative is considered. Fusion is the primary modality in addressing severe sacral arthritis refractory to conservative treatment.

References

1. Carl A, Thomas S. Bilateral sacroiliac joint fracture-dislocation: case report. J Trauma 1990;30(11):1402–1403.
2. Crenshaw AH, ed. Campbell's operative orthopaedics. 8th ed. St. Louis: Mosby, 1992:1356–1357.
3. Chapman M, ed. Operative orthopaedics. Philadelphia: JB Lippincott, 1994:513–540.
4. Dahlin DC, McCarty CS. Chordoma: a study of fifty-nine cases. Cancer 1952;5:1170–1178.
5. Dahlin DC. Bone tumors. 3d ed. Springfield, IL: Charles C. Thomas, 1981:11.
6. Huth JF, Dawson EG, Eilber ER. Abdominal sacral resection for malignant tumors of the sacrum. Am J Surg 1984;48:157–161.
7. Kaiser TE, Pritchard DJ, Unni KK. Clinicopathologic study of sacrococcygeal chordoma. Cancer 1984;53:2574–2578.
8. Localio SA, Eng K, Ranson JHC. Abdominosacral approach for retrorectal tumors. Ann Surg 1980;191, 555–560.

9. Mindell ER. Chordoma. J Bone Joint Surg 1981;63A: 501–505.
10. Mindell ER. Aneurysmal bone cyst. Iowa Orthop J 1987; 7:39–41.
11. Murad TM, Murphy MSN. Ultrastructure of a chordoma. Cancer 1970;25:1203–1215.
12. Patterson FP, Mortar KS. Neurological complications of fractures and dislocation of the pelvis. J Trauma 1972; 12:1013.
13. Rothman RH, Simeone FA. The spine. 3d ed. Philadelphia: WB Saunders, 1992:1022–1040.
14. Sledge C, Harris E, Ruddy S, et al. Arthritis surgery. Philadelphia: WB Saunders, 1994:316–325.
15. Smith J, Ludwig RL, Marcove RC. Clinical radiological features of chordoma. Skeletal Radiol 1987;16:37–44.
16. Sundaresan N, Schmidek H, Schiller A, et al. Tumors of the spine: Diagnosis and clinical management. Philadelphia: WB Saunders, 1990:36–415.
17. Sung HW, Shu WP, Wang HM, et al. Surgical treatment of primary tumors of the sacrum. Clin Orthop 1987; 215:91–98.

SECTION VI

Spinal Procedures and Instrumentations

CHAPTER THIRTY ONE

Spinal Orthoses

Gregory P. Graziano and Lysa M. Charles

Introduction

Spinal orthoses are an important component in the treatment modalities of the clinician managing patients who have spinal pain, deformity, or fracture. One function of a spinal orthosis is to act as an assistive device in order to limit motion and thereby to allow the spine to rest. This provides the injured bone and soft-tissue structures the time required to heal.

In the setting of an acute fracture, muscular injury, or postoperative healing, a spinal orthosis may be prescribed to immobilize, stabilize, or unload the spine. Here the orthosis is used to substitute for or to assist the function of the surrounding musculature. With motion limited, patients also may subjectively feel "supported," both because of the mechanical properties of the brace and a possible placebo effect (17). In addition, orthoses function by acting as a psychological reminder to the patient to limit activities.

Orthotic devices can also be used in an attempt to halt the progression of or to correct spinal deformity and vertebral malalignments (kyphosis, scoliosis). In this setting, orthoses achieve their goal through the biomechanical principles of creep and biological adaptation (24).

For an orthosis to control the spine, it must apply force externally. This force is not applied directly to the spine; rather, forces are transmitted through the adjacent soft-tissue structures or bony prominences. The amount of force applied depends on the stiffness of the structures through which the force is transmitted. Ribs, spinous processes, and other bony structures allow greater force transference than soft tissues such as fat, muscle, and abdominal viscera (2). The transmission of forces through soft-tissue structures relies on increasing the hydrostatic pressure in the surrounding tissues rather than on a direct transmission of force through solid structures.

The ability of an orthosis to transfer force may be limited by the patient's pain and/or the sensitivity of the patient's skin and deep tissues to the forces being applied (40). The resultant discomfort will often affect the patient's compliance with brace use. Compliance can also be limited by the psychological tolerance of the patient. These devices are confining and can aggravate minor claustrophobic tendencies.

Several factors should be considered when prescribing a spinal orthosis. First, the clinician must identify all structurally deficient (fractured bone, ruptured ligaments) or painful elements (arthritic facets) to be immobilized. Once the structures to be immobilized are identified, the clinician can determine which spinal movements are to be restricted. Consideration must be given to the six degrees of motion freedom (rotations and translations around the x, y, and z axes) that characterize spinal motion. The extent of motion in one plane may vary in different areas of the spine. Finally, the clinician must decide on the extent of the area to be immobilized (i.e., cervicothoracic, thoracolumbar, or lumbar). The design and comfort of the orthosis are also taken into consideration in order to balance the patient's comfort and compliance against the immobilization desired.

Orthotic devices may be custom-molded or commercially prepared. Most commercially prepared products are available in a variety of sizes based on multiple average body dimensions. A custom-molded device is prepared for a specific individual on the basis of plaster casting. Although the commercial products are cheaper, they do not always perform or fit as well as a custom-molded product. Communication between the orthotist and the prescribing physician is imperative if the goal of providing a high-quality, durable, functional, and comfortable product is to be achieved.

Cervical Spine

The most commonly used class of orthoses for the cervical spine are the collars. Collars vary in their height and rigidity (1, 18). They act principally to limit flexion, extension, and to a lesser extent, lateral rotation. Fixation points include the chin, occiput, sternum, base of neck, and shoulders. These devices are inexpensive and convenient to use but offer little in the way of immobilization. Indications for the use of cervical collars include the treatment of cervical sprains, strains, spondylosis, and whiplash injury. They are also used in the management of paraspinous muscle spasm and discomfort after cervical decompression procedures. The collar is commonly used along with a spine board to immobilize the unstable cervical spine in the acute setting (7, 23). For this function, the Philadelphia collar system is superior (24). The collar should be removed as soon as possible to avoid complications such as occipital pressure sores (21).

Examples of this type of orthosis are the soft cervical collar (Fig. 31.1) and the newer Canadian collar (Fig. 31.2) (16). The Canadian collar is an adjustable orthosis constructed from polyvinyl chloride tubing clipped together by nylon junctures with chin and sternum supports of a molded nylon rod. This tubular orthosis has the advantage of being cooler and lighter. It is easily assembled and is adjustable to a wide variety of neck sizes and deformities. It is also easily adaptable to a tracheostomy.

In certain situations a greater degree of control of the cervical spine is desired. Lengthening the sleeve of the cervical collar down to the shoulders and chest provides a more effective anchoring mechanism distally, resulting in improved control of flexion and extension as well as additional rotational control (18). Examples of this type of brace include the Philadelphia collar (Fig. 31.3), the four-poster brace, the cervicothoracic orthosis, the SOMI brace (Figure 31.4), and others (4). They are most appropriate for the immobilization of the middle to lower cervical spine.

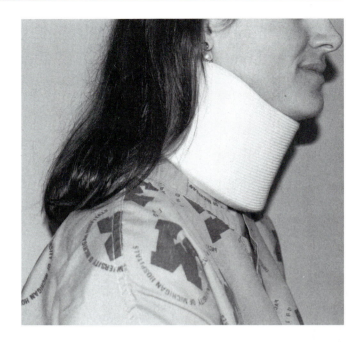

FIGURE 31.1.
Soft cervical collar. This device is constructed of foam rubber covered with stockinet.

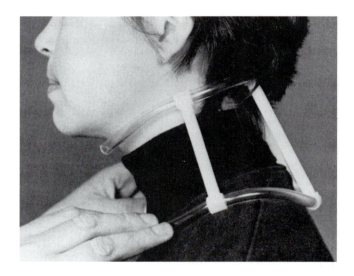

FIGURE 31.2.
Canadian collar. This orthosis is constructed from polyvinyl chloride tubing clipped together with nylon junctions. It is cooler than the soft cervical collar and can be used in patients with tracheostomy tubes. (Reproduced with permission from Hannah R, Cottrill SD. The Canadian collar: a new cervical spine orthosis. Am J Occup Ther 1985;39:3.)

They offer little rigidity to the unstable atlantoaxial region, but they may be appropriate in the treatment of some stable Jefferson fractures and hangman fractures. These orthoses are effective in unloading the neck. However, any body position that alters the shoulder-chest distal fixation may render the orthosis

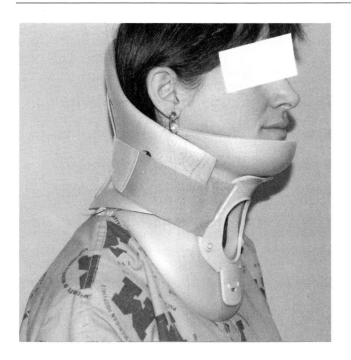

FIGURE 31.3.
Philadelphia collar. Proximally this collar has molded chin and occipital supports; distally it extends to the upper thoracic cage.

less effective. For example, as the patient changes position from upright to supine, the distal anchoring component of the brace (the component resting on the chest or shoulders) is often displaced superiorly and anteriorly. Thus in the supine position this class of devices may only be as effective as a soft collar.

If there has been a significant loss of stability through destruction or removal of supporting structures, then the maximum amount of immobilization and unloading is desirable. Maximum control of the cervical spine is preferred in all six degrees of motion in this situation. The two types of orthosis that offer this level of immobilization are the Minerva cast or body jacket and the halo-vest apparatus.

The Minerva orthosis (Fig. 31.5) or body jacket provides increased rigidity by including the forehead, chin, and high occiput in addition to the chest, sternum, and base of the neck that the collars and poster braces rely on for stabilization. The device is appealing since pins need not be applied to the cranium. It offers considerable control, and recent reports suggest that it is as effective as the halo device for cervical immobilization (6, 14, 22). One limitation, however, is that the orthosis must be applied so that eating and talking are permitted. Opening the mouth requires space for the head to extend and the mandible to move downward. This allows motion at the occiput-C1 and the C1-C2 articulations. Therefore, the Minerva brace is most effective in limiting motion at the middle to lower cervical spine. The Minerva brace or cast should be considered as an option for the immobilization of the cervical spine in pre-school-age children (14).

The halo-vest (Fig. 31.6) apparatus should be considered when distraction or transverse dislocation through ligaments or fractures renders the spine extensively unstable. This device obtains proximal fixation through pins applied to the cranium. Distal purchase is obtained through the chest, sternum, and posterior thoracic spine with a plaster jacket or cast. A recent study by Triggs et al. suggests that the degree of halo immobilization may be independent of the length of the chest support (36). The limiting factor in the degree of immobilization is the extent of sternal and chest-cage contact.

The selection of halo pin sites is critical in halo applications (13). The anterior halo pins are best applied anterior to the temporalis muscle and just lateral to the middle part of the superior orbital rim in order to protect the superior orbital nerves as well as

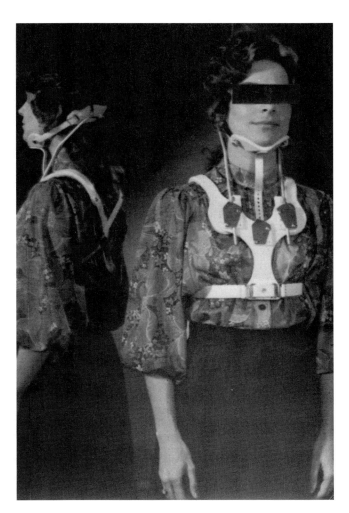

FIGURE 31.4.
SOMI. This apparatus is a cervicothoracic orthosis consisting of a rigid thoracic frame connected to mandibular and occipital supports by metal uprights.

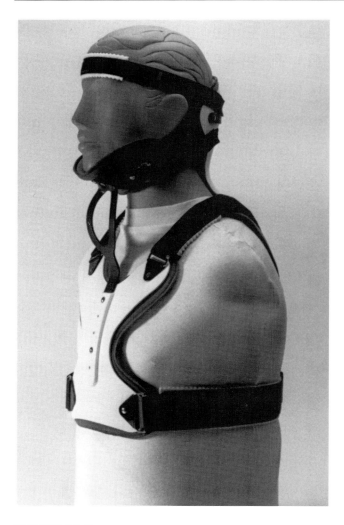

FIGURE 31.5.
Minerva orthosis. This device provides improved cervical immobilization via fixation on the forehead, chin, occiput, and sternum.

phenomenon." In a study by Johnson et al., "snaking" of the cervical spine was defined as a "serpentine movement of the spine whereby a simple overall movement (such as flexion or extension) is accompanied by the unexpected presence of flexion and extension at each intervertebral level" (18). The amount of snaking may be calculated by comparing the difference between the overall measured movement from the occiput to the lowest cervical level, to the sum of movements at each individual intervertebral level. When the sum of movements at each vertebral level is greater than the total movement, snaking is said to be present.

Numerous complications have been reported with the use of the halo device (Table 31.1) (10, 17, 37, 40). Some of these complications can be devastating, and the clinician must be sufficiently aware of them to prevent their development.

the frontal sinus (Fig. 31.7). These pins should be placed as inferiorly as possible, close to the superior orbital ridge, in order to achieve an angle of insertion as perpendicular as possible and thus the most rigid fixation possible (4). The posterior occipital pins should be placed inferior to the largest segmental circumference of the cranium to prevent superior pin migration. The temporal fossa should be avoided because of the relative thinness of bone in this region of the skull. Recent studies (in adults) have found no difference between pin torque applications of 6 and 8 inch-pounds (32). The lower pin torque is now recommended.

Although the halo apparatus is the most effective device for cervical immobilization, some potentially significant motion does occur (32, 41). This motion may occur when the patient changes body position, particularly when moving between the supine and upright positions. This motion is called the "snaking

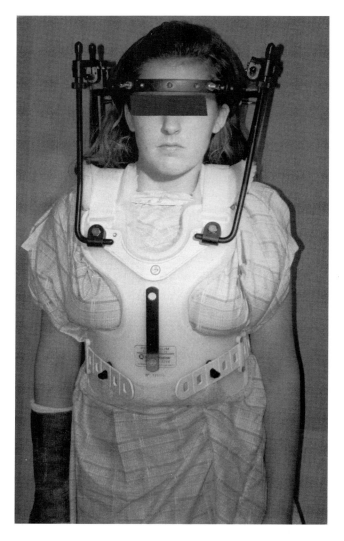

FIGURE 31.6.
Halo-vest apparatus. Consists of a halo ring attached to a prefabricated body vest. The halo ring is fixed to the skull via pins that penetrate the outer table.

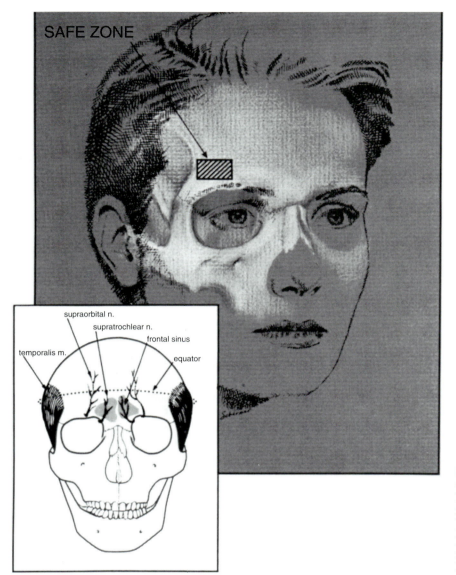

FIGURE 31.7.
Diagram of recommended safe zones for placement of anterior halo pins determined by skull osteology studies. (Reproduced with permission from Garfin SR, Botte MJ, Waters RL, et al. Complications in the use of the halo fixation device. J Bone Joint Surg 1986;68A:320.)

TABLE 31.1.
Halo Complications

Pin loosening (10)
Pin tract infection (10)
Skull perforation (17, 34)
Brain abscess (17, 34)
Depressed in tract scars (10)
Potential for impaired skin integrity (10)
Superior mesenteric artery syndrome (10)
Spontaneous fusion (9)
Facial, abducens, and glossopharyngeal nerve palsies (10)

Numbers in parentheses after each entry refer to the references as listed at the end of the chapter.

Quantitative analyses of the effect of cervical orthoses on the limitation of motion have been performed (18, 40). These studies indicate that no device, including the halo, restricts all cervical motion, and that some devices are better at controlling motion in one plane than motion in another plane. All of the conventional orthoses restrict flexion better than they do extension; and all of the orthoses restrict sagittal plane motion more effectively than they do rotation.

The halo-vest and the Minerva apparatus are the most effective devices for restricting motion in all planes (14, 22). They are most effective in the upper cervical spine. Sagittal plane motion is also controlled by, in order of decreasing effectiveness, the cervicothoracic orthosis, the four-poster brace, the SOMI device, the Philadelphia collar, and the soft collar. The halo-vest and, to a lesser extent, the cervicothoracic orthosis are the most effective devices for controlling cervical rotation. All other braces provide minimal control of rotation. The most effective orthoses for controlling lateral bending (coronal plane motion) after the halo are the four-poster brace and the cervicothoracic orthosis. All other orthoses provide minimal resistance to lateral bending.

In summary, the choice of a cervical orthosis depends on the degree of immobilization required. Cervical sprains and minor ligamentous injuries can be treated with the gentle support of a flexible collar. More rigid immobilization will be called for to limit pain from a ruptured disc or spondylosis, and maximal immobilization is indicated when treating instability from severe bony and/or ligamentous injuries.

Pediatric Halo Considerations

In the application of the halo device in infants and small children, their developmental anatomy must be taken into account. Cranial suture interdigitation may be incomplete and the fontanels may still be open anteriorly in patients less than 18 months of age, and posteriorly in patients less than 6 months of age (12). In children between the ages of 2 and 5 years, significantly lower insertion torques for pin placement are recommended (25).

In children less than 2 years of age, Mubarak recommends 2 inch-pounds of torque per pin (25). Multiple pins are recommended so that the lower torque insertion pressure may be utilized to avoid cortical penetration, cranial distortion, and bone shifting (Fig. 31.8) (8–10).

Although the amount of torque applied per pin is different in children, the desired location of the pins is similar to that in adults. Osteologic studies defining the areas of maximal thickness of the calvaria have confirmed that the anterolateral and posterolateral regions below the equator are the thickest in children (12, 13). Similar findings have been documented in studies of the skeletally mature skull (Fig. 31.9) (13).

Halo-Ilizarov

Halo traction is a well-accepted modality for the correction of severe cervical spine deformity (8, 21, 28, 34). Variations of the technique include countertraction with the use of femoral, pelvic, or clavicular pins as a distal counterforce (19). Distal fixation pins allow the generation of large forces that may be transmitted to the spine. However, when used to treat cervical deformity, the large forces generated by these techniques may affect the lumbar and thoracic spine (9, 35). Pin-tract infection, soft-tissue contractures, osseous disfigurement, joint stiffness, and muscle atrophy may also occur when these methods are used (9, 10, 17, 35, 37). This technique is also limited by its ability to correct deformity in only one plane via vertical traction.

As an alternative, the components of the Ilizarov apparatus have been used to connect a halo to a body cast (Fig. 31.10) (15). The advantages of this device are twofold. First, the use of the Ilizarov components allow multiplanar correction of deformity. Second, the ability to connect the apparatus to a cast facilitates patient mobility during the corrective process.

The body cast is applied using a Risser frame and extends from the sternal notch to the pubic symphysis. It is also carefully molded over the pelvis. Shoulder straps may be added to increase lateral stability. The goal in using the cast is to achieve stability and yet keep the orthotic device's weight as low as possible in an effort to limit hindrance of the patient's mobility.

The Ilizarov components allow a controlled correction of multiplanar deformity while the cervical vertebrae are being distracted. The system can produce translation of one cervical vertebra in relation to another while allowing mobility during the correction process. The Ilizarov apparatus applies force gradually, 1 mm per rotation, so that the soft tissues can adapt and lengthen. Initially, the distractors are turned four, five, or six times daily, in order to place the soft tissues under tension. At this rate, the deformity corrects quickly. When the patient begins to experience discomfort the process is slowed, with the

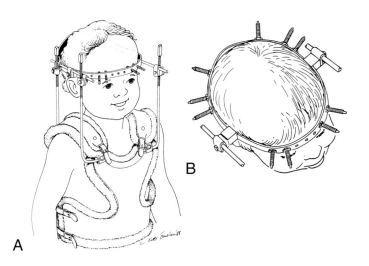

FIGURE 31.8.
Diagram of recommended halo pin placement sites in infants using the multiple-pins, low-torque technique. Four pins are placed anteriorly, avoiding temporal area. Six additional pins are placed in the occipital region. (Reproduced with permission from O'Brien JP, Yau CMC, Smith TK, et al. Halo-pelvic traction. J Bone Joint Surg 1971; 53(B):217.)

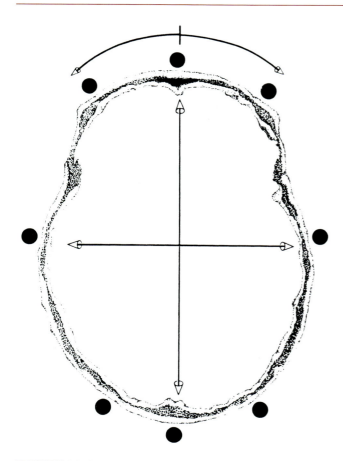

FIGURE 31.9.
Schematic representation of skull anatomy at a level below the equator. Dots indicate the thickest areas recommended for halo pin placement. (Reprinted with permission from Garfin SR, Botte MJ, Centeno RS, et al. Osteology of the skull as it affects halo pin placement. Spine 1985; 10(8):696.)

distractors usually turned twice daily. The speed of correction often depends on the patient's tolerance and the type of deformity being corrected. As the deformity becomes less severe the process is slowed, since the patient can tolerate only small changes at a time. The apparatus may be constructed to perform multiplanar correction of kyphosis, rotation, and translation. Once the desired correction has been obtained, a spinal fusion at the appropriate level is performed to maintain the correction.

In patients with atlantoaxial deformity, overcorrection is recommended, since some of the correction will occur at the occipitoatlantal level. This will prevent the occurrence of deformity rebound during the fusion process.

This technique has a low rate of complications. Minor complications include cast sores and halo pin tract infections (15). All are easily managed with local wound care, oral antibiotics, and pin changes as necessary.

The halo-Ilizarov technique allows the patient to remain ambulatory during correction of the deformity. Careful preoperative planning is necessary to ensure the proper application of corrective forces. If desired, forces may be concentrated through the use of spinous process wires. Wire placement is performed with an open technique.

Thoracic Spine

Thoracic corsets offer a minimal degree of spinal control. This type of orthosis provides a limited amount of immobilization. They may offer some relief for chronic benign thoracic pain. The warmth, massage effect, and possible placebo effect may also help the patient (27, 28).

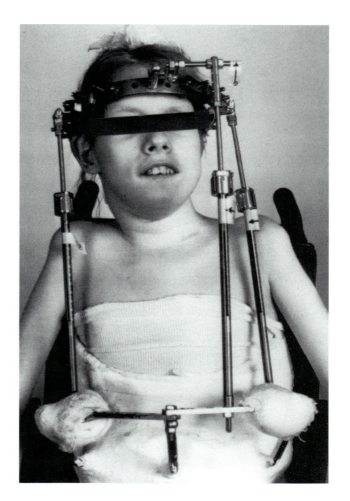

FIGURE 31.10.
Halo-Ilizarov. This device consists of a halo ring attached to a plaster vest by Ilizarov distraction instrumentation. This device allows gradual correction of multiplanar deformity prior to fusion. (Reproduced with permission from Graziano GP, Herzenberg JE, et al. The halo-Ilizarov distraction cast for correction of cervical deformity: report of six cases. J Bone Joint Surg 1993;75A(7):996–1003.)

The hyperextension brace or Jewett brace is an intermediate control brace designed to resist flexion. Its fixation points are the manubrium and the pubic symphysis. Counterpressure is applied between these two points by a posterior strap, thus achieving three-point fixation. This brace is less effective in restricting coronal rotation and offers no resistance to axial rotation. It can be adjusted to obtain some degree of hyperextension and is capable of shifting the weightbearing line over the posterior elements. This may be helpful in relieving stress on the vertebral body and anterior elements. This type of brace is most effective in the immediate region of the thoracolumbar junction (T11–L2). It is only effective in two-column injuries. Despite its effectiveness, many patients find this brace uncomfortable, and compliance with its use is variable (29). The thoracolumbosacral orthosis (TLSO) is an intermediate control brace and is the most commonly used orthotic device for immobilization of the lower thoracic and upper lumbar spine (Fig. 31.11). The region of immobilization is from T5 to L3. It offers control in all planes of motion. This orthosis gains purchase on the sternum, pubic symphysis, middle back, ribs, and soft tissues. This larger area allows the orthosis to spread its forces over a greater surface area than the Jewett device. The result is less irritation of the soft tissues, and thus compliance is greatly improved.

The Taylor brace offers intermediate control (26). It consists of a pelvic band with two vertical posterior bars extending to the shoulders and joined by a transverse bar. Straps pass from these upright bars around the shoulders and under the axillae. A full-length abdominal pad is attached to the upright bars. The points of fixation are the axillae, pelvis, and abdomen anteriorly, thus applying three points of fixation. This brace offers little resistance to lateral bending and poor resistance to axial rotation. It functions mainly to resist excessive motion in flexion and extension. Lateral bending can be controlled by adding lateral upright supports, and rotational control can be gained by adding clavicular pads and straps. The region of maximal effect is the thoracolumbar junction.

The most effective stabilization for the thoracic spine, without using the halo pelvic apparatus, is the Milwaukee brace (Fig. 31.12) (21, 40). This brace is most often prescribed for the correction of deformity in either the sagittal or the frontal plane (kyphosis or scoliosis, respectively). It applies corrective forces to the spine passively through the use of localizer pads. It also aids in active correction of the deformity by acting as a stimulus from which the patient voluntarily moves away.

Several key components of this brace give it its unique ability to correct deformity over time. First, the brace exacts some correction of deformity by dis-

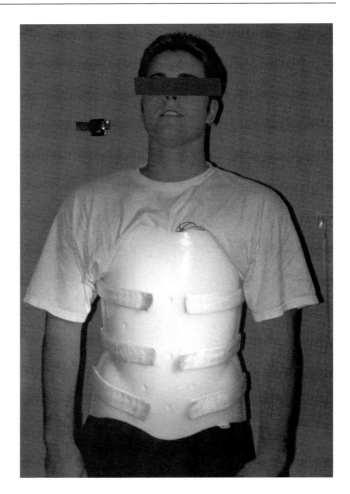

FIGURE 31.11.

Thoracolumbosacral orthosis (TLSO). This device is a clamshell orthosis that provides immobilization from T5 to L3.

tracting the spine between its mandibular-occipital support and its pelvic support. Second, frontal plane correction is achieved through a combination of pads and straps. For example, in a dextrothoracic scoliosis, a localizer pad is placed posterolaterally at the apex of the curve (on the right). This force is counteracted by an axillary sling and pelvic support applied on the opposite side of the thoracic pad, thus providing three-point fixation. Other types of braces, such as the Charleston orthosis (Fig. 31.13) attempt scoliosis correction through positioning and holding the curve at the extremes of bending (31). The brace is usually worn when the patient is sleeping. Deformity correction with either type of brace depends on the remaining growth potential of the spine, and hence they are effective only in skeletally immature patients.

Correction of sagittal plane deformity can also be achieved with the Milwaukee brace. Again, some measure of correction is achieved through distraction between the mandibular-occipital piece and the pel-

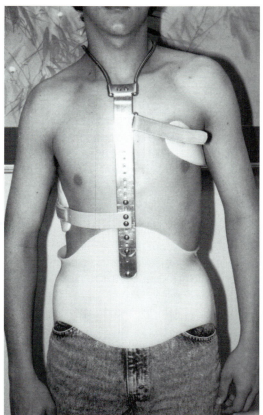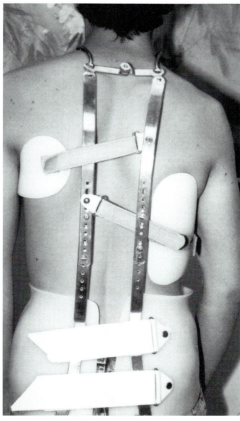

FIGURE 31.12.
Milwaukee brace. This brace is principally used for correction of thoracic deformity through localizer pads.

vic support, and kyphosis is corrected by a posterior pad placed on the apex of the curve. This posterior pad is counteracted by a sternal pad. Experimental studies as well as clinical follow-up studies have proven this brace to be an effective appliance for both correction of deformity in the growing child and immobilization of the thoracic spine.

A well-molded Risser plaster jacket also offers effective control of the thoracic spine (40). Its rigidity counters sagittal plane motion, while molding of the cast about the pelvis prevents axial rotation.

The most effective control of the thoracic spine as well as of all segments of the spine is with the halo pelvic apparatus (8, 28). The skeletal fixation to the skull and pelvis offers maximum control of the spine in all planes of motion. However, distal pelvic fixation with pins is associated with a number of complications. Pelvic disfigurement, infection, and soft-tissue contracture can all result from pelvic skeletal fixation. Since the entire spine and not just the injured segment is immobilized secondary changes may occur in previously normal areas of the spine (9, 10, 35). For these reasons halo-pelvic fixation has generally been abandoned.

Lumbar Region

Lumbar spine orthoses are commonly prescribed to reduce pain. These braces are applied in an attempt to increase abdominal support and to flatten the lumbar lordosis, thereby theoretically limiting motion at the lumbar spine and unloading the posterior facet joints. However, only slightly more than 50% of patients report benefit from the use of a lumbar support, which brings their use into question (30).

Norton and Brown investigated spinal motion and the effect of lumbar braces on that motion (27). They placed Kirschner wires in the spinous processes of volunteers and then, using radiographs, studied the immobilization effect of the various braces. They demonstrated that sitting with a brace, even when sitting erectly, was associated with flexion of the lower two lumbar interspaces. This is presumably a result of the increased lever arm created by a relatively more rigid upper spine and the concentrated movement in the less constrained lower spine. No brace in their study thoroughly immobilized the lumbar spine.

The increase in intra-abdominal pressure pro-

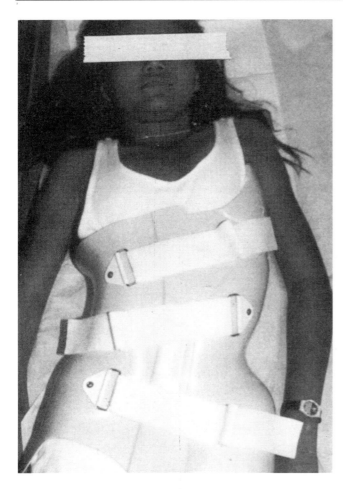

FIGURE 31.13.
Charleston bending brace. This brace corrects and holds scoliosis in extremes of bending.

bar corset provides minimal immobilization. An intermediate level of immobilization can be achieved with the rigid low/short orthoses such as a molded lumbosacral orthosis (LSO) (Fig. 31.14). Additional control is attained by the chairback brace with long paraspinous upright supports. The Taylor brace provides a similar degree of control of the lumbar spine.

Maximal control of the lower lumbar spine and the lumbosacral junction was traditionally thought to require stabilization of the pelvis (33). This is achieved by the inclusion of one hip in a spica component of a body cast or brace (Fig. 31.15). Controversy exists as to the benefits of the unilateral hip spica. Recent stereophotogrammetric studies have demonstrated no difference between the molded TLSO with and without hip spica (3). Finally, as in all regions of the spine, the most rigid stabilization devices involve osseous fixation in the form of a halo pelvic apparatus.

duced by lumbar braces may provide some additional support to the spine. Walters and Morris performed electromyographic studies of the paraspinal and abdominal muscles and demonstrated a decrease in the activity of the abdominal muscle with both the lumbosacral corset and the chairback brace (38). These braces would appear to take over some of the effect of the abdominal muscles by compressing and supporting the abdominal contents and, indirectly, the spine. However, periodically the subjects did demonstrate a paradoxical increase in muscle activity while wearing the brace. This may be due to an attempt on the part of the muscles to overcome the immobilization. This type of brace should obviously be used with caution in patients afflicted with extreme muscle spasms.

A variety of lumbar braces providing variable degrees of immobilization and support are available. The more effective devices are made of rigid materials and incorporate an extended lever arm, either proximally, distally, or both. Specifically, a soft lum-

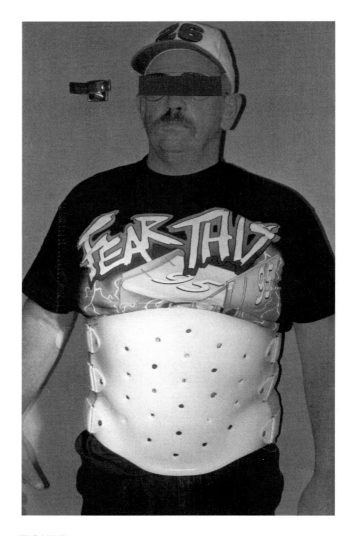

FIGURE 31.14.
Lumbosacral orthosis (LSO). This prefabricated or custom-molded rigid device immobilizes the lower lumbar and the upper sacral vertebrae.

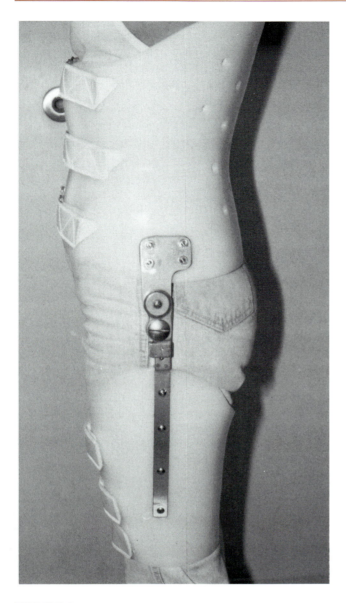

FIGURE 31.15.
Thoracolumbosacral orthosis with hip spica extension. The added spica extension to the TLSO stabilizes the pelvis, thus improving immobilization at the lumbosacral junction.

The disadvantages of this device are discussed in the Thoracic Spine and Halo-Ilizarov sections.

Conclusion

Many factors must be considered in the prescription of a spinal orthosis. The goal of the device (support, correction of deformity, immobilization), the patient's ability to comply with its use, and the cost should be kept in mind. The prescribing physician must be aware of the advantages and the limitations of the appliance in each situation. The proper use of spinal orthoses can offer the treating physician an effective nonsurgical adjunct in the treatment of various spinal conditions.

References

1. Althoff B, Golden IF. Cervical collars in rheumatoid atlantoaxial subluxation: a radiographic comparison. Ann Rheum Dis 1980;39:485–489.
2. Andriacchi T, Schultz A, Belytschko T, et al. A model for studies of mechanical interactions between the human spine and rib cage. J Biomech 1974;7(6):497–507.
3. Axelsson P, Johnsson R, Stromqvist B. Lumbar orthosis with unilateral hip immobilization: effect on intervertebral mobility determined by roentgen stereophotogrammetric analysis. Spine 1993;18(17):876–879.
4. Ballock RT, Lee TQ, Triggs KJ, et al. The effect of pin location on the rigidity of the halo pin–bone interface. Neurosurgery 1990;26(2):238–241.
5. Beavis A. Cervical orthoses. Prosthet Orthot Int 1989;13:6–13.
6. Benzel EC, Hadden TA, Saulsbery CM. A comparison of the Minerva and halo jackets for stabilization of the cervical spine. J Neurosurg 1989;70:411–414.
7. Chandler DR, Nemejc C, Adkins RH, et al. Emergency cervical immobilization. Ann Emerg Med 1992;21(10):1185–1188.
8. Clark JA, Kesterton L. Halo pelvic traction appliance for spinal deformities. J Biomech 1971;4:589–595.
9. Dove J, Hsu LC, Yau AC. Spontaneous cervical spine fusion: a complication of halo-pelvic traction. Spine 1981;6:45–48.
10. Dove J, Yau AC. The cervical spine after halo-pelvic traction: analysis of complications in 83 patients. J Bone Joint Surg Br 1980;62:138.
11. Garfin SR, Botte MJ, Waters RL, et al. Complications in the use of the halo fixation device. J Bone Joint Surg Am 1986;68:320–325.
12. Garfin SR, Roux R, Botte MJ, et al. Skull osteology and its effects on halo pin placement in children. J Pediatr Orthop 1986;6:434–436.
13. Garfin SR, Botte MJ, Centeno RS, et al. Osteology of the skull as it affects halo pin placement. Spine 1985;10(8):696–698.
14. Gaskell S, Marlin A. Custom-fitted thermoplastic Minerva jackets in the treatment of cervical spine instability in children. Pediatr Neurosurg 1991;16(35):35–39.
15. Graziano GP, Herzenberg JE, Hensinger RN. The halo-Ilizarov distraction cast for correction of cervical deformity: report of six cases. J Bone Joint Surg Am 1993;75(7):996–1003.
16. Hannah RE, Cottrill SD. The Canadian collar: a new cervical spine orthosis. Am J Occup Ther 1985;39:171–177.
17. Humbyrd DE, Latimer FR, Lonstein JE, et al. Brain abscess as a complication of halo traction. Spine 1981;6:365–368.
18. Johnson RM, Hart DL, Simmons EF, et al. Cervical orthoses: a study comparing their effectiveness in restricting cervical motion in normal subjects. J Bone Joint Surg Am 1977;59:332–339.

19. Kostuik J, Tooke M. The application of pelvic pins in halo-pelvic distraction: an anatomic study. Spine 1983; 8:35–38.
20. Liew S, Hill DA. Complication of hard cervical collars in multi-trauma patients. Aust New Zeal J Surg 1994; 64(2):139–140.
21. Lonstein JE. Orthotic treatment of spinal deformities: scoliosis and kyphosis. In: Bunch W, ed. Atlas of orthotics: Biomechanical principles and application. St. Louis: Mosby, 1985:371–385.
22. Maiman D, Millington P, Novak S, et al. The effect of the thermoplastic Minerva body jacket on cervical spine motion. J Neurosurg 1984;25(3):363–368.
23. McGuire R, Degnan G, et al. Evaluation of current extrication orthoses in immobilization of the unstable cervical spine. Spine 1990:15(10):1064–1067.
24. Morris JM, Lucas DB. Biomechanics of spinal bracing. Arizona Med 1974;21:170.
25. Mubarak SJ, Camp JF, Vuletich W, et al. Halo application in the infant. J Pediatr Orthop 1989;9(5):612–614.
26. Nagel DA, Koogle TA, Piziali RL, et al. Stability of the upper lumbar spine following progressive disruptions and the application of individual internal and external fixation devices. J Bone Joint Surg Am 1981;63(1):62–70.
27. Norton PL, Brown T. The immobilizing efficiency of back braces. J Bone Joint Surg Am 1957;39:111.
28. O'Brien JP, Yau CMC, Smith TK, et al. Halo-pelvic traction. A preliminary report on a method of external skeletal fixation for correcting deformities and maintaining fixation of the spine. J Bone Joint Surg Br 1971;53(2): 217–229.
29. Patwardhan Ag, Li SP, Gavin T, et al. Orthotic stabilization of thoracolumbar injuries: a biomechanical analysis of the Jewett hyperextension orthosis. Spine 1990; 15(7):654–661.
30. Perry J. The use of external support in the treatment of low back pain. Report of the Subcommittee on orthotics of the Committee on Prosthetic-Orthotic Education. National Academy of Sciences, National Research Council. J Bone Joint Surg Am 1970;52(7):1440–1442.
31. Price CT, Scott DS, Reed FE, et al. Nighttime bracing for adolescent idiopathic scoliosis with the Charleston bending brace: preliminary report. Spine 1990;15(12): 1294–1299.
32. Rizzolo SJ, Piazza MR, Cotler JM, et al. The effect of torque pressure on halo pin complication rates. A randomized prospective study. Spine 1993;18(15):2163–2166.
33. Sharp J, Purser DW. Spontaneous atlantoaxial dislocation and ankylosing spondylitis in rheumatoid arthritis. Ann Rheum Dis 1961;20:47–77.
34. Thompson H. The "Halo" traction apparatus: a method of external splinting of the cervical spine after injury. J Bone Joint Surg Br 1962;44:655–661.
35. Tredwell SJ, O'Brien JP. Apophyseal joint degeneration in the cervical spine following halo-pelvic distraction. Spine 1980;5(6):497–501.
36. Triggs KJ, Ballock RT, Byrne T, et al. Length dependence of a halo orthosis on cervical immobilization. J Spinal Disord 1993;6(1):34–37.
37. Victor D, Bresnan M, Keller R. Brain abscess complicating the use of halo traction. J Bone Joint Surg Am 1973;55:635–639.
38. Walters R, Morris J. Effects of spinal supports on the electrical activity of muscles of the trunk. J Bone Joint Surg Am 1970;52:51–60.
39. Wang G, Moskal JT, Albert T, et al. The effect of halo-vest length on stability of the cervical spine: a study in normal subjects. J Bone Joint Surg Am 1988;70:357–360.
40. White AA, Panjabi MM. Spinal braces: functional analysis and clinical applications. In: Clinical biomechanics the spine. Philadelphia: JB Lippincott, 1990:475–511.
41. Whitehill R, Richman JA, Glaser JA. Failure of immobilization of the cervical spine by the halo-vest: a report of 5 cases. J Bone Joint Surg Am 1986;68:326–332.

CHAPTER THIRTY TWO

Cervical Spine Instrumentation

Howard S. An and Mark Coppes

Introduction

Many different techniques have been developed for fixation of the cervical spine since Hadra first internally fixed an unstable cervical spine in 1891 (31). Since that time a gradual progression toward the use of rigid internal fixation for fusion and stabilization has culminated in the development of some of the newer instrumentation systems available today. The benefits of rigid internal fixation initially popularized by the AO Group in the appendicular skeleton have now been extended to the axial skeleton as well. This includes reduction, maintenance of alignment, early mobilization, and enhanced fusion rates. Although anterior fusion can be accomplished without internal fixation, in most cases it necessitates the use of postoperative immobilization for varying intervals, depending on the pathology of the lesion. The halo-vest orthosis is still widely used for nondisplaced fractures and for postoperative immobilization.

The exact indications for the use of anterior cervical plating and anterior dens screw fixation remain to be defined. Most posterior constructs still use wiring techniques, but newer methods include transarticular C1-C2 fixation, occipitocervical plates, and lateral-mass plating in the subaxial cervical spine. The benefits of internal fixation are well known, but it must be seen as an adjuvant for stabilization rather than as a substitute for fusion. The method chosen should be based on the pathoanatomy of the lesion, the mechanism of injury, and the surgeon's own experience with the technique. A thorough knowledge of the relevant surgical anatomy and precise adherence to the described technique should lead to successful stabilization of the cervical segment with a minimal risk of complications.

The purpose of this chapter is to review the various methods of internal fixation used in the cervical spine, including their indications, surgical techniques, and potential complications.

Anterior Instrumentation

Anterior fusion of the cervical spine can be accomplished mostly by bone graft alone, without any need for additional instrumentation. Odontoid screw fixation and anterior plate fixation may be used in special circumstances. Numerous clinical and biomechanical studies have been performed assessing the stability and efficacy of these implants (1, 2, 7, 11, 16, 21, 27, 56).

Anterior Odontoid Screw Fixation

Indications

Conventional treatment of odontoid process fractures has included traction, Minerva casts, halo application, braces, and operative fixation. Nonunion rates vary from 0 to 64%, depending on the series, with an accepted value of 33% for type II odontoid fractures. Nondisplaced type II fractures or fractures displaced less than 5 mm can be treated successfully with traction and application of a halo orthosis. For fractures with displacements larger than 5 mm, or in patients whose age is more than 60 years or who have had previous loss of reduction, strong consideration should be given for operative fixation.

The advantages of anterior screw fixation over conventional posterior C1-C2 fusion are immediate rigid fixation, preservation of the axial rotation at the C1-C2 facet articulation, minimal postoperative bracing, and the avoidance of the potential complications associated with bone grafting. This operative approach is popular in Europe and Japan, and it is gradually gaining acceptance in the United States as the preferred technique in the management of odontoid fractures (1). Its proponents believe that operative morbidity is lessened by an anterior cervical approach, and blood loss is minimal. The major complication rate of 20% for anterior screw fixation of the dens is comparable to the rates of posterior wiring with less rigid immobilization (1). Böhler, Aebi, and Apfelbaum consider it the procedure of choice for management of acute fractures of the odontoid (1, 7, 11). Fracture patterns in which treatment with this method is indicated include Anderson-Alonzo type II, type III with a shallow base, and combined C1-C2 injuries. Aebi noted that there are two specific situations in which anterior dens screw fixation is contraindicated: *(a)* rupture of the transverse ligament of C1 with concomitant C1 ring fracture with coronal separation of more than 7 mm; and *(b)* type II and type III fractures with an oblique sagittal projection into the C2 vertebral body paralleling the screw (1). This pattern prevents interfragmentary compression with the technique described. This method of treatment should be performed only by experienced surgeons in the appropriate operative facilities.

Technique

Patients are initially placed in the supine position, and awake nasotracheal intubation is performed. Under local anesthesia, the Mayfield headset is applied and then connected to the operating table by means of a crossbar that allows for intraoperative imaging in two planes. If reduction is necessary, maneuvers are performed while the patient is awake, and the neurological examination is repeated before anesthesia is administered. It is important that anatomic reduction be obtained before the beginning of the procedure, for after induction any positional changes are potentially dangerous. Biplanar fluoroscopy with good resolution of the images is essential for correct screw placement. A plastic bite block is used for the intraoperative anteroposterior dens view. This positioning requires some degree of extension to allow for adequate surgical exposure.

The steep approach angle for odontoid screw placement necessitates an initial skin incision at the level of the C5–6 disc space. The standard anteromedial approach to the cervical spine is then used, with the transverse incision extending from midline to the anterior border of the sternocleidomastoid muscle. The platysma is then split in a linear fashion and the carotid sheath identified. The retropharyngeal space is entered by scissor spreading dissection just medial to the palpable carotid pulse. Blunt dissection with the surgeon's finger is performed to clear the prevertebral fascia, extending cephalad to the anterior tubercle of the atlas. An incision is then made through the anterior longitudinal ligament at the inferior portion of C2. The technique varies as to whether the one-screw technique or two-screw technique is utilized. Graziano et al. found that there was no statistical difference between the one- and two-screw techniques in both torsion and bending stiffness (27). They believe that the use of one screw for odontoid fixation would lessen the chances for malposition. If the two-screw method is chosen, then preoperative computed tomography (CT) scanning may be helpful in determining the dimensions of the dens. For single-screw fixation, a 2.0 mm Kirschner wire is inserted midline at the anterior inferior border of C2. It is then advanced under fluoroscopic control, with confirmation of direction in both the anteroposterior and lateral planes through the body of C2 into the odontoid process. A second wire can be utilized for rotational stability while the hole is tapped and then during placement of the 3.5 mm screw, all done under constant fluoroscopic visualization (Fig. 32.1). Cannulated screws can also be used over the Kirschner wire and advanced under fluoroscopy so as to avoid guide wire migration. The tip of the screw should come to rest in the apical portion of the dens for optimum fixation. Biplanar permanent radiographs should be taken for final confirmation of screw placement. Postoperative immobilization varies from 6 to 12 weeks, depending on the surgeon's preference and the degree of expected patient compliance.

The two-screw technique starts 2 to 3 mm lateral to the midline and proceeds in a similar fashion. The use of two screws for insertional stability is recommended for oblique fracture patterns. Ideal mechanical stability would be achieved with short threaded screws and overdrilling the near cortex for lag screw compression.

Montesano et al. advocates the use of a special anteriorly angled curette for debridement of the fibrous tissue of a nonunion (40). In addition, he adds a small amount of graft taken from the body of C3 to the nonunion site. Some surgeons consider nonunion a relative contraindication to the use of this technique. Anterior odontoid screw fixation is technically demanding and requires the use of biplanar high-resolution fluoroscopy for accurate screw placement.

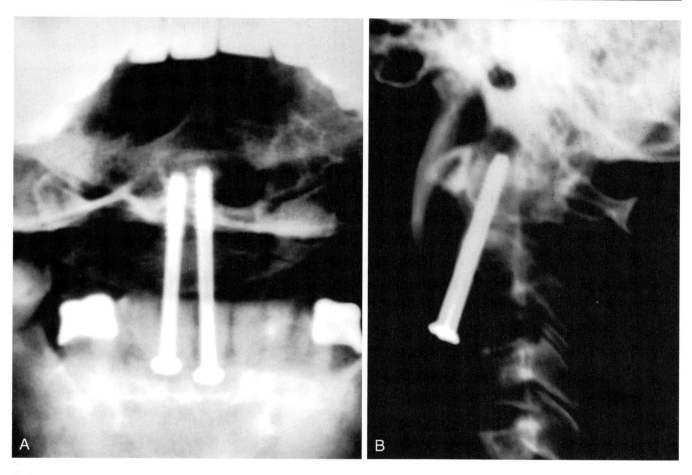

FIGURE 32.1.

A. Anteroposterior radiograph showing two screws in the odontoid process in a patient who sustained a type II odontoid fracture. B. Lateral radiograph shows anatomical reduction and healing of the fracture with screw fixation.

Anterior Cervical Plates

Anterior cervical discectomy and fusion is seen as the standard for treatment of degenerative conditions in the cervical spine. Fusion methods popularized by Bailey and Badgley, Cloward, and Smith and Robinson are widely accepted for the treatment of cervical spondylosis (9, 17, 51). These methods rely on the inherent stability of the bone graft between the involved interspace for fusion to occur in degenerative situations and cannot be the sole method of fixation for the acutely injured spinal segment.

Additional methods of stabilization are necessary for safe and effective treatment of an unstable cervical spine segment. Treatment with prolonged halo-vest immobilization or cranial tong traction may not effectively treat the lesion and are fraught with their own sets of complications. Early mobilization of the patient has been recognized as an important factor in the treatment of acute spinal cord injury patients. Anterior stabilization and decompression can be performed and followed by staged posterior procedures when indicated by the pathology of the lesion.

The precise indications for the use of anterior instrumentation in the treatment of cervical spondylosis have yet to be defined. Many surgeons feel that it is too costly and unnecessary for routine use in degenerative conditions. A detailed study of noninstrumented anterior fusion versus instrumented fusion needs to be performed to define these indications more clearly.

Current recommendations include reconstruction after vertebrectomy for tumor, spondylosis, fracture, or infection (Fig. 32.2). If the intraoperative stability of a strut graft is questionable or the patient will not tolerate a halo-vest orthosis, anterior plate fixation can be an important tool for stabilization. It is also useful in traumatic injuries that involve predominantly the anterior vertebral body or the disc and necessitate stabilization of the anterior column. The use of anterior surgery in the treatment of posterior element pathology is not an established indication, but it may be part of circumferential fusions with complete dislocations. In some cases the use of anterior plate fixation may eliminate the need for a second posterior procedure. A flexion-distraction injury re-

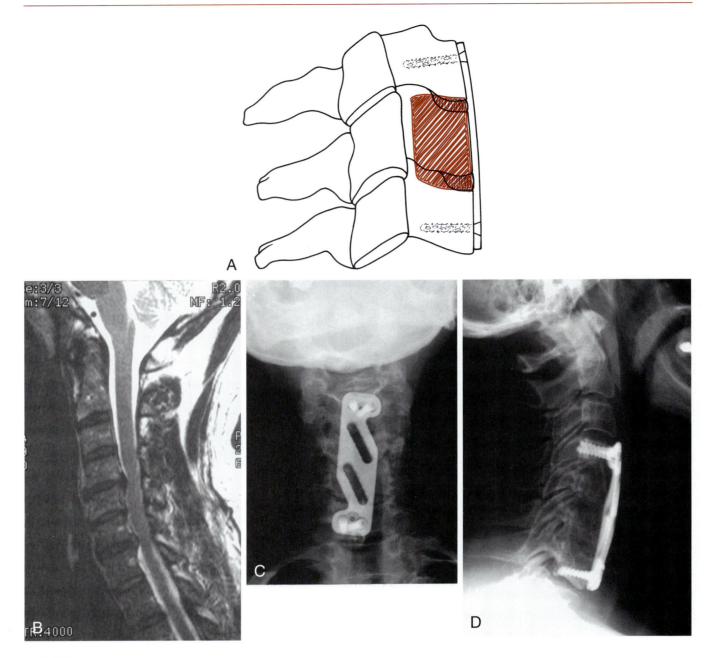

FIGURE 32.2.
A. Diagram showing a strut graft spanning the inferior endplate of the superior vertebra and the superior endplate of the inferior vertebra and plate fixation. **B.** Fifty-five-year-old male with cervical spondylotic myelopathy. Sagittal T2-weighted MRI shows spinal cord compression at C4–5 to C6–7. **C.** Postoperative anteroposterior radiograph shows plate fixation from C4 to C7. **D.** Lateral radiograph shows corpectomy and strut graft from C4 to C7 and proper plate-screw fixation from C4 to C7.

quiring discectomy may be treated by such a single procedure, but posterior element pathology must not be overlooked (Fig. 32.3).

Technique

For a safe and effective surgical approach, proper preoperative positioning is imperative. For most cases, Gardner-Wells tong traction is sufficient to provide intraoperative stability. A small towel-roll is placed between the patient's shoulders, and the arms are secured at the sides with foam protective devices and an overlapping towel. Longitudinal traction with cloth tape applied at the shoulders may be beneficial. The iliac crest is also elevated with the use of a rolled towel or large IV bag. Patients with acute injuries are brought to the operating room in traction on a Stryker frame, which eliminates the need for transfer to an operating table, since the frame allows operative stabilization.

The standard anteromedial Smith-Robinson ap-

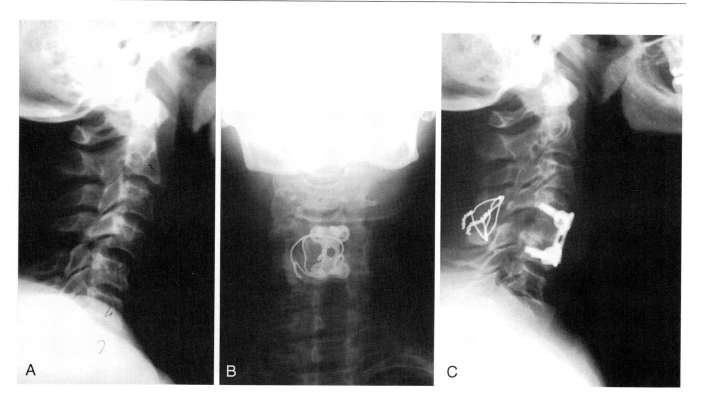

FIGURE 32.3.

A. Lateral view shows fracture-dislocation at C4-C5 in a 60-year-old quadriplegic patient. **B.** Anteroposterior view shows AO-Morscher plating and posterior wiring. **C.** Lateral view shows anatomic reduction, anterior graft, and plate fixation along with posterior triple wiring. (This patient has a combined anterior and posterior fixation because of relatively weak fixation by anterior plating due to osteoporosis.)

proach can be used for one- or two-level fusions (51). It is extremely important to dissect the fascial planes fully for adequate exposure. Occasionally a longitudinal incision along the anterior border of the sternocleidomastoid muscle may be required for longer constructs. Blunt dissection with the finger clears the prevertebral fascia and allows the subperiosteal mobilization of the longus colli muscles. Blunt self-retractor blades are then positioned beneath the reflected longus colli muscles to protect the esophagus and the carotid sheath from injury. Identification of the involved level(s) is usually confirmed with a portable lateral cervical spine film. Decompression or vertebrectomy is then performed according to the character of the lesion. Meticulous preparation of the graft may obviate the need for any supplemental anterior fixation. Anterior plating may avoid the complications of an anterior graft without fixation or staged posterior arthrodesis in cases of vertebral body fracture. If intraoperative stability cannot be achieved with extensive reconstructive grafting for multilevel degenerative or widespread tumor destruction, then plate fixation can be an important adjuvant to stabilization techniques with immediate rigid fixation.

Placement and selection of the size of the plate depends on the instrumentation system chosen for implantation. We favor a system with a convergent screw design for additional safety rather than a divergent design. The plate is positioned just above the graft–vertebral body interface, which also allows for a 15° cephalad and caudal screw placement. This reduces the potential for injury to adjacent healthy cervical disc spaces. The plate is then contoured to fit the anterior surface in order to maximize bony contact. The plate may have a prebent gentle lordotic curve, which can be modified to fit the construct with plate benders, though it must be kept in mind that excessive bending will also change the orientation of the screws at each end. Correct positioning of the plate in the midline must be achieved to reduce the incidence of iatrogenic injury and to provide maximum bone surface for fixation. Contouring of the surface of the plate-bone interface is performed with a rongeur or high-speed burr to increase the stability of the construct. The local anatomy is then reviewed before fixation to ensure that the plate is correctly centered. The uncinate processes can be used as a marker on either side for reference.

The drill guide is then inserted into the plate and drilling is done with appropriate degrees of convergence and cranial/caudal orientation. Preoperative radiographs or CT scans are used to estimate the width of the vertebral body. Depending on the system used, either unicortical or bicortical fixation is used and should provide strong screw purchase to avoid plate loosening. For bicortical systems, specially designed drill bits and drill-stop guides are advanced in sequential fashion in 1 or 2 mm increments until the posterior cortex is reached. Adjustable depth taps and adjustable tap stops can be set at the distance measured, and then advanced. Fluoroscopy can also be used for additional verification in these steps. It is important that intraoperative traction be reduced to 5 pounds before the screws are placed. Proximal and distal screws are placed opposite one another diagonally and partially tightened for initial stability, and then the remaining screws are placed and secured. An intraoperative radiograph is then taken for final verification of screw depth and orientation of the plate. The center screw can be used with long strut graft reconstructions for added stability. Once final positioning of the plate is performed, locking screws are placed to reduce the incidence of screws backing out. The locking screws allow greater stability of the plate with unicortical screw placement. Revision or cancellous screws of a greater diameter can be used if the initial screws do not achieve good fixation. Methylmethacrylate can be used in addition to enhance bony fixation. The wound is then irrigated with copious amounts of saline and closed over suction drainage for approximately 24 hours with perioperative intravenous antibiotic coverage. Care is taken to inspect the esophagus before closure for any evidence of a tear in the muscular wall. External immobilization is applied before transfer to the recovery room or staged posterior procedure if necessary.

In the immediate postoperative period the patient's airway is at risk from the paratracheal edema resulting from the prolonged surgical time and the anatomic exposure. If longer operative procedures are performed, continued intubation perioperatively for 24 to 48 hours may be considered for prevention of acute respiratory compromise. In most cases, however, this is not necessary, and patients can be extubated safely in the recovery room and mobilized immediately with their external orthosis.

The Caspar and AO-Orozco plate systems are made of stainless steel; the AO-Morscher and Orion systems are composed of titanium, which allows postoperative magnetic resonance imaging (MRI) studies to be performed when indicated (33). Other systems are becoming available, and the surgeon should choose an instrumentation system on the basis of biomechanical data, safety, ease of use, and clinical outcome.

Complications in the use of anterior instrumentation systems include the general risks of the Smith-Robinson approach for surgical exposure. Meticulous surgical technique is used for exposure to decrease the potential for complications in this approach and to provide adequate visualization for plate application. Proper placement of the self-retaining retractors beneath the longus colli muscles will protect the esophagus medially and the adjacent lateral carotid sheath. Use of the uncinate processes as an anatomic landmark allow correct medial-lateral placement of the plate. Special drill- and tap-stop guides allow controlled advancement and theoretically decrease potential neural injury. Inadvertent dural penetration may go unnoticed by the operating surgeon and clinically may not represent a significant problem. Exposure and direct repair of the dural tear is not always possible, because of the depth and technical difficulty of the exposure. Sometimes a small piece of absorbable gelatin sponge (Gelfoam) placed across the defect will obviate the need for repair.

Violation of a healthy adjacent disc space is also a potential complication resulting from overestimation of plate length. Intraoperative radiographs are taken before closure so that any modifications in screw length or direction can be performed. Late complications include screw or plate loosening and subsequent injury to adjacent structures. This may be due to osteoporotic bone or technical difficulties encountered in the placement of screws, resulting in the screws having inadequate purchase. Suh et al. reported a 100% fusion rate in 13 patients with no neurologic injuries (54). Although the follow-up was only 13 months on average, serial radiographs failed to reveal screw migration or plate loosening. In a larger series, Meyer reported a hardware failure rate of 2%, which he attributed to improper plate or screw technique intraoperatively (38).

Posterior Instrumentation

Posterior cervical instrumentation can be anatomically categorized into occipitocervical fusion, atlantoaxial fusion, and subaxial (C3–C7) fusion. Occipitocervical stabilization can be accomplished by a number of methods using wire, metal loops, and plate-screw constructs. Bone and methylmethacrylate can be added according to the pathology at hand (52). Posterior C1-C2 fusion is generally performed by wiring techniques, transarticular screw fixation, or combinations of the two. Lower cervical fusion is done by wiring techniques or plate-screw fixation.

Occipitocervical Fusion

Occipitocervical fusion is rarely indicated for trauma since atlanto-occipital injuries are usually fatal. If the patient survives the injury, the clinical presentation may include suboccipital hematoma, respiratory distress, and high quadriplegia (43). Other causes of occipitocervical instability include congenital, post-traumatic, inflammatory arthropathy, infection, and tumor. The surgical treatment is targeted toward adequate decompression of the cervicomedullary junction and solid bony fusion to prevent further neurological deterioration.

Technique

The technique of Wertheim and Bohlman is our preferred method of occipitocervical stabilization (Fig. 32.4A,B) (57). A previously placed halo-vest on a regular operating table or Stryker frame rotation can be used for positioning after nasotracheal intubation. The arms are secured at the sides with foam protective devices, and longitudinal skin traction is used over the shoulders. A radiograph is taken to assure adequate exposure to the occiput, atlas, and axis.

A midline incision is then made extending from the occipital protuberance to the fourth cervical spinous process. The deep incision bisects the nuchal ligament and is carried down to expose the occiput and bony laminae with the use of electrocautery as a dissector. The bony surface of the occiput is exposed subperiosteally, using a small Cobb elevator since the surface can become quite thin, especially in elderly patients. The external occipital protuberance is thick enough to allow the passage of wires without violating the inner table. Approximately 2 cm above the foramen magnum a trough is created with a high-speed burr on each side of the protuberance to decrease the mass effect of the wires and to allow the graft to sit directly on the surface of the skull. A single limb of a right-angle forceps is passed through each side under the outer table of the occiput. A 20-gauge wire is then passed through and looped over the ridge. Wires under the laminae of C1 and through the spinous process of C2 are also passed and bent laterally to avoid inadvertent glove puncture or un-

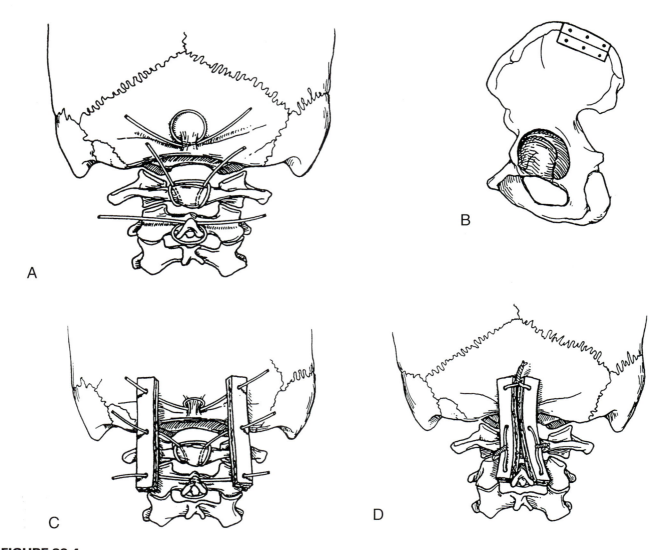

FIGURE 32.4.
Wertheim and Bohlman's method of occipitocervical fusion. **A.** Wires are passed at occiput, C1, and C2. **B.** Bone grafts are obtained from the outer table of the iliac crest. **C.** Wires are passed through holes drilled in the grafts. **D.** The grafts are secured in place.

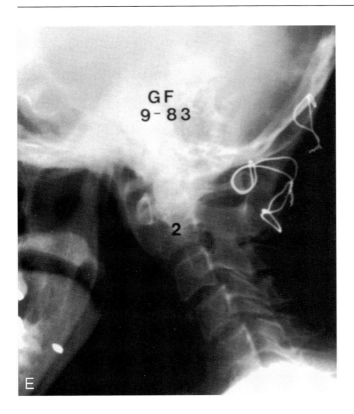

FIGURE 32.4—*continued*

E. Lateral radiograph showing solid occipitocervical fusion in a patient with basilar invagination.

wanted manipulation. The posterior iliac crest site is then exposed and two curved corticocancellous grafts are harvested according to the required dimensions. Three 2 mm holes are then drilled in each graft according to the placement of the wires. The occiput is carefully decorticated along with the posterior laminae of C1 and C2. The three wires are then sequentially tightened over the surface of the graft to secure it in place. After irrigation with saline solution, additional cancellous bone is placed into the fusion bed. Suction drainage is used postoperatively for 24 to 48 hours with perioperative antibiotics. If during the course of exposure small punctate holes in the occiput are encountered, they can be plugged with absorbable gelatin sponge (Gelfoam) or bone wax. Postoperative immobilization in a halo-vest for 10 to 12 weeks is usually adequate.

A trend toward the use of rigid internal fixation for occipitocervical fusion has been suggested by Smith et al., following the previously reported experience of Roy-Camille et al., Grob et al., and others (28, 46, 50). Similar exposure is used for occipitocervical fusion using plate-screw fixation, although lateral dissection must extend 5 to 6 cm from the midline and the lateral masses of C2 and C3 must be adequately exposed. Additional levels can be exposed in a similar manner if fusion requirements so dictate. The use of this method almost dictates pedicle screw placement at C2 for optimum fixation in cases of shorter segment fusion. A CT scan is suggested as an aide to preoperative planning for accurate direction and depth of the screws. Care is taken in exposing the C1–2 interval in order to avoid the large venous plexus laterally. Dissection is the performed with the use of a small curved curette to expose the superior edge of the laminae and allow the passage of a dental elevator to palpate the medial boundary of the pedicle. The direction of placement is 10 to 25° medially and approximately 25° cephalad, starting at the center corner of the upper inner quadrant (Fig. 32.5). After placement of the C2 pedicular screw, the medial wall of the pedicle is checked for any violation of the cortex. If strict adherence to technique is followed with medialization of the C2 screw, then the vertebral artery, which is superior and lateral, is safe from inadvertent injury. Screw placement into the lateral masses of C3 to C7 is performed according to the technique of An et al. (3). The Roy-Camille plate, AO stainless steel reconstruction plates (3.5 mm), or newer plate systems can be used for fixation (Fig. 32.6). The plate modifications for an anatomic fit can be technically demanding, as the curve necessitates transition from kyphosis at the inion to lordosis at the occipitocervical junction and lateral rotation to accommodate the subaxial cervical lateral masses. We suggest placement of the C2 pedicle screw first, as it allows for provisional fixation of the plate to the bony surface. Two or, preferably, three screws are placed into the occiput on each side. A high-speed burr is first utilized to penetrate the outer cortical margin to prevent inadvertent drill spin-off, which may injure adjacent structures. A minimum of 6 to 8 mm of occipital thickness is necessary for safe screw placement, and bicortical fixation is suggested. If cerebrospinal fluid (CSF) is encountered during screw placement, bone wax is used to seal the defect, and screw placement follows. If necessary, wire fixation methods can be used as an adjunct to enhance bony fixation. After decortication has been performed with a high-speed burr, autologous bone graft can be placed into the fusion bed. The postoperative orthosis used depends on the structural integrity of the construct and the quality of host bone determined at the time of surgery.

Complications associated with surgery at the occipitocervical junction can be catastrophic. Extreme care must be taken to minimize injury to the brain or spinal cord when passing wires or placing screws. Knowledge of the surgical anatomy is paramount, as excessive lateral dissection of more than 1.5 cm can lead to injury of the vertebral artery. Exposure of the foramen magnum and the lateral C1–2 margin should be minimized to avoid the potential sources of venous bleeding, which may be difficult to control. Spi-

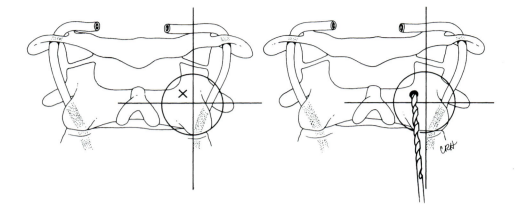

FIGURE 32.5.
The direction of C2 pedicle screw placement is 10° to 25° medially and approximately 25° cephalad, starting at the center corner of the upper inner quadrant. (Reprinted with permission from An HS, Cotler JM: Spinal instrumentation. Baltimore: Williams & Wilkins, 1992.) (4)

nal cord monitoring is suggested for high-risk procedures. Smith and Anderson reported on a series of 14 patients with occipitocervical plate fusion. They noted no neurovascular injuries or CSF fistulas. A screw loosened in four of the patients, but all went on to eventual fusion without further complication (50). In Wertheim and Bohlman's series of 13 patients, all went on to eventual fusion, with complete resolution of pain in 12 of the patients (57). Three of the unsatisfactory results were in patients with severe neurological involvement who did not recover function postoperatively.

Posterior Atlantoaxial Fusion

Indications

The indications for posterior stabilization of the atlantoaxial complex are mostly trauma-related. Atlantoaxial instability caused by rupture of the transverse ligament, type II odontoid fractures in a high-risk patient, or combined injuries can best be treated by posterior stabilization. Atlantoaxial instability can also be caused by a number of nontraumatic causes, including inflammatory arthropathy, metabolic disorders, congenital anomalies, tumor, or infection.

An atlantodental interval of 3 to 5 mm in an adult demonstrates damage to the transverse ligament, and an interval of more than 5 mm indicates insufficiency of the transverse and accessory ligaments (23). Nontraumatic causes of atlantoaxial intervals of more than 3 mm do not necessitate surgery. Patients with rheumatoid arthritis can have severe spinal instability, and when this is coupled with intractable pain and neurologic deterioration, then stabilization is indicated. An evaluation measure used in addition to the absolute atlantodental interval is the space available for the spinal cord. In inflammatory arthropathy associated with rheumatoid arthritis, a canal diameter of less than 14 mm is associated with a worse prognosis and should be considered for decompression and stabilization (10). In traumatic cases with an atlantodental interval of more than 5 mm, atlantoaxial arthrodesis is suggested. In atraumatic cases, review of flexion-extension radiographs and MRI scans can be helpful along with the neurological exam in determining whether fusion is indicated. Recently we have been using flexion-extension MRI sagittal images to determine whether or not neurologic impingement will occur.

The indications for operative treatment of odontoid fractures remains controversial, but prompt reduction and halo-vest application is still our first-line treatment. Patients who are at high risk for nonunion in type II fractures, who have a displacement of more than 5 mm, whose age is more than 60 years, or who have had loss of previous reduction should be considered for operative stabilization (5).

Technique

For nontrauma patients for whom halo-vest immobilization is planned postoperatively, it can be applied in the preoperative area with local anesthesia. For traumatic instability, if traction is necessary to reduce the resultant deformity, it can be maintained during surgery and incorporated into the vest postoperatively.

Stauffer believes that several factors should be considered in the preoperative evaluation to allow safe and effective stabilization of the C1-C2 complex (53). First is the amount of displacement of C1 on C2 and the ease of the reduction. Awake reduction should be performed whenever possible; if reduction is not possible or the deformity is fixed, then wire passage may not be advisable, and consideration

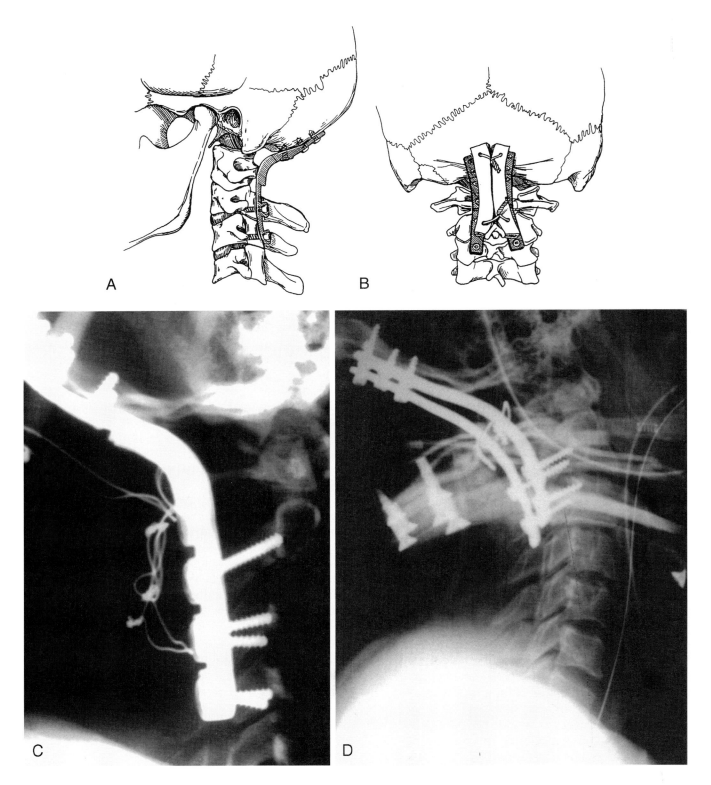

FIGURE 32.6.

Roy-Camille technique of occipitocervical fusion. **A.** Diagram of plate-screw fixation. **B.** Supplemental bone graft may be placed as a strut in the midline or wired as shown. **C.** Lateral radiograph shows Roy-Camille plate-screw fixation from the occiput to C4 in a patient with occiput-cervical instability. **D.** Another lateral radiograph shows custom-made implant fixation from the occiput to C3 in a patient with occiput-cervical dislocation.

should be given to using in situ fusion with external immobilization. Second is the amount of space between the occiput and C1 to allow wire passage. Local anatomy may make the procedure difficult and dangerous to perform. The final consideration is the integrity of the ring of C1. Preoperative CT scans may be more helpful than plain radiographs, as the latter may not show an occult fracture or dysplasia. Other methods of fixation, or treatment in a halo-vest until the ring fracture has healed, may have to be considered as a staged procedure.

Longitudinal skin traction over the shoulders is used along with foam protective devices around the elbows for arm positioning. Cloth tape is used to provide retraction of the patient's hair to facilitate presurgical preparation. A longitudinal midline incision is made, using the spinous process of C2 as a landmark from the occiput to C3. The posterior arch of C1 and the laminae of C2 are dissected subperiosteally, with care being taken to avoid the venous plexus around the C1-C2 articular surface. Lateral dissection is limited to a depth of 1.5 cm to avoid injury to the vertebral artery. Exposure should not reach the C2-C3 facet, in order to avoid iatrogenic instability in that segment.

Posterior atlantoaxial fusion can be performed with wiring techniques using the Gallie method, the Brooks method, or their modifications (13, 24). The Gallie method is easier to perform and is safer, because the spinous process of C2 rather than a sublaminar wire is used for attachment. The Brooks technique has demonstrated greater rotational stability in biomechanical testing (30, 32). The Gallie technique is recommended for most flexion injuries, but the Brooks method is indicated in cases in which greater construct stability is needed in extension and rotation.

We prefer a modification of the Gallie technique performed by Simmons (Fig. 32.7) (48, 49). A Gallie H-graft is fashioned from the iliac crest and contoured to fit over the posterior arches of C1 and C2. A U-shaped 20-gauge wire is then passed from caudal to cranial underneath the laminae of C1 and passed over the bone block and spinous process of C2, and the wires are tightened over the posterior portion of the block.

In the Brooks method, a double wire loop is passed from cranial to caudal beneath the laminae of C1 and C2 (Fig. 32.8). Small rectangular grafts are fashioned from the iliac crest (1.25 cm × 3.5 cm) and bevel-cut to fit wedged into the interlaminar space of C1–2 over the ventral wires. Each double wire is then sequentially tightened by twisting it over the bone grafts.

Although wiring methods have produced satisfactory results for atlantoaxial stabilization, many other methods have been reported in the literature (19, 41, 35). Moskovich and Crockard reported on the use of interlaminar clamps (Halifax) with interposed bone grafts, achieving a fusion rate of 80% within 12 weeks (41). He believed that the major advantage of the technique was the reduced risk of wire passage and the immediate stability provided by the implant. Wire cutout in cases in which osteoporotic or rheumatoid bone was present was reduced by the larger bone surface area in contact with the device.

Posterior transarticular screw fusion was initially reported by Magerl in 1982 (Fig. 32.9) (35). Since that time its popularity has grown both in Europe and in Japan as a method for C1-C2 stabilization but has been slower to gain acceptance in the United States. This technique has the advantage of providing stable fixation of C1 on C2 regardless of the integrity of the posterior arch of C1 or gross instability, and it does not require postoperative halo-vest immobilization. The indications for the use of this technique are the same as for other methods of posterior atlantoaxial fusion, with one exception. Collapse of the lateral masses of C2, seen in inflammatory or degenerative arthropathy, are a contraindication to the use of this technique (29). Destruction of this structure could lead to inadvertent penetration of the vertebral artery with drill bit advancement.

The patient is placed prone with the head maintained in a head holder. A halo is utilized if preoperative traction was necessary for fracture reduction. The occipitocervical joints must be flexed as much as possible with slight flexion of the subaxial cervical spine to facilitate screw insertion. Confirmation of reduction can be checked with fluoroscopy or plain radiographs before surgical preparation. A midline incision is made from the external occipital tubercle to the spinous process of C5 to allow angulation of the drill. Posterior C1 and C2 exposure is performed laterally to allow visualization of the articular facets without exposing the vertebral artery, which enters the canal behind the lateral mass of C2. Care is taken to visualize the inferior articular portion of C2 without destruction of the C2–3 capsule. The crest of the isthmus of C2 and the cranial surface of the laminae are exposed. Magerl and Seeman recommend the use of Kirschner wires to provide soft-tissue retraction for the greater occipital nerve (37). The starting point for the drill is at the inferior aspect of C2 in line with the straight sagittal line passing through the medial aspect of the isthmus and exiting at the posterior aspect of the upper articular process. The exact caudal-cranial angulation is achieved with the use of image intensification. A second drill is used as the first is left to provide direction and rotational stability. The screws are then placed through the facet joints into the lateral masses of C1. In a biomechanical study of posterior atlantoaxial fixation techniques, Grob et al. found that the Magerl technique provided the greatest rotational stability (30). We recommend wiring

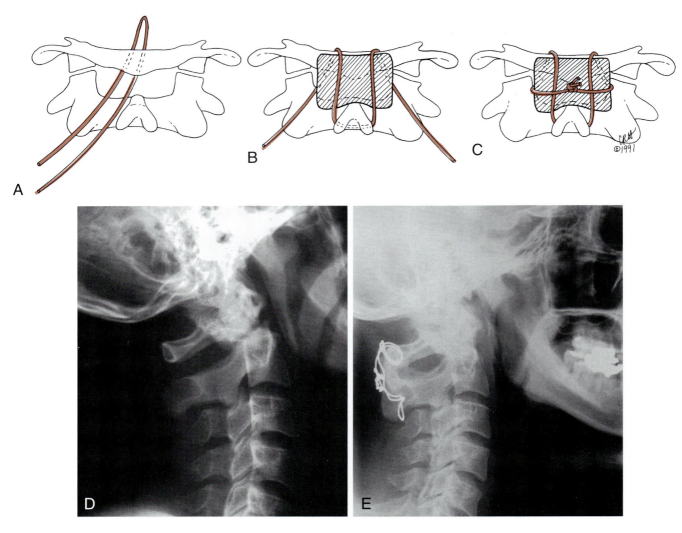

FIGURE 32.7.
Modified Gallie technique for atlantoaxial fusion. **A.** A 20-gauge wire is passed caudal to cranial. **B.** The wire is looped over the spinous process of C2. **C.** The wires are tightened over a contoured bone block between C1 and C2. **D.** Lateral radiograph shows a posteriorly displaced odontoid fracture that redisplaced in halo-vest. **E.** Postoperative lateral radiograph shows solid fusion and wiring at C1-C2.

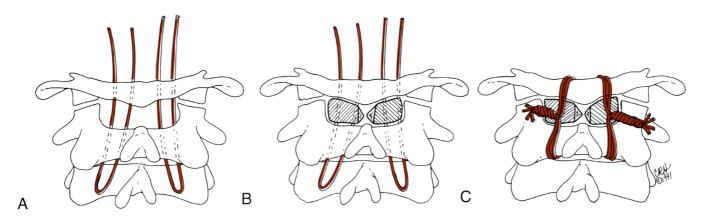

FIGURE 32.8.
Brooks atlantoaxial fusion method. **A.** Two 20- to 22-gauge wires are passed cranial to caudal. **B.** Two rectangular bone grafts are placed between C1 and C2. **C.** The wires are tightened over the grafts.

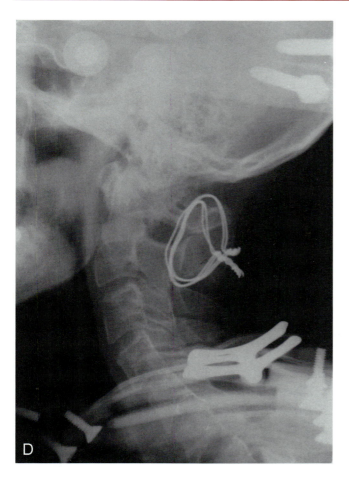

FIGURE 32.8—*continued*

D. Lateral radiograph shows the wiring and fusion construct in a patient with odontoid nonunion. (Reprinted with permission from An HS, Cotler JM. Spinal instrumentation. Baltimore: Williams & Wilkins, 1992.)

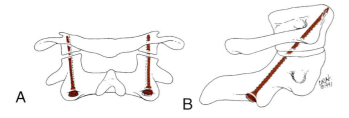

FIGURE 32.9.

Magerl's technique of C1-C2 fixation. **A.** and **B.** Screws enter at the inferior portion of C2, and pass through the facet joints into the lateral masses of C1.

techniques for atlantoaxial stabilization unless the posterior arch of C1 is deficient. Magerl and Seeman recommend additional Gallie wiring to complement the C1-C2 screw fixation (37). This rigid fixation may eliminate the need to use a postoperative halo, but the potential risks and benefits must be considered carefully before choosing a particular method. Other, less commonly used methods include Aprin and Harf's internal fixation of C1 and C2. Two 18-gauge wires are passed beneath the atlas and looped around a threaded Steinmann pin drilled through the base of the spinous process of the axis (8).

The most severe complication of posterior wiring procedures is neurological impairment resulting from the passage of a wire or excessive manipulation of the fracture. Stauffer indicates that sublaminar wires should be passed from cranial to caudal, as he believes that the loop is more difficult to pass around the spinous processes and that the loop is in jeopardy of being pushed into the canal (53). Preoperative reduction of the fracture will negate any excessive manipulation of the fracture site. The potential for wire failure can be reduced by minimizing the manipulation of the strands during placement and careful sequential tightening with the proper tools.

Application of the Halifax interlaminar clamps can be technically difficult. Proper placement of the device and tightening of the screws over the bone grafts is necessary for success. The interlaminar clamp has the potential for rotational instability, and loosening of the screws adds to this problem. Strict adherence to the outlined surgical technique should limit the potential complications. Gebhard and Jeanneret performed a cadaver study on the potential pitfalls of the transarticular screw fusion of C1 and C2 (26). They found that the spinal cord and vertebral artery are not at risk if the surgical procedure is performed as described. Injury to the C2 nerve can be avoided by careful dissection of the soft tissues around the C1-C2 facets. In a multicenter review of the technique, Grob et al. listed the incidence of malpositioning of the screws at 15%, but only 5.9% of the complications were directly related to the screws (29). Pseudarthrosis rate was reported at 0.6%, with eight additional patients having a stable fibrous union.

Subaxial Posterior Cervical Fixation

Posterior fixation of the lower cervical spine (C3–C7) is usually accomplished with wiring techniques or lateral-mass plating. Wire techniques for fusion of the lower cervical spine has been the time-tested method in both biomechanical and clinical studies since initially described by Rogers in 1942 (45). It is safe and easy to perform, and it does not require sophisticated instrumentation for application. Bohlman's triple-wire technique, which is a modification of Rogers's initial method, and the Robinson-Southwick technique have become the main forms of cervical stabilization using wire techniques.

Lateral-mass plate fixation of the cervical spine was initially popularized by Roy-Camille and later modified by Magerl, who used the hook plate (36,

46, 47). This particular technique has recently become a part of the armamentarium for spinal stabilization in the United States. Numerous instrumentation systems have been developed and have been employed in biomechanical and clinical studies (6, 22, 34).

Coe et al. have reported that there is no significant biomechanical difference between wiring and plating constructs as long as the posterior elements are intact (18). Ulrich et al. found that wiring techniques were less effective in resisting rotational and extension forces than plating (56). Sutterlin et al. also found that plating offered superior stability than wiring techniques (55). Roy-Camille et al. found that the plate increased construct stiffness by 92% in flexion as compared to 33% for wire techniques (46).

Indications

Posterior fusion of the lower cervical spine is indicated in traumatic instability, postlaminectomy instability, and destruction of bony anatomy by neoplasm. The goal of internal fixation is to allow for reduction and maintenance of alignment, rigid sta-

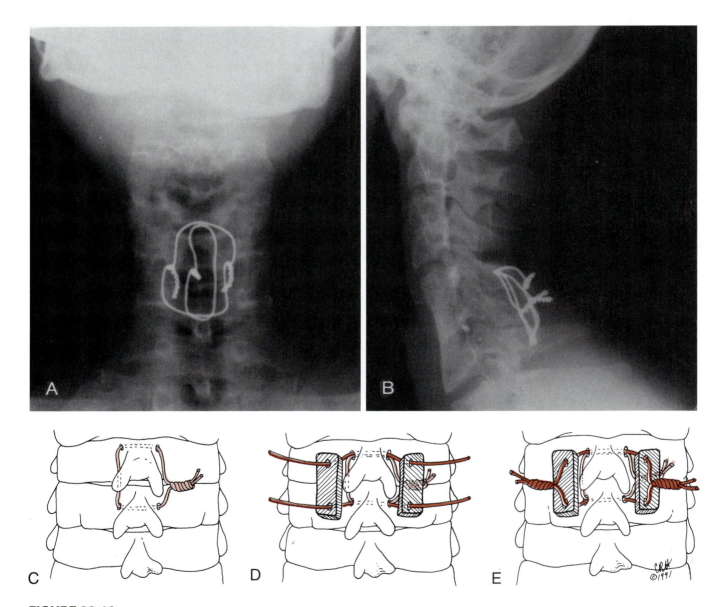

FIGURE 32.10.

Triple-wire technique. **A.** Anteroposterior radiograph shows the triple-wire technique from C5 to C7. (Reprinted with permission from An HS, Cotler JM. Spinal instrumentation. Baltimore: Williams & Wilkins, 1992.) **B.** Lateral radiograph shows the wiring and anterior fusion construct from C5 to C7. (Reprinted with permission from An HS, Cotler JM. Spinal instrumentation. Baltimore: Williams & Wilkins, 1992.) **C.** Diagram shows that the first wire is passed through holes drilled at the base of each spinous process. **D.** The second and third wires are passed through the same holes and through holes drilled in the bone grafts. **E.** The wires are secured over the grafts.

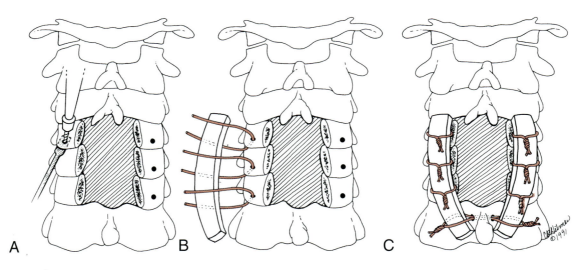

FIGURE 32.11.
Facet wire technique. **A.** Holes are drilled in the facet joint. **B.** Wires are passed through at each level. **C.** The wires are tightened over the grafts.

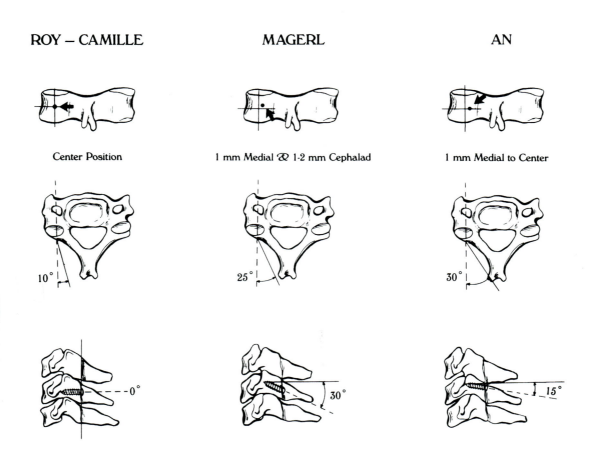

FIGURE 32.12.
Comparison of Roy-Camille, Magerl, and An methods of lateral mass screw orientation.

bilization, and early mobilization. Most cervical fusions can be achieved with simple wiring techniques (14, 15, 20, 25, 42, 44, 45). In cases of postlaminectomy instability or incompetent posterior elements from fracture, simple wiring techniques cannot be utilized. The Robinson-Southwick method or lateral-mass plating can provide stabilization under these circumstances.

In flexion-distraction injuries such as unilateral or bilateral facet dislocation, the involved cervical segments are quite unstable. They are initially managed with prompt reduction and posterior arthrodesis with either wire or plate techniques. In acute injuries associated with a herniated disc, anterior decompression is performed first, prior to posterior stabilization if necessary. Newer anterior plating techniques may decrease the need for circumferential fusions in trauma cases. The indication for treatment of more subtle ligamentous injuries is based on the criteria of White et al. for cervical instability. Eleven degrees of sagittal angulation and 3.5 mm of sagittal translation represent the threshold for stability in the cervical spine (58). More complex deformities may require combined anterior and posterior fusion, depending on the pathology involved. The wiring and plating techniques each have their advantages and disadvantages, and the surgeon should consider these carefully along with his or her own experience when choosing a particular method.

Technique

The triple-wire technique has been shown to be safe and effective in providing immediate stability to an injured cervical segment (Fig. 32.10). The patient is placed prone in traction after rotation on a Stryker frame. Arm positioning at the sides and longitudinal skin traction are established before surgical preparation. A midline incision is then made, using the posterior spinous processes of C2 and C7 as landmarks and carried down through the nuchal ligament. An intraoperative radiograph is taken to confirm the involved level. The posterior cervical muscles are mobilized off of the laminae, and dissection proceeds lateral to expose the facet capsule and lateral mass using the electrocautery. Care is taken not to expose any additional level or facet capsule, in order to avoid unwanted extension of the fusion or iatrogenic instability. A high-speed burr is then used to penetrate the cortex at the base of the spinous process, and the hole is enlarged with the use of a towel clip or single limb of a right-angle clamp. An 18- or 20-gauge wire is passed through the spinous process above and below and sequentially tightened. The second and third wires are passed through the cephalad and caudal holes, respectively. Decortication of the laminae, facets, and lateral masses is then performed with a high-speed burr. Corticocancellous grafts are fashioned from the iliac crest and the two wires are then passed through holes drilled in the surface of the grafts and are tightened in place. The posterior cortex of the grafts should come to rest just beneath the tips of the spinous processes for enhanced stability. Additional cancellous bone graft may be placed within the fusion bed, but not too close to adjacent levels.

The Robinson-Southwick technique involves passing wires after drilling holes in the facets from superior to inferior (Fig. 32.11). These wires are then looped over the bone grafts and tightened. This technique is indicated for use in postlaminectomy or spinous process fractures, when the triple-wire technique can not be used. We prefer to use lateral-mass plating in these instances.

Rigid fixation with the use of lateral-mass plating is indicated in all cases in which wiring techniques are used. In addition, postlaminectomy instability and incompetency of the posterior elements are indications for the use of this technique. In Bohlman's review of 300 acute cervical spine injuries, 23% sus-

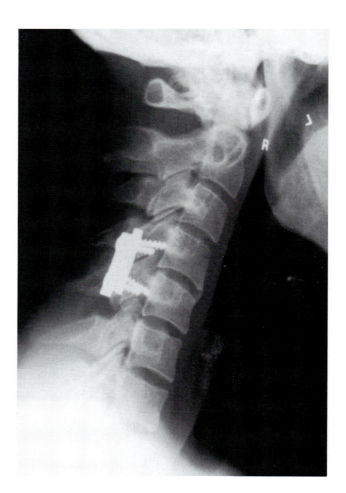

FIGURE 32.13.

Lateral radiograph shows anatomical reduction, solid posterior fusion, and Roy-Camille plate fixation at C4-C5 in a patient with unilateral facet joint dislocation.

tained fractures of the laminae, and 12.6%, fractures of spinous processes (12). Rigid internal fixation allows early mobilization of the patient with minimal postoperative external support.

Patients at risk for neurological injury are nasotracheally intubated and positioned awake with the Stryker frame. The neurological examination is then repeated to check for any changes. For patients who have degenerative conditions or failed anterior fusions and for postlaminectomy patients a Mayfield head rest will suffice. The knees are placed in flexion and the patient is placed in the reverse Trendelenburg position. Surgical exposure is performed exactly as in wiring techniques except that the entire lateral mass must be exposed for accurate placement of screws. A marker is then used to pinpoint the exact center of the lateral mass at each level to be fused. The AXIS plate system is composed of titanium and has plates with interfacet distances of 11, 13, and 15 mm intervals and the choice of two screw positions at each level. A plate template is used over this "road map" to choose the correct interfacet distance and plate length. A small burr is then used to penetrate the outer cortex in order to prevent drill bit spin-off. The orientation of the plate and lateral mass is then checked for proper drill alignment. There are different recommendations for the lateral mass drilling technique (Fig. 32.12); we use the method of An et al. and drill 15° cephalad and 25 to 30° laterally for safe placement of the lateral mass screw (3). A Penfield elevator can be placed within the articular facet to provide additional information as to its orientation. The drill is then advanced sequentially with the use of special drill-stop guides until the opposite cortex is reached. Preoperative radiographs can aide in determining the depth of the screw needed to gain a purchase the opposite cortex. If technical difficulty is encountered in placing the screws or the bone is of poor quality, then larger-diameter revision screws can be placed in a unicortical fashion to reduce the

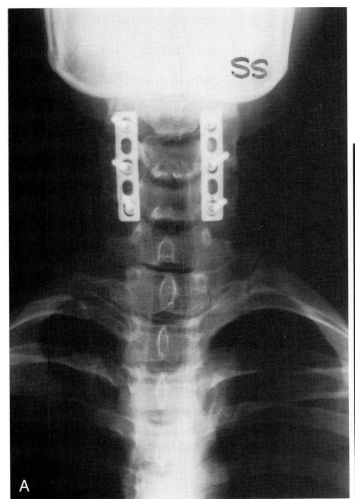
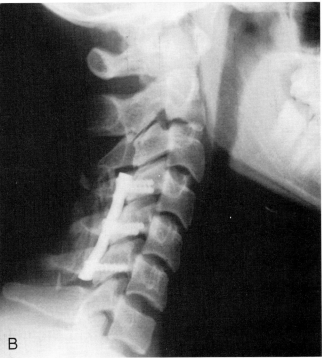

FIGURE 32.14.

A. Anteroposterior and **B.** lateral radiographs show the use of AO semitubular plate and ideal screw placement in a patient with a two-level flexion-distraction injury at C4-C5 and C5-C6.

likelihood of neurovascular injury. Initial tightening of the first screw is performed to give the plate some interface stability while the remaining screws are placed. Traction is reduced to 5 pounds prior to final tightening. There are several plates that could be used for posterior lateral-mass fixation, such as the Roy-Camille plate, the Rene Louise plate, Harms's plate, the AO semitubular plate, the AO reconstruction plate (Synthes, Paoli, PA), the AXIS plate (Danek, Inc, Memphis, TN), and others (Figs. 32.13–32.16).

If C2 screw placement is necessary, then the medial border of the pedicle must be visualized for accurate drilling. The starting point is 3 to 5 mm above the middle part of the C2-C3 facet. The direction of the screw is 10 to 25° medial and approximately 25° cephalad. Palpation of the medial pedicle wall with the use of a dental elevator is performed to prevent inadvertent cord injury with further drilling.

The anatomy at the cervicothoracic junction is highly variable, and preoperative CT scans are suggested for surgical planning if pedicle screws are necessary at C7 to T2. The entry point is at the middle of the facet and the middle of the transverse processes (Fig. 32.13). The medial angulation is about 25 to 30° (Fig. 32.17). A small laminotomy can be performed at the level and the direction checked with a Penfield elevator. Alternatively, the hook-plate designed by Magerl can be used for stabilization at C7 (Fig. 32.18). This plate has a hook that attaches to the inferior lamina of C7, and lateral mass screws are used at C6 and above.

Following instrumentation, decortication is performed with a high-speed burr. Before application of the plate, the articular facets are decorticated, and a small amount of cancellous bone is packed into the defect. Graft is carefully placed into the fusion bed in order to avoid involvement of adjacent levels. The wound is closed over suction drainage for 24 to 48 hours with perioperative antibiotics. A Philadelphia collar is placed before removal of the tongs or Mayfield head rest, and the neck is immobilized for 6 to 8 weeks postoperatively.

Complications associated with posterior fusion of the cervical spine are many. Care is required during passage of the wires or application of the screws to prevent injury to the spinal cord. Complications associated with posterior interspinous wiring in the cervical spine are relatively infrequent. One must avoid unnecessary exposure of the cervical levels beyond fusion areas in order to prevent creeping fusions to adjacent vertebrae. Inadvertent penetration into the ligamentum flavum and the spinal canal can occur if the surgeon is not careful during subperiosteal dissection. Dural penetration can also occur during drilling or passage of wires if the holes are placed

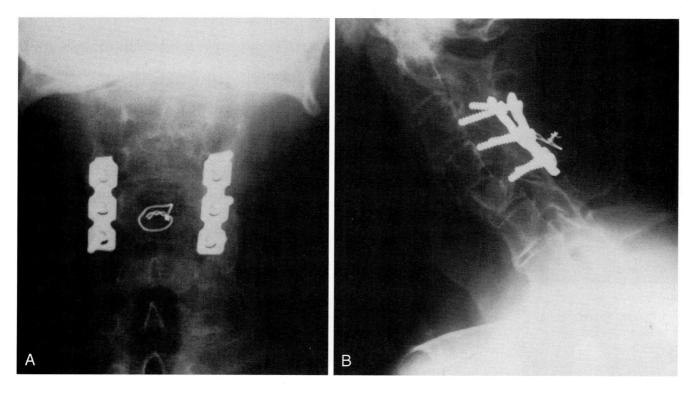

FIGURE 32.15.

A. Anteroposterior and **B.** lateral radiographs show the use of AO reconstruction plate fixation from C3 to C5 and interspinous wiring at C4-C5 in a 62-year-old ankylosing spondylitis patient with fracture-dislocation at C4-C5.

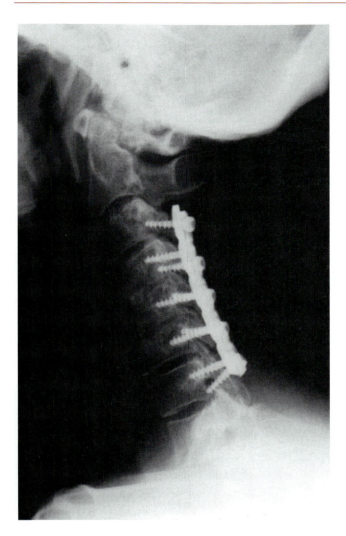

FIGURE 32.16.
Lateral radiograph shows anterior strut fusion from C4 to C6 and posterior laminectomy and plate-screw fixation from C3 to C7 in a 59-year-old patient with cervical spondylotic myelopathy. The spinal cord was severely impinged at C4-C5 and C5-C6 by both ligamentum flavum buckling posteriorly and osteophytes anteriorly. Posterior laminectomy and plating were performed first, followed by anterior corpectomy and fusion. At C7 the pedicle on one side and the lateral mass on the other were used for screw fixation. This patient had a significant improvement of myelopathy, and solid fusion was noted at 1-year follow-up.

too close to the dura. The most common complication associated with wiring procedures in the cervical spine is the loss of fixation and the subsequent recurrence of deformity. This complication is often related to the surgeon's technique and to postoperative external support. If a relatively rigid construct is accomplished, the patient can be treated postoperatively with a cervicothoracic orthosis. However, if the surgical construct is not quite stable, or if the patient's compliance is questionable, a halo-vest orthosis should be used. Complications associated with rigid posterior fixation of the cervical spine may include screw impingement on the nerve root, vertebral artery injury, and hook impingement on the spinal canal. Laminar hooks should be avoided at the injured level, where the spinal cord has already been compromised by edema or mechanical compression.

Conclusion

Cervical spinal fixation is continually evolving, and better and more stable constructs are becoming available. With experience and proper patient selection, the use of such instrumentation may help patients to avoid postoperative halo-vest immobilization, enhance early rehabilitation, and preempt the need for any additional surgical treatment. In stabilizing the cervical spine, the proper fusion remains the most important procedure, and spinal fixation devices may be used to augment the stability of the construct and enhance the fusion rates.

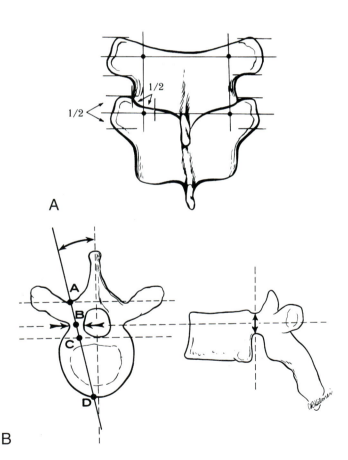

FIGURE 32.17.
A. The entry point for the thoracic pedicle is at the middle of the facet and the middle of the transverse processes. **B.** The pedicle is perpendicular to the vertebral axis, and medial angulation is about 25 to 30° in the upper thoracic region. (Reprinted with permission from An HS, Cotler JM. Spinal instrumentation. Baltimore: Williams & Wilkins, 1992.)

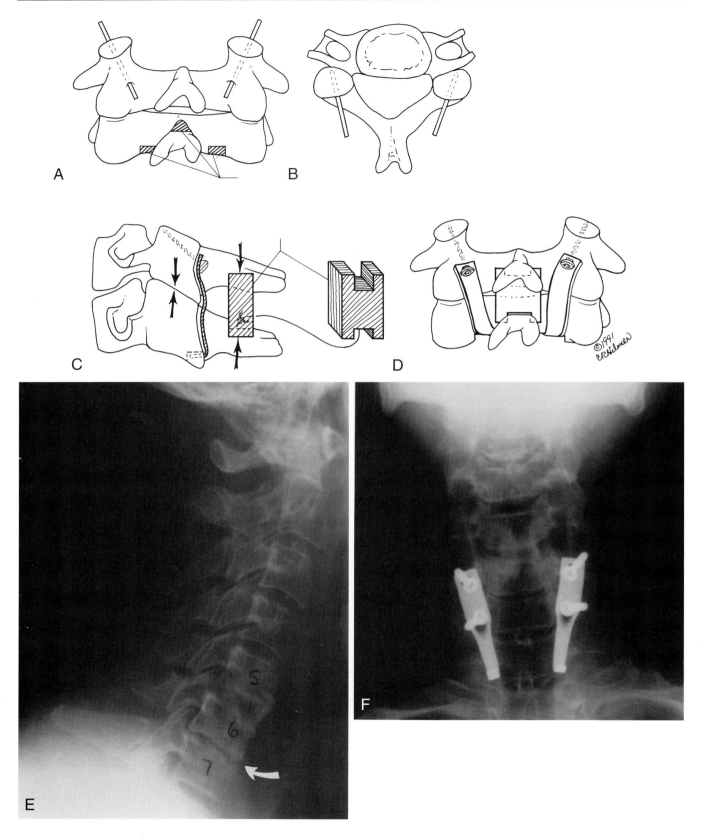

FIGURE 32.18.

Magerl's hook-plate fixation. **A.** The inferior edge of the C7 lamina is prepared for hooks, and the superior edge of the C7 spinous process is prepared for an H-shaped bone graft. **B.** The lateral mass screw is directed laterally and superiorly. **C.** The bone graft is placed first, and screws are tightened to compress the graft. **D.** This construct avoids screws in the thin lateral mass at C7. **E.** Lateral radiograph shows nonunion of C6-C7 in a patient with recurrent C7 radiculopathy (arrow). **F.** Anteroposterior radiograph shows the hook-plate fixation from C5 to C7.

References

1. Aebi M, Etter C, Cosia M. Fractures of the odontoid process. Spine 1989;14(10):1065–1069.
2. Aebi M, Zuber K, Marchesi D. Treatment of cervical spine injuries with anterior plating. Spine 1991; 16(3S):538–545.
3. An HS, Gordin R, Renner K. Anatomic considerations for plate fixation to the cervical spine. Spine 1988; 13:813–816.
4. An HS, Cotler JM. Spinal instrumentation. Baltimore: Williams & Wilkins, 1992.
5. An HS, Simpson JM, eds. Surgery of the cervical spine. London: Martin-Dunitz, 1994;1:383.
6. Anderson PA, Henley MB, Grady MS, et al. Posterior cervical arthrodesis with AO reconstruction plates and bone graft. Spine 1991;16S:S72–S79.
7. Apfelbaum RI. Odontoid screw fixation. Presented at the twentieth annual meeting of the Cervical Spine Research Society, 1992, Palm Desert, CA.
8. Aprin H, Harf R. Stabilization of atlantoaxial instability. Orthopaedics 1988;11:1687–1693.
9. Bailey RW, Badgley CE. Stabilization of the cervical spine by anterior fusion. J Bone Joint Surg 1960; 42A:565–624.
10. Boden SD, Dodge LD, Bohlman HH, et al. Rheumatoid arthritis of the cervical spine: a long-term analysis with predictors of paralysis and recovery. J Bone Joint Surg 1993;75A:1282–1297.
11. Böhler J. Anterior stabilization of acute fractures and non-unions of the dens. J Bone Joint Surg 1982;64A:18.
12. Bohlman HH. Acute fractures and dislocations of the cervical spine. J Bone Joint Surg 1979;61A:1119–1142.
13. Brooks AL, Jenkins EB. Atlantoaxial arthrodesis by the wedge compression method. J Bone Joint Surg 1978; 60A:279–284.
14. Cahill DW, Bellegarrigue R, Ducker TB. Bilateral facet to spinous process fusion: a new technique for posterior spinal fusion after trauma. Neurosurgery 1983;13:1–4.
15. Callahan RA, Johnson RM, Margolis RN, et al. Cervical facet fusion for control of instability following laminectomy. J Bone Joint Surg 1977;59A:991–1002.
16. Caspar W, Barbier DD, Klara PM. Anterior cervical fusion and Caspar plate stabilization for cervical trauma. Neurosurgery 1989;25(4):491–502.
17. Cloward RD. Treatment of acute fractures and fracture dislocations of the cervical spine by vertebral body fusion: a report of 11 cases. J Neurosurg 1961;18:205–209.
18. Coe J, Warden K, Sutterlin CE, et al. Biomechanical evaluation of cervical stabilization methods in a human cadaver model. Spine 1989;14:1122–1131.
19. Cybulski GR, Stone JL, Crowell RM, et al. Use of Halifax interlaminar clamps for posterior C1-C2 arthrodesis. Neurosurgery 1988;22:429–431.
20. Davey JR, Rorabeck CH, Bailey SI, et al. A technique of posterior fusion for instability of the cervical spine. Spine 1985;10:722–728.
21. Doherty BJ, Heggeness MH, Esses SI. A biomechanical study of odontoid fractures and fracture fixation. Spine 1993;18(2):178–184.
22. Ebraheim NA, An HS, Jackson WT, et al. Internal fixation of the unstable cervical spine using posterior Roy-Camille plates: preliminary report. J Orthop Trauma 1989;3:23–28.
23. Fielding JW, Hawking RJ, Sanford RA. Spine fusion for atlantoaxial instability. J Bone Joint Surg 1976; 58A:400–406.
24. Gallie WE. Fractures and dislocations of the cervical spine. Am J Surg 1939;46:495–499.
25. Garfin SR, Moore MR, Marshall LF. A modified technique for cervical facet fusions. Clin Orthop 1988; 230:149–153.
26. Gebhard JS, Jeanneret B. Anatomic assessment of atlantoaxial transarticular screw fixation. Presented at the twenty-first annual meeting of the Cervical Spine Research Society, NY, 1993.
27. Graziano G, Jaggers C, Lee M, et al. A comparative study of fixation techniques for type II fractures of the odontoid. Spine 1993;18(16):2383–2387.
28. Grob D, Dvorak J, Panjabi M, et al. Posterior occipitocervical fusion: a preliminary report of a new technique. Spine 1991;16S:S17–S24.
29. Grob D, Jeanneret B, Aebi M, et al. Atlantoaxial fusion with transarticular screw fixation. J Bone Joint Surg 1991;73B:972–976.
30. Grob D, Crisco JJ, Panjabi MM, et al. Biomechanical evaluation of four different posterior atlantoaxial fixation techniques. Spine 1992;17(5):480–490.
31. Hadra BE. Wiring of the spinous process in injury and Potts disease. Trans Am Orthop Assoc 1891;4:206.
32. Hajek PD, Lipka J, Hartine P, et al. Biomechanical study of C1–2 posterior arthrodesis techniques. Spine 1993; 18(2):173–177.
33. Kostuik JP, Connolly PJ, Esses SI, et al. Anterior cervical plate fixation with the titanium hollow plate system. Spine 1993;18(10):1273–1278.
34. Louis RP. Surgery of the Spine. Berlin: Springer-Verlag, 1983:49–83.
35. Magerl F. Spondylodesen an der oberen halwirbelsaule. Acta Chir Aust 1982;(Suppl):43–69.
36. Magerl F, Grob D, Seeman PS. Stable dorsal fusion of the cervical spine (C2–T1) using hook plates. In: Kehr P, Weidner A, eds. Cervical spine. Vienna and New York: Springer-Verlag, 1987:217–221.
37. Magerl F, Seeman PS. Stable posterior fusion of the atlas and axis by transarticular screw fixation. In: Kehr P, Weidner A, eds. Cervical spine. Vienna and New York: Springer-Verlag, 1987:322–327.
38. Meyer PR Jr. Surgical stabilization of the cervical spine. In: Meyer PR, ed. Surgery of spine trauma. New York: Churchill Livingstone, 1989:11–49.
39. Montesano PX, Juach EC, Anderson PA, et al. Biomechanics of cervical spine internal fixation. Spine 1991; 16S:S10–S16.
40. Montesano PX. Screw fixation of the odontoid process. Techniques in Orthop 1994;9(1):60–67.
41. Moskovich R, Crockard HA. Atlantoaxial arthrodesis using interlaminar clamps. Spine 1991;17:261–267.
42. Murphy MJ, Daniaux H, Southwick WO. Posterior cervical fusion with rigid internal fixation. Orthop Clin North Am 1986;17:55–65.
43. Powers B. Traumatic anterior-occipital dislocations. Neurosurgery 1979;4:12–17.
44. Robinson RA, Southwick WO. Indications and tech-

niques for early stabilization of the neck in some fracture dislocations of the cervical spine. South Med J 1960;53:565.
45. Rogers WA. Treatment of fractures and dislocations of the cervical spine. J Bone Joint Surg 1942;24A:245–248.
46. Roy-Camille RR, Saillant G, Mazel C. Internal fixation of the unstable cervical spine by posterior osteosynthesis with plates and screws. In: Cervical Spine Research Society, ed. The cervical spine. Philadelphia: JP Lippincott, 1989;2:390–404.
47. Roy-Camille RR, Saillant G, Laville C, et al. Treatment of lower cervical spine injuries–C3 to C7. Spine 1992; 17(10S):S442–S446.
48. Savini R, Parisini P, Cevellati S. The surgical treatment of late instability of flexion-rotation injuries in the lower cervical spine. Spine 1987;12:178–182.
49. Simmons EH. Surgery of the spine in rheumatoid arthritis and ankylosing spondylosis. In Evarts CM, ed. Surgery of the musculoskeletal system. New York: Churchill Livingstone, 1983;85–151.
50. Smith MD, Anderson P, Grady S. Occipitocervical arthrodesis using contoured plate fixation. Spine 1993; 18:1984–1990.
51. Smith GW, Robinson RA. The treatment of certain cervical spine disorders by anterior removal of the intervertebral disc and interbody fusion. J Bone Joint Surg 1958;40A:607.
52. Stambough JL, Balderston RA, Grey S. Technique for occipitocervical fusion in osteopenic patients. J Spinal Disord 1990;3:404–407.
53. Stauffer ES. Wiring techniques of the posterior cervical spine following treatment of trauma. Orthopaedics 1988;11(1):1543–1548.
54. Suh DB, Kostuik JP, Esses SI. Anterior cervical plate fixation with titanium hollow screw plate system: a preliminary report. Spine 1990;15:1079–1081.
55. Sutterlin CE, McAfee PC, Warden K, et al. Biomechanical evaluation of cervical stabilization methods in a bovine model. Spine 1988;13:795–802.
56. Ulrich C, Woersdoefer O, Claes L, et al. Comparative study of stabilization of anterior and posterior fixation. Arch Orthop Trauma Surg 1987;106:2326–2331.
57. Wertheim SB, Bohlman HH. Occipitocervical fusion. J Bone Joint Surg 1987;69A:833–836.
58. White AA III, Panjabi MM, Saha S, et al. Biomechanics of the axially loaded cervical spine. Development of a clinical test for ruptured ligaments. J Bone Joint Surg 1975;57A:582.

CHAPTER THIRTY THREE

Posterior Instrumentation of the Thoracolumbar Spine

S. Craig Humphreys and Howard S. An

Introduction

Posterior instrumentation of the thoracic and lumbar spine has evolved tremendously over the past 80 years. Initially, posterior spinal surgery consisted of decompression in the form of laminectomy and rudimentary fixation with single screws and wires. In the late 19th century Hadra, at Galveston, used wires to stabilize a fracture-dislocation of the cervical spine (14). In 1911 Albee and Hibbs reported the first successful fusion (1, 18). In the 1950s facet screws came into wide use. These could achieve reasonable purchase and often initial correction, but failures of fixation and fusion over time were common, leading to the abandonment of facet screws. It has become clear that fusion is the key to success with instrumentation. Over time the powerful forces of spinal motion will eventually cause the most rigid instrumentation system to fatigue and fail.

As our knowledge of the dynamic nature of the spine has grown, more sophisticated and powerful methods have arisen to provide today's spinal surgeon a plethora of instrumentation systems from which to choose. However, as the number and type of these instrumentation systems has multiplied, their effective use has become more difficult. Currently many of the instrumentation systems have only small variations in their design and function, understanding the principles of proper stabilization has become more important in order to achieve adequate fusion before failure of the hardware can occur. Additionally, with the increasing efforts at cost containment many hospitals are limiting the number of systems that are in inventory.

Hooks and pedicle screws allow modern instrumentation to grasp the spine over many segments and to distribute more broadly the forces applied. The instrumentation can be applied to correct a spine in multiple planes of deformity and reliably maintain reduction until fusion can occur. An understanding of the anatomy, pathology, and kinetics of different segments of the spine is paramount in choosing the appropriate treatment option. For example, a traumatic kyphotic thoracic spine resulting from anterior compression forces may be maintained posteriorly by the ligamentous supports and may indeed be correctable through an isolated posterior approach, whereas a kyphosis from Scheuermann's disease often requires an anterior release/fusion and posterior instrumentation.

Currently we are able to manipulate the spine in a multitude of ways with more modern instrumentation systems. A precise understanding of the pathology—whether it be traumatic, congenital, developmental, neoplastic, or degenerative—and of the desired outcome is critical not only in choosing the appropriate instrumentation system but also in order to ensure its intelligent application. As the recognition of pathology expands with our ability to distinguish abnormal anatomy more accurately, and as the variety of instrumentation increases, the spine surgeon is better able to approach each patient's needs and achieve superior results. This chapter provides a presentation of the systems most commonly used and the systems that provide unique approaches to posterior instrumentation of the thoracolumbar spine.

Harrington Instrumentation

Though spinal surgery had been dabbled with early in the century, the revolution in technique began with Harrington in the 1950s and 1960s in Houston. Harrington designed a rod primarily for treating children with poliomyelitis, which was endemic in the United States at the time. The techniques of conservative care such as Stagnara casting were minimally effective, and the operative techniques of the day were fraught with complications and misery for the patients. In this environment Harrington understood the importance of distraction to correct the inevitable collapse of the spine. It was later recognized that fusion must accompany the instrumentation for long-term maintenance of correction. On the basis of this understanding, Harrington developed rods with hooks to maintain and obtain distraction. Initially the attempts were not combined with adequate fusions and resulted in numerous rod breakages and dislodgments. Many revisions of his rod were required before it was widely accepted for general use. It was not until Harrington presented his modified construct of the rod at the American Orthopaedic Association Meeting in 1960 that widespread use of the current Harrington rod system began (15, 16).

The Harrington instrumentation system has stood the test of time. The results of the use of Harrington instrumentation in idiopathic scoliosis have been good even by today's standards. The instrumentation is safe, with a neurologic complication rate of less than 0.5% (26). A disadvantage of the system is its inability to maintain sagittal balance, causing flatback in the thoracic and, more important, the lumbar spine. The loss of lordosis in the lumbar spine can result in significant back pain and gait disturbances. The pseudarthrosis rate is approximately 4%, and the hook dislocation rate is high, reaching as much as 3% in the lumbar spine (26).

New techniques have emerged that improve on Harrington's original design. Modifications by Moe and Edwards assisted in applying forces in different directions. The Harrington rod may be used in treating traumatic injuries with axial loading and flexion compression fractures. Instrumentation usually consists of three segments above and two segments below the injury zone.

Recently methods of treatment based on modern concepts have been presented. The principles outlined by King and associates generally provide excellent curve correction and restoration of trunk balance in patients with spinal deformity (23). The dual compression rod assembly should be used in treating kyphosis, whereas combining compression and distraction with rod assembly should be considered for a scoliotic curve.

Hook placement involves a thorough exposure of the spine, followed by preparation of the facet or lamina. The up-going hook may be inserted under the facet and lamina. The inferior aspect of the facet is removed by an osteotome, and the joint cartilage is removed. Preparation is carried out by removing a portion of the inferior facet and laminar edge with a Kerrison punch to square the edges for a flush fit. Care should be taken to place the hooks under the lamina and not directly into the bone; if the hook is placed between the inner and outer tables of bone, the chances of a laminar or facet fracture with subsequent dislodgment are increased. Down-going hooks are inserted over the top of the lamina. The ligamentum flavum is removed first, and a Kerrison punch is used to prepare the superior part of the lamina to obtain a flush fit. The down-going hook is an intracanal hook, and care must be taken not to compress the underlying spinal cord.

The compression assemblies use multiple hooks configured onto a fully threaded rod. Two sizes of rod are used in the Harrington system: $\frac{1}{8}$ inch and $\frac{3}{16}$ inch. While the smaller rod is easier to contour and thus easier to insert, it also is more likely to fatigue and fail. Two sizes of hooks are available for both rods. Above T11 the hook may be placed over the transverse process of the vertebrae instead of over the lamina. The hooks are placed into appropriate positions first, and then the spine assembly is laid in and attached. Generally three caudad-facing hooks above the apex of the curve and two or three cephalad-facing hooks below the apex are placed, with insertion of the assembly beginning at the upper level and proceeding distally.

In the United States today the Harrington rod has become antiquated, but the results are still good. Many countries still use it because of its ease of assembly and low cost. Traumatic injuries can still be treated effectively with Harrington instrumentation. A thorough understanding of mechanics is necessary. Distraction fractures such as the ligamentous or bony Chance fractures can be treated with compression one level above and one level below.

Axial loading fractures can also be treated with Harrington distraction rods. For most axial loading injuries, a pattern with three hooks above and two below is used. Other systems, such as the Moe square-ended rod and the Edwards modular rod with or without segmental wiring, can be used in a similar fashion.

Luque Sublaminar Wiring

Because of the difficulty in controlling rotation with the Harrington compression/distraction system, the Luque wiring and instrumentation system was developed to help correct rotation and severe curvatures by providing force over many levels of the spine. By distributing the forces, the chances of lamina fracture or rod and/or hook pullout are decreased. The Luque sublaminar wires may be used together with Harrington instrumentation, Luque L-rods, Cotrel-Dubousset instrumentation, and others. After the primary distraction or compression force has been applied, the wires can provide additional translation or derotation.

The Luque sublaminar wiring's most common use today is for neuromuscular scoliosis. It may be used in idiopathic scoliosis for curves greater than 40 to 45° in the skeletally immature patient. It is particularly effective in lordotic deformities in the thoracic and lumbar spine.

Luque wiring has minimal effectiveness in compression or distraction, and its mainstay is in the control of rotation and in providing many points of fixation to distribute the correction force over many levels. Significant correction can be obtained because the multiple points of fixation cumulate to create a tremendous force.

For surgical technique, routine exposure of the spinous processes, lamina, and transverse processes is done, followed by excision of the ligamentum flavum. A double-action rongeur is used to remove the bone overlying the ligamentum flavum in the thoracic spine; the ligamentum flavum is removed until the epidural space is visualized. A Kerrison rongeur may be used to clear the ligamentum flavum for wire passage. Contouring the sublaminar wires is important in preventing damage to the dura and neural elements. Uniform contouring also helps the surgeon to feel where the distal tip of the wire will be during its passage. The end of the Cobb handle works well for the proper curvature, and it also provides a uniform curve that can be duplicated well with different scrub assistants. Zindrick and colleagues developed a mathematical model that indicated that a semicircular model resulted in less canal penetration than the rectangular model (30). He also established that the larger the radius of curvature, the less the penetration of the canal. Goll and associates videotaped the passage of sublaminar wires and came to the following conclusions: *(a)* passage of the sublaminar wire must remain strictly in the midline; *(b)* the tip of the sublaminar wire should not be at an angle greater than 45°; and *(c)* the radius of curvature must be at least the width of the lamina (10).

Passing the wire is a gentle, two-handed maneuver, usually beginning at the inferior end of the lamina and proceeding cephalad. Once the wire is visualized at the proximal end of the lamina, it is grabbed with a large needle holder. While advancing the wire, a constant upward pressure must be applied to avoid inadvertent damage to the dura. Single- and double-stranded wires are inserted in the same manner. After the wires are passed, they are twisted over the lamina to prevent them from migrating into the canal or being inadvertently hit, which could push them into the spinal cord. The rod is then contoured, and the wires are twisted around the rod. As the wires are tightened, the spine, via its laminae, is gradually pulled to the precontoured rod. Wires should be tightened successively to apply the force gradually over many wires, and then time should be given to allow relaxation of the soft tissues before the wires are retightened. Care should be taken not to overtighten the wires and break them. A certain amount of experience helps to cut down on wire breakages (8, 11). Passing wires with the rod in place is much more difficult and should be avoided.

Correction of scoliosis can be performed with several methods, including convex techniques and concave techniques. In the convex technique, the proximal end of the rod is attached to the spine with four or five wires. The opposite end of the spine is then pulled to the relatively straight, stable rod by tightening many wires successively, thereby straightening the curve (Fig. 33.1). Because the rod is contoured, it must be securely fixed at each end and not allowed to rotate. Rotation of the rod will lead to loss of correction. The concave technique is more appropriate in thoracic curves associated with significant thoracic lordosis or lumbar curves. In either technique it is important to tighten the wires slowly and to secure the rod ends. The Galveston technique can be used with segmental wires as well (2, 19). The Galveston technique includes bending the rod so that it can be introduced into the posterior iliac crest for cases in which fusion to the pelvis is desired. Often patients who have neuromuscular scoliosis require fusion to the pelvis for scoliosis combined with severe pelvic obliquity. In this situation the segmental wiring is placed first. The rods are then laid into position on top of the wiring, and the wires are tightened slowly to obtain maximal correction.

Segmental wiring is not often used in trauma patients but can be used for shear injuries or to enhance fixation of the Harrington or similar rods. The

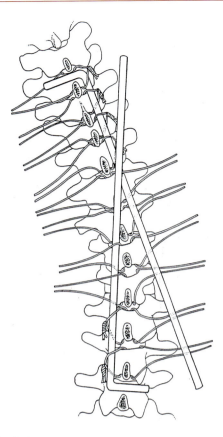

FIGURE 33.1.
A diagram of Luque rods and sublaminar wires. The convex technique involves wiring the proximal end of the rod attached to the spine with four or five wires and correction of scoliosis by gradual cantilever bending and tightening the distal wires.

fracture is then stabilized three levels above and below with segmental wiring. Segmental wiring should not be used at the level of the fracture because of increased risk of dural tear or neural injury.

Drummond Spinous Process Wiring

Segmental spinous process instrumentation with spinous process wires was developed for patients with idiopathic scoliosis as a safer alternative to instrumentation with sublaminar wires. The use of Drummond wiring is similar to that of the Luque sublaminar wiring. It was designed to be used with Harrington instrumentation, Moe instrumentation, and the Luque L-rod (2, 3). Drummond selected the spinous process because it is readily available and accessible to instrumentation, it is safe to work with, and there is usually adequate bone stock (8). The Drummond method uses a button implant made of 316 L stainless steel; an 18-gauge wire is used over the button, which provides surface area for the wire to pull over (2, 17, 25). Because the wires are inserted in pairs, there is a hole in one implant that allows the wires of one implant to pass through another. Because the wire is placed more posteriorly, it gives a greater mechanical advantage to derotation while it provides less force to correct translation. Additionally, the strength of the spinous process should be considered in deciding between Drummond and Luque wires, as the bone quality of the spinous process is not as good as that of the cortical bone in the lamina.

After the spine has been appropriately cleaned and rod placement determined, the facets should be prepared for fusion, because the rods and wires may interfere with later decortication. The wire implants are inserted at the base of the spinous process, ventral enough to maintain good bone stock but dorsal enough to avoid the spinal canal. A curved awl is used to assist in preparation for passage of a wire. After all the buttons are in place, an appropriately

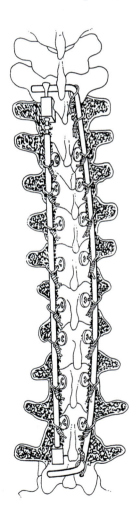

FIGURE 33.2.
A diagram of the Drummond Wisconsin buttons and scoliosis correction construct. After all the buttons are in place, the Harrington distraction rod is placed on the concave side and the Luque rod on the convex side.

contoured rod is inserted through the open loops of wires. The Harrington distraction rod is placed on the concave side, and the Luque rod is placed on the convex side (Fig. 33.2). Again it is important that the rod be fixed securely so that correction is not compromised and the wires can be slowly tightened to the desired correction.

Indications for Drummond wiring are similar to those for the Luque instrumentation system, namely, neuromuscular scoliosis with long curves severe enough to need surgical correction. Some adjustments have been suggested with certain techniques of fixation. In thoracic lordosis or significant hypokyphosis, it is advised that the wire loops around the apex of the curve be twisted. By tightening these wires first, the principal forces of correction are applied to overcome the sagittal deformity rather than the coronal component. For rigid curves the technique is modified by inserting two distraction rods into the concavity of the major curve.

Modular Spinal Segmental Instrumentation

Cotrel-Dubousset Instrumentation

The introduction of the Cotrel-Dubousset (CD) instrumentation at the Scoliosis Research Society in 1984 revolutionized our ability both to correct multiplane deformities with a single instrumentation system and to manipulate the spine in three dimensions. The ability to use multiple hooks allows us not only to distribute the forces more effectively but also to apply both compression and distraction along the same rod (6, 7, 9, 12, 27). Luque and Harrington instrumentation systems were in widespread use and adjuncts to their functions were being developed regularly in the 1970s and early 1980s. However, their use was confined to either compression or distraction forces to achieve reduction. The ability today to control the curve in multiple planes allows the surgeon to correct the spine in the coronal plane, which was difficult with earlier systems.

Instrumentation has become so powerful that the ideas of overcorrection and balance have become commonplace. Consideration of maximum preservation of motion segments, the ability to enhance fusion, and perhaps avoiding overcorrection are weighed against the potential loss of some sagittal or coronal correction to obtain overall coronal and sagittal balance. Often the coronal plane angular deformities do not occur in synchrony with the normal sagittal plane curves, and their apices and radii are different. The principles of deformity surgery are to determine the end vertebrae selection, to define the structural and compensatory curves, and to locate and define the stable and neutral vertebrae. Also important is the avoidance of stopping at the apex of a curve in either the coronal or sagittal plane.

For kyphosis surgery, the end vertebrae should be at least one vertebra beyond the structural curve as described by the Cobb method or as defined by its lying within or anterior to the vertical plumb line. The King classification is a useful way to discuss various curve patterns and will be used as a model in this chapter (23). However, each curve must be evaluated and critically considered independently, both in terms of the patient's history and with the use of appropriate diagnostic studies, to achieve the best clinical results.

In the following discussion some basic instrumentation methods will be covered briefly, using CD as our example. Later we will discuss differences in the TSRH, ISOLA, and Moss-Miami systems. The application of CD instrumentation should be learned from an experienced surgeon. Its technique is not easy for the novice spine surgeon. The rod is more flexible than the Harrington rod and is studded with irregularities that allow the application and strong fixation of either pedicle screws or hooks. Additionally, because of this locking mechanism, the hooks may be applied in either direction and with as many sites of attachment as desired. The addition of intermediate hooks is a powerful addition of force at the area of greatest deformity. The system also contains both lumbar and thoracic hooks in an open- and closed-rod holding design. The availability of low-profile hooks has allowed the instrumentation to be positioned closer to the spine and is less prominent in thin patients. A discussion of hook placement and pattern on all different curves is beyond the scope of this chapter. Consideration will be given to the basic King idiopathic scoliosis patterns and to trauma uses (23).

The King type III curve (right thoracic curve with hypokyphosis) provides a good starting point (Fig. 33.3). The first consideration for hook placement is the end vertebrae for the left concave rod. The upper end vertebra is the neutral vertebra as measured by the Cobb method on standing roentgenograms. The distal end vertebra is usually the stable vertebra. Placement of the hooks should be aimed at creating a balanced spine in the coronal plane. However, consideration of the lateral roentgenograms is important to determine the amount of kyphosis present over the upper segment. The fusion should be extended cephalad if the sagittal deformity is significant. If there is preoperative kyphosis at T12 or L1, the distal hook should be distal to L1 to prevent progressive junctional kyphosis. Additionally, the caudal and cephalad vertebrae should fall within the Harrington sta-

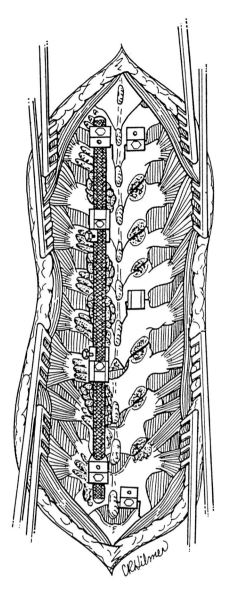

FIGURE 33.3.
A diagram of the Cotrel-Dubousset (Danek, Inc., Memphis, TN) rod and hook configuration for a King type III curve. The proximal and distal end vertebrae are the neutral and stable vertebrae, respectively. The intermediate hooks are placed on the rigid segments of the curve. The rod is distracted or rotated to provide corrections in the coronal and sagittal planes. The end hooks on the convex side are placed for compression. The intermediate hook on the convex side is on the apical vertebra. An additional down-going hook one level above the right distal end vertebra is usually recommended to provide a more stable claw configuration.

ble zone. The position of the intermediate hooks is determined by the right side bending films. Those discs that do not significantly correct and appear most rigid are spanned by an open pedicle hook and an open laminar hook, usually over three or four levels.

On the right convex rod, at the upper end vertebra either a transverse process pedicle claw or a closed thoracic laminar hook in a down-going position may be used. An intermediate open pedicle hook is used at the apex of the curve, primarily to assist as a derotation pressure point with convex rod insertion and to further stabilize the rod itself. A two-segment claw will complete the hook construct at the right lower vertebra with a cranially facing closed laminar hook on the end vertebra and an open laminar hook down-going on the vertebra above. The right rod is contoured into slightly less kyphosis to help with the already counterclockwise rotation. If significant kyphosis is present either at the thoracolumbar junction or at the upper thoracic spine on the lateral view, then the rods must be extended to add a compression force across the kyphosis.

For a King type I curve or primary lumbar curve pattern, hook selection is based on a combination of the right thoracic type III pattern and thoracolumbar curve patterns. The end vertebrae for the left-sided rod are determined by the same criteria as the individual curve patterns. The lumbar or thoracolumbar pattern is chosen with the use of open laminar hooks centered about the apex. In general, six to eight hooks are used on the left-sided rod, or pedicle screws may be substituted for the lumbar hooks. The right-sided rod is inserted with the usual hooks and/or pedicle screws. The intermediate hooks include an open pedicle hook at the apex of the thoracic curve and an open laminar hook opposing the down-going hook on the left-sided rod. Additional open laminar hooks may be placed within the instrumented thoracolumbar or lumbar curve. The left rod is inserted first, with the desired sagittal plane contour. Rotation is achieved and produces simultaneous posterior column lengthening in the thoracic spine and compression force in the lumbar spine. Great care must be taken to ensure that maximum compression is achieved at the apex of the lower curve. Once apical compression has been carried out, distraction is achieved through the intermediate hooks of the thoracic curve. The last hook tightened is that on the left upper end vertebra. Derotation can accomplish correction of the deformities in the coronal plane as well as maintaining thoracic kyphosis and lumbar lordosis. Care must be taken to preserve the transition zone between the thoracic kyphosis and lumbar lordosis at the T12-L1 region. Frequently derotation may create the transition zone at the T10 region by extending lumbar lordosis too proximally, which produces a cosmetically unacceptable high-arched back and protuberant abdomen. Proper rod contouring will prevent this cephalad extension of lordosis.

Type II curve patterns are treated in a fashion similar to curve patterns with right thoracic curves. In type IV curves, the end vertebra usually corresponds to the stable L4 vertebra. The distal end of fusion may be at L3 if bending radiographs reveal the L3 vertebra to be the stable and neutral vertebra. The intermediate vertebrae for the thoracic curve again are chosen as they are for a type III curve. In general, six to eight hooks are used on the left-sided rod. The right-sided rod is inserted with the usual end vertebrae hooks. The left-sided rod is inserted first, with the desired sagittal plane contour. Rotation is achieved and produces simultaneous posterior column lengthening of the thoracic curve and posterior column shortening of the left thoracolumbar curves, if instrumentation extends to the thoracolumbar junction. Great care must be taken at this time to ensure that maximum compression is achieved through the thoracolumbar curves. The right rod is then inserted, with the possibility present for derotation of the thoracic curve. Usually no additional derotation is achieved in the lumbar spine. Several authors have noted that there can be increased decompensation of the entire spine with overcorrection and derotation maneuver. Overcorrection of curve patterns type II, III, and V with derotation frequently result in decompensation. To prevent decompensation, type II curves may be treated by fusing the thoracic curvature only, and the instrumentation should be applied to obtain balance.

The King type V patterns, double thoracic curve patterns, have significant upper thoracic curves. Using the usual type III configuration would produce increasing decompensation and shoulder asymmetry. The left upper thoracic curvature must be included in the fusion to prevent a high-riding left shoulder. A temporary right-sided rod may be placed into the upper curve to distract and increase the kyphosis of the upper thoracic curve, at the same time partially correcting the scoliosis. The hook pattern for the concave rod for the lower right thoracic curve is the same as that for the type III configuration. One or two hooks are added to correct the left upper thoracic curve. In general, an attempt is made to insert the upper left rod as straight as possible, thus diminishing the lordotic moment arm created with rotation and correction of the lower right thoracic curve. The right-sided neutralization rod is configured as for a type III curve, except that there is extension superiorly with a closed pedicle hook at the upper end vertebra.

In juvenile or adult kyphosis, segmental instrumentation with hooks provides compression forces for correction while enhancing the stability of the surgical construct. Sublaminar wires alone should not be used in kyphotic cases, since the compression forces cannot be effectively applied. Segmental instrumentation systems that give apical compression force and additional compressions at the end vertebrae above and below the apex are ideal for kyphotic deformities. With the use of modern segmental instrumentation, compression can be used at several levels of a construct to aid in reduction of the kyphosis. Compression can be used above and below the apex of the curve. By clawing the end two vertebrae with a combination of different claw patterns and compressing the periapical vertebrae, the segments above and below the apex may be corrected initially. The final correction occurs with compression above and below the apex. In addition to compressive forces, cantilever bending correction force should be applied in reducing the kyphosis. One should avoid excessive force to avoid fracturing the lamina.

In most operative cases of kyphosis it is necessary to perform an anterior release of four or five segments around the apex. Traditionally this has been done utilizing a thoracotomy. Modern techniques are allowing minimally invasive approaches to be more readily utilized. Thoracoscopy offers excellent visualization and can provide an alternative to the traditional anterior release.

The CD system may also be used in trauma cases. Smaller and more flexible rods are predominantly used for scoliosis cases because of the ease of contouring that they offer. The stiffer and larger rods are more often used for trauma cases in which strength and rigidity are important. Reconstructive procedures with trauma and tumor invasion are the most common uses. Basic hook patterns involve claws above and below the fracture or defect. In trauma these patterns vary according to the location of the fracture. In the thoracic spine a claw pattern using the two or three vertebrae above and below is often used, and in the lumbar spine it is often accompanied by pedicle screw instrumentation for the inferior vertebrae. Burst type fractures at L1 or L2 often require a combination pedicle screw and hook or double hook claw pattern with a pedicle screw below to provide a stable fixation while preserving distal motion segments. Cross-links stabilize the rods by creating a rigid rectangular pattern and increasing torsional stiffness significantly.

TSRH

The TSRH (Texas Scottish Rite Hospital) instrumentation system was originally designed as an adjunct to the Luque sublaminar segmental instrumentation system. The system provides the original cross-link system using the principles of CD but also expanding on them (20, 21). The ease of revising and removing instrumentations is another advantage. The TSRH instrumentation system allows the linking of one rod to another so that extension of a previously implanted system and revision of a failed system are easier. The addition of pedicle screws with the variable-angle design expands the system's versatility, providing the structural rigidity to stabilize fractures, tumors, and degenerative disorders in addition to deformities (Fig. 33.4).

The cross-link system was designed to prevent migration of the rod. However, studies evaluating the rigidity of the system showed that the cross-links with the TSRH system increased the torsional stiffness and the axial stiffness of the rod-wire construct (20, 21). The rods must adapt precisely in the grooves of the cross-link plate to allow the proper three-point contact for a secure link. During final tightening the nut must be tightened to a minimum of 150 inch-pounds. Gurr and colleagues demonstrated an increased incidence of arthrodesis when spinal fusions were augmented with implants in dogs, but the quality of the fusion mass as a function of the stiffness of the construct is still in question (12). The rod in the TSRH system is smooth. The advantage of a smooth rod is that it offers less friction when the rod is slid into the hooks during insertion and/or rotation. Excessive friction between a knurled rod and hook body may prevent satisfactory rod rotation and displace hooks or cause inadvertent compression of the spinal canal. Three levels of rod stiffness are provided: the 4.8 mm rod, the 6.4 mm (flexible) rod, and the 6.4 mm (stiff) rod. Increased stability has been achieved by widening and deepening the radius between tines so that they more firmly grasp the pedicle. The shape of the axilla of the hook has been modified so that the inferior edge and articular process can be grasped by an anatomic rather than a circular design.

Moss-Miami Instrumentation

The Moss-Miami system was designed by Shuffelbarger and Harms with the goal of segmental fixation and simple instrumentation (Fig. 33.5). The system is designed with top-loading, dual-locking implants, thus eliminating the preloading process. It is designed for universal application in posterior and anterior spinal surgery for deformities, trauma, and degenerative diseases of the spinal column. The smaller 5 mm rods and low-profile design reduce difficulties with instrumentation prominence. Cannulated instruments allow pairs of screws to be placed sequentially and nut heads to be loaded and placed in proper sequence. This system also has the ability to lock rod to rod linkages and for pedicle screw addition. Only six hooks are available for pedicular, laminar, and transverse process constructs. All are open ended for ease of rod placement. The pedicle or sacral screw has a polyaxial screw design to ease the rod placement. The 316-LVM rods provide excellent fatigue resistance and high tensile strength. The benefits of this rod lie in its easy malleability and a lower profile than the larger rods. This system is particularly useful for correcting deformities in which the correction is achieved by cantilever bending as well as segmental correcting forces. However, in large trauma patients or reconstructive tumor patients in which more load-bearing may be needed, it may lack the strength and durability of its larger counterparts.

ISOLA

The ISOLA instrumentation system is much like the TSRH system. Designed in part by Asher, it is an extension of the variable-screw placement system (VSP) developed by Steffee (28). The hook systems attach to the rods in an interference fit, and the ISOLA system provides an end-to-end linkage system. The hook blade tightens against the bone fixation site. Secure connection of the hook to a straight or curved smooth rod is provided by the V-groove. Two rod sizes are available: 6.35 mm (¼ inch) and 4.76 mm (3/16 inch). Four sizes of drop hooks are avail-

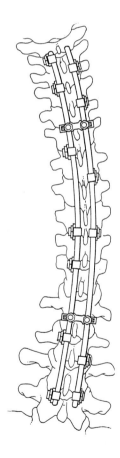

FIGURE 33.4.
A diagram of TSRH (Danek, Inc., Memphis, TN) rods for a King type IV curve. The instrumentation extends from T4 to L4. The distal attachment may be accomplished by hooks or pedicle screws. The correction of this type of curve requires distraction on the concave side of the thoracic spine and segmental application of forces on the lumbar spine to preserve lumbar lordosis and to achieve the balance of the spine.

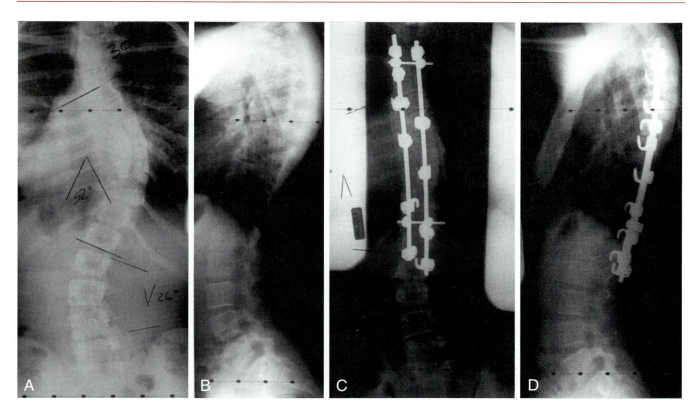

FIGURE 33.5.
Moss-Miami (DePuy-Motech, Inc., Warsaw, IN) instrumentation system in a 14-year-old male with King type V curvature. **A.** Anteroposterior radiograph shows 52° right thoracic scoliosis and compensatory 26° left lumbar scoliosis. The upper thoracic scoliosis was significant at 30° and rigid. This patient had shoulder asymmetry with higher left shoulder. **B.** Lateral radiograph shows hypokyphotic thoracic spine with relatively well-maintained sagittal alignment. **C.** and **D.** Postoperative radiographs show Moss-Miami instrumentation from T2 to L1. The correction of curves and balance were maintained.

able for both rod sizes as well as a variety of new and angled hook-to-rod connectors. Washers of several heights and angles are designed to level the screw rod placement for ease of restoring lordosis and/or kyphosis. Additionally, plate-rod combinations (PRC) are available in a variety of sizes of plates and in 6.35 mm and 4.76 mm rod diameter. Washers for this system are also available in either 3 mm or 5 mm heights, and these have recently become available in wedges for leveling constructs.

A major principle underlying the use of the ISOLA system for deformity surgery is that the coronal plane angular deformities do not occur in synchrony with the normal sagittal plane curves, and their apices and radii are different. Maximal thoracic dorsal displacement normally occurs in the sagittal plane at T5-T6, and maximal lumbar anterior displacement at L4. Thoracic scoliosis most commonly has its apices at T8-T9, and lumbar scoliosis at L2, though this is more variable.

The design of this system is intended to be surgeon-friendly and to maximize versatility with a minimum of components. The implant dimensions are standardized to permit maximum flexibility and versatility in use. The mechanical objectives are the provision of stability, strength, and durability to maintain correction and alignment during the healing of spine arthrodesis. The ISOLA system is designed for adolescent and adult idiopathic scoliosis, burst fractures, degenerative stenosis, and spondylolisthesis (Figs. 33.6–33.9).

Pedicle Screw Instrumentation

Pedicle screw instrumentation is now widely used among spinal surgeons. Pedicle screws provide the ability to manipulate all three columns of the spinal column from a posterior approach. Much debate still exists as to their proper application and placement to achieve the best clinical outcome. Because of the force that can be generated with these devices, normal contours can be changed, and problems such as iatrogenic flat-back are being encountered. Additionally, because the procedure requires precise placement, the structures anterior, medial, and lateral to the spinal canal may be injured. Anterior to the spinal canal are the great vessels and the thorax and abdomen, medial is the spinal cord, and lateral are the

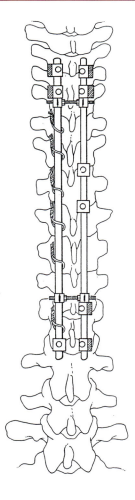

FIGURE 33.6.
A diagram of ISOLA (Acromed, Inc., Cleveland, OH) instrumentation for King type II or III curves. The illustration here spans from T4 to T12. The left rod is used for distraction and the right rod is used for compression. Sublaminar wires are frequently used to apply segmental correction on the concave side of the curve. Rotation maneuver is not routinely used with this system.

nerve roots, thorax and abdomen, and retroperitoneal space.

The pedicle screw is the stiffest construct available today and appears to have the highest fusion rates (13, 28). In addition, its stiffness allows for shorter fusion segments to maintain stability. The pedicle screw can be used with plate and rod constructs as well as with hook combinations. The dimensions of the pedicle vary widely. One study found a mean transverse diameter of 4.5 mm at T4, running to 15 mm at L5, with the inner diameter being approximately 80% of the total. In the thoracic spine the angle of the pedicle, posterolateral to anteromedial, was found to range from 13.9° at T4 to 0.3° at T12 (29). The lumbar pedicles roughly advance from posterolateral to anteromedial at 5° per level. General placement of pedicle screws is 5° at L1, 10° at L2, 15° at L3, 20° at L4, and 25° at L5.

Though averages in pedicle inclination are helpful references, CT, MRI, and roentgenograms should always be looked at before operative pedicular screw placement. Specific inclinations, pedicle widths, and anomalies can be identified and appropriate action taken to place the pedicle screws successfully.

The entrance points and directions are subject to debate. Generally the entrance point for the lumbar spine is crossed by the line that connects the middle of the transverse processes and the lateral edge of the facet (Fig. 33.9A). In the thoracic spine, the entrance point is in line with the middle of the transverse process, which is about 2 mm below the inferior edge of the facet. The thoracic pedicle entry point is also crossed by the vertical line that connects the middle of the facet joint (Fig. 33.9B). Another important consideration in achieving effective placement is to avoid facet injury in segments that are to be unfused. As discussed earlier, bony fusion is the key to successful outcome with instrumentation. Techniques include posterolateral, posterolateral interbody fusion (PLIF), and intertransverse approaches. The pedicle screw's outer diameter is most important in pullout strength, though bone mineral density can also affect pullout strength (24). In trauma patients lumbar fractures can be treated with pedicle screws one level above and below, because the size of the pedicle and the size of the screw can usually stabilize the fracture while it heals. Fractures of T12 and L1 are often better stabilized with a single pedicle screw below and two pedicle screws or a combination of pedicle screws and/or hooks above. Other common indications for pedicle screws are spondylolisthesis, degenerative diseases, adult scoliosis, and pediatric scoliosis.

One disadvantage of pedicle screw instrumentation is that it has a learning curve. Placement of pedicle screws in the lumbar spine should first be practiced in the cadaver and then taught by an experienced surgeon until some degree of comfort is achieved with the technique. The insertion of pedicle screws in the thoracic spine is technically difficult and fraught with complications, including perforation of the esophagus and the aorta. Its use has very specific indications. Only surgeons with a solid understanding of the musculoskeletal structures adjacent to the pedicles should perform this procedure. Rod and hook constructs are usually sufficient to provide adequate stability to allow fusion in the relatively stable thoracic spine. The temptation to apply new adaptations of existing techniques to various clinical situations should be resisted unless less risky, equally effective means of treatment are not available.

Patient positioning for pedicle screw instrumentation is also somewhat controversial. The kneeling position tends to place the spine in a more kyphotic

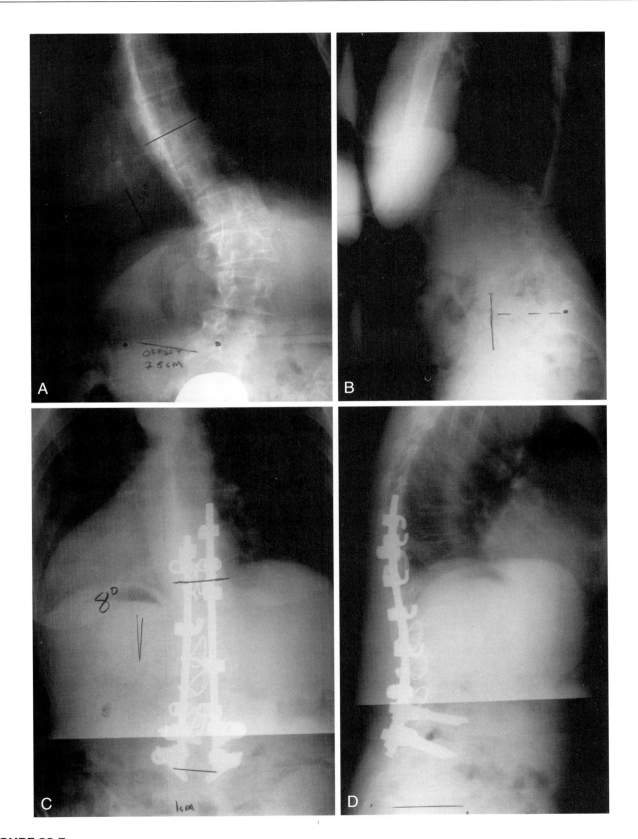

FIGURE 33.7.

Sixty-five-year-old female with progressive right lumbar scoliosis and severe, unrelenting back pain. **A.** Anteroposterior radiograph shows 38° lumbar scoliosis and trunk imbalance of 7.5 cm to the left. **B.** Lateral radiograph shows that the sagittal imbalance is minimal. **C.** Postoperative anteroposterior radiograph shows ISOLA instrumentation from T9 to L4 with good correction of the scoliosis and lateral shift. Sublaminar wires were used on the concave side, with pedicle screws at L3 and L4. **D.** Postoperative lateral radiograph shows the maintenance of lumbar lordosis.

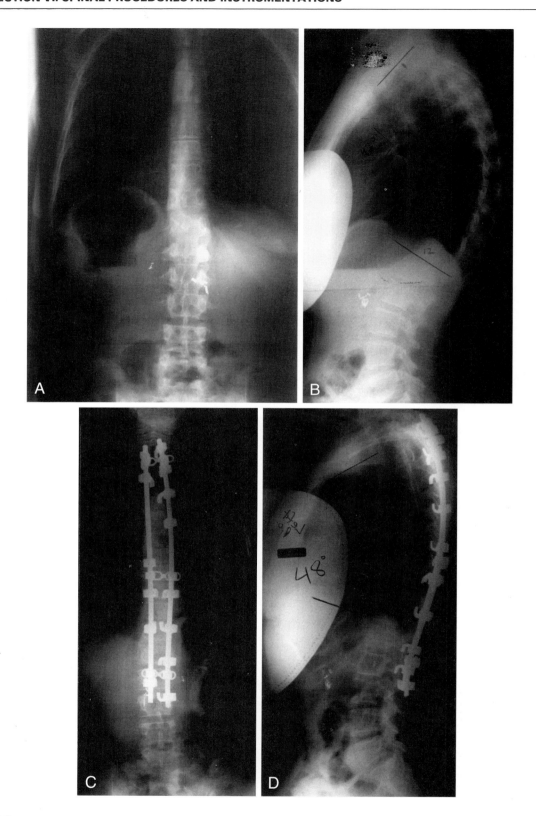

FIGURE 33.8.

Thirty-eight-year-old female with progressive kyphotic deformity of the thoracic spine (Scheuermann's disease) and marked upper back pain underwent anterior thoracoscopic fusion and posterior ISOLA instrumentation. **A.** Anteroposterior radiograph shows no significant scoliosis. **B.** Lateral radiograph reveals 97° kyphotic deformity. **C.** Postoperative anteroposterior and **D.** lateral radiographs show ISOLA rods spanning from T2 to L2. The hooks are placed in compression constructs with two claws above the apex of the kyphosis and two additional claws below the apex on the right rod. The left hooks are placed so that the end hooks oppose the right end hooks. There is one claw above and another claw below the apex on the left rod.

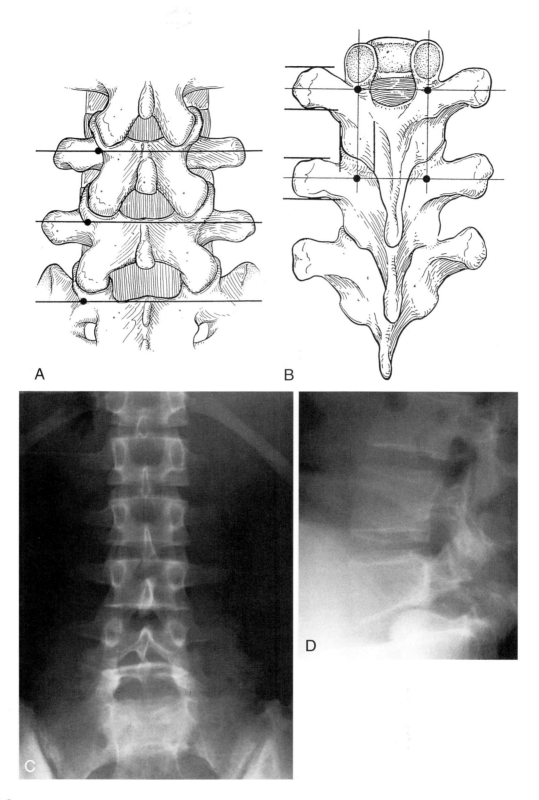

FIGURE 33.9.

A. The pedicle entrance point for the lumbar spine is crossed by the horizontal line that connects the middle of the transverse processes and the lateral edge of the facet. **B.** In the thoracic spine, the entrance point is in line with the middle of the transverse process, which is about 2 mm below the inferior edge of the facet. The thoracic pedicle entry point is also crossed by the vertical line that connects the middle of the facet joint. **C.** Anteroposterior radiograph of 18-year-old male with severe back pain and radiculopathy associated with high-grade L5-S1 isthmic spondylolisthesis. **D.** Lateral radiograph shows grade III spondylolisthesis with lumbosacral kyphosis.

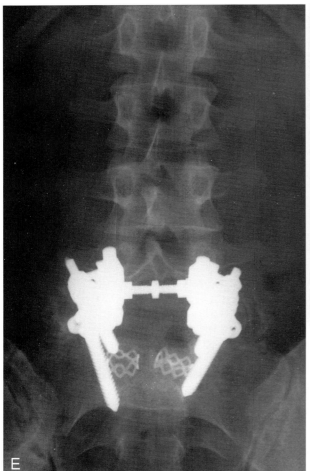
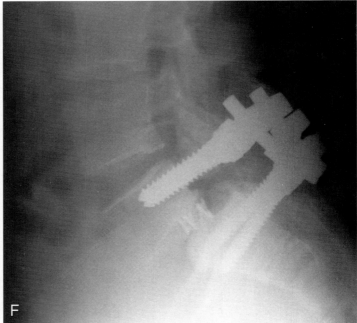

FIGURE 33.9—*continued*

E. Postoperative anteroposterior radiograph shows L5-S1 ISOLA instrumentation and Harms cages that were implanted via a PLIF approach. **F.** Postoperative lateral radiograph shows anterior distraction by the Harms cages, reduction of the slip angle, and pedicle screw instrumentation at L5-S1. Translation was reduced minimally to prevent neurologic deficits. Instrumentation and fusion were performed with application of load-sharing Harms cages anteriorly, followed by posterior compression ISOLA rods. This patient was mobilized immediately, and at 2-year follow-up great pain relief, functional recovery, and solid fusion were noted.

position, which may affect the final lordosis; however, it allows the abdomen to remain free, thus decreasing venous bleeding. The four-poster frame encourages more lordosis and is preferred in cases such as osteotomy for flat-back or fusion in patients with loss of lumbar lordosis.

Surgical technique for pedicle screw instrumentation involves careful cleaning and preparation of the spine—including spinous processes, laminae, facets, pars interarticularis, and transverse processes— and the appropriate landmarks are identified for the placement of the pedicle screws. Roentgenographic, myelographic, CT, and MRI studies should be in plain view in the operating room for reference to help with appropriate placement of the pedicle screws. The midpoint of the transverse process and a point 2 to 3 mm lateral to the pars interarticularis is located. The entrance is then burred, and with the use of a sound or blunt probe the canal of the pedicle is located. Markers are placed and checked intraoperatively with a lateral radiograph for appropriate placement. Adjustments can then be made in the cephalad and caudal directions as needed. With the use of a feeler, the medial, lateral, superior, and inferior walls are felt and checked carefully to be sure no perforations are present. A Penfield elevator works well for this. Other techniques, such as saline injection and visualization with arthroscopy, have been advocated by other authors if any question exists. Tapping is not necessary but may be done with a smaller tap. After tapping is completed, the bone is generally decorticated and bone graft placed before the final placement of the screws. Pedicle screw insertion should be performed using the largest possible screw diameter that can safely be placed in the pedicle as measured on the inner di-

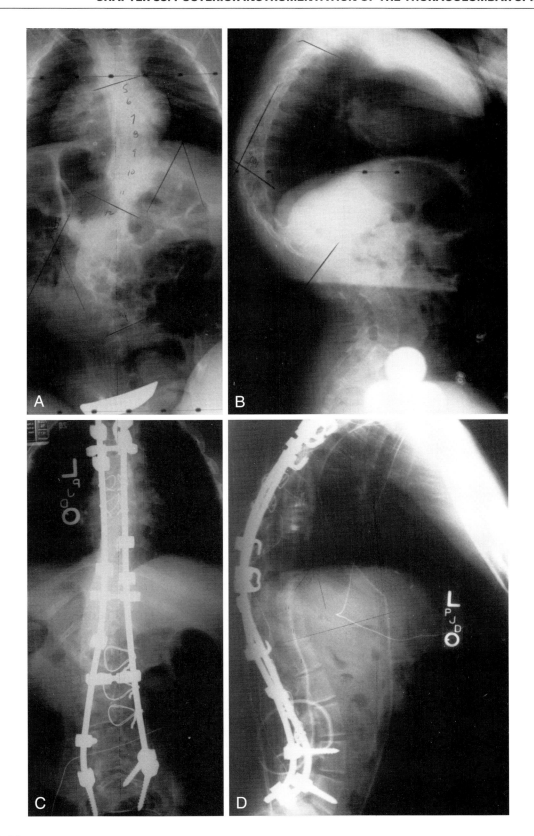

FIGURE 33.10.

Fifteen-year-old cerebral palsy patient with severe paralytic scoliosis and kyphosis. **A.** Anteroposterior radiograph shows scoliosis and pelvic obliquity in patient who underwent anterior thoracic fusion and posterior fusion with Horizon (Danek, Inc., Memphis, TN) instrumentation to the sacrum. **B.** Lateral radiograph shows severe kyphotic deformity of the thoracic spine. **C.** Postoperative anteroposterior radiograph shows segmental instrumentation and fusion from the upper thoracic spine to the sacrum. Good correction of coronal deformity and pelvic balance are noted. **D.** Lateral radiograph shows correction of the kyphotic deformity and pedicle screws in the lower lumbar spine and sacrum.

ameter. The screw should obtain a depth of approximately 80% of the vertebral body as measured from CT or roentgenogram. Screws should be placed parallel to the endplates, or with slightly cephalad angulation, and a screw should be placed at every level if possible. Care should be taken not to injure or impinge facets not involved in the fusion.

Pedicle screw fixation is used most frequently for trauma in the lumbar spine and degenerative disease secondary to instability or spondylolisthesis. Traumatic injuries occur from a variety of mechanisms, including axial load or burst, flexion-distraction, flexion, shear, or any combination of these. The advantage of pedicle screw fixation is the ability to control all three spinal columns and to shorten the fusion segment.

Sacral fixation can be troublesome especially in cases that require longer constructs, sagittal plane realignments, revisions, and in patients who have weak bone (4). The problems of sacral fixation can be attributed to several factors: *(a)* the difficult anatomy in this area; *(b)* the large lumbosacral loads with cantilever pullout forces across this region; *(c)* the posterior position of spinal implants in the sagittal plane; and *(d)* the poor bone quality frequently found within the sacrum even in patients free of significant osteoporosis.

Posterior exposure of the sacrum is done through a vertical midline incision. Care must be taken to avoid dural tear in the midline, particularly in patients who have occult spina bifida. Posterior sacral foramina are richly surrounded by venous structures and can be sources of significant bleeding. The sacrum is most commonly exposed for extension of instrumentation and fusion that extends down to the sacrum.

The most common method of fixation to the sacrum is the S1 screw or ala screw (Fig. 33.10). The entrance point of the sacral screw is at the lower point of the L5-S1 articulation on the elevated ridge of bone. The screw is directed medially about 25° and 10° inferiorly toward the sacral promontory. This sacral screw may be made to gain purchase on the anterior cortex to enhance the fixation. Alternatively, lateral ala screw insertion into the dimple of S1 and directed 35° laterally and parallel to the sacral endplate can be considered. The drill bit will usually rest on the caudal tip of the sacral mass. The drill is pushed anteriorly until it abuts the anterior cortex. The hole is enlarged with larger drill bits or curettes, and the sacral screw is inserted without tapping. This screw may be driven to gain purchase on the anterior cortex as well. The 2 mm hole is enlarged to 3.5 mm and the drill bit advanced just through the anterior cortex of the lateral sacral ala. A depth gauge should be used to select the correct screw length, and the screw should not project more than 2 mm beyond the anterior cortex of the sacrum. This lateral screw may be inserted slightly inferiorly so that both the medial and lateral screws may be inserted into the sacrum. Additionally, an S2 screw may be inserted. The S1 and S2 foramina are exposed. Next, the point is located that is two-thirds distal to the inferior edge of the S1 foramina and two-thirds of the distance from true midline to a line that bisects the midportion of S1/S2 foramina. The posterior cortex is opened with a burr, and the screw is directed 40 to 45° laterally. This screw is pointed toward the anterolateral corner of the S1-S2 ala. The instrumentation system used will also determine the specific technique of sacral screw fixation.

Sacral fixation may be inadequate despite the use of screws, particularly in cases that require longer constructs. Jackson's intrasacral fixation may enhance the stability of sacral fixation by transpedicular endplate screw fixation and intrasacral rod insertion to provide a sacroiliac buttressing effect. Additionally, more anterior and distal insertion of the rods reduces the moment arm acting on the rods and screws. In situ contouring of the rods is made easier by the greater distance between the L5 and S1 screw heads.

There are other types of sacra-pelvic fixation, including iliosacral screws, iliac screws, and Galveston pelvic fixation. These systems are still evolving, and continued research is needed to develop a technique that is biomechanically sound, safe, and easy for the surgeon.

In the Galveston technique, a length of rod is inserted into each ilium (2). The placement of the iliac portion of the rod is intraosseous from a bone entry point at the lower level of the posterior superior iliac spine, across the posterior ilium 10 to 15 mm above the sciatic notch, and into the bone above the acetabulum. The tip of the rod should not be pointed toward the acetabulum. This may occur if the entry point is too cephalad. The optimal rod placement allows a maximum length of rod to be inserted, theoretically reducing stress because of the long lever arm. Insertion of the rod requires a bit of feel. The surgeon must place a finger in the sciatic notch and position the rod with the contralateral hand. The rod should be placed 6 to 9 cm into the pelvis. Shaping the pelvic portion of the rod can be tricky, but with practice it requires two primary bends. The rods should be connected by transverse connectors to improve torsional stability of the construct.

Conclusion

The techniques described in this chapter are meant to serve as a guide to posterior instrumentation of the thoracic and lumbar spine. Many spine fellowships are teaching instrumentation techniques so that the entering classes of spinal surgeons will have a better grasp of instrumentation techniques. However, experience plays an important role in achieving optimum results. Imitations of posterior instrumentation alone should be realized in some situations, and indications for anterior instrumentations are discussed in the following chapter (5, 22).

References

1. Albee FH. Transplantation of a portion of the tibia for Potts disease. JAMA 1911;57:885–886.
2. Allen BL, Ferguson RL. The Galveston technique for L-rod instrumentation. Spine 1982;7:276–284.
3. An HS, Cotler JM. Spinal instrumentation. Baltimore: Williams & Wilkins, 1992.
4. Asher M, Strippgen W. Anthropometric studies of the human sacrum relating to dorsal transsacral implant design and development. Clin Orthop 1986;203:58–62.
5. Been HD. Anterior decompression and stabilization of thoracolumbar burst fractures by the use of the slotted Zielke device. Spine 1991;16:70–77.
6. Cotrel Y, Dubousset J, Guillaumat M. New universal instrumentation in spinal surgery. Clin Orthop 1988;227:10–23.
7. Denis F. Cotrel-Dubousset instrumentation in the treatment of idiopathic scoliosis. Orthop Clin North Am 1988;19:291–311.
8. Drummond DS, Guadagni J, Keene JS, et al. Interspinous process segmental spinal instrumentation. J Pediatric Orthop 1984;4:397–404.
9. Ecker ML, Betz RR, Trent PS, et al. Computer tomography evaluation of Cotrel-Dubousset instrumentation in idiopathic scoliosis. Spine 1988;13:1141–1144.
10. Goll S, Balderson R, Stambough J, et al. Depth of intraspinal wire penetration during passage of sublaminar wires. Spine 1988;13:503–509.
11. Guadagni J, Drummond DS. Strength of surgical wire fixation: a laboratory study. Clin Orthop 1986;209:176–181.
12. Gurr KR, McAfee PC, Warden KE, et al. A roentgenographic and biomechanical analysis of spinal fusions: A canine model. Baltimore: Scoliosis Research Society, 1986:77–78.
13. Guyer DW, Yuan HA, Werner FW, et al. Biomechanical comparison of seven internal fixation devices for the lumbosacral junction. Spine 1987;12:569–573.
14. Hadra BE. Wiring of the spinous process in Potts Disease. Transamer Orthop Assoc 1891;4:206.
15. Harrington PR. The history and development of Harrington instrumentation. Clin Orthop 1988;227:3.
16. Harrington PR. Surgical instrumentation for management of scoliosis. J Bone Joint Surg 1960;42A:1448.
17. Herring JA, Fitch RD, Wenger DR, et al. Segmental instrumentation: a review of early results and complications. Presented at the annual meeting of the Scoliosis Research Society, 1983.
18. Hibbs RA. An operation for progressive spinal deformity. NY State J Med 1911;93:113–130.
19. Johnston CE II, Ashman RB, Sherman MC, et al. Mechanical consequences of rod contouring and residual scoliosis in sublaminar segmental instrumentation. J Orthop Res 1987;5:206–216.
20. Johnston CE II, Haideri N, Ashman RB. Early experience with rigid cross-linking. Presented at the annual meeting of the Scoliosis Research Society, Honolulu, September 1990:23–27.
21. Johnston CE II, Ashman RB, Corin JD. Mechanical effects of cross-linking rods in Cotrel-Dubousset instrumentation. Orthop Trans 1987;11:96.
22. Kaneda K, Abumi K, Fujiya M. Burst fractures with neurologic deficits of the thoracolumbar-lumbar spine: results of anterior decompression and stabilization with anterior instrumentation. Spine 1984;9:788–795.
23. King HA, Moe JH, Bradford DS, et al. The selection of fusion levels in thoracic idiopathic scoliosis. J Bone Joint Surg 1983;65A;1302–1313.
24. Lim T, An SH, Hasegawa T, et al. Prediction of fatigue screw loosening in anterior spinal fixation using dual energy x-ray absorptiometry. Spine 1995;23:2565–2568.
25. Luque ER. The anatomic basis and development of segmental spinal instrumentation. Spine 1982;7:256–259.
26. Renshaw TS. The role of Harrington instrumentation and posterior spine fusion in the management of adolescent idiopathic scoliosis. Clin Orthop 1982;162:41–46.
27. Richards BS, Birch JG, Herring JA, et al. Frontal plane and sagittal plane balance following Cotrel-Dubousset instrumentation for idiopathic scoliosis. Spine 1989;14:733–737.
28. Steffee AD, Biscup RS, Sitkowski DJ. Segmental spine plates with pedicle screw fixation: a new internal fixation device for disorders of the lumbar and thoracolumbar spine. Clin Orthop 1986;203:45–53.
29. Vaccaro A, Rizzolo SJ, Allardyce M, et al. Placement of pedicle screws in the thoracic spine: a morphometric analysis. J Bone Joint Surg 1995;77A:1193–1199.
30. Zindrick MR, Knight GW, Bunch WH, et al. Factors influencing the penetration of wires into the neural canal during segmental wiring. J Bone Joint Surg 1989;71A:742–750.

CHAPTER THIRTY FOUR

Anterior Instrumentation of the Thoracolumbar Spine

Howard S. An and J. Michael Glover

Introduction

In 1956 Hodgson published his preliminary report in the *British Journal of Surgery* discussing a radical approach to the treatment of spinal deformity and neurologic compromise associated with tuberculous spondylitis—anterior spinal fusion (35). Thus began the forty-year time line chronicling the refinement of the anterior approach to the spine for broader applications and the development of anterior spinal instrumentation systems to stabilize the vertebral column.

Dwyer first developed an anterior screw and cable system in 1964, which he applied to the convexity of thoracolumbar scoliosis, thereby shortening the vertebral column (19). He published his preliminary results of eight cases in 1969. Widespread use of Harrington's posterior distraction rods had already begun after 1960, in which the vertebral column was lengthened by distracting the concavity of the curvature (58).

Although excellent correction and fewer fusion levels could be achieved with the Dwyer system, the flattening of the lumbar lordosis and pseudarthrosis were problematic (36, 42). The Dwyer system was best suited to serving as an adjunct to posterior correction and stabilization of complex deformities seen in paralytic scoliosis rather than as a primary application for treatment of idiopathic scoliosis (30). In 1976 Zielke described his modification of the Dwyer system. His ventral derotation system (VDS) used a threaded rod instead of a cable, creating a more rigid device that could be compressed and derotated, preserving lumbar lordosis (75). Moe and associates performed the first Zielke application in North America in 1977 and published their results in 1983, reporting an improved ability to derotate the spine and achieve significant curve correction over a short fusion area (54). However, concern remains about the small caliber of the rod and its kyphogenic potential (9). Newer segmental spinal instrumentation systems developed for posterior applications such as the Texas Scottish Rite Hospital (TSRH) system (Danek, Inc., Memphis, TN), the ISOLA system (Acromed, Inc., Cleveland, OH), the Moss-Miami system (DePuy-Motech, Inc., Warsaw, IN), and others are now being used in the manner of the Zielke system for the treatment of scoliosis. These newer systems are more rigid and less kyphogenic, and they obviate the need for postoperative bracing or casting that was required with the Dwyer and Zielke systems (70).

Instrumentation for spine trauma was pioneered by Dickson and Harrington in 1977 using a long posterior fusion with Harrington distraction rods (16). Modifications of posterior instrumentation systems to include sleeves for rods, better hooks, sublaminar wires, contoured rods, and pedicle screws have improved reduction techniques. However, biomechanical concerns remain about the ability of posterior instrumentation systems to stabilize, reduce, and decompress the spinal canal in certain fracture patterns of the thoracolumbar spine such as burst fractures (24, 25, 62).

With respect to neural decompression in cases of burst fractures, it made intuitive sense to approach the spinal canal anteriorly, particularly since burst fractures are the most common fracture pattern, and anterior debridement of the fracture fragments could be done more effectively (43, 51). The addition of a tricortical strut graft would then provide the needed stability. However, this treatment for acute thoracolumbar fractures often failed because the graft alone could not withstand the compressive forces in this region of the spine (74).

Dunn introduced a device in 1984 for anterior distraction and compression for the treatment of thoracolumbar fractures that consisted of two rods connected to screws and staples placed laterally in the vertebral bodies immediately adjacent to the fracture site (17). This instrumentation, combined with spinal canal decompression and strut grafting, achieved the goals of spinal stability, neurologic decompression, and preservation of motion segments. However, because of this device's prominence and proximity to the great vessels, aortic perforation was reported, and this device is no longer available (38). Other systems have subsequently been developed with lower risk than the Dunn device, and many of these are currently used for anterior applications, such as the Kaneda device (Acromed, Inc., Cleveland, OH), the University plate (Acromed, Inc., Cleveland, OH), the Z-plate (Danek, Inc., Memphis, TN), and several broad, low-profile, multi-holed/slotted plating systems (6, 29, 40, 44, 59, 73).

Anterior instrumentation developed along two lines of application: one for the treatment of scoliosis, and the other for the treatment of unstable spinal fractures. Today anterior spinal instrumentation systems have indications for wide array of spinal disorders, including idiopathic scoliosis (5, 11, 31, 36, 42, 45, 48, 54, 56, 67, 69, 70), congenital scoliosis (5, 45, 54, 67), paralytic scoliosis (5, 8, 45, 46, 50, 53, 54, 56, 57, 67, 68), posttraumatic kyphosis (29, 41, 44, 54, 73), Scheuermann's kyphosis (44), spinal tumors (6, 64, 73), spine trauma (6, 29, 40, 44, 73), degenerative disc disease (6), and pseudarthrosis (6).

Biomechanics

Spinal stability occurs when the osteoligamentous structures successfully resist the physiologic forces applied to the spine and prevent incapacitating pain, deformity, and neurologic injury (72). Denis's development of the three-column spine theory has significantly structured the current thinking on spine instability (15). However, controversy still exists as to whether the intact posterior column or the middle column is the most important factor for resisting deforming forces on the spine (37).

Spinal instrumentation applied anteriorly or posteriorly to the unstable or deformed spine must provide immediate stability and be able to resist the late deforming forces until fusion occurs. Long instrumented fusions are stable but have the disadvantage of losing several motion segments and can cause significant loss of lumbar lordosis. McLain et al. showed that short-segment pedicle instrumentation (one level cephalad and one level caudad) used in treating unstable thoracolumbar fractures had a high rate of failure within 6 months, manifested by progression of deformity and bending or breakage of the screws (52). Most of the injuries in this study were burst fractures, and this effect is secondary to the cantilever bending forces applied to the screws in the absence of a reconstructed anterior column. Others have also shown that short-segment posterior instrumentation alone for the treatment of unstable burst fractures does not restore the necessary stiffness of the intact spine, and they recommend combination with an anterior graft (1, 28, 61).

Gurr et al. compared anterior stabilization and posterior stabilization constructs in a calf spine corpectomy model (27). All constructs except for the anterior Harrington rod and polymethylmethacrylate construct used an anterior iliac crest strut graft. Torsional stiffness was greatest in the anterior Kaneda group and in the posterior transpedicular group using Cotrel-Dubousset and Steffee implants. It was least in the anterior-graft-only group and in the posterior Harrington rod and Luque rectangle groups. This in vitro study evaluated only the effects of initial short-term stabilization, since long-term cyclical loading was difficult to test in this model. Shono et al. showed in a human thoracolumbar spine burst-fracture model that the anterior Kaneda device was the most rigid in axial compression and torsion, restoring stability at or near that of the intact spine and performing better than posterior Harrington rod sleeves and the AO fixateur interne (62). It is also more rigid than other anterior spine systems, such as the Armstrong plate, the Kostuik-Harrington system, and the Zielke system (63, 74). The contoured anterior spinal plate (CASP) developed by Armstrong, although not as rigid as the Kaneda device, is still more stiff axially and torsionally than other anterior constructs, such as the Kostuik-Harrington and Slot-Zielke systems, and it has the advantage of being less prominent (6, 7). Several similar plate systems such as the Z-plate and the University plate have been developed that also allow distraction and compression.

The stability imparted to the spine by these anterior constructs relies on having at least two points of bicortical fixation per vertebral body that are connected either by two rods, as in the Kaneda device, or broad plates placed laterally on the vertebrae, as in the University Plate or the Z-plate. The Kaneda device is further stabilized by two transverse rod-to-rod connectors. Distraction forces can be applied directly to the construct to correct deformity and assist with graft placement, followed by compression to lock the graft in place and enhance fusion.

Single-screw purchase per vertebral body connected by a plate or rod is less stiff, allowing the vertebrae to rotate around the screw (18). Zielke instrumentation is less rigid in torsion and should not be used alone for the treatment of unstable vertebral body defects such as those caused by trauma and tumors. However, this single-point vertebral fixation allows it to be used effectively to derotate the spine in the treatment of thoracolumbar and lumbar scoliosis. The solid rod systems such as TSRH, Moss-Miami, Kaneda rod, and anterior ISOLA rod are applied in a manner similar to that of the Zielke system, but the biomechanical rigidity they impart to the construct is superior (70).

Another point to consider biomechanically when selecting an approach and implant for the treatment of burst fractures with neurologic deficit is canal clearance for adequate neurologic decompression. The neural canal may be cleared indirectly via posterior distraction and ligamentotaxis (21, 24), or directly via posterior transpedicular (32), posterolateral (23), or anterior decompression (51). Edwards and Levine reported an additional 32% of canal clearance using Harrington rod-sleeves applied posteriorly within 48 hours of injury (21). Less clearance was achieved when applied after this time frame. Esses et al. showed reduction from 44% preoperative canal compromise to 16% using the AO fixateur interne (24). Shono et al. reported that the Harrington rod-sleeve and the AO fixateur interne improved the initial canal compromise by only 12% and 18%, respectively (62). They also observed that the success of indirect reduction was predicated upon ligamentous continuity, amount of bony retropulsion, and displacement of the fragments, all of which are difficult to assess preoperatively. Hashimoto et al. have shown that neurologic impairment is probable with canal clearances of less than 65% at T12, less than 55% at L1, and less than 45% at L2 or lower (33). Shono et al. showed that indirect reduction with posterior distraction techniques could not improve the canal clearance beyond the critical value of Hashimoto at the thoracolumbar junction, suggesting that neurologic impairment would persist (62).

Therefore, in patients with major neurologic deficits and canal compromise, a combination of anterior decompression, strut graft, and instrumentation more reliably clears the canal (24, 62) and is biomechanically superior to indirect reduction and posterior instrumentation (1, 47, 62). This technique also has the advantage of a single-stage approach rather than a combined anterior/posterior approach.

Indications/Implants

Several newer anterior spinal systems are available for the management of spinal instability caused by trauma, tumor, severe disc degeneration, and pseudarthrosis. These include the Kaneda device, the Z-plate, the Synthes Thoracolumbar Locking Plate (Synthes, Inc., Paoli, PA), and the University plate. These devices are generally used from T10 to L5, but smaller implants are available to apply to the thoracic spine. The iliac vessels are close to the hardware below L4, and so great care must taken in this region. These modern systems can distract and compress, and they are made of titanium. They use vertebral screws with bicortical purchase, except the Synthes system, which uses unicortical screws with a locking mechanism into the plate. The Kaneda device is the strongest but also the most prominent. The University plate uses fully threaded bicortical 7.0 mm cancellous bone bolts that lock the posterior portion of the plate to the screws with tapered nuts, analogous to the Steffee plate system used in the posterior spine. Additional bicortical 6.25 mm cancellous screws are placed anteriorly in the plate as neutralization screws. The plate is thicker posteriorly than anteriorly for a very low profile near the great vessels.

The indications for anterior spine fusion with instrumentation to treat idiopathic scoliosis are progressive, single thoracolumbar and lumbar curves greater than 40 to 50° that cause significant imbalance of the trunk (48, 69). Double major curves may also be addressed by instrumenting the lumbar curve, though only if the thoracic curve is less than the lumbar curve and is flexible, and correction may be less than in single curves (45, 48, 54, 70). Trammell et al. identified patients over 50 years of age, curves greater than 60°, and rigid curves as groups at high risk for failure of the procedure (69).

The selection of fusion levels is based on the configuration of the disc spaces and the degree of vertebral body translation on the standing posteroanterior radiograph and bending radiographs. All vertebrae bordering disc spaces that are open on the convexity of the curve are included in the fusion as well as vertebrae that are significantly translated more than 5 mm from the vertebra below (54). The distal end vertebra must be neutrally rotated and horizontal to the sacrum on the reverse side-bending posteroanterior radiograph to prevent accelerated disc degeneration distally (9, 48). The average number of levels fused and instrumented is four to five segments.

Surgical Techniques

Anterior Plate (Z-plate, University Plate)

Once the patient's history, physical examination, and radiologic evaluation have been completed and significant neurologic deficit and canal compromise has been found, the patient is indicated for an anterior decompression, strut graft, and plate/screws (Figs. 34.1 and 34.2).

A standard left retroperitoneal or thoracoabdominal approach is preferred because of the ease of locating and manipulating the aorta in comparison with the inferior vena cava. The spine is exposed one level cephalad and one level caudad to the injured segment, which is confirmed radiographically, and the segmental vessels are ligated at all three levels. The disc material and cartilaginous endplate of the cephalad and caudad levels to the damaged vertebra is removed, and a subtotal corpectomy and canal decompression is performed, leaving the anterior and contralateral cortices intact.

A vertebral body spreader is placed inside the corpectomy site against the cephalad and caudad endplates to distract and reestablish tension in the ligamentous structures, correcting the kyphotic deformity. The graft site is then measured from endplate to endplate, and an autologous tricortical iliac crest graft is harvested, shaped, and placed within the distracted corpectomy site. The vertebral body spreaders are removed, allowing the endplates of the cephalad and caudad vertebrae to rest on the graft. Additional morselized graft is placed anteriorly to fill the void between the anterior longitudinal ligament and the strut graft. Meticulous grafting technique is a necessity, because no spinal instrumentation system will compensate for a poor or insufficient graft.

Any ridges or prominences laterally are reduced so that a flat surface is available for the plate. These plate systems use two vertebral screws per vertebra, and compression force can be applied. A drill bit is placed through an appropriate drill guide and a hole is drilled to penetrate both cortices. In general, the posterior screw holes are prepared first, as in Z-plate and University plate systems. After completion of the drilling, the hole may be tapped to the measured depth. Screws of the appropriate length are selected and advanced into the hole, and bicortical purchase is confirmed radiographically or by direct palpation. The plate is placed over the bolts, and the corresponding nut is tightened to secure the plate to the bolts.

While the nut is being tightened the compressor is placed so that the strut graft is loaded in compression. Additional anterior screws are placed so that triangulation is achieved with the two vertebral screws per vertebral body.

Anterior Rod Systems: Zielke Instrumentation

The modification of the Dwyer procedure that Zielke introduced in 1976, also known as ventral derotation spondylodesis (VDS), was designed to correct both the coronal plane deformity and the rotational deformity of scoliosis. This system uses the vertebral body screws that are connected by a threaded rod, providing fine adjustment to the compression force. The Zielke system is primarily used for correcting isolated thoracolumbar or lumbar deformities, and its main advantage over posterior instrumentations is that fewer levels need to be fused, allowing more mobile motion segments to remain distal to fusion. The Zielke instrumentation may be augmented with posterior instrumentation to enhance the rigidity of the construct while saving distal motion segments (Fig. 34.3). This system may also be applied to the anterior aspect of the thoracic spine, but the indications, advantages, and outcomes of anterior rod instrumentations are not well delineated at this time for thoracic scoliosis.

The surgical techniques for VDS are exacting. The exposure of the thoracolumbar spine is made over the convexity of the curve. The bed of the tenth rib is usually used for a thoracoabdominal approach. The vertebral bodies are exposed, and segmental arteries and veins are isolated and ligated individually. The vertebral bodies are exposed circumferentially to the opposite side, and malleable retractors are positioned to protect the great vessels. Radiographs are obtained to confirm the levels of dissection. First, meticulous removal of the intervertebral discs is done. The disc material is removed to the posterior longitudinal ligament, and the annulus fibrosus on the concave side of the curve should be excised as well. The endplates should be fish-scaled to enhance the fusion rate. Zielke screws are placed in the middle of each vertebra from the superior-inferior aspect and the posterior one-third from the anterior-posterior aspect. An awl is used to make the initial entry point, and a screw of appropriate length is inserted to the opposite cortex. The surgeon should palpate the opposite cortex and the tip of the screw to confirm the proper length of the screw. Zielke staples may be used as anchors at the proximal and distal ends of the instrumentation system, and plain washers may be used in the middle segments. The 3.2 mm threaded rod is placed over the screw heads. The derotation and lordosing bridge is attached to the threaded rod, which

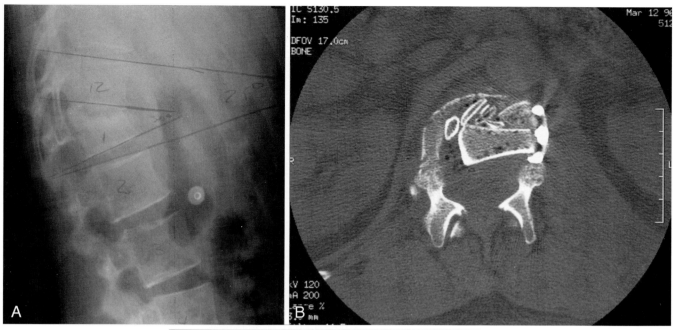
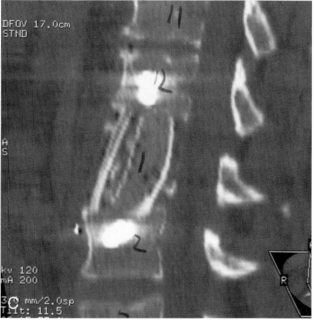

FIGURE 34.1.
A 49-year-old male who sustained an L1 burst fracture with 75% canal compromise resulting in incomplete paraplegia. This patient underwent anterior decompression, strut grafting, and University plate fixation from T12 to L2. His neurologic status improved a Frankel grade, and solid fusion and maintenance of alignment was noted at follow-up. **A.** Lateral radiograph shows the burst fracture and kyphotic angulation. **B.** Postoperative computed tomography scan shows decompression to the opposite pedicle and strut iliac crest graft, rib grafts, and the University plate. **C.** Sagittal reconstruction view shows the strut graft, canal decompression, and correction of the kyphotic deformity.

is anchored to each screw. When the spine is maneuvered into derotation and lordosis, the disc space should open up anteriorly. Morselized bone graft is placed in the disc space. In order to enhance lordosis of the lumbar spine, a structural graft or cage may be placed anterior to the line of the compression rod. Compression is applied in the corrected position, thus locking the spine in the lordotic and derotated position. The excess rod is trimmed, and a chest tube insertion and closure is done as usual. Postoperatively, a thoracolumbosacral orthosis (TLSO) is worn for 5 to 6 months.

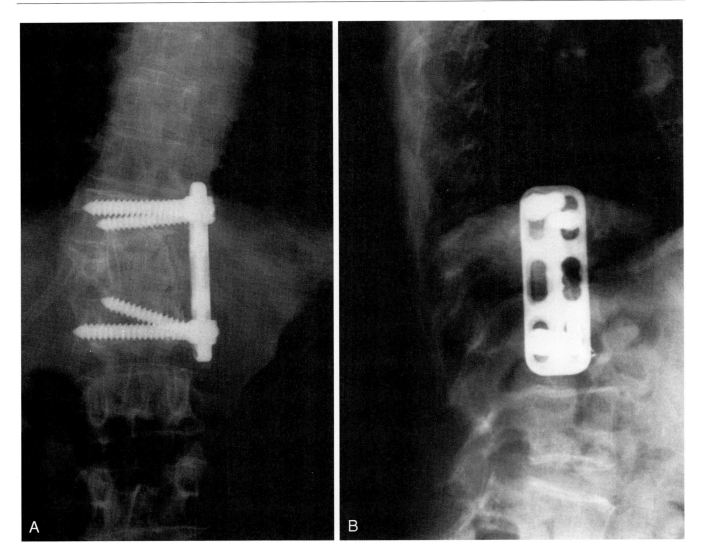

FIGURE 34.2.
A 60-year-old female with plasmacytoma at T12 resulting in significant kyphotic deformity, lower extremity weakness, and conus medullaris syndrome. After failure of radiation and chemotherapy, this patient underwent anterior spinal cord decompression, strut grafting, and University plate fixation. She recovered bladder and sphincter function completely and had significant improvement of motor strength. **A.** Postoperative anteroposterior radiograph shows solid fusion and plate fixation from T11 to L1. **B.** Lateral radiograph shows correction of the kyphotic deformity and plate fixation. There was slight subsidence of the graft and the plate abutting on the T10-T11 disc region, but the patient remained asymptomatic.

Anterior Solid Rod Systems (TSRH, Anterior ISOLA, Moss-Miami, Kaneda, Etc.)

The Zielke system is a flexible rod system that offers fine adjustment capability during instrumentation. The solid rod systems such as TSRH, anterior ISOLA, or Moss-Miami rods are rigid, and they provide more powerful corrective force and more stable constructs (Figs. 34.4–34.6). The indications for rigid rod systems for scoliosis are essentially the same as for the Zielke rod. The TSRH system uses rods of 4.8 mm or 6.4 mm in diameter and screws of 5.5 mm and 6.5 mm in diameter. The screws may be standard or variable-angle types. The ISOLA system uses either 6.35 mm (¼ inch) or 4.76 mm (³⁄₁₆ inch) rods that are connected to vertebral screws with a top-loading set screw mechanism. Moss-Miami rods are 5 mm in diameter, and the connection between the monoaxial or polyaxial screws and the rod is achieved by a top-loading inner set screw and outer nut mechanism.

The Kaneda anterior spinal device consists of the vertebral plate, vertebral screw, paravertebral rod, nut, and transverse fixators. The vertebral plate has tetra-spikes, which are fixed into the lateral vertebral body. The vertebral screw is tapered and self-tapping with a neck diameter of 6.0 mm. The diameter of the paravertebral rod is 5.5 mm. The nuts are fixed into

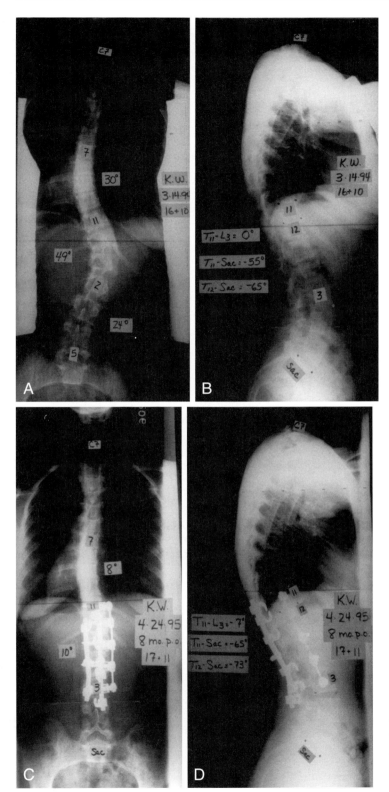

FIGURE 34.3.

A 16-year-old with right thoracolumbar curve at 49°. **A.** and **B.** Upright coronal and sagittal roentgenograms preoperatively. **C.** and **D.** Upright coronal and sagittal roentgenograms at ultimate follow-up. Excellent correction and maintenance of balance was achieved. (Courtesy of Keith Bridwell.)

the screw-head holes on the rod from both sides. The top and bottom vertebral bodies are fixed with an ordinary plate and screws, and the vertebral bodies between the top and the bottom are fixed with the one-hole vertebral plate and screw. The anterior and posterior paravertebral rods are coupled with the transverse fixators. The rod of the multisegmental fixation system is flexible (the rod diameter is 4.0 mm). If the deformity is easily correctable, the rigid paravertebral rod will be applicable.

After exposure, disc excision, and endplate preparation, the screws are placed in the posterior one-

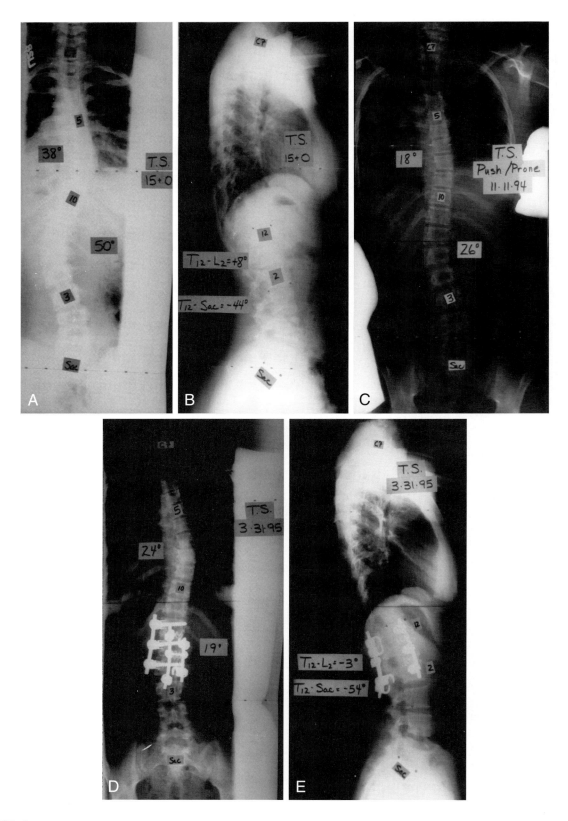

FIGURE 34.4.

A 15-year-old female with left thoracolumbar curve at 50°. **A.** and **B.** Upright coronal and sagittal roentgenograms preoperatively. **C.** A push-prone roentgenogram showing the flexibility of the left thoracolumbar curve. **D.** and **E.** Upright coronal and sagittal roentgenograms in the patient postoperatively. Her parents were very concerned that she maintain spinal flexibility. Excellent cosmetic correction and maintenance of balance have been achieved with a very short anterior fusion and instrumentation. (Courtesy of Keith Bridwell.)

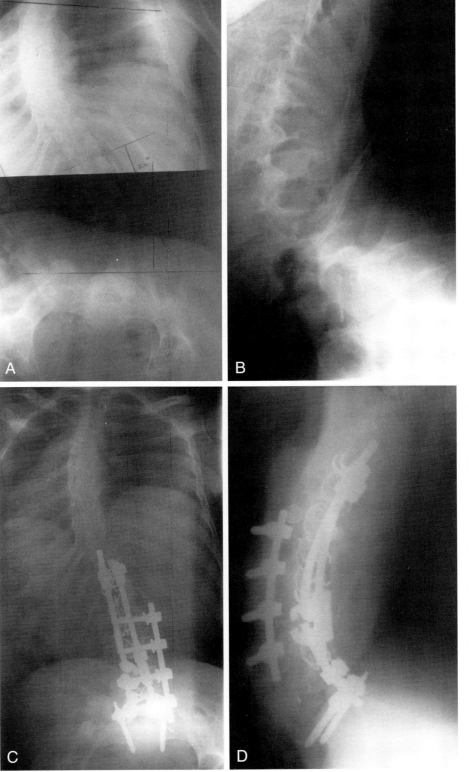

FIGURE 34.5.
A 29-year-old cerebral palsy patient with progressive right lumbar scoliosis and hyperlordosis of the lumbar spine of 110° that causes pain and interferes with sitting. This patient underwent posterior release of the interspinous ligaments, capsules, and ligamentum flavum from T11 to L5, anterior discectomy, fusion, and ISOLA rodding from L1 to L4, and posterior instrumentation and fusion from T11 to the sacrum. **A.** Anteroposterior radiograph shows scoliosis and pelvic tilt due to hyperlordosis of the lumbar spine. **B.** Lateral radiograph shows 110° lordosis of the lumbar spine. **C.** Postoperative anteroposterior radiograph shows good correction of scoliosis and ISOLA instrumentation from T11 to sacrum. **D.** Postoperative lateral radiograph shows correction of lordosis to 68°. The anterior ISOLA rod from L1 to L4 was applied in compression to correct both scoliosis and lordosis. Posterior instrumentation was applied in distraction to correct the hyperlordosis. This patient has good sitting balance and maintenance of correction.

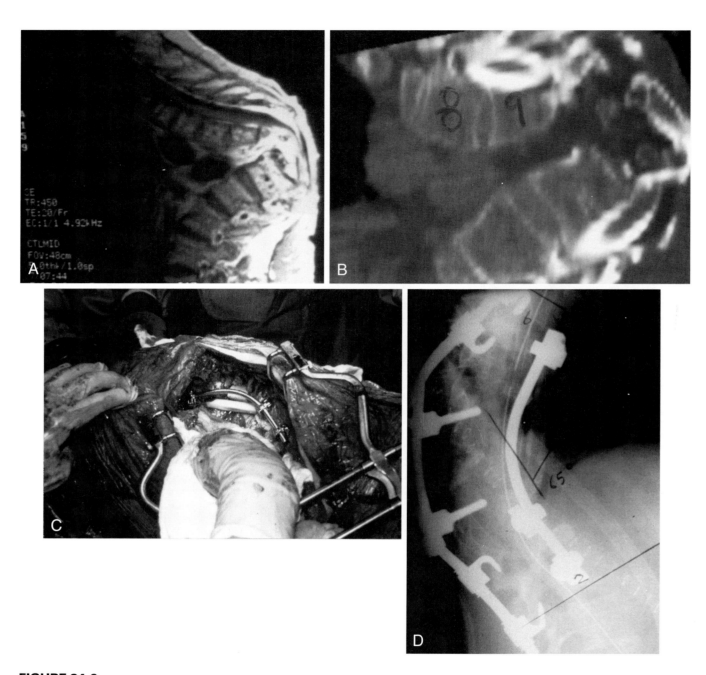

FIGURE 34.6.

A 35-year-old patient with neurofibromatosis presented with severe kyphoscoliosis and paraplegia. The kyphotic deformity was so severe that skin decubitus was developing over the apex of the kyphosis and sitting balance was affected. This patient underwent simultaneous anterior and posterior procedures. The procedures included anterior decompression of the spinal cord over the apex of the kyphosis, anterior vertebral body excision, posterior osteotomy, anterior strut grafting and TSRH rod fixation, and posterior TSRH rod fixation and fusion. **A.** A sagittal T1-weighted magnetic resonance image shows 170° kyphosis and compression of the great vessels anteriorly. **B.** A reconstructed sagittal computed tomography scan shows dystrophic kyphotic deformity with complete myelographic dye. **C.** Intraoperative photograph shows the anterior decompression and fibula strut grafts and TSRH rod fixation. Posterior incision is made simultaneously, and posterior instrumentation was performed as well. **D.** Postoperative lateral radiograph shows correction of the kyphosis to 65° and anterior and posterior TSRH rod fixations. This patient had solid fusion both anteriorly and posteriorly with maintenance of correction at follow-up.

third of the vertebral bodies. If staples are used, the prongs of the staple should go into the endplate. The rod is contoured for lordosis between L1 and L3 and is relatively straight between T11 and L1. The rod is then linked to each screw successively. The rod is usually seated from the caudal to cephalad direction. The rod is rotated 90° into lordosis. The disc spaces are packed with morselized bone grafts or structural grafts, and the instrumentation is compressed and tightened. For the Kaneda system, the vertebral prongs are fixed on the top and bottom vertebral bodies. If the scoliotic curve is rigid, the flexible rod (measuring 4 mm in diameter) is used with the one-hole plates and nuts on the intermediate levels. If the curve is relatively flexible, the semirigid rod (5.5 mm diameter) is used. After inserting the rod into the screw-head holes on the most cephalad and caudal vertebral bodies, a compression force is applied to correct scoliosis. After packing bone chips (usually sectioned rib) into the disc spaces, a screw is inserted into each intermediate vertebral body, and the nuts are tightened on the rod while force is being applied at the scoliotic/kyphotic apex for correction of deformity. Zielke derotator instrumentation can be used as well. Having an assistant push the hump with the palm of the hand can be helpful. An anteroposterior roentgenogram is taken before closure to check the lateral curvature, as overcorrection may occur in a flexible curve. Anterior compression rod systems may also be used for correction of other deformities, such as thoracic scoliosis and hyperlordosis of the lumbar spine. In short, rigid kyphotic deformities, the anterior rod systems are used to distract the anterior column of the spine. Postoperatively, a thoracolumbosacral orthosis (TLSO) is used for 5 to 6 months.

Complications

The anterior approach to the thoracolumbar spine is an extensive exposure and is associated with numerous complications (71). Extensive knowledge of the anatomy, meticulous dissection of the soft tissues, and accurate placement of the instrumentation are absolutely necessary to minimize morbidity and mortality.

Injury to the spinal cord or cauda equina may occur during removal of the intervertebral disc and bone, during insertion of screws into the vertebral bodies, or from vascular insult. Mechanical damage to the neural elements is largely preventable. Screw insertion should be done parallel to the posterior longitudinal ligament and in a posteroanterior direction to avoid penetration of the spinal canal. Avoid ligating segmental arteries close to the intervertebral foramen, especially between the fifth and ninth thoracic vertebrae, which can disrupt collateral circulation to the cord. Temporary occlusion of segmental arteries with observation for somatosensory evoked potential (SSEP) changes may be helpful in preserving key arterial flow to the spinal cord. If paraplegia is noted after surgery, roentgenograms should be taken to rule out penetration of the spinal canal by a screw or bone graft. Spinal cord contusion can be detected by magnetic resonance imaging. Injury to the superior hypogastric plexus or the presacral nerves resulting in impotence and retrograde ejaculation in the male may occur with anterior approaches to the lumbosacral spine.

If a neurologic deficit is noted during or after surgery, corrective force must be reduced immediately. Myelogram, computed tomography, or magnetic resonance imaging may also be helpful in looking for epidural hematoma or cord contusion if the deficit is found postoperatively. If hematoma is present, it should be drained expeditiously. The onset of neurologic deficit as a result of edema or cord ischemia may be delayed for several days (39). Instrumentation should be removed even in late cases in which the clear cause of the neurologic deficit is not found.

Prevention of major vessel injury is a major concern during anterior exposures to the spine. Injury to the aorta or vena cava is most commonly caused by overly vigorous retraction (3). Great caution should be used during removal of the rim of the annulus fibrosus. It is beneficial to have an assistant hold a Chandler elevator between the vessels and the spinal column during disc removal (60). When instrumentation is used, it is important to use screws of the appropriate length so that they will not extend far beyond the opposite cortex and risk penetration of a major vessel (49). Late hemorrhage caused by erosion, leakage, or false aneurysm formation of the vessel has been known to occur (18, 20, 38). If bleeding is encountered during surgery, manual finger pressure or an arterial clamp is used to halt bleeding before formal vascular repair.

In anterior fusions with instrumentation, instrumentation failure may or may not be related to pseudarthrosis. Early screw pullout, rod or plate failure, tilting of the end screw, and vertebral fracture are related to surgical technique and quality of bone. Zielke instrumentation failure is more likely in older adults who have large, rigid curves.

Respiratory complications may include atelectasis, pneumonia, pleural effusion, pneumothorax, chylothorax, hemothorax, acute respiratory distress syndrome, respiratory failure, pulmonary thromboembolism, and fat embolism (2, 10, 26, 71). Chylothorax may follow anterior surgery of the spine (13, 14, 22, 55). Leakage in the lymphatic system should be recognized during surgery, and the stump should be ligated proximally and distally. Treatment of chylothorax consists of chest tube drainage and decreasing the patient's fat intake, although Dehart et al. showed that these patients did well without postoperative drainage (14). Postoperative pulmonary problems such as atelectasis and pneumonia are particularly common in adults, patients with nonidiopathic scoliosis, patients with mental retardation, and in anterior procedures (2). Preoperative medical consultation should be routine in these patients.

Postoperative ileus may occur after anterior spine surgery. Ileus is usually managed with nasogastric suction and delaying oral feeding until bowel sounds return. Narcotics should be used as necessary in the early postoperative period, but prolonged use can disturb gastrointestinal motility. Ileus may be confused with true mechanical obstruction of the bowels. Particularly in the scoliosis patient, superior mesenteric artery syndrome may occur, which gives symptoms of nausea and vomiting due to a high intestinal obstruction (4). This syndrome is a result of a mechanical compression of the third part of the duodenum as it passes between the superior mesenteric artery anteriorly and the aorta and vertebral column posteriorly. When the scoliotic patient undergoes instrumentation, resultant correction of the curve narrows the angle between the superior mesenteric artery and the aorta and compresses the duodenum. Upper gastrointestinal studies with barium swallow are diagnostic. The treatment of this syndrome should consist of nasogastric suction, left lateral decubitus positioning, and occasional modification or removal of the external brace. Surgical intervention is rarely needed, as prolonged nasogastric suction, intravenous hydration, and parenteral nutrition usually corrects this malady.

Urinary tract infections and urinary retention are the most common complications following anterior spine surgery (71). Late hydronephrosis as a result of retroperitoneal fibrosis has been reported (12, 65).

Sympathectomy effect is common after an extensive anterior procedure. The patient reports that the opposite leg is cooler than the leg on the side that was operated on. The sympathetic trunk should be carefully retracted during the procedure and preserved as much as possible. Fortunately, this complication lasts temporarily, typically 3 to 4 months, and is rarely disabling (66). Injury to the spleen has been reported in a patient who underwent left-side anterior surgery for scoliosis (34).

Conclusion

The benefits of anterior instrumentation include a short segment fusion that preserves motion segments; better torsional and axial rigidity in comparison with posterior systems; and decompression and stabilization of the spine via a single approach. However, greater risk is involved, because the anterior approach is more technically demanding than a posterior approach and because of the proximity of the hardware to the great vessels. With meticulous technique, the anterior approach with instrumentation can yield satisfying results with minimal complications.

References

1. An HS, Lim TH, JW You, et al. Biomechanical evaluation of anterior thoracolumbar instrumentation. Spine 1995;20:1979–1983.
2. Anderson PR, Puno MR, Lovell SL, et al. Postoperative respiratory complications in nonidiopathic scoliosis. Acta Anaesthesiol Scand 1985;29:186–192.
3. Baker JK, Reardon PR, Reardon MJ, et al. Vascular injury in anterior lumbar surgery. Spine 1993;18:2227–2230.
4. Barner HB, Sherman DC. Vascular compression of the duodenum. Surg Gynecol Obstet 1963;117:103.
5. Bauer R, Mostegl A, Eichenauer M. An analysis of the results of Dwyer and Zielke instrumentations in the treatment of scoliosis. Arch Orthop Trauma Surg 1986; 105:302–309.
6. Black RC, Gardner VO, Armstrong GWD, et al. A contoured anterior spinal fixation plate. Clin Orthop 1988; 227:135–141.
7. Bone LB, Johnston CE II, Ashman RB, et al. Mechanical comparison of anterior spinal instrumentation in a burst fracture model. J Orthop Trauma 1988;2:195–201.
8. Bonnett C, Brown JC, Grow T. Thoracolumbar scoliosis in cerebral palsy. J Bone Joint Surg 1976;58A:328–336.
9. Bridwell KH. Surgical treatment of adolescent idiopathic scoliosis: the basics and the controversies. Spine 1994;19:1095–1100.
10. Brown LP, Stelling FH. Fat embolism as a complication of scoliosis fusion. J Bone Joint Surg 1974;56A:1764.
11. Byrd JA, Scoles PV, Winter RB, et al. Adult idiopathic scoliosis treated by anterior and posterior spinal fusion. J Bone Joint Surg 1987;69A:843–850.
12. Cleveland RH, Gilsanz V, Lebowitz RL, et al. Hydronephrosis from retroperitoneal fibrosis and anterior spinal fusion. J Bone Joint Surg 1978;60A:996.
13. Colletta AJ, Mayer PJ. Chylothorax: an unusual complication of anterior thoracic interbody spinal fusion. Spine 1982;7:46–49.
14. Dehart MM, Lauerman WC, Conely AH, et al. Management of retroperitoneal chylous leakage. Spine 1994; 19:716–718.
15. Denis F. The three-column spine and its significance in the classification of acute thoracolumbar spinal injuries. Spine 1983;8:817–831.
16. Dickson JH, Harrington PR, Erwin WD. Results of reduction and stabilization in the severely fractured thoracic and lumbar spine. J Bone Joint Surg 1978;60A: 799–806.
17. Dunn HK. Anterior stabilization of thoracolumbar injuries. Clin Orthop 1984;189:116–124.

18. Dunn HK. Anterior spine stabilization and decompression for thoracolumbar injuries. Orthop Clin North Am 1986;17:113.
19. Dwyer AF, Newton NC, Sherwood AA. An anterior approach to scoliosis. Clin Orthop 1969;62:192–202.
20. Dwyer AF. A fatal complication of paravertebral infection and traumatic aneurysm following Dwyer instrumentation. J Bone Joint Surg 1979;61B:239.
21. Edwards CC, Levine AM. Early rod-sleeve stabilization of the injured thoracic and lumbar spine. Orthop Clin North Am 1986;17:121–145.
22. Eisenstein S, O'Brien JP. Chylothorax: a complication of Dwyer anterior instrumentation. Br J Surg 1977;64:339–341.
23. Erickson DL, Leider LL Jr, Brown WE. One-stage decompression-stabilization for thoracolumbar fractures. Spine 1977;2:53–56.
24. Esses SI, Botsford DJ, Kostuik, JP. Evaluation of surgical treatment of burst fractures. Spine 1990;15:667–673.
25. Gertzbein SD, MacMichael D, Tile M. Harrington instrumentation as a method of fixation in fractures of the spine: a critical analysis of deficiencies. J Bone Joint Surg 1982;64B:526–529.
26. Gittman JE, Buchanan TA, Fisher BJ, et al. Fatal fat embolism after spinal fusion for scoliosis. JAMA 1983;249:779–781.
27. Gurr KR, McAfee PC, Shih C. Biomechanical analysis of anterior and posterior instrumentation systems after corpectomy: a calf spine model. J Bone Joint Surg 1988;70A:1182–1191.
28. Gurwitz GS, Dawson JM, McNamara MJ, et al. Biomechanical analysis of three surgical approaches for lumbar burst fractures using short-segment instrumentation. Spine 1993;18:977–982.
29. Haas N, Glauth M, Tscherne H. Anterior plating in thoracolumbar spine injuries: indication, technique, and results. Spine 1991;16(Suppl):S100–S111.
30. Hall JE. Dwyer instrumentation in anterior fusion of the spine. J Bone Joint Surg 1981;63A:1188–1190.
31. Hammerberg KW, Rodts MF, DeWald RL. Zielke instrumentation. Orthopedics 1988;11:1365–1371.
32. Hardaker WT Jr, Cook WA Jr, Friedman AH, et al. Bilateral transpedicular decompression and Harrington rod stabilization in the management of severe thoracolumbar burst fractures. Spine 1992;17:162–171.
33. Hashimoto T, Kaneda K, Abumi K. Relationship between traumatic spinal canal stenosis and neurologic deficits in thoracolumbar burst fractures. Spine 1988;13:1268–1272.
34. Hodge Wa, Dewald RL. Splenic injury complicating the anterior thoracoabdominal surgical approach for scoliosis. J Bone Joint Surg 1983;65A:396–397.
35. Hodgson AR, King FE. Anterior spinal fusion: a preliminary communication on the radical treatment of Pott's disease and Pott's paraplegia. Br J Surg 1956;44:266.
36. Hsu LCS, Zucherman J, Tang SC, et al. Dwyer instrumentation in the treatment of adolescent idiopathic scoliosis. J Bone Joint Surg 1982;64B:536–541.
37. James KS, Wenger KH, Schlegel JD, et al. Biomechanical evaluation of the stability of thoracolumbar burst fractures. Spine 1994;19:1731–1740.
38. Jendrisak MD. Spontaneous abdominal aortic rupture from erosion by a lumbar spine fixation device: a case report. Surgery 1986;99:631.
39. Johnston CE, Happel LT Jr, Norris R, et al. Delayed paraplegia complicating sublaminar segmental spinal instrumentation. J Bone Joint Surg 1986;68A:556–563.
40. Kaneda K, Abumi K, Fujiya M. Burst fractures with neurologic deficits of the thoracolumbar spine: results of anterior decompression and stabilization with anterior instrumentation. Spine 1984;9:788–795.
41. Kaneda K, Asano S, Hashimoto T, et al. The treatment of osteoporotic-posttraumatic vertebral collapse using the Kaneda device and a bioactive ceramic vertebral prosthesis. Spine 1992;17(Suppl):S295–S303.
42. Kohler R, Galland O, Mechin H, et al. The Dwyer procedure in the treatment of idiopathic scoliosis: a 10-year follow-up review of 21 patients. Spine 1990;15:75–80.
43. Kostuik JP. Anterior fixation for fractures of thoracic and lumbar spines with and without neurologic involvement. Clin Orthop 1984;189:116–124.
44. Kostuik JP. Anterior Kostuik-Harrington distraction systems. Orthopedics 1988;11:1379–1391.
45. Kostuik JP, Carl A, Ferron S. Anterior Zielke instrumentation for spinal deformity in adults. J Bone Joint Surg 1989;71A:898–912.
46. Leong JC, Wilding K, Mok CK, et al. Surgical treatment of scoliosis following poliomyelitis: a review of one hundred and ten cases. J Bone Joint Surg 1981;63A:726–740.
47. Lim TH, An HS, Ahn JY, et al. Biomechanical comparison between anterior fixation vs. posterior fixation in an unstable calf spine model. Spine 1997;22:261–266.
48. Lowe TG, Peters JD. Anterior spinal fusion with Zielke instrumentation for idiopathic scoliosis: a frontal and sagittal curve analysis in 36 patients. Spine 1993;18:423–426.
49. Matsuzaki H, Tokuhashi Y, Wakabayashi K, et al. Penetration of a screw into the thoracic aorta in anterior spinal instrumentation: a case report. Spine 1993;18:2327–2331.
50. Mayer PJ, Dove J, Ditmanson M, et al. Post-poliomyelitis paralytic scoliosis: a review of curve patterns and results of surgical treatments in 118 consecutive patients. Spine 1981;6:573–582.
51. McAfee PC, Bohlman HH, Yuan HA. Anterior decompression of traumatic thoracolumbar fractures with incomplete neurological deficit using a retroperitoneal approach. J Bone Joint Surg 1985;67A:89–104.
52. McLain RF, Sparling E, Benson DR. Early failure of short-segment pedicle instrumentation for thoracolumbar fractures. J Bone Joint Surg 1993;75A:162–167.
53. McMaster MJ. Anterior and posterior instrumentation and fusion of thoracolumbar scoliosis due to myelomeningocele. J Bone Joint Surg 1987;69B:20–25.
54. Moe JH, Purcell GA, Bradford DS. Zielke instrumentation (VDS) for the correction of spinal curvature: analysis of results in 66 patients. Clin Orthop 1983;180:133–153.
55. Nakai S, Zielke K. Chylothorax: a rare complication after anterior and posterior spinal correction (report of six cases). Spine 1986;11:830–833.

56. Ogiela DM, Chan DPK. Ventral derotation spondylodesis: a review of 22 cases. Spine 1986;11:18–22.
57. Osebold WR, Mayfield JK, Winter RB, et al. Surgical treatment of paralytic scoliosis associated with myelomeningocele. J Bone Joint Surg 1982;64A:841–856.
58. Roaf R. The basic anatomy of scoliosis. J Bone Joint Surg 1966;48B:4.
59. Ryan MD, Taylor TKF, Sherwood AA. Bolt-plate fixation for anterior spinal fusion. Clin Orthop 1986;203:196–202.
60. Schafer MF. The anterior approach to scoliosis. In: Chapman MW, ed. Operative orthopaedics. Philadelphia: JB Lippincott, 1988:1965–1978.
61. Shiba K, Katsuki M, Ueta T, et al. Transpedicular fixation with Zielke instrumentation in the treatment of thoracolumbar and lumbar injuries. Spine 1994;19:1040–1949.
62. Shono Y, McAfee PC, Cunningham BW. Experimental study of thoracolumbar burst fractures: a radiographic and biomechanical analysis of anterior and posterior instrumentation systems. Spine 1994;19:1711–1722.
63. Shono Y, Kaneda K, Yamamoto I. A biomechanical analysis of Zielke, Kaneda, and Cotrel-Dubousset instrumentations in thoracolumbar scoliosis: a calf spine model. Spine 1991;16:1305–1311.
64. Siegal T, Tiqva P, Siegal T. Vertebral body resection for epidural compression by malignant tumors: results of forty-seven consecutive operative procedures. J Bone Joint Surg 1985;67A:375–382.
65. Silber I, McMaster W. Retroperitoneal fibrosis with hydronephrosis as a complication of the Dwyer procedure. J Pediatr Surg 1977;12:255.
66. Simmons EH, Trammell TR. Operative management of adult scoliosis. In: Evarts MC, ed. Surgery of the musculoskeletal system. New York: Churchill Livingstone, 1983.
67. Stephen JP, Wilding K, Cass CA. The place of Dwyer anterior instrumentation in scoliosis. Med J Aust 1977;1:206–208.
68. Swank SM, Cohen DS, Brown JC. Spine fusion in cerebral palsy with L-rod segmental spinal instrumentation: a comparison of single and two-stage combined approach with Zielke instrumentation. Spine 1989;14:750–759.
69. Trammell TR, Benedict F, Reed D. Anterior spine fusion using Zielke instrumentation for adult thoracolumbar and lumbar scoliosis. Spine 1990;16:1378–1382.
70. Turi M, Johnston CE, Richards BS. Anterior correction of idiopathic scoliosis using TSRH instrumentation. Spine 1993;18:417–422.
71. Westfall SH, Akbarnia BA, Merenda JT, et al. Exposure of the anterior spine: technique, complications, and results in 85 patients. Am J Surg 1987;154:700–704.
72. White AA III, Panjabi MM. The problem of clinical instability in the human spine: a systematic approach. In: White AA, Panjabi MM, eds. Clinical biomechanics of the spine. 2d ed. Philadelphia: JB Lippincott, 1990:277.
73. Yuan HA, Mann KA, Found EM, et al. Early clinical experience with the Syracuse I-plate: an anterior spinal fixation device. Spine 1988;13:278–285.
74. Zdeblick TA, Shirado O, McAfee PC, et al. Anterior spinal fixation after lumbar corpectomy: a study in dogs. J Bone Joint Surg 1991;73A:527–534.
75. Zielke K, Stunkat R, Beaujean F. Ventrale derotationsspondylodesis. Arch Orthop Unfallchir 1976;85:257–277.

CHAPTER THIRTY FIVE

Injection for Diagnosis and Therapy of Back Disease

Quinn Hogan

Introduction

Injection of anesthetic, steroid, or other agents about the vertebral column is performed for therapeutic or diagnostic indications. Pathogenic ambiguity that often accompanies painful conditions of the back is the most frequent motive for diagnostic blockade. Since the patient's history, the physical examination, and imaging studies may fail to isolate a specific anatomic element as the locus of pain, anesthetizing various structures or neural pathways is used to single out the source and hence to guide further therapy. Therapeutic attempts by injection are usually pursued in the hopes of avoiding surgery or of hastening the resolution of a self-limited process and are best used as a component of a rehabilitation program. The relatively low risk in injection procedures and the accelerating pressures for rapid recovery at minimum cost also contribute to the popularity of back pain treatment by injection.

The premise underlying the use of nerve blocks for diagnosis is that relief following injection is due to anesthetic isolation of the nociceptive source from the central nervous system. This is based on certain assumptions about neurophysiology, anatomy, and local anesthetic function that are not entirely reliable and that therefore impose limitations on these methods.

Limitations Due to Sensory Mechanisms

The traditional "hard-wired" model of sensory perception (Fig. 35.1) dictates a consistent response of receptors, invariable pathways of neural signals, unaltered transmission of the unaltered signal to higher centers, and inevitable perception of the stimulus. Each of these assumed steps must be qualified according to new understandings of sensory physiology; the model fits least well in the specific case of chronic pain.

Complex processing of afferent signals from peripheral receptors takes place in the dorsal horn of the spinal cord. The probability that neural activity from a small-fiber pain receptor (i.e., a nociceptive signal) will trigger the second-order spinal cord neuron that transmits to the brain depends on other competing and facilitating input to that cell (Fig. 35.2). Nonpainful peripheral signals traveling on large fibers can block access of the pain signal to the spinal cell, as is described in the gate control theory (113). Descending activity from the brain, such as during stress, may also impede pain transmission in the spinal cord. Finally, neural traffic from other sources, especially deep somatic and visceral structures, converges on spinal cells, so that every dorsal horn neuron has multiple peripheral inputs. Therefore, the re-

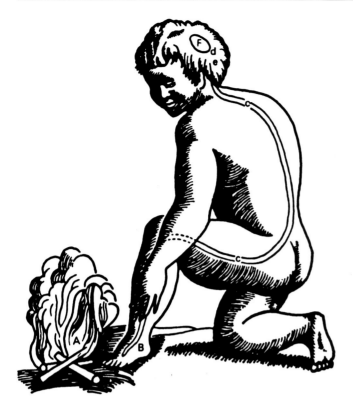

FIGURE 35.1.
Seventeenth-century model of "hard-wired" transmission of pain signals of René Descartes. Transmission of pain is direct, exact, and immutable. (From Melzack R, Wall PD. Pain mechanisms, a new theory. Science 1965;150:971. Copyright 1965, American Academy for the Advancement of Science.)

sponse to a nerve injection will depend on the balance of small- and large-fiber block, convergent signals from other sites, and descending modulation induced by stress. For example, the block of one of the inputs may decrease total stimulation below the threshold for triggering the spinal neuron, producing pain relief even though pathology is widespread. Neural interactions may also lead to reduced perception of back pain secondary to pain from needle insertion and the stress of a block procedure, without blocking the site of pathology.

The likelihood that a spinal neuron will respond to an input is not fixed. These neurons may become sensitized by repeated input, especially from small pain fibers (Fig. 35.3). Once exposed to these conditioning stimuli, they may send a pain signal to the brain even after nonpainful input, a phenomenon termed allodynia. Input from other areas may also produce a signal due to convergence of fibers from different sources on the dorsal horn cell (Fig. 35.3). After sensitization of the cord, blockade of nerves outside the area of primary pathology may result in some relief, spuriously indicating the injured area. Pain relief may be prolonged far beyond the presence of the local anesthetic if spinal sensitization diminishes during the interval of blockade. Surgical nerve ablation rarely duplicates pain relief from blockade because of the spinal sensitization produced by intense conditioning stimuli from neural injury at the time of surgery and from the neuroma afterward.

Limitations Due to Local Anesthetic Effect

Injected local anesthetic rarely results in a physiologic transection of the nerve. Rather, the interruption is variable and partial. Small fibers and rapidly firing fibers are blocked most completely. Therefore, the response to diagnostic block will depend on the relative contribution of large and small fibers to the pain, and on the firing pattern of the nerves. Both of these factors are hard to predict.

Circulating local anesthetic absorbed from the area of injection may be analgesic at distant sites of pathology, especially in injured nerves. Serum levels created by many clinically used blocks are adequate to diminish spontaneous signal generation from injured nerves (Fig. 35.4). This could mistakenly indicate the injected nerve as the pathogenic one.

Limitations Due to Anatomic Considerations

The use of blocks for diagnosis and prognosis depends on an assumption of anatomic consistency: We expect nerve structures to be found in predictable

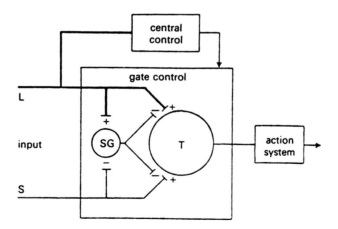

FIGURE 35.2.
Melzack and Wall's gate control theory. Two important components are incorporated into this description of pain signal modulation. First, competition for access to the central nervous system between pain signals transmitted by small fibers (S) and nonpainful input transmitted by large fibers (L) is mediated by interneurons in the substantia gelatinosa of the spinal cord dorsal horn. These segmental interactions determine ascending output by the transmitter (T) cells. Secondly, descending signals from the brain (central control) influence ascending spinal cord output as well. (Reprinted with permission from Melzack R, Wall PD. Pain mechanisms, a new theory. Science 1965;150:971. Copyright 1965, American Academy for the Advancement of Science.)

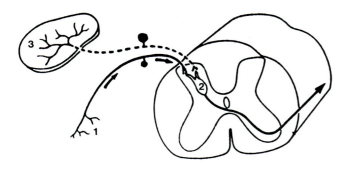

FIGURE 35.3.
Spinal sensitization and convergence. Painful input transmitted by small fibers, especially from deep somatic sites, *(1)* provides conditioning stimuli that can make pain-transmitting second-order neurons of the spinal cord *(2)* more likely to fire, a process termed sensitization. After sensitization, dorsal horn cells may fire after noninjurious low intensity input transmitted by large fibers, which may originate in the area of original stimulation or in distant tissues *(3)* that send convergent input to the dorsal horn cell. (After Fields HL. Pain. McGraw-Hill, 1987:90–91.)

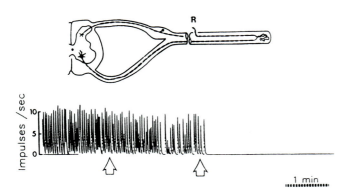

FIGURE 35.4.
Systemic effects of local anesthetics. Section of the sciatic nerve in a rat creates a neuroma, represented by a tangle of nerve fibers at the nerve end in the upper drawing. Recording from distal fibers at R shows spontaneous nerve activity and bursts of activity in response to minimal mechanical stimulation, both absent in normal nerves. These neuropathic pain signals, represented in the tracing below, are suppressed by low circulating levels of local anesthetic from systemic injection at the arrows. (After Devor M, Wall PD, Catalan N. Systemic lidocaine silences ectopic neuroma and dorsal root ganglion discharge without blocking nerve conduction. Pain 1992;48:262.)

places and to have predictable connections. There are important limitations to these expectations. Like any biologic feature, most anatomic parameters show variability about a norm. For example, Tuffier's line between the iliac crests crosses the vertebral column most often at the L4–5 disc (perhaps higher on average in men than in women), but the range is from as low as the L5-S1 disc to as high as the L3–4 disc (Fig. 35.5) (48, 101, 126). A normal distribution also describes the level of the termination of the spinal cord and of the termination of the dural sac (91, 129). This indicates that surface and palpation landmarks are unreliable indicators of deep structures.

The number and location of structures is also variable. The distribution of nerve roots to the intervertebral foramina is anomalous in about 8% of subjects, including, for example cases in which two root pairs exit at one level with an adjacent empty foramen (87, 119, 121). The clinical consequence of anomalous anatomic arrangements is the development of anesthesia in an unexpected distribution after foraminal injection, with resulting diagnostic ambiguity.

The separation of peripheral sensory input into a discernible segmental pattern is a fundamental concept underlying many diagnostic blocks. The distribution of fibers to dermatomes has been mapped using zoster eruptions, residual sensation after sectioning the roots on either side of an intact segment, absent sensation after root section or anesthesia, vasodilatation during stimulation of roots, or pain with nerve root compression and visceral disease (17). The dermatome diagrams these methods produce show considerable disagreement. There is also variability in the formation of segmental spinal nerves and their peripheral distribution. Multiple interconnections of adjacent roots are found within the dural sac in all subjects, with between three and nine such intersegmental anastomoses at the upper cervical region and a similar number at the lumbosacral level (124, 125). Furthermore, extensive overlap between consecutive peripheral dermatomes is evident, since the division of an individual root rarely produces an appreciable loss of sensibility. As a consequence, sensory changes after local anesthetic injections about the vertebral column are variable. There is also segmental inconsistency in the motor innervation of the extremities. Marked departure from the usual distribution of L5 and S1 motor fibers is found in 16% of subjects, in whom stimulation of a nerve root produces movement typical of the other root (158).

Methods

Diagnostic blocks should be performed in a manner that yields the most certain information possible in order not to add to the inherent ambiguity of clinical pain. In many cases, needle position should be confirmed by radiologic imaging. Determination of segmental level is unreliable without confirmation by radiography, and studies of a variety of injection procedures have shown inadequate consistency of needle placement without imaging (54, 130). Since small volumes of local anesthetic must be used in order to minimize spread to untargeted nerves, meticulous needle placement is required to ensure adequate

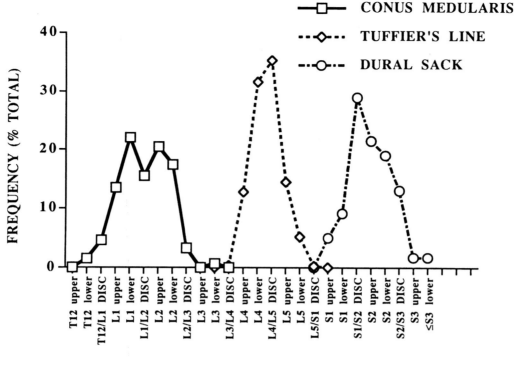

FIGURE 35.5.
Palpation is an unreliable means of determining vertebral level. The frequency distribution of bony segmental levels at which Tuffier's line, which connects the iliac crests, crosses the vertebral column is shown (diamonds/dashed line). Also shown are the distributions for the levels at which the dural sac ends (circles/dot-dash line), and at which the spinal cord ends (squares/solid line). (Reprinted with permission from Hogan Q. Tuffier's line: the normal distribution of anatomic parameters. Anesth Analg 1993;78:194–195.)

blockade of the desired nerve. Injection of a small amount of radio-opaque contrast prior to the anesthetic can identify passage to an undesired nerve or in an ineffective direction. The usefulness of guiding needle insertion by the nature of provoked pain is limited by the lack of specificity of deep sensations (109, 114).

Pain before and after blockade should be evaluated by asking the patient to rate the intensity between 0 (none) and 10 (worst imaginable) to facilitate communication and documentation. Provocative measures such as palpation of a tender area or joint movement may reveal changes in incident pain when compared before and after the block, and spontaneous pain may respond to a block differently than induced pain. If the patient is not feeling his or her usual pain at the time of a diagnostic block, little can be learned about the pain mechanism. When pain is relieved by neural blockade, the duration of analgesia should be determined. Relief lasting only the expected duration of the anesthetic effect (at most 2 hours for lidocaine hydrochloride, 4 hours for bupivacaine) suggests an ongoing peripheral focus of nociception. If relief obviously outlasts the anesthetic, a central process potentiating pain transmission may be involved.

Pain relief, however, cannot be the only measured parameter. Independent confirmation of neural blockade is necessary, since performing the procedure correctly and with care does not guarantee that the intended nerve will be anesthetized and the desired physiologic change achieved. Detailed sensory and motor testing before and after injection can identify somatic nerve block effects. Ability to sense the scratch from a folded corner of a foil alcohol pad wrapper indicates small-fiber (nociceptive) function, while dull touch perception indicates large-fiber function. Stimuli should be performed as consistently as possible, since a stimulus that is more intense, more frequently repeated, or more broadly distributed may be perceived while weaker stimuli are blocked (141).

Pain caused by the procedure itself may result in confused diagnosis, since relief following the injection may be the relief of the iatrogenic pain and not of the preexisting pain for which the block was done. Also, intense pain from the procedure may diminish the perceived severity of the original pain by activating descending pain suppression (Fig. 35.6), creating the illusion that neural blockade effects relieved the pain (140). Judicious use of local anesthetics in the superficial tissues, use of small needles, and careful needle guidance limit the pain of the procedure.

The placebo response is a thorny but central issue in diagnostic blockade. There can never be certainty that pain relief following nerve block is due to the block and not a placebo response. In general terms, placebo responses are incomplete, are inconsistently repeatable, and may lack the appropriate time course for the onset or duration of the active agent. Injections, like surgery, are especially potent placebos (51). No personality features predict a placebo response (94). Saline injection can be used to seek a placebo response. However, individuals are not consistent in being responders or nonresponders, and most individuals will eventually respond to a placebo if administered repeatedly, so it is hard to conclude much from identifying a placebo response (76). Certainly, this is not a means to determine if the pain is real. In a sense, placebos are active agents since an endogenous opioid mechanism is evident (63, 92, 97).

Local Infiltration

The most direct means of identifying a source of pain is by injection of local anesthetic directly into the site, such as in the area of a scar or tender muscle. If relief follows superficial injection, it suggests that deeper sites are not involved. Pain that persists after anesthetizing overlying skin or muscle implies the indirect compression of an inflamed nerve root, joint, or other structure.

Skin that is hyperesthetic in the area of a scar is probably so because of spinal sensitization and mechanical sensitivity of neuromata in the skin. Successful analgesia with local anesthetic injection may be followed by attempts at longer relief by the injection of depot steroids.

Lidocaine 1% or bupivacaine 0.5% is injected through a 22-gauge or 25-gauge needle under the skin along a scar or into the area of tender muscle or fascia. Large tender areas requiring more than about 20 mL injectate are probably best treated by other means. Triamcinolone diacetate or methylprednisolone may be added in the ratio of about 1 mL per 8–10 mL anesthetic. Physical therapy should be consid-

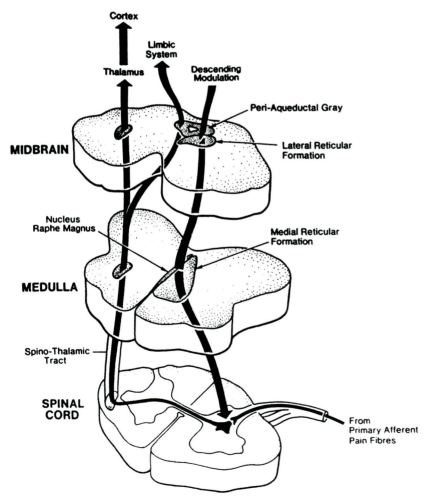

FIGURE 35.6.

Descending modulation. Signals from primary afferent fibers are transmitted to various parts of the brain by axons originating in dorsal horn cells and conveyed in the spinothalamic tract. Ascending pain signals may trigger descending systems in the centers shown, which then suppress activity of the dorsal horn cell and block afferent transmission of pain signals. (Reprinted with permission from Cousins MJ, Phillips GD, eds. Acute pain management. London: Churchill Livingstone, 1986.)

ered during the interval of analgesia to take best advantage of the injection. Repeat injections can be pursued at intervals as short as 2 days but should not be continued unless the period of relief is progressively prolonged, indicating an eventual resolution. Except in the case of injections every few months, continued injection therapy without evidence of progress is not indicated.

Trigger points are a special case of myofascial pain in which the tenderness and pain are focused to one or several small sites in the muscle where a palpable lump is evident. This commonly accompanies other structural or neurologic maladies. Histologic and electromyographic study of these areas has not identified a pathogenic mechanism, but relief following local anesthetic injection may be long lasting. It is possible that the inherent myotoxicity of local anesthetics has a therapeutic role (75). All local anesthetics release calcium from intracellular stores, resulting in activation of proteases and cell destruction. Mature myocytes have such stores in sarcoplasmic reticulum, but nerves, vessels, and immature myoblasts lack calcium reservoirs and are spared. Regeneration of muscle fibers is prompt, and the loss of muscle is rarely evident. The replacement of old muscle cells by new cells might be the means of relieving trigger-point pain by injection.

Some doubt regarding the specificity of the tissue injection is raised by reports showing comparable efficacy from less specific techniques, such as dry needling of trigger points (93) and jet injection of local anesthetic into the skin overlying trigger points (128). Preliminary observations suggest that botulinum toxin in extremely dilute concentrations may give prolonged relief (27). Tissue injection is rarely dangerous, but pneumothorax is possible at thoracic levels. Diagnostic interpretation should consider nearby nerves. For instance, relief after piriformis muscle trigger-point injections could also be the result of the spread of anesthetic to the adjacent sciatic nerve.

Peripheral Nerve Block

The injection of local anesthetic or steroid on a peripheral nerve is occasionally used in the diagnosis and treatment of back pain. Plexopathy following injury may respond to steroid treatment, using standard anesthetic approaches to the brachial, lumbar, or sacral plexus. Block of peripheral branches of the sciatic nerve may relieve pain in well-documented cases of lumbosacral radiculopathy (86, 154). This surprising response perhaps results by blocking antidromic impulses that arise from the nerve root or dorsal root ganglion and are propagated to the periphery, producing changes in nociceptor sensitivity (2).

Sympathetic Blockade

Deep somatic sensation from the vertebral column is supplied by afferent fibers that follow sympathetic pathways (65, 83). Specifically, the costovertebral joints, anterior longitudinal ligament, and much of the annular ligament are directly innervated by branches of the rami communicantes and sympathetic trunks (64). The extensive neural plexus in the anterior epidural space that supplies sensation to the anterior dura, posterior longitudinal ligament, and the posterior portion of the annular ligament of the disc is made of small afferent fibers that enter the vertebral canal as the sinuvertebral nerves, or nerves of Luschka. These originate from the rami communicantes as multiple fine structures and hence enter the intervertebral foramina (Fig. 7A). Connection to their somata in the posterior root ganglia is by way of the paravertebral sympathetic trunks. Fibers from the sinuvertebral nerves may span as many as eight vertebral segments and cross the midline, contributing to the poor somatotopic specification of vertebral sensation.

Sympathetic pathways for vertebral sensations has been documented in experimental settings by electrophysiologic monitoring and in awake human subjects by provoking back pain with electrical stimulation of the sympathetic trunks and rami (6, 60, 142, 150). Local anesthetic blockade of the sympathetic trunk is occasionally used for treatment of back pain, especially in multiply operated backs in which more well-established techniques have been exhausted. If local anesthetic block produces relief, phenol injection may produce a more lasting effect, although the response is usually not permanent and genitofemoral neuralgia may ensue in perhaps 10% of cases. Despite the anatomic and physiologic appeal of this approach, there is only preliminary support so far (19, 32, 50).

Sacroiliac Injection

The sacroiliac joint is well innervated and a probable source of back pain in some patients (145). Injection into healthy joints produces pain in and around the joint, into the gluteal area, and occasionally into the posterior thigh and knee (55). It is often difficult to ascertain the contribution of sacroiliac disease to low back pain. Physical examination maneuvers are only weakly indicative of disease, and anatomic irregularities in the joint space are expected even in asymptomatic individuals, so anesthetic injection may be necessary to distinguish sacroiliac disease from myofascial pain or facet and disc disease (18, 45, 133, 149).

Injection may be performed without imaging at the level of the posterior superior iliac spines (Fig.

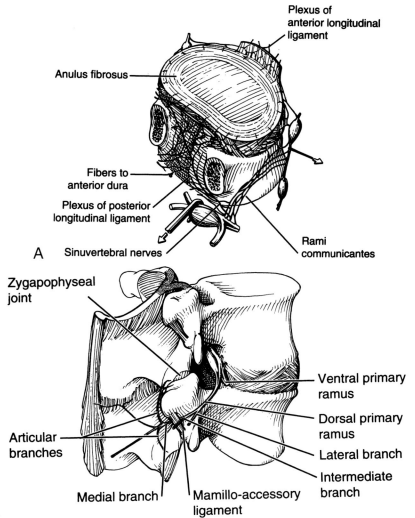

FIGURE 35.7.

Innervation of deep somatic structures of the vertebral column. **A.** The sensory plexus of the anterior dura and posterior longitudinal ligament, as well as the innervation of the outer portion of the annulus fibrosus of the disc, are supplied by afferent fibers that track through the sympathetic chain via the sinuvertebral nerves and the rami communicantes. **B.** Posterior structures are innervated by branches of the posterior (dorsal) primary ramus of the segmental spinal nerve. The facet joint is innervated by ramifications of the medial branch of the posterior primary ramus. (Reprinted with permission from Brown DL. Regional anesthesia and analgesia. Philadelphia: WB Saunders, 1996:62–63.)

35.8A). The needle is inserted at the midline and directed laterally at a 45° angle and advanced through the sacroiliac ligaments until contact is made with bone. Repositioning once or twice is necessary in order to find the deepest point between the ilium and sacrum. Three to 5 mL local anesthetic containing 1 mL depot steroid is injected at this point. Because of the relative inaccessibility of the joint line, this method frequently fails to deliver the injectate into the joint space. However, it is not clear that true intraarticular placement is necessary for a therapeutic response, and benefit may be a result of sacroiliac ligament response or diffusion into the capsule.

More accurate needle placement into the joint space itself (Fig. 35.8B) requires radiologic imaging (55, 70). With the patient prone, a slightly oblique fluoroscopic image is obtained to superimpose the anterior and more medial posterior joint lines of the inferior pole of the joint. Along this axis, a 22-gauge spinal needle is directed anteriorly and laterally into the joint. About 1 mL radiopaque dye is injected and spreads into the joint if the needle is correctly positioned. Tears of the joint capsule may be noted (136). For diagnostic purposes, the nature and distribution of pain elicited by needle contact with the joint and by contrast injection can be compared to the patient's usual pain. This is of unproved value, however, since exact reproduction of the pain is not significantly more frequent in patients who obtain relief following anesthetic injection than in those with a negative response to anesthetic.

A prospective study of the diagnostic use of x-ray controlled injection indicated that 30% of patients with chronic low back pain below L5 were relieved by local anesthetic sacroiliac injection, most of whom exhibited a tear in the joint capsule (136). Most subjects with tears, however did not obtain relief from block. Groin pain was a distinguishing complaint of subjects who obtained relief from injection of the joint. Radiation of pain below the knee was as common in patients relieved by sacroiliac injection as in those with no response. In our clinic (Reynolds AR, Abram SE, unpublished data, 1984), 28 of 35 patients given sacroiliac injections of local anesthetic

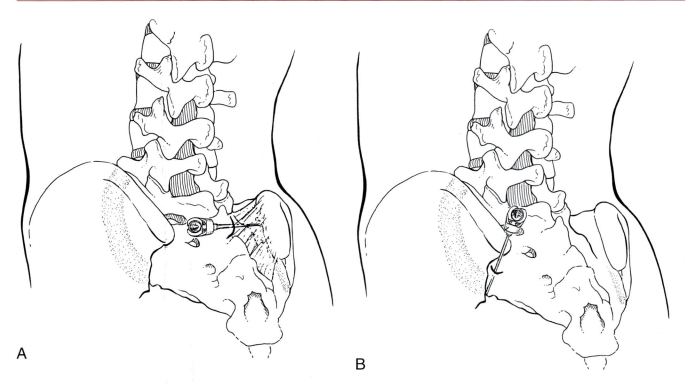

FIGURE 35.8.
Injection into **A.** the area of the sacroiliac joint, or **B.** the joint space of the sacroiliac joint.

without x-ray guidance had pain relief. Seven of 20 patients subsequently injected with triamcinolone diacetate in pursuit of a therapeutic response had more than 75% relief at the end of 6 months of follow-up. In one other uncontrolled study of patients who had seronegative spondyloarthropathy, 81% had more than 70% relief of their pain, and only 26% had a relapse (108). There are no controlled studies testing the value of this therapy.

Facet Injection

There is controversy concerning the frequency with which the facet joints, or zygapophyseal joints, are the source of back pain. There is no doubt that the joint capsule, fibroadipose menisci, and synovial folds are well innervated (59, 112). That these nerves convey pain-producing impulses is evident from the presence in the joint of the neuropeptide substance P, which is associated with nociceptive fibers (49). Also, injection of hypertonic saline into or around the lumbar facet joint capsule produces pain in the back, buttocks, and proximal thigh, while distension of normal cervical facet joint capsules produces unilateral pain ranging from occipital and the upper neck for the atlanto-occipital, atlantoaxial, and C2-C3 joints to scapular pain from the C6-C7 joint (44, 46, 109, 114). Physiologic recordings in laboratory animals have documented mechanoreceptive sensory fields in facet joints (26, 156).

Despite the clear ability of facet joints to produce pain, the incidence of facet pain as the primary pathogenesis of clinical back pain is unclear. First, intervertebral disc degeneration is present in all cases of lumbar facet disease evident by computed tomography (CT) or magnetic resonance imaging (MRI) (22). In addition, stimulation of other vertebral elements by injection or during surgery on awake patients using local anesthesia evokes pain in the back, hip, and buttock indistinguishable from pain produced by facet irritation (47, 53, 71, 85, 89, 116, 143, 151). Therefore, it is difficult on the basis of symptoms to distinguish pathology of the facets from other sources. For the same reasons, the role of facet pathology in generating pain in any particular patient is usually ambiguous. Imaging is also unreliable, since degenerative facet arthritis is seen in CT scans of 10.4% of asymptomatic patients (152). It is in this setting that injection of the joint or the facet nerves leading to the joint is performed to identify their contribution to the patient's pain.

Technique

For the performance of facet blocks, imaging with fluoroscopy is essential. With advanced disease and joint changes, CT imaging may be helpful (117). For lumbar facet joint injection, the patient is placed prone with a pad under the abdomen to lessen the lumbar lordosis. The desired facet is identified with the x-ray beam in a sagittal or minimally oblique angle (Fig. 35.9A) (24). Since the lumbar facets are curved, the joint will also be apparent on more oblique views, but this reveals the joint at its anterior portion, which cannot be directly punctured. After marking the skin and preparing the area, local anesthetic is injected superficially. A 22-gauge spinal needle is inserted along the axis of the beam and directed into the joint space. The bone adjacent to the joint space rises in a ridge, and the needle tip may need to be "walked up" over this ridge before it falls into the joint space. Usually, it can be sensed when the needle slides between the opposing articular surfaces (Fig. 35.9B), and a deviation of the needle tip may also be apparent.

The patient should be asked to compare the distribution of pain created by needle contact with the joint to the usual pain. Injection of 0.5 mL water-soluble contrast (e.g., iopamidol) confirms proper placement by outlining the joint space. Distension of the capsule at the superior and especially the inferior recesses of the joint space create a dumbbell shape, and anterior spread in the joint is seen as a medial sheet. After intra-articular placement is confirmed, 1 mL lidocaine 1% or bupivacaine 0.5% is injected. Steroid (e.g., 20 mg methylprednisolone acetate or 25 mg triamcinolone diacetate) is usually included in pursuit of long-term benefits (23, 95, 100). The prin-

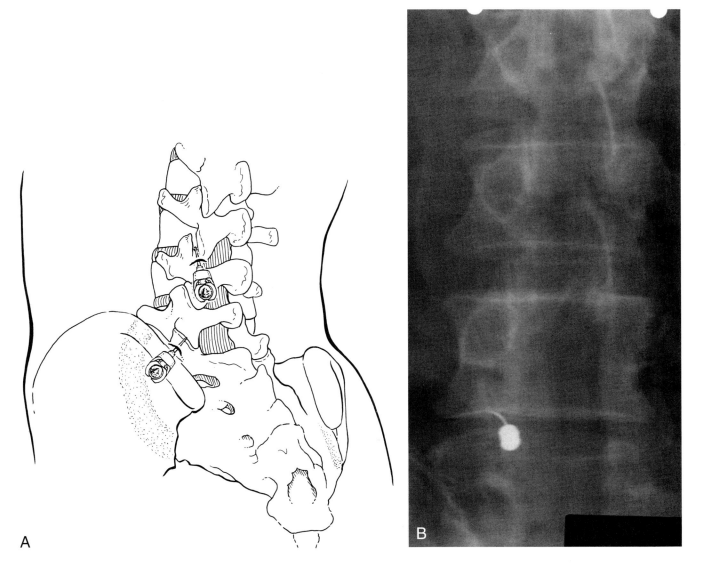

FIGURE 35.9.

A. Lumbar facet joint injection. The plane of the joint space is more coronal in orientation at L5-S1 (lower needle) than at higher levels such as L3-L4 (upper needle). **B.** Needle in place for left L4-L5 facet joint injection.

cipal risk of the procedure is mistaken injection into a nerve root or the subarachnoid space (61). If the patient is not sedated, contact with a nerve root will incite lancinating pain, and aspiration will usually indicate entry into the cerebrospinal fluid (CSF).

To inject into a cervical facet joint, either a lateral or posterior approach may be used. In the posterior method, the patient is positioned prone with a cushion under the chest to allow marked flexion of the neck. The x-ray beam is angled into the plane of the facets, and the needle is directed at the midpoint of the joint. The lateral approach uses a lateral fluoroscopic view achieved with the patient lying on the uninvolved side (Fig. 35.10A). Care must be taken to assure that the images of the right and left joints are superimposed, since it impossible to distinguish the target joint from the contralateral one. The needle is then directed toward the midpoint of the joint, and confirmation of entry is obtained by contrast injection (Fig. 35.10B). Intrathecal or intra-arterial injection is particularly dangerous at cervical levels, so the needle should be advanced cautiously, aspiration should precede injection, and the full dose should only be administered after a test dose of 0.25 mL.

Upper cervical joints may be difficult to image, and the head may need to be turned slightly to one side. Techniques are available for injection of the atlanto-occipital and lateral atlantoaxial joints (44).

Changes in symptoms in response to the block should be monitored by repeating the physical examination within the half hour following the injection, with attention focused on the maneuvers that provoked the pain prior to injection. The patient's pain may be attributed to a facet source if the pain produced by needling is similar to the usual pain, if pain relief is noted in response to local anesthetic injection, and if the postblock sensory exam shows no evidence of segmental spinal nerve block.

As an alternative to injection into the joint space, afferent traffic from the joint may be interrupted by block of the medial branch of the posterior primary ramus of the spinal nerve, which innervates the facet joint (Fig. 35.7B). In the lumbar region, the medial branch of the posterior primary ramus travels caudally and medially from the intervertebral foramen across the junction of the superior articular process and the transverse process (14). It passes along bone between the mammillary process on the base of the

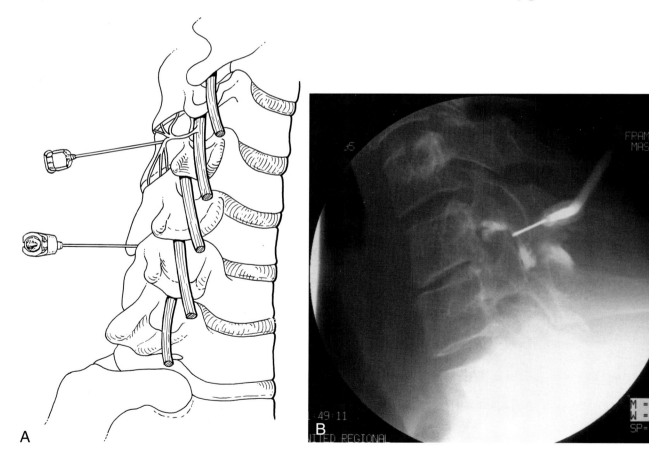

FIGURE 35.10.

A. Cervical facet joint injection (lower needle) using a lateral approach, and for cervical facet nerve block (upper needle). **B.** Arthrogram after left C5-C6 cervical facet joint injection with 0.5 mL contrast medium, showing accumulation in the superior and inferior joint capsule.

superior articular process and the accessory process on the inferior and medial end of the transverse process, enclosed by the mammillo-accessory ligament. At this point it gives off branches to the inferior pole of the facet joint at that level. The nerve continues caudally along the lamina in a medial direction, giving off another set of articular branches to the superior pole of the next joint. The L5 nerve crosses over the base of the sacral ala instead of a transverse process.

By these routes, each facet receives terminal fibers from two posterior rami (e.g., the L4-L5 facet is innervated at its upper pole by branches from L3 and at its lower pole by branches from L4) so two injections are necessary to anesthetize a joint. Blockade of the dorsal primary ramus can be achieved by injection of 1 mL or less local anesthetic on the dorsal aspect of the transverse process at the medial end of its superior edge (Fig. 35.11) (15). Since there is no cutaneous innervation by these branches, adequacy of the block cannot be confirmed by superficial examination. Provocative stimuli of the joint, such as mechanical or chemical irritation, should be repeated after the block to check adequacy of denervation.

Cervical facets may similarly be blocked by injection of the nerves prior to their arrival in the joint capsule (Fig. 35.10A) (7, 13). As in the lumbar region, each joint is innervated by nerves from two levels (e.g., the C5-C6 facet is innervated by branches from the C5 and C6 spinal nerves). From the intervertebral foramen, the medial branch of the posterior primary ramus crosses the middle of the lateral aspect of the articular pillar. At this site, 0.5 mL anesthetic through a needle placed by a lateral approach can effect blockade. The C2-C3 facet differs in having a disproportionate innervation from the C3 medial branch, which crosses over the lateral aspect of the joint space, and minimal contribution from C2 (16). Whereas two injections are required for complete blockade of the other cervical joints, innervation to the C2-C3 articulation can be blocked by injection on the outer surface of the joint capsule at the midpoint of its lateral aspect. Guidance for cervical medial branch injection is best achieved using fluoroscopy in the lateral position, and the risks in these nerve injections are the same as those mentioned for injection into the cervical facet itself.

Evaluation: Diagnosis

The application of block techniques has been used to gain insight into the frequency of the facet as a clinical source of pain. In a noncontrolled and non-blinded study of patients who had chronic low back pain without radiculopathy, 38% had relief after injection into the suspected joint, but 25% of those assigned to receive medial branch nerve blockade of a randomly chosen joint also had immediate relief (106). Both of these rates are comparable to the expected frequency of placebo response. Total absence of pain after injection of local anesthetic into the lumbar facets is less common, occurring in only about 7% of back pain patients (23, 82). Such studies indicate that in typical patient groups suspected of having facet disease, the facets may be an origin of at least part of the patients' pain but rarely the unique or major source.

The ability of blockade techniques to prove facet disease conclusively is uncertain. The are several sources of inaccuracy. Even if mechanical irritation of the joint capsule during facet injection produces discomfort resembling the patient's typical pain, this may not reliably indicate the site of the patient's pathology, since cervical (46, 99) and lumbar (99, 105, 109, 114) facet stimulation produces broadly overlapping areas of pain distribution even into the distal extremity. Patients in whom their usual pain is recreated by facet stimulation are not necessarily the same patients in whom local anesthetic injection in the joint relieves pain (52), and there is a poor correlation between pain provocation and relief from local anesthetic injection (138). In one study, 31% of patients who had a positive response to pain provocation failed to have relief after anesthetic injection into that lumbar facet, and 40% who had relief from injection had not had typical pain during needle

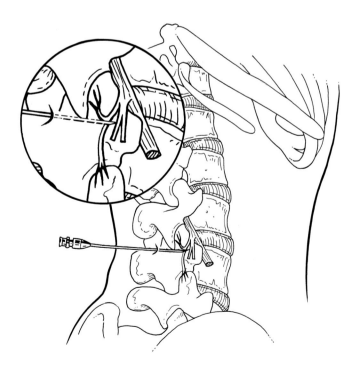

FIGURE 35.11.
Blockade of the lumbar median branch of the dorsal primary ramus for nerve block of the facet joint.

stimulation or distension of the facet capsule with contrast medium (115).

Since the specificity of facet denervation depends on limiting anesthetic spread to the joint or the nerves to the joint, further uncertainty may result from undesired anesthetic spread. The facet joints are not capacious, and rupture during intra-articular injection has been identified after injection of more than 1 mL into cervical facets and after most lumbar injections and also has been demonstrated in cadaver facet injections (37, 42, 43, 115). This spills local anesthetic into neighboring tissues, so pain that is relieved by facet injection could in fact be pain from pathology in muscle, periosteum, or ligaments. Passage of anesthetic into the epidural space or the intervertebral foramen, which occurs routinely with capsule rupture, could interrupt nociception from sensitive structures in the vertebral canal, such as anterior dura and posterior longitudinal ligament, or from any distal site by effects on afferent fibers in the spinal roots (37). Spondylolysis is found in 18% of patients suspected of having lumbar facet pain (103). With this condition, intra-articular facet injection is consistently followed by spread of solution into the epidural space and to adjacent and contralateral facets, and even laterally along a spinal nerve, limiting the specificity of the test (57, 103, 111).

These sources of error limit the diagnostic utility of facet injection. In one study, facet block produced relief in 47% of low back pain patients, but a repeat injection was positive in only 31% of the patients who had initial positive blocks (137). This indicates either a strong placebo component or subtle technical difficulties that cannot be controlled. Relief after facet injection has been evaluated as a prognostic indicator for response to posterolateral lumbosacral fusions, but block results did not reliably predict surgical outcome (81).

Caution must also be used when interpreting blockade of medial branches of the posterior primary rami, since these injections denervate not only the joints they supply but also the muscles, ligaments, and periosteum into which they ramify. Since each medial branch supplies parts of two facets, complete denervation of one facet requires partial blockade of the one above and the one below. Therefore, relief obtained from the blocks cannot distinguish among pain originating at any of the three. Since medial nerve blockade more accurately simulates the effect of radiofrequency denervation than does intra-articular injection, it is the appropriate diagnostic test prior to that procedure.

Because there is no histopathologic standard for confirming facet arthropathy as a source of pain, validation of facet block as a diagnostic measure is ultimately impossible. However, the evidence from multiple studies suggests that facet blockade is useful in resolving back pain pathogenesis if its limitations are borne in mind.

Evaluation: Therapeutic Application

Therapeutic responses have been reported following intra-articular zygapophyseal joint injection, especially if steroid is included, usually about 20 to 40 mg of methylprednisolone acetate or the equivalent. Steroid injected into the lumbar facet joints results in significant relief outlasting the local anesthetic in 30 to 54% of selected patients who have back pain (25, 37, 69, 100, 117). Response rates are lower for patients who have had previous lumbar spine surgery, and after surgery, extra-articular injection is less likely to be therapeutic (99, 100). It should be noted, however, that pain returns by 6 months in many of the steroid responders. Beneficial effects of cervical facet injection with steroid have been reported in 91% of patients, but recurrence occurred in one-half of them (132). In another series, even though there was complete initial relief from cervical facet local anesthetic blockade, there was no lasting benefit from steroid injection (77).

Only two controlled and randomized trials of facet steroid injection have been reported. In one, the results after steroid injection were no different from those after saline injection (95). In the other study, saline injected into lumbar joints produced no discernible difference from steroid injection until 6 months afterward, at which time patients injected with steroid more frequently indicated improvement in their pain (23). This study has been interpreted as showing the inefficacy of steroid facet injections, because of the modest differences between the treatment and control groups and the delay in response (39). However, the selection criteria for facet joint injection candidates included no history, physical examination, or imaging criteria, and all other therapy (except acetaminophen) was discontinued upon injection.

From the available evidence, it should be concluded that the therapeutic efficacy of intra-articular steroid in the facet joint has not been proved. However, if the joint is to be entered for a diagnostic block, steroid injection adds little additional risk and may be beneficial. It is most appropriately used as a component of a rehabilitation program.

Selective Spinal Nerve Injection

Anesthetic injection of a segmental nerve by a paravertebral approach, also known as a foraminal injection (and mistakenly referred to as nerve root injection) has diagnostic as well as therapeutic potential. As with facet blockade, the quality and distribution of the pain produced by needle contact with an individual nerve may be compared with the patient's complaint. Relief following anesthesia of the nerve also further indicates that the nerve is the source of pain.

Selective nerve injection is typically used in the setting of diagnostic confusion, such as when the history, physical examination, imaging, and electromyography are inconclusive or contradictory. Other similar circumstances include the multiply operated back, patients with pathology identified at multiple levels, and back and hip disease occurring in combination. Often, selective spinal nerve block is used for surgical planning, such as for determining the site of foraminotomy.

Therapy for radiculopathy may be attempted by steroid injection in the immediate vicinity of the affected nerve. This approach may be chosen particularly if a midline injection into the epidural space is impossible. Steroid applied outside the foramen by paravertebral injection also may be successful in combination with epidural injection or when epidural injection has failed because of nerve injury within or lateral to an occluded intervertebral foramen.

Technique

This procedure is best performed with radiologic imaging to select the proper level and to confirm needle placement at the lateral aspect of the intervertebral foramen. For lumbar injections (Fig. 35.12A), the patient is placed prone and the skin is marked overlying the pedicle of the same numbered vertebra as the nerve that is to be blocked (e.g., the L5 pedicle for the L5 nerve). The lumbar roots pivot tightly under the pedicles as they enter the intervertebral foramina where the posterior root ganglion sits immediately caudal to the pedicles (30, 72). The target for needle insertion should be at the outer portion of the foramen, in line with the lateral edge of the pedicles. A site for needle insertion is chosen about 3 cm lateral to the skin mark to produce a mesiad angle that will allow the needle to pass under the overhanging lamina. A 22-gauge spinal needle is suitable for most subjects. Local anesthetic in the skin and deeper tissues makes the approach to the vertebra more comfortable, and frequent fluoroscopic checks diminish the need for multiple insertions. The needle can be directed to contact the transverse process first. After determining this depth, the nerve should be identified within 2 or 3 cm of further needle advancement after sliding inferior to the transverse process (88, 146).

Gentle contact of the needle with the nerve confirms exact placement by the production of a paresthesia. The patient is then asked if the quality and distribution of the provoked sensation is similar to the usual pain. A mechanical paresthesia also assures that the needle is within the nerve sheath (epineurium) or close to it, where even a small volume of local anesthetic will be effective. Injection of 0.2 to 0.5 mL non-ionic water-soluble contrast medium (e.g., iopamidol) reveals the extent of solution spread along the nerve if the needle is properly placed (Fig. 35.12B). In an anterior/posterior view, the normal contour of the nerves is straight as they travel laterally and inferiorly. A deformity may offer diagnostic evidence of a lateral extruded fragment of disc material. If contrast outlines the nerve but fails to flow proximally as it usually does, foraminal stenosis may be the cause. Once the needle is suitably placed, 1 mL local anesthetic, typically lidocaine 1% or bupivacaine 0.25%, is injected to anesthetize the nerve. This may be mixed with 20 to 40 mg of methylprednisolone acetate or the equivalent in pursuit of a lasting response.

Successful blockade is evident if a segmental sensory deficit develops. These changes may be subtle, so scratch and cold sensation should be tested as well as touch. Since neural dysfunction is part of the baseline pathophysiology, a careful examination is necessary before injection for comparison. Maneuvers that produced pain prior to the block such as straight-leg-lift or walking should be repeated afterward to evaluate the effect of the block. Optimal insight into the origin of the pain is gained by testing two or three adjacent nerves on separate occasions (135). Possible complications include nerve injury and extensive block, but the risk for these is limited by using only small volumes of local anesthetic, monitoring fluoroscopic images, and aborting injection if it is accompanied by intense pain (58).

The first sacral nerve is blocked by a transsacral approach with the patient prone. Because of the lumbar lordosis, fluoroscopic guidance is improved when the beam is angled caudally, to be perpendicular to the sacrum. With the posterior and anterior sacral foramina superimposed in the image, the needle can be passed to make contact with the spinal nerve in the middle portion of the canal. The rest of the block is done as it is at lumbar levels.

Cervical spinal nerve block is performed with the patient in the supine position and also requires fluoroscopy to be confident that the appropriate nerve is injected. A 22-gauge needle is inserted with a somewhat caudal angle to avoid entry into the intervertebral foramen and is directed to the transverse process (C5 for the C5 nerve, etc.). The brachial plexus overlying the spinal nerves is avoided by entering in a plane anterior to the plexus. A paresthesia can usually be elicited by searching anteriorly and posteriorly along the shelf of transverse process between the anterior and posterior tubercles. The rest of the procedure is the same as that for lumbar injec-

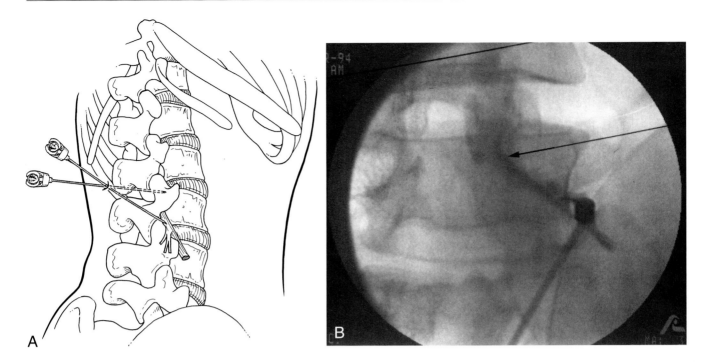

FIGURE 35.12.

A. Anatomy and technique of lumbar selective spinal nerve injection. The needle is first directed to *(1)* the transverse process to ascertain proper depth, and is then redirected *(2)* inferior and just beyond the transverse process where a paresthesia is sought. **B.** Spread of injectate with selective spinal nerve injection. This posteroanterior x-ray image shows the distribution of 0.5 mL contrast medium injected after paresthesia of the right L5 nerve. Contrast medium is seen spreading proximally (arrow), medial to the pedicle into the epidural space, and distally along the nerve. The needle and tubing connected to it are also seen.

tions. Special care in aspirating for blood prior to injection is necessary, since the vertebral artery is in the vicinity of the cervical spinal nerves. Local anesthetic volumes as small as 0.25 mL injected into the vertebral artery can produce a seizure, since it is delivered to the brain undiluted. Needle placement within the foramen risks subarachnoid injection. Even the small volumes of local anesthetic that are used could produce hypotension or respiratory muscle dysfunction if injected into the cervical subarachnoid space.

Evaluation

The pain provocation portion of the spinal nerve injection test examines pain quality and distribution. Duplication of the typical quality of the pain as a criterion is supported by the demonstration that inflamed nerves are more sensitive to manipulation than normal nerves (53, 143). Whereas mechanical stimulation of normal nerves produces paresthesias, an inflamed nerve reproduces characteristic radiating pain when touched. The distribution of the evoked sensation is less certain to be reliable. Since pain with the stimulation of different roots produces overlapping areas of radiation, these patterns may not distinguish the involved root from adjacent ones (143).

Pain relief with blockade of a spinal nerve cannot distinguish between pathology of the proximal nerve in the intervertebral foramen or pain transmitted from distal sites by that nerve. Both tissue injury in the nerve's distribution and neuropathic pain would each be relieved by a proximal block of a nerve. The ability of injection to block vertebral pain without blocking hip pain has not been demonstrated. The accuracy of spinal nerve block depends upon limiting spread of anesthetic to the selected nerve alone. Flow into the intervertebral foramen and epidural space is commonly observed and definitely compromises this assumption (36, 41, 67, 88, 147). Not only will this block pain transmitted by the sinuvertebral nerve from the dura, posterior longitudinal ligament, and annular ligament of the intervertebral disc, but also the spread via the epidural space to other segmental levels could produce misleading results. For instance, injection of a normal nerve S1 with spread to an inflamed L5 nerve could produce relief, with the guilty nerve assumed to be S1. For this reason injection volumes should be limited to only 1 to 2 mL, and the test should not be used outside the context of thorough overall evaluation.

The ability of selective spinal nerve blocks to diagnose disease and predict surgical outcome has been examined in a few retrospective studies. The fraction of patients who have had injections indicating radiculopathy and in whom surgery confirmed radicular pathology at the level indicated by the test (positive predictive values) ranges from 87% to 100% (41, 67, 88, 135). The reliability of a negative response is poorly studied, because few patients have had surgery after a negative test. The proportion of patients who had a negative injection test and who are confirmed at surgery to have normal nerve roots (negative predictive value) is between 27% and 38% in the small number of patients operated on despite a negative test (41, 67). Only one prospective study has appeared, and it showed a positive predictive value of 95% and an untested negative predictive value (146). In general, the accuracy of nerve blocks is better than imaging or electromyography (67, 146). No studies using controls or blinding have been conducted on the diagnostic accuracy of lumbar selective spinal nerve blocks, and the utility of cervical diagnostic spinal nerve injections has not been formally examined in any fashion. A positive paravertebral spinal nerve injection test does not predict success by neuroablative surgery, either by dorsal rhizotomy or by dorsal root ganglionectomy (98, 122, 123).

Despite the lack of conclusive studies and limitations in the interpretation of this technique, a broad group of surgical authorities have found benefits in the use of spinal nerve injection for planning decompressive surgery on complicated patients. There is a need for controlled and blinded studies to refute or support these beliefs. It has no role in evaluating patients for neuroablative procedures. Therapeutic responses are occasionally seen after selective spinal nerve injection, especially if steroid has been used. This may be attributable to steroid effects (see below) or increased blood flow to the compressed root secondary to blockade of sympathetic vasomotor fibers (155). However, no controlled study has been designed to test the value of this treatment.

Epidural Injections

Treatment of radiculopathy and back pain with the epidural injection of steroids is a well-established therapeutic method. Despite its extensive use, however, there remains a vigorous controversy over the suitable application of epidural steroid injections, particularly with regard to indications and complications.

The rationale for steroid treatment of radiculopathy stems from the recognition of the central role of inflammation in the production of pain after leakage of nucleus pulposus from the intervertebral disc. Unlike uninjured roots, inflamed dorsal roots are exquisitely mechanosensitive, generating prolonged repetitive firing upon slight manipulation (78). Dorsal root ganglia are mechanically sensitive even in the absence of injury. As demonstrated in awake patients, manipulation of nerve roots produces the characteristic pain of radiculopathy only when the root is inflamed (89, 143). Histologic studies and intraoperative observations confirm the consistent association of nerve root pain with inflammation (96). Further support for the inflammatory etiology of radiculopathy is derived from the observation that pain resolves despite the persistence of myelographic changes (11). Autogenous nucleus pulposus produces a vigorous inflammatory reaction when injected into the epidural space, by two possible mechanisms (68, 110). A reaction may be provoked directly by the tremendous concentrations of phospholipase A_2 present in nuclear material (134). This enzyme initiates the arachidonic acid cascade central to the inflammatory response. Secondly, because the avascular nucleus of the disc is isolated from the body's immune mechanisms, its proteoglycans are antigenically active in provoking an autoimmune response, contributing to inflammation (12, 107, 118).

The well known anti-inflammatory efficacy of corticosteroids is a logical means of addressing the fundamental pathophysiology of radiculopathy in the presence of disc herniation. Additionally, injured nerves are a source of spontaneous signal generation, which is promptly quelled by topically applied corticosteroid (38). This begins in minutes, far sooner than can be attributed to an anti-inflammatory effect, and it is probably a result of a direct effect on neuronal membrane receptors to produce cell hyperpolarization (79). Furthermore, a probably minor contribution to the analgesic effect of steroids in painful conditions is a result of a selective and reversible conduction blockade of the small, pain-transmitting C-fiber axons (84). A final steroid effect may be modulation of sensory processing in the substantia gelatinosa of the spinal cord dorsal horn (56).

Radiculopathy caused by tumor may also respond to epidural steroid administration. Patients who have conditions other than radiculopathy, such as strain, degenerative joint disease, spondylolisthesis, spinal stenosis, and idiopathic back pain, are additionally frequent subjects for epidural steroid injection. The rationale behind epidural steroid injection for nonradicular back pain is similar to that for radiculopathy, although the target nociceptive sources are structures other than the nerve root, such as the posterior longitudinal ligament, anterior dura, annular ligament, or possibly the sinuvertebral nerves and rami communicantes subserving these structures. The lack of a clear inflammatory causal component in back pain without radiculopathy predicts a less consistent beneficial response.

In addition to steroids and local anesthetics, other agents are occasionally injected epidurally for painful chronic back conditions. Morphine has been added to steroid epidural injections with the apparent result of prolonging the analgesic response in postlaminectomy patients, presumably because of an action upon opioid receptors in the spinal cord (31). Since results have not been encouraging in subsequent controlled studies, this approach has few indications (34, 131). Hypertonic (10%) saline has also been included in epidural injections for the treatment of pain (127). Large volumes of injectate (up to 50 mL) are used, and repeated injections are given on a daily basis. The goal is lysis of epidural adhesions, local anesthetic effect, and reduction of tissue edema, but these outcomes have not been proved. Since hypertonic saline also has neurolytic potential, this utility of this technique is uncertain.

Technique

A thorough physical examination immediately before the injection procedure provides the basis for comparison with a subsequent examination after the block. An intravenous line is not usually necessary, but emergency resuscitation equipment and a physician capable of resuscitative measures must be available. Vital signs should be monitored throughout the procedure. Sedation should be avoided, since an obtunded patient may fail to respond to the contact of a needle or catheter with a nerve or spinal cord. The procedure is contraindicated if there is infection at the injection site, if there is any degree of spina bifida, and if the patient is receiving anticoagulants. Nonsteroidal anti-inflammatory agents probably do not significantly increase the risk of bleeding from the injection.

Epidural needle insertion may be performed with the patient in the sitting or the lateral position. Identification of the midline, a key to success in performing epidural anesthesia, is more easily achieved with the patient sitting, particularly in a stout subject. After sterile skin preparation, local anesthetic is injected in the skin and deeper fascial and ligamentous structures to permit perfection in needle placement without the anguish that repeat insertions may cause. Also, insertion of the large epidural needle is easier after identification of the spinous processes (and therefore the midline) using the smaller-gauge needle for exploration and anesthetic injection.

A 17-gauge or 18-gauge needle is used for epidural placement, usually a standard type with an eccentric orifice and slightly curved tip (Tuohy needle) to lessen the chance of dural puncture. The needle passes in sequence through the skin, subcutaneous tissue, supraspinous and interspinous ligaments, and thence into the ligamentum flavum (Fig. 35.13). Because of the perpendicular orientation of the lumbar and cervical spinous processes, a midline needle must enter at an angle nearly perpendicular to the axis of the dural sac. The depth of the vertebral canal

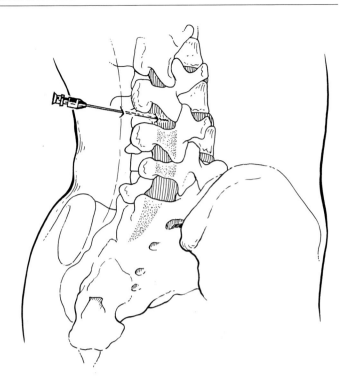

FIGURE 35.13.

Lumbar epidural injection. The patient is usually in a more flexed position than shown here.

from the skin is highly variable, depending on the level in the vertebral column, the amount of subcutaneous fat, body size, and needle angle, such that no safe rule of thumb can be applied.

When the needle tip enters the elastin of the ligamentum flavum, it is possible to discern a change in the texture of the tissues, with a firm homogeneous resistance to advancement rather than the fibrous quality characteristic of the more superficial collagenous ligaments. Compression of the ligamentum flavum will reproduce the pain in some patients with a highly irritable inflamed nerve. Upon passing anterior to the ligamentum flavum, injected air or saline readily passes into the plane between the nonadherent dorsal fat pad and the canal wall. This is the "loss of resistance" noted when the syringe plunger suddenly yields to pressure exerted during needle advancement. Rotation of the needle should be avoided, for this increases the chances of the point's penetrating the dura. Aspiration through the needle is performed to check for return of CSF or blood, in which cases the needle is removed and reinserted at the same or an adjacent level. With age, loss of disc height causes spinous processes to contact one another. Arthritic changes in the facets further complicate entry into the vertebral canal as the space between the laminae of adjacent vertebrae is narrowed. Even in younger individuals, bone may grow into the margins of the ligamenta flava, which may also make needle placement difficult.

After entry of the needle tip into the epidural space has been confirmed, the therapeutic solution is slowly injected. The most common and suitable mix is 2 mL depot corticosteroid (methylprednisolone acetate 40 mg/mL, or triamcinolone diacetate 25 mg/mL) diluted in 5 mL lidocaine 1%. Initial injection may produce a mild temporary provocation of radicular pain by compression of the nerve. When the entire injection has been completed, the patient is placed in a lateral position with the painful side down to assist in distribution of the solution to that side. This position should be maintained for 15 minutes or so, and when the patient first arises there should be assistance available, since lower extremity muscle weakness may temporarily compromise weightbearing. It is advisable not to have the patient drive him- or herself home. The brief interval of relief from the local anesthetic in the injection can be used to further physical therapy. All other therapeutic efforts should be continued during a course of injections.

At cervical levels, the same technique may be used as at lumbar levels, but great care must be taken to avoid excessive depth of needle placement or sudden movement of the patient. An alternative technique uses a drop of saline or anesthetic solution placed in the needle hub, which can be seen to be sucked into the needle as the tip enters the epidural space.

Solution should be injected as close as possible to the suspected site of radiculopathy. At lumbar levels, the line between the iliac crests often crosses the vertebral column at the L4–5 disc. Although this is not totally reliable because of natural variability in anatomic parameters, the error will rarely be more than a one-segment deviation, which is unlikely to matter (73). A greater problem is encountered with injections in patients who have had previous surgery at the intended injection site. Needle placement through the surgical scar cannot be predictably guided to what remains of the epidural space in the operative site. If there is no free space without scar adhesions, the needle may inadvertently be passed into the subarachnoid space.

A more desirable approach in postlaminectomy patients is to pass a catheter through a needle placed in the sacral hiatus. With the patient prone, an epidural needle is passed through the skin and the sacrococcygeal membrane into the sacral epidural space (Fig. 35.14A). If fluoroscopic guidance is not used, failure rates are high, including unrecognized

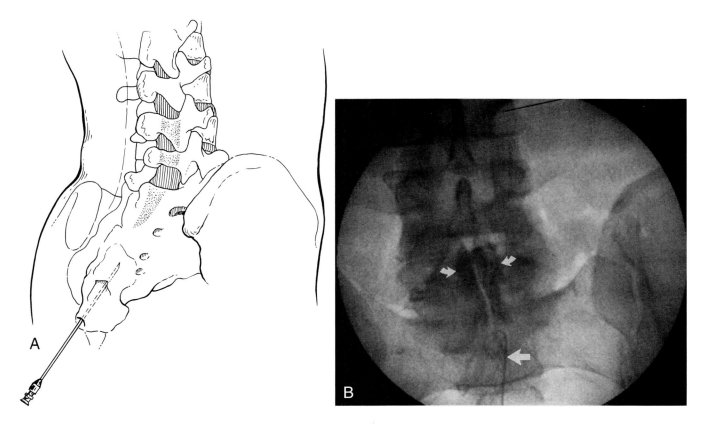

FIGURE 35.14.
A. Caudal catheter technique for epidural steroid administration, showing the needle in place prior to passage of the catheter. The dural sac, also depicted, ends at about the second sacral level. B. Injection of contrast medium and anesthetic/steroid solution (curved arrows) through a caudal catheter (straight arrow) passed to the level of the L5-S1 disc. The lucency in the contrast medium is due to displacement of contrast medium by the midline dorsal epidural fat.

placement of the needle outside the spinal canal or within an vessel (130). After confirming accurate needle entry into the caudal canal, a catheter with a stiffening stylet can be guided cephalad into the proximity of the suspected inflamed root (Fig. 35.14B). Often scarring can be recognized by resistance to further catheter advancement and by the exclusion of contrast injected through the catheter. Using the caudal epidural space as an access route assures that the tip through which the solution is injected will be in the right tissue plane, and fluoroscopic observation confirms that the catheter has passed proximally to the necessary level. Although these measures make sense, the superiority of injection through a catheter over injection through a needle placed just within the sacrococcygeal membrane has not been proved. The great variability in anatomy of the sacral canal and the occasional high volume of the canal is a further incentive not to rely on delivery of solution to the L5 or S1 nerve roots without a catheter (148).

The indications for further injections depends on the response to the first. If adequate relief is provided by a single injection, then additional injections need not be performed. If no response was apparent after the first injection, either the medication did not reach the involved nerve or the problem is not responsive to this regimen. The inclusion of local anesthetic in the injectate allows a distinction to be made between these possibilities. If there is no relief immediately after injection of a solution containing local anesthetic, it is likely that it did not enter the epidural space or was excessively distant from the involved root, and the block should be repeated. If local anesthetic produces a temporary effect, but no response to the steroid is evident within 6 days, then little will be gained by further injection, since most steroid responses should occur within this time frame (62). However, further steroid treatment might be chosen despite an initial negative response in a patient who has a high surgical risk in whom all other options have been exhausted.

The most common pattern of response to the first epidural injection of steroids for radiculopathy pain is relief that begins about 2 to 6 days after the injection and is either incomplete or does not persist. In this setting, a second injection is indicated, usually after an interval of 10 to 14 days. A decision to perform a third injection should be based on the response to the second using the same paradigm. It is unlikely that additional injections after three will contribute any benefit. The indiscriminate practice of three mandatory injections and inappropriate administration of prolonged series of blocks has tarnished the reputation of a technique that should be used on a thoughtful basis.

Evaluation

Several recent reviews weigh the data available regarding the efficacy and risk of epidural steroid injection for back pain and radiculopathy (4, 9, 66). While numerous uncontrolled series have been reported in support of the technique, there are relatively few carefully controlled and blinded studies. Of these, the majority have shown benefits of epidural steroid injection therapy over controls, including lessened pain, decreased analgesic requirements, more prompt return to work, and greater mobility (20, 21, 40, 157). Response rates in the steroid-treated groups are around 60%, about twice the recovery rate in the control groups (20, 40). In another controlled study, epidural steroid injection showed no benefit in pain of short duration, but steroid injection yielded better results than the control-treatment group's response for pain of longer duration (8). Negative studies have also been published that fail to demonstrate any benefit from epidural steroid injection compared to control treatments, adding confusion to the consideration of steroid use for radiculopathy and back pain (33, 144). However, these studies have serious limitations, including the use of only 2 mL solution, injection at the same interspace regardless of the level of pathology, evaluation of the patient after only 24 to 48 hours, the use of no more than one injection, prolonged bed rest, and failure to use other concurrent therapies. All of these factors will tend to produce fewer successes, and they do not reflect conventional practice. Considering treatment a failure if it provides less than 75% relief of symptoms does not acknowledge the desire of chronic pain patients for any degree of relief (33).

The probability of a favorable outcome from epidural steroid injections strongly depends on the underlying disease (3, 9, 66). Radiculopathy is the optimal indication, whereas bony abnormalities such as spinal stenosis, spondylosis, or spondylolisthesis are less responsive to this treatment. The frequency of success is much diminished by previous laminectomy. Other factors associated with diminished efficacy include prolonged duration of pain, loss of work from pain, a persistent pattern of pain, sleep disruption, unemployment because of pain, and low educational level. In general, once the multifaceted chronic pain syndrome has evolved, with emotional, social, pharmacologic, financial, and legal ramifications, even an accurately aimed therapeutic attack upon the ancestral pathophysiologic source may no longer be adequate.

Side effects and complications may occur after epidural steroid injection, either from the needle procedure, local anesthetic effect, or systemic absorption of the corticosteroid (4). Needle injury may include unintended dural puncture with the possible development of headache, hematoma, or the introduction of infection. The incidence of dural puncture should be less than 2% in skillful hands, while bleeding and infection are extremely rare. Hemodynamic or ventilatory compromise might occur if lidocaine is injected in the subarachnoid space, but this malposition of the needle tip should be recognized by aspiration of CSF through the needle. Intravascular injection of these doses have not been reported to be problematic.

Systemic levels of corticosteroid are generated by epidural injections sufficient to suppress plasma cortisol levels for three weeks. Cushingoid side effects have been occasionally reported, including changes in fat distribution, weight gain, fluid retention, hypertension, and even congestive heart failure. These events are also rare, but subjects prone to such complications because of preexisting disease should be treated cautiously.

The most aggressive critique leveled at the use of epidural steroid injections has asserted an unacceptably high risk of neurologic complication (120). It is contended that the polyethylene glycol component of the depot preparations of methylprednisolone acetate and triamcinolone diacetate may cause arachnoiditis, as has occasionally been noted following intrathecal injection of these agents. The evidence for this is anecdotal, and the patients in these cases have typically had preexisting neural disease and received multiple injections into the subarachnoid space. By the most pessimistic estimate, arachnoiditis may occur in as many as 10% of subarachnoid depot steroid injections (120). However, eight series of intrathecal steroid injections encompassing 358 patients failed to produce a single case of arachnoiditis (4). Nonetheless, because of this concern, because intrathecal steroids may also produce transient aseptic meningitis, and because intrathecal injection offers little benefit beyond epidural administration for treatment of sciatica, conventional practice dictates that injection of depot corticosteroids into the cerebrospinal fluid should rarely be done (1). Caution should be exercised to avoid intrathecal placement during intended epidural injection. Testing for aspiration of CSF through the needle is certainly indicated, and some recommend injection of an initial 2 mL dose of local anesthetic alone to seek evidence of intrathecal effect (anesthesia) prior to the injection of steroid.

An alarmist view condemning epidural steroid injections as well as intrathecal injection is based on mistaken evidence. Reports cited by the principal critic as showing the toxicity of the polyethylene glycol component, present in 3% concentrations in depot steroid preparations, in fact studied propylene glycol 80%, (28, 104), or other irritants (80), but not polyethylene glycol alone (120). Examination of the effects of polyethylene glycol on peripheral nerves in concentrations from 3 to 40% showed only temporary conduction block at concentrations of 20% or higher (10). Another study found neuropathic changes after depot corticosteroid only after injection within the neural fascicle, where local anesthetic or even normal saline also produces injury (102, 139). Blind injection of depot steroid preparation around rat sciatic nerves produced pathologic changes without dysfunction, but intrafascicular injection could have been a factor (153). Reassurance is derived from studies showing minimal histologic response to commercial preparations of depot steroids administered in the epidural space and even intrathecally (5, 29, 35). No case of arachnoiditis has been reported following depot steroid injection into the epidural space (4).

It is clear that strongly divergent views are voiced regarding the indications and safety of steroid injections for back pain and radiculopathy (74). A sound approach is to use the technique in the context of other conservative therapies such as physical therapy, mild analgesics, and limited bed rest for acute and subacute disease. A decision to use the technique should include consideration of the likelihood of success as well as the desirability of alternative therapy such as surgery. Finally, it is rarely reasonable to perform more than three injections in a 3- to 6-month interval.

References

1. Abram SE. Subarachnoid corticosteroid injection following inadequate response to epidural steroids for sciatica. Anesth Analg 1978;57:313–315.
2. Abram SE. Pain mechanisms in lumbar radiculopathy. Anesth Analg 1988;67:1135–1137.
3. Abram SE, Hopwood MB. What factors contribute to outcome with lumbar epidural steroids. In: Bond MR, Charlton JE, Wolf CJ, eds. Proceedings of the VIth World Congress on Pain, Amsterdam, Elsevier, 1991: 491–496.
4. Abram SE, O'Connor TC. Complications associated with epidural steroid injections: a review. Reg Anesth 1996;21:149–162.
5. Abram SE, Marsala M, Yaksh TL. Analgesic and neurotoxic effects of intrathecal corticosteroids in rats. Anesthesiology 81:1198–1205.
6. Bahns E, Ernsberger U, Janig W, et al. Discharge properties of mechanosensitive afferents supplying the retroperitoneal space. Pflugers Arch 1986;407:519–525.
7. Barnsley L, Bogduk N. Medial branch blocks are specific for the diagnosis of cervical zygapophyseal joint pain. Reg Anesth 1993;18:343–350.
8. Beliveau P. A comparison between epidural anesthesia with and without corticosteroid in the treatment of sciatica. Rheumatol Phys Med 1977;11:40–43.

9. Benzon H. Epidural steroid injections for low back pain and lumbosacral radiculopathy. Pain 1986;24:277–295.
10. Benzon H, Gissen AJ, Strichartz GR, et al. The effect of polyethylene glycol on mammalian nerve impulses. Anesth Analg 1987;66:553–559.
11. Berg A. Clinical and myelographic studies of conservatively treated cases of lumbar intervertebral disk protrusion. Acta Chir Scand 1952;104:124–129.
12. Bobechko WP, Hirsch C. Autoimmune response to nucleus pulposus in the rabbit. J Bone Joint Surg 1965;47B:574–580.
13. Bogduk N. The clinical anatomy of cervical dorsal rami. Spine 1982;4:319–330.
14. Bogduk N, Long DM. The anatomy of the so-called "articular nerves" and their relationship to facet denervation in the treatment of low-back pain. J Neurosurg 1979;51:172–177.
15. Bogduk N, Long DM. Percutaneous lumbar medial branch neurotomy: a modification of facet denervation. Spine 1980;5:193–200.
16. Bogduk N, Marsland A. On the concept of third occipital headache. J Neurol Neurosurg Psychiatry 1986;49:775–780.
17. Bonica JJ. The management of pain. 2d ed. Philadelphia: Lea & Febiger, 1990:133–146.
18. Bowen V, Cassidy JD. Macroscopic and microscopic anatomy of the sacroiliac joint from embryonic life until the eighth decade. Spine 1981;6:620–628.
19. Brena SF, Wolf SL, Chapman SL, et al. Chronic back pain: electromyographic, motion, and behavioral assessments following sympathetic nerve blocks and placebos. Pain 1980;8:1–10.
20. Brevik H, Hesla PE, Molnar I, et al. Treatment of chronic low back pain and sciatica: comparison of caudal epidural steroid injections of bupivacaine and methylprednisolone with bupivacaine followed by saline. In: Bonica JJ, Albe-Fessard D, eds. Advances in pain research and therapy. New York: Raven, 1976:927–932.
21. Bush K, Hiller S. A controlled study of caudal epidural injections of triamcinolone plus procaine for the management of intractable sciatica. Spine 1991;16:572–575.
22. Butler D, Trafimow JH, Andersson GBJ, et al. Discs degenerate before facets. Spine 1990;15:111–113.
23. Carette S, Marcoux S, Truchon R, et al. A controlled trial of corticosteroid injection into facet joints for chronic low back pain. N Engl J Med 1991;325:1002–1007.
24. Carrera GF. Lumbar facet joint injection in low back pain and sciatica: description of technique. Radiology 1980;137:661–664.
25. Carrera GF. Lumbar facet joint injection in low back pain and sciatica: preliminary results. Radiology 1980;137:665–667.
26. Cavanaugh JM, el-Bohy A, Hardy WN, et al. Sensory innervation of soft tissues of the lumbar spine in the rat. J Orthop Res 1989;7:378–388.
27. Ceshire WP, Abashian SW, Mann JD. Botulinum toxin in the treatment of myofascial pain syndrome. Pain 1994;59:65–69.
28. Chino N, Awad EA, Kottke FJ. Pathology of propylene glycol administered by perineural and intramuscular injection in rats. Arch Phys Med Rehabil 1974;55:33–38.
29. Cicala RS, Turner R, Moran E, et al. Methylprednisolone acetate does not cause inflammatory changes in the epidural space. Anesthesiology 1990;72:556–558.
30. Cohen MK, Wall EJ, Brown RA, et al. Cauda equina anatomy. II: Extrathecal nerve roots and dorsal root ganglia. Spine 1990;15:1248–1251.
31. Cohn ML, Huntington CT, Byrd SE, et al. Epidural morphine and methylprednisolone: new therapy for recurrent low-back pain. Spine 1986;11:960–963.
32. Connally GH, Sanders SH. Predicting low back patients' response to lumbar sympathetic nerve blocks and interdisciplinary rehabilitation: the role of pretreatment overt pain behavior and cognitive coping strategies. Pain 1991;44:139–146.
33. Cuckler JM, Bernini PA, Wiesel SM, et al. The use of epidural steroids in the treatment of lumbar radicular pain: a prospective, randomized, double-blind study. J Bone Joint Surg 1985;67A:63–66.
34. Dallas TL, Lin RL, Wu W-H, et al. Epidural morphine and methylprednisolone for low back pain. Anesthesiology 1987;67:408–411.
35. Delaney TJ, Rowlingson JC, Carron H, et al. Epidural steroid effects on nerves and meninges. Anesth Analg 1980;59:610–614.
36. Derby R, Kine G, Saal JA, et al. Response to steroid and duration of radicular pain as predictors of surgical outcome. Spine 1992;17(Suppl):S176–S183.
37. Destouet JM, Gilula LA, Murphey WA, et al. Lumbar facet joint injection: indication, technique, clinical correlation, and preliminary results. Radiology 1982;145:321–325.
38. Devor M, Govrin-Lippmann R, Raber P. Corticosteroids suppress ectopic neural discharge originating in experimental neuromas. Pain 1985;22:127–137.
39. Deyo RA. Fads in the treatment of low back pain. N Engl J Med 1991;325:1039–1040.
40. Dilke TFW, Burry HC, Grahame R. Extradural corticosteroid injection in management of lumbar nerve root compression. Br Med J 1973;2:635–637.
41. Dooley JF, McBroom RJ, Taguchi T, et al. Nerve root infiltration in the diagnosis of radicular pain. Spine 1988;13:79–83.
42. Dory MA. Arthrography of the lumbar facet joints. Radiology 1981;140:23–27.
43. Dory MA. Arthrography of the cervical facet joints. Radiology 1983;148:379–382.
44. Dreyfuss P, Michaelsen M, Fletcher D. Atlanto-occipital and lateral atlantoaxial joint pain patterns. Spine 1994;19:1125–1131.
45. Dreyfuss P, Dryer S, Griffin J, et al. Positive sacroiliac screening tests in asymptomatic adults. Spine 1994;19:1138–1143.
46. Dwyer A, Aprill C, Bogduk N. Cervical zygapophyseal joint pain patterns. I: A study in normal volunteers. Spine 1990;15:453–457.
47. Edgar MA, Ghadially JA. Innervation of the lumbar spine. Clin Orthop 1976;115:35–41.

48. Edwards E. Operative anatomy of the lumbar sympathetic chain. Angiology 1951;2:184–198.
49. El-Bohy A, Cavanaugh JM, Getchell ML, et al. Localization of substance P and neurofilament immunoreactive fibers in the lumbar facet joint capsule and supraspinous ligament of the rabbit. Brain Res 1988; 460:379–382.
50. El-Mahdi MA, Latif FYA, Janko M. The spinal nerve root "innervation," and a new concept of the clinicopathological interrelations in back pain and sciatica. Neurochirurgia 1981;24:137–141.
51. Evans FJ. The placebo response in pain reduction. In: Bonica JJ, ed. Advances in neurology. Vol. 4. New York: Raven, 1974:289–300.
52. Fairbank JCT, McCall IW, O'Brian JP. Apophyseal injection of local anesthetic as a diagnostic aid in primary low-back pain syndromes. Spine 1981;6:598–605.
53. Fernstrom U. A discographical study of ruptured lumbar intervertebral discs. Acta Chir Scand 1960; S258:10–60.
54. Ferrer-Brechner T, Brechner V. Accuracy of needle placement during diagnostic and therapeutic nerve blocks. Adv Pain Res and Therapy 1976;1:679.
55. Fortin JD, Dwyer AP, West S, et al. Sacroiliac joint: pain referral maps upon applying a new injection/arthrography technique. Part I: Asymptomatic volunteers. Spine 1994;19:1475–1482.
56. Fuxe K, Harfstrand A, Agnati LF, et al. Immunocytochemical studies on the localization of glucocorticoid receptor immunoreactive nerve cells in the lower brain stem and spinal cord of the male rat using a monoclonal antibody against rat liver glucocorticoid receptor. Neurosci Lett 1985;60:1–6.
57. Ghelman B, Doherty JH. Demonstration of spondylolysis by arthrography of the apophyseal joint. AJR 1978;130:986–987.
58. Gilbert J, Bjork K, McAllen A, et al. High cervical epidural blockade complicating thoracic paravertebral block. Clin Int Care 1991;2:241–243.
59. Giles LGF, Taylor JR. Human zygapophyseal joint capsule and synovial fold innervation. Br J Rheumatol 1987;26:93–98.
60. Gillette RG, Kramis RC, Roberts WJ. Sympathetic activation of cat spinal neurons responsive to noxious stimulation of deep tissues in the low back. Pain 1994; 56:31–42.
61. Goldstone JC, Pennant JH. Spinal anaesthesia following facet joint injection. Anaesthesia 1987;42:754–756.
62. Green PWB, Burke AJ, Weiss CA, et al. The role of epidural cortisone injection in treatment of discogenic low back pain. Clin Orthop 1980;153:121–125.
63. Grevert P, Albert LH, Goldstein A. Partial antagonism of placebo analgesia by naloxone. Pain 1983;16:129–143.
64. Groen GJ, Baljet B, Drukker J. Nerves and nerve plexuses of the human vertebral column. Am J Anat 1990; 188:282–296.
65. Groen GJ, Baljet B, Boekelaar AB, et al. Branches of the thoracic sympathetic trunk in the human fetus. Anat Embryol 1987;176:401–411.
66. Haddox JD. Lumbar and cervical epidural steroid therapy. Anesth Clin North Am 1992;10:179–203.
67. Haueisen DC, Smith BS, Myers SR, et al. The diagnostic accuracy of spinal nerve injection studies. Clin Orthop 1985;198:179–183.
68. Haughton VM, Nguyen CM, Khang-Cheng H. The etiology of focal spinal arachnoiditis. Spine 1993;18:1193–1198.
69. Helbig T, Lee CK. The lumbar facet syndrome. Spine 1988;13:61–64.
70. Hendrix RW, Lin PP, Kane WJ. Simplified aspiration or injection technique for the sacro-iliac joint. J Bone Joint Surg 1982;64A:1249–1252.
71. Hirsch C, Ingelmark B, Miller M. The anatomical basis for low back pain. Acta Orthop 1963;33:1–17.
72. Hogan Q. Lumbar epidural anatomy: a new look by cryomicrotome section. Anesthesiology 1991;75:767–775.
73. Hogan Q. Tuffier's line: the normal distribution of anatomic parameters. Anesth Analg 1993;78:194–195.
74. Hogan Q, Abram SE. Epidural steroids and the outcomes movement. Pain Digest 1992;1:269–270.
75. Hogan Q, Dotson R, Erickson S, et al. Local anesthetic myotoxicity: a case and review. Anesthesiology 1994; 80:942–947.
76. Houde RW, Wallenstein MS, Rogers A. Clinical pharmacology of analgesics: a method of assaying analgesic effect. Clin Pharm Ther 1966;1:163–174.
77. Hove B, Gyldensted C. Cervical analgesic facet joint arthrography. Neuroradiology 1990;32:456–459.
78. Howe JF, Loeser JD, Calvin WH. Mechanosensitivity of dorsal root ganglia and chronically injured axons: a physiological basis for the radicular pain of nerve root compression. Pain 1977;2:25–41.
79. Hua S-Y, Chen Y-Z. Membrane receptor-mediated electrophysiological effects of glucocorticoid on mammalian neurons. Endocrinology 1989;124:687–691.
80. Hurst EW. Adhesive arachnoiditis and vascular blockage caused by detergents and other chemical irritants. J Pathol 1955;70:167–178.
81. Jackson RP. The facet syndrome. Clin Orthop 1992; 279:110–121.
82. Jackson RP, Jacobs RR, Montesano PX. Facet joint injection in low-back pain: a prospective statistical study. Spine 1988;13:966–971.
83. Janig W, McLachlan EM. Identification of distinct topographical distribution of lumbar sympathetic and sensory neurons projecting to end organs with different functions in the cat. J Comp Neurol 1986;246:104–112.
84. Johansson A, Hao J, Sjolund B. Local corticosteroid application blocks transmission in normal nociceptive C-fibers. Acta Anaesth Scand 1990;34:335–338.
85. Kellgren JH. On the distribution of pain arising from deep somatic structures with charts of segmental pain areas. Clin Sci 1939;4:35–46.
86. Kibler RF, Nathan PW. Relief of pain and paraesthesiae by nerve block distal to a lesion. J Neurol Neurosurg Psychiatry 1960;23:91–98.
87. Kikuchi S, Hasue M, Nishiyama K, et al. Anatomic and clinical studies of radicular symptoms. Spine 1984; 9:23–30.

88. Krempen JS, Smith B. Nerve root infiltration: a method for evaluating the etiology of sciatica. J Bone Joint Surg 1974;56A:1435–1444.
89. Kuslich SD, Ulstrom CL, Michael CJ. The tissue origin of low back pain and sciatica: a report of pain response to tissue stimulation during operations on the lumbar spine using local anesthesia. Orthop Clin North Am 1991;22:181–187.
90. [Reference deleted.]
91. Larsen JL, Olsen KO. Radiographic anatomy of the distal dural sac. Acta Radiol 1991;32:214–219.
92. Levine JD, Gordon NC, Fields HL. The mechanism of placebo analgesia. Lancet 1978;2:654–657.
93. Lewit K. The needle effect in the relief of myofascial pain. Pain 1979;6:83–90.
94. Liberman R. An experimental study of the placebo response under three different situations of pain. J Psychiatr Res 1964;2:233–246.
95. Lilus G, Laasonen EM, Myllynen P, et al. Lumbar facet joint syndrome: a randomized clinical trial. J Bone Joint Surg 1989;71B:681–684.
96. Lindahl O, Rexed B. Histologic changes in spinal nerve roots of operated cases of sciatica. Acta Orthop Scand 1951;20:215–225.
97. Lipman JJ, Miller BE, Mays KS, et al. Peak B endorphin concentration in cerebrospinal fluid: reduced in chronic pain patients and increased during the placebo response. Psychopharmacology 1990;102:112–116.
98. Loeser JD. Dorsal rhizotomy for the relief of chronic pain. J Neurosurg 1972;36:745–750.
99. Lora J, Long D. So-called facet denervation in the management of intractable back pain. Spine 1976;2:121–126.
100. Lynch MC, Taylor JF. Facet joint injection for low back pain. J Bone Joint Surg 1986;68B:138–141.
101. MacGibbon B, Farfan HF. A radiologic survey of various configurations of the lumbar spine. Spine 1979;4:258–266.
102. MacKinnon SE, Hudson AR, Gentilli G, et al. Peripheral nerve injection injury with steroid agents. Plast Reconstr Surg 1982;69:482–489.
103. Maldague B, Mathurin P, Malghem J. Facet joint arthrography in lumbar spondylosis. Radiology 1981;140:29–36.
104. Margolis G, Hall HE, Nowill WK. An investigation of efocaine, a long acting anesthetic agent. Arch Surg 1953;61;715–730.
105. Marks R. Distribution of pain provoked from lumbar facet joints and related structures during diagnostic spinal infiltration. Pain 1989;39:37–40.
106. Marks RC, Houston T, Thulbourne T. Facet joint injection and facet nerve block: a randomized comparison in 86 patients with chronic low back pain. Pain 1992;49:325–328.
107. Marshall LL, Trethewie ER, Curtain CC. Chemical radiculitis: a clinical, physiological, and immunological study. Clin Orthop 1987;129:61–67.
108. Maugars Y, Mathis C, Vilon P, et al. Corticosteroid injection of the sacroiliac joint in patients with seronegative spondyloarthropathy. Arthritis Rheum 1992;35:564–568.
109. McCall IW, Park WM, O'Brien JP. Induced pain referral from posterior lumbar elements in normal subjects. Spine 1979;4:441–446.
110. McCarron RF, Wimpee MW, Hudkins PG, et al. The inflammatory effect of nucleus pulposus. Spine 1987;12:760–764.
111. McCormick CC, Taylor JR, Twomey LT. Facet joint arthrography in lumbar spondylolysis: anatomic basis for spread of contrast medium. Radiology 1989;171:193–196.
112. McLain RF. Mechanicoreceptor endings in human cervical facet joints. Spine 1994;19:495–501.
113. Melzack R, Wall PD. Pain mechanisms: a new theory. Science 1965;150:971–979.
114. Mooney V, Robertson J. The facet syndrome. Clin Orthop 1976;115:149–156.
115. Moran R, O'Connell D, Walsh MG. The diagnostic value of facet joint injections. Spine 1988;13:1407–1410.
116. Murphey F. Sources and patterns of pain in disc disease. Clin Neurosurg 1968;15:343–351.
117. Murtagh FR. Computed tomography and fluoroscopy guided anesthesia and steroid injection in facet syndrome. Spine 1988;13:686–689.
118. Naylor A. Enzymatic and immunological activity in the intervertebral disc. Orthop Clin North Am 1975;6:51–58.
119. Neidre A, MacNab I. Anomalies of the lumbosacral nerve roots: review of 16 cases and classification. Spine 1983;8:294–299.
120. Nelson DA. Dangers from methylprednisolone acetate therapy by intraspinal injection. Arch Neurol 1988;45:804–806.
121. Nitta H, Tajima T, Sugiyama H, et al. Study of dermatomes by means of selective lumbar spinal nerve block. Spine 1993;13:1782–1786.
122. North RB, Kidd DH, Campbell JN, et al. Dorsal root ganglionectomy for failed back surgery syndrome: a 5-year follow-up study. J Neurosurg 1991;74:236–242.
123. Onofrio BM, Campa HK. Evaluation of rhizotomy: review of 12 years' experience. J Neurosurg 1972;36:751–755.
124. Pallie W. The intersegmental anastomoses of posterior spinal rootlets and their significance. J Neurosurg 1959;16:188–196.
125. Pallie W, Manuel JK. Intersegmental anastomoses between dorsal spinal rootlets in some vertebrates. Acta Anat 1968;70:341–351.
126. Quinnell RC, Stockdale HR. The use of in vivo lumbar discography to assess the clinical significance of the position of the intercrestal line. Spine 1983;8:305–307.
127. Racz GB, Heavner JE, Singleton W, et al. Hypertonic saline and corticosteroid injected epidurally for pain control. In: Racz GB, ed. Techniques of neurolysis. Boston: Kluwer, 1989:73–86.
128. Ready LB, Kozody R, Barsa JE, et al. Trigger point injections vs. jet injection in the treatment of myofascial pain. Pain 1989;15:201–206.
129. Reimann AF, Anson BJ. Vertebral level of termination of the spinal cord with report of a case of sacral cord. Anat Rec 1944;88:127–138.

130. Renfrew D, Moore T, Kathol M, et al. Correct placement of epidural steroid injections: fluoroscopic guidance and contrast administration. AJNR 1991;12:1003.
131. Rocco AG, Frank E, Kaul AF, et al. Epidural steroids, epidural morphine, and epidural steroids combined with morphine in the treatment of post-laminectomy syndrome. Pain 1989;36:297–303.
132. Roy DF, Fleury J, Fontaine SB, et al. Clinical evaluation of cervical facet joint infiltration. J Can Assoc Radiol 1988;39:118–120.
133. Russell AS, Maksymowych W, LeClerq S. Clinical examination of the sacroiliac joints: a prospective study. Arthritis Rheum 1981;24:1575–1578.
134. Saal JS, Franson RC, Dobrow R, et al. High levels of inflammatory phospholipase A_2 activity in lumbar disc herniations. Spine 1990;15:674–678.
135. Schutz H, Lougheed WM, Wortzman G, et al. Intervertebral nerve-root in the investigation of chronic lumbar disc disease. Can J Surg 1973;16:217–221.
136. Schwarzer AC, Aprill CN, Bogduk N. The sacroiliac joint in chronic low back pain. Spine 1995;20:31–37.
137. Schwarzer AC, Aprill CN, Derby R, et al. The false-positive rate of uncontrolled diagnostic blocks of the lumbar zygapophysial joints. Pain 1994;58:195–200.
138. Schwarzer AC, Derby R, Aprill CN, et al. The value of the provocation response in lumbar zygapophyseal joint injections. Clin J Pain 1994;10:309–313.
139. Selander D, Brattsand R, Lundborg G, et al. Local anesthetics: importance of mode of application, concentration, and adrenaline for the appearance of nerve lesions. Acta Anaesth Scand 1979;23:127–136.
140. Sigurdsson A, Maixner W. Effects of experimental and clinical noxious counterirritants on pain perception. Pain 1994;57:265–275.
141. Sinclair DC, Hinshaw JR. A comparison of the sensory dissociation produced by procaine and by limb compression. Brain 1950;73:480–498.
142. Sluijter ME. The use of radiofrequency lesions for pain relief in failed back patients. Int Disabil Studies 1988;10:37–43.
143. Smyth MJ, Wright V. Sciatica and the intervertebral disc. J Bone Joint Surg 1958;40A:1401–1418.
144. Snoek W, Weber H, Jorgensen B. Double blind evaluation of extradural methylprednisolone for herniated lumbar discs. Acta Orthop Scand 1977;48:635–641.
145. Solonen KA. The sacroiliac joint in light of anatomical, roentgenological, and clinical studies. Acta Orthop Scand 1957;27(S):1–27.
146. Stanley D, McLaren MI, Euinton HA, et al. A prospective study of nerve root infiltration in the diagnosis of sciatica. Spine 1990;15:540–543.
147. Tajima T, Furukawa K, Kuramochi E. Selective lumbosacral radiculography and block. Spine 1980;5:68–77.
148. Trotter M. Variations of the sacral canal: their significance in the administration of caudal analgesia. Anesth Analg 1947;26:192–202.
149. Vleeming A, Stoeckart R, Volkers ACW, et al. Relation between form and function in the sacroiliac joint. Part I: Clinical anatomic aspects. Spine 1990;15:130–132.
150. Walker AE, Nulson F. Electrical stimulation of the upper thoracic portion of the sympathetic chain in man. Arch Neurol Psychiatry 1948;59:559–560.
151. Wiberg G. Back pain in relation to the nerve supply of the intervertebral disc. Acta Orthop 1949;19:211–221.
152. Wiesel SW, Tsourmas N, Feffer HL, et al. A study of computer-assisted tomography. I. The incidence of positive CAT scans in an asymptomatic group of patients. Spine 1984;9:549–551.
153. Wood KM, Arguelles J, Norenberg MD. Degenerative lesions in rat sciatic nerves after local injections of methylprednisolone in sterile aqueous suspension. Reg Anesth 1980;5:13–15.
154. Xavier AV, McDanal J, Kissin I. Relief of sciatic radicular pain by sciatic nerve block. Anesth Analg 1988;67:1177–1180.
155. Yabuki S, Kikuchi S. Nerve root infiltration and sympathetic block: an experimental study of intraradicular blood flow. Spine 1995;20:901–906.
156. Yamashita T, Cavanaugh JM, el-Bohy AA, et al. Mechanosensitive afferent units in the lumbar facet joint. J Bone Joint Surg 1990;72A:865–870.
157. Yates DW. A comparison of the types of epidural injection commonly used in the treatment of low back pain and sciatica. Rheumatology and Rehabilitation 1978;17:181–186.
158. Young A, Getty J, Jackson A, et al. Variations in the pattern of muscle innervation by the L5 and S1 nerve roots. Spine 1983;6:616–624.

CHAPTER THIRTY SIX

Percutaneous Procedures in the Lumbar Spine

Hallett H. Mathews and Bruce E. Mathern

Introduction

With the explosion of spinal surgery techniques over the past fifty years there has been a growing interest in less invasive procedures. As was the case with other surgical specialties, the first minimally invasive procedures in spinal surgery were biopsy techniques involving needle biopsy of bony spinal pathology. Though today many of these procedures are of more historical than practical significance, they are important in that they represent the development of percutaneous approaches to the spine that served as the foundation for later developments. These early procedures were for diagnostic purposes, but they rapidly led to the development of therapeutic procedures for the chemical treatment of disc disease and for surgical decompression. With the development of fiberoptic technology and improved visualization there have been significant advancements in diverse areas of minimally invasive spinal surgery, ranging from endoscopic disc removal to combined endoscopic percutaneous fusion techniques.

The benefits of less invasive spinal procedures can be summarized into several basic areas. First is surgical access to the spine without the comorbidities of open spinal surgery. The soft-tissue destruction and potential for biomechanical destabilization are well known in open spinal surgery, and most of this comorbidity can be avoided with minimally invasive techniques. In addition, most of the recovery involved in open spinal procedures is due to the soft-tissue dissection that is necessary in these approaches. Minimally invasive techniques do not involve such extensive tissue dissection, and patients undergoing these procedures are often discharged from the hospital much earlier, resulting in significant cost savings. Finally, current endoscopic techniques allow the surgeon to visualize directly the abnormality that is causing the patient's symptoms as well to confirm the corrective measures taken.

In this survey of percutaneous techniques for the lumbar spine attention will be given to the early development of these techniques, the evolution of therapeutic procedures, and the current state of minimally invasive spinal procedures as well as a forecast for future developments.

Biopsy Techniques

The first percutaneous lumbar spine procedures date from the 1930s with the advent of needle biopsy for spinal pathology (23, 24). In the 1950s Craig developed a percutaneous core biopsy technique that is in use today (10). Since there were few imaging techniques at the time, and radiographic diagnosis of spinal pathology was limited, there was a need for the development of such procedures. As imaging of the spine improved and the use of computed tomography (CT), magnetic resonance imaging (MRI), and nuclear medicine bone scanning became more common, the need to perform needle biopsies of the spine decreased. Interestingly, with the recent resurgence of infectious diseases of the spine such as tuberculosis, the Craig needle biopsy is being used with more frequency.

Patient selection for needle biopsy of the lumbar spine should include patients who have undiagnosed abnormality on imaging for which a diagnosis will guide therapy. Examples of this include the diagnosis of metastatic disease to the spine, which would be treated by radiation therapy, or a culture-based diagnosis of vertebral infection as a guide to antibiotic therapy. It would not be appropriate to perform a biopsy procedure on patients in cases in which the decision has already been made that no further treatment will be used regardless of the diagnosis. In addition, patients who have a suspected or confirmed diagnosis of renal cell carcinoma and patients who have a bleeding diathesis should not have a biopsy, because of the high risk of uncontrollable hemorrhage.

Needle biopsy is usually performed in the operating room with local anesthesia to allow the patient to respond immediately to radicular impingement. The patient is placed in the lateral position and a posterolateral needle approach is used. Fluoroscopy localizes the level of interest and then a needle entry is made 8 to 10 cm lateral to the midline at a 45° trajectory toward the vertebral body. Sequential fluoroscopic images can be viewed as the needle is advanced and directed toward the area of biopsy within the vertebral body. Once the needle is placed on the vertebral body, the position is confirmed with anteroposterior and lateral fluoroscopy. A large dilator/cannula is placed over the needle to expand the tract through the soft tissues, and then a cutting needle with a large bore is placed over the dilator to cut a core-type biopsy from the vertebral body. Gentle aspiration on the needle as it is removed will aid in the retrieval of the sample after it has been cut. If the patient experiences radicular pain that corresponds to the level of the biopsy, then needle location should be confirmed by two-view fluoroscopy and the needle should be checked for cerebrospinal fluid. In addition, it is becoming more common to perform vertebral biopsy procedures under CT guidance to allow the biopsy of much smaller lesions and to aid in needle placement.

The success of needle biopsy in the lumbar spine has been somewhat limited because of small biopsy size and a confined ability to localize small lesions. It has a low complication rate, with local hemorrhage and neural injury the most common.

This technique is best used for patients in whom a tissue diagnosis is required but in whom other, more aggressive surgical treatments are not being considered.

Discography

Discography is another of the early diagnostic percutaneous procedures of the lumbar spine that developed under the conditions of the limited imaging modalities of the 1940s. During a time when radiographic examination of the spine was limited to plain roentgenograms and myelography, discography provided a modality for studying disc abnormalities directly. As myelogram with CT and MRI have become the primary means of imaging the lumbar spine, the role of discography has become controversial. Despite a collection of recommendations on the indications for performing discography relative to defining its role (9, 21, 35, 51, 55), a significant consensus supports the premise that it provides little or no new information beyond MRI (36). We subscribe to the recent position statement of the North American Spine Society that describes discography as an invasive procedure that is indicated as a provocative test to distinguish discogenic pain as the source of a patient's symptoms, for the evaluation of symptomatic discs in patients who have multilevel disc degeneration, and as an adjunct in patients in whom diagnostic testing results are equivocal (12). In addition, discography is excellent at diagnosing annular pathology, such as annular tears (Fig. 36.1), which are a common source of discogenic pain without nerve root compression. Discography is clearly not indicated in every case of lumbar disc disease, but

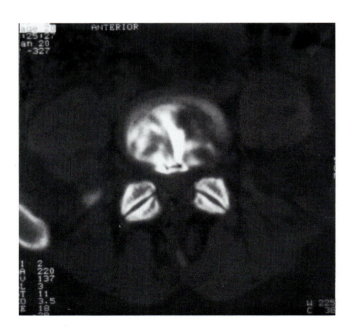

FIGURE 36.1.

Axial computed tomography after discogram injection. Note the large annular tear and extravasation of contrast into the epidural space.

the provocative component can prove to be very helpful in difficult patients when used in conjunction with MRI and CT myelography (2). In fact, Castro and associates have reported the importance of broad-based dye distribution within a disc protrusion as seen on postdiscogram CT scan as a predictor of successful outcome of percutaneous discectomy, specifically for automated percutaneous lumbar discectomy (6, 7).

Despite the controversy surrounding the indications for discography, the contraindications are for the most part limited to patients who have iodine contrast medium sensitivity.

Discography is generally performed either in the operating room or in the radiology department, as many of these procedures are currently performed by radiologists. The most common approach is a posterolateral approach, though a transdural approach has been described. The patient is positioned in the prone or lateral position, and the level of interest is localized using fluoroscopy. Because discography is a provocative test, it is important to use local anesthesia only in the skin and soft tissues above the level of the facet, since anesthesia below this level may anesthetize the annulus fibrosus or the nerve root and blunt any pain response from the intradiscal injection. In the posterolateral approach a needle entry is made 8 to 12 cm lateral to the midline at a trajectory of 45°. As the needle is advanced, sequential fluoroscopic images can guide the needle placement to the appropriate disc level. Once the needle reaches the annulus fibrosus, the placement is confirmed with two-view fluoroscopy (Fig. 36.2A,B). A second needle is placed into the nucleus through the approach needle (Fig. 36.3A). Injection of 3 to 5 mL of contrast medium is done under continuous fluoroscopic view (Fig. 36.3B), and the patient's response to the injection is recorded. The needles are then removed and CT scanning is performed to further define the contrast injection and the disc anatomy. For the potential contribution to diagnosis, discography has a low risk ratio if performed by a skilled practitioner. The chief complication is generally recognized to be discitis. Lesser reported complications include meningitis and arachnoiditis, spinal headache, intrathecal hemorrhage, and serious response to untoward intradural injection. Bowel perforation and retroperitoneal hemorrhage along with disc damage have also been reported.

Diagnostic accuracy and specificity in discography vary, but with the addition of postdiscogram CT scanning, a rate of 94% in the enhancement of the clinical picture has been reported, suggesting that the combined approach may advance the credibility of discography (3).

Chemonucleolysis

The development of chemical degradation for herniated nucleus pulposus is credited to Lyman Smith (53). He performed early work with discography and used this experience to develop the concept of a therapeutic intervention via a posterolateral percutane-

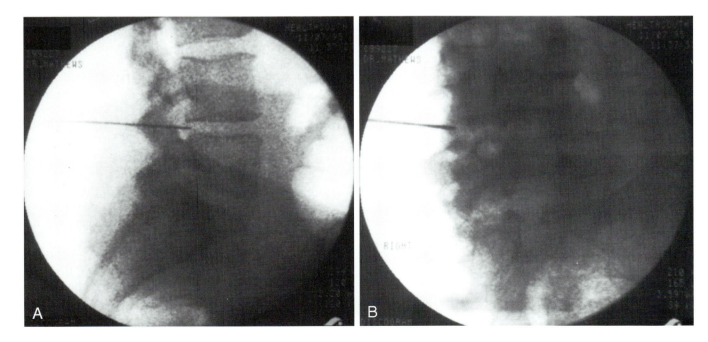

FIGURE 36.2.

A. Lateral fluoroscopic image showing discogram needle on annulus fibrosus. **B.** Anteroposterior fluoroscopic image of discogram needle on annulus.

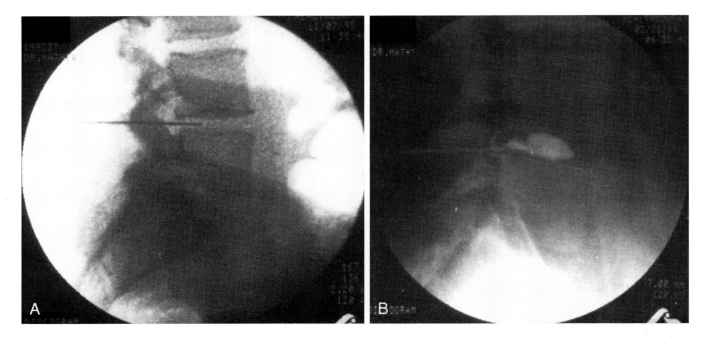

FIGURE 36.3.

A. Advanced inner discogram needle into nucleus pulposus of L4–5 disc. **B.** Extravasation of contrast medium into the epidural space after discography. The patient had a significant pain response to this injection.

ous approach. Thus chemonucleolysis represents one of the first therapeutic percutaneous procedures.

In the mid 1960s chemonucleolysis using the enzyme chymopapain gained enthusiastic acceptance for the minimally invasive treatment of acute disc herniation. While still widely accepted in other areas of the world, the technique underwent a decline in acceptance in the United States during the early 1980s because of the incidence of anaphylactic reactions and transverse myelitis. Transverse myelitis complications have been shown to be related to injection technique rather than to the enzyme. Furthermore, as a result of sensitivity testing and histamine prophylaxis the incidence of anaphylaxis has become quite low (17). Chemonucleolysis remains a minimally invasive therapeutic modality with extensive worldwide use but variable acceptance in this country.

The indications for chymopapain therapy are similar to those for any minimally invasive disc procedure. These include leg pain greater than back pain with possible radicular symptoms and neurologic deficit. Additionally, there should be radiologic evidence of herniated or sequestered disc with nerve root impingement, ideally at only one level, and failure of conservative care management. Patients who have undergone prior lumbar spine surgery are generally not candidates for chymopapain treatment, since scarring may cause anatomic alterations that can make the surgical approach difficult and the therapeutic effect unpredictable.

Contraindications to the procedure include hypersensitivity to chymopapain, structural pathology beyond focal disc pathology such as instability or stenosis, and other medical conditions that would prohibit surgery, such as pregnancy. Alexander has noted that patient medication profiles may be a key to additional contraindications. Patients who are taking beta-blockers may be more difficult to treat in the event of anaphylaxis because of the decreased effectiveness of epinephrine, which is administered to treat the reaction. Because of the ongoing concern for anaphylaxis, many practitioners premedicate patients with a prophylactic regimen of corticosteroids, diphenhydramine, and cimetidine (1).

Via the posterolateral approach with the patient in the lateral or prone position, a small-gauge needle is introduced into the center of the pathologic disc space. Biplanar fluoroscopic verification of needle positioning in the central nucleus is crucial in assuring the appropriate delivery of the enzyme.

Discography has become more common prior to injection as a means of verifying a contained disc and to rule out communication of the nucleus with the epidural space.

Chemonucleolysis has its limitations. It is a nonselective disc debulking technique, and after the procedure the natural history includes disc-space collapse and possible neural compression. Yet the evolution of disc-space collapse in the patient undergoing other percutaneous procedures may be similar. The rapid resolution of radicular symptoms with only transient low back pain provides chemonucleolysis with a high degree of acceptance in the well-selected patient who has the potential for a timely return to quality-of-life activities with minimal restrictions.

The overall success rate for chymopapain therapy in one cohort study was reported at 76% (38). Revel and colleagues have compared chemonucleolysis with automated percutaneous lumbar discectomy, reporting success rates of 66% and 41%, respectively (46).

Chemonucleolysis does not interfere with surgical options in the event of recurrence, and it represents significant cost savings in comparison with open surgery (16).

Percutaneous Nucleotomy

The clinical outcomes of chemical disc degradation by chemonucleolysis stimulated interest in other techniques for minimally invasive therapeutic intradiscal procedures in the lumbar spine. The first technique that evolved was percutaneous nucleotomy, developed independently and almost simultaneously by Hoppenfeld (15) and Hijikata (13, 14). The technique involves uniportal access to the central nucleus for treatment of herniated nuclear pathology (Fig. 36.4). Through manual removal of a measured amount of nucleus pulposus, there is intradiscal depressurization with subsequent reduction in nerve root compression and tension in pain fibers of the annular structure.

With the groundwork laid by chemonucleolysis, experience demonstrated similar selection criteria for what came to be known as percutaneous discectomy. Chief among these are leg pain greater than back pain with root tension signs, radiculopathy, and radiologic evidence of contained disc herniation. Central and paracentral disc herniations are more accessible via the percutaneous posterolateral approach than are far lateral or foraminal herniations.

Patients are usually placed in the right or left lateral position, with variation in surgeon preference. Fluoroscopic guidance provides for placement of a guide-wire in the central portion of the disc. Discography may follow with subsequent advancement of cannulae of increasing size followed by an annular trephine that fits within the largest cannula. With a twisting motion, the trephine fenestrates the annulus and is advanced under fluoroscopic guidance to the predetermined guide-wire location. With the seating of the trephine, manual instruments and suction allow for removal of intranuclear material, with the patient often noting the reduction or relief of radicular symptoms as a result of intradiscal depressurization and diminished irritation of the offending nerve root.

Long-term results of percutaneous nucleotomy techniques alone or of central disc decompression procedures have never been shown to be greater than placebo. In 1994 Mathews and associates reported a 57% overall success rate of percutaneous nucleotomy using laser disc decompression techniques (30).

Manual and suction disc depressurization was advanced with the introduction of percutaneous automated discectomy by Onik and associates (42). This device features a uniportal percutaneous nucleotomy approach with the adjunct of a suction-cutting mechanism intradiscally that shaves nuclear material when it is drawn into the nucleotomy device (11, 26, 27). This instrument has since evolved into a steerable and visual intradiscal device for intradiscal decompression.

Early Visualized Intradiscal Procedures

The success of uniportal nonvisualized intradiscal procedures along with optical advancements associated with large-joint arthroscopy induced Schreiber, Suezawa, and Leu to experiment with discoscopy in biportal percutaneous nucleotomy (48, 50) (Fig. 36.5). The success of their work coincided with the work of Kambin and associates in the development of arthroscopic microdiscectomy (18, 20) and with

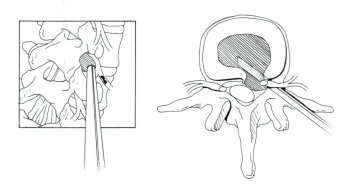

FIGURE 36.4.
Uniportal nucleotomy showing placement of the needle into the central nucleus pulposus. Note the location and direction of the needle in comparison with the disc herniation.

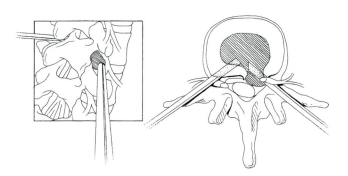

FIGURE 36.5.
Biportal discoscopic nucleotomy showing visualized access to the central portion of the disc.

that of Mayer and Brock, who reported on percutaneous endoscopic discectomy (34). These procedures allow visualized manual, automated, or even laser discectomy aided by irrigation and suction of debris.

In the discoscopic procedure percutaneous nucleotomy techniques are employed, with the patient in the prone position, via the posterolateral approach into the central nucleus for direct or contralateral inspection and visualization of anatomy and central or posterocentral neuropathology (Fig. 36.5). The ability to visualize disc depressurization procedures assists in the correction of abnormality. Key to the success of intradiscal intervention has been the definition of approach parameters and the refinement of instrumentation, both in size and optics, which facilitates the verification of the corrective measures taken.

The posterolateral approach has been the principal mode of access, using cannulae that have ranged in size from 2.5 to 6.8 mm. With the question of approach came that of intradiscal working parameters. Kambin proposed a biportal approach to a triangular working zone with the boundaries being the spinal nerve, the endplate of the inferior vertebral body, and its proximal articulating facet (19).

One additional nucleotomy procedure varying slightly in the mechanism of action is laser disc decompression. First introduced by Choy and colleagues, laser ablation and suction removal of intranuclear material promotes disc depressurization with relief of symptoms (8). Laser wavelengths including Nd:YAG, KTP-532, excimer, and Ho:YAG sidefire laser have provided variable success rates in relief of symptoms, reported to range from 57% with the KTP-532 wavelength to as high as 84% with the Ho:YAG (4, 5, 30, 43, 45, 52). Patient selection on the basis of contained virgin disc pathology seems to be the greatest predictor of successful outcome in percutaneous laser disc decompression with pulsed wavelength delivery via posterolateral cannula access with or without visualization.

For all nucleotomy procedures, success rates are generally accepted to be approximately 70 to 80%, with risks corresponding to earlier percutaneous procedures, including nerve root trauma, infection, bowel perforation, and vascular insult with retroperitoneal hematoma or frank hemorrhage (33).

As with the earliest minimally invasive techniques, patient satisfaction is based on therapeutic effect through percutaneous intervention without biomechanical destabilization and with timely recovery and return to the activities of daily living.

Spinal Endoscopy

Variable-angle lenses and advances in flexible fiberoptics combined to introduce the concept of spinal endoscopy during the late 1980s. The early development featured epiduroscopy concurrent with open surgery employed by Stoll (54). Further evolution of the endoscopic device was pioneered by Mathews along with Stoll and featured the introduction of a flexible steerable endoscope with a working channel providing greater latitude for visualization, resection, and documentation of pathology (32).

The current working channel scope features a 4.5 mm outer diameter with a 2.5 mm working channel. A pair of fiberoptic imaging bundles provides for 30,000-pixel resolution, a 2 to 30 mm depth of field, and a 70° visualization field (Fig. 36.6). The result is imaging with significant clarity and specificity, elements that are essential for the definitive identification and surgical management of anatomic structures at risk and of neuropathology. Differential lensing necessitates a clear understanding of spatial orientation in order to manipulate the scope for appreciation of landmarks and relationships in a safe working zone.

A variety of surgical tools may be employed under visualization for resection and removal of herniated nuclear tissue. Miniaturized manual instruments are commonly used for nerve decompression and disc removal through the working channel. Resection of pathologic nuclear tissue may be provided by motorized instruments such as a Diskector™ (Sofamor-Danek), which resects tissue by a guillotine-like action. The Ho:YAG sidefire laser has also been successfully used for laser vaporization of herniations and fragments, both intradiscally and in the epidural space, under direct visualization (4, 5).

A key component to successful endoscopic visualization in the foramen and the epidural space is the use of high-volume free-flow irrigation, which creates a working space and carries away debris resulting from surgical intervention. In addition, cooling the irrigating solution to 62°F aids hemostasis and provides an anesthetic effect on the nerve roots.

Though spinal endoscopic techniques were launched employing the posterolateral approach into

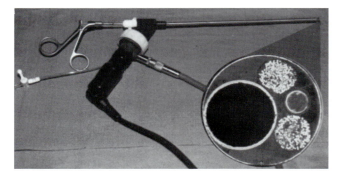

FIGURE 36.6.
Working channel fiberoptic endoscope showing the 2.5 mm working channel and the paired fiberoptic bundles (Sofamor-Danek, Inc., Memphis, TN).

a triangular working zone, a more versatile foraminal approach to the epidural space has evolved (28). A clear understanding of foraminal anatomy is crucial to the approach (Fig. 36.7). The foramen is essentially a dome, the door to which is the foraminal ligament, an extension of the ligamentum flavum that traverses the undersurface of the superior articulating facet and the pars interarticularis. From the dome, access is gained to the safe neural working zone in the epidural space that is defined by the exiting root passing through the approach foramen, the traversing root that courses medially for exit at the subsequent caudal foramen, and the intervertebral disc (Fig. 36.8A). The nerve roots are distinctly recognizable by their associated blood supply, identified as ribbon signs coursing along the respective nerves (Fig. 36.8B).

A clear distinction exists between early percutaneous posterolateral techniques and the foraminal endoscopic approach (Fig. 36.9). Early techniques were exclusively intradiscal procedures that were not pathology targeted. Emphasis was on careful movement of anatomic structures and indirect decompression of posterocentral abnormalities. Since these intradiscal techniques relied on excursion through the annulus fibrosus with withdrawal into the periannular space to search for sequestered fragments, mobility in the epidural space was denied such that sequestered pathologic tissue was inaccessible.

Conversely, the foraminal approach provides direct visualized access to the epidural space with unrestricted navigation. Wide field visualization allows

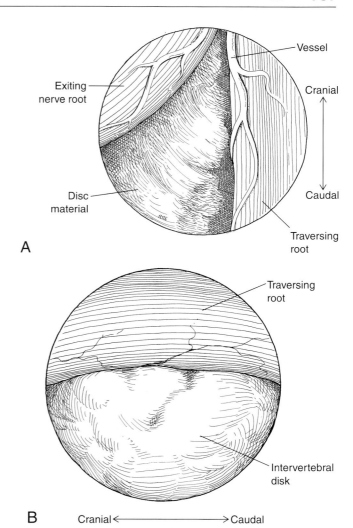

FIGURE 36.8.
A. Endoscopic view of the working zone. Through the endoscope the traversing and exiting nerve roots can be clearly seen as well as their associated blood vessels. **B.** An endoscopic view showing compression of the traversing nerve root by a herniated intervertebral disc.

identification and inspection of structures at risk, which can then be avoided while isolating and addressing neuropathology. Direct field visualization provides for safe, specific resection of contained or free sequestered pathologic tissue and subsequent verification and documentation of surgical effect (Fig. 36.10A,B).

At surgery, the patient is placed prone on a padded radiolucent frame. Local anesthesia with light intravenous sedation by way of monitored anesthesia care allows dialog between the patient and the operating surgeon, a circumstance required so that the patient can respond to sensations that might indicate neural impingement. Monitored anesthesia care also readily allows timely conversion to general anesthesia if conversion to an open procedure is necessary.

The operating room setup is such that the surgeon is positioned on the side of the patient's pathologic

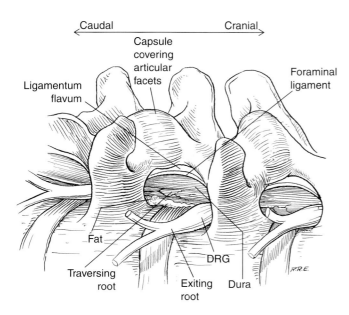

FIGURE 36.7.
Lateral view of the foraminal anatomy. The foraminal ligament, which extends from the superior articulating facet and the pars interarticularis, is shown as well as the exiting and traversing root and their relationship to the intervertebral disc.

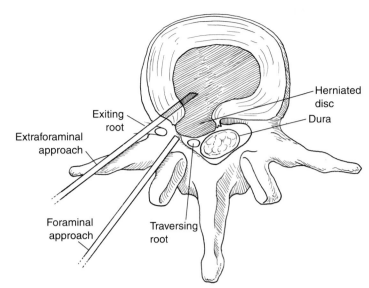

FIGURE 36.9. →

The foraminal approach compared to the percutaneous nucleotomy approach. Note that percutaneous nucleotomy is an intradiscal approach; the foraminal approach allows direct dissection and removal of herniated disc material.

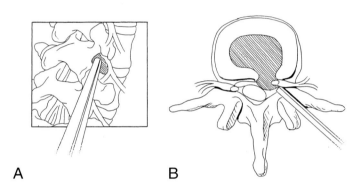

A B

FIGURE 36.10. ←

A. and **B.** The transforaminal approach and the relationship of the endoscope to the foramen, the exiting nerve root, and the herniated disc material.

site with the monitor and endoscopic light source located at the foot of the table so that visualization is unobstructed. The C-arm is located opposite the surgeon and is positioned to allow unobstructed anteroposterior and lateral imaging throughout the procedure. Equipment and endoscopic tools are usually placed on a stand between the surgeon and the video monitor.

The foraminal epidural endoscopic procedure is preceded by verification of the surgical level with fluoroscopic imaging of a needle or Kirschner wire placed at the level of planned surgical intervention. Discography usually follows to verify the contained nature of the disc, although it is not required for the procedure. The foraminal approach begins 9 to 13 cm from the midline with advancement to the pars interarticularis, and then a medial directing of the needle for docking on the foraminal ligament (Fig. 36.11). A cannula is passed over the needle, and the needle is withdrawn (Fig. 36.12A,B). The endoscope is passed through the cannula, and the working channel is used for dissection through the foraminal ligament. Then visualized passage is made through the

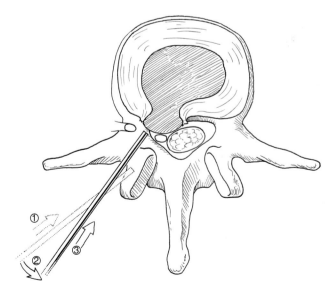

FIGURE 36.11.

Needle placement for the foraminal approach. Starting 9 to 13 cm from the midline, the needle is advanced to the pars interarticularis. The trajectory is then dropped and the needle slides under the pars into the foramen.

foramen until entry into the epidural space (Fig. 36.13).

Cool, free-flow irrigation quickly creates a potential working space, which facilitates the dissection and evacuation of epidural fat and debris as well as a medial pedicular landing, slightly cephalad to the disc, positioned in the safe working zone, as previously defined by the exiting and traversing nerve root and the disc. The irrigation, ideally maintained at 62°F, also promotes intraoperative hemostasis and local analgesic effect. In addition, bubbles generated during irrigation will gravitate posteriorly, resulting in the so-called bubble sign, which aids in maintaining spatial orientation (Fig. 36.14). Free-flow epidural irrigation must have a passive outflow during the surgical procedure. From the foraminal working zone, surgical exploration and intervention can proceed intradiscally or can effectively mimic myeloscopy and microdiscectomy, working within the canal and the epidural space.

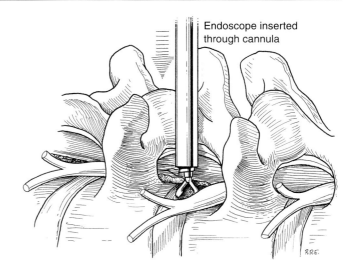

FIGURE 36.13.
The needle has been removed and the working channel endoscope has been placed through the cannula into the foramen. Instruments can then be passed through the working channel to dissect under direct visualization.

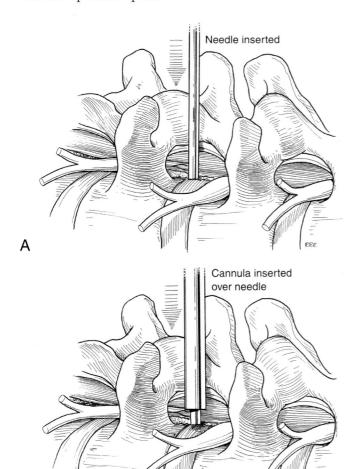

FIGURE 36.12.
A. Needle being advanced through the foramen. B. Cannula being advanced over the needle into the foramen. Instruments can then be passed through the working channel to dissect under direct visualization.

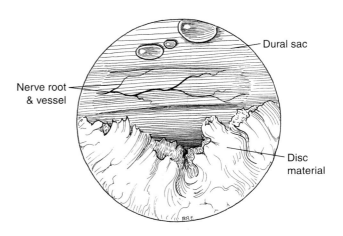

FIGURE 36.14.
Endoscopic view showing the traversing nerve root and the associated blood vessel as well as herniated disc material. Note the air bubble, which serves as a guide for orientation.

The parameters of the foraminal safe zone in the epidural space have allowed access with endoscopes varying in size, but usually limited to 6.3 mm or less, as demonstrated by Mirkovic and colleagues (37).

The unrestricted navigation associated with the foraminal approach into the epidural space allows identification, inspection, and avoidance of anatomic structures and surgical correction with documentation of pathology. The foraminal approach is especially indicated for paracentral, foraminal, and far-lateral herniations, and sequestered free fragments are fair game because of the endoscopic mobility. The foraminal approach is extremely important for foraminal and extraforaminal herniations. Mathews has defined four zones of extraforaminal herniations: zone 1 at pedicle level; zone 2 at disc level; zone 3 is beneath the exiting root; and zone 4 is superior to the exiting root. Fragments in zone 4 are usually not accessible via the foraminal approach and should represent an indication for an open procedure (Mathews HH, Savas PE, Mathern BE, Long BH, Mason S, unpublished work, 1996).

Indications for foraminal epidural endoscopic surgery include lumbar herniations that may be contained but can be uncontained with migration and sequestration but must be limited to less than 50% of the canal diameter to allow navigational access (Fig. 36.15A,B).

Contraindications to the technique are stenosis, epidural fibrosis, gross instability, and multilevel pathology. Relative contraindications to foraminoscopy are obesity, because of the size of instruments relative to the girth of the patient, and previous surgery, which is associated with predictable scar, limiting excursion during endoscopic techniques. Advanced age must also be considered a relative contraindication because of the high probability of stenosis and of degenerated, fibrotic disc material prone to recurrence without more radical discectomy and not amenable to manual endoscopic techniques employing delicate instrumentation.

For contained epidural endoscopic lumbar surgery, neural elements are no longer at high risk since, rather than being moved, they can be seen and

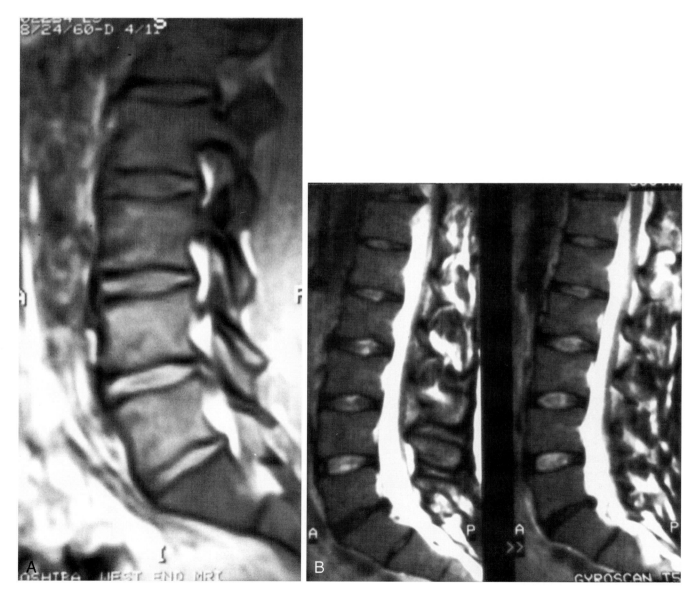

FIGURE 36.15.

A. Sagittal MRI showing large uncontained disc herniation at L4–5. **B.** Postoperative MRI after transforaminal endoscopic discectomy showing complete resection of the herniated disc fragment.

avoided as abnormalities are identified and their correction with manual and/or automated tools can be visualized, verified, and documented. Flexible fiberoptic instrumentation joined with foraminal access has allowed visualized exploration and surgical intervention for neuropathology similar to the technique of microdiscectomy. As such it has been compared to microdiscectomy through a cannula. Intracanal, intradiscal, and epidural space access has resulted in a technique with high specificity and patient satisfaction.

Complications associated with foraminal epidural endoscopic surgery are reduced in comparison with other percutaneous procedures because of the surgeon's ability to visualize all elements of the procedure. The most common surgical event is steep iliac crest anatomic obstruction to approach at L5-S1, which has been well described for all percutaneous procedures even with the aid of curved access cannulae. The incidence of postoperative headache responsive to blood patch has been documented but unexplained in the absence of intraoperative sequelae suggestive of dural insult. Discitis and hematoma are other potential complications. Foraminal epidural endoscopic surgery, though the latest and most promising dimension in minimally invasive access to the lumbar spine, has several deficits; chief among these is the diversity in practitioners' insight into spatial orientation and understanding of anatomy, pathology, and structures at risk. The technique has a significant learning curve for both surgeon and staff, and outcomes are critically linked to patient selection.

Percutaneous Fusion Procedures

Two minimally invasive techniques currently in use for interbody fusion have become recognized for stabilization of the lumbar spine. These are foraminal epidural endoscopy–assisted interbody fusion with or without percutaneous internal fixation, and laparoscopic transperitoneal L4–S1 or laparoscopic retroperitoneal L2–L5 discectomy with anterior lumbar interbody fusion.

Percutaneous Lumbar Interbody Fusion

Foraminal epidural endoscopy–assisted interbody procedures were developed on the basis of the experience of Swiss practitioners Schreiber, Leu, and Hauser, who used percutaneous external fixators as stabilization followed by percutaneous biportal anterior interbody fusions (22, 49). This technique was succeeded by a single-stage procedure reported by Mathews (31).

Clinical indications for percutaneous interbody fusion procedures include gross instability or spondylolisthesis as well as degenerative scoliosis and arachnoiditis. Relative contraindications include spinal stenosis; smoking, as a variable influencing fusion rate and mass; long-term chronic pain, which may affect clinical outcome relative to patient satisfaction and insurance status; advanced age, with potential suboptimum bone integrity; and obesity, in which excessive physical forces may overstress instrumentation. Clinical assessment must be augmented through the evaluation of flexion-extension plain roentgenograms as well as MRI or flexion/extension myelogram with postmyelogram CT and often with the addition of discography.

At surgery, the patient is positioned on a radiolucent frame and provided local anesthesia and intravenous sedation. High-quality fluoroscopy verifies access to the disc via the foramen from a skin starting point 9 to 13 cm from the midline. Following discography and complete discectomy with endplate preparation using manual, automated, or laser tools, spinal anesthesia allows bone graft harvest, pedicular fixation, and arthrodesis.

For instrumentation, the sharp end of a 0.062 guide-wire is advanced through the skin 1 cm lateral to the area for cannulization, followed by anteroposterior fluoroscopic verification. The fluoroscope is then angled at 15° off the AP position in line with the pedicle to be instrumented. Once the guide pin is confirmed as centered within the pedicle and the cortex is palpated, it is tapped into place to prevent "walking" until advancement is desired. Tissue dilators protect muscle until the guide pin is advanced and seated into the vertebral body with anteroposterior and lateral fluoroscopic verification. This procedure is repeated for each pedicle to be instrumented. Small incisions are then made, and the subcutaneous tissue is dissected suprafascially. A three-component tissue dilator serves for drilling, and then placement of 7.0 cannulated self-tapping screws advanced to a 50% depth of all pedicles. Plates are placed, with adjustment of ipsilateral and contralateral screws followed by cross-linking and locking nuts and final biplanar fluoroscopic verification (Fig. 36.16A,B). Bone grafting is done with endoscopic visualization, and then closure is performed.

Potential complications include infection, failure of instrumentation, nerve damage, and failure of arthrodesis, which has been the most significant issue, given soft grafting techniques. With prospective studies and advancement in bone substitutes, foraminal epidural endoscopic lumbar spine stabilization continues to offer the potential for decreased surgical morbidity, diminished hospitalization, and reduced long-term impact on lifestyle, and a higher likelihood of return to the presurgical activities of daily living.

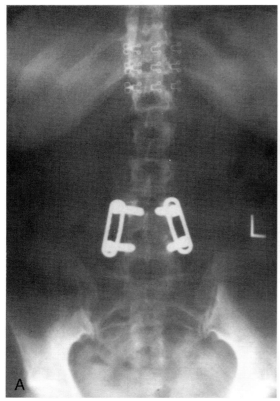
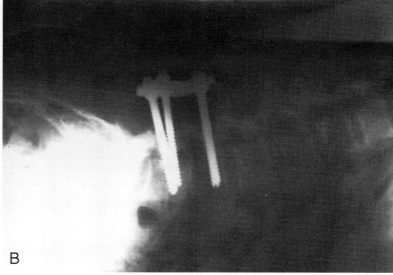

FIGURE 36.16.

A. and **B.** Anteroposterior and lateral roentgenograms showing percutaneously placed suprafascial subcutaneous fixation as part of percutaneous interbody fusion procedure.

Percutaneous Anterior Lumbar Interbody Fusion

For anterior column collapse with early signs, including disc disruption syndrome and disc-space collapse, endplate inflammation, edema, and sclerosis (Fig. 36.17), laparoscopic transperitoneal discectomy with anterior lumbar interbody fusion has shown early promise (29). Other proposed indications have included disc herniation and minimal instability as well as selected deformities and fractures.

Early work with laparoscopic access to the intervertebral disc was done by Obenchain, who reported success with laparoscopic discectomy techniques first at L5-S1, and later at L3–4 and L4–5 (39–41).

Patients present with anterior column pain, radiculitis, and vague pelvic and/or groin pain. Discography may be helpful in determining the true pain generators in the confirmation of the diagnosis. Preoperative MRI staging is highly recommended if not required to determine the location of the aorta and iliac vein confluence and to determine the skin portal of entry, usually 5 cm above the pubic symphysis for parallel access to the endplates and the center of the disc (Fig. 36.18A,B), thus reducing the potential for intraoperative vascular trauma and hemorrhage.

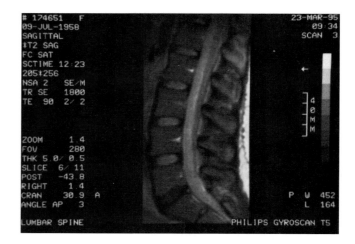

FIGURE 36.17.

Preoperative sagittal MRI showing desiccated and collapsed L5-S1 disc. Discography confirmed that the L5-S1 disc degeneration was the symptomatic pain generator for this patient.

At surgery, the patient is placed in mild Trendelenburg position on a diving board table with excellent fluoroscopic capabilities assured. Adjuncts to surgery include general endotracheal anesthesia, Foley catheter, and nasogastric tube for appropriate de-

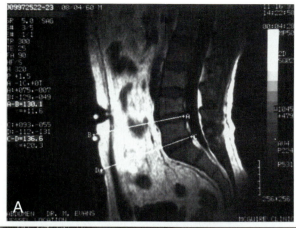

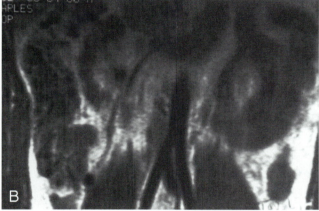

FIGURE 36.18.
A. Sagittal MRI used for preoperative staging prior to laparoscopic anterior lumbar interbody fusion. Skin markers (B and D) correspond to the entry points used to approach the corresponding disc levels. **B.** Bifurcation of iliac vessels, which, when considered in conjunction with axial images, confirms appropriateness of laparoscopic approach.

compressions. Preoperative bowel preparation may also be advised.

It is highly recommended that a general surgeon accomplish the multiportal approach for abdominal laparoscopy. A discogram needle under fluoroscopic view will confirm disc location. With CO_2 seal, cannulated dilators and cannulated drill bits or regular osteotomes facilitate the spine surgeon's preparation of the graft bed following discectomy using manual and/or automated instruments under direct or fiberoptic visualization (Fig. 36.19A,B). Bicortical Cloward-type dowels or rectangular tricortical blocks are then harvested from the iliac crest through a separate incision, and disc height is restored by progressive interspace distraction with delivery and loading of the graft.

Other investigators have pursued a similar surgical technique but with the use of a cage implant for the purpose of restoring disc height and foraminal aperture (56). The procedure has also been performed using cage or bone in retroperitoneal dissection with and without CO_2 insufflation. Theoretical complications for the technique include trauma to the ureter, bowel perforation, and anterior spinal artery syndrome as well as trauma to great vessels and to the hypogastric plexus with transient or permanent retrograde ejaculation. In actual clinical work, there have been reports of vascular laceration with subsequent conversion to open anterior lumbar interbody fusion (ALIF). In such instances the vascular misadventure has been attributed to the surgical learning curve.

Laparoscopic transperitoneal discectomy with anterior lumbar interbody fusion, either instrumented or noninstrumented, seems in its early stages to provide a reasonably safe alternative to traditional ALIF. With surgeon experience, the procedure offers shortening of operative time in comparison with either traditional anterior or posterior fusion procedures with concomitant reduction in anesthesia time. There is also a potential comparative reduction in surgical morbidity, including blood loss, biomechanical destabilization, hospital length of stay, and analgesic requirements. Successful surgical outcome depends on a skilled laparoscopist who is familiar with the anatomy and structures at risk, and on optimum preoperative MRI staging.

MacMillan and colleagues have described a transsacral approach via two 1-inch muscle-splitting incisions. The horizontal position of the sacroiliac joint is entered with a guide-wire traversing the bony sacrum and across the endplate at L5-S1. This is performed bilaterally, creating crossed wires on anteroposterior fluoroscopic views. Discectomy and endplate preparation is then performed via the transsacral intradiscal approach. Bone or screws are inserted after dissection and fusion for fixation. Initial results are promising, and the procedure may carry less risk than laparoscopy for L5-S1 access (25).

Mayer has proposed a microscopic mini-ALIF via transperitoneal and retroperitoneal approaches. The technique appears to advance closer to optimum, less morbid anterior column intervention (Mayer HM, personal communication, 1996).

Long-term prospective outcome studies of noninstrumented as well as instrumented minimally invasive ALIF will be essential to demonstrate and validate efficacy, decreased morbidity, and cost-effectiveness.

The Future of Minimally Invasive Spine Surgery

Currently recognized minimally invasive techniques all continue to have limitations in their applicability and versatility. These relative shortcomings foster the ongoing development of surgical alternatives devoid of the comorbidities associated with open sur-

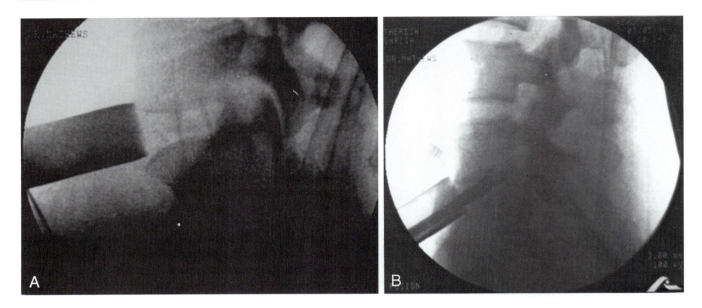

FIGURE 36.19.
A. Large transabdominal cannula docked in the anterior portion of the L5-S1 disc. The placement and securing of this cannula are done in conjunction with a laparoscopic general surgeon. **B.** Lateral roentgenogram showing a large curette in the L5-S1 disc space preparing the graft bed for laparoscopic placement of the bone dowels.

gery. Combining aggressive approaches with advanced technology offers an exciting field of spine surgery that warrants development.

The progressive advancement of fiberoptic technology and working channel endoscopy has provided approaches more aggressively targeted toward pathologic tissues. These advanced techniques offer exciting possibilities for future technology, including the development of disc sealing devices, disc rehydration, and the insertion of carrier mechanisms for bone morphogenic protein.

Technology must continue to address the issue of endoscope size and indications. While smaller endoscopes have allowed entry into the spinal canal for access to extraforaminal herniations, the development of larger scopes will create opportunities to address large collagenized fragments, paramedian herniations, and subarticular stenosis.

Herniated nuclear material and other abnormalities present in many shapes, sizes, and locations. With the development of a family of endoscopes and associated working channel tools, further development and refinement of surgical techniques will expand the indications and interventions for minimally invasive correction of spinal defects and deformities.

References

1. Alexander H. Chemonucleolysis for acute disc herniation. J Musculoskel Med 1995;2:13–24.
2. Aprill C, Bogduk N. High intensity zone: a diagnostic sign of painful lumbar disc on magnetic resonance imaging. B J Radiol 1992;65:361–369.
3. Bernard TN Jr. Lumbar discography followed by computed tomography: refining the diagnosis of low back pain. Spine 1990;15:690–707.
4. Casper GD, Hartman VL, Mullins LL. Percutaneous laser disc decompression with the holmium:YAG laser. J Clin Laser Med Surg 1995;13:195–203.
5. Casper GD, Mullins LL, Hartman VL. Laser assisted disc decompression: a clinical trial of the holmium:YAG laser with side firing fiber. J Clin Laser Med Surg 1995;13:27–32.
6. Castro WHM, Jerosch J, Hepp R, et al. Restriction of indications for automated percutaneous lumbar discectomy based on computed tomographic discography. Spine 1992;17:1239–1243.
7. Castro WHM, Jerosch J, Schilgen M, et al. Automated percutaneous nucleotomy: restricted indications based on CT scan appearance. Neurosurg Clin N Am 1996;7:43–47.
8. Choy DSJ, Ascher PW, Saddekni S, et al. Percutaneous laser disc decompression: a new therapeutic modality. Spine 1992;17:949–956.
9. Colhoun E, McCall IW, Williams L, et al. Provocative discography as a guide to planning operations of the spine. J Bone Joint Surg 1988;70B:267–271.
10. Craig FS. Vertebral body biopsy. J Bone Joint Surg 1956;38A:93–102.
11. Davis GW, Onik G, Helms C. Automated percutaneous discectomy. Spine 1991;16:359–363.
12. Guyer RD, Ohnmeiss DD. Contemporary concepts in spine care: lumbar discography. Spine 1995;20:2048–2059.
13. Hijikata S. Percutaneous nucleotomy: a new concept technique and 12 years' experience. Clin Orthop 1989;238:9–23.
14. Hijikata S, Yamagishi M, Nakayama T, et al. Percuta-

neous nucleotomy: a new treatment method for lumbar disc herniation. J Toden Hosp 1975;5:39.
15. Hoppenfeld S. Percutaneous removal of herniated lumbar discs: 50 cases with ten-year follow-up periods. Clin Orthop 1989;238:92–97.
16. Javid MJ. Chemonucleolysis versus laminectomy: a cohort comparison of effectiveness and charges. Spine 1995;20:2016–2022.
17. Javid MF, Nordby EJ. Lumbar chymopapain nucleolysis. Neurosurg Clin N Am 1996;6:17–27.
18. Kambin P. Arthroscopic microdiscectomy. Arthroscopy 1992;8:287–295.
19. Kambin P. Diagnostic and therapeutic arthroscopy. Neurosurg Clin N Am 1996;7:65–76.
20. Kambin P, Schaffer JL. Percutaneous lumbar discectomy: review of 100 patients and current practice. Clin Orthop 1989;238:24–34.
21. Kinard RE. Diagnostic spinal injection procedures. Neurosurg Clin N Am 1996;7:151–165.
22. Leu HF, Hauser RK. Percutaneous endoscopic lumbar spine fusion. Neurosurg Clin N Am 1996;7:107–117.
23. Lindblom K. Diagnostic puncture of intervertebral disks in sciatica. Acta Orthop Scand 1948;17:231–239.
24. Lindblom K. Technique and results in myelography and disc puncture. Acta Radiol Scand 1950;34:321–330.
25. MacMillan M, Fessler RG, Gillespy M, et al. Percutaneous lumbosacral fixation and fusion: anatomic study and two-year experience with a new method. Neurosurg Clin N Am 1996;7:99–106.
26. Maroon JC, Onik G. Percutaneous automated discectomy: a new method for lumbar disc removal. J Neurosurg 1987;66:143–146.
27. Maroon JC, Onik G, Sternau L. Percutaneous automated discectomy: a new approach to lumbar surgery. Clin Orthop 1989;238:64–70.
28. Mathews HH. Transforaminal endoscopic microdiscectomy. Neurosurg Clin N Am 1996;7:59–63.
29. Mathews HH, Evans MT, Molligan HJ, et al. Laparoscopic discectomy with anterior lumbar interbody fusion: a preliminary review. Spine 1995;20:1797–1802.
30. Mathews HH, Kyles MK, Fiore SM, et al. Laser disc decompression with KTP 532 wavelength: a two-year follow-up. Presented at the annual meeting of the American Academy of Orthopaedic Surgeons, New Orleans, February 1994.
31. Mathews HH, Long BH. Endoscopy assisted percutaneous anterior interbody fusion with subcutaneous, suprafascial internal fixation: evolution of technique and surgical considerations. Orthop (Intl Ed) 1995;3:496–500.
32. Mathews HH, Stoll JE. FDA IDE Study. Sofamor-Danek, 1989.
33. Mayer HM. Spine update: percutaneous lumbar disc surgery. Spine 1994;19:2719–2723.
34. Mayer HM, Brock M. Percutaneous endoscopic discectomy: surgical technique and preliminary results compared to microsurgical discectomy. J Neurosurg 1993;78:216–225.
35. McCormick CC. Radiology in low back pain and sciatica: an analysis of the relative efficacy of spinal venography, discography, and epidurography in patient with a negative or equivocal myelogram. Clin Radiol 1978;29:393–406.
36. Mink JH. Imaging evaluation of the candidate for percutaneous lumbar discectomy. Clin Orthop 1989;238:83–91.
37. Mirkovic SR, Schwartz DG, Glazier KD. Anatomic considerations in lumbar posterolateral percutaneous procedures. Spine 1995;20:1965–1971.
38. Nordby EJ, Wright PH. Efficacy of chymopapain in chemonucleolysis: a review. Spine 1994;19:2578–2582.
39. Obenchain TG. Laparoscopic lumbar discectomy: case report. J Laparoendosc Surg 1991;1:145–149.
40. Obenchain TG, Cloyd D. Laparoscopic lumbar discectomy: description of transperitoneal and retroperitoneal techniques. Neurosurg Clin N Am 1996;75:77–85.
41. Obenchain TG, Cloyd D, Savin M. Outpatient laparoscopic lumbar discectomy. In: Braverman MH, Tawes RL, eds. Surgical Technology II. San Francisco: Surgical Technology International, 1993:415–418.
42. Onik G, Mooney V, Maroon JC, et al. Automated percutaneous discectomy: a prospective multi-institutional study. Neurosurgery 1990;26:228–232.
43. Quigley MR. Percutaneous laser discectomy. Neurosurg Clin N Am 1996;7:37–42.
44. Quigley MR, Maroon JC. Automated percutaneous discectomy. Neurosurg Clin N Am 1996;7:29–35.
45. Quigley MR, Maroon JC, Shih T, et al. Laser discectomy: comparison of systems. Spine 1994;19:319–322.
46. Revel M, Payan C, Vallee C, et al. Automated percutaneous lumbar discectomy versus chemonucleolysis in the treatment of sciatica: a randomized multicenter trial. Spine 1993;18:1–7.
47. Schaffer JL, Kambin P. Percutaneous posterolateral lumbar discectomy and decompression with a 6.9 millimeter cannula: analysis of operative failures and complications. J Bone Joint Surg 1991;73A:822–831.
48. Schreiber A, Leu H. Percutaneous nucleotomy: technique with discoscopy. Orthopedics 1991;14:439–444.
49. Schreiber JA, Leu HJ. Restabilisation intervertébral et arthrodèse intersomatique percutané: possibilités aujourd'hui. Rachis 1989;1:173–189.
50. Schreiber A, Suezawa Y, Leu H. Does percutaneous nucleotomy with discoscopy replace conventional discectomy? Eight years of experience and results in treatment of herniated lumbar disc. Clin Orthop 1989;238:35–42.
51. Simmons EH, Segil CM. An evaluation of discography in the localization of symptomatic levels in discogenic disease of the spine. Clin Orthop 1975;108:57–69.
52. Sherk HH, Black JD, Prodoehl JA, et al. Laser diskectomy. Orthopedics 1993;16:573–576.
53. Smith L. Enzyme dissolution of the nucleus pulposus in humans. JAMA 1964;187:137–140.
54. Stoll JE. Endoscopic spatial orientation and surgical approaches in the epidural space. Didactic Presentation. Current Concepts in Spinal Endoscopy. Williamsburg, VA. April 1993.
55. Walsh TR, Weinstein JN, Spratt KF, et al. Lumbar discography in normal subjects: a controlled, prospective study. J Bone Joint Surg Am 1990;72:1081–1088.
56. Zucherman JF, Zdeblick TA, Bailey SA, et al. Instrumented laparoscopic spinal fusion: preliminary results. Spine 1995;20:2029–2035.

CHAPTER THIRTY SEVEN

Microsurgery for Lumbar Disc Disease

John A. McCulloch

Introduction

Patient selection for surgery for lumbar disc disease largely determines outcome. Whether or not you use the microscope to complete the surgical exercise will have little effect on the outcome (16). In fact, when you first start to use the microscope, your time to complete the surgical exercise will be extended and your complication rate (e.g., dural tears) will increase. So why do we even consider the microscope?

Every surgeon wants to "see better" and "see more," which is why the microscope is so useful in spine surgery. The by-product is a smaller incision and wound (1 inch in length) for single-segment surgery. These wounds have less postoperative morbidity and permit earlier patient mobilization (e.g., outpatient microdiscectomy). In addition, these wounds heal with less scar tissue since there is less muscle dissection and less healing by secondary intention.

In 1913 William Halsted remarked, "I believe that the tendency will always be in the direction of exercising greater care and refinement in operating, and that the surgeon will develop increasingly a respect for tissues; a sense which recoils from inflicting, unnecessarily, insult to structures concerned in the process of repair." This historic observation is becoming more important as more surgery is being performed through limited exposures. The ability to do spine surgery through limited exposure has been brought about by two modern factors. First, there is a much better understanding of syndromes that affect function in the low back. An example is the better distinction between a radicular syndrome resulting from a disc herniation and one resulting from subarticular stenosis. Second, more sophisticated investigative tools, such as computed tomography (CT) scanning and magnetic resonance imaging (MRI), allow an accurate clinical diagnosis on which to base a surgical decision. Not only is an accurate clinical diagnosis possible, but an exact definition and localization of the pathology within the spinal canal is also available, allowing for limited surgical intervention.

Anatomy Essential for Using a Limited Surgical Incision

Anatomy is the foundation of all surgical successes. But the moment you reduce the size of your wound and give up a broad surgical field is the moment you realize the importance of an extremely detailed (millimeter by millimeter) knowledge of spinal anatomy. The following concepts will help you grasp that intimate detail.

Concept 1: The Skeletal Anatomy of the Lumbar Spine

The anatomic unit of the lumbar spine is a vertebral body and a disc below (Fig. 37.1A). Just as the brain needs a skull for protection, the spinal cord and cauda equina need skeletal coverings. To provide this protection, each vertebral segment has attached posterior elements. For a moment, ignore the disc space and concentrate on an imaginary line joining the inferior pedicle borders (Fig 37.1A). There are six named posterior elements, three lying above that line (all paired) and three lying below (two of the three paired). Lying right on that dividing line is the pars interarticularis.

Concept 2: Nerve Root Anatomy

The neural structures in the lower lumbar spinal canal include the dural sheath, containing the cauda equina, and bilaterally exiting nerve roots for each anatomic segment. The exiting nerve root is numbered according to the pedicle beneath which it passes (Fig. 37.1B) (unlike in the cervical spine, where a nerve root is numbered according to the pedicle above which it passes). Lumbar nerve roots are intimately related to the pedicle beneath which they pass; when looking for a nerve root in the spinal canal, a good rule to obey is to locate its adjacent pedicle. Not only does each anatomic segment have paired exiting roots, but also there are the more medial traversing nerve roots (Fig. 37.1B).

Concept 3: Imaging Localization of Pathology

The eyes of today's microsurgeon are the sensitive imaging modalities of MRI and CT. To help localize lesions within the spinal canal, a "three-storied anatomic house" for each spinal segment is proposed (Fig. 37.2A). This concept helps the surgeon reformat in his or her mind the exact location of pathology in the interface between the disc/vertebral column and the neural column (Fig. 37.2B).

Using the inferior border of the pedicles as an artificial division line (Fig. 37.1A), each anatomic segment can be divided into three "stories," as in a house. (The choice of the concept "stories in a house" will become evident in the next few pages).

Now let us reconsider the posterior elements (take another look at Figure 37.1A). Of these six elements, only two are located in a single story—the pedicle and the transverse process are located exclusively in the third story. The superior facet is not only in the third story but it also overlies the disc space (first story) of the segment above. Similarly, the inferior facet straddles the territory of the first and second stories; the cephalad border of the lamina encroaches on the third story of the same anatomic level, and the caudal border overhangs the first story of that anatomic segment.

The next exercise is to "read the stories," an exercise that allows the surgeon to reformat and exactly localize pathology within the interface between the

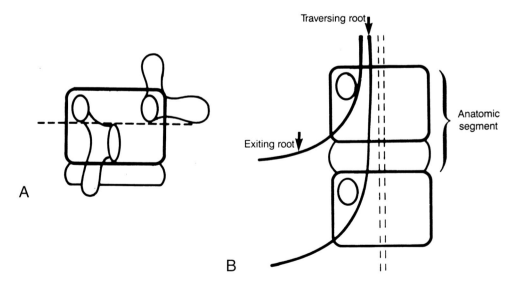

FIGURE 37.1.

A. The anatomic unit of the lumbar spine is the vertebral body and the disc below. The posterior elements are shown, three above the broken infrapedicular line and three (lamina, spinous process, and inferior facet) below this line. **B.** Each anatomic segment has an exiting root and traversing root(s). If this is the fourth anatomic segment, the exiting root would be numbered L4.

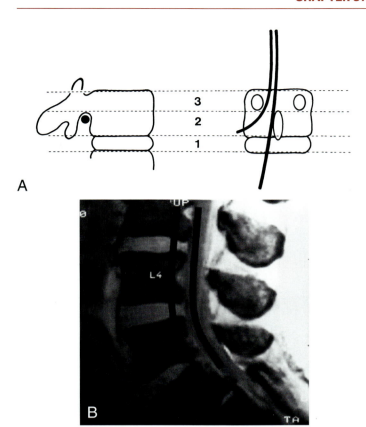

FIGURE 37.2.
A. The "three-storied anatomic house" concept for each anatomic segment: first story—the disc level; second story—the foraminal level; third story—the pedicle level. **B.** This three-storied house concept applies to reading pathology in the interface between the disc/vertebral column and the common dural sac (between the two black lines).

disc/vertebral column and the neural column (Fig. 37.3A–F).

Concept 4: Windows of Opportunity into the Spinal Canal

In linking the anatomic segments and studying the posterior elements, it is possible to construct three "windows of opportunity" into the spinal canal (Fig. 37.4A). You are already familiar with the routine interlaminar window. This unilateral interlaminar window can be used to enter the opposite side of the spinal canal (window 2 in Fig. 37.4A). The third window of opportunity into the spinal canal is the intertransverse window. The use of these three windows of opportunity into the spinal house is facilitated by the magnification and illumination inherent in the microscope.

The Interlaminar Window

The so-called "standard laminectomy" has utilized the interlaminar window. The salient anatomic features of this window are as follows.

1. THE DIMENSIONS OF THE WINDOW

Note on the x-ray that with descending levels in the lumbar spine the dimensions of the interlaminar window become broader and higher (Fig. 37.4B).

This makes entry into the canal for an L5-S1 discectomy a relatively easy procedure—compared to, say, an L2–3 discectomy.

2. LAMINAR OVERHANG

Also note that with ascending levels there is more of the inferior edge of the lamina that overhangs the disc space (Fig. 37.4B). This phenomenon is lessened by surgical frames that flex the lumbar spine and increased by surgical frames that allow positioning of the patient in a neutral or lordotic position. It is an important fact to be aware of when trying to retrieve a disc herniation from the second story of L1, L2, L3, or L4, as a considerable portion of the cephalad lamina has to be removed for a direct view of this pathology.

3. LAMINAR OVERHANG AND WRONG LEVEL EXPOSURES

Laminar overhang and the anteriorly sloping lamina create the setting for wrong level exposures (Fig. 37.4C). Add this to a patient who has degenerative disc disease with a narrowed interlaminar distance, who is short, obese, loose-jointed, and positioned on a kneeling surgical frame (e.g., the Andrew's frame), which cannot reduce lordosis, and it is a reasonable expectation that a limited surgical incision will result in wrong level exposure.

4. CONTENTS OF THE LUMBAR SPINAL CANAL

The more proximal lumbar spinal canal levels have three more salient anatomic features:

1. They contain more neural tissue. L1 has conus medullaris and all of the lumbar and sacral roots, whereas L5 has no cord and only the L5 to S5 sacral roots.
2. The canal space available for neural tissue at L1 is much reduced compared to L5.
3. The proximal lumbar roots take a more horizontal course in exiting through the foramen. This makes the L1 root less mobile than the S1 root.

In summary: An exposure of an L2–3 disc is a much more difficult technical exercise than that of an L5-S1 disc because of laminar overhang, a smaller canal with greater neural contents, and the more horizontally exiting roots. If the disc herniation is up in the second story of a proximal lumbar anatomic segment, you have a real microsurgical challenge.

5. THE AXILLARY DISC RUPTURE

The axilla of the L5 traversing nerve root and the S1 traversing root are related to the disc space as shown in Figure 37.5A. This is an important relationship to appreciate, because an axillary disc, which is more prone to occur at L5-S1 (Fig. 37.5B), can displace a nerve root far into the subarticular region and out of direct view, where it can be damaged by the unwary surgeon.

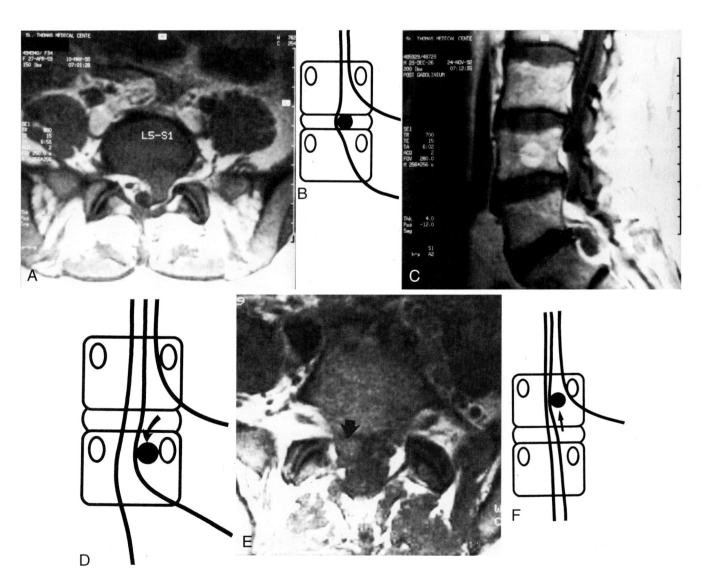

FIGURE 37.3.

A. A disc herniation in the first story of the L5 anatomic segment, and **B.** a schematic for the same. **C.** A disc herniation migrating from the first story of L5 into the third story of the S1 anatomic segment, and **D.** a schematic for the same. **E.** A disc herniation that has migrated up into the second story of L5 (arrow), and **F.** a schematic for the same.

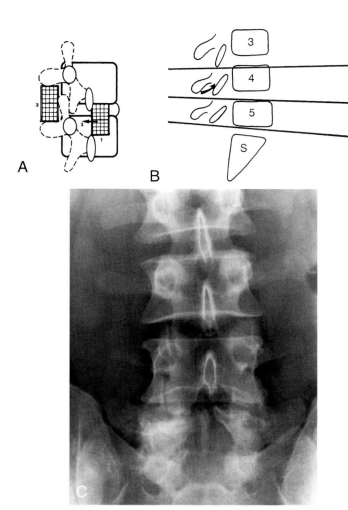

FIGURE 37.4.

A. The windows of opportunity into the spinal canal: *(1)* interlaminar; *(2)* contralateral interlaminar from ipsilateral interlaminar; *(3)* intertransverse. **B.** Note the interlaminar windows (made even larger still at L5-S1 by a spina bifida). **C.** If "laminar overhang" is not appreciated, it is easy to slide cephalad on the lamina of L4 and end up in L3–4 (arrow) instead of L4–5.

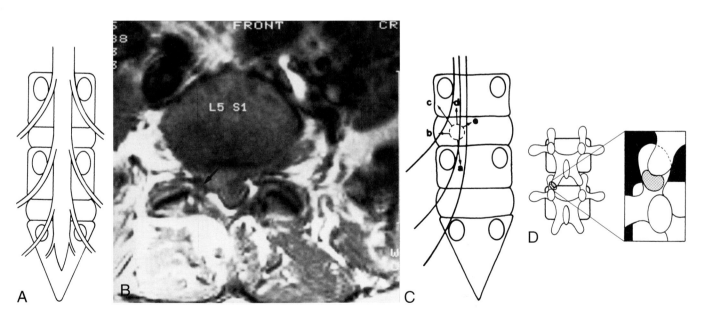

FIGURE 37.5.

A. Note that the axilla of the S1 root is in the first story of L5, whereas the axilla of the L5 root is in the third story of L5—a fact that makes axillary disc herniations more common at L5-S1 than at L4–5. **B.** An axillary disc herniation L5-S1 right. The S1 nerve root is displaced into the lateral recess (arrow). **C.** Migratory patterns of disc ruptures: *(a)* down into the third story of the segment below; *(b)* direct lateral; *(c)* up into the foramen; *(d)* up into the second story within the canal; *(e)* medially. **D.** The "safety net" of "whitish" fat can be found at the inferior edge of the interior facet (inset).

6. THE MIGRATING DISC RUPTURE

Disc herniations usually occur in the posterolateral quadrant of the disc space, but they can migrate as extruded and sequestered fragments (Fig. 37.5C). The MRI scans in Figure 37.3 show migrated disc fragments; the posterior element anatomy has to be utilized to arrive at the exact location of the migrated fragment.

7. LOCATING THE INTERLAMINAR WINDOW— "THE SAFETY NET"

After dissecting soft tissue off of the interspinous/interlaminar windows and positioning the frame retractor, look for the "safety net" (Fig. 37.5D). This area is labeled the safety net because it is marked by the facet fat pad (a "whiter" fat than normal); deep to it lies the joint surface of the superior facet. Plunging a sharp instrument into the safety net is harmless, because the cartilaginous surface of the superior facet protects the nerve root. Once the safety net has been identified, it is then easy to move along the cephalad or caudal laminar borders.

8. ENTERING THE SPINAL CANAL THROUGH THE INTERLAMINAR WINDOW

There are basically three ways to cross the ligamentum flavum to enter the spinal canal:

1. Transligamentous
2. Through the cephalad lamina
3. Through the caudal lamina

Transligamentous. Only if a normal interlaminar space is present is this a viable option. If degenerative changes have narrowed the disc space and/or resulted in facet hypertrophy or shingling of the lamina, this approach should not even be tried. When directly crossing the ligamentum flavum, a word of caution is in order: The L5-S1 ligamentum flavum has a tremendous variation in thickness from patient to patient. It can be very thin, especially in the presence of any congenital lumbosacral anomaly, such as spina bifida; one bold stroke used to cross the midportion of such a ligament may land you in a sea of cerebrospinal fluid because of a dural laceration.

Through the cephalad lamina. Because of the frequency of a narrowed interlaminar space in laminectomy, many surgeons prefer to remove a portion of the proximal (or cephalad) lamina before crossing ligamentum flavum. Often it is recommended that the ligamentum flavum be detached with an elevator before the proximal laminectomy is attempted. Rather, remember that the lamina is thicker (anterior/posterior dimension) laterally and thinner medially. Use this knowledge with the Kerrison medially on the lamina, and dissect sublaminar as you are removing the edge of the lamina.

Through the caudad lamina. Probably the easiest way to enter the spinal canal is through the superior edge of the caudad lamina. This is easy because of two anatomic factors: *(a)* the ligamentum flavum attaches to the posterosuperior edge of the caudad lamina and is easy to remove (Fig. 37.6); and *(b)* the shape of the dural sheath and adjacent nerve root leaves a small, safe area of entry along the midportion of the lamina.

Spinal Stenosis and Window #2

The salient anatomic features of spinal stenosis and the unilateral interlaminar window for bilateral and canal surgery are as follows.

1. THE CENTRAL AND LATERAL ZONES

Spinal stenosis can be divided into central canal stenosis or lateral zone stenosis (Fig. 37.7A). Central canal stenosis is a true circumferential encroachment on cauda equina territory with annular bulging anteriorly (with or without a spondylolisthesis), facet joint hypertrophy laterally, and ligamentum flavum infolding posteriorly (Fig. 37.7B). Note that the predominant location of the lesion in acquired spinal canal stenosis is largely in the first story of the anatomic segment, with some extension of the lesion into contiguous portions of the second story of the same segment and the third story of the adjacent caudad segment.

2. THE ATTACHMENTS OF THE LIGAMENTUM FLAVUM

Using the knowledge of attachment of the ligamentum flavum, it is possible to decompress the lesion in spinal canal stenosis with a limited microsurgical

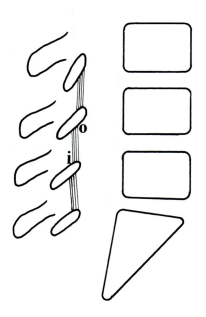

FIGURE 37.6.

The origin (o) of the ligamentum flavum from the anterior half of the cephalad lamina, and its insertion (I) on the superior edge of the caudad lamina.

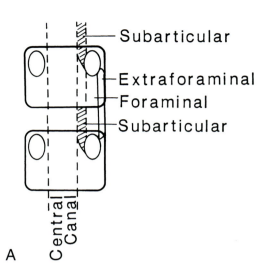
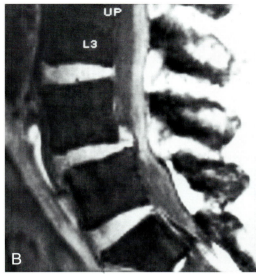

FIGURE 37.7.
A. The lateral canal subzones and the central canal. **B.** A sagittal spin-echo (proton density) MRI in spinal canal stenosis and degenerative spondylolisthesis.

exposure (Fig. 37.8A). The cephalad lamina is removed proximally until the origin of the ligamentum flavum fibers is seen. This is evident as a thinning of the ligamentum flavum proximally and the sighting of the "blue" common dural sac. Next, remove the medial edge of the facet joint. Finally, complete the interlaminar decompression by removing the superior edge of the caudad lamina, which removes the insertion of the ligamentum flavum.

3. THE TWO LEAVES OF THE LIGAMENTUM FLAVUM

Another useful anatomic fact during this decompression is the cleft that usually separates the right and left leaves of the ligamentum flavum. Using this natural division, it is easy to remove the medial portion of the ligamentum flavum, moving cephalad to caudad.

4. THE VIEW OF THE CONTRALATERAL CANAL FROM THE IPSILATERAL INTERLAMINAR WINDOW

By retracting (and saving) the interspinous ligament and rotating the patient away from the ipsilateral side, it is possible to use the magnification and illumination of the microscope to see the contralateral side of the spinal canal. With careful preparation it is possible to do a bilateral decompression of spinal stenosis through a unilateral interlaminar window (Fig. 37.8B,C).

Window #3—The Intertransverse Window

For years spine surgeons have been using the interlaminar window for entry to the spinal canal. With the discovery of the foraminal disc (Fig. 37.9A) by CT and MRI, it seemed only natural to try to retrieve

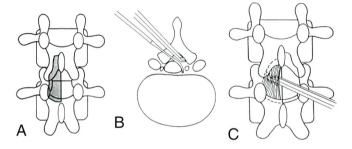

FIGURE 37.8.
A. The shaded area represents the ligamentum flavum that must be removed to decompress one-half of the spinal canal in acquired (degenerative) spinal canal stenosis. **B.** After the ipsilateral side of the canal is decompressed, roll the table away from you and, working anterior to the intact interspinous/supraspinous ligament complex, decompress the contralateral side of the canal. Obviously this is being done without elevating the paraspinal muscles on the contralateral side. **C.** An anterior/posterior schematic to show this technique.

that disc rupture through the "tried-and-true" interlaminar window. These herniations are located lateral to the pars interarticularis in the foraminal zone (Fig. 37.9B). Unfortunately, these disc ruptures lie in Macnab's hidden zone (Fig. 37.9C), and retrieval is difficult through the interlaminar window. All too often in the orthopaedic community the disc fragment was missed, in order to save the facet joint and maintain stability, while in the neurosurgical community the facet was sacrificed to properly see the nerve root and the pathology. To avoid this dilemma, the intertransverse window is proposed as a route to retrieve foraminal pathology.

The Intertransverse Window to the Foramen

The salient anatomic features are as follows:

1. *The foramen.* The boundaries of the foramen are shown in Figure 37.9B.
2. *The roof of the foramen.* At the L1, L2, L3, and L4 anatomic segments, note that the lateral border of the pars interarticularis is on the same sagittal plane as the medial border of the pedicle (Fig.

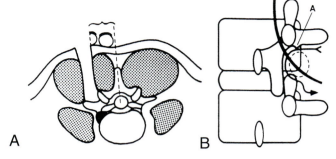

FIGURE 37.10.
A. The Wiltse paraspinal split (one and one-half fingers-breadth off the midline). The disc rupture is the solid black dot anterior to the transverse process. **B.** The foraminal disc herniation (broken circle); the accessory process (A) on the medial/inferior edge of the transverse process.

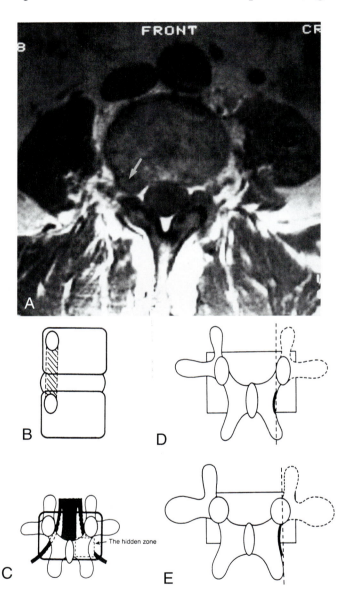

FIGURE 37.9.
A. A foraminal disc herniation (arrow) in the second story of the L4 anatomic segment. **B.** The boundaries of the foramen are from the medial borders of the pedicles to the lateral border of the pedicles, and from the inferior border of one pedicle down to the superior border of the pedicle below. **C.** These disc herniations lie in Macnab's hidden zone. **D.** At all lumbar levels except L5, the lateral border of the pars interarticularis lies on the same sagittal plane as the medial border of the pedicle. **E.** The sagittal-plane relationship between the lateral border of the pars interarticularis and the medial border of the pedicle at L5.

37.9D). The only exception to this lumbar rule is at the L5 anatomic segment, where the sagittal plane for the lateral border of the pars is at mid-pedicle (Fig. 37.9E). If you accept that the foramen is bordered by adjacent pedicles, then the foramen has no bony roof. Rather, the roof of the foramen is the intertransverse ligament. To enter the L1, L2, L3, or L4 foramen from within the spinal canal, it is necessary to cross the pars (sacrificing the inferior facet) to gain a direct view of pathology. Using this anatomic concept, it becomes evident that to retrieve a foraminal disc fragment it is much easier to take the paraspinal approach, crossing the soft-tissue intertransverse ligament roof of the foramen (Fig. 37.10A).

3. *The lateral border of the pedicle.* The little-mentioned accessory process at the proximal inferior border of the transverse process marks the lateral edge of the pedicle (Fig. 37.10B).
4. *The disc lateral to the pars.* In looking at Figure 37.9D it becomes evident that a reasonable portion of the disc space lies lateral to the pars interarticularis. This is more obvious in the proximal lumbar segments, but even at L4 a reasonable portion of the disc space lies lateral to the pars. It is necessary to remove a small portion of the tip of the superior facet to gain entry to the disc space.
5. *The paraspinal surgical approach.* The paraspinal surgical approach to a foraminal disc is shown in Figure 37.11.

Indications for Microsurgery for Lumbar Disc Herniation (LDH)

Herniation

The indications for microsurgery for a lumbar disc herniation are no different from those for a standard lumbar discectomy. The microscope will not "do"

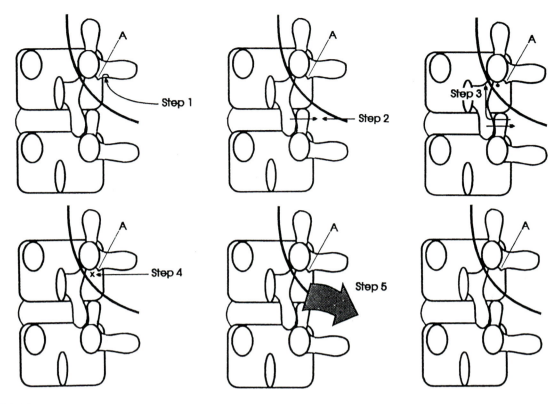

FIGURE 37.11.
The paraspinal approach to a lumbar disc herniation. Step 1: Identify the accessory process and dissect the intertransverse ligament off the transverse process at this level. Step 2: Open the capsule of the facet joint and resect it laterally. Step 3: With a Kerrison rongeur dissect up the anterior lateral border of the pars interarticularis, separating the intertransverse ligament from the fibers of the ligamentum flavum. Step 4: Join steps 1 and 3 to be able to reflect the intertransverse ligament laterally and (Step 5) inferiorly. Step 6: Find the nerve root encased in fat, and then locate the disc rupture that will usually, but not always, be found medial to the nerve root.

the surgery; it is simply a technical aid like a sharp scalpel or your favorite probe. The indications for microdiscectomy are as follows.

A General Statement

One only has to review the natural history of lumbar disc disease to realize that spinal surgeons play a palliative role in the management of this problem. The most outstanding study on the natural history of lumbar disc disease was done by Weber (14). He randomly assigned large groups of patients with unequivocal signs of a disc herniation to surgical and nonsurgical groups. Weber has shown that although surgery initially increases the yields of good results, its advantages disappear on longer follow-up (Table 37.1).

Hakelius also completed a retrospective study of 583 patients with unilateral sciatica (4). His results were similar to Weber's in that the surgically treated patients initially had a better result, but by 6 months there was no difference between the two groups of patients (Table 37.2). He did show that on a 7-year follow-up, the conservatively treated group had more low back pain, more sciatic discomfort, more recurrences, and more lost time from work.

One can only conclude from these and other studies, including those on the natural history of sciatica due to a disc herniation, that it is a transient, self-limiting condition. Satisfactory resolution over time is likely to occur, regardless of the method of treatment intervention, be it surgical or conservative treatment. If one is proposing surgical intervention, it becomes essential to prove that surgery carries with it a high rate of initial success with limited risk to the patient and at the least expense possible to the payers for the service (11).

TABLE 37.1
Weber's Results (1983)

Time Since Surgery	Nonsurgical Results	Surgical Results
1 year	60% better	92% better
4 years	No statistical difference between the two groups	
10 years	No difference between 4-year and 10-year follow-up	

TABLE 37.2
Hakelius's Results (583 patients)

Time Since Surgery	Results
Immediate	Surgical results better
6 months	No difference between surgery and conservative treatment
7 years	Nonsurgical patients had more episodes of low back pain and sciatica and more lost time from work

The following are the indications for surgery in cases of herniated nucleus pulposus (HNP):

Absolute Indications

1. *Bladder and bowel involvement: The cauda equina syndrome.* The acute massive disc herniation that causes bladder and bowel paralysis is usually a sequestered disc that requires immediate surgical excision for the best prognosis (5).
2. *Increasing neurologic deficit.* In the face of progressing weakness, it is wise to intervene early with surgical excision of the disc rupture.

Relative Indications

1. *Failure of conservative treatment.* This is the most common reason for surgical intervention in the presence of a lumbar disc herniation. Ideal conservative treatment is treatment that occurs over at least 6 weeks and not more than 3 months and results in improvement in the patient's symptoms and signs. During that time the amount of complete bed rest that should be prescribed is 2 to 3 days. Other conservative measures such as medication (analgesics, anti-inflammatory agents, muscle relaxants), modalities (heat and cold), and exercises may be used (1). The key to measuring the success of conservative treatment is not only the patient's relief of pain but also the improvement in straight-leg-raising ability. If a patient goes to bed with appropriate medication for 2 to 3 days and there is no improvement in sciatic discomfort or in straight-leg-raising ability, it is likely that the patient is going to follow a protracted conservative course, and surgical intervention is indicated. It is proposed that surgical intervention in the acute radicular syndrome occur before 3 months of symptoms have gone by, in order to try to avoid the chronic pathologic changes that can occur within a nerve root.
2. *Recurrent sciatica.* Conservative treatment can also fail in that the patient experiences recurrences of the sciatic syndrome. Table 37.3 outlines the use of "recurrences of sciatica" as an indication for surgical intervention.
3. *Significant neurologic deficit with significant straight-leg-raising reduction.* This is a relative indication for surgical intervention for an HNP. Again, Weber has shown that these patients eventually recovered just as well with nonsurgical intervention (14). These patients are in extreme pain and often cannot wait for the benefits of conservative care. On the rare occasion, these patients present with severe pain that has resolved as the neurologic deficit has increased; they also should undergo surgery when the MRI demonstrates a large LDH.
4. *A disc rupture into a stenotic canal.* I recommend quick intervention surgically when the neurologic deficit is shown on MRI to be associated with a narrowed spinal canal such as in acquired canal stenosis, subarticular stenosis, or congenital stenosis.
5. *Recurrent neurologic deficit.* If a patient who has sciatica and a neurologic deficit has been successfully treated with conservative care only to have a neurologic deficit reappear with recurrent sciatic symptoms—operate.

Contraindications to Surgical Intervention

Before intervening surgically for the acute radicular syndrome due to a lumbar disc herniation, it is essential to have an accurate clinical diagnosis of the cause of the sciatica, an anatomic level of the lesion, and support for both clinical impressions by some form of investigation. If there is not a perfect consonance between the patient's clinical presentation, the anatomic level, and the structural lesion as demonstrated on myelography, CT scanning, or MRI, the potential for a poor result increases dramatically (Table 37.4).

Patients who have a significant nonorganic component (Table 37.5) to their disability are usually a contraindication to surgical intervention. The presence of a nonorganic component to a disability does not immunize a patient from a disc herniation. On the other hand, few patients with a significant nonorganic component to their disability do in fact have a disc rupture as part of their causative pathology.

TABLE 37.3
Recurring Sciatica[a]: Indications for Surgery

Episode of Sciatica	Prognosis
First	90% of patients will get better and stay better with conservative care
Second	90% of patients will get better, but 50% of the patients will have a recurrence of symptoms; consider surgery
Third	90% of the patients will get better, but almost all will have recurrent episodes of sciatica; propose surgery

[a] This condition is to be distinguished from recurrent HNP (disc herniation recurring after previous surgery).

TABLE 37.4
Contraindications to Surgery for an HNP

Wrong patient (poor potential for recovery, e.g., workmen's compensation patient off work for more than 3 years)
Wrong diagnosis (e.g., other pathology causing the leg symptoms)
Wrong level
A painless lumbar disc herniation (do not operate for primary complaint of weakness or paraesthesias, in absence of pain)
An inexperienced surgeon applying poor technical skills
Lack of adequate instruments

TABLE 37.5
Symptoms and Signs Suggesting a Nonorganic Component to Disability

Symptoms
1. Pain is multifocal in distribution and nonmechanical (present at rest)
2. Entire extremity is painful, numb, and/or weak
3. Exremity gives way (as a result, the patient carries a cane)
4. Treatment response
   a. No response
   b. "Allergic" to treatment
   c. Not on treatment
5. Multiple crises, multiple hospital admissions/investigations, multiple doctors

Signs
1. Tenderness is superficial (skin) or nonanatomic (e.g., over body of sacrum)
2. Simulated movement tests are positive
3. Distraction tests are positive
4. Whole leg is weak or numb
5. "Academy Award" performance

Lumbar Disc Herniation in Special Circumstances

Disc herniations do not always occur in simple, uncomplicated situations. Below are some particular situations that may be related to an LDH causing sciatica.

LDH WITH SPONDYLOLISTHESIS

Patients who have a spondylolisthesis may suffer from a disc rupture, causing an acute radicular syndrome. Most of these will occur at the level above the spondylolisthesis. A disc herniation at the same level of the slip usually occurs into the foramen. For the former situation, simple disc excision or chemonucleolysis is all that is required; for the latter (disc excision at the slip level), discectomy should be accompanied by a stabilization procedure.

LDH IN SPINAL STENOSIS

Spinal stenosis can occur in the central canal or lateral zones. It can be an asymptomatic or a mildly symptomatic condition that can suddenly convert to a significant disability when a disc herniation occurs. Investigation in these patients is somewhat inconclusive, because the stenosis does not allow a clear depiction of the disc rupture. It is only when the presenting symptoms are analyzed and the dominance of the leg pain is ascertained that one will suspect a small disc herniation in the presence of a stenotic canal or lateral zone stenosis.

Simple microscopic removal of the disc herniation along with a local decompression of the stenotic segment is the proposed method of treatment. If it is ascertained in the patient's history that the stenotic component was significantly symptomatic before the occurrence of the LDH, a wider decompression is needed to treat both the stenosis and the LDH.

LDH IN INSTABILITY

Patients who have a long history of back pain and significant degenerative disc disease on roentgenogram may suffer from a disc herniation at the degenerative level. Whether or not this instability should be treated at the time of the disc excision is a difficult question to answer. The author feels that if the disc degeneration and LDH are confined to one level, it is reasonable to consider fusion. If the disc degeneration is present at multiple levels, either on roentgenogram, discography, or MRI, simple disc excision is the best choice.

LDH IN THE ADOLESCENT PATIENT

The younger patient with a disc herniation presents a special problem. As outlined in DeOrio and Bianco's series from the Mayo Clinic, a number of these patients go on to repeat surgical procedures after their initial surgical intervention (2). Because of the high incidence of protrusions rather than disc extrusions, it is proposed that in this age group the optimal treatment is chemonucleolysis rather than surgical intervention (9).

RECURRENT LDH (AFTER DISCECTOMY)

Reherniation of disc material occurs in approximately 2 to 5% of patients. The recurrence may occur at any interval after surgery (days to years) and is most often at the same level and same side. If the recurrence is at the same level and opposite side or another level, it can be considered a "virgin LDH" and the principles discussed earlier in this chapter apply. Unfortunately, most recurrences are at same level and same side, and scar tissue from the previous surgery introduces a whole new element to diagnosis and treatment.

The surgical approach to a recurrent lumbar disc herniation (same level, same side) can be summarized as follows:

- Scarring "tacks" down the dura to the back of the disc space so that a smaller amount of herniated nuclear material is capable of producing a significant amount of pain and neurologic deficit.

- Because of the immobility of the scarred dura, transdural ruptures, although rare, can occur (6).
- Determining the anatomic level by clinical assessment can be difficult because:
  - Some neurologic changes are residual from the prior LDH.
  - The dura may not only be immobilized, it may also be distorted from the scar tissue, leading to lower root involvement than usual for the level of the LDH (e.g., a recurrent L4–5 HNP may affect a number of sacral roots.)
- Investigation can be difficult to interpret because of the scar tissue. To a large extent, this reduces the reliability of myelography and has led to the use of intravenous Conray-enhanced CT and intravenous gadolinium DTPA–enhanced MRI.
- Not only are the clinical assessment and investigation difficult, the surgery is also difficult and prone to complications such as missed pathology, dural tears, and neurologic damage. A basic principle in repeated surgery is to gain as wide an exposure as possible to deal with the recurrent pathology. The microsurgeons are flying in the face of this principle, but with accurate localization of the recurrent pathology by preoperative investigation, microsurgical intervention presents some advantages (3).

THE FORAMINAL DISC HERNIATION

A foraminal disc herniation is depicted in Figure 37.9. It is a disc extrusion or sequestration that lies in Macnab's hidden zone (10). It occurs in the older age group, usually at the L4–5 or L3–4 level, and causes severe anterior thigh pain. In order to live up to the surgical principles of seeing all the pathology that needs to be excised while preventing damage to important structures (the nerve root and inferior facet), this disc herniation should be approached through Wiltse's (17) muscle-splitting paraspinal approach.

THE CAUDA EQUINA SYNDROME

Very large disc ruptures can be approached microsurgically. The magnification and illumination allow clear identification of tissue planes between neural tissue (dura) and disc-annulus. The author has used the microsurgical hemilaminectomy approach in nine cases of cauda equina syndrome with no complication and full recovery for patients seen and operated on in an emergency setting.

Other Indications for Microsurgery for Lumbar Disc Disease

1) Spinal Stenosis
   a) Canal stenosis
   b) Lateral zone stenosis

Problems with the Microscope and Microsurgery

Switching from loupes to the microscope obviously requires a learning curve. This is not a great hurdle to the young surgeon-in-training, but it can be a problem for the established surgeon. The advantages of the microscope over loupes are summarized in Table 37.6.

Problems with the Microscope

Hand-eye coordination. Small wounds leave little room for visualization. This necessitates the use of instruments that are longer (e.g., 8-inch Kerrison) and narrower than standard, in order to keep the operating hand out of the field. Interpose a microscope in this situation, and the only thing visible to the operating surgeon is the working end of the surgical instrument. The loss of hand-eye coordination is a major problem for some surgeons.

Loss of peripheral vision. The microscope delivers excellent visualization within its field, but zero visualization outside its field. This paradox also requires travel along the learning curve.

"Overhang is the enemy." Within the visual field, the surgeon must constantly struggle to be sure that "overhang" does not narrow the field.

The Microscope

The microscope is nothing more than binoculars looking through a magnifying glass. The usual setup for spine microsurgery is:

- Eyepieces = 10 × magnification
- Binocular tube length = 170 mm
- Magnification chamber = 1.6 times
- Objective lens = 350 mm

TABLE 37.6
The Advantages of the Microscope Over Loupes[a]

	Loupes	Microscope
Magnification	Limited in extent and fixed	Relatively unlimited and changeable
Illumination	Not parallel to line of vision (paraxial)	Parallel to line of vision (coaxial)
3-D Vision	Limited with less than 65 mm skin incision	Maintained with 25 mm skin incision
Patient size	The larger the patient, the larger the wound required	Neutralized (every patient is made the same size by the optics)
Teaching	Assistants excluded	Assistants included
Surgeon's neck	Fixed	Sparred

[a] The moment you decide to limit your exposure via the microscope, you will become a much more precise thinker in regard to surgical anatomy and pathology.

The formula for magnification is:

$$\frac{\text{Binocs}}{\text{Objective}} \times \text{eyepieces} \times \text{mag. chamber} = M$$

$$\frac{170}{350} \times 10 \times 1.6 = 7\text{--}8 \text{ times magnification}$$

Problems with Microsurgery

We are all aware of the problems of anesthesia and wounds that are part of any surgical exercise. There are also some general problems particular to spine surgery. But there are problems that are specific to lumbar microsurgery:

- Wrong level exposure
- Retained pathology
- Hemorrhage
- Dural tears and neural injury
- Infection

Wrong level exposure. When you reduce your lumbar wound to a minimum, you give up the ability to count up from the sacrum for level identification, and you immediately expose yourself to the three most common errors in spine microsurgery:

1. *Exposure of the wrong level*
2. *Exposure of the wrong level*
3. *Exposure of the wrong level*

Clearly identify your level of intervention before making the skin incision. I prefer image intensifier localization on lateral view before patient preparation and draping (Fig. 37.12). Secondly, know your pathology and where exactly you will find it; if it is not there, you are at the wrong level and need an intraoperative x-ray.

Retained pathology. Preventing retained pathology requires a clearly thought-out game plan before incision. First, know what pathology you will encounter and where it is located. Second, remember you are doing nerve root surgery, not disc surgery. You are operating because the nerve is "pinched" and you are going to leave the nerve "unpinched" (freely mobile). Third, probe in all directions to be sure that no fragments are left behind.

Hemorrhage. The average blood loss in a simple discectomy performed by an experienced microsurgeon is 25 mL. If the loss rises to 150 to 200 mL and the surgical field is a "bloody mess," the surgeon cannot see, and complications will occur. Prevent this problem with the following steps:

- Patients must cease taking anti-inflammatory medication 7 to 10 days preoperatively.
- Position the patient on the operating table so that the abdomen is free of pressure and there is no vena cava pressure producing backflow through Batson's plexus into the epidural veins.
- Use hypotensive anesthesia when the patient's general health permits.
- Use tamponade frequently and use bipolar coagulation judiciously.

Dural tears and/or neural injury. Excessive hemorrhage and the use of inappropriate instrumentation are the causes of dural tears. Recognize the causes and practice prevention. If a dural tear occurs and is evident (e.g., dorsal dura), it must be repaired. If the tear cannot be seen and will tamponade itself (e.g., ventral dura), do not attempt a repair (you will make it worse). Simply pack the area with absorbable gelatin sponge (Gelfoam) and keep the patient in bed for 48 hours.

Infection. Wilson first pointed out the apparent higher infection rate following microsurgery in comparison with that of conventional laminectomy (16). This is thought to be a result of the presence of undraped, unsterile microscope eyepieces that may be touched by the operating room personnel. Observing very strict sterile technique, performing expeditious surgery, and using prophylactic antibiotics have reduced the incidence of discitis to 3 in 2500 cases in the author's practice.

Technical Complications Meriting Special Mention

Short incision and force. When you have a deep wound with a 1-inch opening and you use force, there is only one way you can go, and that is deep—deep into a spina bifida, and damage the cauda equina; deep into the disc, and damage the vascular tree, the bowel, or the genitourinary system.

Dural tears and root injury. When you are operating in a small wound, force can damage the dura and/or nerve roots. Use the proper instrumentation with precision. If you end up with an inadvertent durotomy, exercise one principle: If the tear will tamponade itself (e.g., anterior dural tears), ignore it; if the tear will not tamponade itself (e.g., dorsal tear in the laminotomy defect), you must repair it with a watertight seal.

Techniques of Simple Microdiscectomy

Anesthesia

The author prefers general anesthesia because of patient comfort, airway control in the prone position, and the potential use of hypotensive anesthesia.

Position

The kneeling frames are the easiest to use and they routinely remove pressure from the abdominal cavity.

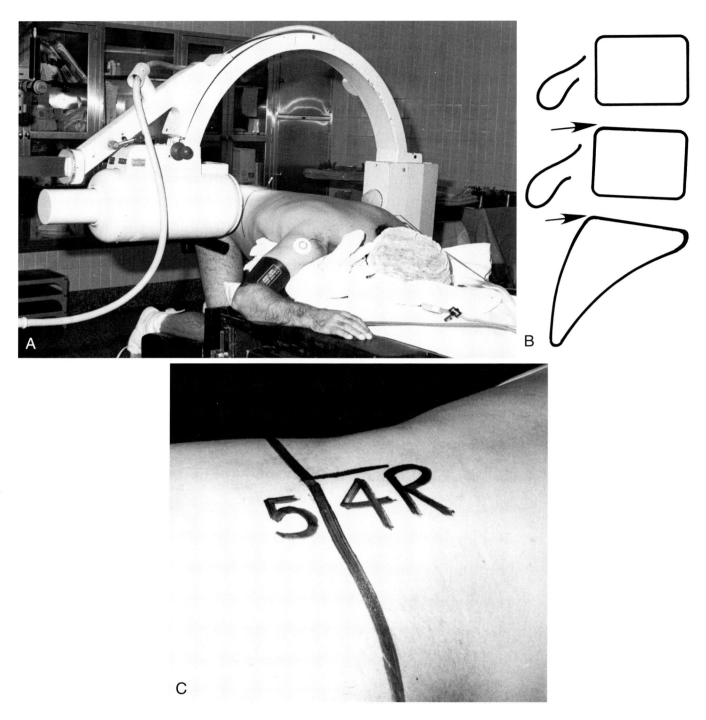

FIGURE 37.12.
A. An image intensifier is used to mark (with a needle) the inferior edge of the disc space. Obviously sterile preparation of the skin is done before the needle is inserted. **B.** The needle is placed in the paraspinal muscles so that it is aligned with the inferior edge of the spinous process and parallel with the inferior edge of the disc space to be exposed. The arrows show proper needle placement for L5-S1 and L4–5. **C.** The skin is marked and the needle removed, and the patient is prepared and draped for surgery.

Level Identification

Do this before patient preparation and draping, using an image intensifier.

Skin Incision and Exposure of Interlaminar Space

The skin incision, ½ to ¾ inch on either side of the marking line, is made beside the spinous processes rather than in the midline. Blunt dissection is used to expose the lumbodorsal fascia, which in turn is opened in a curvilinear fashion (Fig. 37.13A). The skin opening and fascial incision are designed to do the least amount of damage to the interspinous-supraspinous ligament complex. The subperiosteal muscle dissection and elevation are completed and the retractor inserted. At this juncture the microscope is moved into position.

Entry Into the Spinal Canal

The author prefers not to excise the ligamentum flavum but rather preserve it as a flap based medially (Fig. 37.13B).

Extent of Interlaminar Exposure Relative to Pathology

With the knowledge of the location of the pathology in the spinal canal, a plan of cephalad-caudad laminar excision can be followed. For example:

- A third-story HNP in the L5 segment requires removal of some of the cephalad and caudad laminar edges during an L4-L5 exposure.
- A second-story HNP in the L4 segment requires removal of at least one-half of the cephalad lamina.

The Lateral Edge of the Nerve Root

Once in the spinal canal, finding the lateral edge of the nerve root using blunt dissection is the most important step. The pedicle is the key to finding nerve roots. After the lateral border of the nerve root is defined and the root retracted medially, it is possible to become more aggressive with the Kerrison to achieve the cephalad or caudad laminar excision necessary to deal with the pathology.

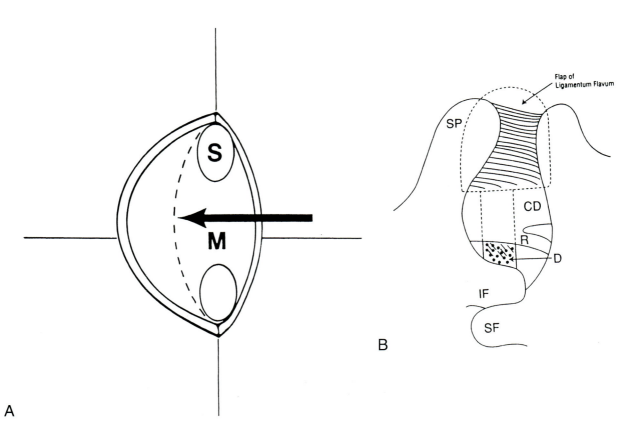

FIGURE 37.13.

A. A flap of lumbodorsal fascia is created to avoid tearing the supraspinous ligament complex with retraction (s = spinous process, m = midline, arrow points to apex of flap, which is 1 cm off midline). **B.** A flap of ligamentum flavum is created. SP = spinous process; CD = common dural sac; R = root; D = disc; IF = inferior facet; SF = superior facet.

If you cannot find the lateral edge of the nerve root, the reason may be one of the following:

- An axillary disc displacing the root laterally
- Failure to remove an osteophytic lipping off the medial edge of the superior facet
- Adhesions
- Anomalous roots

Sharp tools should not be used in the spinal canal until the lateral border of the nerve root has been clearly identified and mobilized.

If you are having trouble finding the lateral edge of the nerve root or are wondering whether there is any root lateral to the root you have identified, remember the following basic rule: Nerve roots are intimately related to pedicles. If you cannot find a nerve root, find a pedicle and the root will be immediately medial to it; if you have a nerve root isolated, check that the medial bony wall of the pedicle is lateral to your probe to prove that no other nerve tissue is lateral to you at that particular point.

Retraction of the Nerve Root

Before retracting the nerve root, be sure that you have its lateral border clearly defined and that no adhesions are present. Microsurgery is a two-handed procedure: One hand holds and manipulates the root, the other hand operates. For this reason, it is best for the surgeon to hold the root retractor, which allows proper positioning of the retractor relative to the operating tool (e.g., pituitary rongeur) and promotes the use of intermittent root retraction during the operation.

Dealing With Canal Pathology

The object of the surgical exercise is to leave a freely mobile nerve root. This requires removal of the obvious portion of ruptured disc and also includes a search of the canal, along with probing of the foramen, for residual disc or bony pathology.

Removing Intradiscal Tissue

How much disc to remove from within the disc cavity is an unanswered question. Removal of as much disc as possible implies curettage of the interspace, including removal of the endplates. Critics of this approach point out the following drawbacks:

- It is not possible to remove all intradiscal material in this manner, no matter how long the surgeon works.
- This aggressive approach increases the risk of damage to visceral structures anterior to the disc space.
- The incidence of the chronic back pain produced by conditions such as sterile discitis and instability is increased.
- Although there are some articles in the literature to suggest that this extensive intradiscal debridement decreases the recurrent LDH rate, there are other articles refuting that position. In the end, the only reasonable prospective controlled study was Spengler's, which suggested that limited disc excision is all that is necessary (12).

Advantages of Limited Disc Removal

The advantages of limited disc removal are as follows:

- Less trauma to endplates and less dissection
- Less nerve root manipulation
- Lower infection rate
- Lower complication rate for structures anterior to disc space (vessel perforation)
- Less disc space settling postoperatively

Microsurgery for Lateral Zone Stenosis

Subarticular stenosis is easily dealt with through a microsurgical approach. Foraminal encroachment is best handled with a surgical approach lateral to the pars interarticularis (Fig. 37.10).

Microsurgery for Spinal Canal Stenosis

Spinal canal stenosis is either congenital or acquired (degenerative). It may also present as a combined congenital and acquired stenosis, which is quite common in men of large stature. In single-segment degenerative stenosis (Fig. 37.7) it is possible to perform a bilateral interlaminar decompression through a unilateral interlaminar window (Fig. 37.8). The procedure is greatly facilitated with the microscope.

Results of Microsurgery for Lumbar Disc Disease

As noted in the introduction to this chapter, spinal surgeons play a palliative role in the management of lumbar disc rupture. The early results of microdiscectomy are no better than those of standard laminectomy-discectomy (7, 13), but the patient is much better off, with less postoperative morbidity, earlier discharge from hospital (e.g., outpatient surgery), and an earlier return to work.

Limited Surgical Intervention for Lumbar Fusion

We have known for a long time that uninstrumented multisegmental lumbar fusions have a high pseudarthrosis rate. Spinal surgeons using instrumentation have shown us that rigid immobilization of the segments to be fused leads to a much higher fusion rate. Unfortunately, it has come at the cost of more immediate complications and long-term breakdown of adjacent unfused segments because of the stress-shielding of rigid instrumentation. Can we learn from their experiences? The reason for the high pseudarthrosis rates in uninstrumented fusions is the usual attendant long incision and muscle elevation in the lateral gutter. On closure, this loose "soft-tissue envelope" offers no immobilization to the bone graft. Use of the soft-tissue envelope concept to elevate only those soft tissues necessary to lay down the bone graft, which in turn will close and rigidly immobilize the bone graft, will likely lead to higher fusion rates without the complications of instrumentation (Fig. 37.14).

Conclusion

Before the contributions of Semmelweis and Lister, infection of the surgical wound was expected. The advent of aseptic techniques, the introduction of antibiotics, and the improvements in surgical techniques changed all that and have made modern surgery possible. Before these advances, avoiding an infection was considered luck; now an infection in a clean wound is rare.

Today's surgeons are at another threshold: We make the incision and we expect scar. Is there some way we can reduce scar—and when its formation is necessary, is there some way we can control its formation? To a certain extent this has been accomplished with such interposition membranes as fat or the ligamentum flavum flap. It appears that the initial proposal by LaRocca and Macnab of using absorbable gelatin sponge (Gelfoam) has not stood the test of time (8). But they did observe that in order to reduce scar tissue, the laminectomy should be as restricted as possible, consistent with thorough decompression of the involved nerve. This is the approach

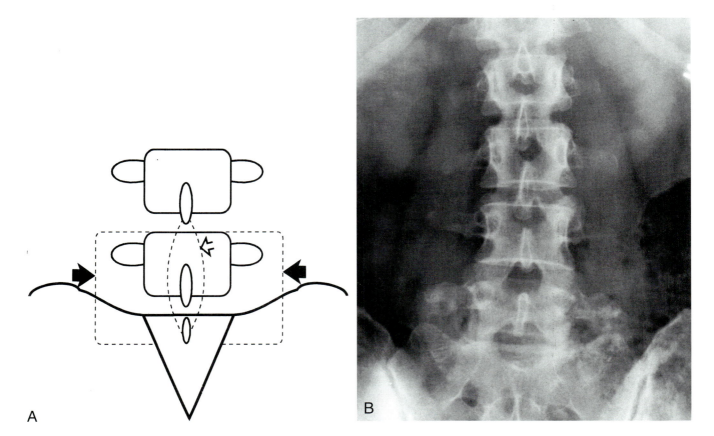

FIGURE 37.14.
A. The limited "soft-tissue envelope" approach to fusion. The open arrow points to the separate fascia incisions to complete the fusion on each side. The heavy arrow points to the extent of muscle elevation to "open the soft-tissue envelope." **B.** An L5-S1 fusion, 2 months after surgery, accomplished through the "limited soft-tissue envelope" approach.

that should be taken to lumbar disc surgery, and the microscope facilitates such a step.

References

1. Bell GR, Rothman RH. The conservative treatment of sciatica. Spine 1984;9:54–56.
2. DeOrio JK, Bianco AJ. Lumbar disc excision in children and adolescents. J Bone Joint Surg 1982;64A:991–996.
3. Goald HJ. A new microsurgical reoperation for failed lumbar disc surgery. J Microsurgery 1986;7:63–66.
4. Hakelius A. Prognosis in sciatica: a clinical follow-up of surgical and non-surgical treatment. Acta Orthop Scand Suppl 1970;129:1076.
5. Hardy RW Jr., David HR Jr. Extradural spinal cord and nerve root compression from benign lesions in the lumbar area. In: Youmans JR, ed. Neurological surgery. Philadelphia: WB Saunders, 1990.
6. Hodge CJ, Binet EF, Keiffer SA. Intradural herniation of lumbar intervertebral disc. Spine 1979;3:346–350.
7. Kahanovich N, Viola K, McCulloch JA. Limited surgical discectomy and microdiscectomy: a clinical comparison. Spine 1989;18:24–27.
8. LaRocca H, Macnab I. The laminectomy membrane. J Bone Joint Surg 1974;56B:24–27.
9. Lorenz M, McCulloch JA. Chemonucleolysis for herniated nucleus pulposus in adolescents. J Bone Joint Surg 1985;67A:1402–1404.
10. Macnab I. Negative disc exploration. J Bone Joint Surg 1971;53A:891–903.
11. Scoville WB, Corkilig G. Lumbar disc surgery: technique of radical removal and early mobilization. J Neurosurg 1973;39:265–269.
12. Spengler DM. Results with limited excision and selective foraminotomy. Spine 1982;6:604–607.
13. Tullberg T, Isacson J, Weidenhielm L. Does microscopic removal of lumbar disc herniation lead to better results than the standard procedure? Spine 1993;18:24–27.
14. Weber H. Lumbar disc herniation: a controlled prospective study with ten years of observation. Spine 1983;8:131–140.
15. Williams RW. Microlumbar discectomy: a conservative surgical approach to the virgin herniated lumbar disc. Spine 1978;3:175–182.
16. Wilson DH, Harbaugh R. Microsurgical and standard removal of the protruded lumbar disc: a comparative study. Neurosurgery 1981;8:422–427.
17. Wiltse LL. Alar transverse process impingement of the L5 spinal nerve: the far-out syndrome. Spine 1984;9:31–38.

CHAPTER THIRTY EIGHT

Bone Grafting Procedures

Lawrence T. Kurz

Introduction

The aim of this chapter is twofold. The first is to present techniques for harvesting autogenous bone from various donor sites, including the iliac crest, the rib, and the fibula. The second is to discuss the complications that may arise from the harvesting procedures themselves.

Harvesting Techniques

Ilium

Many methods have been described for harvesting cancellous and corticocancellous bone from the ilium. However, a number of methods have an inherent disadvantage. The trapdoor method (Fig. 38.1), the cortical subcrestal window (Fig. 38.2), trephine curettage (Fig. 38.3), and oblique sectioning of the crest (Fig. 38.4) all render only a portion of the entire cancellous bed available for harvest (28, 31). Using only a curved gouge may be problematic because the shape and size of the pieces are uneven and inconsistent. In order to bridge the transverse processes, the graft pieces should ideally be 5 to 7 mm in width and at least 6 cm in length. The small width of these pieces increases the total surface area of the graft. Ideally, the cancellous thickness of the graft should be 5 to 10 mm.

Posterior Ilium

The placement of the skin incision for posterior iliac graft harvest depends on the operative procedure being performed. In a midline approach to the lower lumbar spine, the skin incision can be extended distally, and the crest may be exposed through subcutaneous or fascial splitting dissection underneath the lumbodorsal fascia. An alternate method requires a separate oblique or vertical incision made into the skin overlying the posterior iliac crest.

With a paraspinal approach to the lumbar spine with two skin incisions, the extension of only one skin incision distally is needed to directly expose the posterior iliac crest. However, in a paraspinal approach through a single midline incision, distal extension of the skin incision is preferred.

Exposing the posterior ilium begins with incising the periosteum covering the iliac crest. Although using a Cobb elevator for subperiosteal stripping of the outer-table muscles is the most common method of exposure, the surgeon may find that significant bleeding ensues from trauma to the muscle itself. An excellent technique to minimize blood loss is atraumatic "peeling" of the outer-table muscle and periosteum off of the ilium with a pick-up and electrocoagulation. After muscle stripping, a Taylor retractor is placed deep into the wound and is oriented perpendicularly to the floor. The tip of the retractor should not be pointed distally, since this may place

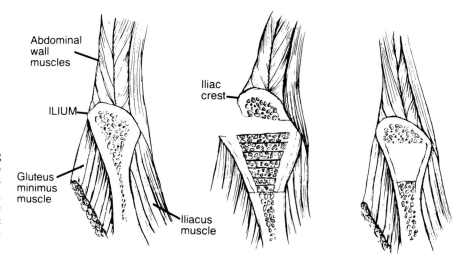

FIGURE 38.1.
Coronal section of the ilium indicating the trapdoor method of harvesting bone graft. The periosteum and fascial attachments of the iliacus and abdominal wall muscles remain intact on the inner edge of the horizontal cut through the iliac crest, thus allowing the crest to be "hinged back" like a trapdoor.

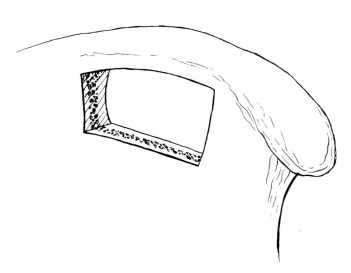

FIGURE 38.2.
The subcrestal window technique of harvesting bone graft. The iliac crest is left completely intact.

the tip close to the sciatic notch. A long piece of gauze (or a sterile metal chain) is placed on the handle of the retractor, from which a 5-pound weight is suspended, thereby leaving both of the surgeon's hands free.

Harvesting the graft with osteotomes requires visualization of the entire width of the iliac crest. The periosteum is peeled off of the medial portion of the crest, all the way over to the edge of the inner table. Beginning at the edge of the crest, a ⅝-inch straight osteotome is then malleted in a ventral direction (Fig. 38.5A). The surgeon should strive to keep the plane of the osteotome perpendicular to the plane of the ilium. About one-half of the blade of the osteotome should project through the outer cortex, while the rest should project into the intramedullary cavity between the two tables. Successive vertical cuts are

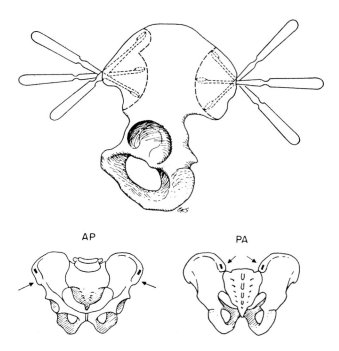

FIGURE 38.3.
Lateral, AP, and PA views of the pelvis depicting the trephine curettage method of harvesting bone graft from the ilium. Small black rectangles indicate the areas with the greatest amount of bone: the iliac tubercle anteriorly, and the posterior superior spine posteriorly.

then made in a similar fashion, about 7 mm apart, parallel to the original cut (Fig. 38.5A). The dorsal (in reference to the patient) edges of the cuts are connected along the crest with a 1-inch curved osteotome (Fig. 38.5B). The plane of the osteotome blade should be parallel to the plane of the ilium, with the curve of the blade facing the outer table. The ventral edges of the cuts are then connected along the outer table to prevent the cuts from propagating into the

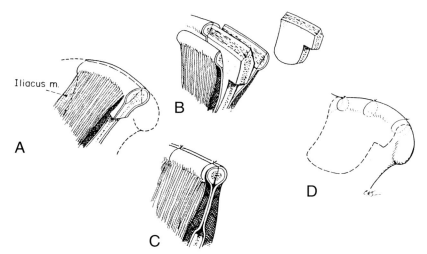

FIGURE 38.4.
The method of Wolfe and Kawamoto for harvesting bone grafts. The iliac crest is obliquely sectioned and reconstituted with wire, thus allowing good cosmesis.

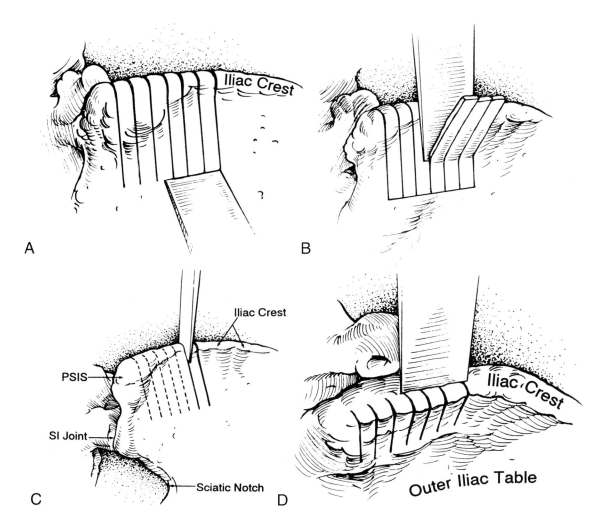

FIGURE 38.5.
Corticocancellous and/or cancellous grafts may be removed from the outer table of the iliac crest. **A.** Longitudinal cuts are made in the outer table of the iliac crest with a 1/2-inch straight osteotome. **B.** A straight osteotome is used to elevate the corticocancellous strips off of the outer table. **C.** A curved osteotome is used along the outer table of the iliac crest along the inferior border of the previously made longitudinal osteotomies. **D.** The bone graft harvesting is completed by removal of the corticocancellous strips.

sciatic notch (Fig. 38.5C). The 1-inch curved osteotome is then placed at the medial edge of the vertical cuts on the crest, in a ventral direction (Fig. 38.5D). Each pass of the osteotome will encompass approximately three vertical strips. These coronal cuts should be continued ventrally until the end of the previously cut strips is reached.

Once these corticocancellous strips have been removed, purely cancellous strips may be taken in the usual fashion with a curved gouge. These strips will be thinner and more uniform in size than corticocancellous strips taken with a gouge. After the inner table has been reached and no more strips can be harvested, small chips of cancellous bone may be harvested with large angled curettes.

Anterior Ilium

Bone graft may be harvested from the anterior ilium in a manner similar to that from the posterior ilium, that is, in strips and chips. More frequently, however, full-thickness grafts are harvested from the anterior ilium. When this is desired, both the outer and the inner tables must be subperiosteally stripped. A skin incision is made just proximal or distal to the anterior iliac crest. Alternatively, if a retroperitoneal or thoracoabdominal approach to the lumbar spine is being performed, subcutaneous dissection over the crest, but superficial to the abdominal musculature, allows the surgeon to avoid a separate skin incision. The next step is to incise the periosteum overlying the anterior iliac crest, thereby releasing the abdominal wall muscles from their insertion on the crest itself (Fig 38.6). Then stripping the inner-table (iliacus) and outer-table (gluteus medius and tensor fascia lata) muscles subperiosteally can be accomplished, thus exposing the full thickness of the ilium for harvest. Full-thickness grafts may be taken using an oscillating saw or an osteotome.

Rib

Ribs are harvested almost exclusively for use during transthoracic or thoracoabdominal approaches to the spine. A rib is frequently removed as part of the exposure. The rib may be harvested after dissection through the latissimus dorsi and trapezius muscles has brought the rib into view (Fig. 38.7). The periosteum over the rib is incised, either sharply with a scalpel or with the use of electrocautery (Fig. 38.8).

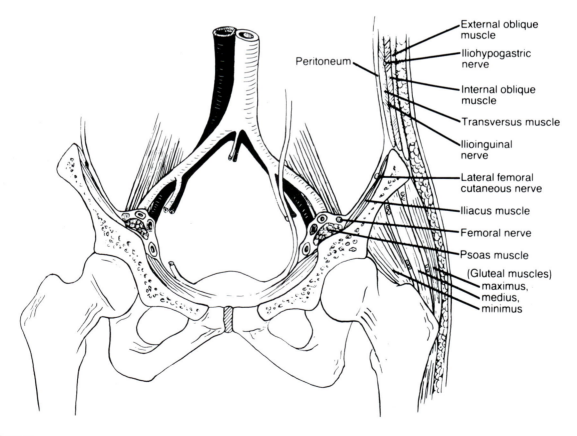

FIGURE 38.6.
Coronal section of the lower abdomen and pelvis showing the neural structures in the iliac fossa and abdominal wall. The peritoneum is closely applied to the inner surface of the abdominal wall and iliacus muscles.

CHAPTER 38: BONE GRAFTING PROCEDURES 769

to excise the rib at its costovertebral and costochondral junctions (Fig. 38.10).

Fibula

Although the fibula is not as commonly used for bone grafting procedures as the ilium, its harvest is certainly no less important. Its donor location in the lower leg necessitates its harvest being meticulous in order to avoid interference with ambulatory function. Fibular harvest is begun by exsanguinating the

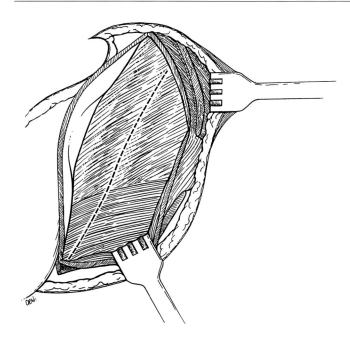

FIGURE 38.7.
Right transthoracic approach divides the serratus anterior muscle after incising the trapezius and latissimus dorsi muscles.

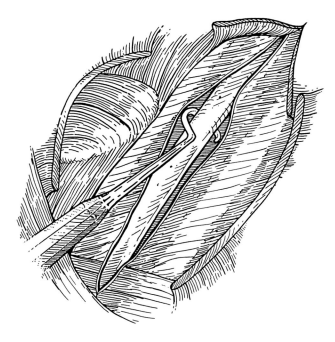

FIGURE 38.9.
Subperiosteal dissection isolates the rib without entering the pleura.

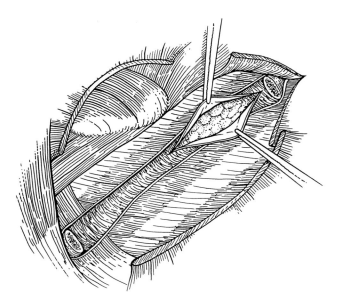

FIGURE 38.8.
Right transthoracic approach continues with a longitudinal incision of the periosteum directly on the rib to be resected.

A periosteal elevator such as a Cobb elevator can then be used to subperiosteally strip the superficial portion of the rib. A rib stripper is then used to subperiosteally strip the pleural surface of the rib (Fig. 38.9). This maneuver is performed all the way to the sternal and vertebral ends of the rib. A rib cutter is then used

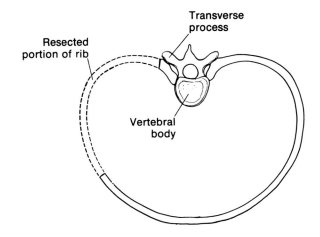

FIGURE 38.10.
Axial view of the thoracic cage showing the region of resection of the rib.

leg by elevating it or by using a compression bandage. A tourniquet is then inflated. The skin incision parallels the posterior border of the fibula and should be centered at the junction of the middle and distal thirds of the bone. The incision is carried down through the intermuscular septum onto the fibula bone itself. Strict subperiosteal dissection will elevate the peroneal muscles located on the anterolateral surface of the bone, the extensor digitorum longus muscle from the anterior surface, the tibialis posterior muscle from the anteromedial surface, the flexor hallucis longus muscle from the posteromedial surface, and the soleus muscle from the posterior surface. While these muscles may not be individually recognizable, it is essential to maintain a subperiosteal cutting depth on the fibula when circumferentially stripping the bone. After the bone is completely stripped, a graft may be harvested with either a Gigli saw or an oscillating saw.

Complications

Ilium Harvest

Pain

No prospective studies have been published demonstrating which harvesting technique is the least painful. Flint, among others, has reported that many patients have discomfort at the donor site long after their recipient sites have become pain free (14). Dawson et al. found that 12% of patients who had undergone posterior iliac bone graft harvest for lumbar arthrodesis had donor-site pain that persisted for more than 3 to 6 months after surgery (10). Bloomquist and Feldman found no difference in pain experienced by patients when comparing anterior and posterior approaches (3). After the removal of even very small bone grafts from the anterior ilium for anterior cervical fusions, De Palma et al. noted that 14% of patients had severe but temporary pain at the donor site, and 36% had severe and persisting pain (11). It therefore seems prudent for the surgeon, whenever possible, to select a method of harvesting that requires as little dissection as possible. Of all the methods of harvesting cancellous bone, trephine curettage (Fig. 38.3) is probably the least painful, as muscle stripping and dissection are minimal.

Nerve Injury

There are seven nerves that may be damaged during the harvesting of bone graft from the ilium; the lateral femoral cutaneous, ilioinguinal, iliohypogastric, and femoral nerves during an anterior approach to the ilium, and the superior cluneal, sciatic, and superior gluteal nerves during a posterior approach.

Injury to the lateral femoral cutaneous nerve can lead to numbness or dysesthesias in a large area of

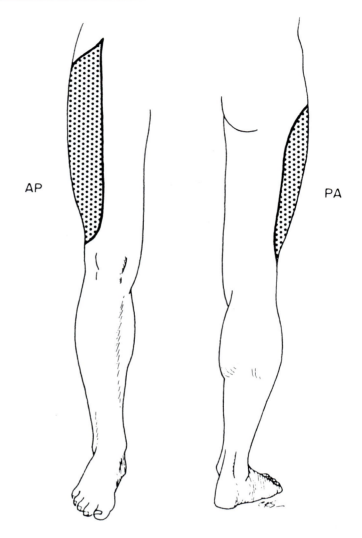

FIGURE 38.11.

AP and PA views of the leg. The dotted area depicts the cutaneous innervation of the lateral femoral cutaneous nerve.

the lateral aspect of the thigh (Fig. 38.11). Its anatomic course, in close proximity to the anterior superior iliac spine, renders the nerve prone to injury when bone grafts are harvested from the anterior ilium. The normal course of the nerve is anterior and inferior to the anterior superior iliac spine, just deep to the inguinal ligament (Fig. 38.12). However, in up to 10% of cases the nerve takes an anomalous course over the anterior crest up to 2 cm lateral to the anterior superior iliac spine (Fig. 38.13) (16). Injury to the nerve has been reported in up to 10% of cases, often presenting as "meralgia paresthetica," which is characterized by pain, paresthesias, or numbness in the distribution of the nerve (17). Resolution often occurs within 3 months without any treatment. Persistent pain or paresthesias that do not resolve on their own may be treated successfully with local nerve blocks or neuroma excision.

The ilioinguinal nerve is mostly a sensory nerve that supplies sensation to a large area of the groin (Fig. 38.14). Its anatomic course takes it between the abdominal wall muscles, and distally it overlies the iliacus muscle (Fig. 38.15). Injury to this nerve has been reported in the form of ilioinguinal neuralgia, which is characterized by pain, paresthesias, or numbness in the distribution of the nerve (29). The cause of this nerve injury is probably a neuropraxia resulting from retraction of the iliacus and abdominal wall muscles when exposing the inner table of the anterior ilium. Treatment with local nerve blocks has been successful.

The iliohypogastric nerve courses slightly proximal to the ilioinguinal nerve and supplies motor fibers to the lowermost portion of the abdominal wall and sensation to the skin surrounding the anterior two-thirds of the iliac crest (Fig. 38.14). Iliohypogastric neuralgia may arise in a fashion similar to that of ilioinguinal neuralgia.

The femoral nerve (L2, L3, and L4) passes behind the psoas muscle, courses over the iliacus muscle, and enters the thigh under the inguinal ligament (Fig.

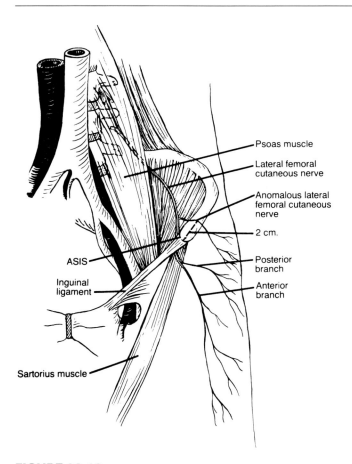

FIGURE 38.12.
AP view of the right hemipelvis showing the normal course of the lateral femoral cutaneous nerve.

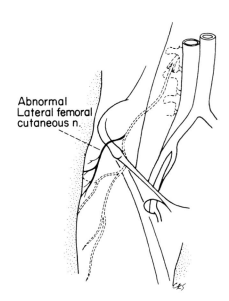

FIGURE 38.13.
AP view of the right hemipelvis showing an anomalous course that the lateral femoral cutaneous nerve may take. It may course over the iliac crest up to 2 cm lateral to the anterior superior iliac spine.

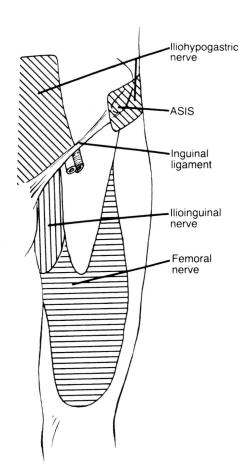

FIGURE 38.14.
AP view indicating the cutaneous innervation of the ilioinguinal, femoral, and iliohypogastric nerves.

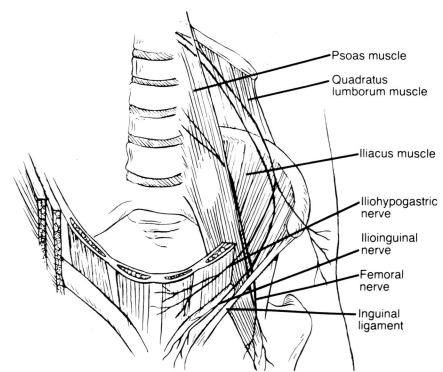

FIGURE 38.15.
AP view showing the normal course of the ilioinguinal and iliohypogastric nerves.

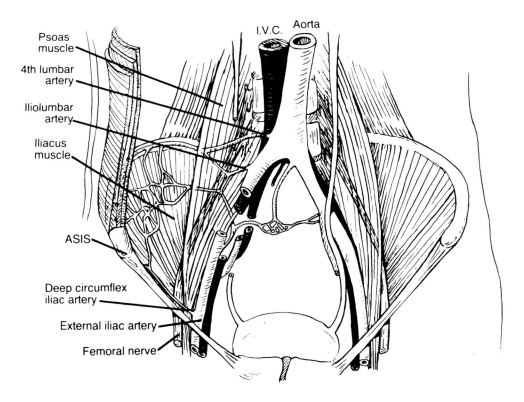

FIGURE 38.16.
AP view of the lower abdomen and pelvis showing the course of the neurovascular structures of the iliac fossa: the femoral nerve and the deep circumflex iliac, iliolumbar, and fourth lumbar arteries.

38.16). It supplies motor branches to the muscles of the anterior compartment of the thigh and medial lower leg and foot (Fig. 38.14). The nerve is in a vulnerable location in the iliac fossa, and avoidance of injury requires careful dissection and retraction during harvesting of bone from the inner table of the anterior ilium.

The superior cluneal nerves (L1, L2, and L3) supply sensation to a large area of the buttocks (Fig. 38.17). They pierce the lumbodorsal fascia and cross the posterior iliac crest beginning 8 cm lateral to the posterior superior iliac spine (Fig. 38.18). A number of patients have formed neuromas at the donor site; unresponsive to cortisone injections, they have been painful enough to require surgical excision. Transient or permanent numbness over the skin of the buttock is a fairly common postoperative complaint from patients who have had bone removed from a posterior site.

The sciatic nerve, a condensation of the sacral plexus (L4 to S3), exits the pelvis to enter the gluteal region through the sciatic notch and courses down

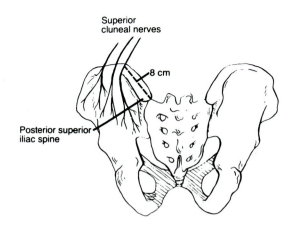

FIGURE 38.18.
PA view of the pelvis showing the superior cluneal nerves as they cross over the posterior iliac crest beginning 8 cm lateral to the posterior superior iliac spine.

the posterior thigh (Fig. 38.19). This nerve may be injured because of its proximity to the sciatic notch. Our cadaver studies show that frequently the sciatic nerve is still manifested as five components of the sacral plexus for a distance of 1 to 5 cm below the proximal border of the sciatic notch. Therefore, injury to the nerve near the notch may mimic a lumbosacral nerve root injury rather than a complete sciatic nerve injury.

The superior gluteal nerve courses with the superior gluteal artery through the sciatic notch to supply motor branches to the gluteus medius and minimus and the tensor fascia lata muscles (Fig. 38.19). Significant injury to this nerve in the region of the notch may manifest itself as weakness of hip abduction.

Arterial Injury

The superior gluteal artery branches off of the internal iliac artery before exiting the pelvis (Fig. 38.19). It then enters the gluteal region through the most proximal portion of the sciatic notch to supply the bulk of the gluteal muscle mass (Fig. 38.20). One reported injury resulted in the formation of an arteriovenous fistula of the superior gluteal vessels, documented by an arteriogram 2 weeks after surgery (13). The fistula was caused by penetration of the sciatic notch with the sharp tip of the Taylor retractor used for exposure during harvesting. Massive hemorrhage deep in the sciatic notch from errant penetration of an osteotome or gouge during harvest from the posterior ilium is a formidable complication to deal with. The injured superior gluteal artery usually retracts proximally into the pelvis. Successful control of bleeding may necessitate removal of bone from the sciatic notch to expose the retracted, injured vessel. In some cases a separate retroperitoneal approach

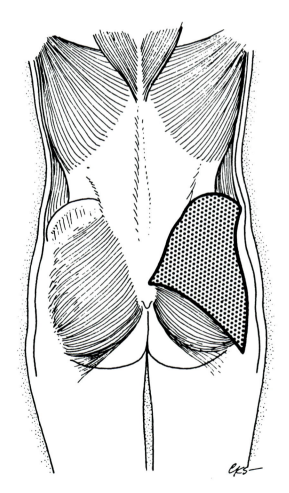

FIGURE 38.17.
PA view of the back in which the dotted area depicts the cutaneous innervation of the superior cluneal nerves.

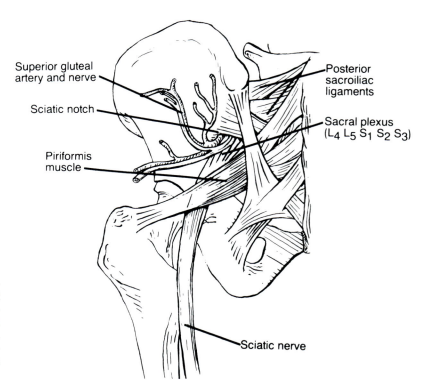

FIGURE 38.19.
PA view of the pelvis showing the neurovascular structures in the sciatic notch. Note that the sciatic nerve may still be manifested as individual components of the sacral plexus for 1 to 5 cm below the superior border of the notch. The superior gluteal artery and nerve course together and are the superiormost structures in the notch.

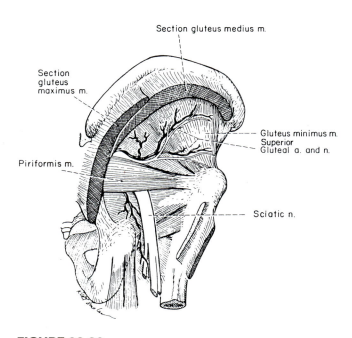

FIGURE 38.20.
PA view of the deep structures of the right buttock. The superior gluteal artery and nerve course together between the gluteus medius and gluteus minimus muscles to send extensive branches to them.

may be required in order to gain access to the vessel for ligation.

There are three major arterial structures that traverse the anterior surface of the iliacus muscle in the iliac fossa: the fourth lumbar artery, the iliolumbar artery, and the deep circumflex iliac artery (Fig. 38.16). They frequently anastomose with each other and provide an extensive supply of blood to the psoas, quadratus lumborum, and iliacus muscles. These vessels can be injured when bone grafts are being harvested from the inner table of the anterior ilium.

Infection

The rate of infection of donor sites is less than 1% and thus no different from that in other orthopaedic procedures. An important aspect of bone grafting in infected recipient sites is to prevent cross-contamination by using separate instruments, gowns, and gloves. In addition, suction drainage and liberal use of topical hemostatic agents will decrease hematoma formation, which might decrease the incidence of infection. Deep donor site wound infections are treated with incision, drainage, and appropriate antibiotic therapy.

Hematoma

Harvesting bone graft can generate substantial blood loss. Cancellous bone bleeding can be profuse, leading to hematoma formation in as many as 10% of patients (11, 27, 30). Posterior wounds have a much lower incidence of significant hematoma formation, probably because of the hemostatic effect of pressure on posterior wounds in the supine position (12). The anterior iliac crest is very superficial, and local hemostasis from tamponade is difficult.

Numerous methods have been used for hemostasis of donor sites, including microcrystalline collagen (6,

23), bone wax (1, 3), thrombin-soaked gelatin foam (28), and injection of an epinephrine and saline solution (18). Thrombin-soaked gelatin foam is most advantageous if removed from the wound prior to closure. In addition, the incidence of donor site hematomas has been reduced to less than 1% through the use of closed suction drainage for 1 or 2 days following surgery. Although theoretically the exposed bone could continue bleeding indefinitely under suction drainage, this is not observed in clinical practice, and all donor site wounds are routinely drained.

Gait Disturbance

As many as 3% of patients exhibit a gluteal gait following bone graft harvest from the posterior ilium (2, 7). Gait analysis can demonstrate that after having bone graft removed from the anterior crest, some patients exhibit a limp or an abductor lurch because of extensive stripping of the outer-table muscles, leading to weakness of the hip abductors, primarily the gluteus medius muscle. A number of patients have also had difficulty climbing stairs and rising from a sitting position. Prevention is the best measure; gluteal fascia must be securely reattached to the periosteum of the crest.

Cosmetic Deformity

Cosmetic deformity has been a problem following full-thickness graft harvest from the anterior iliac crest, which alters the superior contour. Three techniques lend themselves to preservation of the crestal outline. The subcrestal window completely avoids the crest (Fig. 38.2). In addition, Wolfe and Kawamoto described a method of obliquely sectioning the crest (Fig. 38.4) that allows for reconstitution and reportedly excellent cosmesis (31). Furthermore, the trapdoor method (Fig. 38.1) reconstitutes the crest and affords an excellent cosmetic result.

Ureteral Injury

The ureter descends in the pelvis and makes a sharp posterior angle at the sciatic notch (Fig. 38.21). Escalas and De Wald reported on a patient who had postoperative fever, ileus, hematuria, and hydronephrosis after extensive electrocoagulation deep in the sciatic notch in order to control massive hemorrhage from an injury to the superior gluteal vessels (13). The patient had sustained a fulguration injury to the ureter, which resolved within 5 months without any treatment.

Fracture

Stress fractures of the ilium after bone graft harvest rarely occur and have been reported only after removal of full-thickness grafts from the anterior ilium (19). When harvesting large, full-thickness grafts

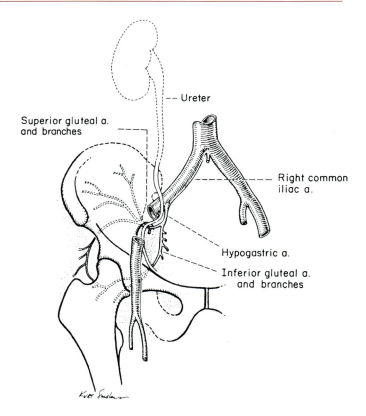

FIGURE 38.21.
AP view showing the course of the ureter. The sharp posterior angle it makes in the pelvis brings it into close proximity to the sciatic notch.

from the anterior ilium, it is important to leave a wide margin of bone from the anterior superior iliac spine to prevent a stress fracture resulting from the downward pull of the rectus femoris and sartorius muscles (Fig. 38.22). The distal bone graft cut should not deviate anteromedially, in order to avoid breaking through the ilium anteroinferior to the anterior inferior iliac spine.

Peritoneal Perforation

The peritoneum is closely applied to the inner surface of the abdominal wall and iliacus muscles (Fig. 38.6). The integrity of the peritoneum may be threatened during bone harvesting from the inner table of the anterior ilium. Peritoneal perforation has occurred after exuberant stripping of the crestal periosteum and of the abdominal wall and iliacus muscles during exposure of the inner table. Repair with primary suture is recommended.

Hernia

The abdominal wall muscles are firmly attached to the iliac crest and prevent herniation of abdominal contents over the crest (Fig. 38.6). The iliacus muscle prevents herniation through defects in the ilium. Routine exposure of the inner table detaches these

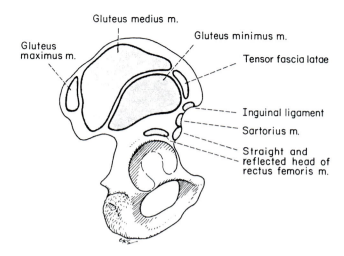

FIGURE 38.22.
Lateral view of the ilium showing three important structures that originate in close proximity to the anterior superior iliac spine: the inguinal ligament and the sartorius and rectus femoris muscles.

muscles and may lead to a weakening of this "retaining wall." Herniation of abdominal contents has been reported only after removal of full-thickness grafts that include the crest (4, 5, 9, 15, 20, 22, 24–26). None have been reported with subcrestal windows. Hernias can be prevented by securely reapproximating the abdominal wall fascia to the ilium by passing heavy sutures through the fascia and holes drilled in the bone.

Sacroiliac Joint Injury

Most of the stability of the sacroiliac joint arises from its strong posterior ligamentous complex (Fig. 38.23). This complex is composed of the short and long sacroiliac ligaments superficially and the deeper the interosseous ligaments (Fig. 38.24) (continuous with the posterior capsule). These ligaments may be damaged during removal of full-thickness grafts from the region of the posterior superior iliac spine. Although most symptoms of sacroiliac joint instability manifest as mechanical and intermittent pain, more serious symptoms, such as those related to dislocation or subluxation of the joint, have been reported (8, 21, 30).

Rib Harvest

Complications of rib harvest are usually limited to pain, lung injury, and intercostal neurovascular damage.

Pain

The pain following rib harvest can be quite severe. It is usually incisional, and tends to radiate from the costovertebral end of the rib resection. Although

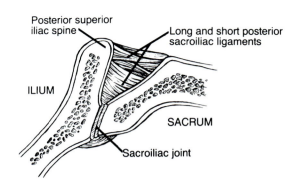

FIGURE 38.23.
Horizontal section of the sacroiliac joint showing the posterior ligamentous complex.

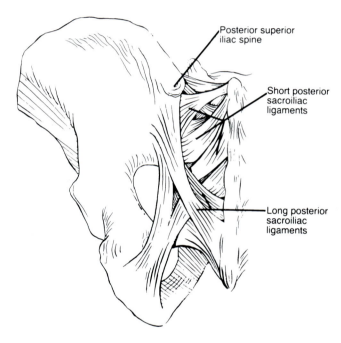

FIGURE 38.24.
PA view showing the posterior sacroiliac ligaments and their proximity to the posterior superior iliac spine.

long-term problems are rare, since symptoms tend to resolve within a few days of surgery, short-term problems are frequent. In the immediate postoperative period, and for up to 48 hours thereafter, patients tend to splint, resulting in shallow respirations and poor drainage of secretions. Pneumonia is not uncommon. The incidence of intercostal pain and its possible sequela of pneumonia may be reduced by nerve block at the costovertebral junction with a long-acting anesthetic. This is usually instituted just prior to wound closure, and it can easily be repeated percutaneously in the early postoperative period.

Lung Damage

Lung damage, if it occurs, is usually in the form of direct fulguration. These burns usually cause only minor problems. However, the lung should be inspected before closure, especially for any overt bleeding.

Intercostal Neurovascular Injury

If this bundle of nerve, artery, and vein is injured, it usually occurs during subperiosteal stripping of the rib. The bundle is located in a groove on the postero-inferior edge of each rib. If hemorrhage ensues from an injury, the vascular structure(s) must be coagulated or ligated.

Fibular Harvest

Fibular harvest may be complicated by injuries to the ankle joint or to the neurovascular structures.

Ankle Joint

Fibular graft should be harvested from the junction of the middle and distal thirds of the fibular shaft. The syndesmosis of the ankle joint ends about 10 cm proximal to the ankle joint itself, so harvest should approach no closer than this 10 cm margin. Disruption of this syndesmosis may cause symptoms of instability of the ankle joint.

Common Peroneal Nerve

The common peroneal nerve runs over the neck of the fibula in the substance of the peroneus longus muscle, and divides into deep and superficial branches. This nerve could be injured if dissection or resection of the fibula is carried out too proximally.

Deep Neurovascular Bundles

There are two deep neurovascular bundles surrounding the fibular shaft that must be avoided. One contains the deep peroneal nerve and the anterior tibial artery and vein. This bundle lies anteromedial to the fibular shaft, on the interosseous membrane. After stripping the extensor digitorum longus and the extensor hallucis longus muscles, if the surgeon strays anteromedially along the interosseous membrane, this bundle may be damaged. The second neurovascular bundle to be avoided contains the tibial nerve and peroneal artery and vein. This bundle lies medial to the fibula. During stripping of the tibialis posterior muscle from the anteromedial surface of the fibular shaft, this bundle can be injured.

Clinical Recommendations

Strict attention to subperiosteal dissection minimizes bleeding and hematoma formation, because all of the muscles have an extensive blood supply. Suction drainage has been shown to decrease the incidence of significant hematoma formation.

Ilium

When approaching the posterior ilium, a limited incision within 8 cm of the posterior superior iliac spine will avoid the superior cluneal nerves and prevent the formation of painful neuromas or bothersome numbness over the buttocks (Fig. 38.18). The sciatic notch should be avoided because the sciatic nerve, the ureter, and the superior gluteal artery and nerve lie close to this region (Figs. 38.19 and 38.21). In addition, when taking full-thickness grafts from the posterior ilium, attempts should be made to preserve as much of the ligamentous structures as possible to avoid sacroiliac joint instability (Fig. 38.24).

When approaching the outer table of the anterior ilium, the incision should stop 2 cm lateral to the anterior superior iliac spine to avoid the sartorius muscle and the inguinal ligament, which attach there, as well as the lateral femoral cutaneous nerve (Fig. 38.25). This will also help to avoid fracture of the ilium. When obtaining bone graft from the outer table, avoid penetrating the inner table to prevent injury to the neurovascular structures that are present in the iliac fossa overlying the iliacus muscle; this includes the deep circumflex iliac, iliolumbar, and fourth lumbar arteries, and the ilioinguinal, iliohypogastric, femoral, and lateral femoral cutaneous nerves (Figs. 38.6 and 38.16). Secure reapproximation of the gluteal fascia helps to prevent a gluteal gait.

When the inner table of the anterior ilium is approached, careful retraction of the abdominal wall

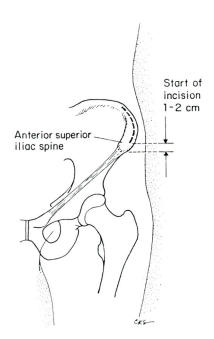

FIGURE 38.25.

Approach to the anterior iliac crest. The skin incision should begin at least 2 cm lateral to the anterior superior iliac spine.

and iliacus muscles may prevent injury to the nerves that overlie the iliacus muscle, including the lateral femoral cutaneous, the ilioinguinal, the iliohypogastric, and the femoral nerves, and also the peritoneum (Fig. 38.6). Secure closure of the fascia of the abdominal wall muscles decreases the risk of herniation of abdominal contents through defects in the iliac crest.

Rib

In harvesting rib grafts, the stripping of the rib must be strictly subperiosteal in order to avoid the most common complications of injury to the intercostal neurovascular bundle and the lung. Postoperative pain and splinting can be minimized by injection of long-acting anesthetic at the costovertebral junction just prior to closure.

Fibula

When harvesting fibular grafts, strictly subperiosteal stripping must be performed in order to avoid injury to the neurovascular bundles (Fig. 38.10). Ankle joint instability may be avoided by resecting the fibula at least 10 cm proximal to the ankle joint, thereby avoiding the syndesmosis.

Conclusion

Awareness of the possible complications, knowledge of the relevant anatomy, and strict attention to the technical details of harvesting autogenous bone grafts will aid the surgeon in planning the approach and minimizing the risk.

References

1. Abbott LC. The use of iliac bone in the treatment of ununited fractures. Instr Course Lect (AAOS) 1944; 2:13–22.
2. Abbott LC, Schottstaedt ER, Saunders JB, et al. The evaluation of cortical and cancellous bone as grafting material. J Bone Joint Surg 1947;29:381–414.
3. Bloomquist DS, Feldman GR. The posterior ilium as a donor site for maxillofacial bone grafting. J Maxillofac Surg 1980;8:60–64.
4. Bosworth D. Repair of herniae through iliac crest defects. J Bone Joint Surg 1955;37A:1069–1073.
5. Challis JH, Lyttle JA, Stuart AE. Strangulated lumbar hernia and volvulus following removal of iliac crest bone graft. Acta Orthop Scand 1975;46:230–233.
6. Cobden RH, Thrasher EL, Harris WH. Topical hemostatic agents to reduce bleeding from cancellous bone. J Bone Joint Surg 1976;58A:70–73.
7. Converse JM, Campbell RM. Bone grafts in surgery of the face. Surg Clin North Am 1954;34:375–401.
8. Coventry MB, Topper EM. Pelvic instability: a consequence of removing iliac bone for grafting. J Bone Joint Surg 1972;54A:83–101.
9. Cowley SP, Anderson LD. Hernias through donor sites for iliac bone grafts. J Bone Joint Surg 1983;54A:1023–1025.
10. Dawson EG, Lotysch III M, Urist MR. Intertransverse process lumbar arthrodesis with autogenous bone graft. Clin Orthop 1981;154:90–96.
11. De Palma A, Rothman R, Lewinnek G, et al. Anterior interbody fusion for severe cervical disc degeneration. Surg Gynecol Obstet 1972;134:755–758.
12. Dick IL. Iliac-bone transplantation. J Bone Joint Surg 1946;28:1–14.
13. Escalas F, De Wald RL. Combined traumatic arteriovenous fistula and ureteral injury: a complication of iliac bone grafting. J Bone Joint Surg 1977;59A:270–271.
14. Flint M. Chip bone grafting of the mandible. Br J Plast Surg 1964;17:184–188.
15. Froimson AI, Cummings AG Jr. Iliac hernia following hip arthrodesis. Clin Orthop 1971;80:89–91.
16. Ghent WR. Further studies on meralgia paresthetica. Can Med Assoc J 1961;85:871–875.
17. Goldner JL, McCollum DE, Urbaniak JR. Anterior disc excision and interbody spine fusion for chronic low back pain. In: American Academy of Orthopaedic Surgeons. Symposium on the spine. St. Louis: Mosby, 1969:111–131.
18. Goldstein LA, Dickerson RC, eds. Pelvis. In: Atlas of orthopaedic surgery. New York: Mosby, 1974:450–453.
19. Guha SC, Poole MD. Stress fracture of the iliac bone with subfascial femoral neuropathy: unusual complications at a bone graft donor site: case report. Br J Plast Surg 1983;36:305–306.
20. Lewin ML, Bradley ET. Traumatic iliac hernia with extensive soft tissue loss. Surgery 1949;26:601–607.
21. Lichtblau S. Dislocation of the sacroiliac joint: a complication of bone grafting. J Bone Joint Surg 1962;44A:193–198.
22. Lotem M, Moor P, Haimoff H, et al. Lumbar hernia at an iliac bone graft donor site. Clin Orthop 1971;80:130–132.
23. Mrazik J, Amato C, Leban S, et al. The ilium as a source of autogenous bone for grafting: clinical considerations. J Oral Surg 1980;38:29–32.
24. Oldfield MC. Iliac hernia after bone grafting. Lancet 1945;248:810–812.
25. Pyrtek LJ, Kelly CC. Management of herniation through large iliac bone defects. Ann Surg 1960;152:998–1003.
26. Reid RL. Hernia through an iliac bone graft donor site. J Bone Joint Surg 1968;50A:757–760.
27. Sacks S. Anterior interbody fusion of the lumbar spine. J Bone Joint Surg 1965;47B:211–223.
28. Scott W, Petersen RC, Grant S. A method of procuring iliac bone by trephine curettage. J Bone Joint Surg 1949;31A:860.
29. Smith SE, De Lee JC, Ramamurthy S. Ilioinguinal neuralgia following iliac bone grafting: report of two cases and review of the literature. J Bone Joint Surg 1984;66A:1306–1308.
30. Stauffer RN, Coventry MB. Posterolateral lumbar spine fusion. J Bone Joint Surg 1972;54A:1195–1204.
31. Wolfe SA, Kawamoto HK. Taking the iliac bone graft: a new technique. J Bone Joint Surg 1978;60A:411.

Index

Italic page numbers indicate figures; page numbers with an italic *t* indicate tables.

Abdominal muscles, 29
Abnormal posture/gait in spondylolisthesis, 252, 253
Abscess
  epidural
    clinical presentation, 581
    diagnostic evaluation, 581–582, *583–584*
    epidemiology and etiology, 580
    management, 582, 585
    microbiology, 581
    pathogenesis and pathology, 581
    prognosis, 585
  intramedullary spinal, 586–587
    clinical presentation, 587
    diagnostic evaluation, 587
    epidemiology and etiology, 586
    management and prognosis, 587
    microbiology, 586–587
  subdural, 585–586
    epidemiology and etiology, 585
    pathogenesis, pathology, and microbiology, 586
Achilles tendon reflex, 432
Achondroplasia, 163, 167
Activities of daily living, 396
Acute cholecystitis as complication of scoliosis surgery, 485–486
Adam's test, 414
Adaptive equipment, 396–397
Adson test, 93
Adult scoliosis, 475–487. (*See also* Scoliosis; Neuromuscular scoliosis.)
  diagnosis, 476–478
  epidemiology and natural history, 475–476
  outcome studies, 486–487
    long fusions to sacrum, 482–483
  surgical treatment, 478–479
    indications for, 478
    management of lumbar curves, *480*, 481–482, *483*
    management of thoracic curves, 479–481, *480*
    medical complications, 485–486
    thoracoplasty, 483, 485
Aerobic conditioning for spinal stenosis, 452
Alar fascia, 29
American Spinal Injury Association (ASIA), 297–324, *324, 325,* 326, *327*
  Impairment Scale, 388, 388*t,* 389, 389*t*
Amyoplasia, 184
Amyotrophic lateral sclerosis, 404
Anesthesia considerations in surgical treatment, 312–313
Aneurysmal bone cysts, 532, 630
  treatment of, 635–636
Angulation, 254–255
Ankylosing spondylitis, 617–618, 639
  cervical osteotomy, 623–625, *624*
  clinical manifestations, 618
  diagnostic evaluation of spinal deformity in, 619, *619*
  fractures, 625
  general surgical considerations in deformity surgery for, 619–620
  low back pain in, 429
  lumbar spine osteotomy, 620–621, *621, 622*
  pathophysiology, 618
  spondylodiscitis, 625
  thoracic spine osteotomy, 621, 623, *623*
Annulus fibrosus, 425–426
Ansa cervicalis, 10
Anterior cervical discectomy and fusion, 406–407, *409,* 409–410

Anterior cervical plate fixation, 316, *317–318*, 319
Anterior cervical plating, 77
Anterior cord syndrome, 389
Anterior corpectomy and strut grafting, 410
Anterior decompression and fusion, 313, *314, 315*, 316
  advantages, 377
  comparative studies, 379
  disadvantages, 377
  instrumentation, 378–379
  techniques, 377–378
Anterior dens screw fixation, 353–354
Anterior epiphysiodesis, *224*, 224–225
Anterior fusion for spondylolisthesis, 258–259
Anterior screw for C1-C2 stabilization, 77
Anterior transthoracic decompression and fusion, 416–417, *418–419*
Anterior transthoracic discectomy and fusion, 417
Anterior triangle, 28
Anterior tubercle, 16
Anterior vertebral screw fixation strength, 80
Anterolateral muscles, 26
Anteromedial retropharyngeal approach to upper cervical spine, 33, *33*, 35
Antibiotic impregnated beads, 571
Anti-inflammatory medications for spinal stenosis, 452
Anulus fibrosus, 22–23
Aorta, 29
Apert's syndrome, 167
Arachnoid cysts, 556
Arachnoid mater, 4
Arachnoiditis, 118
Armstrong plate, 694
Arnold-Chiari malformation, 551
  surgery for, 559
  with and without syringomyelia, 559
Arthritis. (*See also* Rheumatoid arthritis.)
  psoriatic, 639
  sacral, 639
    ankylosing spondylitis, 639
    psoriatic, 639
Arthrodesis
  atlantoaxial, 613–615, *614*
  occipitocervical, 615, *616*
  in treating degenerative lumbar spondylolisthesis, 523
Arthrogryposis, 184
Astrocytomas, 551
  intramedullary ependymoma, 557–558, *558*
  management of high-grade, 557
  management of low-grade, 557
Atelectasis, 175
  as complication of scoliosis surgery, 485
Athletic injuries as cause of cervical injuries, 276
Atlanto axial instability, 279–280
Atlanto axial segment, 279
Atlantoaxial arthrodesis, 613–615, *614*
Atlantoaxial articulation, 13
  impaction, 606
  posterior fusion of, 661, 663, *664*, 665, *665*
  rotatory subluxation of, 280, 338–339
    clinical diagnosis, 339–340
    injury classification, 340–341, *342*

mechanism of injury, 339
radiographic evaluation, 340, *340*, 341
treatment, 341–342
subluxation, 606
surgery for, 611–612
Atlanto-dens interval (ADI) and atlantooccipital motion, *158*, 158–160, *159*
Atlanto-occipital articulation, 12
  abnormalities of, 93
  anomalies, 162–163
  fusion of, 163
Atlas fractures, 279, 334–335
  classification, 335–337, *336–337*
  clinical diagnosis, 335
  mechanism of, 335
  radiographic evaluation, 335
  treatment, 337–338
Atlas hypoplasia, 163
Autonomic dysreflexia, 390–391
Autonomic nervous system, 133
Avascular necrosis, 436
Avulsion teardrop fracture, 305
Axial loading injuries, 305, *306*
  treatment of, 312
Axial loading test, 100
Axial neck pain, 109–110
Axial traction, 341
Axillary disc rupture, 750, *751*
Axis fractures, 346–347
  C2 body, 349
  C2 lamina, 349–350
  C2 lateral mass, 349
  classification, 347, *348*, 349
  diagnosis, 347
  mechanism of, 347
  radiographic evaluation, 347

Babinski's sign, 100
  positive, 96
Back disease, injection for diagnosis and therapy of
  epidural, 721–725, *722, 723*
  facet, 714–718, *715, 716, 717*
  limitations due to anatomic considerations, 708–709, *709*
  limitations due to local anesthetic effect, 708, *709*
  limitations due to sensory mechanisms, 707–708, *708, 709*
  local infiltration, 711–712
  methods, 709–711, *711*
  peripheral nerve block, 712
  sacroiliac, 712–714, *714*
  selective spinal nerve, 718–721, *720*
  sympathetic blockade, 712, *713*
Back pain. (*See also* Low back pain.)
  in spondylolisthesis, 252
Basilar impression, 163–164, *164*
Basilar invagination, 606–607
  surgery for, 612
Basiocciput, visualization of, 332
Beck Depression Inventory (BDI), 469
Bilateral facet dislocations, 305
  treatment of, 311–312

Bilateral laminectomy and facetectomy, 69
Biomechanics
   evaluation of fusion constructs, 75–76
   evaluation of spinal instrumentation, 80
   of fusion graft, 71–72
     biomechanical considerations of graft, 72
     effect of graft size, 74–75, 75*t*
     effect of size, 74–75, 75*t*
     enhancement of bone formation, 75
     materials, 72
     mechanical strength of materials, 72–73, *73*, 73*t*, *74*
   of spinal instrumentation, 76
     cervical spine implants
       anterior screw for odontoid fixation, 76–77
       posterior instrumentation, 77
     thoracic and lumbar spine implants
       anterior instrumentation, 78
       posterior instrumentation, 78–79
   strength of spinal fixation, 79
     pedicle screw, 79–80
Biopsy
   in diagnosing spinal neoplasms, 529–530, *530*
   for lumbar spine, 731–732
   needle, in diagnosing spinal infection, 577
   transpedicular, 48
Biplanar roentgenograms, 67
Bipolar stimulator, 135, 137
Blockade techniques, 717–718
Blount's disease, 239
Blunt trauma, 588
Bohlman triple wire, 321, *322*, 323
Bone cysts
   aneurysmal, 532, 630
     treatment of, 635–636
Bone dysplasias, 163
Bone grafting procedures
   clinical recommendations, 777
     fibula, 778
     ilium, *777*, 777–778
     rib, 778
   complications
     fibular harvest, 777
     ilium harvest, *770*, 770–771, *771, 772, 773*, 773–776, *774, 775, 776*
     rib harvest, 776–777
   harvesting techniques
     fibula, 769–770
     ilium, 765–766, *766, 767*, 768, *768*
     rib, 768–769, *769*
Bone morphogenetic proteins (BMP) in spine fusion, 75
Bone scans. (*See also* Imaging.)
   in evaluating pediatric spine injuries, 275
   in evaluating spinal infections, 579–580
   technetium, 634
Bony landmarks, 67–68
Boston brace, 173
Bowstring test, 100
Brachial plexitis, 404
Bracing in neuromuscular scoliosis, 173
Brooks atlantoaxial fusion method, 663, *664*

Brown-Sequard syndrome, 245, 389
Bubble sign, 739
Burst fractures, 283, 285

C1-C2 stabilization, anterior screw for, 77
C2 isthmus or pedicle screws, 351
C2 pedicle fracture, 281–282
C3 nerve, 94
C4 root, 94
C5 root, 94
C6 sensation, 94–95
C7 sensation, 95
C8 sensation, 95
Calcium phosphates, mechanical strength of, 73–74
Canadian collar, 642, *642*
Cardiac anomalies, 216
Cardiovascular fitness, 466–467
Carotid triangle, 28–29
Carotid tubercle, 16
Carpal tunnel syndrome, 404
Cartesian system, 64
Cartilaginous endplates, 22
Cauda equina, 6, *8*, 446
   compression of, 444
   injury to, 389
   schwannomas of, 553–554, *554*
Cauda equina syndrome, 427, 430, 758
Cause-and-effect relationship of low back pain and scoliosis in lumbar spine, 476
Central canal stenosis, 450–451, *451*
Central herniations, 427
Central stenosis, 446
Cephalad-caudal angulation of pedicle screws, 79
Cerebral palsy, 175–179, *176, 177, 178*
Cerebrospinal fluid, 2, *5*
Cervical collars, 276
Cervical cord, 3
Cervical corpectomy, 410
Cervical disc disease and cervical spondylosis
   clinical presentations, 402–404
   diagnostic evaluation, 404–405, *405, 406*
   differential diagnosis, 404
   nonoperative treatment, 405
   pathophysiology, 401–402, *402*
   surgical indications, 405–406, *407, 408*
   surgical technique
     anterior cervical discectomy and fusion, 406–407, *409*, 409–410
     anterior corpectomy and strut grafting, 410
     posterior procedures, 410–411, *411*
Cervical discography, 404–405
Cervical fixation, subaxial posterior, 665–666, *666, 667, 668*, 668–671, *669, 670, 671, 672*
Cervical lesions, 577
Cervical lordosis, 63, 360
Cervical myelopathy, 111, *112–113*, 114, 403
Cervical nerve root, 4
Cervical neural foramen, 4
Cervical osteotomy, 623–625, *624*
Cervical plates, anterior, 655–658, *656, 657*
Cervical plexus, 9–10

Cervical radiculopathy, 11, 110–111
    Adson test in distinguishing between thoracic outlet syndrome, 93–94
Cervical spinal nerve block, 719–720
Cervical spine
    anterior exposure of lower, 35–37, *37, 38, 39,* 40, *40, 41,* 42*t,* 42–44
    anterior exposure to upper, 32–33, *33,* 35
    assessing strength of, *464, 465,* 465–466, *466*
    axial neck pain, 109–110
    cervicothoracic junction, 44–45, *45, 46,* 47, *47*
    classification of injuries, 300–301, 301*t*
    degenerative disorders of, presenting symptoms, 91–92, 92*t*
    effects of surgical decompression on stability of, 71
    injuries to, 277–280, *278*
    kinematics of
        lower
            functions of anatomic elements, 65
            range of motion and coupling characteristics, 65
        upper
            functions of anatomic elements, 64–65
            range of motion and coupling characteristics, 64, 64*t*
    myelopathy, 111, *112–113,* 114
    orthoses for, *642,* 642–646, *643, 644, 645,* 645*t*
    physical examination of, 92–93, *93*
    posterior surgical exposure of lower, and fusion, 32
    posterior surgical exposure of upper, 31–32, *32*
    provocative tests, *93,* 93–94
        neurologic examination, 94
    radiculopathy, 110–111
    reflex testing, 95–96
    testing by nerve root, 94–95
Cervical spine instrumentation, 653
    anterior
        cervical plates, 655–658, *656, 657*
        odontoid screw fixation, 653–654, *655*
    locking plate, *318,* 319
    posterior
        atlantoaxial fusion, 661, 663, *664,* 665, *665*
        occipitocervical fusion, 658–661, *659, 660, 661, 662*
        subaxial cervical fixation, 665–666, *666, 667, 668,* 668–671, *669, 670, 671, 672*
Cervical spondylolysis, 93
Cervicocranium, traumatic disorders of, 331
Cervicothoracic anomalies, posterior fusion for, 221
Cervico-thoracic brace, 309
Cervicothoracic congenital scoliosis, 217
Cervicothoracic junction, 17–18, 44–45, *45, 46,* 47, *47*
    imaging of, 122
Cervicothoracic lesions, 577
Chamberlain's line, 164, 608, *609*
Charcot-Marie-Tooth, 184
Charleston orthosis, 648, *650*
Chemonucleolysis
    limitations of, 734–735
    for lumbar spine, 733–735
Chemotherapy in treating spinal neoplasms, 539
Chiari malformations, 216
Child abuse, spinal fractures resulting from, 287–288

Cholecystitis, acute, as complication of scoliosis surgery, 485–486
Chondrodysplasia punctata, 167
Chondroitin sulfate, 425
Chondroitin sulfate:keratin sulfate ratio, 110
Chondro-osseous spurs, formation of, 401
Chondrosarcomas, 536, 634–635, *635*
    treatment of, 637
Chordoma, 527, 533–534, *535,* 631, 634, *634*
    treatment of, 636
Chymopapain chemonucleolysis
    indications for, 734
    for lumbar disc disease, 438
Clonidine in treating spasticity, 392
Clonus, 96, 100
Closed reduction of spondylolisthesis, 259–260
Cobb angle, 476–478, *477*
    in adult scoliosis, 475
Cobb technique, 367
Coccydynia, 629
Coccyx, 21
Cognitive-behavioral multimodal disability management program, 470
Collapsing kyphosis, 179
Common iliac artery, 29
Compound muscle action potential (CMAP), 135
Compressed nerve root, diagnosis of, 432
Compression injuries, 361, *361*
Computed tomography (CT) scan, 106, *106,* 111
    in evaluating of spondylolisthesis, 256
    in evaluating pediatric spine injuries, 274
    in evaluating spinal infections, 574, 582, 587, 590
    in evaluating spinal neoplasms, 529
Concomitant L5/S1 spondylolisthesis, 196
Conduction distance, 135
Congenital anomalies, 551
    of cervical spine
        craniofacial syndromes, 167
        craniosynostosis syndromes, 167
        familial cervical dysplasia, 165–166
        fetal alcohol syndrome, 167
        Klippel-Feil syndrome, 166
        normal embryology, growth, and development
            of occiput-axis-atlas complex, 157
            of vertebrae C3-C7, 157
        normal growth and development
            atlas, 158
            axis, 158
            C3-7, 158
        normal radiographic parameters
            Atlanto-dens Interval (ADI) and atlantooccipital motion, *158,* 158–160, *159*
            normal lower cervical spine motion, 161
            pseudosubluxation, *160,* 160–161
        Os odontoideum, 165
        Sandifer's syndrome, 166–167
        skeletal dysplasias, 167–168
        torticollis
            Atlanto-occipital anomalies, 162–163
            basilar impression, 163–164, *164*
            congenital muscular, 161–162
            unilateral absence of C1, 164–165

Congenital curves, 213
Congenital kyphosis, 216
Congenital muscular torticollis, 161
Congenital spine deformities, 213
    classification of, 213, *214*, 215
    genetics, 215
    kyphosis
        natural history, 228–229, *229*
        nonoperative treatment, 229, *230*
        surgical treatment, 229, 231, *232*, 233
    lordosis, 233
        nonoperative treatment, 233
        surgical treatment, 233, *234*, 235
    patient evaluation
        cardiac, 216
        genitourinary, 215–216
        neurologic, 216
        radiographic, 217
        respiratory, 217
        spinal dysraphism, *216*, 216–217
    scoliosis
        natural history, 218*t*, 218–219
        nonoperative treatment, 219
        surgical treatment of, 220
Congenital Wryneck, 161
Contralateral straight leg raise, 100
Conus medullaris, 1
    injury to, 389
    lesions to, 144
Conventional pluridirectional tomography (CPT), 104
Convex growth arrest, *224*, 224–225
Cordectomy, radical, 557
Cord-meningeal complex, 369
Coronal imbalance, treatment of, 219
Corticosteroids, anti-inflammatory efficacy of, 721
Costotransverse lamella, 16
Costotransversectomy, 416, 578
Cotrel-Dubousset instrumentation, 243–244, 479, 483, 679–681, *680*
    configuration, 480–481
Cranial settling, 606, 607
Cranial suture interdigitation, 646
Craniofacial syndromes, 167
Craniosynostosis syndromes, 167
Crankshaft effect, 221, 223
Cremasteric reflex, 96
Crouzon's syndrome, 167
Cushinoid syndrome, 436
Cybex Trunk Modular Component (TMC), 465, *465*
Cybex Trunk Rotation (TR) device, *466*
Cyclic fatigue tests, 80
Cyclic loading tests, 81

Dantrolene in treating spasticity, 392
Decompensation, 206–207, *208*
Decompression
    without fusion for spondylolisthesis, 257
    of spinal cord, 48
    for spinal injuries, 289–290
Decompressive laminectomy in treating degenerative lumbar spondylolisthesis, *523*, 523–524
Deconditioning syndrome, 462, 463

Deep venous thrombosis and pulmonary embolus, 390
Deep wound infections, 569
Degenerative disc disease, 110, 115
Degenerative lumbar spondylolisthesis, 455, 517–526, *518*
    diagnosis, 518–521, *519, 520, 521*
    nonoperative treatment, 521
    pathogenesis, 517–518, *518*
    spinal instrumentation, 524–526, *525*
    surgical treatment, 521–524, *522, 523, 524*
Denis classification, 360–361, *637*, 637–638
Dentate ligament, 2
Dermatomal evoked potentials (DEPs), 143
Dermatomes, 11, *11*
Dermoid cysts, 551
Diabetic patients, neurologic deficits in, 578
Diaphragm, 29
Diastematomyelia, *560*, 560–561
Diazepam in treating spasticity, 392
Diffuse idiopathic sclerosing hyperostosis (DISH), 110
Digastric triangle, 28–29
Diminution of pulse, 94
Disability, 385
Disc bulging, 426–427
Disc degeneration, 444–445
Disc herniation, 291, 427, *427*
    intraneural, 563–564
Disc nutrition, 426
Disc protrusion, 426
Disc space narrowing, 66
Discectomy, 52–53, 69
    for lumbar disc disease, 438
    and spine stability, 69
Discitis, 569, 571
    pediatric, 578–580
    septic, 568
Discogenic pain, anatomic basis of, 426
Discography, 104–105
    controversy over, 434–435
    for lumbar spine, *732*, 732–733, *733*
Displacement in spondylolisthesis, 254, *254*
Disseminated intravascular coagulation (DIC) as complication of scoliosis surgery, 486
Distraction injuries, 361–362, *362, 363*, 364
DMSO for thoracolumbar spine injuries, 371
Dorsal nerve plexus, 9
Dorsal root ganglion (DRG), 21
Dorsal sensory rootlets, 4, 6, *6*
Double crush syndrome, 145, 404
Down syndrome, 280
Drug therapy in treatment of lumbar disc disease, 435–437
Drummond spinous process wiring, *678*, 678–679
Dual energy x-ray absorptiometry (DEXA), 80
Dual rod systems, 379
Duchenne's muscular dystrophy, 181
    natural history of spinal deformity in, 181–182
Dunn system, 379, 694
Dura mater, 2, 4, *5*
Dural arteriovenous fistulae and true arteriovenous malformations, 561–562
Dwyer instrumentation, 199, 207, 693

Dysphasia, 92
Dysreflexia, autonomic, 390–391
Dyssynergia, 394

Edwards modular rod, 677
Electrodiagnosis, 129
    applied anatomy and physiology, 132–134
    in clinical practice, 129–132, 130*t*, 131*t*
    electrodiagnostic findings in diseases of spinal cord and nerve roots, 143–146, 145*t*
    late responses, 135–136, *136*
    motor conductions, *134*, 135, 135*t*
    needle electrode examination, 131*t*, 137–138, *138, 139,* 140
    normal studies, 146–147
    pathophysiology of denervation/reinnervation in motor nerve fibers, *139, 140,* 140–141
    sensory conductions, 136–137, *137*
    SEPs, 141–143, 142*t, 143*
    techniques in, 134–135
Electromyography (EMG)
    in diagnosing degenerative lumbar spondylolisthesis, 521
    in rheumatoid arthritis, 611
Endochondral ossification, longitudinal growth of, 269–270
Environmental factors in development of spondylolisthesis, 251–252
Eosinophilic granuloma, 531–532, *533*
    low back pain in, 429
Ependymomas, 551
    intramedullary, 557–558, *558*
Epidermoid cysts, 551
Epidural abscess
    clinical presentation, 581
    diagnostic evaluation, 581–582, *583–584*
    epidemiology and etiology, 580
    management, 582, 585
    microbiology, 581
    pathogenesis and pathology, 581
    prognosis, 585
Epidural injections, 721–725, *722, 723*
    for degenerative lumbar spondylolisthesis, 521
    for lumbar disc disease, 437
Epidural space, 2
Epiphysis, 268
Erector spinal muscles, 25
Escherichia coli in spinal infections, 572
Esophageal perforation, 567
Ewing's sarcoma, 533, *534*
Extension injuries, 271, *307,* 307–308, 362, *363*
    treatment of, 312
Extramedullary arteriovenous malformation, 562

F wave, 133
Facet cysts, 116–117
Facet degeneration, 445
Facet injection, 714–718, *715, 716, 717*
Facet joints, 14, 65, 66
Facet wire technique, 323, *323,* 667, *668*
Facetectomy and spinal stability, 70
Facial joint injections for lumbar disc disease, 437

Familial cervical dysplasia, 165–166
Far-out syndrome, 455
Fasciculus cuneatus, 1
Fasciculus gracilis, 1
Fast spin-echo (FSE) imaging, 108
Fatigue tests, 80–82
Femoral stretch test, 100
Ferguson view, 217
Fetal alcohol syndrome, 167
Fibula
    harvesting of bone from, 769–770
        clinical recommendations in, 778
        complications of, 777
Filum terminale, myxopapillary ependymoma of, 555
Finger escape sign, 96
Fischgold liens, 608, *609,* 610
Fixed thoracic hyperkyphosis, 201–202
Fixed thoracic lordosis, 201, *203*
Flatback syndrome, 509
Flexion distraction injuries, *284,* 285
Flexion rotation injuries, 271
Flexion-compression fractures, 282–283
    treatment of, 372
Flexion-compression injuries, 361, *363,* 369
Foot-drop, 431
Foramen magnum, 1, 64
Foraminal disc herniation, 758
Foraminotomy, *320,* 321
Forestier's disease, 110
Forward bending test, 97–98, *98*
Fracture dislocation injuries, 285
Fractures
    atlas, 279, 334–338, *336–337*
    avulsion teardrop, 305
    axis, 346–350, *648*
    burst, 283, 285
    hangman's, 281
    of lumbar spine, 289
    occipital condyle, 331–333, *332*
    odontoid, 280–282, 343–346, *345*
    in patients with ankylosing spondylitis, 618
        treatment of, 625
    spinal
        imaging of, 272–274
        resulting from child abuse, 287–288
        treatment of pediatric, 288–289
Friedreich's ataxia, 183
Functional electrical stimulation, 397–398
Functional Independence Measure (FIM), 396
Functional restoration of back and neck work-related injuries, 461–472, 462*t*
    outcome monitoring, 470–472
    psychosocial barriers to recovery, 468–469
    quantification of physical and functional capacity, 463
        cardiovascular fitness, 466–467
        cervical and trunk strength, *464, 465,* 465–466, *466*
        range of motion, 463–465, *464*
        task measurements, 467–468
    tertiary care treatment plan for, 469–470
Functional retraining, 396
Functional spinal unit (FSU), 63

Functions of anatomic elements, 65
Fusion biomechanics, 71–72
   constructs, 75–76
   grafts, 72
      effect of size, 74–75, 75*t*
      enhancement of bone formation, 75
      materials, 72
      mechanical strength of materials, 72–73, *73*, 73*t*, *74*

Gadolinium-DTPA/dimeglumine, 118
Gait abnormalities in spondylolisthesis, 252, 253
Gallic fusion techniques, 351
   for atlantoaxial fusion, 663, *664*
Gallium scans, 108–109
   in diagnosing spinal infections, 574
Galveston technique, 482–483
Gangliosides in treating traumatic spinal cord injury, 389–390
Gardner-Wells tong traction, 656
Gate control theory, *708*
Genitourinary tract, congenital anomaly in, 215
Giant cell tumors, 531, *532*, 630, 631, *632–633*
   treatment of, 636
Glycosaminoglycan ratio, 425
GM-1 ganglioside for thoracolumbar spine injuries, 371
Goldenhar's syndrome, 167
Goniometric spine mobility, 463
Gradient-echo imaging, 108
Greater occipital nerve, 10
Grisel's syndrome, 280
Guillford brace, 309
Gunshot wounds, transpharyngeal, 588

H reflex, 133
Halifax interlaminar clamps, 665
Halo application, 290–291
Halo immobilization, 279
Halo-Ilizarov, 646–647, *647*
Halo-vest, 31, 309, 643, *644*, 645
Hamilton Depression Rating Scale, 469
Handicap, 385
Hangman's fracture, 281
Hard collar, 309
Harre-Luque technique, 374
Harrington compression, 374
Harrington distraction, 373
Harrington instrumentation, 543, 676–677
   development of, 173–174
   modifications, 373–374
   rod-hook construct, 374
Heel walking, 403
Hemangiomas, 531, 558
Hematocolpos secondary to imperforate hymen, 96–97
Hematogenous vertebral osteomyelitis and disc-space infection, 572–578
   clinical presentation, 573
   diagnostic evaluation, 573–577, *574*
   epidemiology and etiology, 572
   management, 577–578
   microbiology, 572
   pathogenesis, *572*, 572–573
   prognosis, 578

Hemiatrophy, 97
Hemihypertrophy, 97
Hemilaminectomy, 552–553
Hemimetameric segmental displacement, 215
Hemivertebra, 215
   contralateral, 218
   excision, 225
   incarcerated, 215
   nonsegmented, 215
   segmented, 215
   semisegmented, 215
Herniation, 754–758, 755*t*, 756*t*, 757*t*, 758*t*
   intradural lumbar disc, 563
Heterotopic ossification, *391*, 391–392
High thoracic kyphosis, 195
HLA-B27 in pathogenesis of ankylosing spondylitis, 617–618
Hoffmann's sign, 404
   positive, 96
Hofmann's ligament, 24
Holdsworth slice fracture, 362
Hong Kong procedure, 594
Horizontal traction spurs, 426
Horizontal translation on flexion/extension, 279
Horner's syndrome, 92, 333
Hydronephrosis, 394
Hydroxyapatite ceramics, mechanical strength of, 73–74
Hyperextension brace, 648
Hyperextension injuries, 274
Hyperflexion injuries
   axial loading, 305, *306*
   bilateral facet dislocations, 305
   controversies and current trends, 308–309
   extension, *307*, 307–308
   general treatment, 308
      history, 308
   ligamentous, 301, *302*, 303
   nonoperative treatment, 309
   surgical treatment
      anesthesia considerations, 312–313
      anterior cervical plate fixation, 316, *317–318*, 319
      anterior decompression and fusion, 313–314, *315*, 316
      facet wire technique, 323, *323*
      interspinous wire technique, 321, *322*, 323
      lateral plate mass fixation, 323–324, *324*, *325*, 326, *327*
      posterior cervical fusion, 321
      posterior decompression, 319, *320*, 321
   treatment of, 309–310
      axial loading, 312
      extension, 312
      hyperflexion, 310–312
      minor, 310
      unilateral facet dislocation, 303, *304*, 305
Hyperflexion ligamentous injuries, treatment of, 310–311
Hyperkyphosis
   fixed thoracic, 201–202
   thoracic, 196
Hyperlordosis of lumbar spine, 369
Hypermobility, 66

Hypermobility compensatory subluxation, 403
Hyperreflexia, 100, 403
Hypochondroplasia, 163
Hypokyphosis, mid-thoracic, 195
Hypolordosis, lumbar, 195–196

Iatrogenic infections, 567–572
  clinical presentation, 569
  diagnostic evaluation, 569–570, *570*
  epidemiology and etiology, 567–568
  management, 570
  microbiology and prophylactic antibiotics, 568–569
  prognosis, 571–572
Ileus as complication of scoliosis surgery, 485
Iliac crest for bone grafts, 72
Iliocostalis muscle, 9, 25
Iliolumbar ligaments, 21
Ilium
  clinical recommendations in bone harvesting, *777*, 777–778
  harvesting cancellous and corticocancellous bone from, 765–766, *766, 767,* 768, *768*
  harvesting of bone complications in, *770,* 770–771, *771, 772, 773,* 773–776, *774, 775, 776*
Imaging, 103. (*See also* Bone scans.)
  in evaluating spinal infections, 119–120, 570
  fast spin-echo, 108
  gallium, 108–109
    in diagnosing spinal infections, 574
  general considerations, 109
  gradient-echo, 108
  modalities
    cervical spine, 109–111, *112,* 113
    computed tomography, 106, *106*
    discography, 104–105
    general considerations, 109
    lumbar spine, 114–117
    magnetic resonance imaging, 106–108, *107,* 107t
    myelography, *105,* 105–106
    plain film tomography, 104
    plain radiographs, 103–104
    radionuclide, 108–109, *109*
  of postoperative lumbar spine
    back pain predominant, 118–119
    leg pain predominant, 117–118
  radionuclide, 108–109, *109*
    in evaluating spinal infections, 574, 590
    in evaluating spondylolisthesis, 255–256
    technetium 99 in, 115
  of spinal fractures, 272–274
    bone scintigraphy, 275
    cervical injuries, 277–280, *278*
    computed tomography (CT) scanning, 274
    differential diagnosis, 275
    early management, *276,* 276–277
    infection, 275
    magnetic resonance imaging (MRI), 274
    metabolic disease, 275
    myelography, 274
    neoplasm, 275
    normal variance, 274
    odontoid, 280–282
    plain tomography, 274
    in Scheuermann's disease, 276
    in spondyloepiphyseal dysplasia, 275
    thoracic and lumbar injuries, 282–283, *284,* 285–288
  spine trauma, 122–123, *123*
  tumors, 120–122, *121, 122*
Impairment, 385
In vivo spinal motion measurement methods, 67–68
Incarcerated hemivertebra, 215
Inclinometers, 463–464
Indium-111-labeled leukocyte scan, 109
Infections. (*See* Spinal infections; Wound infections.)
Inheritance, role of, in development of spondylolisthesis, 251
Instrumentation. (*See also* Cervical spine instrumentation.)
  anterior, 378–379
  Kaneda
    anterior spinal device, 694, 698–699, 703
    solid rod system, 379, 693, 695, 698–699, *700, 701, 702,* 703
  Luque, 181, 543, 546
    segmental spinal, 174
    sublaminar wiring, 677–678, *678*
  Moss-Miami, 682, *683,* 693, 695, 698–699, *700, 701, 702*
  pedicle screw, 78–79, 374–376, *375,* 546, 683–684, 688, 690
  Texas Scottish Rite Hospital (TSRH) instrumentation system, 681–682, *682,* 698–699, *700, 701, 702*
Interbody fusion in treating degenerative lumbar spondylolisthesis, 523
Intercostal nerves, 6
Interlaminar clamp for C1-C2 fixation, 77
Interlaminar window, 749
  entering spinal canal through, 752, *752*
Intermediolateral horn, 2
Interspinales muscles, 25
Interspinous ligament, 25
Interspinous wire techniques, 321, *322,* 323
Intertransversarii muscles, 25
Intervertebral disc, 65, 66, 425, 444–445
  stabilizing role of, 69
Intervertebral disc and ligaments, 21–25, *22, 23*
Intervertebral foramen, 3, *16,* 17, *19,* 19–20, 21
Intervertebral foraminal stenosis, *447,* 451
Intradural lesions of spine, 551–564
  congenital anomalies of
    Arnold-Chiari malformation with and without syringomyelia, 559
    diastematomyelia, *560,* 560–561
    dural arteriovenous fistulae and true arteriovenous malformations, 561–562
    surgery for Arnold-Chiari malformation, 559
    syringomyelia, 559–560
    tethered cord syndrome, 561
  diagnosis of abnormalities, 551
  inadvertent opening of dura, 564
  transdural removal of herniated disc, 562–564
  tumors of spinal cord and nerves, 552
    extradural tumors, 552

intradural-extramedullary, 552–556
intramedullary tumors, 556–559, *558*
Intradural lumbar disc herniation, 563
Intradural meningiomas, 554–555, *555, 556*
Intradural-extramedullary tumors, 552–556, 555–556, *556*
operative procedures, 552–553
Intramedullary arteriovenous malformation, 562
Intramedullary ependymoma, 557–558, *558*
Intramedullary spinal abscess
clinical presentation, 587
diagnostic evaluation, 587
epidemiology and etiology, 586
management and prognosis, 587
microbiology, 586–587
Intramedullary tumors, 551, 556–559, *558*
Intraneural disc herniation, 563–564
Intraoperative monitoring (IOM), 129
of evoked potentials during spine surgery
interpretation of findings in, 149–153, *150, 151, 152*
methodology, 147*t*, 147–149, 148*t*, *149*
Intraspinal lipomas, 631
Intrinsic muscles, 25
Inverted radial reflex, 95–96
Isokinetic devices, 467
Isokinetic strength tests, 467
ISOLA instrumentation system, 682–683, *684, 685, 686, 687–688, 689,* 693, 695, 698–699, *700, 701, 702, 703*
Isthmic spondylolisthesis, 116–117, 517

Jaw reflex, 95
Jefferson burst type fracture, 271
Jewett brace, 648
Joints of Luschka, *14, 16,* 269
Juvenile kyphosis, 239
diagnosis, *240,* 240–241
nonoperative treatments, 241, *241*
pathogenesis, 239
surgical treatment, 241–245, *243, 244*
complications, 245–246
thoracoscopy, 246

Kaneda instrumentation
anterior spinal device, 694, 698–699, 703
solid rod system, 379, 693, 695, 698–699, *700, 701, 702,* 703
Keratin sulfate, 425
Kerrison rongeurs, 410–411
in treating spinal stenosis, 453
Kinematics
of cervical spine
lower
functions of anatomic elements, 65
range of motion and coupling characteristics, 65
upper
functions of anatomic elements, 64–65
range of motion and coupling characteristics, 64, 64*t*
of lumbar spine
functions of anatomic elements, 66
range of motion and coupling characteristics, 65–66
of spine, 63–64

of thoracic spine, range of motion and coupling characteristics, 65
Kinetic beds, 372
Klippel-Feil syndrome, 162, 163, 166, 167, 217, 275, 280
Kostuik-Harrington system, 379, 694
Kyphosis, 213
congenital, 216
high thoracic, 195
natural history, 228–229, *229*
nonoperative treatment, 229, *230*
progressive, 595
sagittal plane abnormalities in, 513*t*, 513–514, 514*t*
segmental, 367
surgical treatment, 229, 231, *232,* 233
thoracolumbar, 195
Kyphotic deformity after flexion-compression injuries, 372
Kyphotic segmental deformity, 369

Laboratory tests in evaluating spinal infection, 569, *570*
Laminar facet screws, 78
Laminar overhang, 749, *751*
Laminectomy, 319–320, 376, 585
decompressive, in treating degenerative lumbar spondylolisthesis, *523,* 523–524
posterolateral decompression, 376–377
and spinal stability, 70
for spinal tuberculosis, 594
Laryngeal nerve, 29
Lateral access syndrome, 446
Lateral extracavitary approach, 416
Lateral plate mass fixation, 323–324, *324, 325,* 326, *327*
Lateral recess, 19, 21
Lateral retropharyngeal approach, 354
Lateral (rotatory) subluxation, 606
Lateral stenosis, 446
microsurgery for, *754, 762*
Latissimus dorsi, 25
Leg pain in spondylolisthesis, 252
Legg-Calve-Perthes disease, 239
Lesser occipital nerve, 10–11
Leukemia, 537
Ligamentous injuries, 301, *302,* 303
treatment of, 310–311
Ligamentum flavum, 7, 24–25, 65
Ligamentum nuchae, 25, 65
Lipomas, 551, 558
Load sharing mechanism in spinal instrumentation, *82,* 82–84, *83,* 84*t*
Longissimus muscle, 9
Longus capitis, 27–28
Longus colli, 27
Lordoscoliosis, 213
Lordosis, 233
cervical, 360
changes in lower lumbar segmental, following fusion, 507, 509*t*, 509–511
lumbar, 360
nonoperative treatment, 233
surgical treatment, 233, *234,* 235
Low back pain
in ankylosing spondylitis, 429

Low back pain—*continued*
    cause-and-effect relationship of, and scoliosis in lumbar spine, 476
    in eosinophilic granuloma, 429
    incidence of, 427
    in osteoblastomas, 429
    in osteoid osteoma, 429
    risk factors associated with, 427
    and scoliosis in lumbar spine, 476
    smoking in, 428
    in spondylolisthesis, 252, 429
Lumbar curves, management of, in adult scoliosis, *480*, 481–482, *483*
Lumbar disc disease, 425–438, 447
    anatomy of, 425–427, *427*
    clinical evaluation, 428–430
    conservative treatment of, 435–437, *436*
    epidemiology and patient population, 427–428
    microsurgery for, 747
        anatomy essential for using limited surgical incision, 747–754, *748, 749, 750, 751, 752, 753, 754, 755*
        indications for, 754–758, 755*t*, 756*t*, 757*t*, 758*t*
            herniation, 754–758, 755*t*, 756*t*, 757*t*, 758*t*
        for lateral zone stenosis, *754*, 762
        limited surgical intervention for fusion, 763, *763*
        problems with microscope and, 758*t*, 758–759
        results of, 762
        for spinal canal stenosis, *753*, 762
        techniques of simple microdiscectomy, 759, *761*, 761–762
    natural history, 428
    physical examination, 430–432
    radiologic evaluation, 432–435, *433, 434*
    studies of patients with degenerative, 498
    surgical treatment of, 437–438
Lumbar fusion, limited surgical intervention for, 763, *763*
Lumbar hypolordosis, 195–196
Lumbar intervertebral foramen, 7, *8*, 9, *9*
Lumbar lordosis, 1, 59–60, 63, 360, 432
Lumbar nerve roots, 6
Lumbar pseudo-radicular syndrome, 414
Lumbar spine, 98, 99*t*
    acute low back pain, 114–115
    anterior exposure of, 55–59, *56, 57, 58*
    chronic low back pain, 115–116
    effects of surgical decompression on stability of, 69–71, *70*
    fractures of, 289
    history of, 98–99
    imaging of postoperative, 117
        back pain predominant, 118–119
        leg pain predominant, 117–118
    injuries to, 282–283, *284*, 285–288
    kinematics of
        functions of anatomic elements, 66
        range of motion and coupling characteristics, 65–66
    leg pain predominant, 116
    orthoses for, 649–651, *650, 651*
    percutaneous procedures in, 731
        biopsy techniques, 731–732
        chemonucleolysis, 733–735
        discography, *732*, 732–733, *733*
        early visualized intradiscal, *735*, 735–736
        fusion, 741–743, *742, 743, 744*
        future of minimally invasive surgery, 743–744
        percutaneous nucleotomy, 735
        spinal endoscopy, *736*, 736–741, *737, 738, 739, 740*
    physical examination, 99–100
    skeletal anatomy of, 748, *748*
    thoracoscopic and laparoscopic exposure of, 59–60
Lumbar spine osteotomy, 620–621, *621, 622*
Lumbar spondylolisthesis
    classification of, 249
        congenital, 249, *250*
        degenerative, 250
        isthmic, 249–250, *250*
        pathologic, 250
        post-surgical, 250–251
        traumatic, 250
    clinical evaluation
        physical findings, 252–253, *253*
        presenting complaints, 252
    definition of, 249
    imaging studies
        adaptive changes, 255, *255*
        angulation, 254–255
        anteroposterior radiograph, 253
        computerized tomography, 256, *256*
        displacement, 254, *254*
        dynamic radiographs, 255
        lateral radiograph, 253–254, *254*
        magnetic resonance imaging, 256
        myelography, 256
        oblique radiographs, 255, *255*
        radionuclide scanning, 255–256
    natural history
        congenital, 251
        environmental factors, 251–252
        genetic factors, 251
        isthmic, 251
        risk of symptoms, 252
        slip progression, 252
    nonoperative treatment, 256
    surgical treatment, 256
        classification of techniques, 257–259
        combined anterior-posterior procedures, 262
        indications, 256–257
        posterior procedures, 260–261, *261*
        reduction of, 259–260
Lumbopelvic alignments, 489
Lumbosacral articulation, 1
Lumbosacral facet, 19
Lumbosacral kyphosis in spondylolisthesis, 253
Lumbosacral orthosis, *650*
Luque instrumentation, 181, 543, 546
    segmental spinal, 174
    sublaminar wiring, 677–678, *678*
Lymphoma, 528, 536

Magerl method of lateral mass screw orientation, *667*
Magnetic resonance imaging (MRI), 106–108, *107*, 107*t*, 111, 114, 115
    in evaluating degenerative lumbar spondylolisthesis, 521

in evaluating herniated discs, 116
in evaluating pediatric spine injuries, 274
in evaluating spinal infections, 574–575, *575–576*, 576–577, 579–580, 582, 586, 587, 590
in evaluating spinal neoplasms, 529
in evaluating spine, 450
in evaluating spondylolisthesis, 256
Mannitol for thoracolumbar spine injuries, 371
Marfan's syndrome, 97
McGregor's line, 164, 608, *609*
McRae's line, 164, 608, *609*
Mechanical thoracic disc disease, 414
Mediastinitis, 567
Medical Outcome Study (MOS) Short-Form 36 (SF-36), 486–487
Medulla oblongata, 1
Meningiomas, 551
    intradural, 554–555, *555, 556*
Mesenchymal syndromes, 163
Methacrylate for spinal neoplasms, 547
Methyl methacrylate in enhancing spinal stability, 568
Methylprednisolone
    for thoracolumbar spine injuries, 371
    for traumatic spinal cord injury, 389–390
Metzger liens, 608, *609*, 610
Meurig-Williams plates, 373
Miami J collar, 309
Microdiscectomy, 567
    techniques of simple, 759, *761*, 761–762
Microsurgery. (*See also* Surgery.)
    for lumbar disc disease, 747
        anatomy essential for using limited surgical incision, 747–754, *748, 749, 750, 751, 752, 753, 754, 755*
        indications for, herniation, 754–758, 755*t*, 756*t*, 757*t*, 758*t*
        for lateral zone stenosis, 754, 762
        limited surgical intervention for fusion, 763, *763*
        problems with microscope and, 758*t*, 758–759
        results of, 762
        for spinal canal stenosis, *753*, 762
        techniques of simple microdiscectomy, 759, *761*, 761–762
Mid-thoracic hypokyphosis, 195
Migrating disc rupture, 752
Million visual analog scale, 469
Milwaukee brace, 173, 648, *649*
    for congenital scoliosis, 219
    for juvenile kyphosis, 241, *241*
Minerva orthosis, 309, 643, *644,* 645
Minimally invasive spine surgery, future of, 743–744
Minnesota Multiphasic Personality Inventory (MMPI), 469
Minor spinal fractures, 285
Moe square-ended rod, 677
Mononeuritis multiplex, 404
Morquio syndrome, 167, 275
Moss-Miami instrumentation, 682, *683*, 693, 695, 698–699, *700, 701, 702*
Motor unit (MU), 132
Motor unit action potential (MUAP), 132, 138, *139*, 140, *140*, 141
Mucopolysaccharidoses, 167

Multilevel stenosis, 446
Multiple epiphyseal dysplasia, 167
Multiple myeloma, 536–537
Muscle relaxants for lumbar disc disease, 437
Muscular triangle, 28–29
Myelography, *105*, 105–106, 111, 114
    in evaluating degenerative lumbar spondylolisthesis, 521
    in evaluating pediatric spine injuries, 274
    in evaluating spinal canal stenosis, 449–450, *450*
    in evaluating spinal infection, 586, 587
    in evaluating spinal infections, 582
    in evaluating spinal neoplasms, 529
    in evaluating spondylolisthesis, 256
Myeloma, 528
Myelomeningocele–kyphosis, *179,* 179–181, *180*
Myelopathy, 92, 413
Myofascial pain, 712
Myotome, 132
Myxopapillary ependymoma of filum terminale, 555

Naik's values, 274
Naloxone for thoracolumbar spine injuries, 371
Nash-Moe method, 195
Near-field potentials, 142
Needle biopsy in diagnosing spinal infection, 577
Neoplasms. (*See* Spinal neoplasms.)
Nerve root anatomy, 748, *748*
Nerve root canal stenosis, 446
Nerve root groove, 17
Nerves, spinal, 3–4, *6,* 6–7, *7, 8,* 9–11
Neural events, 142
Neurocentral joint osteophyte, 92
Neurofibromas, 631
Neurofibromatosis, 163, 168, 430
Neuroforamen, 445
Neurogenic claudication, comparison of vascular with, 448*t*
Neurogenic shock, 371–372
Neurologic amyotrophy, 404
Neurologic bladder, *394,* 394–396, *395*
Neurologic compromise, risk of, with kyphosis surgery, 245
Neurologic deficits
    in rheumatoid arthritis, 617
    in spondylolisthesis, 252, 253
Neurologic problems, 216
Neuromuscular scoliosis. (*See also* Scoliosis; Adult scoliosis.)
    arthrogryposis, 184
    cerebral palsy, 175–179, *176, 177, 178*
    Charcot-Marie-Tooth, 184
    Duchenne's muscular dystrophy, 181
        natural history of spinal deformity in, 181–182
    Friedreich's ataxia, 183
    general principles, 173–175, *174, 175*
    myelomeningocele–kyphosis, *179,* 179–181, *180*
    poliomyelitis, 184
    Rett's syndrome, 183–184
    spinal muscular atrophy, 182–183
Neutral vertebra, 194
Night pain, 528

Nonoperative treatment
    for juvenile kyphosis, 241, *241*
    for pediatric spine injuries, 283
    for spondylolisthesis, 256
Nonorganic physical sign testing, 100
Nonorganic tenderness, 100
Nonsteroidal anti-inflammatory drugs (NSAIDS) for degenerative lumbar spondylolisthesis, 521
Nucleus pulposus, 21–22, 69, 270
    composition of, 425

Obliquus capitis inferior, 26
Obliquus capitis superior, 26
Obliteration of pulse, 94
Obstetrical trauma, 277
Occipital condyle, 12
    fractures, 331
        classification, *332*, 332–333
        clinical diagnosis, 331–332
        mechanism of, 331
        radiographic evaluation, 332
        treatment, 333
Occipital triangles, 28
Occipitoatlantal injuries
    clinical diagnosis, 333
    injury classification, 334
    mechanism of, 333
    radiographic evaluation, 333–334, *334*
    treatment of, 334
        dislocation, 279
Occipitocervical arthrodesis, 615, *616*
Occipitocervical fixation
    plates and screws for, 77
    wiring for, 77
Occipitocervical fusion, 658–661, *659, 660, 661, 662*
Occipitocervical synostosis, 162–163
Occipoatlantal dislocations, 277–279, *278*
Occult sacroiliitis, 431
Odontoid abnormalities, 163
Odontoid fractures, 280–282
    classification, 344, *345*
    clinical diagnosis, 343–344
    mechanism of, 343
    radiographic evaluation, 344
    treatment, 344–346
Odontoid hypoplasia, 167
Odontoid process, 13, 269
Odontoid screw fixation, anterior, 76–77, 653–654, *655*
Omohyoid muscle, 28
Open reduction in spondylolisthesis, 260
Opiate antagonists for thoracolumbar spine injuries, 371
Oppenheimer's sign, 96
Orthogonal system, 64
Orthotic treatment for congenital scoliosis, 219
Os odontoideum, 165, 344
Osseous structures and articulations, *12*, 12–14, *13, 14, 15, 16*, 16–19, *17, 18, 19, 20*, 21
Ossification centers of atlas, 268, *268*
Osteoblastomas, 527, 531, 631
    low back pain in, 429
    treatment of, 635–636
Osteochondromas, 530–531, 631
Osteogenesis imperfecta, 163, 275

Osteoid osteoma, 531
    low back pain in, 429
Osteomyelitis
    pyogenic, 578
    vertebral, 572, 573, 578
Osteopenia, 275
Osteophytes, 66
Osteosarcoma, 532–533
Osteotomy
    lumbar spine, 620–621, *621, 622*
    thoracic spine, 621, 623, *623*
Outcome monitoring in functional restoration of back and neck work-related injuries, 470–472

Paget's disease, 163
Pain
    anatomic basis of discogenic, 426
    axial neck, 109–110
    leg, in spondylolisthesis, 252
    low back
        in ankylosing spondylitis, 429
        cause-and-effect relationship of, and scoliosis in lumbar spine, 476
        in eosinophilic granuloma, 429
        incidence of, 427
        in osteoblastomas, 429
        in osteoid osteoma, 429
        risk factors associated with, 427
        and scoliosis in lumbar spine, 476
        smoking in, 428
        in spondylolisthesis, 252, 429
    in lumbar spine
        acute, 114–115
        chronic, 115–116
    myofascial, 712
    night, 528
    Pennsylvania Plan algorithm for low back and leg, 435, *436*
    radicular, 92, 476
    in thoracic disc disease, 414
Pain syndrome, connection between lumbar disc disease and, 426
Paralumbar spasm, 569
Paraparesis, 388
Paraplegia, 228, 292, 359, 388
Paraspinal musculature, 7
Pars defect repair for spondylolisthesis, 257
Pars interarticularis, 7, 21
Pars lateralis, 629
Partial discectomy, 69
Passive modalities, 462
Patellar tendon reflex, 432
Pediatric discitis
    clinical presentation, 579
    diagnostic evaluation, 579–580
    epidemiology and etiology, 578–579
    microbiology and pathogenesis, 579
Pediatric idiopathic scoliosis, surgical treatment of
    bone grafting techniques, 202–203, *204*, 205
    clinical evaluation, 187
    complications
        decompensation, 206–207, *208*
        instrumentation prominence, 209

neurologic, 207, 209
pseudoarthrosis, 206
wound, 206
curve classification
double major curve, 191, *192*
double thoracic curve, 189, 191, *191*
false double major curve, 189
left thoracic curve, 192, *195*
long thoracic curve, 189, *190*
lumbar/thoracolumbar curves, 191–192, *193*
single thoracic curve, 189, *190*
decision-making regarding indications for, 187, 189
indications and techniques of anterior and posterior approach
crankshaft, 201, *202*
fixed lumbar kyphosis T12 to sacrum, 202
indications and techniques of posterior approach
instrumentation without fusion, 198–199
orientation of hooks, 196
rod rotation maneuver, 196
role of pedicle fixation, 196, *197*, 198
three rod, 196, *197*
translation with segmental wiring, 196
very, very short anterior instrumentation, 198, *199*
indications for anterior approach and anterior instrumentation
anterior instrumentation alternatives for thoracolumbar lumbar curves, 199–200
determining fusion levels, 199
thoracic curves, 200
thoracolumbar and lumbar curves, 200–201
use of structural grafts or cages, 200, *201*
postoperative management
immediate postop, 205–206
post-hospitalization and beyond, 206
principles of where to start and stop fusion, 192, 194–195
radiographic evaluation, 187
sagittal considerations
concomitant L5/S1 spondylolisthesis, 196
high thoracic kyphosis, 195
lumbar hypolordosis, 195–196
mid-thoracic hypokyphosis, 195
thoracic hyperkyphosis, 196
thoracolumbar kyphosis, 195
Pediatric spine injuries, 267
anatomy, *268*, 268–270, *269*
biomechanics, bone properties, 270
complications
late deformity, 291–292
paraplegia or quadriplegia, 292
decompression, 289–290
diagnosis, 271–272
disc herniation, 291
etiology, 267–268
halo application, 290–291
imaging of fractures, 272–274
bone scintigraphy, 275
cervical, 277–280, *278*
computed tomography (CT) scanning, 274
differential diagnosis, 275
early management, *276*, 276–277
infection, 275
magnetic resonance imaging (MRI), 274
metabolic disease, 275
myelography, 274
neoplasm, 275
normal variance, 274
odontoid, 280–282
plain tomography, 274
Scheuermann's disease, 276
spondyloepiphyseal dysplasia, 275
thoracic and lumbar, 282–283, *284*, 285–288
pathomechanics, mechanisms of, 270–271, *271*
prevention, 291
return to activities, 291
SCIWORA, 291
traumatic spondylolysis, 290
treatment of, 288–289
operative, 289
thoracic and lumbar spine fractures, 289
Pedicle screw instrumentation, 78–79, 374–376, *375*, 546, 683–684, 688, 690
fixation strength, 79–80
Pennsylvania Plan algorithm for low back pain and leg pain, 435, *436*
Percutaneous procedures in lumbar spine, 731
biopsy techniques, 731–732
chemonucleolysis, 733–735
discectomy for lumbar disc disease, 438
discography, *732*, 732–733, *733*
early visualized intradiscal, *735*, 735–736
fusion, 741–743, *742*, *743*, *744*
future of minimally invasive surgery, 743–744
nucleotomy, 735, *735*
percutaneous nucleotomy, 735
spinal endoscopy, *736*, 736–741, *737*, *738*, *739*, *740*
Peripheral nerve block, 712
Peripheral nerve entrapment syndromes, 404
Peripheral vascular disease, 447
Perivascular plexus, 9
Pfeiffer's syndrome, 167
Philadelphia collar, 309, 642, *643*
Pia mater, 2
Placebo response, 711
Plain film tomography, 104
in evaluating pediatric spine injuries, 274
Plain radiographs, 103–104, 114
Plasmacytoma, 527
Plates and vertebral screws, 78
for lower cervical spine fixation, 77–78
for occipitocervical fixation, 77
Platysma muscle, 26–27, 29
Platyspondylisis, 275
Plica mediana dorsalis durae matris, 2
Pneumonia as complication of scoliosis surgery, 485
Pneumothorax as complication of scoliosis surgery, 485
Poliomyelitis, 184
Porous tricalcium phosphate (TCP) in bone grafts, 72
Posterior atlantoaxial fusion, 661, 663, *664*, 665, *665*
Posterior atlantoaxial subluxation, 606
Posterior atlantodental interval (PADI), 607–608, *608*
Posterior autogenous iliac harvesting, 203
Posterior C1-C2 facet screw fixation, *352*, 352–353
Posterior cervical fusion, 321
Posterior decompression, 319, *320*, 321

Posterior fusion for spondylolisthesis, 258
Posterior hemiarthrodesis, *224,* 224–225
Posterior interbody fusion for spondylolisthesis, 258
Posterior occipital screw placement, 353
Posterior procedures for spondylolisthesis, 260–261, *261*
Posterior segmental fixation, 374
Posterior triangle, 28
Posterolateral costotransversectomy, 48–49, *49*
Posterolateral decompression, 376–377
Posterolateral fusion for spondylolisthesis, 257–258
Posterolateral herniation, 427
Postlaminectomy kyphosis, 71, 537
Posture, abnormality of, in spondylolisthesis, 252
Powers ratio, 278, *278,* 334
Pressure ulceration, 393–394
   as cause of morbidity in spinal cord injury, 398
Prevertebral fascia, 29
Primary treatment, 462
Progressive kyphosis, 595
Prone straight leg raise test, 100
Proteus species in spinal infections, 572
Pseudoachondroplasia, 167
Pseudoarthrosis, 52, 206, 617
Pseudomeningocele, 553
Pseudomonas aeruginosa in spinal infections, 572
Pseudosubluxation, *160,* 160–161
Psoriatic arthritis, 639
Psychosocial barriers to recovery, from back and neck work-related injuries, 468–469
Pulmonary embolism as complication of scoliosis surgery, 485
Purser's sign, 606
Pyogenic disc-space infection, 573–577, *574*
Pyogenic osteomyelitis, 578

Quadriparesis, 388
Quadriplegia, 292, 388
Quantified pain drawing, 469
Quantitative computed tomography (QCT), 80

Radical cordectomy, 557
Radicular arteries, 3
Radicular pain, 92, 476
Radiculopathy, 144, 403, 721
   treatment for, 437
Radiographs
   in evaluation of spondylolisthesis, 253–254, *254,* 256
   plain, 103–104
Radionuclide scanning, 108–109, *109*
   in evaluating spinal infections, 574, 590
   in evaluating spondylolisthesis, 255–256
   technetium 99 in, 115
Radiotherapy in treating spinal neoplasms, 539
Ranawat's criteria for basilar invagination, 610, *610*
Range of motion in quantification of physical and functional capacity, 463–465, *464*
RARE (Rapid Acquisition Relaxation Enhanced), 108
Reconstructive upper extremity surgery, 397
Recording electrode, 141–142
Rectilinear tomography, 104
Rectus capitis anterior, 28
Rectus capitis lateralis, 28

Rectus capitis posterior major, 25–26
Rectus capitis posterior minor, 26
Redlund-Johnell values, 610, *611*
Reference electrode, 135
Rehabilitation of traumatic spinal cord injury
   adjustment, 398
   areas of concern, 396
   automatic dysreflexia, 390–391
   deep venous thrombosis and pulmonary embolus, 390
   distribution of impairments, 389
   effects upon marriage, 398
   epidemiology, 386–387
   general approach to improving function, 396
   heterotopic ossification, *391,* 391–392
   long-term morbidity, 398
   maintenance of range of motion, 396–398, 397t
   neurogenic bladder, *394,* 394–396, *395*
   neurologic assessment, 387–389
   neurologic prognosis, *389,* 389–390
   pressure ulceration, 393
   residence, 398
   scope of, 385–386
   spasticity, 392–393
Respiratory problems and congenital spine deformation, 217
Retrograde ejaculation as complication of scoliosis surgery, 486
Retropulsed bone, 372
Retropulsion of middle column, 361
Rett's syndrome, 183–184
Reverse straight leg raise test, 100
Reverse Trendelenburg positioning, 32–33
Rheumatoid arthritis. (*See also* Arthritis.)
   atlantoaxial arthrodesis, 613–615, *614*
   clinical manifestations, 606–607
   complications
      mortality, 616–617
      neurologic deficit, 617
      progression of instability, 617
      pseudoarthrosis, 617
   electrophysiologic testing, 611
   general surgical considerations, 612–613
   indications for surgery
      atlantoaxial subluxation, 611–612
      basilar invagination, 612
      subaxial disease, 612
   occipitocervical arthrodesis, *616*
   pathophysiology, 605–606
   radiologic evaluation, 607–608, *608, 609, 610,* 610–611, *611*
   subaxial subluxation, 616
   transoral decompression, 615–616
Rheumatoid pannus, 605–606
Rheumatoid spondylitis, 606
Ribs
   harvesting of bone from, 72, 768–769, *769*
      clinical recommendations in, 778
      complications in, 776–777
Risser frame, 646
Risser plaster jacket, 649
Robinson-Southwick technique, *667,* 668
Rod and vertebral screws, 78

Rods and hooks, 78
Rods and wires, 78
Roentgenograms in diagnosing spinal infections, 573–574, 574
Romanus lesion, 618
Rotation, 64, 362, 363, 364
Rotation test, 100
Rotator cuff tendinitis, 404
Rotatores muscles, 25
Rotatory subluxation, 340
   of atlantoaxial joint, 338–339
      classification, 340–341, 342
      clinical diagnosis, 339–340
      mechanism of, 339
      radiographic evaluation, 340
      treatment, 341–343
Roto-Rest bed, 372
Roy-Camille technique
   of lateral mass screw orientation, 667
   of occipitocervical fusion, 660, 662

Sacral anatomy, 629
Sacral arthritis
   ankylosing spondylitis, 639
   psoriatic, 639
Sacral cornua, 21
Sacral foramina, 21, 629
Sacral fractures, 285–286, 637, 637–638
   treatment, 638
Sacral hiatus, 21, 629
Sacral kyphosis, 63
Sacral median crest, 629
Sacral meningiomas, 631
Sacral promontory, 629
Sacral tumors, 629–630
   benign, 630–631, 632
      aneurysmal bone cyst, 630
      giant cell, 631, 632–633
   chondrosarcoma, 634–635, 635
      metastasis, 635
   malignant, 631
      chordoma, 631, 634, 634
   results, 637
   treatment, 635–637
Sacroiliac injection, 712–714, 714
Sacroiliac joint, 20, 21
   fracture-dislocation problems, 638–639
Sacrum, bony structures of, 20, 21
Sagittal plane
   abnormalities of, in disorders of adult spine, 489–515
      changes in lower lumbar segmental lordosis following fusion, 507, 509t, 509–511
      definitions and determinants of balance, 493, 495–497, 496, 497
      fixation and manipulation with instrumentation, 507, 508
      kyphosis, 513t, 513–514, 514t
      normative data studies for alignments, 489–492, 490, 491, 492, 494, 495
      positioning studies in patients under anesthesia and in awake volunteers, 504, 505, 506t, 506–507
      scoliosis, 512–513
      in specific, 497–504, 499t, 500, 503t
      spondylolisthesis, 511–512
      thoracolumbar burst fractures, 514–515
   correction of deformities in, 648–649
   restoration of, 374
   spinal contours, 360
   translation, 65–66
Sagittal spinal balance
   center of gravity for, 507
   definitions and determinants of, 493, 495–497, 496, 497
Salmonella osteomyelitis in spinal infections, 572
Sandifer's syndrome, 166–167
Scalenus anterior, 28
Scalenus medius, 28
Scalenus posterior, 28
Scanning. (*See* Imaging.)
Scapula, 29
Scapulohumeral reflex, 95
Scheuermann's disease, 97, 229, 276
   incidence of, in general population, 239
Scheuermann's kyphosis, 240, 414
Schmorl's nodes, 239
Schober test, 431
Schwannomas, 551, 552, 552, 558–559
   of cauda equina, 553–554, 554
Sciatica
   incidence of, 427
   natural history of, 428
   risk factors associated with, 427
SCIWORA (spinal cord injury without radiologic abnormality) syndrome, 286, 291, 369
Sclerosis, amyotrophic lateral, 404
Sclerotomes, segmentation of, 572
Scoliosis, 184, 213, 455. (*See also* Adult scoliosis; Neuromuscular scoliosis; Pediatric idiopathic scoliosis.)
   association with osteoblastoma, 528
   association with osteoid osteoma, 528
   cervicothoracic congenital, 217
   correction of, 677
   natural history, 218t, 218–219
   nonoperative treatment, 219
   sagittal plane abnormalities in, 512–513
   secondary to spasm, 569
   surgical treatment of, 220
   thoracolumbar, 693
Scoliosis fusions, 567
Screw fixation, 351–354, 352
Secondary treatment, 462
Segmental fixation systems, 489
Segmental kyphosis, 367
Segmental pointer muscles, 132
Segmental sensory nerve evoked potentials (SSEPs), 143
Segmentation, error of, 213
Semispinalis muscle, 25
Sensory evoked potentials (SEPs), 141–143, 142t, 143
Sensory nerve action potentials (SNAPs), 137
Septic discitis, 568
Sequestered disc fragment, 426
Serratus posterior inferior, 25
Serratus posterior superior, 25
Severe compression fractures, 283

Shear injuries, 364, *364*
Short-latency sensory evoked response, 142–143
Sibson's fascia, 44
Sickle ligament, 629
Sinuvertebral nerves, 9
Skeletal dysplasias, 167–168
Slip progression in spondylolisthesis, 252
Smoking and low back pain, 428
S/N ratio, 108
Snaking phenomenon, 644
Soft cercical collar, 309
Soft cervical collar, 642, *642*
Soft disc herniations, 403
Solitary plasmacytoma, 536, *536*
Somatomotor neurons, 2
Somatosensory evoked potentials (SSEP) monitoring, 31, 32
  in rheumatoid arthritis, 611
Somatosensory neurons, 2
SOMI brace, 642, *643*
Spasm, paralumbar, 569
Spasticity, 392–393
Spencer's ligament, 24
Spinal alignment
  and deformity, 477
  normative data studies for, 489–492, *490, 491, 492, 494, 495*
Spinal artery, 3
Spinal canal stenosis, microsurgery for, *753,* 762
Spinal cord, 133
  anatomy of, 1–3, *3, 4*
  arteries of, 3
  compression of, 403–404, 537–539, 538t
    death due to, 607
  injuries
    hyperflexion, ligamentous, 301, *302,* 303
    pathophysiology of, 297–298, *299,* 300
    without radiographic abnormalities (SCIWORA), 270
    without radiologic abnormality syndrome, 286, 291, 369
Spinal dysraphism, *216,* 216–217, 430
  treatment of, *234,* 235
Spinal endoscopy, *736,* 736–741, *737, 738, 739, 740*
Spinal fixation
  biomechanical strength of, 79
    pedicle screw, 79–80
  and manipulation with instrumentation, 507, *508*
Spinal fractures
  imaging of, 272–274
  resulting from child abuse, 287–288
  treatment of pediatric, 288–289
Spinal fusion, 76, 456
Spinal infections, 275, 567–596
  granulomatous, tuberculosis, 588–590, *591–593,* 593–596
  infections of canal
    epidural abscess, 580–585
    intramedullary spinal abscess, 586–587
    subdural abscess, 585–586
    from traumatic injuries, 587–588
  magnetic resonance imaging (MRI) of, *119,* 119–120
  plain radiography of, 119
  pyogenic
    hematogenous vertebral osteomyelitis and disc-space infection, 572–578
    Iatrogenic, 567–572
    pediatric discitis, 578–580
  radionuclide studies of, 119
  from traumatic injuries, penetrating trauma, 587–588
Spinal injuries
  evaluation of, 295
  physical examination of, 295, *296,* 297, 297t
  radiographic examination of, 297
Spinal instability, 66
  definition of, 66–67
  in vivo spinal motion measurement methods, 67–68
  diagnosis of, 68t, 68–69
Spinal instrumentation
  biomechanical evaluation of, 80
  biomechanics of, 76
    cervical spine implants
      anterior screw for odontoid fixation, 76–77
      posterior instrumentation, 77
    thoracic and lumbar spine implants
      anterior instrumentation, 78
      posterior instrumentation, 78–79
  load sharing mechanism in, *82,* 82–84, *83,* 84t
  in treating degenerative lumbar spondylolisthesis, 524–526, *525*
Spinal muscular atrophy, 182–183
Spinal neoplasms, 275, 527–547
  benign primary tumors, 530–532
  diagnosis, 528, 528t
    biopsy techniques, 529–530, *530*
    imaging techniques, 528–529
  indications, 539
  malignant primary tumors
    consistency, 532–534, *534, 535,* 536, *536*
    metastatic, 536–537
    pediatric, 537
  nonoperative treatment, 539
  pathogenesis, 527
    age, 528
    incidence, 527
    location, 528
    presentation, 527–528
  primary tumors of bone, 530
  spinal cord compression, 537–539, 538t
  surgical treatment, 539–540
    anterior approach, 543
    metastatic disease, 541–542, *542*
    posterior approach, 542–543, *544*
    reconstruction, 543, *545,* 546–547, *546*
    resection, *540,* 540–541, *541*
Spinal nerve injection, 718–721, *720*
Spinal nerves, 3–4, *6,* 6–7, *7, 8,* 9–11
Spinal orthoses, 641–642
  for cervical spine, *642,* 642–646, *643, 644, 645,* 645t
    Halo-Ilizarov, 646–647, *647*
    pediatric halo considerations, 646, *646, 647*
  for lumbar region, 649–651, *650, 651*
  for thoracic spine, 647–649, *648, 649, 650*
Spinal stability, effects of surgical decompression on cervical region, 71

lumbar region, 69–71, *70*
thoracic and thoracolumbar regions, 71
Spinal stenosis, 2, 25, 431, 443–457, 444*t*
  acquired, 443
  clinical presentation
    history, 447–448, 448*t*
    physical examination, 448
    radiologic findings, 448–451, *449, 450, 451, 452*
  congenital, 443
  nonoperative treatment, 451–452
  pathoanatomy
    facets, 445
    intervertebral disc, 444–445
    zones of stenosis, 445–447, *446, 447*
  pathophysiology, 443–444
  surgical treatment, 452–457, *453, 454, 455, 456*
Spine
  anatomy of, 1, *2*
  biomechanical functions of, 63
  functions of, 1
  kinematics of, 63–64
  motion segments in, 63
Spine trauma imaging, 122–123, *123*
Spinous processes, 25
Splenius capitis muscles, 25
Splenius cervicis muscles, 25
Spondylitis
  rheumatoid, 606
  tuberculous, 567
Spondylo- or retro-listhetic deformities, 66
Spondylodiscitis, 625
Spondyloepiphyseal dysplasias, 275
Spondylolisthesis, 97. (*See also* Degenerative lumbar spondylolisthesis.)
  concomitant L5/S1, 196
  low back pain in, 429
  sagittal plane abnormalities in, 511–512
Spondylolysis, 718
  traumatic, 290
Spontaneous fusion, 578
Sprengel's deformity, 217
Spurling's maneuver, 403
Stability tests, 81
Stagnara casting, 676
Stagnara wake-up test, 207
Standards for assessing and classifying spinal cord injuries, 297
Standing sagittal balance, 489
Staphylococcus aureus in spinal infections, 568–569, 572, 581
Staphylococcus epidermidis in spinal infections, 581
Sternocleidomastoid, 26–27
Sternohyoideus muscles, 27
Sternothyroid muscles, 27
Sternum-splitting approach, 44–45, *45*
Straight-leg raising test, 432
Strength tests, 80–82
  devices for, 466
Structured Clinical Interview for DSM-III-R diagnosis (SCID), 469
Subarachnoid space, 2
Subaxial disease, surgery for, 612
Subaxial injuries, 282
Subaxial posterior cervical fixation, 665–666, *666, 667, 668,* 668–671, *669, 670, 671, 672*
Subaxial subluxation, 616
Subdural abscess
  epidemiology and etiology, 585
  pathogenesis, pathology, and microbiology, 586
Sublaminar wiring, 79, 350–351, *351*
Submental triangle, 28–29
Suboccipital muscles, 25–26
Suboccipital nerve, 9
Suction-irrigation system, 571
Suicide rates for victim of spinal cord injury, 398
Superficial fascia, 29
Superficial infection, 569
Superior facet syndrome, 446
Supraclavicular triangle, 28
Suprascapular nerve palsy, 404
Supraspinous ligament, 25
Surgery. (*See also* Microsurgery.)
  for adult scoliosis, 478–479
  anesthesia considerations in, 312–313
  for congenital scoliosis, 220
    combined anterior and posterior fusion in, *222,* 223–224
    convex growth arrest, *224,* 224–225
    hemivertebra or wedge excision, 225, *226–227,* 228
    posterior fusion in, 220–221, *221,* 223
    principles in, 220
  for degenerative lumbar spondylolisthesis, 521–524, *522, 523, 524*
  effects of decompression, on spinal stability
    cervical region, 71
    lumbar region, 69–71
    thoracic and thoracolumbar regions, 71
  exposure and fusion techniques
    anterior
      of lower cervical spine, 35–37, *37, 38, 39,* 40, *40, 41,* 42*t,* 42–44
      of lumbar spine, 55–59, *56, 57, 58*
      of thoracic spine, 53–54, *53–54*
      of thoracolumbar junction, 54–55, *55*
      of upper cervical spine, 32–33, *33, 34, 35*
    cervicothoracic junction, 44–45, *45, 46,* 47, *47*
    posterior
      of lower cervical spine, 32
      of upper cervical spine, 31–32, *32*
  indication for, in thoracolumbar spinal injuries, 367, 369–371
  for juvenile kyphosis, 241–245, *243, 244*
  for kyphosis, 229, *230,* 231, *232,* 233
  for lordosis, 233, *234,* 235
  for lumbar disc disease, 437–438
  for lumbar spondylolisthesis
    operative treatment
      classification of techniques, 257–259
      combined anterior-posterior procedures, 262
      indications, 256–257
      posterior procedures, 260–261, *261*
      reduction of, 259–260
  for lumbar spondylolisthesis
    operative treatment, 256

Surgery—continued
  for management of spinal tuberculosis, 590, 593–596
  for occipital condyle fracture, 333
  for pediatric idiopathic scoliosis
    bone grafting techniques, 202–203, *204,* 205
    clinical evaluation, 187
    complications
      decompensation, 206–207, *208*
      instrumentation prominence, 209
      neurologic, 207, 209
      pseudoarthrosis, 206
      wound, 206
    curve classification
      double major curve, 191, *192*
      double thoracic curve, 189, 191, *191*
      false double major curve, 189
      left thoracic curve, 192, *195*
      long thoracic curve, 189, *190*
      lumbar/thoracolumbar curves, 191–192, *193*
      single thoracic curve, 189, *190*
    decision-making regarding indications for, 187, 189
    indications and techniques of anterior and posterior approach
      crankshaft, 201, *202*
      fixed lumbar kyphosis T12 to sacrum, 202
    indications and techniques of posterior approach
      instrumentation without fusion, 198–199
      orientation of hooks, 196
      rod rotation maneuver, 196
      role of pedicle fixation, 196, *197,* 198
      three rod, 196, *197*
      translation with segmental wiring, 196
      very, very short anterior instrumentation, 198, *199*
    indications for anterior approach and anterior instrumentation
      anterior instrumentation alternatives for thoracolumbar lumbar curves, 199–200
      determining fusion levels, 199
      thoracic curves, 200
      thoracolumbar and lumbar curves, 200–201
      use of structural grafts or cages, 200, *201*
    postoperative management
      immediate postop, 205–206
      post-hospitalization and beyond, 206
    principles of where to start and stop fusion, 192, 194–195
    radiographic evaluation, 187
    sagittal considerations
      concomitant L5/S1 spondylolisthesis, 196
      high thoracic kyphosis, 195
      lumbar hypolordosis, 195–196
      mid-thoracic hypokyphosis, 195
      thoracic hyperkyphosis, 196
      thoracolumbar kyphosis, 195
  for spinal infection, 577–578
  for spinal neoplasms, 539–540
  for spinal stenosis, 452–457, *453, 454, 455, 456*
  for spondylolisthesis, 256–259
  for upper cervical spine injuries
    instrumentation, 350–351, *351*
    screw fixation, 351–354, *352*
    technical considerations, 350
Surgical decompression, 582, 585
Swischuk's posterior cervical line, 281
Sympathetic blockade, 712, *713*
Synchondroses, 268
Synchondrosis, 158
Syndrome of inappropriate antidiuretic hormone secretion (SIADH) as complication of scoliosis surgery, 486
Synthetic bone graft, development of, 72
Syringomyelia, 216, 404, 559–560

Taylor brace, 648
Tear-drop fracture, 305
Technetium bone scans, 108, 634
Tectorial membrane, 64
Telangiectatic osteosarcoma, 630
Tertiary care treatment, 462
  for functional restoration, 469–470
Tethered cord syndrome, 180, 561
Tetraplegia, 388
Texas Scottish Rite Hospital (TSRH)
  rod system, 693, 695
  screws, 200
Texas Scottish Rite Hospital (TSRH) instrumentation system, 681–682, *682,* 698–699, *700, 701, 702*
Thecal sac, 21
Thoracic curves
  management of, in adult scoliosis, 479–481, *480*
  requiring anterior releases, 201
Thoracic disc, transdural removal of, 563
Thoracic disc disease, 413
  complications, 417, 421, *422*
  diagnosis and presentation, 413–414
    discography, 415
    localization problems, 415
    localized pain, 414
    lumbar pseudo-radicular syndrome, 414
    myelopathy, 414
    physical examination, 414–415
    radiculopathy, 414
  indications for operation, 415–416
    operative approach, 416
  nonoperative treatment, 415
  operative technique
    anterior transthoracic decompression and fusion, 416–417, *418–419*
    anterior transthoracic discectomy and fusion, 417
  results, 417, *420, 421*
Thoracic discography, 415
Thoracic hyperkyphosis, 196
Thoracic kyphosis, 1, 63, 360
Thoracic laminectomy, 48
Thoracic myelopathy, 414
Thoracic outlet syndrome, 404
  Adson test in distinguishing between cervical radiculopathy, 93–94
Thoracic radiculopathy, 413, 414
Thoracic spine, 23–24
  anterior exposure of, 53–54, *53–54*

effects of surgical decompression on stability of, 71
fractures of, 289
injuries to, 282–283, *284,* 285–288
kinematics of, range of motion and coupling characteristics, 65
nerves in, 6
orthoses for, 647–649, *648, 649, 650*
posterior approaches to, 47–53, *48, 49, 50, 51, 52*
thoracoscopic and laparoscopic exposure of, 59–60

Thoracic spine osteotomy, 621, 623, *623*
Thoracic vertebrae, *17,* 18
Thoracolumbar burst fractures, sagittal plane abnormalities in, 514–515
Thoracolumbar junction, anterior exposure of, 54–55, *55*
Thoracolumbar kyphosis, 195
Thoracolumbar scoliosis, 693
Thoracolumbar spine, 96–97
    anterior instrumentation of, 693–694
        biomechanics, 694–695
        complications, 703–704
        indications/implants, 695–696
        plate (Z-plate, university plate), 696, *697, 698*
        solid rod systems, 698–699, *700, 701, 702*
        Zielke, 696–697, *699*
    effects of surgical decompression on stability of, 71
    injuries to, 359
        anterior decompression and fusion
            advantages, 377
            comparative studies, 379
            disadvantages, 377
            instrumentation, 378–379
            techniques, 377–378
        diagnosis, *366,* 366–367
            radiographs, *366,* 367, *368, 369, 370,* 366–367
        laminectomy, 376
            posterolateral decompression, 376–377
        nonoperative treatment
            closed reduction and immobilization, 372
            early medical management, 371–372
        pathogenesis
            anatomic classification, *360,* 360–361
            late neurologic change, 366
            mechanistic classification, *361,* 361–362, *362, 363, 364, 364*
            morphologic classification, 364
            musculoskeletal, 359–360
            neurologic injury, 364–366, *365*
        surgical treatment
            indications for
                complete neurologic deficit, 369
                incomplete neurologic, 371
                neurologically intact, 367, 369
        surgical treatments
            Harrington compression, 374
            Harrington distraction, 373
            Harrington modifications, 373–374
            pedicle screw segmental instrumentation, 374–376, *375*
            posterior segmental fixation, 374
            posterior techniques, 373
    physical examination of, 97–98

posterior approaches to, 47–53, *48, 49, 50, 51, 52*
posterior instrumentation of, 675–676
    Cotrel-Dubousset, 679–681, *680*
    Drummond spinous process wiring, *678,* 678–679
    Harrington, 676–677
    ISOLA, 682–683, *684, 685, 686, 687–688, 689*
    Luque sublaminar wiring, 677–678, *678*
    Moss-Miami, 682, *683*
    pedicle screw, 683–684, 688, 690
    TSRH (Texas Scottish Rite Hospital), 681–682, *682*
Thoracolumbosacral orthosis (TLSO), 577, 648, *648, 651*
Thoracoplasty, 483, 485
Thoracoscopy for juvenile kyphosis, 246
Thyrotropin-releasing hormone (TRH) for thoracolumbar spine injuries, 371
Tirilazad mesylate in treating traumatic spinal cord injury, 390
Titanium cages for spinal neoplasms, 547
Toe walking, 403
Toe-to-heel tandem gait, 403
Torticollis, 161–162
    Atlanto-occipital anomalies, 162–163
    basilar impression, 163–164, *164*
    congenital muscular, 161
    unilateral absence of C1, 164–165
Total spondylectomy, 50
Transarticular screw for C1-C2 fixation, 77
Transdural removal of herniated disc, 562–564
Translation, 63–64
Translational instabilities, 279–280
Transoral decompression, 615–616
Transpedicular approach, 51–52
Transpedicular biopsy, 48
Transpedicular bone grafting, 377
Transpharyngeal gunshot wounds, 588
Transplantation therapy, 390
Transverse processes, 25
Transversospinalis muscle, 25
Trapezius, 25
Traumatic disorders of cervicocranium, 331
Traumatic spinal cord injury, rehabilitation of
    adjustment, 398
    areas of concern, 396
    automatic dysreflexia, 390–391
    deep venous thrombosis and pulmonary embolus, 390
    distribution of impairments, 389
    effects on marriage, 398
    epidemiology, 386–387
    general approach to improving function, 396
    heterotopic ossification, *391,* 391–392
    long-term morbidity, 398
    maintenance of range of motion, 396–398, 397t
    neurogenic bladder, *394,* 394–396, *395*
    neurologic assessment, 387–389
    neurologic prognosis, *389,* 389–390
    pressure ulceration, 393
    residence, 398
    scope of, 385–386
    spasticity, 392–393
Traumatic spondylolysis, 290
Tricortical strut grafting for spinal neoplasms, 547

Trigger points, 712
Triple-wire technique, *666,* 668
Trunk motion, 463
Trunk shortening in spondylolisthesis, 253
Trunk strength, assessing, *464, 465,* 465–466, *466*
Tuberculosis, 588–590, *591–593,* 593–596
   clinical presentation, 589
   diagnostic evaluation, 589–590, *591–593*
   epidemiology and etiology, 588–589
   management, 590, 593–596
   pathogenesis and pathology, 589
Tuberculosis spondylitis, 595, 693
Tuberculous spondylitis, 567
Tumor imaging, 120–122, *121, 122*
Tumors. (*See also* Sacral tumors.)
   giant cell, 531, *532,* 630, 631, *632–633*
     treatment of, 636
   intradural-extramedullary, 552–556, 555–556, *556*
     operative procedures, 552–553
   intramedullary, 551, 556–559, *558*
Turner's syndrome, 97

Ulceration, pressure, 393–394
Ulnar cubital tunnel syndrome, 404
Uncinate process, 22
Unilateral absence of C1, 164–165
Unilateral facet dislocations, 303, *304,* 305
   treatment of, 311
Unilateral injury, to vertebral basilar system, 333
University plate, 694
Upper cervical spine injuries in adult, 331
   atlas fractures, 334–335
     classification, 335–337, *336–337*
     clinical diagnosis, 335
     mechanism of, 335
     radiographic evaluation, 335
     treatment, 337–338
   axis fractures, 346–347
     C2 body, 349
     C2 lamina, 349–350
     C2 lateral mass, 349
     classification, 347, *348,* 349
     diagnosis, 347
     mechanism of, 347
     radiographic evaluation, 347
   lateral retropharyngeal approach, 354
   occipital condyle fractures, 331
     classification, *332,* 332–333
     clinical diagnosis, 331–332
     mechanism of, 331
     radiographic evaluation, 332
     treatment, 333
   occipitoatlantal
     clinical diagnosis, 333
     injury classification, 334
     mechanism of, 333
     radiographic evaluation, 333–334, *334*
     treatment, 334
   odontoid fractures
     classification, 344, *345*
     clinical diagnosis, 343–344
     mechanism of, 343
     radiographic evaluation, 344
     treatment, 344–346
   rotatory subluxation of atlantoaxial joint, 338–339
     classification, 340–341, *342*
     clinical diagnosis, 339–340
     mechanism of, 339
     radiographic evaluation, 340
     treatment, 341–343
   surgical treatment of
     instrumentation, 350–351, *351*
     screw fixation, 351–354, *352*
     technical considerations, 350
Upward migration of odontoid, 606
Urinary retention as complication of scoliosis surgery, 486
Urinary tract infection
   as cause of morbidity in spinal cord injury, 398
   as complication of scoliosis surgery, 486
   after spinal cord injury, 395–396

Vacuum disc, 110
Valsalva maneuver, 93
Vascular claudication, 429, 448
Vascular disease, 447
Venous plexus, 2, 3
Ventral derotation spondylodesis, 696–697
Ventral derotation system, 693
Ventral rami of lumbar spinal nerves, 11
Vertebra prominens, 13
Vertebra-disc-vertebra motor unit, 425
Vertebral anomaly, classification of, 213
Vertebral apophysis fractures, 286–287, *287, 288*
Vertebral arteries, 3
Vertebral basilar system, unilateral injury to, 333
Vertebral body
   longitudinal growth of, 269–270
   in lumbar spine, *18,* 18–19
Vertebral centrum, 269
Vertebral osteomyelitis, 572, 573, 578, 588
Vertebrectomy, 410
Vertebrobasilar artery insufficiency, 332
Vertebrobasilar insufficiency, 606
Vertical compression, 271
Vertical subluxation, 606
Virchow's triad, 390
Visceral fascia, 29

Wackenheim, 610, *610*
Wackenstein, basilar line of, 334
Waddell signs, 100
Wallenberg's syndrome, 333
Wechsler Adult Intelligence Scale-Revised (WAIS-R), 469
Wedge excision, 225, *226–227,* 228
Weiss Springs, 373
Wholey dens-basion method or distance, 334
Windshield-washer phenomenon, 482
Wiring
   for C1-C2 stabilization, 77
   for lower cervical spine fixation, 77
   for occipitocervical fixation, 77

Wisconsin wires, 374
Work-related injuries, functional restoration of back and neck, 461–472, 462t, 464, 465, 466
Wound infections, 569, 570–571, 571t

Yale brace, 309

Zielke instrumentation
  derotator, 192, 199, 207, 695, 696–697, *699,* 703
  rod system, 693, 694, 695
Z-plate, 379, 694
Zygapophyseal joints, 7, 9